fifth edition

MARY W. FALCONER, R.N., B.A. M.A.

Formerly Instructor of Pharmacology
O'Connor Hospital School of Nursing, San Jose, California

ANNETTE SCHRAM EZELL, R.N., B.S.N., M.S.

Associate Professor and Curriculum Coordinator
University of Nevada, Reno, Nevada; Formerly Assistant
Professor, School of Medical Sciences, University of
Nevada, Reno, Nevada

H. ROBERT PATTERSON, B.S., M.S., Pharm.D.

Professor of Bacteriology and Biology
San Jose State University, San Jose, California

EDWARD A. GUSTAFSON, B.S., Pharm.D.

Pharmacist, Valley Medical Center, San Jose, California

THE DRUG THE NURSE THE PATIENT

1974 W. B. SAUNDERS COMPANY · PHILADELPHIA · LONDON · TORONTO

W. B. Saunders Company: West Washington Square
Philadelphia, PA 19105

12 Dyott Street
London, WC1A 1DB

833 Oxford Street
Toronto, Ontario M8Z 5T9, Canada

The Drug, The Nurse, The Patient ISBN 0-7216-3548-2

Press of W. B. Saunders Company. Library of Congress catalog card number 66-15620.

Last digit is the print number: 9 8 7 6 5 4 3 2 1

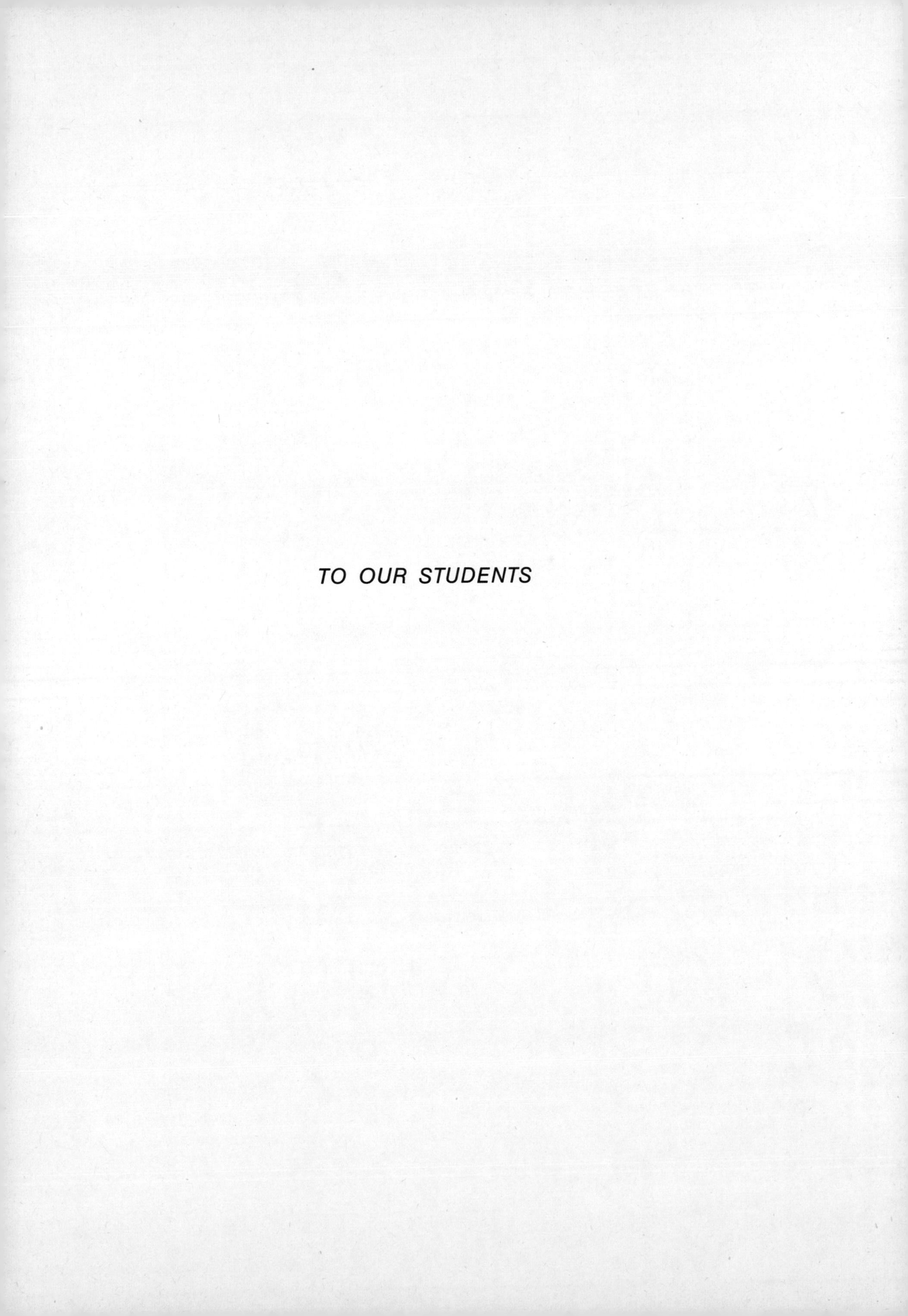

TO OUR STUDENTS

PREFACE TO THE FIFTH EDITION

Those who have used previous editions of this book will find extensive changes which we feel are important and will be helpful. There has been considerable rearrangement of material and updating of information. However, the same patient-centered approach has been maintained. There has been increased emphasis in the areas marked "The Nurse" and "The Patient." Since many of the technical aspects of medicinal therapy are now done by other personnel (the pharmacist, technical specialists, and the like), the nurse is able to concentrate on drug therapy as it relates to the patient.

A short chapter entitled "The Actions and Interactions of Drugs in the Body" has been added in the first part of the book. This topic is expanded throughout the book. A new subheading, "Interactions," has been added where pertinent. The nurse will need to continually expand her knowledge and awareness of problems involving these relationships.

The two chapters previously entitled "Arithmetic Review" and "Posology" have been combined and shortened. The nurse now is rarely called upon to calculate dosage. Of course, this very fact makes some inclusion all the more important. Knowledge—what is used daily is easy to remember; when not used, it is often forgotten. The chapter should be a good reference source, and answers to problems given will be found in the Appendix.

The chapter previously entitled "Variations in Drug Therapy to Suit Patients of Different Age Groups" has been expanded and divided into two new chapters: "Changes in Drug Therapy for Infants and Children" and "Changes in Drug Therapy for the Older Patient." This places emphasis on two important medical specialties, pediatrics and geriatrics.

The reference bibliography in the Appendix has been deleted and a list of references now follows each chapter. This change had been requested by several instructors. It is hoped that having the references nearer the material being studied will be helpful to the instructors and will introduce the student to literature pertinent to the profession.

As in previous editions, the most recent revision of the Current Drug Handbook has been included. As before, it is also published as a separate book and is revised every two years.

THE AUTHORS

PREFACE TO THE FIRST EDITION

The teaching of pharmacology by the teacher and its learning by the student has always been one of the most difficult accomplishments in the nursing school curriculum. Students, generally, have seemed to be unable to crystallize the subject clearly in their minds, and there has been attendant difficulty in translating classroom theory into bedside nursing. Everyone agrees that rote memory with parrot-like answering is inadequate. The administration of medicines must include not only remembering, but understanding and critical thinking as well. A student who thinks critically, uses and applies facts and principles. In giving medicines, the nurse must recall facts and principles which apply to the situation, and use these in acting upon and evaluating the results. She must be able to select information about her patient which is relevant and pertinent, see the significance of these data and be able to act upon them. It cannot be denied that the theoretical study of drugs, to be effective and thorough, cannot be separated from practical application.

A variety of different methods of teaching this subject have been tried with varying degrees of success; but no one method ever seemed to carry with it what could be considered a full measure of success. Some years ago, the answer yielded itself to teachers who had deliberated and struggled with the problem for so long a time. The answer embodied the desirability and the necessity of approaching the teaching of the subject from the clinical viewpoint—using the patient and his recovery as the central theme of the course. Since then, this approach has been used by an ever-increasing number of teachers, and results have brought assurance that it is the correct one, the logical one, the practical one. It encourages the student and the teacher to focus attention and emphasis on the chief motive of nursing—helping the patient. It is the most valuable method, for it finally bridges the gap between classroom theory and bedside nursing. It should enable the nurse to use the problem-solving technique in the administration of medications.

This book has been prepared to present the study of drugs from this more interesting aspect. It is important to note that because the book describes this subject through the medium of the patient, it is automatically adapted for use in the academic program which correlates the various classroom subjects in the area of treatment, as well as where pharmacology is taught as a separate subject.

The limitation on the number of hours that can be devoted to the teaching of this subject precludes encompassing all the facts of pharmacology that have usually been included in the course in years gone by, as well as all of the material which automatically makes up the clinical approach to the subject. The time limitation necessitates the elimination of some of "the old" because of the necessity of including "the new." Those teachers who feel that the correlated program is the correct approach appreciate that the over-all improvement, resulting from presentation of the material from the clinical viewpoint, more than overshadows the loss of some of the strictly pharmacologic material.

For practical reasons, the book has been divided into two parts. The first part provides a comprehensive basis for the clinical study which follows in Part II. The clinical section is neither entirely nor primarily concerned with the study of drugs as such. Rather, the study of drugs is in balance and in relation to those other equally important aspects of the total picture, the nurse and the patient. The extensive index provides a quick means of finding data about drugs.

Because an understanding of the educational assets and the method of using a book is a sensible prerequisite to its use, the authors have prepared a brief summary of suggested means of obtaining the most value from this book. It is suggested that those using this book carefully read the "Suggestions to Teachers and Students."

A wide variety of references has been used in the preparation of the manuscript. The authors have relied heavily on the United States Pharmacopeia XV and the British Pharmacopoeia not only to insure the most up-to-date list of drugs, but also to offer drug standards. Information on the more recent drugs has been secured from several different sources, all of which are ethically and scientifically acceptable and regularly used.

A bibliography of books which the authors have found useful is included. It is not intended to be all inclusive. Some of these are official publications, others are general reference books, while still others are publications from the field of pharmacy. This last group will be needed to keep the student abreast of the latest information in the field of drugs.

The authors are deeply grateful for the assistance of all the many people who have helped to bring this work to completion. All clinical chapters have been checked for accuracy by physicians who are specialists in their fields. Special thanks go to Sister Leander, R.N., B.S., for the aid she has given, both material and spiritual. We would like to express our grateful appreciation to Miss June Roslund, R.N., M.S., and Dr. N. A. Hall for their valuable critical appraisal of the manuscript.

MARY W. FALCONER

MABELCLAIRE R. NORMAN

SUGGESTIONS FOR THE USE OF THE BOOK FOR BOTH TEACHERS AND STUDENTS

This book is the result of much thought about the ways and means of making the subject of Pharmacology more meaningful to the student and of bringing into closer contact the formal study of drugs and the actual care of the patient. The authors have attempted to keep the book patient-centered at all times. It would seem unnecessary to emphasize that "drugs are used to treat people—not diseases," but many nurses become so enthusiastic over the scientific and therapeutic value of drugs for specific conditions that they forget that it is an individual person who is being treated and that, no matter how good a certain drug may usually be, it can be wholly ineffective for the patient under treatment.

The book itself is patient-centered, but all the major drugs that nurses are usually called upon to administer have been collected for reference in the Current Drug Handbook. It has been planned that the text will be used throughout the student's entire preclinical and clinical experiences, and that it may also be retained as a reference after graduation.

The book is divided into three parts:

I. Material of basic general interest which will be needed in all clinical areas.

II. Material about the administration of drugs.

III. Material on drugs and their use in the treatment of patients, divided according to the usual clinical divisions of most hospitals and medical books.

The first part of the book does not deviate markedly from a standard pharmacology textbook, though the authors have tried to eliminate nonessential details in order to make this area more interesting to the student.

Chapter 5 covers the mathematics of pharmacology. It has been kept as simple as was consistent with the material involved. Only those areas which are usually difficult for the student to understand have been included. Any student seriously deficient in basic arithmetic processes should take a remedial course before attempting posology. The number of practice and review problems is small. Some have been added at the end of various clinical chapters. The instructor should use those which are pertinent to the practice in her area. Calculation of dosage is becoming less and less the nurse's responsibility. However, when it is required, she must be able to do the calculations accurately.

The third part of the book is planned for use in conjunction with the various clinical experiences of the student. There are chapters discussing drugs used in specialized areas, such as in the treatment of the obstetric patient, as well as chapters discussing drugs for the general medical and surgical patient.

A regular chapter plan has been used in the development of this part of the text, varying only as needed to suit the different materials presented. At the beginning of each chapter there is a list of basic scientific information important in the understanding of the material in the body of that chapter. These are very brief, but the student should study (from an appropriate reference source) any she feels she does not fully understand. A somewhat arbitrary coding has been used to secure uniformity. The sciences have been numbered with Roman numerals as follows:

I. Anatomy and Physiology
II. Chemistry
III. Microbiology
IV. Physics
V. Psychology
VI. Sociology

The subheadings have been given Arabic numerals, thus 1, 2, 3, and so on. This plan has been followed even though, in some cases, a heading has only one subheading. References have been placed at appropriate places in the body of the chapters, thus, I-3, V-1, III-4, etc. It is expected that the student will refer back to the beginning of the chapter to aid her understanding of the subject matter presented. Naturally, some chapters will need far more basic scientific background than others and, in some cases, there will be only one or at most two sciences used as reference.

The body of each chapter in which clinical material is included contains, first, a brief discussion of the typical clinical picture, with the predominant symptoms as they are usually encountered. Following this is a consideration of which drugs are used to alleviate these symptoms or to cure the condition, how they are administered, and what action is likely to take place. Only information about drugs directly pertinent to the proper care of the patient is given. If further information is desired, the student is expected to refer to the last section of the book or to other appropriate references.

The following outline has been maintained throughout the clinical section, varying, as mentioned before, according to change in subject material.

Definition (of the disease or condition, usually with a brief discussion of it)
Major Symptoms
Drug Therapy
  The Drug
  The Nurse
  The Patient

The basic divisions have been further subdivided as follows:

THE DRUG NAME

The Drug. Here is a brief statement as to source, historical significance of the drug or any other pertinent fact not covered in the other areas.

Physical and Chemical Properties: A very brief coverage of the physical and chemical properties of the drug under consideration, especially those that are of significance to the nurse.

Action: This covers the action of the drug in the body insofar as this is known.

Therapeutic Uses: Conditions for which the drug is used.

Absorption and Excretion: How the drug enters the body, its fate within the body, how, where and in what form it is excreted. Again, this insofar as it is known.

Preparations and Dosages: Various preparations of the drug, how given, the average dose and usually how often it is administered. In this area are included the generic and major trade names, both of the United States and Canada. The letter designation is also given, such as U.S.P., N.F., B.P.

THE NURSE. There may or may not be a short introductory statement of the place of the nurse in the administration of this drug, depending upon the contents of the subheadings under this main heading.

Mode of Administration: Here is given how the drug is administered, why that route is used, if pertinent, and any problems the nurse is likely to encounter in giving this drug. The next four headings may be combined or one or more may be omitted depending upon the specific drug being discussed. They are:

Side Effects: Effects to be expected from this drug other than those for which it is given. What, if anything, can and should be done about them.

Toxicity and Treatment: If the side effects are all undesirable, this heading may merge with the one above. However, usually serious toxic symptoms and their treatment are discussed here.

Interactions: Effect this drug has on other drugs given at or about the same time, and also their action on the drug being discussed.

Contraindications: Contraindications are given if there are any.

Patient Teaching: This heading is self-explanatory, what the nurse should tell the patient and/or his family about the medicine, especially if the drug is to be taken at home without direct medical or nurse supervision.

In some instances under the heading THE NURSE no subdivisions are given, since a brief overall coverage seemed more appropriate.

THE PATIENT. Under this heading is considered the psychologic, emotional, social, economic and spiritual aspects of the particular drug and/or disease being discussed. Some phases of patient teaching may be included here. In some instances the material under this heading may be applicable to several drugs. Where this is the case, the information is given only once to avoid repetition. There are cross references to cover this contingency.

Each major drug has been covered in detail only once. This is to avoid repetition. In the index, in bold type, will be found the reference for this. Since many drugs are used for a number of different disorders, but in most cases there is one main use, cross references are again used to show this and to designate other uses.

At the end of each chapter the authors have included a section labeled "It Is Important to Remember." Very briefly, this gives some of the more important facts brought out in the chapter, especially facts which are somewhat contrary to the layman's belief. Lastly, there is a section marked "Topics for Study and Discussion." It is hoped that these will serve to stimulate the student to further investigation of drugs and their place in helping people to "get well" and to "keep well." Among these topics will be found problems which the student may encounter in giving the drugs, discussed in the body of the chapter. The authors feel that even though the subject of the mathematics of drugs may be covered early in the nursing program, it is well to refresh the memory with up-to-date problems. Many instructors ask this type of question at each class as a teaching aid.

It is planned that each chapter will be taught with the clinical classes covering that specific material and/or the clinical experiences in that particular subject. Thus, the chapter "Drugs Used During Pregnancy, Delivery and Lactation" would be studied while the student is doing practical work in obstetrics. If the school curriculum is not planned so that this is possible, the student should review the chapter when studying the clinical material to which it relates.

Some of the chapters can be covered in a single class, but most of them have been planned for several classes. For instance, the chapter just mentioned contains discussion of the drugs used during pregnancy, labor, delivery and the puerperium. This might be four separate classes or parts of several classes dealing with these areas in the general course in obstetric nursing. Or, the instructor might feel that there is insufficient material for more than two classes. These are things that will be decided by the number of hours devoted to the entire subject.

When pharmacology is taught as a separate subject preceding or concurrent with the first clinical courses, this text will prove very valuable, since there is sufficient coverage of the various diseases and conditions to show the reasons for the drugs used in treating them.

The fourth and last part is a revision of the Current Drug Handbook, published by the same authors. This part was also included at the request of the instructors using the text. The authors have tried to list all the old drugs still in relatively common use and, at the same time, to include many of the newer ones. It is impossible for any book to comprise all drugs or to be completely up-to-date. There are a great many new drugs marketed each year, and some of them become important adjuncts to pharmaceutical therapy. Because of the time lapse between writing and publication, those of recent origin will not be found. The student is advised to augment the information found in the text with a notebook or card file system of her own. Most pharmaceutical firms will gladly give information about their products, and many new drugs come with printed material telling of their use, dosage, toxicity, etc. Excellent reference information for the library and classes can be obtained from the same sources. The instructor, if she has not already made this discovery, will find that drug companies will gladly place her on their mailing lists, and this will g ve a constant source of information about new drugs and new uses for old drugs.

A glossary has not been included since most students find it more convenient and helpful to use a regular medical dictionary for words not understood or not properly explained in the text.

THE AUTHORS

CONTENTS

PART ONE INTRODUCTION

PART TWO CLINICAL PHARMACOLOGY

Section 1 Drugs Used in a Variety of Clinical Conditions

Current Drug Handbook (1974–76) follows the Index.

PART ONE

INTRODUCTION

CHAPTER 1

THE DEVELOPMENT OF PHARMACOLOGY

Fire properly controlled is man's best friend—uncontrolled, it is his worst enemy. This same statement might well be applied to drugs. Properly used, drugs are a great blessing to mankind; indiscriminately or improperly used, they could destroy the race.

The nurse will find the study of drugs a fascinating pursuit. There is real romance in the origin of many medicines, and a real thrill in the dramatic recoveries some drugs produce. However, as with most important subjects, the study of pharmacology is accompanied by many less interesting details. The student must be able to see the final goal—the lessening of human suffering—to appreciate the need for understanding these seemingly minor points. It is the fact that most drugs can kill as well as cure that makes the full understanding of all the details essential.

The history of pharmacology is as old as the story of mankind. Man has always experienced sickness and injury and has searched for means of combating disease and caring for the wounded. This search for therapeutic measures marks the progress of civilization.

Man's earliest medicinal remedies were the result of several divergent factors. One was his observation of the activities of animals, both wild and those he early domesticated. He was able, by watching them, to learn some of the therapeutic properties of various plants, waters and muds. Most primitive peoples believed that the world was filled with invisible spirits which were either good or bad. Disease was the manifestation of the evil spirit. Therefore, to cure disease it was essential to "drive out" these spirits by giving the patient all sorts of noxious materials. The experimentation with these substances led to the beginning of medicine, for some of the "medicines" actually did help the patients to recover. Combining the information gained from these, and no doubt other sources, with his own observations of the effects of certain herbs, other plants, and animal products, led early man to the discovery of the real value of many substances used in medicine today. Savages in widely separated areas knew the effects of certain poisons such as curare, veratrine, ouabain and nux vomica. They used these poisons on their arrows and spear tips to paralyze or kill the victim, animal or man. Curare, which causes temporary paralysis, was used mainly for hunting, as the agent did not affect persons eating the meat of animals on which it had been used. Today curare is used as a skeletal muscle relaxant. Veratrine, ouabain and nux vomica usually killed and in the latter case the meat was apt to be poisonous. Strychnine is obtained from nux vomica. It is a strong muscle stimulant causing convulsions in large doses. It is not in common use now since other less toxic drugs are available. Veratrine derivatives are now used to reduce high blood pressure and ouabain is used in the treatment of certain forms of heart disease.

Primitive men also knew of the beneficial effects of many drugs which are still used. Probably the most important of these was the latex (milk) of the capsule of the poppy—opium—which is still used to relieve pain.

PRE-CHRISTIAN MEDICINE

Egyptian

Some of the oldest written records of drugs are the Egyptian papyri, the most important of which is the Ebers papyrus written about the sixteenth century B.C.

This is a scroll over 20 yards long which contains clinical reports, a collection of prescriptions and formulas covering a wide range of materials. Many of the recipes include drugs that are still in use. Among these are castor oil, wormwood, aloe, peppermint, opium and henbane. Minerals and metals used by the Egyptians were iron, copper sulfate, magnesia, niter, sodium carbonate, sodium chloride and precious stones finely pulverized. The animal products included such extraordinary substances as lizard's blood, swine's teeth, asses' hoofs, goose grease, animal fat and animal excreta; other weird things listed were the thigh bone of a hanged man and moss grown on a human skull.

The pharmacist of the period made pharmaceutical preparations of these drugs in the form of pills, powders, infusions, decoctions, salves, plasters and confections. Some of the recipes contained as many as 35 ingredients. It is believed that the Egyptians used the juice of the poppy and Indian hemp to make the patients drowsy before surgical operations were performed. Since physicians were also priests, the healing art was closely associated with the spiritual life; no doubt there were many patients healed by "psychosomatic" means. Many of the Egyptian drugs found their way later into the materia medica of the Greeks and, through them, were passed on to other nations.

Asia Minor

Babylonia, Assyria, Palestine and Persia (the "Fertile Crescent") were all, at one time or another, important historically. In general, these countries contributed more toward the prevention than the cure of disease. Moses gave the Hebrews excellent rules for community sanitation which may be found in the Bible in the Books of Leviticus and Numbers. Here are discussed means of obtaining clean food and water, the proper disposal of waste and the isolation of people with communicable diseases. King Hammurabi's Code listed many fine rules of hygiene and sanitation for the people of Babylon. There is not much in these writings, however, concerning actual drugs.

Other Areas

In the New World, the various Indian tribes had their "medicine men" who used incantations and many herbs to cure diseases. As with other primitive peoples, their medicine was a mixture of religion, mysticism, superstition and actual knowledge of the medicinal properties of various substances. Specifically, in South America, the Peruvians used cinchona for malaria and coca (from which cocaine is derived) to relieve fatigue. Cocaine and its derivatives are now used as local anesthetic agents. Brazilians used ipecac for amebic dysentery. The North American Indians knew of the value of cascara as a laxative, arbutus for rheumatism, lobelia for colds, sassafras leaves for wounds and the root of this plant for "cooling and purifying" the blood.

Other countries early contributed to the realm of medicine. Indians (Hindus) used rauwolfia to calm the restless and to treat heart diseases. It is still used for these and other conditions. The Chinese used ma huang, from which ephedrine is obtained, to treat asthma centuries before the birth of Christ. The alkaloid ephedrine, responsible for the effectiveness of ma huang, was first isolated in 1924, and it is still used extensively in the management of asthma and other conditions.

Greco-Roman

In Greece, as in all ancient countries, the healing art was a part of the religious practices of the people. Temples to Aesculapius, the god of healing, were built. Since these temples were usually situated in the hills and mountains near mineral springs, they virtually became sanatoria. The patients were treated first by prayer and sacrifices for spiritual perfection. Then came physical cleansing in the mineral baths and internal cleansing by catharsis. Further treatments were massage, inunctions and the taking of medicated wines. Soft music was used to induce restful sleep. If the treatments were successful and the patient recovered, a votive tablet giving the history of the case and the treatment was hung in the temple where anyone who wished might consult it. In this way, a considerable body of empirical knowledge was assembled, and these temples of health took on some of the characteristics of medical schools.

Hippocrates, often called the father of medicine, lived in Greece in the fifth century B.C. He denied the supernatural origin of disease. He felt that treatment should be by natural means and not by magic, and his therapeutic measures were decidedly modern. He believed that nature had the power to cure disease, and that the physician should aid natural recuperative powers by sunlight, diet, baths, massage and drugs. Although he mentioned over 400 drugs in his writings, there is evidence that he used a relatively small number of them in actual practice. Among the preparations used by Hippocrates were poultices, suppositories, pills, lozenges, ointments, cerates and gargles.

Dioscorides, in the first century B.C., wrote a materia medica which was an important reference for many years. He was a Greek physician who followed the lead of Hippocrates but enlarged upon his work. He described many drugs now used, such as opium, arsenic and aspidium. Some of the 600 drugs he discussed are still listed in the present pharmacopeias.

With the Roman conquest of Greece, Greek medicine was introduced into Rome. Some of the physicians were taken to Rome as slaves, and others went voluntarily as freemen in search of better opportunities. One of the Greek doctors who went to Rome was Galen (A.D. 131-201). He based his teachings and practices very largely on the work of Hippocrates and established a system of medicine and pharmacy which made him the supreme authority for several hundred years. Galen held that drugs should be used to counteract the symptoms of the disease. He originated many preparations of vegetable drugs which even now are spoken of as "galenicals."

EARLY MIDDLE AGES

With the downfall of Rome and the ensuing "Dark Ages," the progress of medicine, in common with most of the arts and sciences, came almost to a standstill. There was little change in the old established customs. The practices of the Greek and Roman doctors were kept alive during this period by various means, the most important of which were the work of the monastic orders and the Arabian physicians.

The monks, particularly those of the Benedictine monasteries, used a wide variety of medicinal substances. Treatment of the sick and injured was a part of their mission in life and was both spiritual and physical. They prescribed rest, good food and herbs grown in the monastery gardens. Many of the substances used by them are familiar to us, such as colchicum for gout, cantharides as a vesicant and others that are still in use. Since the monks were not allowed to shed blood, blood letting and surgery were done by barbers; thus, the barber-surgeon came into being.

Superstition still held considerable sway, especially among the laymen. Charms were worn to ward off disease. Many people believed that disease was the punishment for "sin," hence prayers and penance were used in the treatment of various disorders.

MEDIEVAL MEDICINE

In the eighth century A.D. the Arabs swept over Asia Minor and northern Africa and into Spain. They absorbed the medicine of Hippocrates and Galen, and during the 500 years of their supremacy advanced the science of medicine and pharmacy in many ways. One of the greatest of the Arabian physicians was Avicenna (A.D. 980-1037), whose "Canon of Medicine" was in use centuries after his death. Rhazes, whose real name was Abu Bakr Muhammad ibn Zakariyya (A.D. 860-932), also contributed greatly to the Arabian knowledge of medicine.

The Arabians not only contributed many new plant drugs, but they also made great strides in the chemistry of medicines. Some of the plant drugs they used were senna, camphor, cubeb, aconite, cannabis and sandalwood. Mineral substances employed by them in the treatment of diseases included antimony, iron, nitrates, nitric acid and mercuric chloride. The Arabs compiled the first pharmacopeia and they are also considered to be the first to separate pharmacy from the other healing arts.

During the fourteenth and fifteenth centuries, medicine was brought to the foreground by the repeated "plagues" of the times. Severe epidemics were common; bubonic plague and various forms of dysentery brought widespread terror. Ergotism, a type of poisoning produced by fungus-infected grain, was frequent.

It was during this period that alchemy, the forerunner of chemistry, was popular. The alchemists were searching for the "elixir of life," which would ward off or cure all diseases, and for the "philosopher's stone," which would turn base metals into gold. Although they did not realize their objectives, they did discover many important things, and their work formed the basis for modern chemistry.

MEDICINE DURING THE RENAISSANCE

Our modern medicine and pharmacy had its beginning during the sixteenth century renaissance. Many of the physicians, barber-surgeons and other medical workers began to question the established methods. One of the most notable of these was Theophrastus Paracelsus (1493-1541), a Swiss physician, who traveled and studied extensively and who believed strongly in knowledge gained by experience. He was contemptuous of the "old school," and publicly burned Avicenna's Canon and the works of Galen and Hippocrates. He tried to get the alchemists to direct their attention to medicinal formulas rather than gold. A number of new remedies were introduced by Paracelsus, such as calomel, sulfur and the mercurial compounds for syphilis.

A collection of formulas by Valerius Cordus which was adopted by the governing body of the city of Nuremburg, Germany, in 1546 was the first official pharmacopeia. It mentioned such pharmaceutical preparations as confections, syrups, pills, lozenges, plasters, ointments and cerates.

In 1618 the first pharmacopeia in Britain was published in London. It was based largely on the works of Galen and the Arabian physicians, and included more than 1900 remedies. One formula called for 130 ingredients.

Although several cities had pharmacopeias, the first national one was not published until 1818 (the French Codex). It was soon followed by one in the United States, 1820, and later by one in Great Britain, 1864, and in Germany, 1872.

During the seventeenth century many new drugs came into use. Some of these are still popular, such as laudanum (tincture of opium), Rochelle salts (potassium sodium tartrate), Epsom salts (magnesium sulfate) and boric acid. In 1638 cinchona was introduced from Peru for the treatment of "ague" (malaria). It had been used by the South American Indians for generations. Other such importations included coca from Peru, ipecac from Brazil and jalap from Mexico.

Belladonna, from the deadly nightshade, and mandrake, a related plant, were used for many purposes by Arabian, Greek and Roman physicians. Later, belladonna was used by the Spanish ladies to dilate the pupils of the eyes for its beautifying effect. It thus obtained its name (bella—beautiful, donna—a lady). Belladonna and its derivatives form an important segment of drug therapy today.

EIGHTEENTH CENTURY MEDICINE

In the latter part of the eighteenth century, Edward Jenner (1749-1823), an English physician, gave the world a method for preventing smallpox by vaccination. There have been numerous dramatic episodes in the history of medicine, and many men have contributed lifesaving drugs to the long list of effective medicines used today, but probably one of the most sensational was the result of the keen observation of a country doctor. Jenner saw what others before him had seen, namely, that milkmaids were very pretty because they were not marred by pox marks, but he went beyond that, noting that it was because these girls had had cowpox that they did not get smallpox. The conclusion was obvious. After studying the problem thoroughly, he was able to prove conclusively that inoculation with cowpox would prevent smallpox. In 1779 (in England) 15,000 people died from smallpox; in 1823 the number of deaths from the same disease was only 37. This was the first of a long list of diseases now effectively controlled by the proper use of preventive measures such as inoculations.

Digitalis, the purple foxglove, was an herb added to many remedies used during the late Middle Ages. About the middle of the eighteenth century, William Withering, an English physician, associated this herb with the relief of dropsy, a generalized edema, which is a symptom of heart failure. This led to the realization that digitalis could be used to treat heart disease. It is still one of the leading drugs used for disorders of cardiac origin.

About the same time Thomas Dover originated his "Dover's Powder," a mixture of equal parts of opium powder and ipecac. It is said that he used such large doses that the pharmacists advised his patients to make their wills before taking the drug. It is also said that he was not a regular physician but what, today, would be called a "quack." Dover's Powder was used to treat any number of diseases.

NINETEENTH CENTURY MEDICINE

With the advent of the germ theory of disease, as demonstrated by the work of such men as Leeuwenhoek, Pasteur and Koch, medical treatment was directed toward a new line of attack. It became evident that medicines must be found that would kill these tiny organisms without injuring the patient, and from this time on medical discoveries have been numerous.

Louis Pasteur of France (1822-1895) developed the preventive for rabies, and this treatment still bears his name. His theory of antitoxins is the basis for much of present preventive medicine. Pasteur also did a great amount of work in the field of microbiology and the prevention of various animal diseases, such as anthrax in sheep. During this period, attention was directed to the use of antiserums to control such infections. A very notable contribution was the discovery of diphtheria antitoxin by von Behring in 1890.

Joseph, Lord Lister (1827-1912), a Scottish surgeon, applied Pasteur's finding to the field of surgery. He used phenol (carbolic acid) as a means of destroying microorganisms in the operating room. Several antiseptic solutions had been discovered earlier; among these were potassium permanganate, hydrogen peroxide and iodine. These, with the use of anesthesia, made modern surgery possible.

Early in the nineteenth century Justus von Liebig synthesized chloral hydrate, chloroform and some other drugs. Sir James Simpson, in England, demonstrated the effectiveness of chloroform as an anesthetic agent. About the same time, working in the United States. Dr. Crawford Long and Dr. William T. Morton showed that ether was useful in producing anesthesia. Some other important advances during this period were:

The demonstration of the value of *Strophanthus* in heart diseases by Sir Thomas Fraser.

The discovery of the property of the nitrites in the reduction of blood pressure by Sir Thomas Brunten at St. Bartholomew's Hospital, London. He also used the nitrites in the treatment of angina pectoris. Nitrites are used for this purpose today.

Frederick Sertürner's isolation of the first active principle of a drug—the alkaloid morphine from opium—was a real contribution to the family of medicines. There have followed a long line of such discoveries, which even now is continuing. To mention a few: Pierre Pelletier isolated quinine from cinchona and François Magendie, strychnine from nux vomica.

With increased knowledge of chemistry, more and more drug compounds were broken down into simpler substances. This analytical chemistry led to many pharmaceutical discoveries, both directly and indirectly. In 1850, the French Society of Pharmacy offered a prize of 4000 francs for an artificial method of preparing quinine. Although this was not accomplished until nearly a century later, William Henry Perkins in trying to solve that mystery discovered the first coal tar dye—the first of an almost endless list of coal tar preparations, medicinal and otherwise.

Late in the nineteenth century there were discoveries in chemistry and physics that were to become very important to medicine. These were the discovery in 1893 of radium by Madame Curie and the discovery in 1895 of the x-ray by Wilhelm Roentgen.

TWENTIETH CENTURY MEDICINE

During the first part of the twentieth century there have been enormous strides in the field of pharmacology. Of the old drugs, many have been discarded, many more purified and many entirely new ones have been found. Even the concept of drug therapy has changed in many ways. This will be enlarged upon in subsequent chapters. However, some of the more important discoveries should be mentioned here.

In 1907, Paul Ehrlich in his six hundred and sixth experiment perfected salvarsan (or 606), an arsenic preparation, used against the spirochetal and protozoal infections that plague man. Later Paul Hanslite made Sobisminol, an oral bismuth compound, for the treatment of diseases caused by the same organisms. Chaulmoogric acid, obtained from chaulmoogra oil, which has been used to treat Hansen's disease (leprosy) was the work of Frederick Power.

Numerous drugs are the result of several people's work and cannot be credited to any one person. A few such are the changing of resorcinol to hexylresorcinol; the perfection of carbon tetrachloride, a remedy for various helminthic infestations; the reduction of strong mercury compounds into milder and very useful antiseptics. Near the turn of the last century various fever reducing drugs came into use. These include the coal tar derivatives, notably antipyrine and salicylic acid and its derivatives.

Food deficiency as a cause of disease was first demonstrated conclusively by the Dutch physiologist Christian Eijkman in 1886. Somewhat earlier a Japanese named Takaki had made the same observation, but it was not widely publicized. He showed that beriberi resulted from a diet of polished rice. In 1911 Casimir Funk showed that the substance lacking in that diet was vitamin B_1. That lime juice prevented scurvy had long been known, but the reason for this or its real significance was not shown until after the isolation of vitamin C.

Charles Edouard Brown-Séquard on June 1, 1889, started the quest for knowledge about hormones that is still going on. He thought that he had found a substance that would prevent aging. He was wrong, but he had pointed the way to a new field of research.

Insulin was first used for diabetes by Dr. Frederick Banting and Dr. Charles H. Best of the University of Toronto, Ontario, Canada, in 1922. This has given hope and life to many thousands of diabetics. Discovery of two other hormones preceded that of insulin; epinephrine, first isolated in 1897 by Abel and Crawford, and thyroxin, isolated by Kendall in 1914. The first gonadal hormone isolated was estrogen in 1923 by Allen and Doisy.

The value of liver in the treatment of pernicious anemia was shown by George R. Minot and William P. Murphy a few years after the discovery of insulin. It has since been shown that the vitamin B_{12} in liver is the active principle.

Penicillin (the wonder drug) was discovered, by accident, by Sir Alexander Fleming at St. Mary's Hospital, London, in 1929. Fleming noted that in a culture of staphylococci contaminated with the mold *Penicillium notatum*, the growth of the bacteria was inhibited. Further research led to the development of the drug, which came into general use during World War II. Penicillin was the first in a long line of antibiotic drugs, and the end has not yet been reached.

There are many other men whose work has been of importance in the field of pharmacy. Among those whose work has had a profound effect upon medicinal therapy are:

Sydenham, who taught that the body had the ability to repair itself. He used drugs sparingly and only to aid nature.

Hahnemann, who founded homeopathy, used only one drug at a time. This he gave well diluted in small amounts at frequent intervals. He directed this medicine at the principal symptom of the disease. He stressed dietary and hygienic regimens to aid nature to overcome disease.

Skoda repudiated the use of drugs indiscriminately. He advocated using only those medicines scientifically proved to be effective.

In recent years, with the rapid advances in many sciences, medicines are often first conceived as chemical formulas directed at specific disease agents or bodily functions. This is then produced as a chemical entity, tested for purity, tested on animals for effectiveness and lack of toxicity and then given clinical trials in humans. *Rationalism* has replaced *empiricism*. Older biological drugs are broken down into their component parts and only the effective portions, the active principles, are used. Often these active principles can then be produced synthetically.

Many new drugs have appeared during the middle of the twentieth century, but there have been no dramatic breakthroughs. No single individual has perfected the newer preparations, since most new drugs are the result of the work of a team of scientists. Often, the team works toward a specific goal, such as the elimination of certain undesirable side effects of an existing drug, replacement of a medication no longer effective or discovery of a drug to combat a recently identified disorder.

The quest for beneficial remedies had its beginnings with the earliest man and the search goes on. Man continues to strive, not only for a longer life span, but for a healthier one as well. He has gone a long way in realizing this goal, but as he overcomes one obstacle, another arises, so the task is never ending.

IT IS IMPORTANT TO REMEMBER

1. That man has been seeking ways and means of lessening his suffering, and curing his ills since the beginning of time, and the search is still going on.
2. That in each age some new preparation or treatment has been hailed as a "panacea," and then has been found to be limited in its action.
3. That no one drug can ever cure all ills, since there are so many and almost all have different causes. The medicine that will cure one disease may be useless in the treatment of another.
4. That the end of drug discoveries has no more been reached than the end of any other scientific research.
5. That though it is of interest to know how, when, where and by whom the various medicines were discovered, it is vastly more important to know how, when and why they are used for the benefit of the patient.

TOPICS FOR STUDY AND DISCUSSION

1. What superstitions about medicine, health and disease exist today? Make a survey among your acquaintances and bring the results to your class for a general discussion.
2. Where might primitive medicine exist today? Why could this be possible?
3. What was the basis for primitive man's treatment of disease? What were the causative factors behind these treatments?
4. Why might it be helpful to understand the treatments and medications used by primitive people living today as well as the traditional lore of earlier cultures (such as the American Indians or mountain people of Appalachia).
5. What effect did Christianity have upon medicine and pharmacy? Were the effects good or bad or both? Justify your answer.
6. What events in history have had especially profound effects upon drugs? Name at least two, and tell why you selected these.
7. Make a list of men of the nineteenth century who made important pharmacological discoveries, and tell what each discovered.
8. Make a list of men of the twentieth century who made important pharmacological discoveries, and tell what each discovered.
9. What advances or discoveries in chemistry and physics have produced marked effects upon medicines and their use? Give at least two and tell what the effect was.

CHAPTER 2

GENERAL INFORMATION ABOUT DRUGS

CORRELATION WITH OTHER SCIENCES

II. CHEMISTRY

1. An alkali or base will react with an acid to form a salt. This process is called neutralization.
2. A catalyst is a substance which hastens or aids a chemical reaction without entering into that reaction.

VI. SOCIOLOGY

1. Standards of various products are set by law. These laws may be local, state, national or international. Experts in each field give the lawmakers data which determine the standards. These standards are then set forth in legal publications.
2. The United States government maintains a patent office where new products, discoveries, inventions, etc., can be protected for a specified length of time against duplication by others.

INTRODUCTION

In order to understand any new subject it is essential to have a working acquaintance with the words used in discussing it. This is especially true of pharmacology. Few laymen have occasion to learn the definitions of many pharmacological terms. Although the nurse does not need to know so many as does the pharmacist or the physician, nevertheless she must be familiar with those which are applicable to her field. In this and other chapters such definitions will be given as seem essential for the nurse to know in order to fulfill her duties successfully.

The words drug and medicine have already been used. They are, for all practical purposes, synonymous terms. There are many definitions of these words, but the following will suffice for our uses:

A *drug* (or *medicine*) is, broadly speaking, any substance other than food which, when taken into the body, affects the living protoplasm.* This definition, like most definitions, does not entirely satisfy all types of drugs but does cover the more important medicinal products. The word drug is derived from the Dutch word "droog" meaning dry, since most early drugs were dried plants and plant products.

Pharmacology is the science which treats of the origin, the nature and the effects of drugs. It is the most common term now used to cover the entire subject.

---

*The United States Pure Food and Drug Act defines a drug as follows: "The term drug as used in this act shall include all medications and preparations recognized in the United States Pharmacopeia or the National Formulatory for internal or external use and any substances or mixtures of substances intended to be used for the cure, mitigation or prevention of disease of either man or animals."

Toxicology is the science which treats of the nature and effect of poisons, including the poisonous effects possible from a medicinal drug.

Therapeutics is the treatment of disease, medicines being only one small portion of the entire subject.

Poison is any substance which when taken into the body, usually in small amounts, will endanger life.

Posology is the science of the dosage of drugs.

SOURCES OF DRUGS

Almost all types of drugs were originally prepared by grinding and mixing dried plants or parts of plants (Fig. 1). Although these are still used, most drugs today are prepared in the pharmaceutical laboratories and do not even faintly resemble the substances from which they are derived. It must be realized that, even though most of the preparations are manufactured products, they are secured from basic sources, and many of these are the same as the original drugs. It has become more important in many instances to understand the chemical formula and the properties of a medicinal substance than to know its source. Since most nurses have only a limited knowledge of organic chemistry, the chemical formulas of the drugs will not be stressed, but the properties of each drug will be emphasized. However, some basic knowledge of the sources of drugs is desirable.

Organic Sources

PLANT SOURCES

All portions of plants are used as drugs—stem, wood, bark, roots, bulb, corm, rhizome, leaves, buds, blossoms, seeds, fruit and sap. If the product is used without much refinement, such as the ground leaves or powdered dried sap, the substance is called a crude drug. In such form it will contain much that is extraneous and not of a medicinal nature and, although most of this material is inert, it may be somewhat irritant to the body tissues. In these crude drugs there are substances known as *active principles* which are responsible for the major action of the drug. Active principles vary greatly in nature and effect. The more important types will be given.

Alkaloids form one of the largest groups of active principles. As the name implies, they act like an alkali. Alkaloids are organic substances that react with an acid to form a salt (II-1). It is this neutralized, or partially neutralized, form that is usually used since salts are more readily soluble in body fluids. The names of alkaloids and their salts usually end in *ine:* for example, atrop*ine*, code*ine* and strychn*ine*.

Glycosides are active principles which when decomposed form sugars and an aglycone. The names of glycosides usually end in *in:* for example, digitox*in*, gital*in* and strophanth*in*.

Other active principles of plant drugs include saponins, oils, tannins, resins, balsams and organic acids. For further information refer to the Appendix.

Fungi and *bacteria* are also sources of drugs, mainly the antibiotics which are the secretions or excretions of the organisms.

ANIMAL SOURCES

Drugs derived from this source are becoming increasingly important. In most

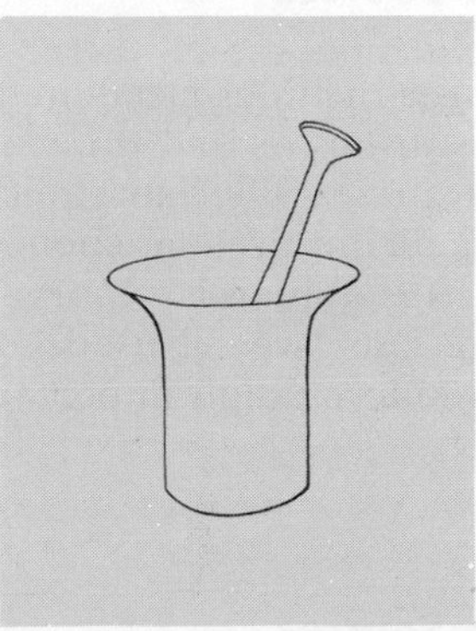

FIGURE 1. The mortar and pestle. These are used by the pharmacist to grind and mix drugs. This is the symbol of the pharmaceutical profession.

cases the medicinal substances are derived either from the animal's body fluids or glands. However, any or all parts of the animal may prove to be sources for various useful drugs. Like the plant products, the drugs from animal sources may be the crude (unrefined) form or the refined material.

The active principles of animal drugs include the following:

Proteins are various compounds of amino acids.

Oils and fats are similar to the plant oils. Most animal oils are fixed oils.

Enzymes are substances produced by living cells which act as catalysts (II-2).

Other biological products include the following:

Serum is the clear fluid portion of the blood. It is similar to plasma but does not contain fibrinogen.

Vaccines are suspensions of killed, modified or attenuated microorganisms.

FROM EITHER PLANTS OR ANIMALS

Microbiological agents, in addition to those mentioned previously, may be the sources of drugs. These agents may be either plant or animal.

Certain substances are secured from both plants and animals. The most important of these are the vitamins. Vitamins are constituents of natural foods essential to normal growth, development and the maintenance of life.

Inorganic Sources

This source includes metal, metalloid and nonmetal substances and the various compounds of these. The inorganic materials used in medicine are the chemically pure forms of the minerals. Inorganic acids, alkalis and salts are all used. Radioactive isotopes are increasingly important in medicine.

Synthetic Sources

Synthetic drugs are those drugs that are prepared (synthesized) in the pharmaceutical laboratories. They may be organic or inorganic or, as is often the case, a combination of organic and inorganic compounds. Many of these are important by-products of other industries. These drugs form an ever-increasing proportion of the products used in medicine.

Additional information on drug sources will be found in the Appendix.

DRUG PREPARATIONS

The types of drug preparations, like their sources, have changed greatly in recent years. Many forms once in regular use are rarely seen now. The pharmaceutical houses today prepare the drug in the form the patient will use, often in the exact dose to be given. This makes the work of the nurse much easier. Injectable medications even come in disposable hypodermics or disposable units for use in especially prepared metal hypodermic frames. These may or may not have the needles attached. If the needle comes with the unit it is used only once and destroyed. If no needle is supplied with the hypodermic or unit, regular needles are used.

A summary of the various preparations may be found in the appendix. The more commonly used ones are discussed briefly here with the method of administration involved.

In the past, medicines were thought to be of value in direct proportion to their unpleasantness, and this led to the use of all sorts of noxious materials as drugs. Refer to Chapter 1. This view is no longer considered correct, for medicinal substances are now used primarily for their chemical action in the body. Since this is true every attempt is made to make the drug as palatable as possible. Various flavoring and coloring agents are used in the preparation of drugs to be given orally so as to make them more attractive. Bitter and sour ingredients are sweetened or better tasting substances added. If the drug can be given in small enough amounts it is put into capsules, pills or tablets. Pharmacists try to make the dispensed drug attractive, pleasant to take and easy to administer.

In hospital practice, it is increasingly common for medications to be dispensed by the "unit system." Drugs are put in individual dose containers and sent to the floor in the exact number of doses required by a particular patient for a given time. The system facilitates the nurses' work and aids greatly in preventing medication errors, since each patient's drugs are entirely separate from all other drugs.

For more information about various drug preparations refer to the Appendix.

OFFICIAL AND NONOFFICIAL DRUGS

All drugs may be divided into two groups – official and nonofficial. By far the majority fall into the latter class. It should be understood that because a drug is listed as nonofficial does not mean that it is a drug of inferior quality or that it is ineffective therapeutically.

Official drugs are those listed in the official publications: the *United States Pharmacopeia* and the *National Formulary*. Drugs listed in these publications are written with the proper initials U.S.P. or N.F. after the name of the drug and they must conform to the standards set by the publication. These publications are revised every four or five years. U.S.P. is revised by a committee of representative medical, pharmaceutical and scientific experts, including officials of the Food and Drug Administration of the federal government (VI-1). For each drug it gives the source, chemical and physical composition, method or methods of assay, usual dosage, primary use and other pertinent information. N.F. is published by the American Pharmaceutical Association and gives similar information about the drugs included in it.

Drugs are occasionally seen on the American markets with the initials B.P. or Ph.I. after the name. These refer to the *British Pharmacopoeia* and the *Specifications for the Quality Control of Pharmaceutical Preparations* (formerly *Pharmacopoeia Internationalis*) (VI-1). The former, which is the official British publication, corresponds to the *United States Pharmacopeia*. The *Specifications for the Quality Control of Pharmaceutical Preparations* is published by the World Health Organization, an agency of the United Nations. This is a relatively new organization, and its standardization of important drugs used by many countries is a great step forward in the control of drugs on the international level.

Since the official publications are revised only every four or five years, and since many very useful drugs come into common use each year, an interim publication is needed. This was previously supplied by the yearly edition of *New and Nonofficial Drugs* published by the Council on Drugs of the American Medical Association. However, in 1965 the American Medical Association published in its place a book called *New Drugs*. Then in 1968 this was replaced by a book called *The A.M.A. Drug Evaluation*. It has been stated that this book should be of considerable clinical value to the physician.

There are many other publications that give valuable information about drugs. *The United States Dispensatory* is a general reference book on botany, chemistry, pharmacology and therapeutics of medicinal substances (VI-1).

These publications are some of those available to the nurse as source material for information on medicinal preparations. In addition, most of the pharmaceutical houses furnish material about the drugs which they sell. The nurse will also find in the library various textbooks of pharmacology, and other books dealing with specific aspects of the subject such as toxicology and therapeutics. The physician and the pharmacist will always remain the nurse's best source of information concerning a specific drug being given to a particular patient.

Each patient has a problem which is different from all other patients' problems. The same drug, given to several patients, may exert a different influence on each. Since human beings are being dealt with, no generalizations can be made even in the case of medicines. The nurse must realize that, though the pharmacology book can give the correct information for the average, usual or expected condition, it does so in an entirely impersonal way. However, the patient to whom the nurse is giving the drug may not be an average case and, therefore, the book's information may not apply. The doctor will be able to explain the use of the medication in any specific instance.

There are many definitions of the word *proprietary*, but one will suffice. According to the American Medical Association Council on Drugs: "The term 'proprietary article' shall mean any chemical, drug, or similar preparation used in the treatment of disease, if such article is protected against free competition, as to name, product, composition, or process of manufacture by secrecy, patent, copyright, or in any other manner" (VI-2). Many useful drugs are proprietary preparations. Such substances vary from simple harmless chemicals to very potent therapeutic agents. Proprietary drugs may become official; they may continue to be used but never be entered in an official publication; or they may eventually be dropped from use.

The word *patent* has been used, but it is not an accurate term for medications. Drugs, except as new chemicals, cannot be patented; but the name or trademark can and often is protected by registration. It is possible for a company, by using a specific name as a trademark, to hold virtually perpetual rights to the use of the name. This was done with the name Adrenalin—the original trade name for epinephrine. The company which introduced this drug has the exclusive rights to the use of the name Adrenalin. The registration is renewable every 20 years. Since under the provisions of the Federal Food, Drug, and Cosmetic Act, the pharmacist may not substitute any other drug where a trade name is used—even though the substances are chemically identical—when the physician uses the name Adrenalin in the prescription, Adrenalin must be provided, unless the physician gives the pharmacist permission to make substitution.

The student should remember that a drug may have more than one name. Actually, most drugs have at least three names: proprietary (trade, common, popular), chemical and official or generic (pharmaceutical, medical). For example, Demerol is the proprietary name for the chemical N-methyl-4-phenyl-4-carbethoxypiperidine hydrochloride. The official name is meperidine, U.S.P. Often the proprietary name is the most commonly used because of the advertising done by the company which sells the product. Since several companies may put out the same drug, each with its own trade name, the nurse should be familiar with the generic name as well as the trade name or names. It is not usually essential for the nurse to know the chemical name. The generic name serves as the medical or pharmaceutical name if and until the drug becomes official. The generic name may or may not be adopted by the official publication. If a new name is given, the previous generic name is usually discarded.

DRUG STANDARDIZATION

All drugs must meet certain rigid standards. These standards are established by the federal government to assure the physician and his patient the receipt of the exact medicinal material ordered. The drug must be what it is represented to be and nothing else. If inert materials are used these must be entirely harmless (VI-1).

Drugs must first be physically pure; that is, there must be no extraneous ingredients. For instance, ground digitalis leaf must not contain parts of the blossoms, stalk or roots. This is the simplest form of purification and standardization.

The second type of purification and standardization is chemical. There must be a definite chemical compound, and this must be of the strength stated. For drugs that are simple chemicals or even some very complex chemical compounds this method of assay is very efficient. For instance: 95 per cent ethyl alcohol must contain 95 parts of ethyl alcohol (C_2H_5OH) and 5 parts of distilled water (H_2O). If the drug is a solid, similar conditions must be fulfilled. If the tablet is marked aspirin gr. 5, it must actually contain five grains by weight, plus or minus 10 per cent of acetylsalicylic acid ($C_6H_4OHCOOC_2H_5$). This is *chemical assay*, and drugs so standardized are measured by weight, if the drug is a solid, and per cent, ratio or amount of solute to solvent, if a liquid. In some cases the removal of the last minute particle of inert substances may prove impractical and cause excessive increase in price. The official publications set definitive limits for such conditions. The vast majority of all the drugs in common use are in these forms. For all drugs whose chemical composition is known, this is the basic method of assay.

There are many drugs whose basic chemical composition is not known. Often it is difficult or impossible to standardize these by chemical means, so some other process must be used. Since the composition of the substance is not known, it cannot be stated that it contains so much of a given material.

Instead, these drugs are administered to a laboratory animal under controlled conditions and the effect or effects noted; this is called *biological assay*. These drugs are measured in units instead of by weight or per cent of the active ingredient. The unit is the amount of the medicine needed to bring about certain changes in laboratory animals of a specific kind and size. It is stated either according to the type of animal used, as in the Rat Unit, or a standard set by a governmental agency, as the International Unit. Some unit drugs meet the standards set by many countries or by an international council, or they may meet the standards of only one country. The basic fact for the nurse to understand is that the unit is the amount of the drug that is known to produce a definite effect. Units are used mainly for hormones and vitamins. Often a drug that originally was standardized in units is later reported in grains or grams. This happens when research discloses the chemical composition of the drug or when a drug previously obtained from an animal or vegetable source is later synthesized.

Some drugs are standardized by their clinical use. This does not mean that new drugs are used indiscriminately on patients to see what the results will be. New drugs are used very cautiously on the human patient and only after extensive research has been done. However, they do not always produce the same effect in the human that they do on the laboratory animals. Some drugs prove much more efficient than had been anticipated; others prove to be relatively useless. The results of the use of the drug on the human patient are known as *clinical assay*. Only one or two drugs now available were standardized by this method.

DRUG CONTROL

Before this century there was no effective government control of drugs. Many herbs were grown in home gardens and were used by the families alone. Much of this was valuable medicine and, as we have seen, gave to the medical profession some of its most important drugs. As long as it remained a "family" affair, there were no major complications, since the older members of the household usually understood enough about these herbs to prevent excessive use, and their knowledge was handed down from generation to generation. However, as time went on the herbs were given to others—at first only to the immediate neighbors—later to more distant people. As their use increased, they were often added to harmless, or mildly harmful, preparations and sold as "cure-alls." Thus developed the "patent" medicine of the latter part of the nineteenth century and its salesman became a well-known figure of that period. His product was usually a mixture of various vegetable substances in a rather strong (high percentage) alcoholic solution. When the sale of such preparations became popular and the spreading of home remedies common, some form of control became necessary. A few states passed laws designed to protect their residents from fraudulent claims and injurious preparations (VI-1). However, if the neighboring states did not have similar laws, enforcement was difficult and often ineffective. A national law was needed to cope with the situation adequately; in 1906 the first such law was enacted. It was titled the *Pure Food and Drug Act*. There was great opposition to this law, and in its final form it was not too efficient. Even so it was a step in the right direction. The final version listed 11 narcotic and habit-forming drugs and prohibited the sale of any preparation containing any of these drugs or their derivatives without use of a label stating what the drugs contained and the amount. The law also prohibited the making of false claims of cures for any drug or medicinal substance and provided penalties for the adulteration of any product—food or drug. *Adulteration* is the substitution of one product for another without stating this on the label. Usually it is the use of a cheap, inferior substance in place of a superior and more expensive product.

All federal laws apply only to those products that are transported in interstate commerce. They do not apply to drugs produced, sold and used intrastate. Because of the complexity of our present social system, most drugs do come under the provisions of the federal laws. In addition, most states enact laws that conform to the provisions of the federal laws.

The 1906 Pure Food and Drug Act had many loopholes. In fact, it was so ineffective that there was widespread demand for its revision; and in the early thirties the demand became so great that Congress began the consideration of changes in the law (VI-1). People objected to the various proposed provisions of the new law; each succeeding year brought debates and changes; amendments followed amendments in a long procession. Then, in 1937, a tragic event occurred. A drug sold under the name of "Elixir of Sulfanilamide" caused the deaths of an estimated 100 or more people throughout the country. The deaths were due not to the sulfanilamide but to the solvent—diethylene glycol—that was used. Following these deaths, popular demand for legal means of preventing the recurrence of such a tragedy greatly strengthened the law which was passed in 1938. This law is the *Federal Food, Drug, and Cosmetic Act*. It has a very broad coverage with many specific provisions. The more important requirements, insofar as the nurse is concerned, are:

1. The contents must be clearly stated on the label in words understandable to the average person.
2. Any preparation containing habit-forming drugs or their derivatives must be specially labeled with the name of the drug and the amount or per cent strength given. The bottle must show the precaution "Warning—may be habit forming." The drugs considered habit forming are listed in the text of the law.
3. Any drug designated as U.S.P. or N.F. must conform to the standards set by the publication indicated.
4. Labels must bear adequate directions for the use of the drug, and proper statements concerning dosage if used by infants or children. The label must also indicate the limitations or contraindications, if any, of the drug's use in specific conditions.
5. There must be no false or misleading labeling.

Additional requirements have been added by amendments from time to time.

The Federal Drug Administration controls the release of drugs both for general use and for clinical trial. Recent amendments to the basic rules have strengthened the safeguards covering experimentation.

Drugs dispensed by prescriptions from licensed physicians, dentists and veterinarians are exempted from certain provisions of the law as listed under numbers one and two above.

It was mentioned earlier that some state drug laws preceded the first national law. At the present time, most states have laws covering the manufacture and distribution of drugs, and many of these are much more stringent than the federal laws. Many state laws are intended specifically to restrict the "over the counter" (OTC) without a prescription sale of certain drugs as hypnotics, antibiotics and glandular derivatives. Some of the laws have been enacted in response to popular demand when abuses have brought about unnecessary suffering or death. Most states follow closely any revision of the federal laws, enacting legislation of their own to keep the state in line with the national trend.

In a few instances, local communities—counties or municipalities—have special drug regulations. In such cases the nurse must be familiar with the local ordinances. Thus, the nurse must understand not only the federal drug laws but state and local ordinances as well.

It should also be mentioned that, with the increase in international cooperation, many drugs have come under international control. Narcotic drugs have been under such jurisdiction for many years, but lately many other potent drugs have been added to such coverage.

THE NARCOTIC PROBLEM AND ITS CONTROL

(The specific control of narcotics and other abused drugs will be discussed at greater length in Chapter 6, The Problem of Drug Abuse.)

Narcotic drugs have been a problem for ages the world over. Sporadically through the centuries there have been efforts to control the use or, more aptly, the abuse of these drugs. Since most of the early attempts at control were local in character, they proved of little value. Smuggling was too easy.

The first major attempt to control the use of narcotic drugs came in 1912 with the convening of a conference at The Hague, in The Netherlands. This meeting was called "The Hague Opium Conference" and it set regulations for the sale of opium on international markets. In 1914 the United States government passed a law designed to bring this country in line with the regulations of The Hague conference. The law, which became known as the *Harrison Act* after Senator Patrick Harrison of Mississippi, its sponsor, became effective in 1915. It controls the manufacture, importation and sale of opium and its derivatives and coca (cocaine) and its derivatives. The law has had several revisions, and various synthetic drugs similar to the two original drugs have been added so that it now covers all the opium products, the coca drugs and many synthetic preparations. As new synthetic narcotics appear they are added to the provisions of the law.

These drugs require special prescriptions. The physician, or other professional person, must have a special license to write such prescriptions. The pharmacist must also be licensed to dispense such drugs. In the hospital such drugs are recorded on special blanks, and the nurse administering the drug must sign the blank indicating what drug was given, the amount, the time, by whom it was ordered and to whom it was given. Exact details will vary a little from one institution to another, but the main procedure will be the same in all cases.

In 1937 an act similar to the Narcotic Act was passed pertaining to the use of the plant *Cannabis sativa* (Indian hemp) or marihuana. Historically, marihuana is very old. It was the hashish of Asia Minor, from which we derive the word assassins. Since groups of criminal bands often took hashish before they went out on excursions the name "hashishins" eventually came to be assassins. Marihuana is called bhang in India. Bhang is stronger than marihuana owing to the variety of the plant and to the area of cultivation. Since this plant will grow throughout the United States and smuggling from Mexico is easy, its control is especially difficult.

In 1970, a new law was enacted to replace the original narcotic act and its amendments. This law, called "The Controlled Substance Act," covers narcotics and dangerous drugs. Parts of this act did not become effective until January 1, 1972.

The act sets up schedules for the various controlled substances, and these schedules are similar to those of the Canadian system which has been in effect for some time. The following is a very brief review of the schedules. Complete information can be obtained from the Regional Office of the Drug Enforcement Agency (DEA).

Schedule I. Drugs in this schedule are those that have *no accepted medical use* in the treatment of diseases in the United States. Some examples are: heroin (and some other opium derivatives), marihuana (active principles are tetrahydrocannabinols), D-lysergic acid diethylamide (LSD), peyote (mescaline), psilocybin and others.

Schedule II. Drugs in this schedule include those previously known as "Class A Narcotics" with the addition of amphetamine and similar drugs. Some examples are opium, morphine, codeine, oxycodone (Percodan), opium alkaloid hydrochloride (Pantopon), dihydromorphinone (Dilaudid), cocaine, methadone hydrochloride (Dolophine), meperidine (Demerol), analeridine (Leritine), oxymorphone (Numorphan), levorphanol tartrate (Levo-Dromoran), piminodine (Alvodine), amphetamine (Benzedrine), methamphetamine (Methedrine), dextroamphetamine (Dexedrine), phenmetrazine (Preludin) and methylphenidate (Ritalin).

Schedule III. Drugs in this schedule include those formerly known as "Class B Narcotics." Some examples are various drugs or combinations of drugs containing codeine, such as the combination aspirin, phenacetin, caffeine and codeine (A.P.C. with codeine, Empirin Comp. with codeine, many trade names), aspirin with codeine (Codasa), acetaminophen with codeine (Tylenol with codeine), phenaphen with codeine (a combination of phenacetin, hyoscyamine, phenobarbital and codeine), carisoprodrol with codeine (Soma with codeine). Other narcotics include dihydrocodeinone with homatropine (Hycodan), dihydrocodeinone with homatropine, pyrilamine, phenylephrine and ammonium chloride (Hycomine), hydrocodone and phenyltoloxamine (Tussionex) and camphorated tincture of opium (paregoric), formerly an exempt narcotic.

Non-narcotics included under Schedule III are methyprylon (Noludar), chlorhexadol (Lora), glutethimide (Doriden), aprobarbital (Alurate), amobarbital (Amytal), secobarbital (Seconal), pentobarbital (Nembutal), butabarbital (Butisol), amobarbital and secobarbital (Tuinal), carbromal and pentobarbital (Carbrital). Also all amphetamine and methamphetamine combinations not listed under Schedule II.

Schedule IV. Drugs in this schedule include barbital (Veronal), phenobarbital (Luminal), chloral hydrate, ethinamate (Valmid), paraldehyde, methohexital (Brevital), chloral betaine (Beta-Chlor), petrichloral (Periclor), ethchlorvynol (Placidyl), meprobamate (Equanil, Miltown). Chlordiazepoxide (Librium) and diazepam (Valium) have been added to Schedule IV.

Schedule V. Drugs in this listing include preparations formerly known as "Exempt Narcotics." There are any number of medications under Schedule V, mainly cough preparations containing codeine.

Special regulations cover the manufacturing, transporting, storing, prescribing, dispensing and administering of the drugs in each schedule.

The use of narcotic drugs of one kind or another has been known throughout the world as long as there has been any recorded history. The actual drugs have varied from place to place and from time to time, but the problem has remained much the same. Many narcotic drugs are interesting mainly because of their social significance. These will be discussed in other courses. The nurse is most concerned with the use of the pain-relieving narcotic drugs which are used frequently in medicine and are, therefore, of major importance. Cocaine addiction is also on the increase here. There are many new synthetic analgesics that now must be included with the habit-forming drugs.

CONTROL OF DRUGS IN CANADA

Canadian drug laws have all antedated those in the United States, but like the United States, in most cases provincial laws have preceded the dominion or federal laws.

The first Canadian drug law was enacted in 1874 and was patterned after a British law which became effective in 1872. Its major purpose was to prohibit the adulteration of both drugs and foods. It has been called The Adulteration Act. It was a rather weak law which, though it helped, did not fulfill its function too well. It was amended in 1884 and several times since. The last major revision was in 1953–1954. However, the law has been amended frequently since that time. It is now called the Food and Drug Act. This law is similar to the Federal Food, Drug, and Cosmetic Act in the United States; it covers the manufacture, importation and sale of drugs, cosmetics, vitamins and foods. Drugs that come directly under the jurisdiction of this act are those whose ingredients are listed on the label. Narcotics, proprietary or patent medicines and certain others called controlled drugs have additional laws which specifically apply to these preparations. However, all drugs of whatever nature come under the general provisions of this act.

There are no "official" drugs in Canada as the term is used in the United States. However, any drug listed in any of the publications listed on p. 19 is considered to be "standard" so long as it conforms to the requirements listed in the publications as on p. 19. The Food and Drug Act prohibits adulteration, false labeling and advertisement, unsanitary preparation, use of substandard material and so forth for drugs, cosmetics, vitamins and foods. It contains several lists (schedules) of drugs with specific requirements for each category, and it also includes a list of drugs that may not be used in Canada at all. These lists are revised from time to time as new drugs appear and older ones prove to be dangerous or ineffective.

Before the last major revision, many provincial laws differed considerably from the dominion or federal laws and from each other. This made for discrepancies. A drug might be sold "over the counter" in one province and require a prescription in another. Or, one requiring a prescription in one province might be refillable in that province but require a repeat prescription in another. Now all provincial laws are in line with the dominion or federal laws. The latter in all cases supersede the provincial laws.

In 1908 the Narcotic Control Act was enacted. It was revised in 1919 and from time to time since. The last major revision was in 1961. The original law applied only to opium and its derivatives. Later cannabis (marihuana) and its derivatives were added, and still later, coca and its derivatives. Lately the synthetic analgesics have been included under this act; there is a long list of them and additions are made each year as new drugs appear on the market. Heroin importation and manufacture is now pro-

NAME OF PUBLICATION	ABBREVIATION	EDITION
Specifications for the Quality Control of Pharmaceutical Preparations (formerly Pharmacopoeia Internationalis)	(formerly Ph.I.)	1967 (2nd edition)
Supplement		1971
The British Pharmacopoeia	(B.P.)	1968
Addendum		1971
The United States Pharmacopeia	(U.S.P.)	1970 (18th edition)
Supplement		1971
Pharmacopée Française; Codex Français, rédigé par ordre du gouvernement	(Codex)	1965 (8th edition)
The Canadian Formulary	(C.F.)	1949
The British Pharmaceutical Codex	(B.P.C.)	1968
Supplement		1971
The National Formulary	(N.F.)	1970 (13th edition)
Supplement		1973

hibited. The supply has long since been expended.

The narcotic act is directed mainly against the illicit drug traffic and the addicts from this trade. The act indicates three types of addicts: professional (medical and paramedical personnel), medical (patients who become addicted from taking drugs during sickness) and the illicit drug addict who takes the drug without any medical need for the sensations it produces. The first two groups are cared for by the doctors and are neither numerous nor a serious problem. However, the illicit trade does pose a problem and stricter measures have been put into the law to discourage the activities of the smugglers and pushers (sellers). Practically all illicit drugs are smuggled into the country. Compared with many other countries, Canada has a relatively small number of addicts.

A prescription is required for the dispensing of all narcotic drugs, unless the amount is very small and it is prepared in combination with other drugs, as in cough syrups.

In 1961 the Controlled Drug Act was enacted. It is similar to the Narcotic Control Act, but it deals with drugs that are not narcotics. The major drugs listed under this act are the amphetamines (derivatives and similar preparations) and the salts of barbituric acid. The act notes that all drugs are under control in Canada, but the drugs listed in the act have been shown to be dangerous with indiscriminate use, though they are not narcotics in the international use of the term. Controlled drugs require the same type of prescription as do the narcotics. Drugs are added to the list covered by the act as is deemed advisable to avoid the use of dangerous drugs without medical supervision.

In 1908 the Proprietary and Patent Medicine Act was enacted. It has had several revisions, the last major one in 1952. The law controls the so-called "secret formula" drugs. It requires that each drug be registered and a license be secured before it can be sold to the public. This license must be renewed each year and it is revocable at any time if the product is found to be harmful or not to meet the specifications made at the time of registration. For registration, the manufacturer must present complete information to the authorities, giving chemical formulas, method of preparation, dosage to be advised and other information. There must be no fraudulent claims made for the drug. Certain drugs may not be used in the formula, certain others must be listed on the label and still others must be listed with the actual amount of the drug contained in the preparation or in each dose. These lists are added to as is deemed advisable.

There is no law in the United States that is comparable to the Proprietary and Patent Medicine Act in Canada.

The entire control of drugs in Canada is under the direct supervision of the Department of National Health and Welfare.

IT IS IMPORTANT TO REMEMBER

1. That drug forms change from time to time, and the nurse must be alert to these changes. She will need to learn new things about drugs, and also to forget some of her previous knowledge. Pharmacology and pharmaceutical preparations are subject to great variation at any given time.

2. The letters following a drug refer to the publication whose standards the drug fulfills. She should recognize U.S.P., N.F., and B.P.

3. Though "official" drugs are known to be effective for the conditions for which they are used, many proprietary drugs are equally valuable.

4. That drugs covered by Schedule I are not used legally in the United States or Canada.

5. That drugs are added, deleted and moved from one schedule to another, and that the nurse must be aware of these changes so as to properly record their use.

TOPICS FOR STUDY AND DISCUSSION

1. Make a list of 15 or 20 drugs from a textbook on medical or surgical nursing. Look up the sources of these drugs. Where do they come from? Does this indicate the need for international, national or state control?

2. What is the difference, in general, between the sources and preparations of drugs in 1970 and 1870? How do you account for such a change?

3. What is an active principle? Of the list of drugs obtained under Topic 1, which are active principles? What kinds of active principles are they?

4. Do any of the drugs in the list from Topic 1 have more than one name? List the generic and proprietary names for all that you can.

5. Secure lists of drugs from various sources such as those found in (a) a hospital division, (b) home medicine cabinet, (c) nursing school infirmary or health office. Check the list to see how many are "official." What makes a drug official? Of the nonofficial drugs, how many are listed in any of the schedules? How many are proprietary drugs? What is the significance of the findings?

6. Using the above or a similar list of drugs—secured from sources such as the hospital pharmacy, a drug store, drug salesman or a drug price list—find out as nearly as can be determined the cost of the drugs. Remember that it is the retail price that the patient pays for his medicines.

7. Take a survey of drug advertisements by television, radio, newspapers or magazines. Compare these with the lists secured under Topic 1. Are the advertised drugs the ones appearing most commonly on the various lists? What is the significance of your findings?

8. Write to your state department of health for a list of the state drug laws. How do these compare with the federal laws? What are the important provisions of these laws? How are they helpful in preventing the abuse of medicines? What other means of control exist? How may these controls be made more effective?

BIBLIOGRAPHY

Books and Pamphlets

American Medical Association Council on Drugs, *Drug Evaluations, 2nd Ed.*, Chicago, 1973, American Medical Association.

American Pharmaceutical Association National Formulary Board, *National Formulary, 13th Ed.*, Washington, D.C., 1970, American Pharmaceutical Association.

Bureau of Narcotics and Dangerous Drugs, *The Controlled Substance Act of 1970* (Several bulletins covering details of the act), Washington, D.C., 1970, Department of Justice.

Canadian Pharmaceutical Association, *Compendium of Pharmaceutical Species, 7th Ed.*, Toronto, 1972, Canadian Pharmaceutical Association.

Committee of Revision, *The United States Pharmacopeia, 18th Ed.*, Washington, D.C., 1970, Trustees of the United States Pharmaceutical Committee Inc.

Duhamel, R., *The Food and Drug Act and Regulations 1964–1967 and Amendments*, Ottawa, 1967, Queen's Printer, Controller of Stationery.

Falconer, M., Patterson, H. R., and Gustafson, E., *Current Drug Handbook, 1974–76*, Philadelphia, 1974, W. B. Saunders Co.

Food and Drug Administration (*Various bulletins*), Washington, D.C., 1970–1973, Department of Health, Education and Welfare.

Goodman, L., and Gilman, A., *Pharmacological Basis of Therapeutics, 4th Ed.*, New York, 1970, The Macmillan Co.

Goth, A., *Medical Pharmacology, 6th Ed.*, St. Louis, 1972, The C. V. Mosby Co.

Lehner, E., and Lehner, J., *Folklore and Odyssey of Food and Medical Plants*, New York, 1962, Tudor Publishing Co.

Lewis, A., *Modern Drug Encyclopedia*, New York, 1970, The Yorke Medical Group.

Journal Articles

Dowling, H. F., "Today's dilemma—Will drugs work?" *J. Am. Pharm. Assoc.* NS 11:6:331 (June, 1971).

CHAPTER 3

METHODS OF ADMINISTERING DRUGS

CORRELATION WITH OTHER SCIENCES

I. ANATOMY AND PHYSIOLOGY

1. The gastric juice is acidic because of the presence of free hydrochloric acid.
2. The intestinal contents become neutral or alkaline when mixed with bile and other intestinal secretions which are alkaline and, therefore, neutralize the acid from the stomach.
3. The physiologic activities of the human body vary with different ages. Most authorities consider the adult between ages 25 and 35 as the average person.
4. During the period from conception to maturity the changes in the human being are progressive. From maturity to death the changes are regressive.
5. Overweight and underweight may be physiologic or pathologic. The former is the more common form. In making estimates based upon weight, it is often better to use the amount the individual should weigh rather than what he actually does weigh. The optimum weight is determined by statistical averages obtained by securing the weights of a large number of persons who are in apparently good health.
6. The rate of absorption through the body membranes depends upon many factors. The more important of these factors are the type of membrane, the strength of the solution and the hydrogen ion concentration of the fluid. Absorption is rapid wherever there is a large supply of blood and lymph capillaries.
7. There are two main layers in the skin, the dermis and the epidermis. The epidermis is further divided into four layers: the stratum corneum, stratum lucidum, stratum granulosum and the stratum germinativum. Below the dermis is a layer of adipose tissue known as the subcutaneous layer.

II. CHEMISTRY

1. An acid and a base or alkali will react with each other to form a neutral salt, if both the acid and the base are either weak or strong. A weak acid and a strong base will form a basic salt. A strong acid and a weak base will form an acid salt.

IV. PHYSICS

1. Capillary attraction is the elevation or depression of liquids in capillary tubes.
2. Surface tension is the tendency of the molecules of a liquid to adhere closer together on the surface of the liquid. This tends to form a sphere of the liquid when the pressure is equal on all sides.
3. In mixtures of a solid and a liquid, or of two liquids of differing specific densities, the two will separate, the lighter rising to the surface. This lighter upper liquid is called the supernatant fluid.

V. PSYCHOLOGY

1. Temperament is a variable factor in the organization of the individual which is probably more the result of heredity than of environment. Temperament is relatively stable during the lifetime of a person. It changes much less than many other factors which go to make up the total personality.
2. Habit is the process of conditioning responses until the course of the nerve impulses is established. The more a habit is exercised the deeper it is fixed, and the harder it is to eradicate.

VI. SOCIOLOGY

1. People with the same or similar occupations often tend to have similar physical make-up insofar as occupation tends to influence physical condition.
2. Some occupations are known to be hazardous, and special precautions should be used to prevent the occurrence of accidents or illnesses associated with these occupations.

INTRODUCTION

Before the physician decides upon the type and amount of a drug to be used in the treatment of a patient, certain basic factors must be considered. Each patient presents a particular problem. It is not enough to presume that because a special drug is recommended for this disease it will be of value in the case being treated. The automobile mechanic can add liquid graphite to the oil or gasoline of an engine that is not performing as it should and he will be able to predict accurately what effect the graphite will have. The mechanic is working with particular metals. The physician, on the other hand, is dealing with a living human being, a person unlike any other person in the whole world. The doctor must take into account all possible factors that might influence the effect of the drug on the patient being treated. Of course, it is impossible for us to discuss all these factors, but the nurse should be aware of the more important ones.

The first things the physician will consider are what drugs to use and in what amounts. Since these two factors are discussed in detail elsewhere they will only be touched upon here.

GENERAL PURPOSES FOR WHICH DRUGS ARE USED

PREVENTIVE OR PROPHYLACTIC. Preventive or prophylactic drugs are used to prevent the occurrence of a disease or to lessen its severity if it does occur.

More and more drugs are being used for this purpose. The old adage, "An ounce of prevention is worth a pound of cure," is still valid, especially when applied to disease. Many conditions once common have all but disappeared because of preventive medications. One classic example is the drastic reduction in the incidence of smallpox since the first use of the vaccine by Jenner in 1796. Each year new names are added to the long list of diseases which can be prevented by the proper use of the prophylactic measures now available.

DIAGNOSTIC. Drugs used to aid the physician in deciding what is causing the patient's symptoms are known as diagnostic drugs.

These drugs not only help the doctor to determine the reason for the patient's illness but they are also often of benefit in locating the exact area of the body affected.

THERAPEUTIC. The noun therapy and the adjective therapeutic both mean treatment; therefore, therapeutic drugs are those drugs used in treating the patient's illness. There are many kinds of therapeutic drugs; the more common ones are:

CURATIVE. For certain diseases there are medicines which will remove the causative agent of the disease. These are called specific or curative drugs.

In some instances, one drug is effective against only one disease; in other cases, one drug may be effective in the treatment of several diseases.

PALLIATIVE OR SYMPTOMATIC. Drugs used to relieve the distressing symptoms of disease are palliative or symptomatic drugs.

Whether or not the disease can be eradicated, its severity lessened, or its progress checked, the most important thing to the patient is the relief of the pain or other undesirable manifestations of the disease. In other words, what the patient seeks is to feel better. To a great extent this is the prime purpose of medicine and nursing.

SUPPORTIVE. Supportive treatment is used to sustain the patient until other measures can be instituted which will either cure or alleviate the condition.

The human body's normal recuperative

powers will overcome most illness, but with help they will do the job more effectively and in less time than alone. Supportive treatment is designed to accomplish this.

Substitutive. Drugs used to replace substances normally found in the body but which, because of disease, injury or other factors, are absent or diminished in amount, are substitutive or replacement drugs.

These drugs may be given to tide the patient over temporary diminution of the body product until his own tissues are again manufacturing the substance in adequate quantity, or they may be required throughout the patient's entire life.

Restorative. Drugs used to help return the body to its normal healthy state are called restoratives. These drugs are usually used during convalescence to aid nature in its reconstructive processes.

DRUG SELECTION. The selection of the right type of drug for the right disease forms the material for the major part of this textbook. Consequently, it will not be emphasized here.

DOSAGE. How much medicine to give, how often, and for how long? These are questions to be decided in each case. They are based upon many factors, some of which will be discussed in Chapter 4 and throughout the book. The frequency of the dosage may be changed from time to time as circumstances change; and a drug originally intended to be given for only a few days may be continued for many weeks. Such changes arise from circumstances that add information that was not available when the original estimate was made. It is obtained from watching the effect of the drug on the patient being treated.

Other factors governing the use and the dosage of drugs follow.

FACTORS RELATED PRIMARILY TO THE PATIENT

GENERAL FACTORS

Age. Obviously the dose of the drug given an adult must be reduced for a child or infant. Much less obvious, but equally important, is the change in dosage necessary when treating the adolescent, a patient during the climacteric and the elderly (I-3, 4). As far as drugs are concerned, we recognize roughly about six age groups—infancy, childhood, adolescence, adulthood or maturity (early and late) and senility. The dosage must be adjusted to each group. The adult dose is used as the standard.

Sex. Sex is of importance as a determining factor only at certain stages of development and under specific conditions.

Size. Height and weight are, of course, factors to be considered. Certainly the patient weighing 200 pounds would be apt to need more of a given medication than one weighing only 100 pounds. However, experience has shown that the dose would be much less than the weight differential would indicate. Dosage is usually based upon the optimum (not the actual) weight of the patient. One hundred and fifty pounds is accepted as the standard adult weight (I-5). In certain situations, the dosage is estimated according to surface area of the patient. This is especially valuable for use with infants and small children.

CONDITION OF THE PATIENT

General Physical Condition. There are many ways of describing the physical condition of the patient. Expressions such as excellent, good, fair, and poor are common terms used to denote the health status. Obesity and emaciation also indicate general physical condition.

Temporary Physical Condition. Not only is the general physical state a factor in determining the choice and amount of the drug to be used, there are also temporary circumstances that must be taken into consideration. Among these are pregnancy and lactation. Obviously in these cases the baby as well as the mother must be considered. In patients with gastrointestinal disorders the channel of administration as well as the drug may need to be changed; the patient with nausea may not be able to retain medications given orally. If the patient has increased peristalsis, as occurs in diarrhea, the drug may not remain in the intestinal tract long enough for absorption to take place.

Pathological Conditions. This factor needs no explanation. It is clear that the type and the amount of the drug used will depend primarily upon the disorder from which the patient is suffering. See Part II, Section III.

Emergency. Naturally, in many cases, dosage will be modified to suit the urgency of the condition. The dosage of a drug given to relieve pain may be doubled when the patient is in acute pain caused by either traumatic injury or severe illness.

FACTORS REFERABLE TO THE INDIVIDUAL PATIENT

It has been emphasized that in all cases it is the patient who is being treated. However, some factors are referable to any patient and some only to the individual being treated. Of the latter the following are important.

Temperament. It is easy to see that the amount of sedative needed to quiet a patient would have to be greater for the individual with a nervous disposition than that required for a quiet, phlegmatic person (V-1).

Idiosyncrasy. In certain people drugs act in totally unexpected ways. This deviation from the usual response is called idiosyncrasy. If the patient has had the drug previously he will be able to tell the doctor or nurse what is apt to happen. However, the nurse must be alert at all times to note early signs of unanticipated reactions to drugs.

Occupation. This factor applies not only to the specific types of occupations but also to general kinds inasmuch as they tend to influence the physical condition of the patient. Thus, the office worker might be given a different amount of a drug from that given the professional athlete (VI-1). This might be a factor in itself, or it might influence the administration of medicine by changing the general condition of the patient, as discussed in an earlier paragraph. Certain occupations have a direct influence on drugs and dosage. For instance, the painter, who is exposed consistently to lead, probably would need a different amount of any preparation containing lead than would the person who had not been so exposed (VI-2).

FACTORS RELATED PRIMARILY TO THE DRUG

GENERAL

Purpose of the Drug. This is the first and most important factor. The physician is thinking mainly of what the drug should accomplish for this particular patient.

Nature of the Drug. The administration of any medicine is greatly influenced by the physical and the chemical properties of the drug. Its form will dictate the mode of administration and may even change the actual choice of drug.

Form of the Drug. This refers to the physical characteristics of the drug. Is it a solid, liquid or gas? Is it in powder, tablet, capsule or any of the various forms listed in the Appendix? The form of the drug especially influences the mode of administration and may change the choice if the channel by which the drug usually is given is not usable in the particular patient being treated.

ACTION OF THE DRUG IN THE BODY

Rate of Absorption. A rapidly absorbed drug will usually act quickly, but its action may be short. Such drugs must be given at frequent intervals if continuous effect is desired (I-6). Drugs absorbed very slowly will probably not have any immediate action, but the action, once established, may last for many hours.

Rate and Amount of Metabolism. Some drugs are changed by the body into substances quite different from the original. The drug may be effective only after this metabolic change has taken place. Other drugs are rendered ineffective by the body. These factors influence the time, amount and channel of administration.

Duration of Therapeutic Effect. This has already been touched upon in the preceding paragraphs. It is clear that the length of time the drug will be therapeutically valuable will influence the type, amount and especially the frequency of administration. The duration of therapeutic effectiveness is often associated with the amount of drug in the circulating fluids; hence the term *blood level* has become very important. In some cases it is essential that, once the drug is started, it be continued at frequent enough intervals to maintain, at all times, a certain amount of the drug in the blood. This makes the time of administration a very important matter. A half hour variation may greatly decrease the efficiency of the drug.

Excretion of the Drug. There are

three points to consider here: the time of excretion, the organ of excretion and the form of the medicine when excreted. Any given drug may be excreted by all or only one of the excretory organs. Some drugs are not changed by the body and are excreted in the form in which they were administered. All these matters influence the estimation of the type, amount and frequency of administration.

FACTORS RELATED TO THE ACTION OF THE DRUG IN THE BODY

Some of these factors will be discussed in Chapter 4, namely, cumulative synergistic and antagonistic action.

Many drugs tend to become less effective the longer they are taken. This is called *tolerance.* Tolerance may be due to any number of causes, some of which are physiological and some of which appear to be more emotional (psychic).

The terms addiction, habituation and dependency will be further discussed in Chapter 6. However, a brief coverage here may be helpful. *Addiction* is usually applied to those drugs which cause, upon withdrawal, severe or serious physical symptoms. *Habituation* refers to any drug used long enough to become a habit. It may or may not cause physical symptoms when stopped, but it usually does cause emotional (psychological) disturbances. *Dependency,* the term now preferred, covers both addiction and habituation. Drug dependency may be physical, emotional or both.

FACTORS RELATED PRIMARILY TO ADMINISTRATION

The Major Channels of Administration

Medicinal substances have been used by human beings since time immemorial. In fact, animals use many of the same drugs that man uses and for much the same purposes. Until relatively recently most drugs were taken orally. At present, however, oral administration is only one of many ways of giving medication; in fact, some very useful drugs cannot be given orally.

The action of drugs in the human body may be divided into two main types—local and systemic (pp. 39 and 40).

LOCAL CHANNELS OF ADMINISTRATION

SKIN

Spraying or *painting* the drug (for example iodine or Mercurochrome) on the skin for direct action at the point of contact. These may be watery solutions, lotions or alcoholic solutions (tinctures).

Inunction or the rubbing of a drug into the skin. This may be for either local or systemic action, depending on the drug used.

Ointments are oily preparations of drugs that may be rubbed in as an inunction, or may simply be applied to the skin for local action on skin lesions of various kinds. *Creams* and water-soluble substances are used for the same purpose. *Liniments* are fluid drugs used in a similar manner.

Plasters and *poultices* may be used for local action or they may contain substances which when absorbed will affect other areas of the body.

Moist dressings or *local baths* may be used for either local or systemic action, though the former is much more common. Some medicinal baths are used to improve the general "health" and are often of value in relieving the pains of arthritis.

MUCOUS MEMBRANES

Sprays or *nebulae* are fine particles of a drug usually suspended or dissolved in water and inhaled. They are used for the nose, throat and lungs and may be effective locally at the point of contact or systemically after absorption through the mucous membranes.

Aerosols are a suspension of fine solid or liquid particles in air or gas. They may be drawn into the respiratory tract on air or forced into the tract on a flow of gas such as oxygen from a tank.

Steam is also used as a vehicle to carry drugs into the lungs. In this case it is the water vapor that is inhaled. The vapor may be the important substance or it may carry needed drugs.

Inhalation is also accomplished by *smoking* the drug. The medicine may be burned and the patient inhales the smoke, or it may be smoked in the form of a cigarette.

Irrigation or flow of water containing the drugs may be a means of reaching the mucous membranes. Irrigations are used in body cavities that communicate directly with the exterior such as eyes, nose, throat, bladder, vagina and rectum.

Drugs may be *dropped directly* on the mucous membranes. A relatively small amount of the drug is used, but it may be very potent. Places where drops are often used include the eyes, nose and ears. (Technically, the ears are not lined with mucous membrane, but skin.)

Drugs may be placed upon an absorbent material (often cotton) and inserted in a body cavity. These are called *packs* or *tampons*. They are used in the nose, ears, and vagina.

Gargles or *mouthwashes* are similar to irrigations and are used for much the same conditions. They are useful for the mouth and the throat and can be employed without any special equipment.

Swabbing and *painting* are used for direct action at the point of contact. The drugs are usually in watery solutions.

SYSTEMIC CHANNELS OF ADMINISTRATION

ALIMENTARY TRACT

Suppositories are drugs in a base that is solid at ordinary room temperature but which will melt at body temperature or dissolve in body fluids. These are inserted into the various body cavities. They may be used for either local or systemic action.

The *sublingual* or *buccal* route is used when the drug needed cannot be given orally, rapid action is desired or professional help is not available for parenteral administration. The tablet, which must be readily soluble, is placed under the tongue. It dissolves readily and is absorbed directly into the blood stream.

Drugs given *orally* come in contact with mucous membranes. In this case it is the membranes lining the digestive tract, either the stomach or the intestines or both. Some preparations are absorbed by the lining of the stomach and some are so coated that they will dissolve only in the intestines. Drugs may be given orally for direct action on the membrane of the stomach or the intestines, or they may be given for systemic action after absorption.

Oral drugs are of many and varied forms: solids include powders, tablets, capsules or pills (uncoated, coated, enteric coated, delayed action); liquids include syrups, elixirs, tinctures, spirits, emulsions, magmas, mixtures. Refer to the Appendix for details concerning these and other preparations.

Many oral drugs are designed for immediate action, some for delayed action, and others for a more or less sustained action over a given period of time. Drugs which can be dissolved in an acid medium are usually absorbed from the stomach (I-1). These act quickly, but the action is usually of short duration. Those which dissolve in an alkaline medium (enteric coated) are absorbed from the small intestines (I-2). The action of these is necessarily somewhat slower but it is apt to be effective for a longer time.

PARENTERAL ROUTES

The term parenteral is used to indicate all methods of systemic administration of

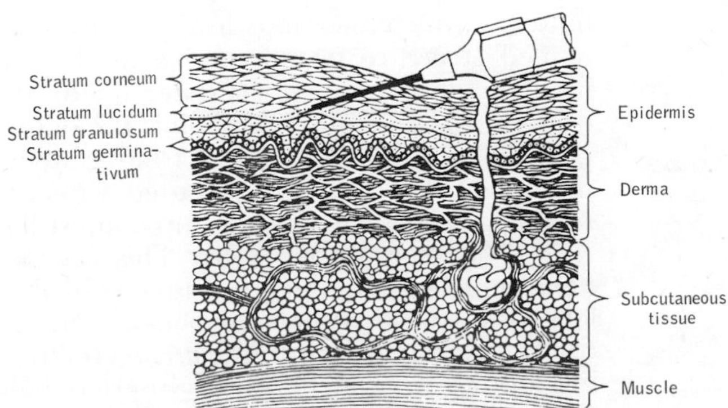

FIGURE 2. Intradermal administration. Note length and bevel of the needle, angle of administration and point at which fluid would enter. Intradermal medication should enter either the stratum lucidum or at the upper portion of the papillary layer, where the epidermis and the dermis meet. There should not be any rupturing of blood vessels.

drugs other than the alimentary tract. Parenteral administration requires special equipment and training.

Intradermal administration (Fig. 2) is the introduction of the drug between the layers of the skin. This method is used mainly for diagnostic purposes, and for very potent medicines. The skin of the palmar surface of the forearm and the skin on the back are most commonly used (I-7). This method has definite limitations. The amount of the drug that can be given this way is very small, and absorption is relatively slow.

Subcutaneous administration (Fig. 3) is one of the most useful parenteral routes. The drug is deposited in the subcutaneous layer of fat (I-7). This is the channel selected when:

a. It is inadvisable to give the drug orally.

b. The drug is rendered ineffective by the digestive juices.

c. A more rapid effect is desired than can be obtained by the oral route.

The most common area used for this method is the outer portion of the upper arm, though almost any area may be used where there is ample subcutaneous tissue to allow for introduction of the drug.

In *intramuscular* administration (Fig. 4) the drug is placed in the layers of the muscles. This method is used when:

a. Immediate effect is desirable and it is inadvisable or impossible to inject the medicine directly into the vein. Muscle tissue is richly supplied with blood vessels hence absorption is relatively rapid.

b. The drug is not suitable for subcutaneous or intravenous injection.

c. It is desirable to place a relatively large amount of the drug into the tissues at one time for absorption over a long period of time—a so-called "pool" of the drug.

There are many areas of the body which may be used for intramuscular administration of drugs. It is essential that the drug be placed in the muscle and not in the subcutaneous layer of the skin. With the young athletic person this is usually easy. However, with some, such as the elderly, this may be difficult. Some areas that may be used are the upper arm (deltoid muscle), the lateral anterior portion of the thigh (the lateral portion of the quadriceps muscle) and the buttocks (the glutei muscles). In the last-named structure two parts are used: the inner angle of the upper, outer quadrant (the gluteus maximus) and below the outer portion of the iliac crest (the gluteus minimus). This last can be used without turning the patient, but the nurse must be careful to measure correctly. This can be done by placing the first two fingers of the left hand (for right-handed persons) along the angle of the iliac with the fingers following the crest. The needle is inserted between the outstretched fingers.

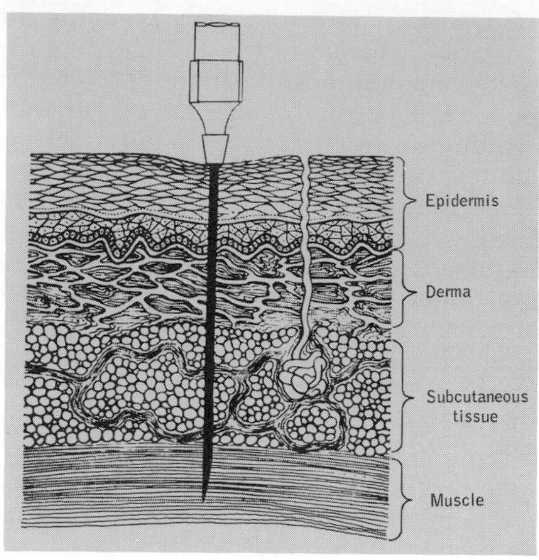

FIGURE 4. Intramuscular administration. Note the length of the needle, the angle of administration and the point at which fluid would enter. Intramuscular medication should enter the main body of the muscle. The needle should pass the skin, the subcutaneous adipose tissue and the fascia.

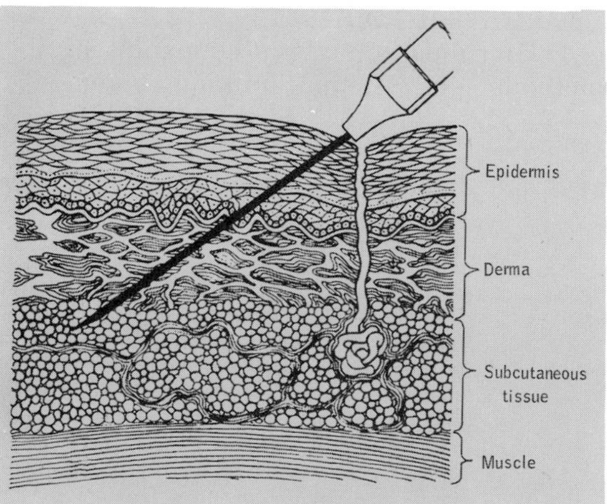

FIGURE 3. Subcutaneous administration. Note length of needle, angle of administration and point at which fluid would enter. Subcutaneous medications should enter the subdermal adipose layer.

There are two common methods of giving intramuscular injections, the pinch and the Z method. For the Z technique, the three middle fingers of the left hand (for right-handed persons) are placed on top of the area selected and lifted upward. This slides the upper layer over the underlying tissues. While maintaining this hold, insert the needle with a quick motion and at a right angle to the skin. Pull the plunger back slightly to ascertain whether the needle has entered a vein. If blood appears, withdraw the needle and select another site. If no blood appears, push the plunger in slowly until cylinder is empty. Withdraw the needle rapidly on the line of insertion and at the same time release the left hand. This allows the tissue to slide back into place and seal the fluid in.

The pinch method is similar. However, the tissue is pinched instead of being slid as with the Z process.

Some nurses prefer the Z technique for repository drugs and the pinch method for rapidly used drugs. For repository drugs the area is not massaged, but it usually is for drugs whose action is required quickly.

The Z technique is often preferred for the obese patient, whereas the pinch method is usually better for the emaciated patient. Great care must be used in each of these conditions to see that the drug is put into the muscle. For the obese patient this may require a longer than normal needle. Change of sites is of vital importance for these patients as their tissues are not normal and may easily break down. It is also important when this route is used for repeated injections.

No intramuscular drug should be given into the buttocks of a patient with dependent edema. The drug will be absorbed improperly and will concentrate additional water in an area that already has excess fluid.

In dehydration, it will probably be necessary to select the site for the injection with more care than with the "normal" patient as here again the tissues are not in good condition.

Hypodermoclysis is the injection of a large quantity of fluid into the subcutaneous tissue. This method is used when fluid as well as some medicinal substance is needed. It may be used for fluid alone. The most common sites are the upper surfaces of the thighs, under the breasts, under the shoulder blades and under the arms. This last is called "axillary seepage."

Intraperitoneal administration is the introduction of the fluid and/or drug directly into the peritoneal cavity.

Intravenous administration (Fig. 5) is the injection of the drug directly into the vein. Small or large quantities may be given by this method. There are many veins that may be used. For a single injection, the veins of the bend of the elbow are often used. Others include the veins of the ankle, the back of the hand and in the very young infant the longitudinal sinus. For this vein, the needle is inserted through the anterior fontanel. If there is to be continuous intravenous infusion, plastic materials are used and the veins of the forearm (the accessory cephalic and the median anterior brachial) are often used. This allows the patient to move more freely. Of course, these same veins can be used for a single injection.

The term intravenous *infusion* means administering a relatively large amount of fluid whereas an intravenous *injection* means administering a relatively small amount of fluid. An intravenous infusion may or may not contain any medication as such, whereas an intravenous injection most often involves giving medication via the veins. Various electrolytes, as well as glucose, dextrose or total alimentation, are administered by intravenous infusion.

It is not uncommon to introduce a medi-

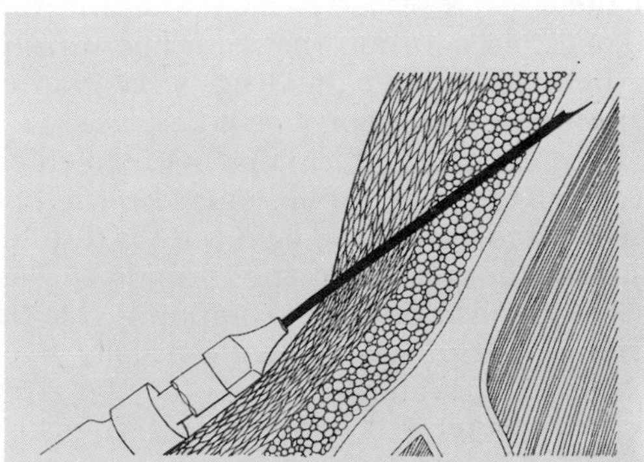

FIGURE 5. Intravenous administration. Note length and bevel of the needle, angle of administration and point at which fluid would enter. It is important to have the point of the needle free in the vein and the complete bevel inside the vein, otherwise the fluid may partially pass into the tissue outside the vein or into the wall of the vein.

cation into an ongoing intravenous infusion. Plastic tubing, which is not self-sealing, is often used for infusion. It is therefore important to insert a short length of rubber tubing at a point in the plastic tubing close to its site of entry to the patient's body. Medication can be added by introducing a needle into the rubber tubing. When the needle is removed, the rubber tubing seals itself.

Intra-arterial administration is occasionally used to put a drug directly into a part of the body. This method is used primarily to introduce a drug into a tumor and is not usually used for systemic purposes.

A look at the illustrations will show the angle of needle insertion and the area of medicinal instillation for the major channels of parenteral administration. The length of the needle, the length and the angle of the bevel as well as the gauge of the needle are important factors in each procedure.

Other channels of administration include:

Intracardial administration, used only in emergencies, is introduction of the drug directly into the heart.

Intrapleural administration is the introduction of the drug into the pleural cavity (between the lungs and the chest wall).

Drugs are also placed in the spinal canal, under the outer covering of the spinal cord, but outside the cord itself. This is called *intraspinal, intrathecal* or *subarachnoid* injection.

Tablet *implants* are used for certain types of drugs. A small specially prepared tablet of the drug is placed in the tissues through a small incision into the skin. The incision is then closed over the drug. Very gradual dissolution and absorption take place.

Except for the tablet implants, all medications given parenterally must be in fluid form. Frequently, the fluid used is distilled water with, or without, the addition of various electrolyte or buffer compounds. If the drug is "viscid" in nature, it is usually given I.M. or I.V. Watery solutions may be given by any route. For intraspinal administration, the physician may withdraw spinal fluid and dissolve the medication in this fluid and then reinsert. The patient receives only the drug without any extraneous diluent.

OTHER FACTORS INFLUENCING TYPE AND DOSAGE OF DRUGS

TIME OF ADMINISTRATION. In addition to factors already considered, others of importance include:

Time in relation to meals. The drug may be given before, after, during or between meals. For instance, appetizers are given before meals, digestants after meals.

Time in relation to sleep. A drug may be given several hours before the expected time of sleep, directly before retiring or directly upon awakening.

Time in relation to excretory functions. Drugs may be given at a time when excretion is expected or after it has occurred.

ATTRACTIVENESS OF THE DRUG. Under this heading are considered such things as color, taste and form. Attractiveness, always a factor in any case, is of utmost importance in giving drugs to children. For instance, dulcets are tablets that are sweetened and flavored and may be eaten by the child as candy. Medicines in the form of chewing gum are also available, as are liquids which look and taste like a milk shake.

CLIMATE. This has long been known to influence the effectiveness of some drugs. What is valuable in a cold climate may be wholly ineffectual in the tropics.

ALTITUDE. The real significance of altitude in relation to medicine has been brought to light with the advent of the "air age." Doctors and nurses have had to "relearn" pharmacology as it is influenced by changes in air pressure. Oxygen scarcity and changes in atmospheric pressure in the upper atmosphere are potent forces in the usefulness of certain drugs. They also make changes in dosage essential.

DRUG PREPARATION

The preparation of drugs for administration is usually done by the pharmacist or the pharmaceutical company selling the drug. However, the nurse must know how to vary dosage or form to suit the individual situation. It is important that the student review at this time the general subject of solutions, definitions, component parts, and other pertinent data (Chapter 5).

The calculation of dosage is less and less an important activity of the nurse, but it is dangerous to overlook it. If the nurse is not regularly required to change dosage she is apt to forget how it is done. Many times she is taught dosage calculation as the need occurs on the clinical division, but Chapter 5 should serve as a reference to augment this if a specific course in posology is not given.

The administration of medicines has changed greatly through the years. It is still changing, at perhaps an accelerated rate. The nurse must be prepared to meet new methods and to acquire new skills. She should also be prepared to help initiate new methods and to aid in their perfection. Until very recent times most drugs were given by mouth or were applied directly to the skin or mucous membranes. Parenteral administration came into popular use with the advent of aseptic techniques and the invention of the hypodermic syringe. It is interesting to note that the first parenteral method used was the tablet implant, which only recently has been revived. This method was used before the invention of the hypodermic syringe and the introduction of aseptic techniques. Since it was used without asepsis, it often resulted in infection and, therefore, was not popular. Modern methods have eliminated this danger. It is now used when long-delayed absorption is desirable, such as with the administration of hormones. The effects may last weeks or even months.

The Role of the Nurse in the Administration of Drugs

This area heading might be the title of the entire book, since the role of the nurse in drug therapy permeates the whole volume. However, some specific points need emphasis early in the student's study of this important subject.

Professional nursing today requires that the nurse have an understanding of her place on the health team. She must also be familiar with the duties of all other members of the group. This division will endeavor to show the student the nurse's place as it relates to the administration of medicines. The first thing the nurse must know is what drug to give, when to give it and how it is to be given.

HOW DRUGS ARE ORDERED FOR THE PATIENT

There are many ways of ordering drugs for patients. In the hospital the method of ordering for inpatients will differ from that used in the home or doctor's office. It will also differ from the method used in the clinics or outpatient departments of the hospital and other institutions. The nurse should be aware of all these methods and she should understand the language and abbreviations used in making the orders.

Outside the hospital, the prescription is the usual method of ordering medicines. The prescription is actually an order to the pharmacist telling him what medicines to give the patient, how to prepare them and the directions to be given the patient for taking them. Generally speaking, prescriptions are much simpler now than they once were, since pharmaceutical supply houses prepare many drugs for delivery in such form that the pharmacist has merely to measure the desired amount, label correctly and give to the patient.

The following sample is included to acquaint the student with the parts of a prescription. It is rare now to see all four elements of the inscription in any one prescription. The parts of the prescription follow rather closely the parts of a letter, thus:

SUPERSCRIPTION. The superscription includes the patient's name and address, the date and the symbol R.

INSCRIPTION. The inscription is the body of the prescription, containing the names and the amounts of the drugs to be used. If several ingredients are included the following is the usual order:

a. Basic—the most important and usually the most potent drug

b. Adjuvant—the drug used to assist the basic drug

c. Corrective (corrigent)—the ingredient used to disguise the taste of an unpleasant tasting drug

d. Vehicle (excipient, menstruum)—the substance in which the others are dissolved or mixed

SUBSCRIPTION. The subscription is the directions to the pharmacist.

SIGNATURA. The signatura is the directions to be given to the patient, usually begun with either Sig. or S.

SIGNATURE. The signature includes the doctor's name (signature), address and registration number.

The physician's name, address and number are usually printed on his prescription blanks. The prescriptions may be written in English or Latin, or a combination of English and Latin, and the measurements used may be either metric or apothecary. It is not customary to mix the systems in any one prescription.

The sample prescription given below is written mainly in English. The system used is the metric. This is designated by the line drawn through the numbers where the decimal points would be. The words gram or milliliter (cubic centimeter) are not written, as the student (and the pharmacist) should know that fluid ingredients will be measured in milliliters and solid ones in grams or parts thereof.

This prescription is read as follows:

For Mrs. A. J. Jenkens of 1011 Marlor Street, Centreville, Ohio, March fifth, 1974.

Take thou:

Of Tincture of hyoscyamus	5 milliliters
Tincture of lobelia	10 milliliters
Aromatic elixir	10 milliliters

And enough distilled water to make 100 milliliters.

Mix and write on the label

One teaspoonful in water three times a day for three days then once a day.

By order of Dr. H. L. Kelter of 880 Medical Building, this city, whose federal registration number is AK 7890215.

The number is a federal narcotic license number. It is essential in all prescriptions containing any drug listed in the federal narcotic law. Some doctors' prescription blanks also give their state license number.

In the hospital, doctors usually do not use prescription blanks for their orders. Instead, these are given directly to the nurse or the hospital pharmacist by one of several means, the most common being:

VERBAL ORDERS. Verbal orders are used in emergencies when there is insufficient time to write the order, or when the physician is treating a patient and cannot stop to write his orders. Verbal orders are confirmed in writing as soon as circumstances permit.

PHONE ORDERS. Phone orders are those given by the doctor to the nurse or the pharmacist over the telephone. These also are confirmed in writing when the doctor next visits the patient.

WRITTEN ORDERS. Written orders are those which the physician writes and signs

Sample:

Mrs. A. J. Jenkens 1011 Marlor Street Centreville, Ohio	3-5-74		Superscription
℞			
Tincture hyoscyamus	5|00	(basic)	Inscription
Tincture lobelia	10|00	(adjuvant)	Inscription
Elixir aromatica	10|00	(corrective)	Inscription
Distilled water q.s. ad	100|00	(vehicle)	Inscription
M et Sig.			Subscription
5 ml. in water t.i.d. for 3 days then o.d.			Signatura
# AK 7890215	H. L. Kelter, M.D. 880 Medical Building City		Signature

himself. These are the most common orders.

In the first two instances the nurse writes the order for the doctor, signs his name and then her initials after it. Custom has made it proper to add V.O. for verbal orders and P.O. for phone orders. Thus an order might read:

"Coramine 1 cc. by hypodermic stat. V.O. Dr. Graham per L.C.D." The date and time would be included. The physician is requested to verify the order by placing his initials beside the order when he can do so.

Hospitals vary as to where and how orders are written. Usually they are written on a special form on each patient's chart, but other methods are also employed. The important thing is not the method used, but how accurately it is used. Some general rules can be considered.

1. The nurse may take the order directly from the sheet and carry it out. She should check the order carefully to be sure she is giving exactly what the doctor has ordered and in the amount and the way he has ordered it.

2. The charge nurse, team leader or clinical nurse may copy the order on a file and/or a medicine card for each patient and the nurse then uses this as her guide. If in doubt the nurse should refer to the original order.

It should not be necessary to re-emphasize that great care must be taken to make sure that the order is accurately copied at each step. It should be checked each time.

Each individual nurse is considered responsible for:

1. Making sure of the order she is carrying out.

2. Charting the drug in the proper place.

3. Signifying, by whatever means is customary, that she has carried out the order.

In some institutions, drug orders are initialed by the nurse giving the drug, but in other hospitals the initials are not required. Drugs which come under the jurisdiction of special state and federal laws need to be recorded according to the requirements of the law. The charge nurse will assist the student in becoming familiar with such routines. Each hospital and geographic area varies a little, but all require special recording of these drugs.

The nurse will often need to help the patient in the interpretation of drug orders, especially when the patient is leaving the hospital. Care must be taken to make sure that the patient or some responsible relative has a full understanding of how the drug is to be taken. Often a brief explanation of why the drug is used will aid the patient in understanding the importance of any special directions. The student should consult the charge nurse, instructor or doctor as to how much detail should be given in each individual case. Proper instruction for home care is an important duty every nurse has to perform, and the student should take every opportunity to gain experience in teaching patients.

A nurse does not give medications by all the various channels discussed in this chapter. She is expected to be able to administer drugs by local and by oral routes, but some of the parenteral methods are used only by the physician. However, there is an increasing tendency for doctors to delegate duties to nurses, and many procedures formerly done only by doctors are now considered routine for the nurse; this same tendency applies to the giving of medications. That this will gradually increase the scope of the nurse's work appears certain. Furthermore, even though the nurse may not actually give the medicine by a specific route, for example intraspinally, she must understand the entire procedure, for she is the one who must prepare the patient both physically and emotionally for the treatment, secure the proper equipment, see that it is ready for use, have the correct drug available in the exact amount needed and assist the physician with the actual administration.

Accuracy has been, and will continue to be, stressed. Although it seems obvious that it is necessary to be absolutely sure of the right medication, in the right amount, being given to the right patient, still, because of human failure, errors in medication do occur. These are relatively infrequent, but since the patient's life may be at stake, all possible means of preventing such mistakes must be taken.

How can the possibility of errors be minimized? There is an old adage in nursing which says, "Read the label three times—once before removing the container from the shelf, once before removing the drug from the container and once upon returning the container to the shelf." This still applies, especially where stock drugs are kept on the hospital floors or when more than one dose of a drug is on hand. It is absolutely essential in any case that the drug name be carefully checked with the order for the patient and the dosage verified. The nurse should give her entire attention to the preparation of the medication and, insofar as is possible, she should not be disturbed for any other duties.

Most institutions have a definite system for the administration of medications. Some hospitals use cards, with different colors designating different hours. The patient's name, location, drug and dosage and any other pertinent information are written on the card, which is then placed on or under the medicine container, such as the medicine glass, paper cup or hypodermic syringe. Other hospitals merely use pieces of paper upon which the name of the patient is written, together with his location. This is then placed under the medicine container. When the nurse is securing only one medication at a time and it is to be taken directly to the patient, less labeling is needed. However, if the nurse is preparing medications for several patients, some means of differentiation is essential. A word of caution here—*no nurse should chart a medication as given unless she personally gave the drug.* There is one exception: when the drug is administered by the physician, the nurse assisting in the administration charts the drug as given by the doctor. Insofar as possible, the nurse caring for the patient should give that patient his medications. The nurse should never leave a patient until the drug has been taken. Patients have been known to hoard drugs until a toxic or lethal amount is on hand and then take the entire amount at one time with serious, even fatal, results. Many patients who appear perfectly rational are not so well as their conversation would indicate.

When pouring liquid medications (Fig. 6), the nurse should be careful to hold the cup at eye level, pour away from the label to avoid soiling it and read the measure at the lowest point of the meniscus (IV-1). The meniscus is the curve of the top of a fluid in a narrow container (IV-2). Fluid drugs should be thoroughly shaken before pouring, unless special instruction to the contrary is given. Sometimes the supernatant fluid only is to be given (IV-3). The nurse

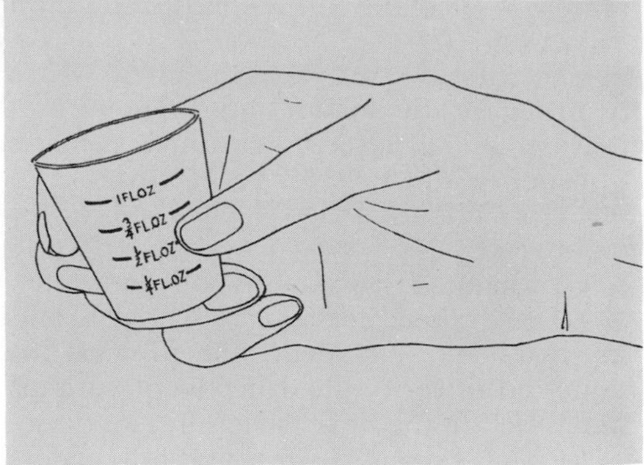

FIGURE 6. Measurement of medication. This glass is marked with household measurements. The thumb should be placed at the bottom of the meniscus (fluid curve) and the glass or paper cup held at eye level to get the correct amount of the fluid.

should wipe the top of the bottle, restopper it, and return it immediately to its proper place in the cupboard. If the label has become illegible or is missing, wholly or in part, or the drug has changed color or consistency, it should not be used. In the hospital such drugs should be returned to the pharmacy. At home it is best to destroy the contents of the bottle.

There are many innovations in the administration of medicines. Some hospitals use unit carts sent from the pharmacy with each day's drugs ready for delivery to the patients. Extra drugs are sent as ordered. Few if any drugs are kept on the division. Usually, those that are on the wards are emergency drugs. In other cases the pharmacist brings the drugs to the division and directly supervises their dispensation. These and similar procedures are intended to increase the efficiency and to decrease the margin of error in the administration of drugs. The nurse must be alert to all such possibilities.

The nurse must always be extremely careful to use accurate measures. The type of measure ordered must be used—thus, minims for minims, drops for drops (Fig. 7). If it is essential to change from one type of measure to another, and if the nurse has any doubt as to dosage, the physician should be consulted for the exact amount he wishes used. If dosage must be changed—from one system to another, for example—the nurse should check carefully and, if in any doubt, have the charge nurse check the order. If

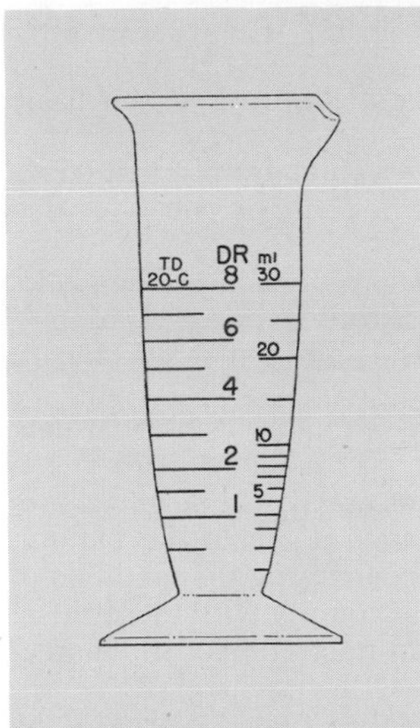

FIGURE 7. Dual calibrated glass for measuring drugs. It is marked for both the metric and the apothecary systems and used to measure the drug which is then placed in the cup to be given to the patient. If the dose is small, a little water can be used to rinse the measuring glass and this added to what is in the cup to make sure that the patient receives the full amount.

there is any question about dosage, she should not guess—a mistake may mean death. It is better not to give the drug at all than to give the wrong one or the wrong amount.

Hospitals and homes vary in their manner of caring for drugs, but certain procedures remain essential. Some system must be used and certain basic principles observed. Oils and similar substances should be kept in a cool place. Vaccines, sera and some other preparations must be kept under refrigeration. If the refrigerator is also used for food, the medicinal substances must be kept separate, for which purpose a small locked box, such as a metal strong box, is very good. Drugs to be used externally should be kept in a separate place from those to be taken internally. Narcotic drugs and any drugs under special legal regulations should be kept in a definite place under lock and key. Poisons should be kept entirely away from other drugs and clearly marked POISON. In the home, all drugs and poisons should be kept where children cannot possibly get them.

There is an increasing tendency in hospitals to keep each patient's medicines separate, with no stock drugs being used. This has its advantages and, as might be expected, its disadvantages. A few precautions seem indicated. First, the nurse should be very sure that she has the right patient's cupboard or shelf area—she must check carefully. Then, if a patient leaving the hospital does not take his drugs with him, she should return the unused medicines to the pharmacy promptly so that there can be no possible confusion with the next patient's drugs. Second, the patient's name, not the room number, should be used to designate the medicines. Room numbers do not change; patients do. Since it is almost impossible not to become impersonal when dealing with room numbers, the good nurse will always use the patient's name, correctly spelled and pronounced.

In the administration of drugs the individual patient is always the first consideration. Many persons are averse to taking medicines. To them the word "drug" means drug addiction, or the use of narcotic or habit-forming drugs, and they feel that once they begin it will be impossible to stop. Patients may be fearful of hypodermic or intramuscular administration of drugs; they are afraid of "needles" or "shots." They may be alarmed by the equipment used for an intravenous infusion or an inhalation drug. The nurse should explain in simple understandable terms what is being done and why. She should try to allay fears. She should also promote the patient's confidence in the physician's decision, both as to the drug selected and the method of administration. If in doubt as to what should be told the patient, the student should consult the instructor or the charge nurse on the floor.

Unless the physician expressly orders otherwise, the nurse should remain with the patient until the drug is taken. The nurse should record all medications promptly after they are given. She should, when leaving the ward or division, tell her relief what has been given.

The nurse should know the medication she is giving, understand its use, its toxic symptoms, the results expected from its use and any other pertinent facts about it. The effects of the drug on each individual should be recorded accurately on his chart. The nurse must watch for early symptoms of poisoning, cumulative action, untoward effect and idiosyncrasy and should report them to the physician promptly so that adequate measures may be taken to prevent the development of any serious complications.

IT IS IMPORTANT TO REMEMBER

1. That most of the material in this chapter is factual and important basic information.

2. That drugs are given to help patients and are valuable only insofar as they do help, though the method of doing so may be not only physical but also through emotional or psychologic means.

3. That purposes for which drugs are used are prophylactic, diagnostic, therapeutic (curative or palliative), supportive, substitutive and restorative.

4. That the type and dosage of each drug used by the physician is selected on the basis of many varied factors.

5. That drugs are administered by a wide variety of methods and that new means are constantly being perfected.

6. That errors in the administration of medications are avoidable and therefore inexcusable and that they can spell injury or even death to the patient.

7. That each hospital has its own specific rules concerning the methods of ordering and caring for drugs, and that the nurse must comply with these rules.

8. That the nurse is responsible for the over-all administration of all medications, even those actually given by the physician.

9. That patients or relatives must be given proper directions for drugs to be taken after the patient goes home. This is often an excellent time for health teaching.

10. That proper instructions for the home care of drugs will eliminate, or greatly reduce, the number of accidental poisonings which occur.

TOPICS FOR STUDY AND DISCUSSION

1. Explain the paragraph written to define "palliative" drugs. Do you agree with the authors? How may the nurse explain to the patient the value of a palliative medication if the patient becomes aware of the fact that the medicine is not an actual "cure"?

2. List the general factors relating to the patient which modify the dosage of a drug. Can you add to those given in the text? What additional explanations of those might be made?

3. Answer Topic 2 with reference to a specific patient.

4. List all the solid forms of drugs you can. Check with Chapter 2 and the Appendix. Did you miss any? Did you add some not found in the text? What are some of the important inferences for drug selection which are referrable to the form of the drug?

5. If a certain drug is changed in the body to an inert substance in six hours and another remains effective for 12 hours, what effect would this have on the ordering of the drugs? Why?

6. What is meant by blood level? How is it maintained? What is the significance for the nurse?

7. A certain person has been taking a "headache remedy" for some months. He tells the nurse and doctor, "I can't get along without it." What is the probable condition? How would you attack the problem?

8. List as many channels of drug administration as you can. Divide them into those which may be used by the nurse and those which only the physician may use. Check with your text, your nursing arts text and with your instructors. Did you include all? Did you separate them correctly? Can you describe briefly the procedure for each? Write out an explanation you could give to a patient if one of the more unusual methods were to be employed.

9. Parenteral administration of drugs is relatively recent. What discoveries have contributed to the effective use of this method?

10. Secure a few prescriptions from whatever source may be available. Can you read them? Divide these into their various parts. Note especially the directions to the patient. Take two or three and write out how you might explain them to the patient who is to take the medicine home.

11. What routine is used for medicinal orders in your hospital? What safeguards have been taken to avoid accidents?

12. Secure from the hospital one or more patient's drug lists. Suppose the patient is going home and is taking these drugs with him. Write out in detail how you would explain to the patient the methods to be used in taking the medicines in his home.

13. How would you secure the patient's cooperation when he does not want to take a medicine? (Assume you are to give a narcotic drug to a patient who is afraid of becoming a drug addict.)

14. You are to give an intramuscular injection to a child eight years of age. How would you explain the procedure to him? How might you procure his cooperation?

15. Write a skit showing a good and a bad approach in the giving of a drug to a patient. This might be a project for two or three students to present to the class.

16. List a few possible ways in which a mistake might be made in the giving of medications. Show in every case how the mistake might have been avoided.

BIBLIOGRAPHY

Books and Pamphlets

American Medical Association Council on Drugs, *Drug Evaluations, 2nd Ed.*, Chicago, 1973, American Medical Association.

Bergersen, B., *Pharmacology in Nursing, 12th Ed.*, St. Louis, 1973, The C. V. Mosby Co.

Du Gas, B. W., *Kozier-Du Gas' Introduction to Patient Care, 2nd Ed.*, Philadelphia, 1972, W. B. Saunders Co.

Goodman, L., and Gilman, A., *Pharmacological Basis of Therapeutics, 4th Ed.*, New York, 1970, The Macmillan Co.

Rodman, M., and Smith, D., *Pharmacology and Drug Therapy in Nursing*, Philadelphia, 1968, J. B. Lippincott Co.

Watson, J. E., *Medical-Surgical Nursing and Related Physiology*, Philadelphia, 1972, W. B. Saunders Co.

Journal Articles

Teitelbaum, Ann C., "Intra-arterial drug therapy," *Am. J. Nurs.* 72:9:1634 (September, 1972).

Weiblem, J. W., "Why we need better medication systems," *Calif. Pharm.* XIX:12:12 (June, 1972).

Wilmore, D. W., "The future of intravenous therapy," *Am. J. Nurs.* 71:12:2334 (December, 1971).

CHAPTER 4

ACTIONS AND INTERACTIONS OF DRUGS IN THE BODY

CORRELATION WITH OTHER SCIENCES

I. ANATOMY AND PHYSIOLOGY

1. The stomach receives all swallowed material. Its slow rhythmic waves (peristalsis) gradually propel its contents toward the pyloric opening to the small intestine. Substances vary in the length of time they remain in the stomach; fluids leave fairly rapidly, fatty material leaves slowly.
2. Some absorption takes place in the stomach, but by far the greater amount is through the walls of the small intestine.
3. Although in anatomy and physiology we learn the body structure and function of the average person, few people fit that average in all areas. People vary widely in individual traits but are alike in the majority of characteristics.

II. CHEMISTRY

1. The gastric juice, which is a clear fluid, normally contains about 99% water and 0.2 to 0.5% hydrochloric acid as well as mucus and enzymes.
2. The pancreatic juice (from the pancreas) and bile (from the liver) are both alkaline (basic) in reaction. This causes the fluid from the stomach gradually to become basic in reaction. They are both secreted into the duodenum (the upper portion of the small intestine).
3. The hydrogen ion is a standard electrochemical unit.
4. The pH of a solution is determined by its hydrogen ion concentration. A pH of 7.0 is neutral, over 7.0 is basic (alkaline) and below 7.0 is acid.
5. The pH of urine is usually 6.0, or slightly acid.
6. An alkali (base) will react with an acid to form a salt. This process is called neutralization.
7. A catalyst is a substance which hastens or aids a chemical reaction without entering into that reaction.

IV. PHYSICS

1. A permeable membrane is a membrane which will allow dissolved particles to pass through.
2. Osmosis is the passage of a solvent through a membrane separating regions of different solvent concentrations.

INTRODUCTION

In the very beginning of the study of drugs and their actions, the student must be aware of the fact that *drugs are given to people.* Nurses are apt to lose sight of this fact and think of drugs in relation to the diseases or symptoms for which they are given. For example, Nurse A thinks of insulin as a drug used to make life possible and happier for the person suffering with diabetes, while Nurse B thinks of insulin as being a drug used to treat diabetes. The difference in their viewpoints is obvious.

In this chapter and those that follow, drugs will be considered in relation to their usual or expected actions. It must be remembered that each individual is different, and though a drug usually acts in a specific way, it may not act as expected in the patient being treated (I-1). Even the same patient may react differently to a given medicine from time to time. These facts are not intended to frighten the student, but to explain many unexpected situations that may arise. It is essential to be aware of such possibilities and to recognize them when they occur.

GENERAL TERMINOLOGY DESCRIBING DRUG ACTION

It was mentioned earlier that drugs act differently in different individuals, but the actions of most drugs can be accurately predicted. Some of the major types of drug action are as follows.

ACCORDING TO THE LOCATION OF THE ACTION

Local or Topical. Drugs whose major effect takes place at the point of contact with the body are local or topical drugs.

Systemic Action. Drugs whose major effect occurs after absorption into the body fluids are systemic in action. These drugs must be soluble in the body fluids and be able to pass through a permeable membrane (IV-1).

Selective Action. Systemic drugs that affect a specific organ or organs are said to have selective action. These drugs have an affinity for certain body tissues.

General Action. These drugs appear to affect the body as a whole.

ACCORDING TO THE EFFECT UPON ALL ACTIVITY

Stimulation. Drugs which increase the functional activity of the cells are said to stimulate or to have stimulating action.

Depression. Depression is the opposite of stimulation; hence, drugs that decrease cell activity are called depressants.

Stimulation or depression may be secured by action either directly upon the organs involved or upon the nerve centers controlling those organs.

Irritation. Irritation is stimulation causing excessive or undue cell activity. This causes some cell damage which is usually mild and temporary; prolonged irritation depresses the activity. Severe irritation may produce vesicant action (blistering) or even escharotic action (destruction of tissue).

Demulcent. Demulcent drugs coat and protect the tissues. The word *emollient* is also used for this type of action if the drug is fatty.

Salt Action. Certain solutions, especially neutral salts of alkalis in water, exhibit varied physical properties which have been called "salt action." These may change the osmotic pressure, surface tension and electrical potential of the cells (IV-2).

ACCORDING TO THE CONDITION OF THE PATIENT

Physiologic Action. Physiologic action is the action of a drug on normal tissue.

Therapeutic Action. Therapeutic action is the action of a drug on diseased tissue.

VARIOUS TERMS USED TO DESCRIBE THE ACTION OF DRUGS

Side Effect. Action of a drug in the body other than the main effect for which the drug was given is called its "side effect." Side effects may be beneficial, harmful or neither. A harmful side effect usually is called an *untoward action.* To illustrate: morphine sulfate given for the relief of pain will also relax tension and aid in inducing sleep, which would be beneficial. It would probably also contract the pupils of the eyes, which would do no harm, or it might cause nausea and vomiting, which would be undesirable.

Idiosyncratic Action. Idiosyncratic action is an unexpected effect produced by a drug in a given individual. For example, a drug which usually causes stimulation, may cause depression.

Toxic Action. Toxic action is a poisonous effect, either from a regular dose or an overdose of a drug.

Cumulative Action. When a drug is excreted slowly, it tends to accumulate in the system, giving rise to toxic symptoms—this is cumulative action. Cumulative action may also occur when a subsequent dose of the medicine is given before the effects of the first dose have disappeared.

Antagonistic Action. When one drug counteracts the action of another drug it is said to have antagonistic action. For example, the action of a depressant and stimulant given at the same time would be antagonistic. There are several mechanisms by which antagonism may happen, but the two most common are opposite action or inactivation of one or both drugs wholly or in part by chemical action.

Synergistic Action. When two or more drugs are given at the same time and they increase the potency or reduce the undesirable side effects of the drugs, the action is called *synergistic*. The giving of large numbers of drugs, although once popular, is now largely in disrepute, but there are many times when two drugs given together are more effective than either one given alone, even in dosage equivalent to the combined dosage of the two.

The action of any single drug in a specific instance may or may not follow the pattern expected. A drug may cause a specific reaction repeatedly in the chemist's test tube but may not produce that same action when tried on the living animal. Again, it may produce the expected results in the experimental animal and not in the human being. Still again, it may produce the expected result in most patients but not in all patients. The reason for this last is the fact that each person is an individual; his body metabolism is different from that of others; and, therefore, he reacts differently. Drug action is not the same in every disease. Thus, one drug may produce several effects, depending upon the conditions being treated.

ACTION OF DRUGS IN THE BODY

The fate of the individual drug in the body (insofar as it is understood at the present time) is discussed throughout this book and will be found in column four of the Current Drug Handbook. However, a brief general consideration of the subject early in the course may be of value to the student.

Topical drugs, those applied directly to the surfaces of the body for action at the point of contact, will not be covered here, since they do not usually enter the body fluids in significant amounts.

ABSORPTION. It is obvious that any drug given for internal use must pass through at least one membrane or cell wall. Most will pass through the wall of the gastrointestinal tract, and into and out of the capillaries, into the interstitial spaces, and then through the cell membrane. If the drug is given subcutaneously or intramuscularly, it will bypass the gastrointestinal wall and enter the capillaries directly. If given intravenously, it will need only to leave the blood stream to enter the interstitial spaces.

By far the larger portion of drugs is administered orally. Most oral drugs now are either tablets or capsules. The tablets may or may not be coated. Pills are usually smaller than tablets and generally ovoid in shape and coated.

Before any substance can pass through a membrane it must be in solution. Drugs given parenterally are already dissolved, as are some given orally. Dissolution of capsules, tablets or pills depends upon a number of factors, including:

1. Hardness of the outer coating.
2. Rate at which the tablet or capsule disintegrates—the smaller the particle, the more readily it can be dissolved.
3. Dissolution rate. Some drugs are more readily soluble than others. The pH of the surrounding medium can cause a change in rate, making it either slower or faster (II-4).
4. Excipients or binders used, chemical stability and complex formations.

These and other conditions will determine the *availability* of the drug for absorption. The so-called delayed release drugs and other similar medicines are designed to take advantage of these factors. They allow some of the drug to be quickly available but delay other portions for varying periods of time. Drugs given sublingually or buccally are in a form that dissolves rapidly and is readily available for absorption.

Just how medicinal substances pass

through the cell wall (membrane) is, as yet, only imperfectly known. There are several theories, and certain facts have been fairly well established, but much is yet to be determined. Detailed explanation is beyond the scope of this book but a brief discussion of some of the pertinent facts should aid the student in understanding some of the complex actions and reactions of drugs.

Absorption of medicine from the gastrointestinal wall is the same as the passage of drugs across any biologic membrane. Absorption is favored (see preceding factors determining availability) by (1) a low degree of ionization, (2) a relatively high lipid/water partition coefficient of the nonionized form, and (3) a small molecular radius of the dissolved particles. Lipid-soluble substances are believed to pass through the cell membrane without aid. Other substances require what is called "active transport" or "carriers." (See Figure 8.)

Some substances are destroyed by the digestive enzymes and cannot be given orally. Examples include insulin and epinephrine. Any substance which forms an insoluble precipitate or which is not soluble either in water or in lipid cannot be absorbed.

DISTRIBUTION. Once a drug is in the blood stream, it may be taken to any or most parts of the body. The point at which it leaves the blood stream may be of prime importance. Drugs given orally may leave the gastrointestinal tract via either the blood capillaries or the lymph capillaries. If the drug goes by the former route, it will pass through the liver before reaching the systemic circulation. The liver may or may not change the composition of the drug.

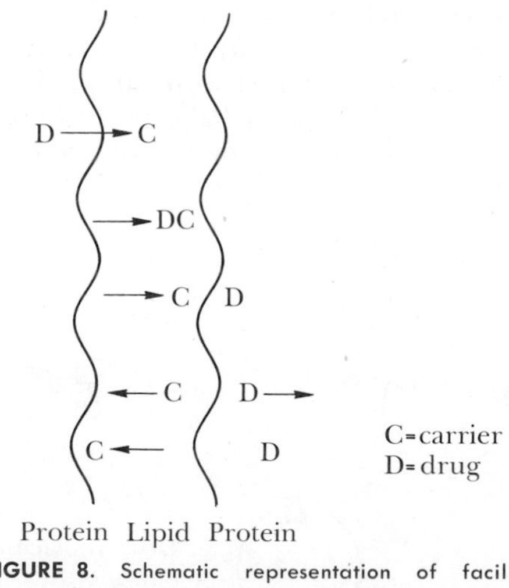

FIGURE 8. Schematic representation of facilitative transport of a drug across a lipid cell membrane by means of a carrier.

To be effective, the drug must reach the site of action where it is needed. It may or may not enter the cell. In the blood stream some drugs become bound to the blood proteins (protein-bound). This binding may be very unstable or moderately stable. Usually these bound forms set up an equilibrium with the unbound form of the drug and are released at either regular or irregular intervals. The slower the release, the longer the drug will be effective. The degree of that effectiveness, however, may be greatly diminished by this binding to the extent of being ineffective.

The point at which a given drug will leave the blood stream depends upon the chemical composition of the drug and the type of tissue it passes. When the drug leaves the blood stream and enters the interstitial spaces it may remain there, become attached to the cell or pass through the cell membrane wholly or in part. Certain medicinal substances have an affinity for specific body tissues, and as the blood carries them past these tissues, they leave the blood stream. This tissue may not be the diseased part or the target area. If it is not, the rapidity of the withdrawal of the drug from the blood at these locations will probably necessitate changes in the amount and frequency of dosage. Areas where drugs commonly tend to concentrate include the liver, lungs, kidneys, bones and other connective tissue. There may be a *redistribution* of the drug upon its release from these organs as it re-enters the circulation.

The term blood-brain barrier refers to the barrier which may or may not prevent substances in the circulation from entering the cerebrospinal fluid and thus reaching the brain. It is mainly those drugs which are lipid soluble, either originally or after metabolic changes in the body, which will pass this barrier.

The placenta also acts as a barrier to some substances, drugs included, thus the term placental barrier.

THEORIES OF DRUG ACTION. To date, little is known of the cellular biochemistry and physiology of drug action. However, there are several theories given to explain the mechanism of action of certain drugs.

Generally, it is thought that drugs produce their effects by:

1. Altering the permeability of the cellular membrane and/or interfering with the passage of the drug across the cell membrane.

2. Interfering with protein synthesis within the cell or with other cellular metabolic activities.

3. Interfering with enzyme function at the so-called receptor sites. (See Figure 9.)

According to the receptor site theory, drugs are classified as

1. Agonists—drugs which combine with receptors and initiate a response. They are said to have affinity (attraction to the site) and efficacy (effective action).

2. Antagonists—drug action which is the result of affinity without efficacy. This means that the drug compound may resemble the chemical structure necessary to occupy the receptor site, but the usual pharmacological effect is not obtained.

METABOLISM OF DRUGS. There are only a few medicinal substances which enter and leave the body without some chemical change; most are changed (metabolized) in some manner. The body enzymes initiate various chemical reactions. These reactions that metabolize drugs include deaminization, acetylation, oxidation, hydroxylation and conjugation. If the metabolites are inactive, the medicine will be effective only as long as it remains unchanged. However, in certain instances, the drug is effective only after the change has taken place. Again, a drug may be therapeutically useful both before and after metabolic changes in the same or varying degrees of activity. These facts in relation to a specific drug will affect the dose and the schedule of administration.

EXCRETION OF DRUGS. Drugs may be excreted by any of the excretory organs—lungs, skin, intestines or kidneys. In the majority of cases, the kidneys are the site of excretion. As noted above, the drug may leave the body unchanged, but in most cases it is the metabolites that are excreted. The metabolite may be active, and the drug may be given because of its action on the kidneys. If the drug is active in an acid medium, a second drug may not be necessary, since urine is normally acidic. But if the drug acts best in an alkaline medium, it may be essential to give an alkalinizing agent to insure an alkaline urine. It may also be necessary to check the patient's diet to be sure that most of the food taken will result in an alkaline ash residue. The metabolite excreted may also be inactive.

DRUG INTERACTIONS

Interactions between drugs may occur in vitro (outside the body) or in vivo (inside the body). Usually, the term *incompatibility* is used in reference to interactions in vitro; *interactions* are drug reactions in vivo.

Incompatibility may be either *physical*, as when two or more fluid drugs change color and/or consistency when mixed together, or *chemical*, as when the drugs react with each other to form an entirely different chemical compound.

Interaction is the modification of the action of a drug by one or more other drugs given concurrently or sequentially. This may be beneficial, neutral or detrimental. Drugs may also interact with various foods, with chemicals used in laboratory tests or with certain endogenous physiological agents.

With the multiplicity and complexity of

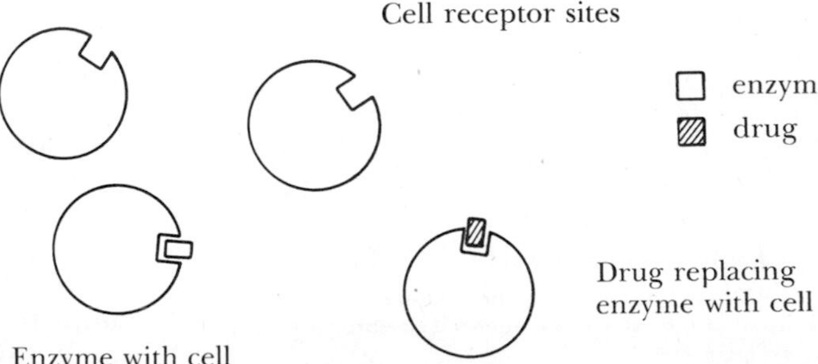

FIGURE 9. Schematic representation of the receptor theory of drug action. The drug replaces the enzyme at the receptor site.

modern medicines, the subject of drug interactions is extremely intricate. Much research is being done on the subject, but it is a difficult and time-consuming process. In this chapter, the student can be given only a glimpse of the possible interactions. These interactions will be covered in later chapters in the discussions of particular drugs used in specific therapeutic situations.

It is thought that many interactions are due to a change in the body's enzyme systems (biotransformation), especially the microsomal enzyme systems of the liver, and the monoamine oxidase enzyme. It is presumed that many other enzyme systems are involved also.

Interactions may occur during absorption, transportation, metabolism, storage, at receptor sites or excretion. The interaction of one drug with another may enhance, retard or negate the action of one or both drugs, or the result may be an entirely different action. In some cases the interaction is desirable and expected. In others, despite a possible undesirable reaction, two drugs may be given together because it is believed that the net result will be beneficial to the patient. In long-term use, a drug may interact with itself in the body.

Some other terms used in describing drug interaction are as follows:

1. Heterergy when only one of a pair of drugs produces an effect.

–*Synergism* is the combined effect of heterergic drugs that is greater than that of the active components alone. It often results from alteration of the distribution or inactivation of the active component.

–*Antagonism* is the effect of heterergic drugs that is less than the effect of the single active component.

–*Chemical antagonism* refers to the interaction of an agonist and an antagonist to form an inactive complex.

–*Competitive antagonism* occurs when an antagonist acts reversibly at the same receptor site as an agonist.

–*Non-equilibrium* occurs when a receptor antagonist acts irreversibly.

–*Non-competitive antagonism* occurs when the agonist and antagonist act at different receptor sites.

2. Homergy when two drugs produce the same overt effect.

–*Summation* is a situation in which the combined effect of two drugs is equal to the sum of their individual effects.

–*Additive effect* is the combined action of the two drugs which is greater than the sum of their individual effects.

–*Supraadditive effect* is much greater than summation or additive effect.

–*Infraadditive effect* is the action of two combined drugs which is less than additive.

3. Physiologic or functional antagonism refers to the antagonism between two drugs having overtly opposite effects.

Drug interactions (the effect of one drug on the activity of another) are becoming more important as sophisticated drugs become widely available and frequently used. The nurse must be ever alert to the possibility that a second drug may either increase or decrease the effect of the first.

Throughout the book each major drug or drug group and its more important and known interactions, if any, will be discussed. The discussion will include those facts which are pertinent to nursing care but does not presume to be complete in a general sense.

The nurse, no matter where she works, is in a unique position to help prevent, or detect early, complications resulting from drug interactions. Since there are so many non-prescription (over the counter, OTC) drugs sold that are actually potent medications, the layman may unknowingly take combinations that can be detrimental. Many times the patient does not tell the doctor the names of the medications he is taking because he may not think of the OTC drugs as medicines. However, he may let the nurse know, especially if she does a bit of judicious detective work. One illustration might clarify this. The patient on oral anticoagulant therapy is taking an "arthritic compound" for his arthritis even though his physician had told him not to take aspirin. Aspirin has limited anticoagulant properties, and most arthritic drugs sold without a prescription contain aspirin; however, few people read the fine print on the label.

The accompanying diagram will indicate some of the ways drugs interact. The actual physiologic processes are varied and complex. Some are well understood, some partially known, but others act in ways not yet determined. Just a few of the possibilities include changing the activities of the body's enzyme systems, competing for receptor sites and increasing or decreasing excretion of one or the other of the drugs. (See Figure 10.)

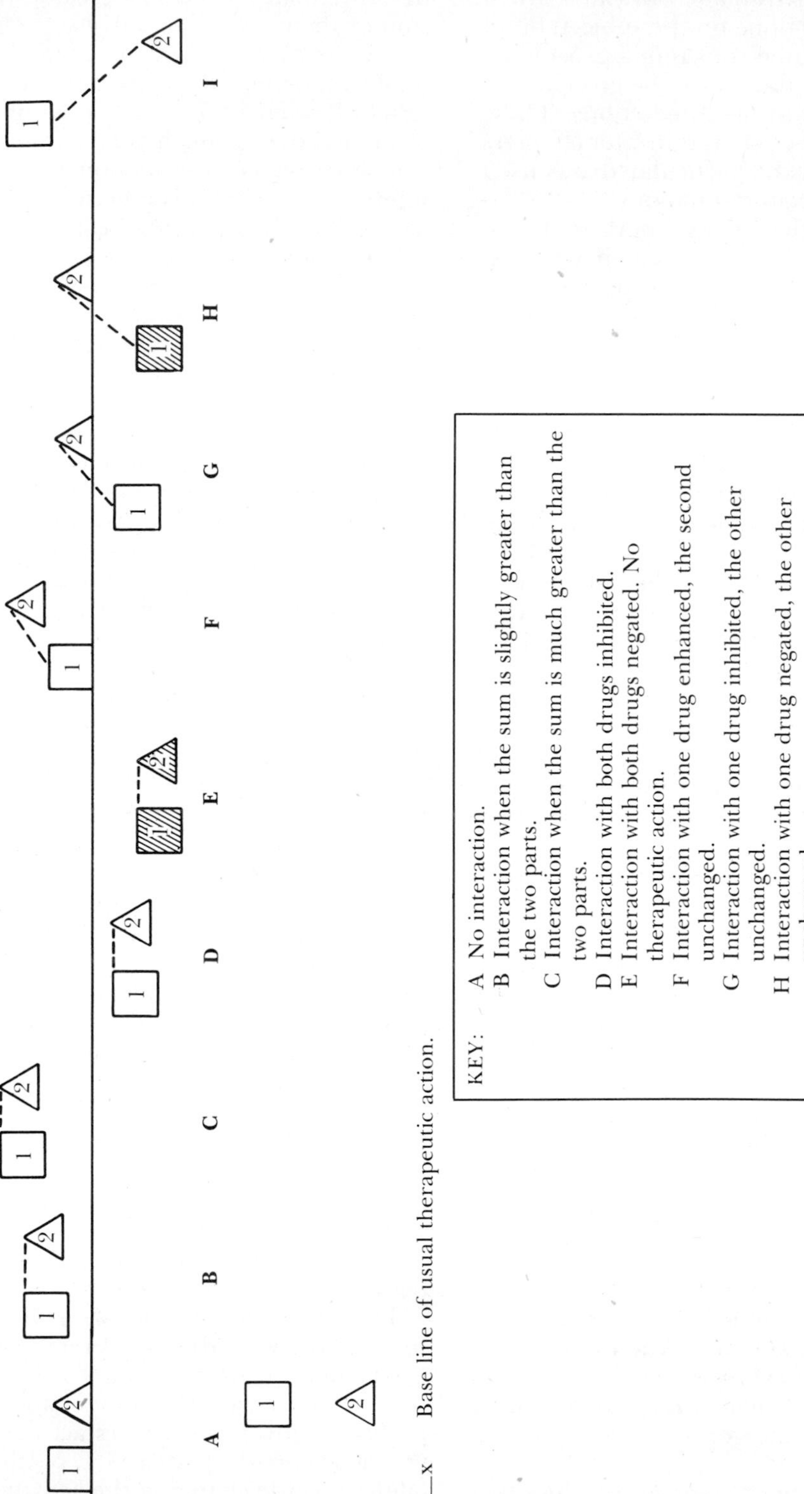

FIGURE 10. Some of the possible interactions of drugs.

IT IS IMPORTANT TO REMEMBER

1. That drugs are given to patients and are valuable only insofar as they do help, whether they are used as physical aids or as emotional or psychological aids.
2. That there are many types of action which drugs produce in the body and that much research is being done in this field. The nurse must keep up with the new findings.
3. That as research discloses new facts, the nurse must be ready to exchange the older facts she has known for newer information.
4. That the drug interactions known at present are probably only a small per cent of the total. The nurse must be ever alert for symptoms of the unknown as well as the known.
5. That as new drugs are formulated there will be new actions and interactions to be learned.

TOPICS FOR STUDY AND DISCUSSION

1. Some oral preparations are so arranged that part of the material will dissolve in an acid medium and some in an alkaline (basic) medium. What is the significance of this? Would the patient with hyper- or hypoacidity in the gastric juice have the same results as the patient with a normal gastric acid content? Defend your position.
2. Take one common drug (such as aspirin) and see what other drugs might interact with it. Several students could work on this, each taking a different drug.
3. Make a list of at least 10 or 12 drugs. Give the action of each in the body and tell what purposes each is used for.

BIBLIOGRAPHY

Books and Pamphlets

American Medical Association, *Drug Evaluations, 2nd Ed.*, Chicago, 1973, American Medical Association.

Goldstein, A., Aronow, L., and Kalman, S. M., *Principles of Drug Action*, New York, 1969, Harper and Row, Publishers.

Goodman, L. S., and Gilman, A., *Pharmacological Basis of Therapeutics, 4th Ed.*, New York, 1970, The Macmillan Co.

Goth, A., *Medical Pharmacology, 6th Ed.*, St. Louis, 1972, The C. V. Mosby Co.

Hartshorn, E. A., *Handbook of Drug Interaction*, Cincinnati, 1970, Donald L. Francke.

Korolkovas, A., *Essentials of Molecular Pharmacology*, New York, 1970, Wiley-Interscience (John Wiley and Sons).

Meyers, F. H., Jawetz, E., and Goldfine, A., *Review of Medical Pharmacology, 3rd Ed.*, Los Altos, California, 1970, Lange Medical Publications.

Pfeiffer, J., *The Cell*, New York, 1964, Life Science Library.

Rodman, M. J., and Smith, D. W., *Pharmacology and Drug Therapy in Nursing*, Philadelphia, 1968, J. B. Lippincott Co.

Journal Articles

Brodie, B., "Physiochemical and biochemical aspects of pharmacology," *J.A.M.A.* 202:7: 148, (1967).

DiPalma, J. R., "The why and how of drug interaction," *R.N.* March, April and May, 1970.

Hassar, D. A., "Drug interaction—The pharmacist's opportunities and limitation," *J. Am. Pharm. Assoc.* NS 12:9:467 (September, 1972).

Lachman, L., and Roemer, W. C., "Pharmaceutical properties of drugs and dosage forms affecting physiological availability," *J. Am. Pharm. Assoc.* NS 5:215 (May, 1972).

Milne, M. D., "Disorders of amino acid transport," *Br. Med. J.* 1:327:336, 1964.

Smyth, D., and Whitten, R., "Membrane transport in relation to intestinal absorption," *Br. Med. Bull.* 23:3:231.

Ward, D. R., "Pharmaceutical receptors," *Pharmacol. Rev.* 20:2:49:88.

CHAPTER 5

DRUG MATHEMATICS AND POSOLOGY

Arithmetic Review; Weights and Measures

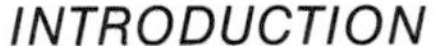

INTRODUCTION

To an ever-increasing degree, medicines come to the nurse ready to administer. The tablet, capsule, liquid or pill is in the exact dose to be given. The plastic hypodermic or the hypodermic cartridge with metal frame contains the amount of the drug to be used for a single dose. These things make the nurse's work easier and the calculation of dosages rare. However, this increases rather than decreases the possibility of error. The more a technique is used, the easier, better and more accurate the results will be, provided the technique used is good. Disuse makes for forgetting and ineptness. Since recovery of health, even life, may depend upon the correct measurement of drugs, the nurse's responsibility is clear.

Before attempting to calculate dosage, the student must have an adequate understanding of basic arithmetical processes. Women tend to say, "I can't learn mathematics," but, at the same time, they drive the hardest bargains, are the holders of most of the country's wealth and make many, if not most, of their families' financial transactions. "It just does not add up." Before giving up, the student should think how much she uses mathematics each and every day.

There is not time in a course of this length (usually 16 hours or 1 unit) to teach arithmetic, but a review is helpful. The major processes used that may have been forgotten will be covered very briefly in the next few pages. The student should check them over and study any that do not seem too familiar. Addition, subtraction, division and multiplication of whole numbers have not been included. Rules for various arithmetical processes involving common and decimal fractions are given to refresh the student's memory and for reference. One example is given in each case to illustrate the process involved.

SOME BASIC ARITHMETICAL RULES

Fractions

COMMON FRACTIONS

ADDITION AND SUBTRACTION

RULE: ADDITION AND SUBTRACTION: Find the least common denominator, change the terms of the fractions to this and proceed as with whole numbers. Change the resulting fraction to whole or mixed numbers, as indicated.

EXAMPLE: ADDITION:

$1/3 + 7/10 + 3/5 + 5/12;$

LCD 60;

$$\frac{20 + 42 + 36 + 25}{60} = \frac{123}{60} =$$

$$\frac{41}{20} = 2\ 1/20$$

EXAMPLE: SUBTRACTION:

$$7/8 - 2/9 = \frac{63 - 16}{72} = \frac{47}{72}$$

$$\text{LCD} = 72$$

There are many ways of finding the least common denominator, but all have the same objective: reduce all the denominators to their prime numbers, eliminate duplicates and then multiply the remaining numbers. In the fractions for addition as given: $1/3 + 7/10 + 3/5 + 5/12$ the least
$3 \quad 2 \times 5 \quad \cancel{5} \quad \cancel{2} \times 2 \times \cancel{3}$
common denominator is $3 \times 2 \times 5 \times 2$ or 60.

For the problem in subtraction it is necessary to multiply both denominators since there are no duplications.

MULTIPLICATION AND DIVISION

Cancellation, where possible, reduces the amount of the calculations. It is the elimination of numbers common to both the numerator and the denominator. Remember, dividing or multiplying both terms of a fraction by the same number does not change the value of the fraction. Thus: ${}^{1}\cancel{2}/3 \times 7/\cancel{12}_{6} = 7/18$

EXAMPLE: 4/12 = 1/3 both divided by 4. 0.1/20 = 1/200 both multiplied by 10.

RULE: MULTIPLICATION: Multiply the numerators and the denominators. Reduce and change to whole or mixed numbers as indicated. Cancel where possible.

EXAMPLE: ${}^{1}\cancel{2}/\cancel{9}_{3} \times {}^{1}\cancel{3}/\cancel{10}_{5} = 1/15$

RULE: DIVISION: Invert the terms of the *divisor* and proceed as in multiplication.

EXAMPLE:

$16/27 \div 2/3 = {}^{8}\cancel{16}/\cancel{27}_{9} \times {}^{1}\cancel{3}/\cancel{2}_{1} = 8/9$

DECIMAL FRACTIONS

Decimals, as the name indicates, are a matter of "tens"; the decimal fraction is indicated by the period. Whole numbers are to the left and fractions are to the right of the point. Thus 12.6 is twelve whole numbers (10 + 2) and 6/10 of one whole number.

Where there are no whole numbers, it is good practice to place a zero before the decimal point. This will avoid the chance that the decimal point may be overlooked.

ADDITION AND SUBTRACTION

RULE: Place the numbers in columns with the decimal point in exact line. Proceed as with whole numbers. If need be for clarity, zeros may be added to the right of last numeral to the right of the decimal point. This does not change the value.

EXAMPLE: ADDITION

1,072.8
27.004
1.7652 OR
120.01
9.3
1,230.8792

1,072.8000
27.0040
1.7652
120.0100
9.3000
1,230.8792 or rounded to 1,230.88

EXAMPLE: SUBTRACTION

1,072.8
27.004 OR
1,045.796

1,072.800
27.004
1,045.796 or rounded to 1,045.80

MULTIPLICATION AND DIVISION

RULE: MULTIPLICATION: Proceed as with whole numbers. Count off the *total* number of decimal points from the right.

EXAMPLE:

238.46
1.213
71538
23846
47692
23846
289.25198

Answer can be written: 289.25198
or if rounding permitted: 289.252

RULE: DIVISION: Change the divisor to a whole number by moving the decimal point the required number of places to the right. Move the decimal point in the dividend an equal number of places to the right. Place the decimal point in the quotient above this point. Proceed as with whole numbers.

EXAMPLE:

1.0 ÷ 0.25

4.
0.25‸ ⟌ 1.00‸
1 00

Percentage, Ratio and Proportion

Percentage and ratio refer to relationships of one number to another. Proportion also is a matter of relationships but of more than one number. To determine how to change one to another, refer to the section "Changing from One Number Form to Another Form."

PERCENTAGE: Percentage is the relationship of a number to 100 (per centum).

EXAMPLE: 2 per cent is equal to 2:100.

RATIO: Ratio is the relationship of one number to another. The first should be 1, if possible. A colon is placed between the two numbers.

EXAMPLE: 1 to 4000 is written 1:4000, or using the numbers above 2:100 or preferably 1:50.

PROPORTION: Proportion is the relationship of two ratios to each other. In other words, the ratio of the first two numbers is the same as the ratio of the second two numbers. This is the formula used for most problems in dosage and solution. The multiplication of the means (inner numbers) and the extremes (outer numbers) together produces the same number. It is wise regularly to place the X either to the right or to the left of the double colon or times sign.

EXAMPLE: 1:100::2:200, 1 × 200 equals 200 and 2 × 100 equals 200 and 200 equals 200. If the letter X is substituted for any one of the four numbers, its value can be determined by the above process. Thus:

1 : X :: 2 : 200, 2X equals 200,
X equals 100 or 200 ÷ by 2.

Proportion also may be written as a common fraction. Thus: 1/X = 2/200

Changing from One Number Form to Another Form

This is very easily done, and it is often helpful to be able to do this quickly.

COMMON FRACTIONS TO DECIMALS: Divide numerator by denominator. Place decimal point in the correct position.

EXAMPLE:

$$2/3 = 3\overline{)2.000}\ \text{with quotient}\ .666 \text{ or } 0.666\ (0.67)$$

COMMON FRACTIONS TO PER CENT: Proceed as above. Move the decimal point 2 places to the right and add the per cent sign (%).

EXAMPLE: 0.666 equals 66.6%

COMMON FRACTIONS TO RATIO: Write the terms of the fraction with a colon between, numerator first, denominator second. Reduce if possible.

EXAMPLE: 2/3 equals 2:3

DECIMAL TO COMMON FRACTION: Place the figure over the proper number of zeros with a 1 to the left. Omit the decimal point. Reduce if indicated.

EXAMPLE: 1.027 equals $\frac{1027}{1000}$ or $1\frac{27}{1000}$

DECIMAL TO PER CENT: Move the decimal point 2 places to the right, thus multiplying by 100; add per cent sign.

EXAMPLE: 0.02 equals 2.0%

DECIMAL TO RATIO: Write the number as the first term and the proper number of zeros with a 1 to the left as indicated. Separate with a colon. Reduce if possible.

EXAMPLE: 0.02 equals 2:100 or 1:50

PER CENT TO DECIMAL: Move the decimal point 2 places to the left, thereby dividing by 100 and omit the per cent sign.

EXAMPLE: 16% equals 0.16

PER CENT TO RATIO: Write the number as the first term and 100 as the second term with a colon between. Reduce if possible. Omit per cent sign.

EXAMPLE: 16% equals 16:100 or 4:25

PER CENT TO COMMON FRACTION: Write the number as the numerator, 100 as the denominator. Omit per cent sign. Reduce if possible.

EXAMPLE: 16% equals $\frac{16}{100}$ or $\frac{4}{25}$

RATIO TO DECIMAL: Divide the first term by the second.

EXAMPLE: 1:20 equals 0.05

$$20\overline{)1.00}\ \text{with quotient}\ 0.05;\ 1.00$$

RATIO TO PER CENT: Proceed as above. Move the decimal point 2 places to the right and add the per cent sign.

EXAMPLE: 1:20 equals 0.05 or 5.0%

RATIO TO COMMON FRACTIONS: Write the two numbers with a horizontal line where the colon was. Reduce if possible.

EXAMPLE: 1:20 equals $\frac{1}{20}$

Roman Numerals

This system of numerals was used throughout the Roman Empire and was only gradually replaced by the Arabic numerals.

In the Roman system, letters are used in place of what we know as numerals. Each letter is assigned a numerical value. These numerals are still used in many areas—chapters or other book divisions, clock dials and the like.

They are used in prescription writing when the apothecaries' system is used and with the symbols. It is customary to use capital letters for the numbers, but in the writing of prescriptions, lower case letters are often used and the letters i and j are dotted as is correct. Where several (2 or 3) i's are in a row, the last one is written as a j; otherwise the j is not used.

ROMAN NUMERALS AND THEIR VALUES IN ARABIC NUMERALS

I (i) =	1
V (v) =	5
X (x) =	10
L (l) =	50
C (c) =	100
D (d) =	500
M (m) =	1000

RULES: A smaller value letter (number) placed to the left of a larger one is subtracted from the larger one. Only one may be so placed.

EXAMPLE: XL = 40 (50 − 10) XXL would be incorrect for 30, which is written XXX.

A smaller value placed to the right of a larger number is added to the larger one. As many as three may be so placed, but no more than three.

EXAMPLE: LX = 60 (50 + 10), LXX = 70 (50 + 10 + 10), LXXX = 80(50 + 10 + 10 + 10). LXXXX *does not* equal 90; this is written as XC (100 − 10).

It is possible to do arithmetical calculations in Roman numerals, but it is better to change to Arabic with which we are all familiar.

WEIGHTS AND MEASURES

Medicines and solutions used in medical and nursing practice in the United States and Canada are measured by more than one system, and this often leads to confusion. The nurse must learn these measures and their relationships to be able to administer drugs intelligently. The systems used are the apothecaries' or English and the metric or French. In addition, household measures may be needed, especially when nursing in the home. It is the system commonly used in cooking and the household arts. Only those weights and measures most often used by the nurse are given here. More complete tables will be found in the Appendix.

Where the symbols are used, the distinction between drams and ounces must be clear. Small Roman numerals (lower case letters) are used after the symbols. Common fractions are used with the exception of one-half which is written ss, usually with a line drawn over the two letters. The following examples will clarify this: ʒ iss reads, drams one and one-half; ℥ iii 1/3 reads, ounces three and one-third; m.xv reads, minims fifteen. It is becoming increasingly common to use the abbreviations and Arabic numerals for the apothecaries' system. The symbol or abbreviation should always precede the numeral.

Metric System

This system was invented by French scientists at the time of the French Revolution and is based, as is our monetary system, on multiples of ten. The system is based on the *meter* which is a measure of length and is the approximate length of our yard—specifically, 39.37 inches. More complete tables will be found in the appendix.

NOTE: Abbreviations used include the initial letter and the letter following which is indicative of the item. The numerals always precede the letter abbreviations, and decimal fractions are always used.

EXAMPLES: 1.5 kg. equals or reads, one and five-tenths kilogram (not 1½ kg. or kg. 1.5).

3.25 Gm. equals or reads three and twenty-five hundredth grams.

NOTE: Approximate equivalents vary from region to region. Those given are only suggestions. The instructor should indicate any changes common in her area.

Apothecaries' Table of Weights

APOTHECARIES'	APPROXIMATE METRIC EQUIVALENT
	60 to 65 milligrams (mg.) = 1 grain
60 grains (gr.) = 1 dram (dr. ʒ)	4 grams = 1 dram
8 drams = 1 ounce (oz. ℥)	30 to 32 grams = 1 ounce
12 ounces = 1 pound (lb.)*	370 to 375 grams = 1 pound
	0.37 to 0.375 kilograms = 1 pound

*Note that in the avoirdupois table there are 16 ounces in one pound. In the Troy table there are 12 ounces in one pound as with the apothecaries'.

Metric System of Weights

METRIC	APPROXIMATE APOTHECARIES' EQUIVALENT
1000 microgram (mcg.) = 1 milligram (mg.)	gr. 1/60 = 1 mg.
1000 milligrams = 1 gram (Gm.)	gr. 15-16 = 1 Gm.
1000 grams = 1 kilogram (kg.)	2.2 lb. (avoir.) = 1 kg.

Apothecaries' Table of Volume

APOTHECARIES'	APPROXIMATE METRIC EQUIVALENT
1 minim (m.)	= 0.06 ml.
60 minims = 1 fluid dram (fdr.)	4 ml. = 1 fdr. (fl. dr.)
8 fluid drams = 1 fluid ounce (foz.)	30 ml. = 1 foz. (fl. oz.)
16 fluid ounces = 1 pint (pt. or O.)	500 ml. = 1 pint or 0.5 liter
2 pints = 1 quart (qt.)	1000 ml. = 1 quart or 1 liter
4 quarts = 1 gallon (gal. or C.)	4000 ml. = 1 gallon or 4 liters

Metric Table of Volume

METRIC	APPROXIMATE APOTHECARIES' EQUIVALENT
1000 milliliters (ml.)* = 1 liter (l.)	15 minims = 1 ml.
1000 liters = 1 kiloliter (kl.)	1 quart = 1 liter or 1000 ml.

*One cubic centimeter (cc.) is often used in place of one milliliter (ml.). A milliliter of water occupies one cubic centimeter of space.

HOUSEHOLD MEASURES
Volume (Wet)

60–75 drops (gtt.)	= 1 teaspoonful (t.) (4 cc.)
3-4 teaspoonfuls*	= 1 tablespoonful (T.)
2 tablespoonfuls 6–8 teaspoonfuls	= 1 ounce (oz.)
6 ounces	= 1 teacupful
8 ounces	= 1 glassful or one measuring cupful
16 ounces	= 1 pint (pt.)
2 pints	= 1 quart (qt.)
4 quarts	= 1 gallon (gal.)

*Latest U.S.P. gives 3 teaspoonfuls to 1 tablespoonful.

No table of weights is given for household measures since it is not usual to use such in the home. However, if used, these would be the same as the apothecaries' or the avoirdupois.

Approximate Equivalents to be Memorized

Since the nurse will not always have ready access to conversion tables, it is essential that the more commonly used equivalents be memorized. If the basic table and certain important key equivalents are known, it is usually not difficult to convert to any needed numbers.

One method of remembering the various equivalents is to try to find out how many things are equal to each of the major measures. For example: one teaspoonful equals one fluid dram, 60 minims, 60 drops, 4.0 milliliters (cc.), 1/8 ounce, 1/2 of a dessertspoonful or 1/4 of a tablespoonful. Similar relationships should be found for other measures.

Conversion of One System to Another

RULES: To change
GRAINS TO GRAMS: Divide by 15
Example: 60 grains equals 60 ÷ 15 or 4 grams.
GRAMS TO GRAINS: Multiply by 15
Example: 3 grams equals 3 × 15 or 45 grains.
GRAMS TO OUNCES: Divide by 30

Approximate Equivalents To Be Memorized

Household	*Apothecaries'*	*Metric*
	Volume, Liquid or Wet	
60 drops or 1 teaspoonful	60 minims or 1 fluid dram	4 milliliters (cc.)
2 tablespoonfuls	1 fluid ounce	30 milliliters (cc.)
1 measuring cupful (1 glassful)	8 fluid ounces	240 milliliters or 0.25 liter
1 pint	1 pint	500 milliliters or 0.5 liter
1 quart	1 quart	1,000 milliliters or 1.0 liter
1 gallon	1 gallon	4,000 milliliters or 4.0 liters
	Weight or Dry	
	1/60 grain	1.0 milligram
	1 grain	60.0 milligrams
	15 or 16 grains	1.0 gram
	1 dram	4.0 grams
	1 ounce	30.0 grams
	2.2 pounds (avoirdupois)	1.0 kilogram

Example: 80 grams equals 80 ÷ 30 or $2\frac{2}{3}$ ounces.

OUNCES TO GRAMS: Multiply by 30

Example: 2 ounces equals 2 × 30 or 60 grams.

MILLIGRAMS TO GRAINS: Divide by 60

Example: 30 milligrams equals 30 ÷ 60 or $\frac{1}{2}$ grain.

GRAINS TO MILLIGRAMS: Multiply by 60

Example: 10 grains equals 10 × 60 or 600 milligrams. (This also equals 0.6 gram.) A more complete table of approximate equivalents will be found in the Appendix.

The nurse should be very careful in the abbreviations of the words grams and grains. Gram should be written Gm. with a capital G and a small m. Grain should be written gr., a small g followed by a small r. Mistakes in this could be dangerous. Also, it is usual to put the number before the Gm. and after the gr., using, if required, decimal fractions with the Gm. and common fractions with the gr. If these precautions are taken routinely, mistakes should not occur.

Fahrenheit and Centigrade Temperature Scales

There are two systems for the measurement of heat. These are used in medical and nursing practice, though not primarily in pharmacology. However, inclusion here seems appropriate. The student is no doubt familiar with these systems since Fahrenheit is used in our everyday life and centigrade is used in science. The conversion of one to the other may not be familiar.

CONVERSION RULES

To convert centigrade to Fahrenheit

$$\frac{9 \times \text{C.}}{5} + 32 = \text{F.}$$

EXAMPLE:

70° C. to F. $\frac{9 \times 70}{5} + 32 =$

$$\frac{630}{5} + 32 = 126 + 32 = 158° \text{ F.}$$

To convert Fahrenheit to centigrade

$$\text{F.} - 32 \times \frac{5}{9} = \text{C.}$$

EXAMPLE:

80° F. to C. $80 - 32 \times \frac{5}{9} =$

$$48 \times \frac{5}{9} = \frac{240}{9} = 26.6° \text{ C.}$$

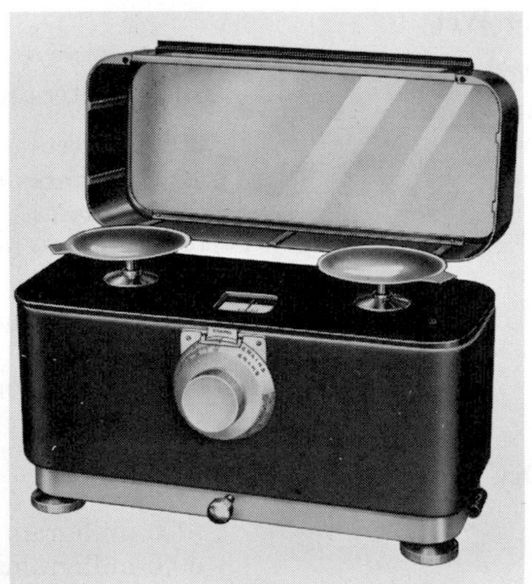

FIGURE 11. Balance scale. This is one type of scale used to weigh drugs, chemicals and other materials when it is essential to have accurate measurements. (Courtesy Arthur H. Thomas Co., Philadelphia, Pa.)

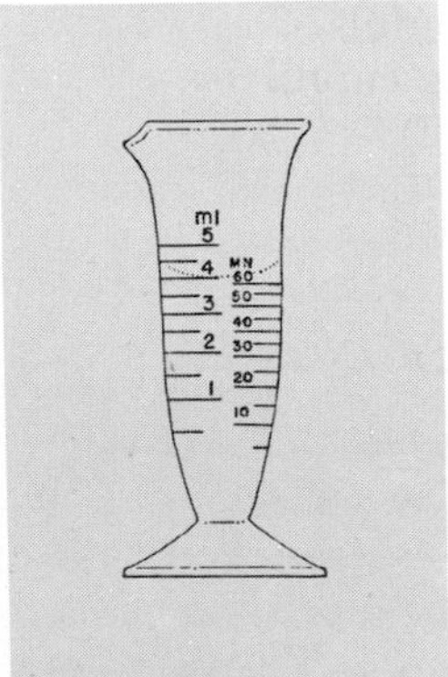

FIGURE 12. Dual scale glass for measuring small amounts of fluid drugs. The dotted line indicates the meniscus (fluid curve). The reading should be made from the bottom of the curve. In this particular case it is 4 ml., slightly over 60 minims.

COMPARISONS

Centigrade	*Fahrenheit*	
0° C.	32° F.	Freezing point of water
20° C.	68° F.	Room temperature
37° C.	98.6° F.	Body temperature
40° C.	104° F.	Fever
100° C.	212° F.	Boiling point of water

Posology

DOSAGE AND SOLUTIONS

Posology has customarily been divided into two broad categories; dosage and solutions. This is not too accurate since many substances considered under dosage are solutions. However, it seems wise to continue this procedure of separation since the terms are understood by most medical and nursing personnel. The term solutions is intended here to refer to those that are used as disinfectants, antiseptics and relatively large amounts of fluids administered to the patient, usually intravenously. Dosage then refers to medicinal substances (solids, liquids, gases) given to the patient by any one of a number of methods such as oral, topical, parenteral.

A few sample problems are given for homework. These are by no means complete or sufficient. Since the popularity of sample problems varies widely from one area to another, the instructor should add or subtract from those given to suit the needs of her students.

Solutions

A solution is the combination of a solvent and a solute. In most cases the solvent (liquid) is water and the solute (substance dissolved) is a salt. Pharmaceutically, many other liquids are also used as solvents, such as alcohol, acetone, ether, etc. If not designated, the solvent is water. The solute may be a solid, another liquid, or a gas. Solutions may be classified in many ways, but the following will suffice for use here:

ISOTONIC. One which has the same osmotic pressure as a given standard. The standard used in medicine is that of the body fluids, 0.85–0.9 per cent sodium chloride.

HYPERTONIC. One which has a greater osmotic pressure than a given standard. Medicinally this is one that is greater than 0.9 per cent sodium chloride.

HYPOTONIC. One which has a lesser osmotic pressure than a given standard. Medicinally this is one that is less than 0.85 per cent sodium chloride.

SATURATED. One in which the solvent holds all of a given solute it can under ordinary circumstances.

SUPERSATURATED. One in which the solvent holds more of the solute than it would under ordinary circumstances. This is an unstable solution. It is usually obtained by increasing the temperature of the solvent. Dissolving the solute into the solvent can usually be speeded by increasing the temperature of the solvent and by agitation.

PROBLEMS IN SOLUTIONS

No drug names have been used in these and other problems. This will allow the instructor to employ those most often used in her area. It will also emphasize the mathematics. This is not to imply that the actual drug is not of prime importance for, of course, it is. However, most students taking the course in dosage and solutions know few if any drugs. Often valuable time is lost trying to explain the type of preparation, especially if the preparation is not in common use.

Before attempting to solve any problems, the student should observe the following rules:

1. **READ THE PROBLEM CAREFULLY.** Think it through. What is wanted? What is available? What relationships exist?

Try to solve by logical reasoning. Now check your answer arithmetically.

2. **SEE THAT ALL ITEMS ARE IN THE SAME SYSTEM OF MEASUREMENTS AND ARE COMPARABLE.** Example: Use drams with drams, not drams with minims, or milliliters or (if solid) grams.
3. **WHEN THREE NUMBERS ARE KNOWN AND ONE UNKNOWN, PROPORTION IS THE SIMPLEST METHOD OF SOLVING THE PROBLEM.** Exceptions to this do occur and they will be dealt with later. It will be helpful if the proportion is always set up the same way. Thus: Drug:Solution::Drug:Solution. Preferably the X or unknown is always on the same side of the colon or times mark.
4. **WORK THE PROBLEM.** Prove your answer. Write out an explanation of what should be the actual procedure.
5. **UNLESS OTHERWISE INDICATED,** it is best to use ***the metric system,*** converting as indicated. The use of ratio for weaker solution and percentage for stronger solution is advisable. Those less than 1 per cent or 0.5 per cent by ratio, those stronger than 1 or 0.5 per cent by per cent.

   Example: A solution in which there is 1 gram of solute to 1 liter of water would be written 1:1000 (1000 milliliters).

   A solution in which there is 1 gram of solute to 100 milliliters of water would be expressed as 1%.
6. **NOTE:** Grams and milliliters are comparable since 1 milliliter of water weighs 1 gram. In the same way grains and minims correspond.

SAMPLE PROBLEMS

A. Determine the amount of powder that will be required to prepare 1 liter of a 10 per cent solution. In a 10 per cent solution there are 10 parts of solute to 100 parts of solvent, or in this case 10 grams of solute in 100 milliliters of water.

Solute to solvent as solute to solvent
Grams : ml. (cc) :: Grams : ml. (cc)

10 : 100 :: X : 1000
100X = 10000
X = 100

proof:
10 : 100 :: 100 : 1000
10000 = 10000

Therefore, 100 grams of powder will be required to prepare 1000 milliliters (1 liter) of a 10 per cent solution.

B. To determine the strength of a solution when the amount of the solvent and the solute is known.

EXAMPLE: There are 10 grams of a drug dissolved in 2 liters of water. What is the strength of the solution?

10 : 2000 :: X : 100 (If percentage is desired)
2000 X = 1000
X = 0.5 Therefore, the solution is 0.5 per cent in strength.

10 : 2000 :: 1 : X (If ratio is desired)
10X = 2000
X = 200 Therefore, the solution is a 1:200 solution.

EXAMPLE: There are 10 grains in 1 fluid dram. What is the strength of the solution? Since there are 60 minims in 1 fluid dram and minims and grains are comparable the proportion would be as follows:

10 : 60 :: X : 100
60X = 1000
X = 16⅔ Therefore, the solution is 16.6 or 16⅔ per cent in strength.

EXAMPLE: If 1 liter of water contains 30 grains of drug, what is the strength of the solution? 15 grains = 1 gram, therefore, 30 grains = 2 grams. 1 liter equals 1000 ml. and grams and milliliters are comparable. The amounts are now in a form that can be put into a proportion.

2 : 1000 :: 1 : X (Note: Since this appears to be a weak solution, we start with ratio.)
2X = 1000
X = 500 Therefore, the solution is 1:500 in strength.

PRACTICE PROBLEMS (Answers to all practice problems will be found in the Appendix.)

Determine the strengths of the following solutions:

1. Solvent 5.0 ml. (cc.), solute 0.1 Gm.
2. Solvent ℥ss, solute ʒss
3. Solvent 1 liter, solute ounce i
4. Solvent 100 ml. (cc.), solute gr. v
5. Solvent quarts 1, solute 6 Gm.
6. Solvent 50 ml. (cc.), solute 0.1 mg.
7. Solvent 30 ml. (cc.), solute 1.0 Gm.

8. Solvent ℥ iv , solute ʒ ii
9. Solvent 1000 ml. , solute 1 Gm.
10. Solvent 1 gallon , solute grains iii

C. To prepare a solution when the solute is 100 per cent in strength. The solute may be a solid (powder or crystal), a solution or a tablet.

Note that when the solute is a liquid, the amount of the solute must be subtracted from the total amount desired to secure the amount of the solvent to be used. This is because the fluid will not dissolve in the solvent as does the salt but mixes evenly.

Note, also, that when the solute is a tablet, there will need to be two problems. First, to secure the amount of the solute required and then, second, to determine the number of tablets that will give the required amount. Thus, if the tablets are 5 grains each and 30 grains are required, 6 tablets will be needed.

PRACTICE PROBLEMS

1. Prepare 1 gallon of a 1:8000 solution from tablets grains iiss each.
2. Prepare 500 ml. of a 1:500 solution from crystals.
3. Prepare 1000 ml. of a 1:200 solution from a full strength liquid.
4. Prepare 1 ounce of a 2 per cent solution from tablets grains 10 each.
5. Prepare 1 pint of a 0.5 per cent solution from crystals.
6. Prepare 150 ml. of a 1.0 per cent solution from a full strength liquid.
7. Prepare 1 quart of a ¼ per cent solution from a full strength liquid.
8. Prepare 3 pints of a 1:100 solution from powder.
9. Prepare 15 gallons of a 1:6000 solution from crystals.
10. Prepare ½ glass (4 ounces) of a 0.5 per cent solution from tablets grains v each.

D. To prepare a weaker solution from a stronger one. Since there are more than three knowns in these problems, it is easier to use another rule. This rule can be a short cut for almost all problems, but most students find that proportion is easier to understand. The rule is: express all terms as common fractions. Invert the terms of the solution or drug on hand. Multiply by the terms of the solution desired and by the amount desired. (The short cut is simply: want over have, times amount.)

EXAMPLE: How much of a 10 per cent solution will be required to make 1 liter of a 2 per cent solution? On hand 10 per cent, wanted 2 per cent, wanted 1 liter or 1000 ml. (cc).

$$\frac{\overset{1}{\cancel{100}}}{\underset{\underset{1}{\cancel{5}}}{\cancel{10}}} \times \frac{\overset{1}{\cancel{2}}}{\underset{1}{\cancel{100}}} \times \frac{\overset{200}{\cancel{1000}}}{1} = 200$$

The answer then is 200 ml. Since this is a liquid, it must be subtracted from the total. Therefore: 200 ml. of the 10 per cent solution and 800 ml. of water will make 1000 ml. (1 liter) of a 2 per cent solution.

$$\text{Short cut: } \frac{2}{\cancel{10}} \times \frac{\overset{100}{\cancel{1000}}}{1} = 200$$

PRACTICE PROBLEMS

1. Prepare 15 liters (1 average bathtubful) of a 0.1 per cent solution from a 25 per cent solution.
2. Prepare 1 gallon of a 5 per cent solution from a 50 per cent solution.
3. Prepare 5 liters of a 0.25 per cent solution from a 5 per cent solution.
4. Prepare 1 quart of a 1:5000 solution from a 10 per cent solution.
5. Prepare 1 ounce of a 1 per cent solution from a 20 per cent solution.

E. To find the amount of required solution that can be secured from a given amount of a drug.

EXAMPLE: How much of a 2 per cent solution can be made from 1.0 gram of the drug?

$$2 : 100 :: 1 : X$$
$$2X = 100$$
$$X = 50$$

Therefore: 50 ml. (cc.) of solvent will be required to make a 2 per cent solution from 1.0 gram of the drug.

PRACTICE PROBLEMS

1. How much 5 per cent solution can be made with 1 ounce of drug?
2. How much 1:5000 solution can be made with 10 grams of drug?

3. How much 1:800 solution can be made with 1 dram of drug?
4. How much of a 25 per cent solution can be made with 1 ounce of drug?
5. How much 0.5 per cent solution can be made with grains X of drug?

F. To find the amount of water to be added to a given amount of drug to make a specific strength solution.

Example: How much water must be added to 1.0 gram of pure drug to make a 2 per cent solution (when the drug is a solid)?

$$2 : 100 :: 1 : X$$
$$2X = 100$$
$$X = 50$$

Therefore: 50 ml. of solvent will be required to make a 2 per cent solution from 1 gram of pure drug.

How much water must be added to 1 ml. of drug to make a 5 per cent solution (when the drug is a liquid)?

$$5 : 100 :: 1 : X - 1$$
$$5X - 5 = 100$$
$$5X = 100 + 5$$
$$5X = 105$$
$$X = 21$$

$$21 - 1 = 20$$

Therefore: 20 ml. is the amount of water to be added.

Practice Problems

1. How much water must be used to make a 1:500 solution from 1 fluid ounce of drug?
2. How much water must be used to make a 12 per cent solution from 10 ml. of drug?
3. How much water must be used to make a 3 per cent solution from 2 grams of drug?
4. How much water must be used to make a 1 per cent solution from drams 4 of drug?
5. How much water must be used to make a 1:1000 solution from 100 mg. of drug?

Dosage

The calculations here involve much smaller amounts than in solutions. Medicines are given to patients as solids or liquids, and in either case dosage changes may be required. Gases and radiation are also administered as medicinal agents, but the calculation of dosages in these areas is not usually the responsibility of the nurse.

Dosages for drugs to be given by mouth (oral) and those to be given by hypodermic (parenteral) will be considered separately as there are major differences in the calculations.

ORAL DOSAGE

As was stated earlier, many drugs come to the nurse in the exact form and dosage to be given, but this is far from being universally true. It is the exceptions that must be understood.

Solid drugs come in tablets, capsules, pills, powders, etc. Some of these are so prepared as to be released over an extended period of time. These may not be divided since this would defeat the purpose for which they are designed. Usually delayed-release preparations are either tablets or capsules and are made in such a manner that part of the medication dissolves in an acid medium, giving immediate action, and part in an alkaline medium, giving later action. Usually capsules and pills are not divided, but multiples of them may be and often are used. Some tablets are prepared so as to be divided easily. These are *scored* tablets. They may be scored to be divided into two or four portions. There is a depression and the tablets break easily into fairly even portions. (See Fig. 13.)

In measuring liquid dosages, the form in which the drug is ordered should be used insofar as is possible. Thus, minims should be measured in a minim glass, drops with a medicine dropper and milliliters (cc.) into a glass calibrated in the metric system. Many

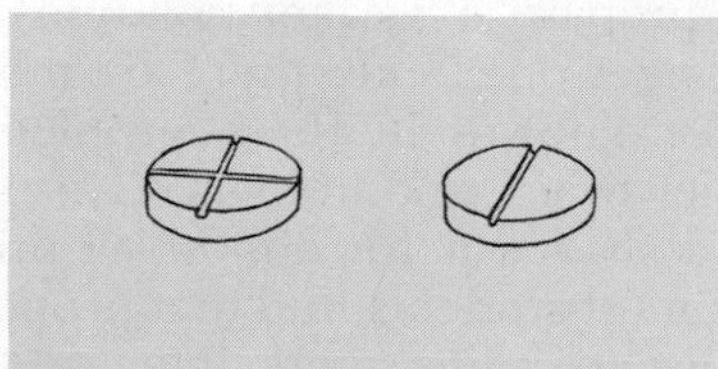

FIGURE 13. Scored tablets which break readily into fairly accurate dosage divisions, one-half or one-quarter.

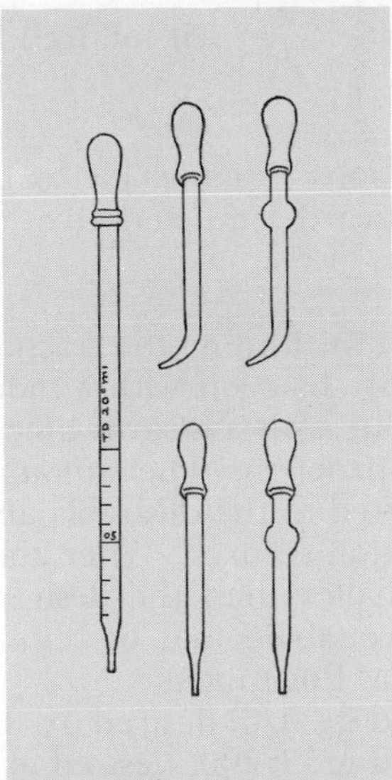

FIGURE 14. Medicine droppers vary widely in size and shape. Some are calibrated to show the minim or the milliliter equivalent. The majority are not marked. The amount in a "drop" depends upon the size and shape of the dropper as well as the surface tension and density of the fluid being measured. All other things being equal, the greater the viscosity of the fluid, the larger the drop.

measuring graduates have two or even three calibrations and can be used for any system.

In most cases the rules for the calculation of dosages are the same as those for solutions. Remember: THINK THROUGH THE PROBLEM before you attempt to solve it. Most of the problems are very easy and require very little arithmetical calculation. One thing to be sure of in all cases is that the various numbers are in comparable forms. If conversion is needed, it is better to use the system in which the stock drug is found.

A. SOLID PREPARATIONS FOR ORAL ADMINISTRATION

Example: The physician's order is for 0.2 Gm. The capsules on hand are marked gr. iss each. The nurse should proceed as follows:

System "on hand" is the apothecaries', so the order should be changed to this system. 0.2 Gm. equals gr. 3 (15 grains equals 1 gram).

The capsules contain grains iss each; grains 3 was ordered. Therefore, give 2 capsules $(3 \div 3/2 = \not{3} \times \frac{2}{\not{3}_1} = 2)$ Note the arithmetic is minor; reasoning, major.

Practice Problems

1. On hand scored tablets marked 0.5 mg. The order is for 0.25 mg. How should the nurse proceed?
2. The order is for 1.0 Gm. The tablets on hand are marked gr. v each. How should the nurse proceed?
3. The tablets on hand are marked 0.1 mg. each. The order is for gr. 1/300. How should the nurse proceed?
4. The doctor orders ʒss and the drug is in capsules grain xv each. How many or what part of a capsule will be needed?
5. The order is for grains 1/100. The scored tablets on hand are marked 0.6 mg. each. How many or what part of a tablet should be used?

B. ORAL FLUID DRUGS

Unless the fluid has a known strength (such as the standard tincture which is 10 per cent), the strength is indicated on the label. It may be expressed as per cent, ratio or solute to solvent as 1 per cent, 1:100 or 1.0 gram to 100 milliliters (cc.).

Example: The order reads 75 mg. The bottle is marked "50 mg. per ml. (cc.)." How much should be given?

$$50 : 1 :: 75 : X$$
$$50X = 75$$
$$X = 1\frac{1}{2}$$

Therefore, 1½ ml. should be given. (1 ml. or cc. equals 15 minims)

$$\text{or } 50 : 15 :: 75 : X$$
$$50X = 1125$$
$$X = 22\frac{1}{2}$$

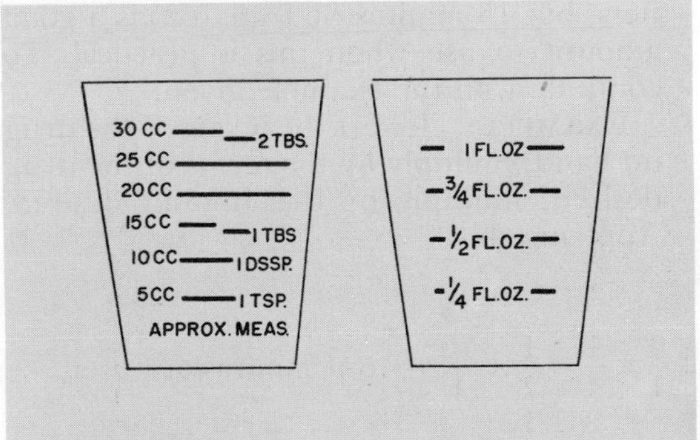

FIGURE 15. Medicine glass showing three measuring systems: metric, household and apothecary. This is one of the most common types of containers for dispensing fluid drugs. It comes in glass, plastic and also in paper. The paper or plastic ones are used only once and then discarded.

Therefore 22½ minims should be given.

Practice Problems

1. Give 5 grains from a 10 per cent solution.
2. Give 0.5 Gm. from a 1:200 solution.
3. The drug is marked as a 50 per cent solution. You are to give 5 grams. How much of the drug will be needed?
4. The order is for grains 1/100. The drug is a 1 per cent solution. How much of the drug should be used?
5. Prepare 10 grains from a 1:50 solution.

PARENTERAL DOSAGE

Drugs given parenterally (subcutaneous, intramuscular, intravenous, etc.) are usually in solution when given. However, the medication may come as a crystal, powder or tablet to be dissolved in the correct amount of solvent (distilled water, saline or buffered solution) before administration.

C. PARENTERAL DOSAGE FROM TABLETS

As with the making of a solution from a stronger solution, there are more than three known and, therefore, proportion is apt to be difficult. The rule given for the solution problems should be used here. Therefore, a two-stage problem is best. An example will clarify this. The order is for grains ¼ of the drug. The tablet on hand is marked grains ½. Obviously, one-half a tablet should be used. If the drug is to be given either subcutaneously or intramuscularly, the total amount of fluid should not be too small or too large to be given with the usual 2 ml. (cc.) (32 m.) hypodermic syringe. The amount of solution used may vary up or down a few minims without losing effectiveness, but 15 minims or 1 ml. (cc.) is a good amount to use when this is practical. To continue with the example given:

Example: Invert the terms of the drug on hand, multiply by the terms of the drug desired, multiply by the amount desired. Applying this:

$$\frac{\overset{1}{\cancel{2}}}{1} \times \frac{1}{\underset{2}{\cancel{4}}} = \frac{1}{\underset{1}{\cancel{2}}} \times \frac{\overset{15}{\cancel{30}}}{1} = 15 \text{ if minims are used.}$$

Reads: Dissolve 1 tablet gr. ½ in 30 minims of solvent. Discard 15 minims and give 15 minims which will contain gr. ¼.

$$\frac{\cancel{2}}{1} \times \frac{1}{\underset{2}{\cancel{4}}} = \frac{1}{\underset{1}{\cancel{2}}} \times \frac{\cancel{2}}{1} = 1 \text{ if ml. (cc.) is used.}$$

Reads: Dissolve 1 tablet gr. ½ in 2 ml. of solvent. Discard 1 ml. and give 1 ml. which will contain gr. ¼.

The reason for finding the fraction first can more readily be seen with a more difficult problem, but it always saves time to use the two-stage problem. The amount selected can be related to the desirable amount and to the fraction secured. When the tablet on hand is smaller than the desired amount, two or more tablets may be required.

Practice Problems

1. On hand gr. 1/6, desired gr. 1/8.
2. On hand gr. 1/200, desired gr. 1/120.
3. On hand gr. 1/32, desired gr. 1/12.
4. On hand gr. 1/300, desired gr. 1/100.
5. On hand gr. 1/4, desired gr. 1/6.

D. Often the dosage of the tablet is in the metric system, and the fractions, if any, are decimal. There are several ways of solving this type of problem, but the easiest is to change the fractions into common fractions and proceed as above.

Example: The order is for 0.2 mg. The tablet is marked 0.5 mg.

0.2 = 2/10 or 1/5,
and 0.5 = 5/10 or 1/2

$$\frac{2}{1} \times \frac{1}{5} = \frac{2}{\underset{1}{\cancel{5}}} \times \frac{\overset{5}{\cancel{25}}}{1} = 10$$

Dissolve 1 tablet 0.5 mg. in 25 minims of water. Discard 15 minims and administer 10 minims which will contain 0.2 mg. of the drug.

Practice Problems

1. To give 0.2 mg. from 0.6 mg. tablet.
2. To give 0.5 mg. from 1.5 mg. tablet.
3. To give 32 mg. from 40 mg. tablet.
4. To give 0.1 Gm. from 0.2 Gm. tablet.
5. To give 80 mg. from 0.08 Gm. tablet.

E. Many drugs come already dissolved in sterile vials or ampules. These are marked as to the amount of drug in a given amount of solution, usually per milliliter or cubic centimeter. It is necessary to determine how much fluid should be used.

EXAMPLE: The order is for 0.5 mg. The vial is marked 0.25 mg. per ml. (cc). In this type of problem there are three known and one unknown and, therefore, proportion is the simplest means of determining the answer.

0.25 : 1 :: 0.5 : X
0.25X = 0.50
X = 2 2 ml. will be required

0.25 : 15 :: 0.5 : X
or 0.25X = 7.50
X = 30 30 minims will be required

PRACTICE PROBLEMS

1. A 10 ml. vial contains a total of 1.0 gram (1000 mg.) of the drug. How much will be required to give 50 mg.?
2. A vial is marked "2 ml. (cc.) contains 100 mg." How much will be required to give 75 mg.?
3. A vial is marked "1 ml. (cc.) contains gr. 1½." The order is for 0.3 Gm. How much should be used?
4. A vial is marked "30 minims contains 1 grain." The order is for gr. 1/5. How much should be used?
5. A vial is marked "1 ml. contains 2.5 mg." How much should be used to give 1.0 mg.?

F. Not all drugs are measured by weight or volume. Some are measured by what the drug can do under given conditions. These are called units, a unit equaling the amount of the drug required to obtain a specific reaction. Mathematically the same procedure is used.

EXAMPLE: The vial is marked "1 ml. (cc.) contains 20,000 units." The order is for 30,000 units. Obviously, 1.5 ml. will be required.

20,000 : 1 :: 30,000 : X
2X = 3
X = 1.5

In the preparation of insulin several strengths are used and these are marked as to the number of units per ml. (cc.). Thus: U-40 means 40 units in each ml.; U-100 means 100 units in each ml.; and so on. The more commonly used preparations are U-40, U-80, U-100.

EXAMPLE: The order is for Units 24, the vial is marked U-40.

40 : 1 :: 24 : X
40X = 24
X = 0.6 0.6 ml. would be required

or 40 : 15 :: 24 : X
40X = 360
X = 9 9 minims will be needed

PRACTICE PROBLEMS

1. Prepare 40 units from a U-100 vial of insulin.
2. Prepare 48 units from a U-40 vial of insulin.
3. Prepare 30 units from a vial marked "U-40 insulin."
4. The order is for 15,000 U. The vial is marked 10,000 U per ml. (cc). How much should be used?

CHAPTER 6

THE PROBLEM OF DRUG ABUSE

CORRELATION WITH OTHER SCIENCES

I. ANATOMY AND PHYSIOLOGY

1. Dilation of superficial blood vessels leads to diaphoresis and a lowering of the body temperature. The reverse is also true.

V. PSYCHOLOGY

1. An emotionally unstable individual or one with personality defects tends to rely upon various "crutches" to bolster his ego.
2. The psychologically inferior person is very apt to be led easily into undesirable habits.
3. No two individuals are alike, yet all people have some characteristics in common.
4. Most people tend to be followers, to want to belong to the group and to do what others are doing.
5. The prepsychotic person may appear to be normal, but he may harbor many abnormal feelings and emotions.

VI. SOCIOLOGY

1. The emotionally unstable person often becomes a public charge since he is unable to compete with others who are psychologically better equipped to do the job.
2. The individual who is dependent upon drugs (especially alcohol) is a menace in the present machine age since he is accident prone. He is unable to judge speed and distance. His reflexes are slow and unreliable. These things combine to make him dangerous to himself and others when attempting to operate a machine.
3. All drug dependent persons are an economic loss to the nation. Such an individual produces nothing, spends his money for materials that are not constructive and requires a great deal of care.
4. Radio, television, magazine and newspaper advertising is responsible for many common fads, including the abuse of certain drugs.

DRUG ABUSE

The terms *habituation* and *addiction* have previously received brief mention. There are many different ways of defining them. Habituation simply means habit forming. The habit may be good or bad, but when applied to drugs it usually means the use of the drug after the therapeutic need for it is over or when there never was any genuine medicinal reason for its use. Addiction has been used to indicate dependence on a drug which produces adverse physical symptoms on withdrawal. The distinction between the two is difficult and at times almost impossible to delineate. Lately, the term "drug dependency" has come into use to replace both habituation and addiction. It includes physical as well as emotional or psychological dependence upon drugs.

Before the problem of the abuse of

specific drugs is examined, a few words concerning the type of person apt to abuse drugs may be helpful. This will be further discussed in sections or areas of importance. The social and psychological aspects of drug abuse, to be sure, will be dealt with in other courses. Here the emphasis will be on the drug and its pharmacological effects.

Drugs have been abused in all countries and in all recorded time. Specific drugs have changed with time and place, but no country is entirely immune.

Most drug abusers are young, experimenting with drugs as they experiment with other things. Most youthful experimenters do not become habitual users. They try it and then give it up, an encouraging situation. However, many continue to use drugs. The reasons are varied and probably not identical for any two users. However, the majority fall into five categories:

1. An inability to face the realities of life.
2. A desire to live in a dream or "fantasy" world, i.e., a desire to remain "the child." Fear of adult responsibilities may be one reason.
3. Rebellion against authority or "the establishment."
4. A feeling that life is too monotonous and needs zest, verve and excitement.
5. A basic emotional disorder or a prepsychotic condition (V-1).

Possibly this last is, more or less, the basis of the entire problem.

Those who persist in the use of drugs often "drop out" of general society. They tend to congregate and to live together, often in very unsanitary conditions. Many turn to burglary, pandering and prostitution to secure money for their "fix." The drug habit can be very expensive since the drugs are illegally obtained.

Such young people feel that they cannot be bothered by the humdrum routine of life. They are above such mundane affairs. They are likely to be undernourished, even ill, because of not eating properly or taking decent care of themselves. These things are especially true of those using the hallucinogenic drugs, the "hard" narcotics, alcohol, marihuana and similar drugs. Such individuals often become public charges (VI-2).

It should be emphasized that although most drug abusers, especially of the drugs just mentioned, are in their late "teens" and early "twenties," drug abuse is by no means limited to this age group. It is appalling to realize that the use of dangerous drugs is increasingly common among younger children, even the "subteen" group. Taking drugs is the "in" thing to do. Often the habit begins with the child's stealing drugs from the family medicine cabinet and taking them to "see what will happen."

The older person taking drugs excessively often started by taking the drug for therapeutic use. Any number of drugs may fall into this category, but stimulants, depressants and analgesics predominate. Since these drugs are all used in the treatment of many diseases and disorders, their abuse is often difficult to determine. The patient may continue to take the drug after he no longer needs it. However, it may be difficult to prove that the patient no longer requires the drug. The number of drugs that may be so abused is inordinately high. Most of them will be discussed in the area of their importance in therapy.

It is difficult to explain or condone the disproportionately high number of addicts among physicians, dentists, nurses and paramedical personnel. Of course, they do have easier access to drugs than most people, but they should know better the value and the danger of drugs. Like many other drug users, they usually begin by taking small doses of a relatively harmless drug and gradually become dependent upon it. This leads to stronger drugs and greater dosage until the habit is established. The moral is "don't start." Never take a drug of any kind unless ordered to do so by the physician who is caring for you, and never continue taking a drug after the therapeutic need for it has ceased.

Drug abuse is not confined to any social or economic group. It is seen most often in the emotionally unstable person regardless of his social status (V-1).

The hazards of drug abuse need not be discussed in detail here; they are common knowledge. It is well known that the use of drugs leads to physical deterioration, mental apathy, and loss of moral values and ambition. For the older person it may also mean the loss of his job and even his family.

However, one hazard the public knows little about is the danger of contracting serum hepatitis (infection of the liver) from poorly sterilized hypodermic equipment which has been used by several persons. Since the incubation period of serum hepatitis is long (often three or four months), it is often impossible to confirm the source of the infection. This condition will be discussed under infectious hepatitis in Chapter 17.

THE NARCOTIC PROBLEM

Included in this discussion are opium and its derivatives, mainly morphine and heroin, and the major synthetic narcotics such as meperidine (Demerol) (pethidine, Pethidone [C]).

Opium

Opium—the dried latex of the ripe capsule of *Papaver somniferum*—was probably used in prehistoric times. Certainly it has been used medicinally as long as history has been recorded. It and its derivatives are effective pain killers. However, it gives a false sense of well-being. At first, the user needs only a small amount to control pain—real or imaginary, and it is also possible to do without the drug, at least for short periods. As time goes on, ever-increasing amounts are needed, and the individual is more and more dependent upon the drug, until he cannot be without it. The habit may have begun in many ways. A few of these are:

1. The continued therapeutic use of the drug during a long illness (perhaps even when other measures may be equally effective).
2. The use of the drug as an attempt to escape from failure, poverty, conscience, etc., just as the alcohol-dependent person uses alcohol; many times the drug-dependent person was an alcoholic first (V-1).
3. The use of the drug as a cure for insomnia or other minor condition.
4. The use of the drug in a dare or as an experiment, especially by the youth who wants to prove himself "strong."

The Synthetic Analgesics (Narcotics)

The abuse of these products is an outgrowth of their synthesis (see Table 1). The original hope that they would be nonaddictive has proved to be false. At first, their misuse was confined to medical and paramedical personnel, having as they did easy access to them and understanding their value. Then, at some point, patients treated with these drugs continued to use them after they no longer needed to. Recently, since illicit trade in them has increased, their misuse has spread. How the layman procures them is difficult to explain. Possibly, acquisition is through smuggling, clandestine laboratories and diversion from legitimate sources. Drugs from clandestine laboratories are especially dangerous since they may be heavily contaminated or grossly inferior in quality. Incidentally, these same means of procurement apply equally to any misused drug, not just narcotics. Symptoms vary with the preparation. Refer to the Current Drug Handbook for details.

Problems Relating to All Abused Narcotics

The way the drug is taken depends somewhat upon how the habit started. The drug may have been snuffed or inhaled or put under the tongue or swallowed. In any case, it soon becomes necessary to introduce the drug subcutaneously and, later, intravenously. The addict usually is in too much of a hurry to bother with sterility, even if he knew how to maintain surgical cleanliness; therefore, abscesses and infections are common and may be severe. The picture of the addict is anything but happy. He is an absolute slave to the drug. When he has had his customary dose, he is a happy, contented, amiable person. All seems well, though one may see the tell-tale signs of his condition if one watches carefully enough. Pupils of the eyes are apt to be pinpoints and muscular coordination unstable; he may be drowsy or a little hysterical. Often, however, no symptoms are apparent even to the observant person. The picture is entirely different when he is denied his regular dose. He then becomes restless, has vague aches and pains and various gastric and intestinal disturbances. He gradually becomes worse until, after a day or two without the drug, he is the picture of abject misery. He is in constant pain, has abdominal and muscular cramps and, in fact, pain of almost every kind. He is nauseated, will vomit if he tries to take any food, cannot sleep and is apt to be delirious. In this condition the addict will do anything—steal or even kill—to procure his drug.

Commonly, because the eyes become photophobic and the pupils constrict to pinpoint size, the addict affects dark glasses, even when not in the sun. He may take to wearing long-sleeved shirts, when short-sleeved ones would be the rule, to conceal telltale needle marks on his arms. Emotionally, he is either erratic or unresponsive. It is easy to see why the "pusher" or dope peddler has control over the addict.

The federal government maintains two hospitals, one at Lexington, Kentucky, and one at Fort Worth, Texas (VI-3). These hospitals are maintained for research into the problems of drug abuse.

The nurse has a direct responsibility in the administration of narcotics. There are some addicts who get their start from indiscriminate or excessive administration by doctors and nurses of pain-relieving medications. Even if this were true for only a very few, it is a challenge to the medical professions. Surely no nurse wants to feel that she has in any way contributed to drug dependency. It is, therefore, of utmost importance that each nurse do all in her power to reduce the amount of narcotic drugs used by patients under her care. This does not mean that the nurse should deny the medicine to those needing it or that she should question the physician's orders. It does mean that she should use all nursing measures possible before giving narcotic drugs, especially those that are ordered p.r.n. (whenever necessary). Many times the busy nurse will give a restless, uncomfortable patient a "hypo" when a back rub, smoothing of the bed and rearrangement of pillows would have the same effect. It is this type of situation that the thoughtful nurse can handle well. Of course, there are cases in which induced drug addiction is almost inevitable. These are primarily terminal cancer cases. It is important that the nurse comprehend the patient's condition, the physician's desire and her own responsibility in each case. In the giving of any habit-forming drug, especially the narcotics, the nurse should ask herself: 1. Is this a direct order? 2. If not, is it really needed? 3. Am I doing the best thing for this patient by giving this medicine? 4. Could the same relief be secured equally well by other means? If she can conscientiously answer these questions, she need have no fear that she is doing anything to further drug dependency in her patients.

Of course, the nurse's responsibility is not solely to the immediate patients under her care. She has a general social obligation to do anything that is within her power to prevent drug dependency of any kind. Probably she can help best by dispelling superstition and discrediting false information.

Crude opium and the products of opium containing the entire drug are not used extensively in this country. Abuse centers almost entirely around the derivatives (alkaloids), morphine and heroin, especially the latter. Heroin is derived from morphine. Originally, it was thought not to be habit forming, but it has, in fact, proved to be even more habituating than crude opium or morphine. The manufacture, importation and sale of heroin are prohibited in the United States and Canada. Heroin is smuggled into these countries directly or indirectly from those countries which grow opium. The drug is often "cut" or diluted with other substances. Adulteration, of course, forces the addict to require larger amounts of the drug to obtain relief, making the profits to smugglers and "pushers" even higher. Morphine—but not heroin—is used medicinally in these countries (VI-3).

In recent years, there has been a marked increase in the number of heroin addicts in this country. Among the many reasons for this increase are

1. The general tendency of a large segment of society to feel that there is a pill, capsule or chemical to cure all of life's troubles. Once started, the drug habit progresses.

TABLE 1. COMPARISON OF VARIOUS NARCOTICS AND OTHER DANGEROUS DRUGS

NAMES (Generic and Proprietary)	Slang	SOURCE	THERAPEUTIC USE	HOW TAKEN	DOSE
Narcotics					
Diacetylmorphine (heroin)	H., horse, scat, snow, joy powder, Harry	Opium	Depressant (Not used in U.S. or Canada)	Snuffed, parenterally	Varies
Morphine sulfate	M., white stuff, Miss Emma, dreamer	Same	Analgesia	Orally, parenterally	15 mg.
Methylmorphine (codeine)	Schoolboy	Same	Analgesia	Orally, parenterally	30 mg.
Methadone (Dolophine, Amidone)	Dolly	Synthetic	Analgesia	Orally, parenterally	10 mg.
Other synthetic analgesics		Same	Analgesic	Orally, parenterally	Varies
Cocaine	Speed balls, gold dust, coke, Bernice, Corine, flake, star dust	Coca plant	Local anesthesia	Snuffed, orally, parenterally	Varies
Marihuana	Pot, grass, locoweed, weed, Mary Janes, tea, gage, reefers, hashish, bhang	Cannabis sativa plant	None	Smoked, orally, snuffed	Usually 1 or 2 cigarettes
Depressants, barbiturates (Nembutal, Seconal, Amytal, phenobarbital)	Barbs, blue devils, candy, yellow jackets, phennies, peanuts, blue heavens, pinks	Synthetic from barbituric acid	Sedative and hypnotic	Orally, parenterally	50 to 100 mg.
Other depressant drugs such as chloral hydrate, paraldehyde and even bromides may be used, but their use is much less common than is the barbiturates.					
Stimulants					
Amphetamines, amphetamine (Benzedrine), dextroamphetamine (Dexedrine), methamphetamine (Methedrine)	Bennies, dexies, co-pilots, wake-up, lid proppers, hearts, pep pills, speed	Synthetic	Cerebral stimulation, narcolepsy, and treatment of hyperkinetic children	Orally, parenterally	2.5 to 5 mg.
Hallucinogens					
Lysergic acid diethylamide (LSD)	Acid, sugar, big D, cubes, trips	Synthetic; originally from ergot	None	Orally	100 μg.
Dimethyltryptamine (DMT)	Businessman's high	Synthetic; also from certain plants	None	Parenterally	1 mg.
Peyote (mescaline)	Cactus	Peyote cactus	None	Orally	350 μg.
Psilocybin (psilocyn)	Mushrooms	Mushrooms	None	Orally	25 mg.

TABLE 1. COMPARISON OF VARIOUS NARCOTICS AND OTHER DANGEROUS DRUGS (Continued)

Effect (About)	DURATION OF SYMPTOMS Immediate	Long Term	DEPENDENCY Physical	Psychological	TOLERANCE	REMARKS
4 hours	Euphoria, drowsiness	Addiction, constipation, anorexia, convulsions with heavy dosage	Yes	Yes	Yes	
6 hours	Same	Addiction, constipation, respiratory distress	Yes	Yes	Yes	
4 to 6 hours	Drowsiness	Addiction (but much less and slower produced than above)	Yes	Yes	Yes	
4 to 6 hours	Similar to, but less acute than, morphine	As above	Yes	Yes	Yes	
4 to 6 hours	Similar to morphine, but varies with preparations	Similar to morphine, but varies with preparations	Yes	Yes	Yes	Such drugs as Demerol, Lisentil, Leritine
Varies	Excitation, talkativeness, tremors	Depression, convulsions with heavy dosage	No	Yes	?	
4 hours	Relaxation, euphoria, alteration of perception and judgment	?	No	?	?	
4 hours	Drowsiness, relaxation	Addiction with severe withdrawal symptoms. (Possibly convulsions; even death)	Yes	Yes	Yes	Very dangerous when taken with alcohol; phenobarbital least addictive
4 hours	Alertness, activeness	Delusions, hallucinations	No	Yes	Yes	Phentermine (Ionamin) and phenmetrazine (Preludin) are similar products
10 hours	Exhilaration, excitement, disturbed speech	?	No	?	?	
4 to 6 hours	Exhilaration, excitement	?	No	?	?	DET is a similar substance
12 hours	Exhilaration, anxiety, gastric distress	?	No	?	?	
6 to 8 hours	Nausea, vomiting, headache	?	No	?	?	

2. The ease with which our military service personnel were able to secure pure or nearly pure heroin in Southeast Asia.

Numerous methods of control have been instituted, but none has been completely successful. The same can be said for the treatment of narcotic (mainly heroin) addiction. There are many approaches to the problem, but it is agreed by most authorities that the heroin addict must be treated for the physical dependence (the short-term effect) and then rehabilitated (the long-term effect). This rehabilitation should include physical, psychological, and vocational readjustment to society.

The two main forms of physical treatment are "cold turkey" and detoxification. In the former, the patient is taken off the drug without being given anything to make the withdrawal symptoms less severe. In detoxification, the patient is given an analgesic (usually methadone) which is then gradually withdrawn by decreasing the dosage. It must be understood here that methadone is a synthetic narcotic and is also addictive. With some patients, if a good rehabilitation program is begun early, heroin addiction will not recur and the patient will become a useful citizen again. Regrettably, the number of these successes is small, and many resume their heroin habit within a few days or a few weeks. This type of program has been used in hospitals, jails and clinics, and it was found that the clinic approach was the least successful. An additional approach was definitely needed.

Several approaches to the problem of rehabilitation have been tried and have been more or less successful. Among the more promising are the following.

1. The group (communal) living of ex-addicts. These groups, such as Synanon, Daytop, Phoenix House and others, have been very successful. However, the number of addicts they are able to reach is very limited.

2. Methadone maintenance is probably the most widespread of the various long-term rehabilitation programs. Although under investigation by the Federal Drug Administration, methadone treatment is being used throughout the country. In this program the addict is detoxified and a methadone dose sufficient to allay his craving for heroin is established for him. The dosage is such that if heroin is taken, the addict will not get the euphoric feeling which makes heroin so attractive. This program is based on the fact that although methadone is addictive, its use does not prevent the individual from becoming a useful member of society. The patient receives his dose daily, usually in fluid form taken in a small amount of fruit juice. In most cases a urine specimen is obtained and tested for heroin to assure that the patient is not taking both. The program may be under the control of the pharmacist, as is the case in Oregon, or under the control of a general or special clinic, as is more commonly done. Since the use of methadone is still considered investigational, the person or persons administering such a program must first obtain permission from the F.D.A.

3. The third program, which is relatively new, is the use of the narcotic antagonists to control the patient's craving for heroin. Nalorphine (Nalline), a synthetic drug derived from morphine, naloxone (Narcan), also a synthetic drug similar to nalorphine, and cyclazocine (an analgesic) have been used. The effects of nalorphine are of too short duration (4 to 6 hours) to be of much value. Although the effects of naloxone and cyclazocine are not of long duration and are consequently shorter-lived than the effect of methadone, they do last longer than that of nalorphine.

Because of their limited supply, their use is as yet not widespread, but it does give promise of being an important step in the control of heroin addiction. Unlike methadone, naloxone and cyclazocine are not narcotics and are not in themselves addictive, hence, there are no physical withdrawal symptoms when they are discontinued.

The doctors using these various programs use other medicines as adjunct therapy to control adverse symptoms as they arise. However, most physicians use as few of these as is possible. They are aware that most heroin addicts are drug oriented and they avoid giving a drug no matter how innocuous it may seem, lest the patient begin to feel he must have more drugs.

Much research is being done in the area of drug addiction, and no doubt many more approaches to this problem will be tried. Nevertheless, it remains more important to prevent addiction than to try to cure it.

PROBLEMS WITH DRUGS OTHER THAN NARCOTICS

Cocaine

There has been an increase in the abuse of cocaine in recent years, although no plausible reason has been advanced for this. Cocaine is an alkaloid obtained from the coca plant which grows in Peru and other Andean countries of South America. It has been and still is used extensively by the natives of these countries who chew the leaves to aid in overcoming hunger, fatigue and cold. Their euphoria is, of course, false, and the continued use of coca often leads to physical debility and an increased tendency toward disease.

Cocaine is used medically as a surface, local anesthetic. However, for most local anesthesia, its derivatives or synthetic preparations are usually used.

Cocaine (called "snow" or "happy dust" by the drug users) is a central nervous system stimulant. As used by the addict, it may be snuffed, taken orally or injected, but the last route is the most commonly used. Cocaine gives the user a sense of well-being and of having superior physical strength and improved intellectual ability. Long-term use may result in various toxic symptoms including paranoid ideation, persecutory delusion and/or visual, auditory and tactile hallucinations. Since cocaine is rapidly detoxified by the liver, tolerance is not thought to develop. However, the person using cocaine tends to increase the dose, probably to gain an increased sense of well-being. Withdrawal symptoms, which include depression, fatigue and lassitude, are not usually severe.

Marihuana

Not a narcotic, marihuana is more appropriately classified as a hallucinogenic drug. In recent years its abuse has become a major problem in the United States. Known by many names including "pot," "reefers," "Mary Janes" and "Mary Warners," the product is derived from the plant *Cannabis sativa,* which grows easily and in widely different geographic areas (Fig. 16). The strength of the drug depends upon the region where it is cultivated and upon the type of plant from which it is extracted. The product grown in India, called *bhang,* is relatively stronger than its counterpart in the Americas. In Asia Minor it was called hashish, from which the word "assassins" is derived. Bands of men who smoked or chewed hashish and then undertook expeditions of rape and murder were called hashishins. The word came into English as assassins.

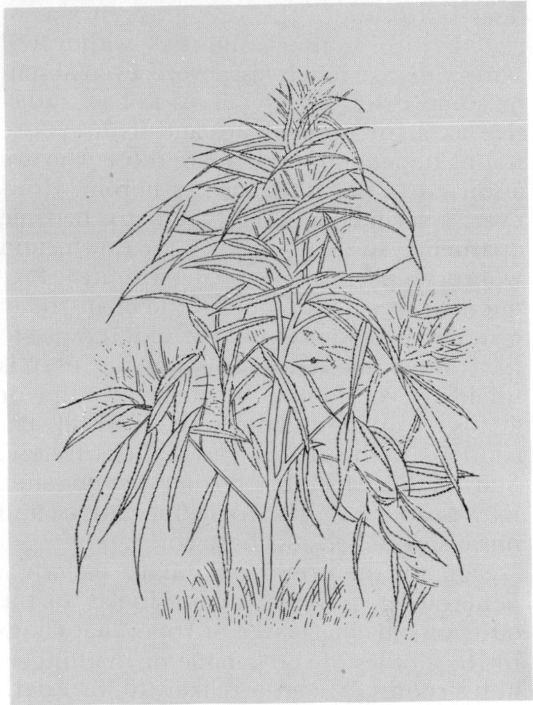

FIGURE 16. *Cannabis sativa* (hemp), commonly called marihuana. This is an attractive plant which grows easily in the United States. Used commercially to produce hemp for rope, the plant has hallucinogenic action when taken internally, especially the flowering portion. It is unlawful to grow it in the United States without specific permission from the federal government.

Because the plant, *Cannabis sativa,* can be grown in many areas of North America, its control is particularly difficult. Smuggling the product into the United States from Mexico provides a regular source of income for the criminal and unscrupulous. Marihuana—the leaves and the flowers of the plant—is usually smoked in pipes or in hand-rolled cigarettes. Marihuana, per se, does not produce the strong urgency associated with opium, and the withdrawal symptoms are much less severe, even absent in some cases. Marihuana is not as addictive as many other drugs and its users are not as dependent on it as are those who are addicted to narcotics such as heroin. However, marihuana users tend to become apathetic; students' grades go down, and workers' performances deteriorate. Frequently users "drop out" of the mainstream of daily living owing to their indifference to the things about them. Often the user is unable to continue in his normal routine or at his occupation. There are, however, exceptions to the generalities laid down here. Marihuana, which has no therapeutic value, may produce confusion, hallucinations and impulsive or reckless behavior.

Signs of the use of marihuana include a penetrating, pungent odor (similar to the odor of burning leaves or rope) that clings to the clothes of the habitué or that lingers in his rooms. The user is likely to wear dark glasses owing to photophobia. Sleep habits are disturbed, since the user sleeps and remains awake for longer than normal intervals. Inattention, apparent daydreaming, listlessness and general behavioral changes often occur with the habitual use of marihuana.

Tobacco

Tobacco is not used medicinally, but since its use plays a part in so many undesirable physical conditions, it is important for the nurse to know some pertinent facts about the drug. She will minister to patients who use tobacco. If the patient is denied its use for medical reasons he may develop additional problems.

Nicotine, the active principle of tobacco, is responsible for many of the symptoms of tobacco poisoning. Tobacco also contains various other substances such as tars which probably add to its toxic effect. The constant tobacco user is apt to exhibit some or all of the following: gastrointestinal disturbances, especially a tendency to nausea; headache; insomnia; anxiety; irritability; tremors; neuralgias; cardiac arrhythmias; palpitation; coldness of the extremities and many other symptoms. Nicotine is a strong vasoconstrictor which causes spasmodic contractions of the peripheral arterioles with reduction in blood to various areas of the body, mainly the extremities. It is especially dangerous to any patient with a circulatory disturbance such as arteriosclerosis, coronary disease, diabetes mellitus and peripheral vascular diseases. Nicotine depresses the autonomic nervous system. When the habitual tobacco user is denied his regular tobacco (as is often the case when he is sick in the hospital), he will show various symptoms such as restlessness, craving, discomfort and other vague symptoms similar to those of opium removal. However these usually subside more quickly than the latter and much more easily. It is necessary to explain to the patient why the tobacco may not be used and to assure him that withdrawal will not have harmful results. If later during the course of the illness the physician does allow tobacco, it must be introduced gradually. The physician may designate the amount that the patient may have, but if he does not the nurse should advise the patient to return to smoking slowly.

The nurse must be extremely watchful if a patient is allowed to smoke in bed. This is a great fire hazard, and many people have been burned to death because they fell asleep while smoking. There is the added danger that it might start a general fire.

If asked about the deleterious effects of tobacco and its effect upon longevity, the nurse should be able to give specific information. Accurate figures are difficult to obtain, but certain diseases are found more often in smokers than in nonsmokers. These diseases include endarteritis obliterans, primary pulmonary carcinoma, carcinoma of the lips and tongue and certain heart diseases. The life expectancy of the heavy smoker appears to be considerably less than that of the nonsmoker.

Alcohol

The use of alcohol, like that of tobacco, is very common in this country. Those who drink vary in their habits from the person who takes an occasional beer or small glass of wine to the chronic alcoholic. Alcoholism and its effects on the individual and society will be discussed more in detail in other courses, but some discussion here should be helpful.

Many people think that alcohol is a stimulant, but this is not true. The apparent stimulation from alcohol is due to the depression of higher centers which are usually of an inhibitory nature. Thus, the person who is usually quiet and reserved may become noisy and loquacious after drinking an alcoholic beverage. Alcohol is a descending depressant starting with the higher cerebral centers and affecting other areas as the amount of the intake is increased until, finally, the lower nerve centers are involved—and the user is in a drunken stupor.

When nursing a patient who is known to take alcohol regularly, the nurse should first find out what procedure the physician wishes to be followed. Like tobacco it is usually withheld during the acute stage of an illness. The patient should be assured that he will be physically better for not having had his usual "nip" even if he does show some physical symptoms of its withdrawal. These symptoms are similar to those of tobacco withdrawal mentioned earlier. If symptoms indicative of delirium tremens and cardiac involvement are noted, the physician should be notified.

The chronic alcoholic not only will have the symptoms produced by the alcohol but also, in most cases, will show signs of qualitative and quantitative food deficiency. He has no real desire for food and so seldom takes time to eat properly. If he does eat at all it is in insufficient quantities and often not really nourishing foods. These patients rarely obtain enough vitamin B, and many of the symptoms attributed to alcoholism may actually be a result of vitamin B deficiency. One of the most important treatments for the alcoholic is an adequate diet. In addition to this, supplementary vitamins, especially vitamin B, are usually ordered. It is important for the nurse to understand these factors since many alcoholics fall ill with other afflictions. These patients will need special consideration as far as food intake is concerned.

Alcohol also causes dilation of the superficial blood vessels. This may necessitate extra warm surroundings to prevent colds, pneumonia or other respiratory disorders. Alcohol also causes excessive perspiration which calls for more careful skin care (I-1).

While the individual who takes excessive amounts of alcohol or tobacco is in the hospital there may be many opportunities to help the patient to understand his problem and to guide him toward a solution. Naturally, the nurse must not become a "temperance preacher." She must confine her remarks to answering questions and giving such information as may be useful. If in doubt it is always best to refer the patient to his physician.

THE PROBLEM OF THE CONTROLLED (DANGEROUS) DRUGS

In 1970 a new law was enacted to cover all previous legislation relative to narcotics and dangerous drugs. (See Chapter 2.) Of the various schedules listed, the first contains the names of drugs not used medicinally in the United States. (A Canadian law has similar schedules and lists.) The second and third schedules list those narcotics, stimulants and depressants for which accurate accounts must be kept and which, unless specifically exempted, require a prescription. Naturally, it is easier to obtain and thus easier to abuse those substances in Schedules 2 and 3 than those in Schedule 1.

The users of all narcotic, dangerous drugs and similar products are very clever at securing their drugs. Alcohol and tobacco, of course, can be bought on the open market since they are not prohibited by law. Some of the methods used for obtaining the "illegal drugs" have already been mentioned such as smuggling and clandestine laboratories. For the stimulants and depressants which may be secured by prescription, and some of the narcotics, the situation is different. Prescriptions are altered and blanks are stolen from the doctor's office and used illegally. Drugs are stolen directly from the physician's office and from the pharmacy. In a few cases unscrupulous personnel give the individual drugs. Then there is "the prescription collector." He goes from one doctor to another collecting prescriptions as he goes until he has sufficient product for his immediate needs. He then waits an interval and repeats the procedure. The actual ways of securing the needed drug are almost legion.

THE HALLUCINOGENIC DRUGS

Marihuana might have been placed here since it is primarily a hallucinogen; however, it was described earlier because it has been under legal control for a much longer time than the drugs given in this discussion.

The hallucinogenic drugs have no proven value in therapy. Most of them act on the autonomic nervous system, either intensifying or blocking its action. They do have some effects on the central nervous system, a factor of greater importance for the purpose of this discussion.

The hallucinogenic drugs are obtained mainly from clandestine laboratories, although some are smuggled into the country. The product which the user receives may or may not be pure. It may be "cut" or adulterated with other substances, or it may be contaminated through unclean handling. This is true of all illegally used drugs.

The hallucinogens distort or intensify the sense perceptions. Colors are increased, sounds are changed and the sense of time and space is altered. Mental effects are unpredictable. Sometimes the user has a happy experience or, in the parlance of the initiated, a "good trip." At other times, he may be subject to fear, abject terror or severe depression—a "bad trip." The users of these drugs are, in the main, young people. Among them, it has become popular to "expand" the mind with drugs. Often parties are held at which each member takes the drug being offered. If the drug is very potent, one of the members will refrain from taking the drug so as to stand guard lest any of the party have a bad trip. It is not uncommon for a person to become violent or even suicidal under the influence of the more potent hallucinogenic drugs. Those taking these drugs, if they had a good trip, feel that the experience is vastly rewarding, and they may become proselytes for the use of the drug. However, they are often unable to articulate convincingly the reasons that their experience was so valuable to them.

Most of the hallucinogenic drugs do not produce physical dependence, but may and often do cause psychic dependence. Especially is this true if the user has had good trips, and if he is trying to escape the unpleasant aspects of life. Some hallucinogens have produced psychoses after as little as one dose. Many people who take these drugs require psychiatric treatment, some for long periods of time.

L.S.D. OR D-LYSERGIC ACID DIETHYLAMIDE (lysergide; lysergamide, Delysid [C])

The diethylamide derivative of lysergic acid (L.S.D.) is produced synthetically from lysergic acid. Its therapeutic value has not been proved. An extremely potent chemical, a dose of 50 to 200 micrograms is sufficient to produce a "trip" lasting as long as eight hours. This amount is so small that it is scarcely visible to the naked eye. L.S.D. is usually taken orally. Since the amount taken is so small it has to be contained in some medium, which may be a cube of sugar, a bit of food or a beverage.

The physical symptoms elicited by L.S.D. include lowered temperature, nausea, diaphoresis, dilated pupils, incoherent speech and tachycardia. Psychological changes are profound with changes in mood, distortion of sensations (illusions) and hallucinations. The mental symptoms may recur after days, weeks or even months following a single dose. Experiments seem to prove that L.S.D. may produce changes in the brain, spinal cord and the chromosomes. This last could conceivably be detrimental to the children of those using the drug. L.S.D. is called "acid" by its users who then become "acid heads." Psychotic conditions have developed after the use of L.S.D.; they may occur after only one dose and be immediate or they may become manifest only after months or years. The complete story of L.S.D. and its results probably has not yet been told. What it will be can only be conjectured. However, the fact remains that it is a very dangerous drug. The person who takes L.S.D. frequently shows wide personality changes from elation to depression and loss of motivation.

S.T.P. (A PREPARATION FROM AMPHETAMINE)

Although claimed to be stronger than L.S.D., it in fact takes much more S.T.P. to secure the same results. The usual dose is 1 to 3 milligrams. S.T.P. is not found in nature but is produced synthetically. Symptoms are similar to those of L.S.D. Like L.S.D., the preparation is taken orally and little is known of its long-term effects.

MESCALINE (PEYOTE)

The buttons of the peyote cactus and its derivative, mescaline, have been used in religious rites by Indians for many years. It is a hallucinogenic drug that produces illusions and hallucinations lasting from five to 12 hours. Like most of these drugs it is taken orally.

PSILOCYBIN OR PSILOCYN

Psilocybin or psilocyn is obtained from certain mushrooms generally grown in Mexico. As with mescaline it has been used in certain religious rites. Its effects are similar to those of mescaline, causing illusions and hallucinations.

D.M.T. (DIMETHYLTRYPTAMINE) AND D.E.T. (N_2N-DIETHYLTRYPTAMINE)

D.M.T. and D.E.T. are closely related. The former is obtained from the seeds of certain plants native to the West Indies and parts of South America. The latter is prepared synthetically. Both are taken by snuffing or more commonly by inhaling the smoke given off by burning the drug with tobacco, parsley leaves or other substance. These drugs are relatively short acting preparations. D.M.T. is effective for about one hour, D.E.T. for from two to three hours. As with others of this group they produce illusions and hallucinations.

BUFOTENINE

Another drug related to D.M.T. is bufotenine. It is secured from the glandular secretions of certain toads or from the amanita fungus. It is injected and produces severe and stressful physical symptoms, especially those associated with the cardiovascular system. The mental disturbances include illusions, hallucinations and distortion of time and space.

IBOGAINE

Still another in this series is ibogaine, which is derived from all parts of a particular African shrub. It, like many others of this group, has been used a long time by the natives where it is found. Its use in the United States is recent. It causes excitement, mental confusion, hallucinations and intoxication.

THE DEPRESSANT DRUGS

Of the many depressant drugs available, the short acting barbiturates are the most commonly abused. However, other drugs are also misused such as chloral hydrate and its derivatives, other barbiturates, paraldehyde or bromide. The abuse of these drugs will be discussed in the areas of their main therapeutic use, but some consideration is essential here.

The barbiturates have various nicknames by which they are identified: "barbs" for any of them, "yellows" or "yellow jackets" for pentobarbital (Nembutal), since it usually comes in yellow capsules, "reds," "pinks" and "red devils" for secobarbital (Seconal) for the same reason and "blues," "blue birds" and "blue devils" for amobarbital (Amytal). These are taken orally. Of course, it is possible to secure the sodium salts of some of these for injection, but the oral route is more common for the drug abuser.

Concerning the abuse of these medications, it is important that the nurse recognize their symptoms. They include slurring of speech, loss of balance, changes in disposition and lethargy. Patients often become fractious and quick-tempered. A change from happy or quiet relaxation to depression and temper tantrums may indicate that too much of the depressant drugs, especially the barbiturates, has been taken. For paraldehyde, the only indication may be the offensive breath odor. For the bromides, the appearance of a skin rash is characteristic.

The nurse should keep firmly in mind that a grave potential hazard exists in the unrestrained use of barbiturates. Taking a barbiturate after imbibing alcohol may cause unconsciousness and even be fatal. Although the amount of the individual products may not be deadly, the combination may well be. Physical dependence develops with the excessive use of barbiturates, and withdrawal symptoms are severe. Abrupt or very rapid withdrawal can cause death.

STIMULANTS

The stimulant drugs most often used to excess include amphetamine and its various salts and isomers. Medicinally they are used primarily for the treatment of narcolepsy, a disorder characterized by an overwhelming desire for sleep, and for the treatment of the hyperkinetic child.

These drugs produce tolerance; consequently the person requires an ever increasing amount to secure the same effects. The mental sequelae (not seen in their medical use owing to the lower dosage) are excitability, garrulousness, tremors of the hands, dilated pupils and inordinate sweating. In serious cases, a drug psychosis may occur attended by illusions and hallucinations. The use of the stimulant drugs by the automobile driver to ward off sleep may result in serious accidents or in severe fatigue due to overexertion.

The amphetamines have many nicknames such as "pep pills," "wake-ups," "eye openers," "co-pilots" or "bennies." This last sobriquet is derived from the proprietary name of amphetamine sulfate which is "Benzedrine." Methamphetamine is called "speed."

Some people use both the stimulants and the depressants. They take a depressant at night because without it they "can't sleep." Then in the morning they need a stimulant to "get going."

OTHER ABUSED DRUGS

Many drugs are used to excess. It is hard to draw a line between use and abuse. Some people take too much of the nonprescription (over the counter, O.T.C.) drugs such as mild analgesics, cough medicines, cathartics and so forth. These people cannot be called "drug addicts," yet in a sense they are drug dependent. Of course, the vast majority of them do not and will not become so dependent upon their drugs as to be classified in this way, but a few do go on to a relative drug "addiction."

Some of these nonprescription drugs are definitely being abused. Instances of the use of excessive amounts of the sympathomimetics, primarily those used for allergy (asthma) have been reported. They are used by persons who have no physical need for the drug. One such instance is the use of Asthmador, a mixture of stramonium and belladonna, by the teenagers and even the subteenagers. Severe and serious symptoms result from the use of such preparations. Symptoms include confusion, disorientation, hyperactive agitation, slurred speech and terror. Physical symptoms are flushed face, dry skin and mucous membranes and dilated pupils.

What other drugs will be abused and when cannot be predicted. There seems to be a tendency on the part of many people to try anything for "kicks." How strong the "kick" will be is impossible to say, but continued use often depends upon just that.

GLUE SNIFFING

Glue, of course, is not a drug. Its inclusion here is to give the nurse a quick look at the problem, since it is a serious one in some areas. The use of model airplane glue is widespread and dangerous to health and even to life.

Most glue sniffers are minors and in many cases below average in intelligence. Many, although by no means all, are from the lower socioeconomic stratum. Some are from higher social levels and possess average or above average intelligence. Those who indulge in sniffing glue are often "loners." They do not mix well with the crowd, and often have trouble in school.

The symptoms of glue sniffing can easily be detected in most cases. The odor of the breath is distinctive. Other symptoms include unusually silly actions, watery eyes, a dreamy look, dilated pupils, staggering, "runny" nose, dizziness, incoherent speech, anorexia and weight loss.

Treatment varies but is directed mainly toward alleviating underlying emotional problems. Improving the environment, when possible; placing the youth in a more congenial school; group therapy; counseling; providing adequate health care; and helping the individual achieve a sense of self-worth are some of the measures employed. Treatment, however, especially for those who refuse to throw away their "crutch," is not always successful.

Other substances in addition to glue that are used to provide release include volatile solvents, gasoline and propellants contained in hair sprays and oven cleaners. Symptoms vary with the preparation but are roughly analagous to those observed in glue sniffing. Since the appearance of some of these preparations is so recent, symptoms are still incompletely defined.

SOME GENERAL SYMPTOMS OF THE DRUG USER

The individual who takes drugs excessively will commonly manifest some or all of the following symptoms: change in mood, lowered performance at school or work, unusual temper outbursts, physical deterioration, anorexia, loss of weight, the wearing of sunglasses when not needed to conceal changes in the pupils and other eye symptoms (photophobia), the continuous wearing of long-sleeved shirts by those who take their drugs by injections (called "main lining" if they take them by vein), borrowing excessively or stealing money and association with confirmed drug users.

SELF-MEDICATION

Between the area of medically prescribed drugs and drug abuse, is one that may be called "self-medication." It refers to the individual who prescribes for himself. It may also be the person, not a physician, who tells his friends what medicines to take. The habit of self-medication has become nationwide. Almost everyone has his own remedy for a cold, indigestion, headache, constipation or other "mild" disorder. Sometimes the drug has been previously prescribed by a doctor, but many have merely heard its merits extolled through advertising and communications media (VI-4). The drug companies constantly publicize the value of their products for the treatment of various ailments. In the susceptible person, this often prompts a feeling that he should have this specific drug, since his "symptoms" are the same as those publicized. Such preparations are sold without a prescription, and this may initiate the habit of self-medication. It is appalling to realize how widespread the practice is. By far the vast majority of medicaments sold in the United States are over the counter (O.T.C.—nonprescription) drugs. Of the drugs sold by prescription, the majority are for refills. Of course, the refills may be entirely legitimate. However, refills are often obtained when the medication is no longer really needed.

Preparations most commonly sold without prescription are vitamins, cough medications, cold remedies, cathartics, analgesics, tonics, antihistamines, tranquilizers, antiseptics, sunburn lotions and eye washes.

The American public has received so much information (and sometimes misinformation) about drug products that it feels well qualified to judge the merits or demerits of a given substance and the circumstances under which the substance should be used (VI-4). The old adage, "A little knowledge is a dangerous thing," certainly applies here. So many things must be considered before any drug is administered that one is shocked at the thought of the number of individuals who take medications without the advice of a physician. The nurse has a grave responsibility in teaching the public about "no-self-medication." To begin the crusade she should start at home by never taking any medication that has not been prescribed by a physician. Nurses are just as prone as any one else to think that they "know it all" about drugs. Because they study pharmacology and handle drugs continuously, it is only natural that nurses should feel that they know a great deal about medicines. They may actually be very well informed, but the difficulty lies in the fact that each patient is different, and although the textbook says one thing, the individual may react in an entirely different manner (V-3). With her limited knowledge of medicine the nurse cannot cope with this type of situation. The nurse's second responsibility is to those with whom she comes in contact: her family, friends and patients. Many people will ask the nurse questions which they would hesitate to ask the physician. There are several reasons for this. In some cases, the person may be trying to secure medical information without having to pay a physician's fee. He may be trying to find out if a nonprescription (over-the-counter) drug can be used, since many have been told that prescription drugs are more expensive than the same drug bought directly over the counter. In certain cases this is true, but usually the physician will give the patient the name or tell the pharmacist what he wishes used without a regular prescription. He then gives the instructions for taking the drug directly to the patient. In this case the doctor is responsible, and the drug is being taken under circumstances which are entirely satisfactory to all.

It might be asked, "What are some of the arguments against self-medication?" The entire list would take many pages, but the following should supply the nurse with sufficient "ammunition" to win most arguments:

1. If the substance is harmless it probably is also worthless and, therefore, the patient is merely throwing away good money. This is true of many of the vitamin preparations on the market. Few people need more vitamins than are secured by an adequate diet. Excessive intake does not produce added vigor as the excess is excreted by the body. Moreover, some vitamins in excessive amounts can be harmful.
2. If the drug is not harmless, what are the main reasons for advising against its use without a physician's order?
   a. The drug may relieve the symptoms the patient notes, but it may also mask the symptoms and signs of a serious underlying condition. Thus the "stomach sweetener" may cover the symptoms of peptic ulcer or gastric carcinoma for several months. By the time the "sweetener" no longer gives relief it may be too late to treat the disease effectively.

      The drug may relieve the patient's immediate pain, but it may not in any way help the real trouble. Relief of pain may or may not be a desirable thing. Suppose the patient is complaining of pain under the right shoulder blade. He decides it is muscular rheumatism and treats it as such with various drugs he has heard advertised for rheumatism. This goes on until he suddenly becomes acutely ill with severe pain, jaundice, gastrointestinal disturbances and possibly other symptoms. His original subscapular pain was, in reality, the referred pain of a gallbladder disorder.

      Almost everyone is familiar with the undesirability of using laxatives for abdominal pain. Many such cases have ended with the death of the patient. How many times has Mrs. R. been overheard telling Mrs. S., "Oh! Johnnie has just what Tommie had last month (or year). Dr. B. gave me this for Tommie and I didn't use it all. You can give it to Johnnie. The directions are right on the bottle." Possibly Tommie may have eaten something which disagreed with him, while Johnnie may have acute appendicitis. At times the symptoms are not unlike in such cases.
   b. The drug may be a potentially dangerous preparation, such as a hormone. In most states it is not possible to obtain these except by prescription. However, the patient may not take all of the drug ordered. The remainder is set aside until a relative or friend develops the "same symptoms." Then these very potent drugs become a real hazard. The extent of damage they may do is almost endless. This also holds true for many other drugs.
   c. Another difficulty lies in the emotional or psychologic effect of the drug. Drugs can become "emotional crutches." The patient leans upon his "medicine" which he "cannot do without." In short, he becomes habituated to the drug in much the same way that a person becomes habituated to any excess such as coffee, "cokes," tobacco, etc. It often marks the person as the subject of undue emotional stress.
   d. There may be actual toxic reaction to the drug. This may be the direct result of an overdose or the reaction to a normal dose administered improperly or under the wrong circumstances. This toxic reaction varies from a simple easily remedied condition to one resulting in death. It must also be remembered that excessive amounts of drugs may be taken by a person attempting suicide or by children or adults accidentally. It cannot be said too many times that all drugs should be kept away from infants and children. Many a child has suffered, and some have

died, from eating candy laxatives or sweet-tasting children's preparations of other drugs. Too often the parents will say, "But it was only baby aspirin," or some such preparation. It can still kill if taken in sufficient quantity.

"Old" medications should be destroyed carefully. The garbage can is usually a poor place for these, since many children and animals "pick" over garbage. The child may be intrigued by the "little pills" or the "pretty capsules" to his own great harm. They probably are best flushed down the toilet.

e. One other danger of self-medication that few people consider is the possibility of an allergic or idiosyncratic reaction. There are case histories of patients who died from anaphylactic shock after taking a single aspirin tablet. Of course, this is not common, but other and less drastic allergic reactions are common. Many very efficient medications produce allergic reactions in a relatively large number of persons. If the patient is under the physician's care, the doctor is aware of this possibility and prescribes accordingly. However, if the patient is treating himself, he will not anticipate any untoward symptoms and will often let the early indications go unnoticed until it is difficult or impossible to prevent organic damage.

The whole subject of self-medication is extremely complicated. Much has been written on the matter. What has been said here is in no way complete, but it should furnish the nurse with some of the answers to the questions she is apt to meet. It is hoped that it will also stimulate her interest to such a degree that she will study more about this topic on her own. If in doubt, the nurse should refer the patient to his physician. The nurse should say as little as possible, especially about controversial subjects, but still show a personal interest in the patient's problem. She should explain, briefly, what the problem is and why a nurse cannot answer that particular question. Most patients have great respect for the technical knowledge of the nurse; they feel that her advice is the very best they can receive next to the doctor's. The nurse must do all in her power to warrant such confidence. If there is one all-important qualification for the nurse, it is to be a good listener always. Patients like to feel that they can talk freely to the nurse. Often they think that the doctor is too busy to listen to all of their problems, but the nurse who is with them so much longer can give the time. The nurse who is willing to give this time may be giving the patient the very best treatment possible.

IT IS IMPORTANT TO REMEMBER

1. That the most important medicinal drug producing addiction is opium—in all its forms. The nurse should always endeavor to prevent addiction, and to aid in overcoming the habit once it has become established.
2. That "self-medication" is dangerous, and the nurse should do all in her power to discourage it. The nurse should answer all the questions the patient asks that she is qualified to answer, but she should not hesitate to say, "I do not know." It takes great skill and tact to know what to say and when to say it, but the nurse must try to do just that. When in doubt—always refer the patient to someone with more knowledge, usually the physician.
3. That the nurse has a great social responsibility in this area and she should accept it. The social and emotional care of the patient is just as important as the physical care and vastly more difficult. No nurse should shirk her responsibilities in these matters.
4. That controlled drugs are also known as dangerous drugs.

TOPICS FOR STUDY AND DISCUSSION

1. Drug addiction has been a problem in all lands and all ages. What drugs constitute the most serious problem in the United States? In what ways may the nurse aid in the prevention of drug addiction? What can the lay person do to help? Why do drug addicts often return to the use of drugs after a so-called "cure"? How can this be prevented?

A panel discussion of drug addiction might be very helpful. The discussion might cover the various drugs, and the different phases of the problem such as medical, economic, social, psychologic, etc.

2. A survey of your own families and friends will reveal the prevalence of self-medication. Find out how many are taking any drug preparations, including vitamins, tonics, laxatives, cough medicines, headache remedies, sleeping pills and antacids. Ask why they started using the particular preparation. Did a doctor prescribe the remedy? If so was there any time limit? Has this time limit been exceeded?

3. Make a list of the sources of information concerning medicines that are available to the nurses in your school. Tell what type of information is found in each source.

BIBLIOGRAPHY

Books and Pamphlets

American Medical Association Committee on Alcoholism and Drug Dependence, *The Crutch That Cripples*, Chicago, 1967, American Medical Association.

American Pharmaceutical Association, *Drug Abuse Education—A Guide for the Professions, 2nd Ed.*, Washington, D. C., 1969, American Pharmaceutical Association.

Bowen, H., Hill, L., and Hoffman, G., *Drug Abuse Information—Teacher Resource Material*, San Jose, California, Santa Clara Office of Education.

Bureau of Narcotics and Dangerous Drugs, *The Pharmacist, Drug Safety, Drug Abuse* (Fact sheets and pamphlets) Washington, D.C., 1970–1972, United States Department of Justice.

Dole, V. P., *Detoxification of Sick Addicts in Prison*, Paper presented at the 4th National Conference on Methadone Treatment, San Francisco, January 8–10, 1972. Taken from proceedings published by the National Association for the Prevention of Addiction to Narcotics, New York.

Goodman, L., and Gilman, A. *Pharmacological Basis of Therapeutics, 4th Ed.*, New York, 1970, The Macmillan Co.

Lasher, L. P., *L.S.D., the False Illusion, Part II*, Washington, D.C., September, 1967, Reprint from Food and Drug Administration Papers, United States Department of Health.

The New York Times, "The Drug Scene," Reprint of Series, January 8–12, 1968.

Penna, R., and Roberts, C., "Advertising contributing to the drug abuse problem," *American Pharmaceutical Association News Letter*, Washington, D.C., July, 1972.

Smith, Kline and French Laboratories, *Drug Abuse—Escape to No Where*, Philadelphia, 1967, Smith, Kline and French.

Journal Articles

Bensel, J., "Methadone maintenance of narcotic addicts," *J. Am. Pharm. Assoc.* NS 11:7 (July, 1971).

Canada, A., and Flenkow, S., "Narcotic addiction—A methadone program," *J. Am. Pharm. Assoc.* NS 11:7 (July, 1971).

Condon, A., and Roland, A., "Drug abuse jargon," *Am. J. Nurs.* 71:9:1738 (September, 1971).

Done, A. K., "A physician looks at non-prescription medication," *J. Am. Pharm. Assoc.* NS 7:9 (September, 1967).

Fink, M., et al., "Narcotic antagonists. Another approach to addiction therapy," *Am. J. Nurs.* 71:7:1359, (July, 1971).

Foreman, N., and Zerwek, J., "Drug abuse crisis intervention," *Am. J. Nurs.* 71:9:1736 (September, 1971).

Fort, J., "Comparison chart of major substances used for mind alteration," *Am. J. Nurs.* 71:9:1740 (September, 1971).

Leary, J., Vasella, D., and Yeaw, E., "Self-administered medications," *Am. J. Nurs. 71*:6:1193 (June, 1971).

Lipp, M., Benson, S., and Allen, P., "Marijuana use by nurses and nursing students," *Am. J. Nurs.* 71:12:2339 (December, 1971).

Miller, D. E., "Methadone maintenance—Toward a rational approach," *J. Am. Pharm. Assoc.* NS:11:7 (July, 1971).

Musgrave, L. C., "Hot line takes the heat off," *Am. J. Nurs.* 71:4 (April, 1971).

Office of Drug Abuse, "Drug antagonists," Report of White House Special Action Committee, *Sci. News* 102:3:58 (July 19, 1972).

Rodman, M., "Drugs used against addiction," *R.N.* 33:10:71 (October, 1970).

Rogers, P. G., "Drug abuse in our society," *J. Am. Pharm. Assoc.* NS 8:3 (March, 1968).

PART TWO

CLINICAL PHARMACOLOGY

SECTION I

DRUGS USED IN A VARIETY OF CLINICAL CONDITIONS

DRUGS USED TO PREVENT AND CONTROL INFECTION

DRUGS USED FOR DIAGNOSTIC PURPOSES

DRUGS ACTING ON THE CENTRAL AND THE AUTONOMIC NERVOUS SYSTEMS

DRUGS USED TO MAINTAIN FLUID AND ELECTROLYTE BALANCE

TOXICOLOGY

THE PSYCHOLOGICAL ASPECTS OF DRUG THERAPY

CHAPTER 7

DRUGS USED TO PREVENT AND CONTROL INFECTION

CORRELATION WITH OTHER SCIENCES

II. CHEMISTRY

1. Ionization is the process of producing ions. An ion is an atom or group of atoms which has lost or gained one or more orbital electrons and has thus become capable of conducting electricity.

2. Saponification is the conversion of an ester into an alcohol and a salt; in particular, the conversion of fat into a soap and glycerin by means of an alkali.

III. MICROBIOLOGY

1. Microbiology is the science which treats of living organisms which are too small to be seen without magnification. These organisms are plants (fungi and bacteria), animals (protozoa), and other forms whose status has not been determined, such as rickettsiae and viruses.

2. The gram-positive organisms are those organisms that appear dark blue under the microscope when stained with Gram's stain. The gram-negative organisms appear pink when stained by Gram's method.

Streptococci, staphylococci and pneumococci are gram-positive. The Neisseria and Escherichia are gram-negative.

3. Microorganisms, like the higher organisms, have their enemies. One group is antagonistic to another. In certain cases, one organism excretes a poison which will destroy another; on the other hand, some organisms assist each other, one group helping another to live.

4. Immunity is the condition of being nonsusceptible to a specific disease.

5. Immunity is active if the individual has built up his own antibodies. This is a relatively long immunity.

6. Immunity is passive if the individual has been given antibodies from some other person or animal. This is a relatively short immunity.

7. An antigen is a substance which when taken into the body causes the production of antibodies.

8. A toxin is a biologic poison. Certain microorganisms excrete (or secrete) powerful poisons as exotoxins. Others have a poison in their bodies which is released only after the organism has been killed (endotoxins). The toxins may be poisonous to many types of organisms or only one or a few.

An antitoxin is a substance (an antibody) which will counteract the action of a toxin or destroy the toxin.

9. Viruses are minute living organisms so small they can be seen only with the aid of the electron microscope. They are parasites which proliferate only upon living tissue.

10. Rickettsiae are small organisms intermediate between viruses and bacteria. Like viruses they live only on living tissue. Some are large enough to be seen under high magnification of the ordinary microscope; others can be seen only by use of the electron microscope.

11. Bacteria are minute plant-like organisms that can be seen under high magnification of the ordinary microscope.

IV. PHYSICS

1. Surface tension is the tendency of the molecules of a liquid to adhere closer together on the surface of the liquid. This tends to form a sphere of the liquid when the pressure is equal on all sides.

2. A colloid is a state of matter in which the individual particles, of submicroscopic size, are distributed in some medium called the dispersion medium. The particles consist either of a single large molecule, as a protein, or an aggregate of smaller molecules. The dimensions of the particles of a colloid lie in a specific size range.

INTRODUCTION

"An ounce of prevention is worth a pound of cure." No one will deny the importance of this fact. Certainly, every physician, nurse and patient would prefer to prevent a disease rather than to have to try to cure it. Prophylactic (preventive) measures are now being used for an ever-increasing number of diseases, and although this is especially true of the communicable diseases, even certain of the noncommunicable diseases are responding to preventive measures. This field of medicine is expanding so rapidly that only an introduction can be given here.

Prevention of disease is accomplished in a number of ways, some of the more important methods being:

1. Prevention of the susceptible individual from coming in contact with the disease agent. This may be done by:

a. Isolating the patient.

b. Quarantine of exposed persons during the period of incubation.

c. Keeping the infecting agent away from the person—as by supplying clean food and clean water and screening windows and doors to prevent the entrance of mosquitoes, flies and other insects.

d. Disinfecting or cleaning of articles that have become contaminated by disease organisms.

2. Production in the individual of a passive immunity by the introduction of the antibodies specific for the infecting organism (III-4, 6).

3. Production in the individual of an active immunity by the introduction of antigens that will stimulate the production of antibodies (III-5, 7).

4. Giving drugs to the individual which will kill the offending organism if and when it enters the body.

5. Giving drugs to the individual in the early stages of an infection to lessen the severity of the original infection and to prevent complications.

These will be considered in the following sections.

Biological Medications Used to Prevent Communicable Disease

ISOLATION AND SANITATION

Discussions of isolation and quarantine (1, a and b) are not within the scope of this book. They are in the field of epidemiology and public health, and the student is referred to books dealing with these subjects for further information.

Various chemical substances generally referred to as antiseptics and disinfectants are used to destroy disease organisms which might contaminate drinking water, food or articles which come in contact with people (1, c and d). These will be discussed later.

PASSIVE IMMUNITY

Passive immunity is that immunity received from some outside source. The antibodies are not produced by the individual (III-6). Passive immunity may be acquired naturally from the mother through the placenta and from the mother's milk.

Passive immunity is acquired artificially through various serums. Artificial passive immunity, usually of relatively short duration, is important in several conditions, but the most common use is during an epidemic to prevent exposed persons from becoming ill or to lessen the severity of the disease (III-6). Usually introduced into the exposed individual by parenteral means, the antibodies used are of two varieties—*antitoxic serums* and *antibacterial serums.*

Toxins can be chemically treated so that they lose their toxicity but are still able to stimulate antibody production; these treated toxins are called *toxoids.* Antitoxin serums are prepared by injecting suitable animals, usually horses because of their large size and blood volume, with increasing doses of toxoid until the maximal amount of antibody (antitoxin) is produced. A non-lethal amount of blood is then drawn, and the serum is separated, processed for sterility and standardized. Antibacterial serums are prepared in a similar manner, using killed or altered bacterial injections that are unable to initiate disease in the animal.

Passive immunity is also obtained by the use of human blood plasma or serum fractions. Two types are available—*high titer serum* from a person recently immunized against the disease, and *immune serum globulin* and/or *gamma globulin.* The latter is used for some of the so-called childhood diseases. Since most adults have had, or been exposed to, the various communicable diseases of childhood, their blood contains antibodies against these diseases. By using the serum of many adults mixed together it is reasonable to assume that it will contain antibodies of the disease or diseases in question.

Antitoxic serums are available for the prophylaxis of *diphtheria, tetanus, gas gangrene, scarlet fever streptococcus* and *botulism* (III-8). These serums are given to exposed persons during the incubation period. They either entirely prevent the occurrence of the disease or reduce the severity. These same serums are also used in the treatment of the diseases. The use of the serums in the prevention and treatment of scarlet fever and botulism has not been so successful as in the other conditions mentioned. However, they are still used in most cases, especially in botulism, since there is always the hope that they will prevent the disease. There are also *antitoxic serums (antivenin)* for use against the poisons of certain snakes and the black widow spider, but these are more often used in treatment than they are in prevention.

Antibacterial serums have not proved very successful in the prevention of disease. They are used mainly for treatment.

Human immune globulin (gamma globulin) is used for the prevention or modification of such conditions as measles and infectious hepatitis. It is also employed in the treatment of agammaglobulinemia to provide the patient with the normal adult antibodies.

Convalescent serums are available for the treatment of such diseases as mumps, measles, poliomyelitis and scarlet fever. They are used to lessen the severity of the disease or, during incubation, to prevent the development of the disease.

Before administering any serum, a skin test for sensitivity should be done unless the physician expressly directs otherwise. This is done by injecting a minute amount of the serum, about 0.1 ml. intradermally—usually into the ventral surface of the forearm. After about 20 minutes the area is checked. If there is a raised, reddened wheal, the physician should be consulted before the serum is administered.

ACTIVE IMMUNITY

Active immunity is that immunity produced by the individual himself; the person builds antibodies in the blood stream in response to the introduction of an antigen (III-5). This may result from having an attack of the disease or be secured by immunization. Active immunity, produced artificially by the introduction of various antigens such as *vaccines*, *toxin-antitoxins* and *toxoids*, has many advantages over the use of serums to produce passive immunity; some of these follow:

1. The antibodies are produced in the individual's own blood stream and remain in it rather than being eliminated (as is true of foreign antibodies introduced into the blood stream).

2. An actively immunized individual is less apt to develop the disease.

3. The immunity produced by the individual himself lasts much longer than does the passive immunity.

There is one disadvantage of active immunization that must be considered—it takes some time to develop the antibodies essential for the immunity. The length of time differs with various antigens but it is usually about six weeks. Thus, for a disease with a short incubation period active immunization cannot be secured between the time of exposure and time the patient would become ill. It is necessary in such cases to use passive immunity or to immunize before exposure.

Immunizing agents are available for the production of active immunity to a long list of conditions, and the list is constantly growing. These antigens are of various types. The more important ones are:

1. *Living virus* that has been attenuated by some means. Example—smallpox virus attenuated by passage through the cow.

2. *Dead* or *attenuated bacterial cells*. Example—typhoid vaccine.

3. *Bacterial toxins* that have been *partially detoxified*. Example—diphtheria toxin-antitoxin or toxoid.

Active immunizing agents are available for certain diseases caused by viruses, rickettsiae and bacteria (III-9, 10, 11).

For viral diseases the oldest universally used antigen is the smallpox vaccine. The vaccination for smallpox has reduced the malady from a severe plague to a disease seen only rarely, and in those areas where vaccination is compulsory it has been practically eliminated. Smallpox vaccine is very effective, producing a relatively long immunity. Although the exact length of time for which it is effective has not been proved, it does immunize for a period of from one to several years, and some people receive lifetime immunity from one vaccination. The United States Public Health Service no longer recommends routine vaccination for smallpox except for those traveling to countries where the disease is endemic. The possibility of exposure in this country is so low that there appears to be more risk from vaccination than from the disease. The only cases appearing here for a long time have been imported. The Public Health Service requires vaccination before entry of anyone coming into the United States from a country where the disease still exists in order to prevent spread of the disease by anyone traveling during the incubation period. Some countries require vaccination for everyone entering that country. The Public Health Service will provide specific information regarding vaccination to any would-be traveler.

There are vaccines available for some of the more common strains of the *influenza virus*. Although not used universally, they are of importance for persons especially susceptible to the disease, for people who are likely to be excessively exposed and when an epidemic threatens.

Vaccine for *rabies* has been known and used since the time of its discovery by Louis Pasteur. It is regularly used only after exposure to the disease since the incubation period of rabies is long, and it is therefore possible to build up the immunity during this time. Persons bitten by rabid animals must have the Pasteur treatment, for once clinical symptoms appear, the disease is always fatal. At the present time, the vaccine used is prepared from duck embryo (dried, inactivated virus). It is much less painful than the previously used vaccine which was treated with formalin. The vaccine is given to any person who has been bitten by an animal which is suspected or known to be rabid. The number of individuals exposed, especially in the United States and Canada, is relatively small. The vaccine is used for the production of active immunity in animals, particularly dogs, which naturally reduces the incidence of the disease in humans.

Yellow fever vaccine, also a viral vaccine, is used in those areas where the disease is endemic. Any person who is traveling to such places should receive the vaccine before he goes into the country.

Other viral vaccines include *mumps*, *measles* and *poliomyelitis vaccines*. Mumps vaccine may or may not be given to the small child. Some pediatricians give it routinely as with other immunizations. Some doctors feel that this is not the best practice. Mumps in the small child is usually a mild disease and the immunity produced is of long standing, often life-time. However, if the child approaching puberty has not had the disease, the vaccine is given. Complications of mumps in the youth or adult can be very serious.

Measles (rubeola) vaccine is useful in the prevention of this serious childhood disease. It is not always given with the early routine immunizations, but is used later in the first year. If used, the vaccine will reduce the severity of the disease, if it does not prevent it. Immune serum globulin may be given with the vaccine. This covers the period necessary to produce antibodies to prevent the occurrence of the disease.

There is a vaccine for rubella (German measles). The infant or small child may or may not have the vaccine since in this age group the disease is not severe or serious. However, it is used for the girl approaching the child-bearing age, if she has not had the vaccine or the disease earlier. Rubella contracted in the first trimester of pregnancy can cause serious congenital deformities. As with most vaccines, it is not usually given during pregnancy.

Another vaccine is the Salk vaccine for poliomyelitis. It is named for the physician mainly responsible for its perfection. This vaccine has greatly reduced the incidence of paralytic poliomyelitis. The Sabin oral poliomyelitis vaccine, named for the physician who perfected it, is now being extensively used in the prevention of this crippling disease. Since it is given orally, it is much easier to administer than the Salk vaccine, which must be given parenterally. Some doctors give both of these vaccines; since poliomyelitis is such a serious disease, they do not want to leave anything to chance. The Sabin vaccine is given in three doses at about four week intervals.

Bacterial vaccines are available for a number of diseases. Typhoid vaccine has been used successfully for many years. It is especially important in situations where there is danger of a contaminated water supply.

Pertussis vaccine is now routinely given to infants and small children since pertussis (whooping cough) is a serious infection in the small child. It sometimes fails to prevent the disease when the child is later exposed, but it will reduce severity. Thus, having the disease in a mild form produces a prolonged immunity for the child.

Combination preparations are available which allow immunization for more than one disease at a time. One that has been used for a number of years is D.P.T. (diphtheria toxoid, pertussis vaccine and tetanus toxoid). Another more recent combination is M.M.R. (measles, mumps and rubella virus vaccine, live). Schedules vary, but these vaccines may be given at any time from infancy until puberty. There is also a combination of diphtheria and tetanus toxoid vaccines which is given to older children who have not been previously inoculated against diphtheria and tetanus.

BCG or *bacille Calmette-Guerin* is a vaccine for *tuberculosis*. It has been used extensively in Europe for several years and recently has been used in this country. Although statistics and opinions vary as to the safety and effectiveness of the vaccine, its use seems indicated in areas where tuberculosis is very prevalent. It is given mainly to children, as they are more readily susceptible to tuberculosis than is the adult. It is used only for tuberculin-negative individuals. If the tuberculin test is positive, the person already has developed antibodies against tuberculosis.

Vaccines are available for *cholera, bubonic plague, tularemia* and *brucellosis* (undulant fever). These, like many of the other vaccines, are of importance in areas where these diseases are endemic. Any person going into such an area should have the vaccine prior to the trip.

Bacterial vaccine can be secured for certain strains of *staphylococcus* and *pneumococcus*, but these have not proved very successful. If immunity is produced it is of short duration. However, vaccines are sometimes used for treatment.

Rickettsial vaccines for *typhus* and *Rocky Mountain spotted fever* have been used successfully. Again, these are used mainly in areas where the disease is endemic or for persons who are apt to be exposed to the disease.

In some cases the toxins produced by the organisms of the diseases are used to secure immunity (instead of the organisms themselves), the toxin first being detoxified, wholly or partially, by various means. The most common preparations are toxin-antitoxins, toxoids and alum precipitated toxoids. The *toxin-antitoxin* is exactly what its name implies, a combination of the toxin with enough antitoxin to avoid unduly severe reactions, but not enough to completely neutralize all the toxin. The unneutralized toxin will stimulate the formation of the antibodies in the individual.

The *toxoids* are produced by treating the toxin with formalin and incubating until the toxicity is lost.

Toxoids and toxin-antitoxins are available for use in the prophylaxis of *diphtheria, tetanus* and *gas gangrene*. These are marketed separately and also in various combinations.

Dermatemycol is a preparation used for immunization against *ringworm*. Available also are polyvalent vaccines for various fungi such as trichophyton, microsporum, achorion, endodermophyton and epidermophyton. Their efficiency has not been proved.

The *undenatured bacterial antigens* (UBA) are preparations produced from bacterial cultures by mechanical processes. They contain only the antigens of the disease (III-7). They appear to be very efficient in producing active immunity quickly; however, the immunity is not so lasting as that secured by other means.

For infants, who have not had the opportunity to build up any active immunity of their own, immunization is usually begun without testing, but for the older child or the adult, susceptibility tests are given before immunization when possible.

Amantadine hydrochloride, N.F. (Symmetrel) is a drug used only for the prophylaxis of Asian (A_2) influenza. It appears to act by preventing penetration of the virus into the host cell. It is given orally (capsule or syrup) in doses of 200 mg. once or twice a day. Side effects include ataxia, nervousness, insomnia, inability to concentrate, psychological reactions, dry mouth, gastrointestinal disturbances and skin rashes. Amantadine should be given cautiously, if at all, to patients with central nervous system disorders, or epilepsy (or history of any seizures), geriatric patients with arteriosclerosis, or patients who are taking psychopharmacologic agents or central nervous system stimulants. It is for prevention of disease only and should not be given if the patient has active influenza or other respiratory disorders.

PREVENTIVE MEDICATION

For some diseases active immunization cannot be secured by inoculations. If a person must go into areas where such diseases are endemic, other means must be undertaken to prevent illness. One way is to give the individual small doses of a nontoxic drug which will kill or inhibit the multiplication of the organism on contact. The best illustration of this method is the use of such a drug as *chloroquine* (Aralen) or *quinacrine* (Atabrine) in the prevention of *malaria*. Our troops going into malarious areas in the South Pacific during World War II were given small daily doses of one of the drugs. Then, if and when they were bitten by malaria-carrying mosquitoes, the drug was in their blood streams in sufficient concentration to inhibit the malarial parasite.

Chemicals Used to Control Microorganisms in the Environment and on Body Surfaces

INTRODUCTION

Most of the discussion in the first portion of this chapter dealt with biological medications used to prevent various communicable diseases. In this portion we will consider some of the chemical preparations that are usually classified as antiseptics and disinfectants. These are used to destroy or retard the growth of microorganisms in the environment and on body surfaces.

Before the actual drugs are discussed, certain terms should be defined. *Sepsis* is the presence of pathogenic microorganisms. *Infection* is a similar word but is usually limited to actual disease conditions in an individual. An *antiseptic* is a substance which inhibits the growth of microorganisms. A *disinfectant*—to remove infection—is a substance which destroys pathogenic microorganisms. *Germicides* or *bactericides* are chemicals which will destroy all microorganisms, both pathogenic and nonpathogenic. The word chemical has been used in connection with these terms. It should be understood that physical conditions may also be disinfectant or germicidal but that only chemicals will be discussed in this chapter. It has become common practice to consider the three terms disinfectant, germicide and bactericide as synonymous. *Fungicides* are substances used to destroy fungi (yeasts and molds). *Parasiticides* are materials that will destroy parasites—organisms of the animal kingdom that are larger than bacteria. A *bacteriostatic agent* is one which tends to retard or stop the multiplication of bacteria. The organisms are not killed but remain in a condition that might be described as suspended animation. *Astringents* are chemicals which act as osmotic or protein precipitant influences. They are not usually used for their action on bacteria but often are bacteriostatic, antiseptic or disinfectant in action. *Deodorants* are agents used to overcome undesirable odors; they may or may not have an effect upon bacteria. *Anti-infectives* are substances used to fight infection (microorganisms) on or in the human body. They may be specific, acting against one or a limited number of microorganisms, or general, acting against a variety of organisms.

Substances used to destroy microorganisms are many and varied. Some are harmful to man and others are harmless. Most of the chemicals are used in solution. (A review of solutions is advisable.) Some of the chemicals used kill all the microorganisms (sterilization); some kill the pathogens but not all the organisms (disinfection); while others merely stop the multiplication of the organisms (bacteriostasis or antisepsis); still others simply remove the organisms from the part.

The effect a chemical has in a given situation depends upon many factors, the more important of which are:

1. Type of chemical
2. Its strength or concentration
3. The length of time the chemical is in contact with the material to be disinfected
4. The temperature of the solution
5. The degree of ionization of the solute, and the hydrogen ion concentration of the solution (II-1)
6. The amount of organic material present
7. The consistency of the material to be disinfected

Antiseptics, disinfectants and anti-infectives may be arranged in several groups, the most important of which are those used to keep the environment of the patient free from harmful organisms, those used on the body surfaces and those used to combat diseases after they are absorbed into the body fluids. In

*ANTISEPTICS AND DISINFECTANTS IN COMMON USE**

ACTIVE INGREDIENTS	PREPARATIONS	USES ON BODY SURFACES AND STRENGTHS USED	USES IN THE ENVIRONMENT AND STRENGTHS USED	REMARKS
Alcohol	Ethyl alcohol.	70% used for skin antisepsis before injections and some surgical procedures	Not effective against spores, therefore unsuited for environmental use.	Solutions stronger or weaker than 70% are usually less effective.
	Isopropyl alcohol.	50 to 70% as above.		
Chlorine	Sodium hypochlorite solution diluted (Zonite).	0.5% solution (modified Dakin's solution) used for infected wounds.	5% (household bleach) used for utensils.	When Dakin's solution is used, skin must be protected against irritation.
	Oxychlorosene (Clorpactin XCB).	0.5% solution topical to kill cancer cells in an operative field.		
	Oxychlorosene sodium (Clorpactin [WCS–90]).	0.1 to 0.4%, topical,–antiseptic.		
	Halazone.		4 to 8 mg. to 1 liter of water to render it potable.	
Iodine	Iodine solution.	2% antiseptic.		Tincture of iodine, 7%, too irritating; no longer used.
	Povidone-iodine (Betadine, Isodine).	0.1 to 1.0% for various areas–antiseptic.		
	Undecoylium chloride-iodine (Virac).	0.2 to 3.2% solution–antiseptic.		
Mercurial	Nitromersol sodium (Metaphen).	0.04% solution, topical. 1:200 tincture, topical.		May cause skin irritation.
	Phenylmercuric nitrate acetate (Nylmerate).	1:1500 ointment. 1:3000 tincture, topical.		
	Thimerosal (Merthiolate).	Various strengths and preparations–topical.	Used in dilute solution to preserve various biologic substances.	

Silver	Silver nitrate.	Topical (fused or solid form), used to cauterize. 1% solution, topical, used in the eyes. Also 1% used on other surfaces.		
	Silver picrate.	1 to 2% solution, topical.		
	Silver protein mild (Argyrol).	5 to 25% solution, topical.		
	Silver protein strong (Protargol).	0.25 to 1.0% solution, topical.		
Quaternary Ammonium Compounds	Benzalkonium chloride (Zephiran).	1:1000 to 1:40,000 solution, topical.	1–1000 to 1:5000 solution, environmental.	These are all "detergents."
	Benzethonium chloride (Phemerol).	1:1000 to 1:5000 solution, topical.	Same strength, environmental.	
	Cepylpyridinium chloride (Cepacol).	1:1000 to 1:5000 solution, topical.		
	Methybenzethonium (Diaparene).	0.1% ointment, topical.	1:25,000 solution, environmental.	
Aldehydes	Formaldehyde (Formalin).		37% solution, environmental.	Formaldehyde is a gas (formerly used for fumigation). Now used in solution almost exclusively.
	Glutaraldehyde (Cidex).		2% solution, buffered with 0.03% sodium bicarbonate.	Said to be an excellent disinfectant with few toxic effects. After solution is made up, should be discarded after 2 wks.
Others	Phenols.			Seldom used.
	Boric acid.			Seldom used.
	Hydrogen peroxide.	3% solution, topical, used straight or diluted with water.		Main use is to loosen tissue debris and pus.

*For names of other antiseptics and disinfectants and for further details on those mentioned here, see Current Drug Handbook.

many instances the same basic substance is used for all three purposes. The strength and the chemical formula will vary with the purpose for which the chemical is to be used.

SUBSTANCES USED TO MAINTAIN A HEALTHY ENVIRONMENT FOR THE PATIENT

Substances used by the nurse to maintain a biologically clean environment for the patient fall into four main classes:

A. Substances used to disinfect the things which come in contact with the patient—such as surgical instruments and dressings, various nursing appliances, room furnishings and linens.

B. Chemicals used to render human excretions noninfective.

C. Substances used to remove or destroy microorganisms found on the skin.

D. Substances used to remove or destroy microorganisms found on exposed mucous membranes.

Since, in most instances, the same basic chemicals are used for all of these purposes, they can be discussed together. It must be remembered that the strength and the form of the preparation used will vary with the use for which it is intended.

Most of the substances used on the body surfaces are antiseptic in action. However, some are strong enough to destroy most of the pathogenic organisms and, therefore, approach the disinfectant in action. It is very difficult to produce actual sterility of any of the body surfaces, but in surgical procedures a relative sterility is reached.

Patients differ greatly in their ability to withstand various chemicals. The nurse should be alert for any undesirable developments. She should make note of any allergy or idiosyncrasy about which the patient may tell her. Many times the patient has had an unhappy experience previously, and he should not be subjected to a repetition. If the preparation is one that the physician has specifically ordered, it will be necessary to acquaint him with the patient's inability to use that drug. The doctor can then decide upon a substitute.

New synthetic antiseptics and disinfectants are numerous. Every drug company tries to produce a good disinfectant that is not hard on the skin of the user and that will not damage metal or various surface finishes of furniture and walls. Most of these are effective. Their strength, best uses and toxicity are given by the pharmaceutical houses that release them. The nurse should familiarize herself with those used in the hospital where she is working and should also try, by reading pharmaceutical literature, to keep informed of the newest developments in this and other fields of medicine.

The selection of the proper disinfectant may or may not be left to the individual nurse. Some institutions are very liberal in such matters, while others have a regular routine which every nurse is expected to follow. In cases where the nurse is expected to make her own choice, the following questions may help her to decide which of any number of preparations is the best to use:

1. Which preparation will be most effective?
2. In what strength should it be used?
3. Will it damage the material to be disinfected?
4. Is it hard on the skin?
5. If so, will rubber gloves overcome this difficulty?
6. How long must the disinfectant be in contact with the material to be disinfected to be effective?
7. Is a quicker and yet equally efficient preparation available?
8. Does it have any disagreeable odor?
9. How long will such an odor last?
10. Is it economical?

The nurse will often be called upon to advise others as to the use of these products. Since this is true, the nurse should be informed about the antiseptics and disinfectants which are currently in use in her area.

Anti-Infectives

INTRODUCTION

In the previous portion of this chapter antiseptics and disinfectants used on the surfaces of the body and upon the surroundings of the patient have been discussed. The next group to be considered are drugs which act within the human body. As explained earlier, these drugs are called anti-infectives (meaning "against infection"). Anti-infectives can be further divided into those that act only on one or a limited number of organisms and those that act upon many different organisms. The term "specific" has been used to designate the first group. These will be discussed with the appropriate material later in the book. Those anti-infective drugs that act on several different organisms are called "general" anti-infectives.

There are two main divisions of the general anti-infectives—the sulfonamides and the antibiotics. The discoveries of these drugs, touched upon briefly in the historical sketch in Chapter 1, represent a very dramatic breakthrough in man's long struggle to overcome the diseases that beset him. They have been effective in so many conditions that they have changed the therapeutic picture of medicine in many respects. It is wrong, however, to think that these drugs will immediately cure all disease. They are not panaceas but are very valuable additions to the list of therapeutic drugs.

SULFONAMIDES

(See Current Drug Handbook for additional information.)

The Drugs. The sulfonamides are all synthetic compounds. The first of these compounds was *Prontosil*, a red dye which was found to have bacteriostatic properties. Research disclosed that it was the liberation of a substance called *sulfanilamide* which gave the compound its anti-infective value. Since the early 1930's when Prontosil was first tried as an anti-infective agent many different sulfonamides have been synthesized.

The sulfonamide drugs have been found to be most effective against the gram-positive bacteria such as the streptococci, pneumococci, staphylococci and such gram-negative organisms as the *Neisseria* (meningococci, gonococci), the *Escherichia coli* and others (III-2).

Physical and Chemical Properties. All the sulfonamide drugs have similar structural formulas. They are all derivatives of p-amino-benzenesulfonamide. The substitutions, which are either on the amine or the amide group, can change the physical properties as well as the therapeutic effectiveness.

Many of the synthesized sulfonamide compounds have been found to be therapeutically ineffective or too toxic for use. The sulfonamides are white crystalline powders that are relatively insoluble in water except for their sodium salts which are easily dissolved in water.

Action. The exact action of the sulfonamides in the body is unknown. It is thought, however, that their ability to compete with para-aminobenzoic acid for incorporation into folic acid or pteroyl glutamic acid plays a part.

Therapeutic Uses. The sulfonamide drugs were used to a much greater extent before the advent of penicillin and other antibiotics. Most of the sulfonamides are relatively more toxic than the antibiotics. However, for certain conditions they remain the agents of choice.

Absorption and Excretion. Varying greatly in their rates of absorption, most of the sulfonamides are administered orally and reach a high blood level. Others are so poorly absorbed as to render them useless for therapeutic use outside the gastrointestinal tract. They are changed (acetylated, conjugated) in the body, some more than others. The extent and rapidity of acetylation are important, for in this form they are less effective and more difficult to eliminate. The readily absorbed sulfonamides are usually distributed throughout most or all of the body fluids, and excreted by the kidneys.

Preparations and Dosages. (Refer to the Current Drug Handbook.)

THE NURSE

Mode of Administration. Most of the sulfonamides are administered orally; a few are prepared for intravenous use. Sulfanilamide powder, or any of the powdered forms, may be applied directly to a wound.

If the drug is to be absorbed into the blood stream, or if it is to be injected directly into it, the time interval between doses is important. If the drug is not given at the time ordered, the organism may build up a tolerance to it, and subsequent doses will be ineffective. Thus, maintaining drug levels in the blood is important. It is not uncommon to give a double or even a quadruple dose when administration is initiated in order to reach the desired level in the blood stream quickly, subsequent doses being just sufficient to maintain that level. Thus, if the first dose is 2.0 Gm., later doses may be 0.5 to 1.0 Gm.

The sulfonamides are commonly formulated in tablet form, relatively large and difficult to swallow. Scoring and dividing the tablet, or crushing and placing it into a capsule are ways of overcoming this difficulty, many people being able to swallow a capsule more easily than a tablet. It is important that the nurse maintain intake and output records on patients receiving absorbable sulfonamide preparations because the drugs sometimes form crystals in the kidneys, blocking normal urine flow.

It is usually wise to see that the fluid intake is about 2500 ml. Unless the physician orders otherwise, alkaline fluids, or foods that will produce an alkaline urine should be used, since the sulfonamides tend to form crystals less in alkaline than in acid urine. Some physicians routinely order sodium bicarbonate with these drugs to insure an alkaline urine. Unless specifically directed, it probably is not wise to let the intake exceed 3000 ml. The urine output should not be allowed to fall below 1500 ml. If it does fall below this point, the physician should be notified. With some of the sulfonamide preparations such as sulfamethizole (Thiosulfil), the fluid intake may be restricted so as to concentrate the drug in the urinary tract for treatment of infections of these organs.

Side Effects, Toxicity and Treatment. All the sulfonamides are potentially toxic, but this is particularly true of those that are readily absorbed from the gastrointestinal tract. The toxic symptoms are often more alarming than actually dangerous, especially the rather common early symptoms of nausea and vomiting, which result from the effect of the drug upon the vomiting center in the brain. Cyanosis is common with sulfanilamide but is not apt to occur with the other preparations. It is not a persistent symptom and usually clears rapidly once the drug is withdrawn. Dizziness, lack of coordination and temporary mental lapses are also common during sulfanilamide therapy. When these drugs are being used the patient should be aware of the dangers of such activities as driving a car or working at a dangerous machine. Usually these patients are in bed, but occasionally the drugs are taken by ambulatory patients. The nurse must not "scare" such a patient but should judiciously advise him to remain inactive and stay near home if not actually in bed. Mild anemia, stomatitis and swollen joints are other symptoms that may occur during the course of sulfonamide therapy, but these are usually transitory. Drug fever, rashes, severe or persistent anemia, hepatitis and agranulocytosis are more serious toxic reactions. Because of their toxicity, the sulfonamide preparations have been largely replaced with other, less toxic, anti-infective compounds.

The nurse must be alert to the very earliest signs of any of the untoward reactions. When the usually mild and transitory symptoms appear, it may be sufficient to reassure the patient that this is not a serious condition and that it will not last long. If the patient worries, his condition will only be aggravated.

Toxic symptoms have been much less frequent since the introduction of the practice of giving two or more sulfonamides together, as this allows for a lower dosage than would be possible when one is given alone and usually gives better results. There are many such preparations and many combinations of the drugs. Each has its specific place. When two or three of the sulfonamide drugs are given together, the total dosage is the same or less than it would be for one alone. Thus, if the physician wishes to start the patient with 2.0 Gm. of sulfonamide he might give:

1. Sulfadiazine 2.0 Gm., or
2. Sulfadiazine 1.0 Gm. and Sulfamerazine 1.0 Gm., or
3. Sulfadiazine 0.66 Gm. and Sulfamerazine 0.66 Gm. and Sulfathiazole 0.66 Gm.

Since each is being given in relatively small dosage, there is less chance for a drug in the combination to produce toxic changes, especially kidney blockage, than one drug given alone would have.

Interactions. The action of the sulfonamides is enhanced by urinary acidifiers which decrease the excretion of the drug. Their action is also enhanced by the oral anticoagulants, phenylbutazone and the salicylates. With these drugs there is displacement from the binding site. The sulfonamides are inhibited by antacids which cause a decrease in absorption and by urinary alkalinizers which hasten the excretion of the drug. The sulfonamides potentiate the action of the oral anticoagulants, Methotrexate and the salicylates by displacement at the binding site.

Patient Teaching. This topic has already been partially covered. The patient should be advised of possible side effects if he is to take the drug at home, and also of the necessity for taking the drug at the exact times ordered. He should also understand that while taking these preparations he should be under the direct supervision of the physician and to report promptly to him any untoward symptoms.

Exposure to direct sunlight for prolonged periods is undesirable for any patient taking the sulfonamides.

THE PATIENT. The nurse should consult the attending physician before administering sulfonamides to a patient with known allergy to them. Usually the allergy is to one and not to all sulfa preparations. Patients should understand that the unpleasant side effects are transitory and will disappear, even if the drug is continued. The sulfonamide drugs are relatively inexpensive and lay no undue financial burden on the patient or his family.

Other Information of Interest. Sulfanilamide was the first of this group to achieve widespread use. It is very effective but, possessing high toxicity, is not now in common use.

Many forms, preparations and kinds of sulfonamide drugs are available. Some of these include the so-called sustained-release preparations which allow the drug to enter the blood stream slowly. However, some are relatively toxic. Some of the sulfonamide medications are combined with the azo dyes for more effective microbiologic action. The azo dyes also exhibit some analgesic effect in the genitourinary tract. Also some of the drugs are prepared in lipid solutions, which is believed to increase their effectiveness. The attempt to find a sulfonamide product that is effective and nontoxic continues, each new preparation having some advantages but usually also some disadvantages. These drugs are effective in the treatment of a large number of diseases, and most patients are able to tolerate some, if not all, of them. They form a most important segment of modern drug therapy.

Antibiotics

The phenomenon of antibiosis (III-3) has been recognized since the 1890's but it was not until the late 1930's that it was applied to medicine. Alexander Fleming's observation of the antibiotic activity of a mold contaminating a culture of staphylococcus led to the isolation and production of penicillin, the first antibiotic widely used for systemic infections. Since the discovery of penicillin any number of other organisms have been found to excrete substances that are bactericidal or bacteriostatic, and these substances form the ever-expanding list of antibiotics. The antibiotics are useful for treating a great number of diseases. Some are administered several ways; others can be given by only one route; still others can be given by a few means, but there is usually one preferred method.

Some antibiotics are useful in the treatment of infections caused by only one or a limited number of organisms. Other preparations can be used for a much greater number of conditions caused by a variety of microorganisms. These latter are called "broad spectrum antibiotics."

The selection of the antibiotic or other anti-infective drug by the physician in any specific case depends upon many factors such as known sensitivities of the patient to a particular drug, the type of organism involved and a selective sensitivity test of the organism. A culture of the organism is tested with a number of anti-infective drugs to determine which will be most effective in destroying the organism.

PENICILLIN

The Drug. Penicillin is still the drug of choice in a wide variety of conditions (III-2). Penicillin, like most of the sulfonamide drugs, is most effective against the gram-positive organisms and the pathogenic Neisseria. It is useful, as well, in the treatment of certain diseases caused by spirochetes. Consequently, diseases caused by the pyogenic organisms—streptococcus, staphylococcus, pneumococcus, gonococcus and meningococcus—as well as syphilis, diphtheria, tetanus and many other diseases may be successfully treated with penicillin.

Physical and Chemical Properties. The basic chemical form of penicillin is a thiazolidine ring connected with a beta lactam ring to which is attached a side chain. This last moiety varies with the different forms of the drug. Penicillin is produced by the mold, *Penicillium chrysogenum*, which is the naturally occurring drug. It is used in this form, but is also changed (semisynthetic) by various means to increase its effectiveness. It can be entirely synthetic. Most of the changes are in the side chains, not in the basic rings.

Penicillin is prepared in a number of compounds, of which the potassium and sodium salts are the most common. It also exists in several natural types: G, F, O, X and K. Type G is the most effective and is therefore more commonly used than the others.

Penicillin is soluble in water and in body fluids, but the solubility of the various preparations varies considerably.

Action. The action of the penicillins in the body is imperfectly understood, but they are believed to block the synthesis of the bacterial cell wall. They are not effective against viruses or protozoa.

Therapeutic Uses. Penicillin is the drug of choice in most diseases caused by gram-positive bacteria (e.g., pneumonia, bacterial endocarditis, streptococcal sore throat and puerperal fever). It is also effective against infection caused by gram-negative cocci (gonorrhea) and spirochetes (syphilis and yaws). It is used in viral diseases to prevent complications of secondary infection by gram-positive bacteria.

Absorption and Excretion. Penicillin is not metabolized by the body. Some preparations—penicillin V, especially—combine with blood proteins, thereby losing some of their effectiveness. In its naturally occurring form, penicillin is poorly absorbed from the gastrointestinal tract. However, some of the newer semisynthetic forms are readily absorbed and adequate blood levels can be obtained from oral administration. Since penicillin is not metabolized by the body, it is excreted unchanged by the kidneys.

Most penicillins are widely distributed throughout the body. Some, however, do not enter the cerebrospinal fluid.

Preparations and Dosages. To make the discussion of the penicillins easier, it is best to separate them into groups according to their activity against susceptible organisms. Some newer preparations have a much broader spectrum of activity than the original natural penicillin.

Only representative preparations will be given here. For additional information see Current Drug Handbook.

Group 1. These are the naturally occurring penicillins, types F, G, K, O and X which differ in side effects only, and the synthetic penicillin V. Of these, only types G, O and V are available in the United States and only G and V in Canada. Penicillin G is the most effective of the group. It is available in sodium and potassium salts. Procaine penicillin G, U.S.P., B.P. 200,000 to 1,200,000 units q 12 to 24 h I.M. (Note B.P. gives dosage in milligrams. Approximate equivalent is 400,000 units equals 250 mg.) This is a penicillin modified to prolong its effectiveness.

Phenoxymethyl penicillin, U.S.P., B.P. (Penicillin V) 200,000 to 800,000 units oral q.i.d. This is a synthetic penicillin.*

Group 2. These are the semisynthetic penicillins which are phenoxyalkyl derivatives. Phenethicillin is the main drug in this group. It is well absorbed orally. Even though higher blood levels can be obtained,

*The student should review in Chapter 5 the material on unit dosage if she is unsure of the meaning.

these compounds have reduced activity against susceptible organisms as compared with penicillin G.

Potassium phenethicillin, N.F. (phenoxyethylpenicillin [C]) 125 to 250 mg. q.i.d. orally.

Carbenicillin disodium (Geopen; Pyropin [C]) 200 to 500 mg. per kg. per day I.V. in divided doses or by continuous drip. It is also prepared in tablet form for oral administration.

Carbenicillin indanyl sodium (Geocillin) 1 to 2 tablets four times a day orally. Each tablet contains 382 mg. of carbenicillin.

These preparations are used mainly in infections due to *proteus* or *pseudomonas* organisms or to *E. coli.* Carbenicillin should not be mixed in the same intravenous solution as gentamicin (Garamycin) because it will inactivate the gentamicin. The same applies to kanamycin (Kantrex) or colistin (Coly-mycin), since both drugs are inactivated in the latter case.

Group 3. This group includes compounds designed to be effective against penicillinase-producing organisms such as resistant staphylococci. Penicillinase acts to hydrolyze the penicillin molecule and these compounds, because of their chemical composition with substituted side chains, delay or reduce the action of the penicillinase enzyme long enough for the drugs to have their bactericidal effects. These drugs have only about one-tenth the activity of penicillin G against susceptible organisms and are not effective against sensitive gram negative organisms such as the Neisseria.

Methicillin sodium, U.S.P. (meticillin [C]) 1 Gm. q 4 to 6 h I.M. or I.V.

Oxacillin sodium 250 to 500 mg. q.i.d. orally, 250 to 1000 mg. q 4 to 6 h I.M. or I.V.

Nafcillin sodium (Unipen) 250 to 500 mg. q 4 to 6 h orally, 500 to 1000 mg. q 4 h I.V., 500 mg. q 6 h I.M.

Group 4. The fourth group of penicillins is known as the cephalosporins. They have an amino acid side chain, greatly increasing the spectrum of their activity. They are effective not only against the usual organisms susceptible to penicillin but in addition can be used for infections caused by many other organisms such as *Streptococcus faecalis, Hemophilus influenzae* and some strains of *Escherichia coli, Salmonella, Shigella* and *Proteus.*

There are no specific contraindications for the use of these drugs, but they should not be given to individuals known to be sensitive to penicillin. Cephaloridine is used with caution in cases of known renal damage.

Because of their increased activity, these drugs are used frequently. However, excessive dosage should be avoided. It is recommended that for cephaloridine the dosage should not exceed 4 Gm. per day, because of the possibility of renal tubular necrosis. With cephalothin not more than 12 Gm. per day should be used. For specific directions, the commercial brochure should be consulted.

Ampicillin (Omnipen, Penbritin, Polycillin) 250 to 1000 mg. q 6 h I.M. or I.V. (This is not a true cephalosporin, but it has similar activity.)

Cephaloridine (Loridine, Caporin, Cephalomycin [C]) 250 to 1000 mg. I.M. or I.V. 2 to 4 times a day.

Cephalothin (Keflin) 500 to 1000 mg. q 4 h I.M., 2 to 6 Gm. I.V. daily.

Cephalixin monohydrate (Keflex) 250 mg. to 1.0 Gm. orally q 6 h.

Cephaloglycin dihydrate (Kafocin) 250 to 500 mg. orally q.i.d. for urinary tract infections only.

The cephalosporin drugs are all semisynthetic derivatives of Cephalosporin C, derived from Cephalosporium sp. They are broad spectrum antibiotics used in the treatment of a variety of diseases, especially urinary infections, since most of the preparations are excreted either unchanged or as active metabolites. If the patient is sensitive to penicillin, care should be taken in giving the cephalosporins because cross-sensitivity occurs in some cases. If at all possible, a sensitivity test of the organism should be performed before any one of these drugs is used. Toxicity varies with the different drugs. Those given orally may cause gastrointestinal disturbances. When the drugs are given intramuscularly, pain at the point of injection is not uncommon. Refer to the Current Drug Handbook for further details.

THE NURSE

Mode of Administration. Penicillin is marketed in an endless number of preparations and is administered in any number of ways. For severe infections intramuscular or intravenous injection is the preferred route since the desired blood level can be maintained best by this method. When the drug is given orally much larger dosages are required as absorption is incomplete. Blood levels are more difficult to maintain because individuals differ in their ability to absorb the drug by the oral route. However, for home use and when the infection is not too severe the oral route is used. With the antibiotics, as with the sulfonamides, regular and punctual administration is important so as to maintain the proper blood level. In giving the patient these intramuscular preparations, especially when they are given at frequent intervals, the nurse must be careful to indicate on the chart the exact site at which the injection was given. This should prevent another nurse from giving an injection in the same spot. This is especially important for the emaciated or elderly patient. It is also very important to be sure the drug is given intramuscularly and not intravenously, since the intravenous administration of some intramuscular preparations is very dangerous and should always be carefully avoided. The subcutaneous administration of an intramuscular preparation is not so dangerous as the intravenous administration, but it can cause a "sterile abscess" or a very sore area.

While penicillin is most commonly given intramuscularly for systemic effect, it is available for oral use in both tablet and liquid form. These preparations are given at regular and usually frequent intervals. Unless the physician directs otherwise, the doses are given night and day, with the patient being awakened for the night doses.

Side Effects, Toxicity and Treatment. Penicillin is a biologic product and produces in some patients an allergic reaction which varies from some stinging or burning sensation at the point of contact to a severe dermatitis or even anaphylactic shock and death. The nurse should be on the watch for symptoms of allergic reactions. It is also important to relay to the physician any information gained concerning previous reactions the patient may have had.

Occasionally these preparations will cause gastrointestinal disturbances (the most common of which is diarrhea) and, if symptoms of such disorders occur, the physician should be notified. The drug should not be stopped until the doctor gives specific orders to do so, since he will usually change the method of administration, rather than discontinue the drug entirely. In very high dosage some preparations may cause bone marrow depression; this has been reported with methicillin. Occasional cases of renal involvement have been noted.

Penicillin, when applied locally or topically, may induce an allergic reaction. For this reason, many physicians avoid this method of application. Another antibiotic is used, reserving penicillin for what are often more serious, systemic diseases. Penicillin may at times be given as an aerosol for diseases of the respiratory tract. If so, it is usually combined with other medications and given by nebulizer, with oxygen or by use of the intermittent positive pressure apparatus.

The dosage of penicillin varies widely according to the preparation, mode of administration and purpose. Because of the tendency of organisms to build up a resistance to the drug, the initial dose of penicillin is often very high, with the subsequent doses either the same or much less. Some physicians order only one large dose of penicillin and, if the symptoms persist, another drug is used. Because of this tendency of the organism to build up resistance to penicillin, the drug should be reserved for those conditions which *require* its use.

Penicillinase (Neutrapen) is a biologic product which is used to neutralize (inactivate) penicillin in the treatment of allergic reactions to penicillin. It has proved to be most effective in the treatment of pruritus. It aids in overcoming delayed reactions but is ineffective in acute, emergency conditions. It has no preventive properties.

Interactions. The action of penicillin is enhanced by aspirin, phenylbutazone and probenecid because of displacement from the binding sites. It is inhibited by tetracycline because of interference with the mechanism of action. Penicillin is antagonized by chloramphenicol and antacids.

Patient Teaching. Ordinarily, there is no great need for patient teaching: most patients are already acquainted with the drug. Some of their information, however, may be incorrect. If the patient is to take the drug orally at home, the nurse should stress the importance of taking the medication exactly as prescribed. If the occasion arises, the nurse should inform the patient that surplus tablets or capsules should not be used for any other illness or given to another individual without specific direction of the prescribing physician. The patient should be aware of the possibility of intestinal disturbance following ingestion of penicillin.

THE PATIENT. Penicillin, being a biological product, can cause allergic reactions. The reaction, if it occurs, is more apt to occur after more than one dose of the drug has been taken. Early stages of allergic reaction may be overlooked; subsequent stages can lead to death. It is important that the doctor be apprised of any untoward reaction, however slight.

STREPTOMYCIN

(See Current Drug Handbook.)

THE DRUG. Streptomycin is derived from an organism called *Streptomyces griseus*. Streptomycin was introduced after penicillin and was of much interest as it extended the spectrum of action to include the gram-negative and the acid-fast bacteria (III-2, 3).

Physical and Chemical Properties. Streptomycin is an organic base which contains an amino and a sugar group. It is made up of three component parts as follows: streptidine, streptose and n-methyl-l-glucosamine. Streptomycin and its salts are soluble in water and in body fluids.

Action. Extensive research into the action of streptomycin continues. The latest hypothesis suggests that the drug interferes with the protein synthesis in the bacterial cell causing it to make proteins that are unusable. The filling of the cell with useless proteins to the exclusion of the useful ones eventually kills the cell. Some microorganisms develop tolerance to the drug rather quickly; others are slower in their efforts at resistance.

Therapeutic Uses. Streptomycin is used in the treatment of diseases caused by gram negative and acid fast bacteria including tuberculosis, leprosy, typhoid and paratyphoid fever, tularemia, plague and brucellosis. Streptomycin may be combined with penicillin in the treatment of conditions of mixed or undetermined origin.

Absorption and Excretion. Streptomycin is administered parenterally since it is poorly absorbed from the gastrointestinal tract, the intact skin or mucous membranes. It is widely diffused throughout the body in the extracellular fluid, except in the spinal fluid. It does not enter the healthy meninges and in meningitis enters only incompletely so that it is necessary to introduce the drug intrathecally. Some streptomycin is bound to the blood proteins. Maximum blood levels are reached in two to four hours. After this the level gradually drops and is much lower by the end of eight hours. Excretion is slow but is usually complete by the end of 24 hours. Streptomycin is excreted unchanged, unless there is severe renal impairment.

Preparations and Dosages. To overcome streptomycin's toxicity, a synthetic preparation called dihydrostreptomycin was developed. However, it proved in some ways to be more toxic than the parent compound and has gradually been abandoned. The preparation now used is streptomycin sulfate, U.S.P., B.P., given 0.5 to 2.5 Gm. I.M. daily. This amount may be divided into four or six doses or given in one dose depending upon conditions. The amount and frequency of administration are reduced as soon as possible due to toxicity.

THE NURSE

Mode of Administration. Streptomycin is given intramuscularly, except in meningitis when it is administered intrathecally. Since injections are commonly repeated, it is essential that the sites of needle placement be changed. Keep a record of the sites used so that no one locus is used too often. Sometimes, streptomycin is given orally preoperatively to decrease the bacterial count in intestinal tract surgery. If required to give streptomycin often, the nurse is advised to wear rubber or plastic gloves, since severe dermatitis has been reported from the handling of the drug.

Side Effects, Toxicity and Treatment. Streptomycin, moderately toxic, produces adverse symptoms running the gamut from headache to severe blood dyscrasias. However, two toxic symptoms resulting from its use are more common than the others. One is an allergic reaction. Especially vulnerable are those who have had streptomycin previously and those with a history of allergies. As in other allergies, the symptoms are skin rashes, headache, nausea, vomiting and drug fever. In severe cases anaphylactic shock may occur.

The second common adverse reaction to

streptomycin occurs in the vestibulocochlear portions of the inner ear. Symptoms are dizziness, vertigo, tinnitus, and partial or complete loss of hearing. Streptomycin is more apt to cause vestibular disorders while dihydrostreptomycin exerts its adverse action mainly on the cochlear portion of the inner ear. Symptoms may appear either during or after use of the drug. Either form of the drug may cause symptoms resembling Meniere's disease: dizziness, vertigo, lessening of auditory acuity. One dose of dihydrostreptomycin has been known to cause permanent deafness. It is wise to test the patient's hearing before starting streptomycin therapy and frequently during its administration. At any sign of hearing loss, the drug should be discontinued.

It is essential that the nurse report any adverse symptoms, since reducing dosage will usually be sufficient to control them. This, of course, does not apply to allergic reactions since even a small dose of the drug can cause this.

Contraindications. Streptomycin is contraindicated in severe renal impairment.

Patient Teaching. Patient teaching is especially important when medication is to be continued for extended periods, as in tuberculosis or leprosy. The patient must understand that adverse symptoms may occur and that *any* unusual condition, no matter how trivial, should be reported to the physician immediately. The nurse should convey to the patient the importance of reporting immediately to the physician any sign of dizziness or loss of hearing. Of course, the nurse should not frighten the patient with long, detailed enumerations of potential symptoms. She should, however, remind him to communicate frequently with his doctor and to report any new condition that develops.

THE PATIENT. The nurse should alert the patient that he may feel depressed during the first few days of streptomycin therapy; the symptom, however, is transient, disappearing within a short time. A solid advantage of this drug is its allowing the patient, who might otherwise be confined to bed, to be ambulatory. In combating tuberculosis and leprosy, the drug is commonly combined with other compounds, all of which are essential, all of which enhance the efficacy of the others. The patient should expect no miracles; like penicillin, the drug is a valuable and important antibiotic, but it is not a cure-all.

THE TETRACYCLINES

(See Current Drug Handbook.)

THE DRUGS. The tetracycline drugs are the result of extensive research into the antimicrobial action of the secretions (excretions) of various soil bacteria. Some are semisynthetic, but all are derived directly or indirectly from various members of the *Streptomyces* organisms. The tetracyclines are known as broad spectrum antibiotics, being effective against a large variety of organisms.

Physical and Chemical Properties. Similar in chemical formula, they are congeneric derivatives of polycyclic naphthacenecarboxamide. The parent drugs are not readily soluble in water, but their salts are. All are stable in dry form, but relatively unstable in liquid form. Raising the pH and temperature increases the instability of these drugs. Demethylchlortetracycline is more stable than others of this group.

Action. The exact mechanism of the action of these drugs is not known. They may interfere with the synthesis of the organism's proteins. In moderate dosage they are bacteriostatic; in large doses they may be bactericidal.

Therapeutic Uses. The tetracyclines are used singly or in combination with other antibiotics such as penicillin in a large number of infections. Their effectiveness varies with the preparations, but all have wide antimicrobial activity. The tetracyclines have been used effectively in the Rickettsial diseases such as Rocky Mountain Spotted fever, typhus, Q fever; those diseases caused by the "large viruses" such as psittacosis, lymphogranuloma venereum; mycoplasma infections; atypical pneumonia; bacterial diseases, brucellosis, tularemia; some infections caused by the hemolytic streptococci and staphylococci, subacute bacterial endocarditis, gonorrhea, some infections of the urinary tract, the eyes and the peritoneum; chancroid; and various diseases caused by other organisms such as granuloma inguinale, syphilis and amebiasis.

Absorption and Excretion. These drugs are readily absorbed from the gastrointestinal tract, especially from the stomach and the upper portion of the small intestines. The absorption from the lower part of the small intestines is much less and there is almost no absorption from the colon. The tetracyclines are widely distributed throughout the body fluids, but there is relatively less in the spinal fluid than in the others. The tetracycline drugs pass the placental barrier and thus may affect the fetus. Therapeutic blood level is reached, after oral administration, in roughly two to four hours and persists for about six hours. Considerable amounts of the drugs are extracted by the liver and excreted into the bile, although some is reabsorbed. Most of the drug is removed by the kidneys, a lesser amount in the feces. Because of the action of the liver, effects of these drugs may continue for some time after administration has stopped. Calcium tends to decrease the absorption of these drugs.

Preparations and Dosages

Chlortetracycline hydrochloride, N.F., B.P. Aureomycin. 250 to 500 mg. q 6 h orally or I.V.

Demethylchlortetracycline, N.F., B.P. (Declomycin) 150 to 300 mg. q 6 h orally.

Doxycycline hyclate (Vibramycin) 200 mg. first day then 100 mg. q 12 h, 100 mg. q 12 h orally or I.V.

Methacycline hydrochloride, N.F. (Rondomycin) 150 mg. q 6 h or 300 mg. q 12 h orally.

Minocycline (Minocin), initial dose 200 mg., then 100 mg. q 12 h orally or I.V. Dosage should not exceed 400 mg. in 24 hours.

Oxytetracycline hydrochloride, U.S.P., B.P. (Terramycin) 250 to 500 mg. q 6 h orally, 100 to 250 mg. q 6 h I.M., 250 to 500 mg. q 12 to 24 h I.V.

Rolitetracycline, N.F. (Syntetrin, Syntetrex [C]) 150 to 350 mg. q 6 h I.M. 350 to 700 mg. o.d. I.V.

Tetracycline hydrochloride, U.S.P., B.P. (Achromycin, Cefrecycline [C]) 250 to 500 mg. q 6 h orally, I.M., I.V. Also used as an ophthalmic ointment.

Tetracycline phosphate complex (Panmycin phosphate, Sumycin, Tetrex) 250 to 500 mg. q 6 h orally, I.M.

THE NURSE

Mode of Administration. The tetracyclines are given by many means such as intramuscular, intravenous, in the eyes, and so forth, but the main route is oral. It is extremely important that these drugs be given at the times ordered since maintaining blood level is essential. Most of the preparations produce microbiologically resistant forms; the process is accelerated by a lowering of the amount of the drug in the body fluids. When repeated doses are given intramuscularly, the locus of injection must be changed, since the drugs are irritating to the tissues. In giving these drugs intravenously, infiltration must be avoided for the same reason.

Side Effects, Toxicity and Treatment. The tetracyclines are not without side effects and toxicity. Side effects vary from one preparation to another, the variations being more of degree than of kind. Main symptoms are associated with the gastrointestinal system. Heartburn, nausea and vomiting, which may occur early in the administration of the drug, can usually be avoided by giving the medicine with food. Diarrhea is a common symptom, occurring either during the course of the treatment or several days after the drug has been stopped. These drugs tend to change the flora of the intestinal tract. Thus toxic bacteria and fungi are allowed to grow excessively in the absence of the normal microorganisms. For the overgrowth, some other drugs may be used depending upon type of organisms in the overgrowth and the condition of the patient.

As with any such preparations, the tetracyclines can cause an allergic reaction. These are treated as any allergy is treated.

Intravenous therapy with the tetracyclines can cause thrombophlebitis, especially if repeated doses are given in the same area.

With prolonged usage some blood changes have been reported; however, severe granulocytopenia does not develop and blood changes are reversed when the drug is discontinued. In some cases, discoloration of the teeth has been observed when the drug was used during the development of the teeth pre or postnatal. For this reason, these drugs are used cautiously in the latter part of pregnancy and during early childhood.

Demethylchlortetracycline may cause light sensitivity producing mild to severe skin rashes if the patient is exposed to the sun during therapy.

These drugs are used with caution in renal or hepatic disorders. High dosages for extended periods can cause hepatic impairment.

Interactions. The tetracyclines are inhibited by di- and trivalent ions forming an inactive complex. They antagonize penicillin because of their mechanism of action. Tetracycline is incompatible with methicillin in the same intravenous solution. Antacids inhibit the action of tetracycline.

Contraindications. Contraindications, as previously noted, include renal or hepatic disorders, late pregnancy and early childhood.

Patient Teaching. The patient on these drugs at home should take them exactly as prescribed. Any untoward symptoms, no matter how trivial, should be reported to the attending physician.

The Patient. The tetracyclines are among the so-called "wonder" drugs and in many cases do produce wonders—almost miracles. However, they are not "cure alls." They will not in all cases produce the miraculous cures the patient may wish for and this can be very depressing. Some patients know of the value of these drugs, but may not realize their limitations. They may be very upset if their physician does not order one of these drugs for them when they or their friends think that he should have done so. The nurse can be helpful in explaining these things to the patient.

CHLORAMPHENICOL. Chloramphenicol (Chloromycetin), originally obtained from *Streptomyces venezuelae* but now produced synthetically, is a broad-spectrum antibiotic which is readily absorbed after oral administration, but can be given intravenously if necessary. Chloramphenicol reaches a peak concentration in the blood in from one to three hours after oral administration. Chloramphenicol is distributed throughout the body, but the concentration differs; it is highest in the liver and kidneys and lowest in the brain and the cerebrospinal fluid.

The dosage rate for chloramphenicol is relatively high. For children and adults it should be 50 mg. per kilogram of body weight per day in divided doses given every six hours. This dose should be reduced in persons with impaired liver or renal function. Care should be exercised in the use of chloramphenicol in very young or premature infants and the dose should not exceed 25 mg. per kilogram per day. Toxic reactions have occurred in premature infants and full term babies under two weeks of age.

The side effects of this drug have received a great deal of publicity and have occurred from both short- and long-term therapy. When the drug is used, adequate blood studies should be carried out. The following warning is given by the manufacturer:

WARNING

Serious and even fatal blood dyscrasias (aplastic anemia, hypoplastic anemia, thrombocytopenia, granulocytopenia) are known to occur after administration of chloramphenicol. Blood dyscrasias have occurred after both short and prolonged therapy with this drug. Bearing in mind the possibility that such reactions may occur, chloramphenicol should be used only for serious infections caused by organisms which are susceptible to its bacterial effects. Chloramphenicol should not be used when other less potentially dangerous agents will be effective, or in the treatment of trivial infections such as colds, influenza, or viral infections of the throat, or as a prophylactic agent.

PRECAUTIONS

It is essential that adequate blood studies be made during treatment with this drug. While blood studies may detect early peripheral blood changes, such as leukopenia or granulocytopenia, before they become irreversible, such studies cannot be relied on to detect bone marrow depression prior to the development of aplastic anemia.

There are other side effects from chloramphenicol, such as gastrointestinal disturbances, neurotoxic reactions and dermatitis, both vesicular and maculopapular.

The use of chloramphenicol is still justified in certain conditions. These are mainly in the treatment of typhoid fever and other salmonella infections and certain rickettsial diseases, such as scrub or epidemic typhus and Rocky Mountain spotted fever. It is also recommended for use in certain urinary tract infections such as those caused by *Escherichia coli, Aerobacter aerogenes, Pseudomonas aeruginosa, Proteus* species, *Streptococcus faecalis* and *Staphylococcus aureus.* Most physicians feel that, due to its toxicity, chloramphenicol should be reserved for severe infections that do not respond to other therapy.

ANTIFUNGAL ANTIBIOTICS. *Amphotericin B* (Fungizone) is a polyene type antibiotic which can be used to treat systemic fungal infections. It can be given only by intravenous administration as it is not absorbed to any appreciable degree on oral use. Demonstrable blood levels are seen 18 hours after intravenous injection, indicating that it is slowly excreted by the kidneys.

The drug is used for disseminated mycotic or protozoal infections, such as coccidioidomycosis, cryptococcosis, candidiasis (moniliasis), histoplasmosis, South American leishmaniasis and North and South American blastomycosis.

The drug is given by slow intravenous infusion over a period of approximately six hours. The recommended concentration for the infusion is 0.1 mg. of the drug in each ml. (cc.) of the fluid. Dosage range is from 0.25 mg. per kilogram of body weight at the start of therapy to 1.0 mg. per kilogram. In rare cases as much as 1.5 mg. per kilogram can be given provided no toxic symptoms have occurred. The dosage under no circumstances should exceed this amount.

The side effects seen with the administration of amphotericin B include headache, vomiting and rise in blood urea nitrogen and nonprotein nitrogen.

Griseofulvin (Fulvicin, Grifulvin) is an orally effective agent used for the treatment of certain types of fungal infection, especially the ringworm infections of the hair, skin, and nails. It has the following spectrum of action: It is effective against *Trichophyton rubrum, T. tonsurans, T. mentagrophytes, T. interdigitalis, T. verrucosum, T. sulphureum, T. schoenleini, Microsporum audouini, M. canis, M. gypseum* and *Epidermophyton floccosum.* It is not effective against the Candida, tinea versicolor or the systemic fungal infections.

Griseofulvin is absorbed from the gastrointestinal tract and is deposited in the keratin of the skin, hair and nails. It is deposited in a concentration sufficient to be fungistatic. Cure is complete only when the keratin containing viable but inactive fungi is gradually exfoliated and replaced by noninfected tissue. It must be remembered that griseofulvin is fungistatic and not fungicidal.

The drug is given in daily doses of 1.0 gram and continued for four to six months, depending on the location of the infection and the rate of growth of the infected part.

Interactions. Griseofulvin is potentiated by the concurrent use of diphenylhydantoin (Dilantin). The exact mechanism of action is not known. Phenylbutazone (Butazolidin), the barbiturates and orphenadrine decrease the effectiveness of griseofulvin. Griseofulvin decreases the activity of the oral anticoagulants because of enzyme induction.

Nystatin (Mycostatin) is another polyene antibiotic which is used locally as a cream, ointment and dusting powder and vaginally as a tablet. It is also available in a suspension for the treatment of children with thrush in the mouth. It is used mainly in treating local mycotic infections caused by *Candida (Monilia) albicans.*

VARIED ANTIBIOTICS. There are any number of other antibiotics. The following are some of the more commonly used ones. The student is referred to Current Drug Handbook.

Neomycin, N.F. (Mycifradin) is an organic base containing an amino sugar. It has a spectrum of activity similar to that of streptomycin. Since it is not absorbed after oral administration it is used primarily for the antisepsis of the intestinal tract before surgery or for local application in the form of ointments, powder or solution. It is not only ototoxic but also has nephrotoxicity when given by injection. For these reasons its use is limited to treatment of resistant infections, such as penicillin-resistant staphylococcic infections or severe gram-negative infections which fail to respond to the less toxic agents. Dosage is 0.5 to 1.0 gram orally or 200 to 250 mg. intramuscularly. Neomycin, if given with oral penicillin, tends to block the absorption of the penicillin.

Kanamycin, U.S.P. (Kantrex) is another organic antibiotic containing an amino sugar, and derived from *Streptomyces kanamyceticus.* A broad spectrum antibiotic whose range is closer to streptomycin and neomycin than to penicillin, it is effective against gram-negative and gram-positive organisms, acid-fast bacteria and *Neisseria.* Resistance develops slowly except against the acid-fast organisms, when it occurs rather rapidly. Kanamycin is used to combat tuberculosis, intestinal infections caused by *Salmonella* and *Shigella*, preoperative intestinal and postoperative peritoneal sepsis and infections resistant to other antibiotics.

Kanamycin is poorly absorbed from the gastrointestinal tract and is given orally only to achieve local antisepsis. After intramuscular injection, the drug is rapidly absorbed, reaching a peak blood level in about one hour and remaining in the body in therapeutically active amounts for about eight hours. It diffuses into all body fluids except the cerebrospinal fluid, and is excreted by the kidneys.

In the ordinary dosage levels the incidence of side effects (nausea, vomiting and diarrhea) is not high. However, kanamycin is not without danger. It, like streptomycin, is both ototoxic and neurotoxic, and can cause irreversible damage to the eighth cranial nerve. If the drug is to be used for any length of time a pre-therapy hearing test with frequent tests during the course of the treatment should be given. Any evidence of hearing impairment or ear disorder should cause immediate cessation of the drug. Kanamycin should not be used for patients with renal impairment, since it will not be excreted properly and repeated doses can cause a toxic blood level. It is wise to consult the commercial brochure for other warnings and information before administering this drug.

Dosage: 1 Gm. q 4 to 6 h oral, 15 mg./kg. I.M. (not more than 1.5 Gm. per day) in divided doses, Kanamycin is also prepared for intravenous and intracavity use. Kanamycin should not be mixed in the same intravenous solution as carbenicillin (Geopen) since this will inactivate both drugs.

Erythromycin (Erythrocin, Ilotycin) is an antibiotic used as a substitute for penicillin in patients who have sensitivities to penicillin and for organisms that are resistant to that drug. It is mainly effective against gram-positive bacteria. It is well absorbed orally and well distributed throughout the body with the exception of the spinal fluid. This drug is relatively free from serious side effects. Gastrointestinal disturbances are sometimes seen with dosage greater than 0.5 gram. Usual dosage is 100 to 250 mg. orally every six hours. Erythromycin is also available for I.M. use (100 mg. q 8 to 12 h), but this form is very irritating and painful to the patient.

Polymyxin B (Aerosporin) is an antibiotic derived from *Bacillus aerosporus* or *B. polymyxa* and is a polypeptide type antibiotic. It is effective against gram-negative bacteria such as *Escherichia coli* and some strains of *Pseudomonas.* It is not absorbed to any great extent after oral administration. In order to treat systemic infections it must be given by intramuscular or intravenous injection. It does not appear in the spinal fluid after such injection and is rapidly excreted in the urine. It is used only when less toxic agents are not effective. It is also used in irrigations and in ointments which are applied topically. The most frequent side effects encountered after systemic use are neurological; these include ataxia and paresthesias. The dose is 1.5 to 2.5 mg. per kilogram of body weight daily in three divided doses or 0.1 to 0.25 per cent when used topically.

Colistin (Coly-Mycin) and *Colistimethate* (Coly-Mycin injectible) are other polypeptides of the polymyxin group and are effective against the same organisms. They have the same type of side effects as polymyxin. Dosage is 100 to 200 mg., given either intramuscularly or intravenously. Children's dosage is 3 to 5 mg. per kilogram of body weight given orally for its effect on the intestinal flora. Colistin and carbenicillin should not be mixed in the same intravenous solution because this will cause inactivation of both drugs.

Gentamicin sulfate (Garamycin) is a bactericidal antibiotic effective against a wide variety of organisms including *Pseudomonas aeruginosa.* Patients receiving this drug should be under close clinical supervision because of its toxicity. It has been known to have ototoxicity, especially in patients with pre-existing renal impairment. It is administered intramuscularly 0.8-3.0 mg./kg. daily in divided doses usually t.i.d. or q.i.d. It is also prepared for intravenous administration. Administration should extend beyond 7 to 10 days only in severe cases. Gentamicin and carbenicillin should not be mixed in the same intravenous solution, since this will inactivate the gentamicin.

Bacitracin is also a polypeptide which has bacteriostatic effects against gram-positive organisms. It is poorly absorbed from the intestinal tract. It is used in ointments for local application and can be used for systemic infections when given by injection. The major toxicity seen with this antibiotic is renal tubular necrosis. Because of its toxicity, its parenteral use is limited to organisms which are resistant to other antibiotic therapy. The intramuscular dosage is 10,000 to 20,000 units.

Tyrothrycin (Soluthricin) is a polypeptide antibiotic made up of two polypeptides, gramicidin and tyrocidin. It is bactericidal to gram-positive organisms but it can only be used topically as it is hemolytic when given parenterally. It comes in ointments, creams, and solutions.

IT IS IMPORTANT TO REMEMBER

1. The distinctions between vaccines, toxoids, toxins and antitoxins.
2. The distinctions between active and passive immunity and also between natural and artificial immunity.
3. That a skin sensitivity test should be done before *any serum* is administered.
4. That human immune globulin (gamma globulin) contains the antibodies of not just one but many diseases.
5. That the number of diseases for which active immunization is possible is increasing so rapidly that the entire picture of communicable disease therapy is changing.
6. That the drugs listed in this chapter are only a representative few of the almost limitless number of substances used for the purpose of destroying harmful microorganisms.
7. That the various terms used have similar, but often definitely distinct, meanings and all should be understood.
8. That the term "antibiotic" has been given to a large number of drugs which are derived from living organisms. They are substances which an organism excretes or secretes which destroy other organisms.
9. That antibiotics appear to lose their effectiveness. Certain organisms gradually build up a resistance to a certain drug so that succeeding generations of the organism are unaffected by the medication.

TOPICS FOR STUDY AND DISCUSSION

1. What are the routine prophylactic drugs used in the school health program? Make a survey of your class (or the entire student body) to find out what preventives have been given to each individual. What reasons can you give for the variations? Why have some students had more than others?
2. Discuss the subject "All children entering the first grade in school should be immunized against poliomyelitis, diphtheria, measles and pertussis (whooping cough)." Be sure to present both the affirmative and the negative sides of the question.
3. Is immune serum globulin specific? That is, does it immunize against one disease only? Defend your answer.

   What type of immunity does immune serum globulin confer—active or passive? Defend your answer.
4. List some of the diseases which may be prevented by means of medicines. Were these diseases ever serious scourges? What effect have drugs had on longevity?
5. From either a medical or nursing history book try to locate the names of people who have aided in the prevention of diseases by positive means such as Jenner used. What effect have their discoveries had on the course of history?
6. Secure a list of the disinfectants and antiseptics used in the hospital in which you secure your experience.
   a. Are these trade names? If so look up the generic names and the active ingredients.
   b. What is the special value for each preparation? How and why is it used?
7. Have each student bring a list of the antiseptics and disinfectants found in her home. Repeat Topic 1 for this list. Separate the drugs into those used outside the human body and those used on the skin or mucous membranes.

8. An order for penicillin is 400,000 units I.M., O.D. The vial contains 10 ml. of penicillin 600,000 units per ml. How much should be given at each dose? How long will the vial last?

9. The nurse is to prepare 1 liter (1 quart) of saponated cresol solution 1/4 per cent strength. The stock solution is 5 per cent in strength. How should the nurse proceed?

BIBLIOGRAPHY

Books and Pamphlets

American Medical Association Council on Drugs, *Drug Evaluations*, Chicago, 1971, American Medical Association.
American Pharmaceutical Association National Formulary Board, *National Formulary, 13th Ed.*, Washington, D.C., 1970, American Pharmaceutical Association.
Beeson, P. B., and McDermott, W., *Cecil-Loeb Textbook of Medicine, 13th Ed.*, Philadelphia, 1971, W. B. Saunders Co.
Canadian Pharmaceutical Association, *Compendium of Pharmaceutical Specialties, 7th Ed.*, Toronto, 1972, Canadian Pharmaceutical Committee, Inc.
Chatton, M. J., Margen, S., and Brainerd, H., *Handbook of Medical Treatment, 12th Ed.*, Los Altos, California, 1970, Lange Medical Publications.
Committee of Revision, *United States Pharmacopeia, 18th Ed.*, Washington, D.C., 1970, Trustees of the United States Pharmaceutical Committee, Inc.
Conn, H. F., (Ed.), *Current Therapy, 1974*, Philadelphia, 1974, W. B. Saunders Co.
Duhamel, R., *The Food and Drug Act and Regulations 1964–1967* and *Amendments*, Ottawa, 1967, Queen's Printer, Controller of Stationery.
Falconer, M. W., Patterson, H. R., and Gustafson, E. A., *Current Drug Handbook, 1974–76*, Philadelphia, 1974, W. B. Saunders Co.
Goodman, L. S., and Gilman, A., *Pharmacological Basis of Therapeutics, 4th Ed.*, New York, 1970, The Macmillan Co.
Goth, A., *Medical Pharmacology, 6th Ed.*, St. Louis, 1972, The C. V. Mosby Co.
Lewis, A., *Modern Drug Encyclopedia*, New York, 1970, The Yorke Medical Group.
Sollman, T., *A Manual of Pharmacology, 8th Ed.*, Philadelphia, 1957, W. B. Saunders Co.

Journal Articles

Au William, Y. W., "Broad spectrum antibiotics," *Am. J. Nurs.* 64:10:105 (October, 1964).
Bodansky, M., and Perlman, D., "Peptide antibiotics," *Science* 163:3865:352 (1969).
Brachman, P. S., "Symposium on infection and the nurse," *Nurs. Clin. North Am.* 4:141 (December, 1968).
Ferguson, D., "Paréian and Listerian slants on infection in wounds," *Perspect. Biol. Med.* 14:1:63.
Gorini, L., "Antibiotics and the genetic code," *Sci. Am.* 214:102:109 (June, 1966).
Hillman, R. M., "Toward control of viral infections," *Science*, 164:3879:506 (1969).
Smith, M. I., "Death of staphylococci," *Sci. Am.* 218:2:84 (February, 1968).
Stewart, R. B., and Deal, W. B., "Streptococcal infections—The pharmacist's responsibilities," *J. Am. Pharm. Assoc.* NS 12:12:516 (December, 1972).
Utz, J., and Benson, M., "The systemic mycosis," *Am. J. Nurs.* 65:9:103 (September, 1965).
Watanabe, T., "Infectious drug resistance," *Sci. Am.* 217:6:19 (June, 1967).

CHAPTER 8

DRUGS USED FOR DIAGNOSTIC PURPOSES

CORRELATION WITH OTHER SCIENCES

I. ANATOMY AND PHYSIOLOGY

1. The gastric juice is secreted by various small glands in the mucous membrane lining the stomach. These glands secrete hydrochloric acid and certain enzymes such as pepsin, rennin and gastric lipase.

2. The kidney has many functions. One of the more important of these functions is the removal from the blood of poisonous or inert materials. It also aids in maintaining proper fluid balance.

3. A substance introduced into the venous circulation will eventually be carried by the blood stream to all parts of the body. It will go first to the heart, then through the pulmonary circulation, back to the heart and then out through the arterial system to the various body tissues.

II. CHEMISTRY

1. The solubility of any substance depends upon many factors. Materials soluble in one solvent may be insoluble in another. Each element or compound differs from every other in this respect.

2. A catalyst is a substance that initiates or alters the rate of a chemical reaction without being changed as a result of the reaction. Enzymes are proteins produced by living organisms that mediate biologic chemical reactions and are frequently described as "biological catalysts."

IV. PHYSICS

1. X-rays, discovered by Wilhelm Konrad Roentgen, are invisible rays which penetrate certain substances but not others.

2. A radioactive element or compound is one that gives off invisible chemically active rays. Some elements, such as radium, are naturally radioactive. Other elements can be made radioactive by exposure to the process of nuclear fission. Artificial radioactivity is usually of short duration. Each element remains radioactive for a definite length of time. During this time it will emit the rays. When it has lost one-half of this activity it is said to have reached its "half life."

V. PSYCHOLOGY

1. An individual is more cooperative, more willing to give aid, if he understands thoroughly the need for the effort. On the contrary, most people resist any procedure or any change in status for which they see no accruing benefit.

2. Memory is the ability to recall things which happened in the past. It is often dependent upon the pressure of the immediate thoughts. That is, if the thoughts are very insistent, very important, they push some past ideas into the subconscious mind. Sometimes it is possible to recall forgotten events by reducing the persistence of the present mental activity.

INTRODUCTION

Drugs used for diagnostic purposes, like those used for the prevention of disease, can be divided into two groups:

I. Those used outside the body
II. Those used directly on or in the human body

The first group is of interest mainly to the laboratory technician. Since these drugs and chemicals are used on various body secretions or specimens removed from the body, they are outside the general province of the nurse and will not be discussed in this chapter. The student will learn more of these later in this and other courses. Suffice to say that this would include all the drugs and the chemicals used by the pathologist in aiding the physician in making a correct diagnosis. The discussion here will be confined to those medicinal substances used diagnostically either on or in the human body.

CLASSIFICATION OF DIAGNOSTIC DRUGS

A. X-ray opaque drugs used to aid in the demonstration of abnormal conditions inside the body in organs not normally visible without this.

B. Drugs used to stimulate the secretion of various glandular substances.

C. Radioactive drugs used to locate diseased areas because of their affinity for specific body tissues.

D. Miscellaneous drugs which are used as diagnostic agents.

DRUGS USED IN CONJUNCTION WITH X-RAY. Certain substances such as *iodine, bromine, barium* and *bismuth* are opaque to the x-ray, and this property can be used to indicate the condition of internal structures that are not in themselves x-ray opaque (IV-1). Two conditions are essential before a drug can be used for this purpose: (1) the drug must be relatively harmless, and (2) it must be put into the organ or part that the physician wishes to examine.

In the preparation of the patient for these examinations the nurse plays a very important part since much of the success of the test depends upon the pre-examination orders being carried out exactly as directed. When the directions seem unduly severe to the patient, the nurse must explain the reason for each order and its importance to the success of the examination (V-1). The nurse is expected to secure the patient's cooperation in the carrying out of the pre-examination orders and also in the testing procedure itself. If the patient understands fully why the tests are being done, he will usually be much more cooperative.

For the visualization of the gastrointestinal tract, *barium sulfate* or *bismuth subcarbonate* is given orally, with the drug suspended in some liquid such as malted milk for actual administration. The tract must be empty for best results. It is usual, therefore, to give some form of catharsis and no food before the examinations are made. These drugs are not soluble in body fluids, hence are not absorbed and pass through the intestinal tract unchanged (II-1). By using the x-ray (fluoroscope or film) an outline of the alimentary tube, showing any abnormality in the contour of the tract and any abnormal positions of the organs, may be obtained. It is also possible to judge the speed of peristalsis by taking pictures at regular intervals.

If the doctor wishes to have a picture of the large bowel, the barium or bismuth is given by enema. When the drug is taken orally it is broken into small portions in its passage through the small intestines. It enters the large bowel in such small amounts that it does not fill the lumen of the bowel and thus does not show the abnormalities so well as is desired to secure an accurate diagnosis.

Many conditions may be demonstrated by a series of gastrointestinal x-rays (G.I. series). Among the more important are gastric and duodenal ulcers, carcinomas, adhesions, some forms of appendicitis, diverticuli and diverticulosis.

Iodine in various combinations is used to visualize parts of the body. The drug can be injected into many cavities or areas, and is excreted readily. It is used to test for possible disease of many internal organs.

When iodine is used for liver and gallbladder visualization, the drug containing the iodine is given either orally or intravenously, and an x-ray examination is made to determine: (1) speed and completeness of its removal by the liver, and (2) the excretory power of the gallbladder. By noting the dye in the gallbladder, stones may be detected. It is also possible, after giving the patient food containing fat, to determine whether the gallbladder is emptying normally. Thus, the one drug will often determine several factors. When the drug is given orally, it is usually administered at night after a light, fat-free supper. Exact orders, of course, may vary with the preparation and other conditions. Nothing else is given by mouth until after the x-rays have been taken in the morning, although water may be allowed for a part of the night. If the drug is to be administered by the intravenous route, it is given when the x-rays are to be taken.

Organic compounds of iodine used in the diagnosis of urinary disorders include: iodopyracet injection, iodohippurate sodium, iodomethamate sodium and other similar drugs. There are two methods employed for the administration of these:

1. The drug is given either orally or intravenously, the latter being the more common route. Since the iodine is normally rather rapidly excreted in the urine, the x-ray can be used to test the effectiveness of the kidneys. It will also show the contour of the urinary tract, and this aids in determining abnormalities. Since the rate of excretion by the normally functioning kidney is known, a comparison of the patient's rate will give a good indication of the effectiveness of the kidneys. As the drug is excreted it will, in turn, outline (partly or completely) the kidney pelves, the ureters and the bladder.

2. If the physician is more interested in possible kidney stones, neoplasms or other obstructions, the drug may be introduced by a catheter into the ureters. This will outline the kidney pelves and the ureters above the end of the catheter (providing a complete obstruction is not present) but will not, of course, demonstrate the secretory powers of the kidneys.

Various forms of iodized oils (iodized oil, iodobrassid and chloriodized oil) are used as x-ray opaque material to show abnormalities in other portions of the body such as the bronchial tree and the alveoli of the lungs, the brain and spinal cord and the gynecologic passages.

For the diagnosis of abnormal conditions of the lungs, such as bronchiectasis, emphysema or neoplasms, the drug is introduced into the bronchial tree by means of bronchoscopy.

To show lesions of the central nervous system, the drug may be injected by any of three methods. It may be introduced into the subarachnoid space by means of either a lumbar or a cisternal puncture or be placed directly into the ventricles of the brain by means of a ventricular puncture. The last is a major surgical procedure.

Iodine compounds are used to test the patency of the fallopian tubes. The drug is inserted into the body of the uterus under slight pressure. If the tubes are open, the fluid will pass through them into the abdominal (pelvic portion) cavity. The passage of the fluid can be watched by means of the fluoroscope. This is one test for female fertility. Refer to Chapter 28.

To test for abnormal conditions of the cardiovascular system angiograms are made. Drugs that may be used include diatrizoate (either the sodium or the magnesium salt) or sodium iothalamate. Diatrizoate, in a suitable medium, is also used for the diagnosis of various gastrointestinal conditions. For other uses, these compounds are usually introduced into the circulation by means of either a needle or a catheter in one of the superficial blood vessels.

Nursing Implications. The psychologic preparation of the patient for these procedures is most important. It is necessary for the nurse to explain to the patient, and to his relatives, the value of the examinations, why they are done and what help they will be in aiding the physician in the treatment of the condition (V-1). The nurse need not go into detail as to the procedure or try to explain the neurologic findings that may be secured. She should limit her discussion to a simple explanation of the reasons for the examination. The physician will give a more complete statement if he deems it advisable. Sometimes the nurse will be asked to amplify the doctor's remarks. This is because some doctors use terms that the patient does not understand. In this case, the nurse will as simply as possible give the physician's ideas in words which the patient, or his relatives, will understand. She should not try to explain anything that the physician has not covered or anything she herself does not clearly understand.

DRUGS USED TO STIMULATE THE SECRETION OF VARIOUS GLANDS. In the discussion of the x-ray opaque media, it was mentioned that the secretory power of the liver and the kidneys could be tested by this means. The iodine compound is removed from the blood stream by the gland, the rapidity and completeness of its removal being checked by the x-ray. It is thus possible to find out how well the organ is functioning by comparing the results with the known normal.

There are also other means of testing the functioning of the glands by the use of medicines. The secretory power of the stomach is determined in a number of ways. A test meal may be given, the amount and kind of food being carefully gauged. When the meal has been in the stomach a certain length of time, it is removed by gastric expression; the food is then examined for the type and amount of digestion that has taken place. Since no drug is used this is not a pharmacologic procedure.

Simple and accurate diagnostic procedures using drugs have been evolved which give the same information as the test meal. One method employs chemically pure *ethyl alcohol* 7 per cent. A stomach tube (small caliber) is passed, and a given amount of the alcohol (usually 2 ounces) is inserted. At stated intervals samples of the gastric contents are removed. These samples are then tested for the amount and type of acid they contain. The alcohol stimulates the secretion of water, acid and inorganic materials but not enzymes (II-2). It has been found that the determination of the power of the stomach mucosa to secrete acid is the best diagnostic indication of its condition (I-1). This method, though effective, has several disadvantages. Probably the main difficulty with the use of alcohol is the rapidity with which it is absorbed. This leads to the possibility of the patient's showing symptoms of inebriation, which naturally may be embarrassing to the patient, especially after the effects wear off. The nurse should explain the whole procedure to the patient and warn him of what may happen.

The more common drug used to test the secretory power of the stomach is *histamine* (either the *phosphate* or the *dihydrochloride*). Histamine is a natural body product thought to be the same as gastrin, which is secreted by the gastric mucosa. Histamine, a strong gastric stimulant, is given parenterally. Like alcohol, it does not stimulate secretion of the enzymes. Histamine does not produce symptoms of inebriation as does alcohol and it is relatively more efficient. The stomach contents are removed by gastric expression at the time or times ordered following the administration of the drug. This is a procedure needing special explanation to the patient as it is most unpleasant. The nurse must watch for the toxic symptoms of excess histamine which are not uncommon and include headache, dizziness, flushing of the face, local irritation at the site of the injection and sometimes a severe drop in blood pressure. The physician should be advised of the condition. Epinephrine (Adrenalin) with a hypodermic syringe should be ready. Betazole hydrochloride (Histalog) is a product similar to histamine and is used for the same purposes.

Quinine carbacrylic resin (azuresin [C]) is a synthetic drug used to estimate gastric acidity by testing the urine. It is given orally and stimulates the secretion of gastric juice. The urine is carefully collected according to specific directions and sent to the laboratory for analysis. By testing the urine it is possible to determine the amount of acid secreted by the gastric glands.

Several drugs are used to test kidney function in addition to the x-ray opaque drugs mentioned previously (I-2). One of those commonly used is a nonpoisonous dye called *phenolsulfonphthalein* (PSP). It is given parenterally, and then specimens of urine are taken by catheterization if necessary, at appointed intervals. Since the dye is excreted by the kidneys, the amount excreted by the patient can be compared with the amount expected from a normally functioning kidney. The results indicate the condition of the patient's kidneys, at least insofar as their excretory function is concerned (I-2). At times a retained catheter is inserted and many specimens are taken. In this case, the time the dye first appears is noted and is reported to the laboratory when the specimens are taken there.

There are other drugs that test a specific type of kidney function. *Para-aminohippuric acid* to test urine flow is one of these. *Mannitol* is used to test the functioning of the glomeruli. There are also kidney function tests performed without drugs similar to the test meal for gastric function. These will be covered in other courses.

Liver function tests have already been partially considered in the discussion of x-ray opaque media. However, there are other means of testing the efficiency of the liver. Of the drugs used the most common are the choline group. These include *Sodium dehydrocholate* and *dehydrocholic acid*. They are given intravenously and the rate of bile secretion noted. These drugs also test circulatory function. *Sulfobromophthalein sodium* (Bromsulphalein–BSP) is used to test the function of the liver. The drug is given intravenously, and the dose is usually estimated in relation to body surface area. Previously it was 2 mg. per kg. of body weight. A blood sample is taken at five and again at 30 minutes after the injection. The amount of the drug remaining in the blood is determined, and this is compared with known norms. The efficiency of the liver is then computed.

Another drug used to test liver function is indocyanine green (Cardio-Green). It is also used to test circulation time (considered later in this chapter). Indocyanine green is cleared from the circulation very rapidly, usually within twenty minutes. The parenchymal liver cells transfer nearly 100 per cent directly into the bile. The drug is not effective in testing any other excretory function. It is somewhat less accurate than sulfobromophthalein sodium in testing minimal liver damage, but appears to be more accurate in assessing severe liver damage. It is less toxic than sulfobromophthalein and takes less time for the testing process. Ear lobe densitometry is reported to be quite accurate and this avoids venipuncture. The solutions are unstable, so the drug must be prepared for each test. The dose is 0.1 to 0.5 mg. per kg. of body weight.

Another drug used to test glandular efficiency is cosyntropin (Cortrosyn). This is a synthetic preparation, structurally similar to corticotropin (ACTH), that is used to test adrenal cortex activity. It is used in any case of suspected adrenal cortical insufficiency. Since the drug is synthetic, it very seldom produces serum sensitivity reactions which occur much more often with either the animal or human corticotropin. The drug is given intravenously either by one injection or by infusion over a 6-hour period. The dose is 25 mg. dissolved in saline or glucose. It should not be dissolved in plasma or blood if the infusion method is used, since the enzymes in these substances might deactivate the drug. A control blood specimen is taken. The drug is then injected and a second blood specimen is taken exactly thirty minutes later. The two specimens are compared for cortisol level. If the infusion method is used, the blood specimen is taken at the end (after six hours) of the infusion. The following is considered to be the normal response.

1. Control plasma cortisol level should exceed 5 mcg. per 100 ml.
2. The thirty-minute level should show an increase of at least 7 mcg. per 100 ml. above the basal level.
3. The thirty-minute level should exceed 18 mcg. per 100 ml.

RADIOACTIVE TRACERS. Another diagnostic procedure involving drugs is the use of *radioactive isotopes* in the location of disease conditions within the human body (IV-2).

A discussion of the radioactive isotopes is beyond the scope of this book; however, a brief word of explanation is in order. A radioisotope is a chemical–usually an element–that has been made radioactive itself for a definite length of time. It is either attached to a compound, such as albumin, or given by itself. The isotope can be given to the patient and by use of a scanner, its travel through the body can be traced. There are certain criteria which must be met before the isotope can be of diagnostic value: First, the element must be one that is not harmful to the human body. Second, the isotope must retain its radioactivity long enough to be given to the patient and its progress traced. Third, the isotope must be made from an element that has an affinity for a definite type of body tissue. If the last condition is not met, the element will be evenly distributed throughout the body and will be valueless as a diagnostic agent. Several radioactive isotopes are used for diagnosis, and the number is increasing constantly. Many of these same isotopes are also used for the treatment of diseases, mainly neoplasms.

One of the more important uses for radioactive tracers is the location of tumors. Iodine, for example, has an affinity for the cells of the thyroid gland. Cells from a malignant tumor of the thyroid may be transmitted by way of the blood stream or the lymphatic system to another part of the body and there start a new tumorous growth. Since the iodine will be attracted to the thyroid tissue wherever it is in the body, the iodine will locate every tumor. The patient is given the radioactive iodine, usually orally, and its course through the body is traced with a scanner. It is possible to locate very accurately the position of any thyroid tumors—large or small. Even the size of the tumor can be fairly well judged.

Further discussion of the use of radioisotopes for treatment as well as diagnosis will be found in Chapter 29.

MISCELLANEOUS TESTS USED FOR DIAGNOSIS. Under this category are grouped a number of somewhat unrelated tests in which drugs are used for the purpose of diagnosis.

Various skin tests form one large segment of this group, and this is an area which is expanding rapidly. To many nurses such tests as the *Schick* and the *tuberculin* test will be familiar. Both are diagnostic skin tests, but their use is very different. The *Schick* test is a test which indicates susceptibility of the person to *diphtheria.* This test is not truly diagnostic since it determines susceptibility to, and not the presence of, the actual disease. The Schick test reaction occurs because the susceptible individual has no antibodies against the toxins secreted by the organism which causes diphtheria. A minute portion (0.1 ml.) of the toxin is injected into the layers of the skin. If the person's blood contains the antibodies they will neutralize the toxin and nothing will happen. This constitutes a negative result and indicates that the individual is resistant to diphtheria. If, however, the person's blood does not contain such antibodies the toxin will produce a local irritation. This is a positive reaction. It indicates that the individual being tested is susceptible to diphtheria and would, in all probability, contract the disease upon exposure. This is a very valuable test for screening of a group of people so that only those who actually need immunization receive it. There is also a skin test that is used to diagnose scarlet fever, the so-called *Schultz-Charlton* test. In this case a minute portion of the antitoxin is injected into the layers of the skin where the rash is heavy. If the rash is that of scarlet fever, the antitoxin will neutralize the toxin in the area surrounding the point of injection, and the rash will disappear. Since there are many rashes that look like the rash of scarlet fever this is of importance in differential diagnosis.

The tuberculin test differs from the foregoing in that it demonstrates a sensitivity to products of the tubercle bacillus resulting from previous infection which may have been subclinical. Protein extracts of the bacillus (tuberculin) are injected intradermally, through skin scratches or by the application of a "patch" which resembles a Band-Aid. A positive reaction is characterized by an area of induration and redness that appears 24 to 48 hours after the application. Patients who have not been infected are not sensitive to the product and thus are "tuberculin negative." Various preparations of the organisms are used. In all of them the organisms are killed or changed in such a way as to make the test accurate but prevent the development of the disease. These tests will be further discussed in other courses.

Tests of a similar nature are available for the diagnosis of trichinosis, brucellosis, lymphogranuloma venereum and certain fungal infections such as histoplasmosis, coccidioidomycosis, etc.

Tests for hypersensitivity are available for a large number of possible materials, including foods, pollens, animal products and miscellaneous substances. These are also intradermal skin tests in which a small portion of the allergen is introduced and the results noted. A wheal is a positive reaction, indicating that the patient is allergic to the substance. Refer to Chapter 25.

Antihuman chorionic gonadotropic serum (Gravindex) is a urine test for pregnancy. It depends upon the fact that the urine of pregnant women contains chorionic gonadotropin. The level of this hormone is usually sufficiently high to give a positive reading 13 days after the first missed period or 41 days after the onset of the last menstrual period. It is a relatively easy test to perform and takes only a short period of time. A false positive may result if the patient has either a hydatidiform mole or chorionepithelioma, since in these conditions a high level of chorionic gonadotropin is produced.

The location of lesions and/or foreign bodies in the eye is often very difficult. Many procedures are used to aid the doctor. One relatively simple one, which will quickly show local lesions, is the dropping into the eye of a weak solution of *fluorescein sodium.* This solution, because of its chemical content, will produce a greenish iridescent circle around the lesion or foreign body, thus marking its location clearly. It is, of course, of value only in surface conditions.

The diagnosis of various emotional (psychologic) disturbances involves many factors and, in most cases, drugs do not aid in such diagnoses. However, there is one instance where drugs are of value in arriving at the cause for the patient's psychotic or psychoneurotic behavior. The patient is given a *sedative*, usually a *barbiturate*, in an amount sufficient to make him drowsy but not enough to produce unconsciousness. While in this stage of narcosis, the patient will often reveal thoughts and feelings ordinarily locked in the subconscious mind, giving the skilled psychiatrist a clue to the background cause of the disturbance and guiding him to the correct type of treatment (V-2). It takes adroit questioning by a highly trained person to elicit valuable information, but it is many times very successful. Refer to Chapter 30.

In the discussion of the liver function test, the testing of circulatory adequacy was mentioned. Some of the drugs used for the testing of the function of the liver can be used to determine circulation time, but there are also drugs used specifically for this purpose. In one of these tests the drug Fluorescein potassium or sodium (Fluorescite) is used (I-3). The drug is introduced intravenously and then the room is darkened. A small light (flashlight or ophthalmoscope) is turned on, and in the dim illumination the drug will show as a soft greenish light in the lips. The time the light takes to appear after the drug is introduced intravenously is the patient's circulation time. For some patients this may be a very frightening experience, and the nurse must be ready and able to reassure the patient of the complete harmlessness of the procedure, not only before the test is started but also while it is being done.

Another circulatory test depends upon the feeling of excessive warmth. A compound composed of *magnesium sulfate*, *magnesium carbonate* and *copper sulfate* is given intravenously (I-3). It produces feelings of heat in the throat, perineum, hands and feet, in that order. The time, again, is accurately checked and the patient's time compared with the norm.

In the timing of these circulatory tests a stop watch is the best mechanism to use. However, if one is not available a watch with a sweep second hand can be used. The seconds must be noted as well as the minutes.

IT IS IMPORTANT TO REMEMBER

1. That drugs are used in most laboratory and x-ray procedures, as well as in diagnostic tests in the physician's office and the hospital.
2. That the main responsibility of the nurse in these diagnostic procedures is not the administration of the drug but the physical and emotional care of the patient before, during and after its administration.
3. That the nurse may be called upon to aid in giving these medications, and she may also be responsible for giving the patient adequate instructions preceding and following the treatment.
4. That the nurse is often responsible for the administration of various intradermal tests, and she must be extremely careful that the drug is administered into and not below the skin.

TOPICS FOR STUDY AND DISCUSSION

1. What specimens are used to aid in the establishment of an accurate diagnosis? Are drugs used in connection with any of these?

2. How may the nurse prepare a patient psychologically for a G.I. series? Presume the patient is afraid of the procedure and also is fearful that cancer may be found.

3. What routine is followed in your hospital for each of the diagnostic procedures described? Write out detailed instructions that might be given to the patient, or home attendant, to carry out these procedures. Most of these patients are outpatients and are not admitted to the hospital until the diagnosis has been made. Presume in writing your instructions that the patient is not acquainted with medical terms and with hospital rules. Several students might work together on this topic, each taking a separate procedure.

BIBLIOGRAPHY

Books and Pamphlets

American Medical Association Council on Drugs, *Drug Evaluations, 2nd Ed.*, Chicago, 1973, American Medical Association.

Beeson, P. B., and McDermott, W., *Cecil-Loeb Textbook of Medicine, 13th Ed.*, Philadelphia, 1971, W. B. Saunders Co.

Chatton, M. J., Margen, S., and Brainerd, H., *Handbook of Medical Treatment, 12th Ed.*, Los Altos, California, 1970, Lange Medical Publications.

Conn, H. F., (Ed.), *Current Therapy, 1974*, Philadelphia, 1974, W. B. Saunders Co.

Falconer, M., Patterson, H. R., and Gustafson, E., *Current Drug Handbook, 1974–76*, Philadelphia, 1974, W. B. Saunders Co.

Goodman, L. S., and Gilman, A., *Pharmacological Basis of Therapeutics, 4th Ed.*, New York, 1970, The Macmillan Co.

Miller, B. F., and Keane, C. B., *Encyclopedia and Dictionary of Medicine and Nursing*, Philadelphia, 1972, W. B. Saunders Co.

CHAPTER 9

DRUGS ACTING ON THE CENTRAL AND THE AUTONOMIC NERVOUS SYSTEMS

CORRELATION WITH OTHER SCIENCES

I. ANATOMY AND PHYSIOLOGY

1. The central nervous system consists of the brain and spinal cord, the cranial and spinal nerves and the receptors and effectors attached to the nerves. The central nervous system controls all mental processes, the skeletal muscles and many body functions.
2. Reflex action is the bodily response to a sensory stimulus without the interference of consciousness.
3. A sphincter muscle is a somewhat circular bundle of muscle fibers around an opening, whose contractions close the opening.
4. The autonomic nervous system is that part of the general nervous system which controls autonomic or involuntary action. It is mainly connected with the activities of the visceral organs. The autonomic nervous system maintains body metabolism and takes command of bodily functions in time of emergency.

V. PSYCHOLOGY

1. Euphoria is a condition in which the individual feels well and happy though the physical or psychologic situation may not warrant such feelings.
2. The emotionally immature or disturbed individual needs something or someone to lean on. Many such people use drugs as a "crutch."

DRUGS ACTING ON THE CENTRAL NERVOUS SYSTEM

Drugs which act upon the nervous system have two effects: first, they affect the nervous system itself and, second, they affect the organs controlled by that area of the nervous system (I-1). Thus, a central nervous system depressant will decrease mental activity and, if the motor control centers are involved, will also decrease muscular activity. Often the secondary effect is the prime reason for giving the drug. For instance, a medicine given as a cerebral stimulant will aid in more rapid mental activity, but most cerebral stimulants are given to improve respiration or cardiac function.

Drugs Which Increase the Activity of the Central Nervous System

There are several drugs which will increase the activity of the central nervous system. They are called "cerebral or central nervous system stimulants." Some of these are not used extensively, but their inclusion is necessary since they are still ordered in some areas. Central nervous system stimulants include such drugs as caffeine, strychnine, amphetamine, methylphenidate, pentylenetetrazole and nikethamide. Since these medicines stimulate the higher nervous system centers, they are useful in many conditions in which there is a depression of these centers; for example, shock and collapse, respiratory or cardiac failure and depressant drug poisoning. Central nervous system stimulants are not usually used in general debility, as this condition may best be corrected by treatment for the underlying factor. Furthermore, these drugs are not used routinely for the purpose of increasing mental activity. It is never wise to depend on any drug for the long continued use that such a purpose would demand.

As might be expected, some drugs of this group act better under certain conditions. A brief discussion of each of the important drugs with their principal uses follows. For additional details see the Current Drug Handbook. Caffeine and strychnine are included here because of their historical significance and because they show rather clearly the distinction between ascending and descending nervous system stimulants.

CAFFEINE. Caffeine is one of the active principles—alkaloids—of several plants, of which coffee and tea are the best known. It is also found in the kola plant and to a limited extent in cacao—cocoa. Caffeine is one of three "xanthine" drugs, the others being theophylline and theobromine. They have similar properties, but the level of effectiveness varies. Theophylline and theobromine will be discussed later in the book, since their main action is not central nervous system stimulation. Theophylline is used primarily in respiratory disorders such as asthma, and the main action of theobromine is diuresis. Caffeine has largely been replaced as a stimulant by newer, more effective drugs, but it is still used occasionally.

Caffeine is a general descending central nervous system stimulant. Except in massive doses, it does not affect the spinal cord. It increases mental activity and lessens drowsiness and depression, although the action is not prolonged. Caffeine may be administered orally or parenterally, but absorption from the gastrointestinal tract is erratic. When administered by the oral route, caffeine does not affect the medulla, but when given parenterally, it does stimulate the cardiac and respiratory centers. Its main therapeutic use is to combat the after effects in the arousal period of patients suffering from drug-induced coma. For this purpose, it is given parenterally. Though not a true analgesic, caffeine seems to have a synergistic action which enhances the action of other analgesics when combined with them. Many of the orally administered compounds used for minor aches and pains contain caffeine.

Toxic reactions to caffeine are rare in the adult, though some side effects such as transient flushing, tachycardia, palpitation and insomnia, especially after large doses, may occur. Most adults drink coffee in varying amounts, and the average cup of coffee contains roughly 100 to 200 mg. of caffeine. Thus, it is easy to see that the average adult gets some caffeine each day. Tea also contains caffeine, but because of the method of preparation, the usual cup of tea contains less caffeine.

Children may accidentally ingest caffeine, either as the drug or as coffee. They may be seriously poisoned, since they have not built up any tolerance to the drug. Symptoms then include extreme restlessness, delirium, tachycardia and hyperpnea.

The use of caffeine to keep awake to drive long hours at night or to cram for examinations is very poor practice, since it may mask fatigue. The result may be an accident if driving, or confusion and failure if "cramming." (See Current Drug Handbook.)

STRYCHNINE. Strychnine is an active principle of the plant nux vomica. Like caffeine, it has been used for many years. However, unlike caffeine, it is not an ingredient of any commonly used food product, nor is it a xanthine drug. The other important distinction between caffeine and strychnine is that, while caffeine is a descending stimulant, strychnine is an ascending stimulant; where caffeine acts first on the higher centers, strychnine acts first on the lower centers. These facts explain rather quickly why strychnine has never been used so commonly as caffeine and why it is now rarely used in medical practice.

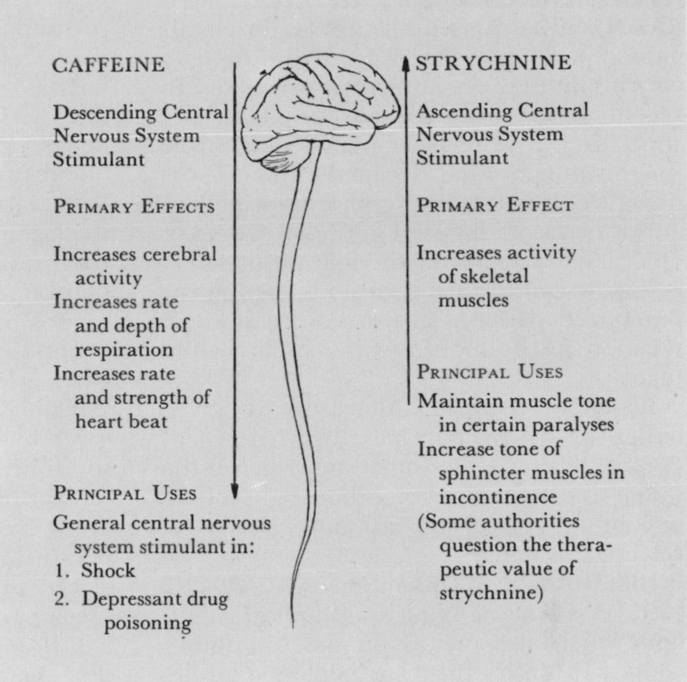

CAFFEINE
Descending Central Nervous System Stimulant
PRIMARY EFFECTS
Increases cerebral activity
Increases rate and depth of respiration
Increases rate and strength of heart beat
PRINCIPAL USES
General central nervous system stimulant in:
1. Shock
2. Depressant drug poisoning
STRYCHNINE
Ascending Central Nervous System Stimulant
PRIMARY EFFECT
Increases activity of skeletal muscles
PRINCIPAL USES
Maintain muscle tone in certain paralyses
Increase tone of sphincter muscles in incontinence
(Some authorities question the therapeutic value of strychnine)

FIGURE 17. Comparison of caffeine and strychnine.

Previously, it was an ingredient in many "tonics," in which its main value was to stimulate the appetite. Since strychnine is an extremely bitter substance, it seems, when taken before meals, to increase the secretion of the digestive juices, which increases the patient's appetite. He then eats more and is better able to digest his food because of the increased amount of digestive enzymes. Thus, the patient is better nourished, gains weight, has increased energy and looks and feels better. However, strychnine is not the only substance that can produce these results. Any bitter substance that may be taken in the same way will bring about the same desirable condition, and other less toxic drugs are usually preferred for this purpose.

The major symptoms of acute strychnine poisoning are restlessness, tremors and an increase in sensory reactions. The patient reacts violently to minor stimulation. A sudden noise or light may cause jerking, jumping movements and crying out; later, convulsions may occur.

Severe poisoning from strychnine is all too common! Strychnine is an ingredient of many rodent poisons and, since these poisons are often so compounded that they taste good, it is not unusual for them to be eaten by children with serious, if not fatal, results. This condition is much easier to prevent than to try to treat. The nurse must explain to those who may ask that insect and rodent poisons are also poisonous to man as well as to animals and must be kept away from children.

Reference to Figure 17 will show graphically why caffeine is the preferred drug for general stimulation.

DRUGS USED TO STIMULATE THE RESPIRATORY AND CARDIAC CENTERS

Analeptic Agents

The analeptic agents are those stimulatory agents used primarily in the treatment of depressant drug poisoning or respiratory depression. They do have other uses which will be discussed later.

PENTYLENETETRAZOLE (LEPTAZOL, METRAZOL). *Pentylenetetrazole*, N.F., originally gained wide popularity from its use as a convulsant in the treatment of psychoses. In recent years, with the advent of electric shock therapy, the use of pentylenetetrazole for this purpose has declined until its use is now rare. It is a strong respiratory stimulant and is occasionally used in the operating or emergency room, but the margin of safety is low. It can cause convulsions even in the narcotized patient. This is one reason it is not now in common use as a cerebral stimulant.

Pentylenetetrazole (Metrazol) is given either orally or parenterally in doses of 100 to 200 mg. The nurse must be on the watch for twitching or other signs of an oncoming convulsion in any patient receiving this drug.

NIKETHAMIDE (CORAMINE; ANACARDONE [C]). *Nikethamide* N.F. is a cerebral stimulant which acts mainly on the respiratory center. It is a useful drug in all types of depression and in shock and collapse. It causes vasoconstriction and a reflex rise in blood pressure. Nikethamide is used in some types of cardiac conditions.

Nikethamide (Coramine) comes in ampules for parenteral administration or in a liquid for oral use. In emergencies it is given either intravenously or intramuscularly. The average dose is 1.0 ml. of a 25 per cent solution. The oral preparation is given to maintain an adequate blood pressure level in such cases as cardiac decompensation. The drug is relatively safe, and toxic symptoms are not common. However, where heavy doses are given—as in emergencies—the patient should be watched for symptoms of excessive stimulation. Convulsions have occurred after a number of large doses. Nikethamide is not as efficient an analeptic agent as the other drugs discussed in this group.

BEMEGRIDE (METHETHARIMIDE [C]). *Bemegride* is another of the synthetic analeptic drugs. It is used primarily for barbiturate poisoning but is also valuable in the relief of depression caused by barbiturates including anesthetic agents. It is administered intravenously in 50 mg. doses, repeated as circumstances warrant.

DOXAPRAM HYDROCHLORIDE (DOPRAM). *Doxapram hydrochloride*, N.F., is used in operative and postoperative respiratory depression and to increase arousal in the recovery stage. It is a non-specific analeptic, but has not been used as such. Hyperactivity, muscle twitching, increased deep tendon reflexes, laryngospasm, tachycardia, increased blood pressure and convulsions may occur. It is contraindicated in convulsive disorders, hypertension, cerebral edema, hyperthyroidism and pheochromocytoma. It should not be given to patients who are taking monoamine oxidase inhibitors or adrenergic agents. This drug is given intravenously when close monitoring of vital signs is available. There is no fixed dose. It may be given by intravenous infusion in dextrose or sodium chloride solution, usually at a rate of approximately 5 mg. per minute. If given by intravenous injection, the dose is 0.5 to 1.5 mg. per kg. of body weight, either as one injection or in divided doses, 5 minutes apart.

ETHAMIVAN (EMIVAN). *Ethamivan* is a non-specific analeptic agent similar in action to doxapram hydrochloride. It is used in respiratory depression due to depressant drug toxicity and in chronic lung diseases when adequate ventilation is not maintained by other means. Its toxic symptoms and contraindications are the same as those for doxapram hydrochloride. Ethamivan can be given either intravenously or orally. The size of the dose depends upon the response of the patient. With intravenous administration close monitoring of vital signs is required. Recommended starting doses are 20 to 60 mg. orally 2 to 4 times daily; intravenous infusion, 1 Gm. in 250 ml. of dextrose or sodium chloride solution administered at a rate of approximately 10 mg. per minute; and intravenous injection, 0.5 to 5.0 mg. per kg. of body weight, given slowly over a period of several minutes.

THE AMPHETAMINE DRUGS. This group of drugs includes several closely related synthetic compounds. They are derived from ephedrine and show some ephedrine-like action. The main drugs in this group are amphetamine sulfate, N.F. (Benzedrine), dextroamphetamine sulfate, U.S.P., (many trade names) and methamphetamine hydrochloride, U.S.P., (many trade names). For doses and other preparations refer to the Current Drug Handbook.

These drugs have a direct stimulatory action on the central nervous system and also, to a greater or lesser degree, on the sympathetic nervous system. These drugs tend to raise blood pressure and produce a distinct euphoria.

The amphetamines have been widely used in a variety of conditions including obesity, depressive syndromes, parkinsonism, in conjunction with other therapy in the treatment of depressant drug poisoning, in narcolepsy, and for the hyperkinetic child. Only the last two conditions are now regularly treated with amphetamines.

The side effects and toxicity are mainly an exaggeration of the expected clinical effects—increased activity, restlessness, talkativeness, headache and vertigo. There may also be cardiac arrhythmias and gastrointestinal disturbances. The amphetamines are contraindicated in hypertension and in some cardiac conditions and are usually avoided in thyrotoxicosis.

The problems of drug abuse were discussed in Chapter 6. Possibly no drug has been abused so much so rapidly. Since amphetamines induce tolerance, increasing doses are required. As obesity is a common problem, and since the drugs were used along with a diet in weight reduction, their use and subsequent abuse became widespread. Their use in weight reduction has not proved to be successful in most cases.

Other similar drugs are diethylpropion hydrochloride (Tenuate, Tepanil, Derpon and Regenon [C]), phenmetrazine hydrochloride (Preludin, Metrazine, Probese P. and Willpower [C]), phentermine and phentermine hydrochloride (Ionamin, Wilpo and Duromin [C]). See the Current Drug Handbook for details.

These drugs are no longer used for weight reduction by order of the Federal Food and Drug Administration, and are controlled by the Drug Enforcement Agency. See Chapter 2 for further information.

Methylphenidate hydrochloride (Ritalin) has been used as an analeptic agent both orally and parenterally. The parenteral form is no longer available, but the oral tablets are still manufactured. Like the amphetamines, its use now is primarily for the treatment of narcolepsy and for the hyperkinetic child. Side effects are similar to those of the amphetamines, since they are both central nervous system stimulants. Refer to the Current Drug Handbook for details.

STIMULANTS ACTING BY REFLEX ACTION. Many drugs exert a stimulating action when they come in contact with the nerve endings. The most important of these are camphor and ammonia (I-2). The stimulation brought about in this way is of short duration; therefore, these drugs are used mainly in emergency situations.

Ammonia is most commonly used in fainting. The preparation of choice is the aromatic spirits of ammonia. It may be placed on a piece of gauze or cotton and inhaled or, if the patient is conscious, given in water orally. One-half to one teaspoonful in about a half ounce of water is the adult dose. It should not be too dilute or the desired stimulation will not result. In a home emergency where none of these drugs is available, household ammonia may be used—*but it must be only by inhalation*. Even with inhalation care must be taken not to give the patient too much. One method is to let the patient smell the cap. Another method is to open the bottle for an instant near the patient but not directly under the nose. If held too close, the patient may choke, and this might defeat the purpose.

Antidepressants

Antidepressants, also called psychic energizers or psychomotor stimulants, are drugs whose main use is to fight depression, especially psychosis. Their use has been the subject of much discussion. Some doctors believe that they have a definite place in the treatment of such patients and that they help the patient to have a more normal outlook. Other physicians feel that the drugs do not achieve this purpose.

Antidepressants are divided into two groups, those which inhibit the action of the enzyme monamine oxidase and those which act in other ways. The amphetamine drugs, discussed previously, are included in the latter group. Some of the more important drugs are:

Tricyclic compounds:
  Imipramine (Tofranil)

Amitriptyline (Elavil)
Desipramine (Norpramin, Pertofrane)
Doxepin (Sinequan)
Nortriptyline (Aventyl)
Protriptyline (Vivactil)
Monoamine oxidase inhibitors:
Isocarboxazid (Marplan)
Nialamide (Niamid)
Phenelzine (Nardil)
Central nervous system stimulants:
(largely replaced by the above drugs)
Amphetamines
Dextroamphetamines
Methamphetamines
Methylphenidate (Ritalin)

See the Current Drug Handbook for information concerning these drugs, especially toxicity and precautions.

Dosages of these drugs are individually adjusted and vary rather widely. Liver damage may occur from the use of these preparations so symptoms suggestive of this should be watched for closely. Further discussion of these drugs will be found in Chapter 30.

Central Nervous System Depressants

Central nervous system depressants include a wide variety of drugs. Everything from a mild sedative or simple analgesic to a general anesthetic comes under this heading. Some of these are rather specific in their use, having only one or two purposes, while others are useful in a number of conditions. Those that have specific action will be discussed later.

Central nervous system depressants are generally classified as analgesics, sedative-hypnotics, anticonvulsants and anesthetics. Since the last two groups are limited in action they will be discussed with the areas of major use: the anticonvulsants (Chapter 32) and the anesthetics (Chapter 15).

Drugs Used to Relieve Pain—Analgesics

See Current Drug Handbook and accompanying chart.

Analgesics, drugs used to relieve pain, probably have the widest use of any group of drugs (see Table 2). Pain in varying amounts is an accompaniment of almost all disease and disorders and, in addition, minor aches and pains occur during what appears to be normal health. The prevalence of the use of pain-relieving medicines is well known. One cannot read a magazine or paper, listen to radio or watch television without being told of the merits of this or that "pain killer." This problem has been mentioned in the discussion of self-medication in Chapter 6. Here, the analgesic as the medical profession uses it will be discussed. To the patient, pain is his worst symptom and relief from it his most immediate need. The patient is not too interested in how that relief is obtained, except that the easiest method from his point of view is best. Nursing measures other than drugs can often be used to relieve minor pain and these should be employed wherever possible. It is inexcusable for the nurse to give an analgesic if the same results can be obtained without a drug.

OPIUM

THE DRUG. Since the dawn of civilization, opium has been one of the most important drugs for the relief of pain. Its origin lost in antiquity, it was used in its crude form in China and in other parts of the world many centuries before the Christian era. Opium is the juice of the unripe seed capsule of the white poppy, *Papaver somniferum*.

Physical and Chemical Properties. Opium contains several alkaloids and from these others have been synthesized. The more important ones occur in two groups: the phenanthrenes, morphine, codeine and thebaine; and the benzylisoquinolines, papaverine, noscopine (formerly called narcotine) and narceine. Thebaine and narceine are not used medicinally separately, but they do occur in the preparations containing the complete drug. Papaverine has little analgesic action and is used mainly as a smooth muscle relaxant. Noscopine's principal use is as an antitussive agent.

Opium is a gray or brownish powder; the purified alkaloids are white. The alkaloids are relatively insoluble, but their salts are readily soluble in water and body fluids.

Action. Most of the action of opium

derives from the morphine it contains, hence it is best to place the main discussion on the action of morphine. A depressant of the central nervous system, it seems to act primarily on the corticothalamic pathways and on the preceptive areas of the brain (Fig. 18). It causes only limited depression of the higher centers, but does produce euphoria and some sedation, both directly and indirectly through its relief of pain (V-1).

It has a selective action on the medulla, depressing respiration and cough, but stimulating the vagus and the vomiting centers. It causes marked pupillary constriction and tends to decrease the basic metabolic rate. Morphine does not have a profound effect on circulation, but superficial dilation of blood vessels may occur attended by flushing and increased perspiration. Stimulation of the vagus center produces a slowing of intestinal peristalsis with resulting constipation.

The action of codeine is similar to, but in most cases less pronounced than, morphine. It produces less euphoria, is a weaker analgesic, rarely causes vomiting or flushing and does not constrict the pupils.

Therapeutic Uses. Opium and its derivatives, used mainly for the relief of pain, are also used to reduce cough, control diarrhea and induce pre and postoperative analgesia. The preparation to be used in a specific case will depend upon the purpose of the drug, the route of administration and the severity of the pain, if given as an analgesic.

Morphine and powdered opium are used for severe pain. Codeine is used to relieve milder pain and cough. Laudanum and paregoric are used primarily for the relief of diarrhea.

Dilaudid and Pantopon are used for the same purposes as morphine, especially in patients who cannot tolerate morphine. Oxymorphone is also used as is morphine, but since it is no more effective and appears to be more addictive than morphine, it is not often used. Methadone (discussed in more detail later), since it can be administered orally, is usually the analgesic given to terminal cancer patients who are cared for at home.

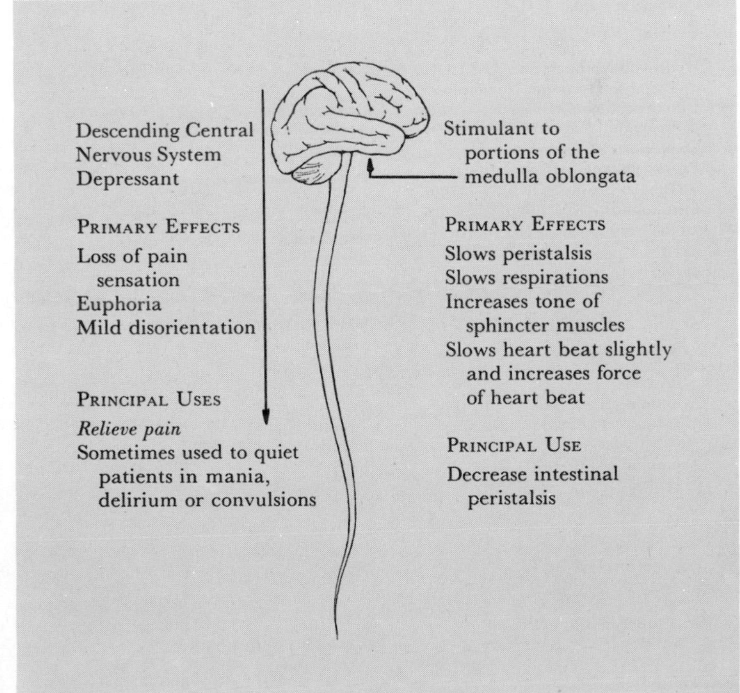

FIGURE 18. Opium (morphine sulfate) as a therapeutic agent.

TABLE 2. COMPARISON OF VARIOUS ANALGESIC DRUGS

GENERIC NAME (TRADE)	SOURCE	DOSAGE	MODE OF ADMINISTRATION	USUAL TIMES ORDERED
Morphine sulfate, U.S.P., B.P.	Opium	8 to 16 mg.	Oral or parenteral	p.r.n. (q 3 to 4 h)
Opium, powdered, U.S.P.	Opium	60 mg.	Oral or rectal	Same
Opium, tincture, U.S.P., B.P. (Laudanum)	Opium	0.6 ml.	Oral	p.r.n.
Opium, camphorated tincture, U.S.P., B.P. (Paregoric)	Opium	4 to 8 ml.	Oral	p.r.n.
Pantopium hydrochloride, U.S.P. (Pantopon)	Opium	5 to 20 mg.	Oral or parenteral	p.r.n. (q 3 to 4 h)
Hydromorphone hydrochloride, U.S.P., L.P. (Dilaudid)	Synthesized from morphine	2 to 4 mg.	Oral or parenteral	p.r.n.
Oxymorphone (Numorphan hydrochloride)	As above	1 to 1.5 mg. 2 to 5 mg. 10 mg.	Parenteral Rectal Oral	p.r.n.
Meperidine hydrochloride, U.S.P. (Demerol) Pethidine hydrochloride, B.P. (Pethidone)	Synthetic	25 to 100 mg.	Oral or parenteral	p.r.n. (q 3 to 4 h)
Alphaprodine hydrochloride, N.F. (Nisentil)	Synthetic	40 to 60 mg.	Subcutaneously or I.V.	p.r.n. (q 3 to 4 h)
Anileritine, N.F. (Leritine)	Synthetic	25 to 50 mg.	Oral or parenteral	p.r.n. (q 3 to 4 h)
Methadone hydrochloride, U.S.P., B.P. (Adanon, Dolophine)	Synthetic	5 to 10 mg.	Oral or parenteral	p.r.n. (q 3 to 4 h)
Levorphanol tartrate, U.S.P. (Levo-Dromoran, Levorphan)	Synthetic	2 to 3 mg.	Oral or parenteral	p.r.n. (q 3 to 4 h)
Methotrimeprazine (Levoprome, Levomepromazine, Nozinan [C])	Synthetic	20 mg.	Parenteral	q 4 to 6 h
Pentazocine, N.F. (Talwin)	Synthetic	50 to 100 mg. 50 mg.	Parenteral Oral	p.r.n. (q 4 to 6 h)
Phenazocine (Xenazol)	Synthetic	2 mg.	Parenteral	p.r.n. (q 4 to 6 h)
Piminodine ethansulfonate (Alvodine)	Synthetic	10 to 50 mg. 25 to 50 mg. 10 to 20 mg.	Oral Subcutaneously I.V.	p.r.n. (q 3 to 4 h)
Fentanyl citrate (Sublimaze)	Synthetic	0.25 to 0.1 mg.	Parenteral	Depends on usage
ANALGESICS THAT ARE LESS POTENT AND USED FOR LESSER PAIN				
Codeine phosphate, U.S.P., B.P., Codeine sulfate, N.F.	Opium	15 to 60 mg.	Oral or parenteral	p.r.n. (q 3 to 4 h)
Hydrocodone bitartrate, U.S.P. (Dicodid, Hycodan, Naideine)	Synthetic	5 to 15 mg.	Oral or parenteral	p.r.n. (q 3 to 4 h)
Dihydrocodeine, (Drocode, Paracodin, Rapacodin)	Synthetic	5 to 15 mg.	Oral or parenteral	p.r.n. (q 3 to 4 h)
Oxycodone	Synthetic	10 to 15 mg.	Oral	p.r.n.
Propoxyphene hydrochloride, N.F., (Dextro-Propoxyphene, Darvon)	Synthetic	32 to 65 mg.	Oral	p.r.n. (q 3 to 4 h)
Ethoheptazine (Zactane)	Synthetic	75 mg.	Oral	p.r.n. (q 6 to 8 h)
ANALGESIC-ANTIPYRETICS				
Aspirin, U.S.P., acetylsalicylic acid, B.P.	Synthetic from salicylic acid	600 mg.	Oral	p.r.n.
Acetaminophen, N.F. (Tempera, Tylenol, Tralgen)	Synthetic, para-aminophenal derivative	300 to 600 mg.	Oral	p.r.n.
Acetanilid (Antifebrin)	Same	200 mg.	Oral	p.r.n.
Phenacetin, U.S.P., B.P. (Acetophenetidin, Phenidin)	Same	300 mg.	Oral	p.r.n.
Aminopyrine (Pyramidon, Amidopyrine)	Synthetic pyrazolone derivative	300 mg.	Oral	p.r.n.
Antipyrine, N.F.	Same	300 mg.	Oral	p.r.n.
Dipyrone	Same	300 mg., 500 to 1000 mg.	Oral Parenteral	t. or q.i.d. p.r.n. (q 4 h)

TABLE 2. COMPARISON OF VARIOUS ANALGESIC DRUGS (Continued)

THERAPEUTIC USES	SIDE EFFECTS, TOXICITY	TOLERANCE, ADDICTION, DEPENDENCY, REMARKS
Analgesia, diarrhea, cough, pre and postoperative	Respiratory depression, miosis, constipation, diaphoresis, nausea, vomiting, skin itching	Tolerance and addiction produced; withdrawal symptoms severe
Same and for local rectal pain	Same	Same
Analgesia, but mainly for diarrhea	Same	Same as above, but not now in common use
Analgesia, for diarrhea	Same	Dependency can occur, but this is rare due to usage
Analgesia (as morphine)	Same	Same as morphine
Analgesia (as morphine)	Same	Same as morphine
Analgesia	Same	Same as morphine, but use limited as it appears to produce more tolerance and addiction
Analgesia	Depresses respiration (tidal volume, not rate), diaphoresis, syncope, dizziness, dry mouth, euphoria, palpitation, nausea	Produces tolerance and dependency, but not as rapidly or as severely as morphine
Analgesia, especially for short quick relief	As above, but respiratory depression rare	Tolerance may occur, but dependency is not common
Analgesia	Similar to meperidine	Similar to meperidine
Analgesia in trauma, dysmenorrhea, myalgia, cancer and for opium withdrawal	Similar to morphine, but less euphoria and no constipation	Tolerance and dependency do occur, but more slowly than with opium and withdrawal symptoms are less severe
Similar to morphine when given parenterally and to methadone when given orally	Similar to morphine, but much less severe	Tolerance may develop with prolonged use
Analgesia, obstetrics, postsurgery, general	Main—orthostatic hypotension. Long-term use with heavy dosage may cause agranulocytosis or liver damage	Do not give with ephedrine (severe hypotension may result). A phenothiazine derivative, so may show similar effects
Analgesia (general), surgical and obstetrical use	Similar to morphine, but less severe	Appears to be nonaddictive; it is a mild narcotic antagonist
As above	Similar to morphine	Tolerance and dependency occur
As above	More like meperidine than morphine, but less severe; produces less euphoria than morphine; is not constipating	Tolerance and dependency do occur
Used in conjunction with anesthesia. May be given pre- or postoperatively I.V. or I.M., but is used most with anesthesia intravenously	Similar to morphine	The most common use of this drug is in conjunction with the antipsychotic agent droperidol. The trade name is Innovar
(NOT INCLUDING DRUGS USED PRIMARILY FOR ARTHRITIS)		
Analgesia for slight to moderately severe pain, diarrhea, dysmenorrhea	Similar to morphine, but much less severe	Tolerance and dependency occur with long continued use; withdrawal symptoms much less severe than those of morphine
As above	As above	As above
As above	As above	As above
As above	As above	Main ingredient in Percodan
Analgesia for slight to moderate pain	Side effects are not common, but drowsiness, nausea, vomiting and skin rash may occur	Nonaddictive and non-narcotic
As above	Side effects are not common, but may include nausea, vomiting, dizziness	Is not as effective alone as in combination with aspirin 325 mg.; it is nonaddictive and is non-narcotic
(See also drugs used for arthritis)		
For arthritis and all minor pain, headache, myalgia, neuralgia, dysmenorrhea	Side effects are not common, but irritation of the intestinal mucosa may occur, especially with prolonged use; some people are allergic to aspirin	Development of dependency is rare
As above	Side effects are not common; toxicity is low	Prepared in flavored liquid for children; development of dependency rare
As above	Side effects and toxicity much more common than with others of this group; may cause weakness, palpitation, anorexia, dizziness, nausea, numbness, blood dyscrasias	Can cause dependency; anti-anemic treatment may be required with prolonged use
As above	As above, but less toxic; blood dyscrasias and kidney damage have been reported with prolonged use	Development of dependency is not common
As above	Can cause depression, tachycardia, cyanosis, diaphoresis and hypotension; may cause blood dyscrasias	Can cause dependency. Formerly a common ingredient of various headache remedies, now prohibited
Used mainly as an antipyretic	Same as above, but is somewhat less toxic	
Antipyretic, analgesic and antirheumatic	May cause skin rashes, dizziness, chills; with prolonged use may cause blood dyscrasias	

Absorption and Excretion. The salts of the alkaloids of opium and their derivatives are readily absorbed from the intestinal tract. They are well distributed in the body fluids, are inactivated wholly or in part by the liver and excreted through the kidneys.

Preparations and Dosages. See Table 2. This lists the main opium preparations still in common use, the main opium alkaloids, the drugs synthesized from morphine and the important non-opium analgesics.

THE NURSE

Mode of Administration. Powdered-opium in a proper base is used as a suppository for pain, local or general. It is very effective in relieving the discomfort of rectal surgery and rectal disorders but is also valuable in the treatment of the patient who is suffering from pain anywhere in the body. The opium suppository is especially useful when the patient is unable to take medications by mouth and when the parenteral route is deemed inadvisable. Often, especially in the geriatric patient, the body tissues do not absorb instilled fluids well. This patient may be either emaciated or edematous, or both, and the nurse may hesitate to give the drug parenterally for several reasons. First, it is apt to be poorly absorbed, preventing the patient from obtaining the desired effect. Second, the danger of a sterile abscess is ever-present. If, in addition, the patient is nauseated and reluctant to take drugs orally, the administration of medications poses a real problem, and the opium suppository is often the best possible answer. Powdered opium may also be given orally, but this is rare.

Tincture of opium (Laudanum) is also given orally but, as with powdered opium, its use now is uncommon. However, camphorated tincture of opium (Paregoric) is frequently used to relieve diarrhea in children and adults. It may be given alone or added to other drugs to enhance their effectiveness. Distinction between these drugs, Laudanum and Paregoric, is very important since Laudanum is roughly 25 times stronger than Paregoric. A mistake in giving Laudanum for Paregoric could have serious or even fatal results.

Pantopon, Dilaudid, morphine and codeine may be administered either orally or parenterally. In home practice these drugs may be given sublingually to secure quicker results than the oral route. Of course, to be used sublingually, the tablet must be of the kind that dissolves easily. This route is almost as rapid as the subcutaneous one.

Codeine is often the ingredient in cough mixtures and in combinations for analgesia such as aspirin, phenacetin, caffeine and codeine. These are administered orally only.

Side Effects. These have already been touched upon under ACTION. Briefly, opium and its main alkaloid, morphine, produce euphoria, relaxation and sedation. They also cause constipation, respiratory depression, pupillary constriction, increased perspiration and sometimes nausea and vomiting. In some patients excitement rather than relaxation occurs and in some there is itching of the skin.

Codeine acts in much the same manner, but its side effects are much milder. It does not cause constriction of the pupils and rarely nausea, vomiting or diaphoresis.

Acute Toxicity and Treatment. The most serious toxic effect of opium is respiratory depression with a rate below 12 per minute. However, other symptoms usually precede. First occurs tachycardia, then dizziness, nausea, slow weak pulse, pinpoint pupils and slow respiration. Later cyanosis and Cheyne-Stokes respiration may be present. Nalorphine (Nalline) or another narcotic antagonist is always given parenterally. Lavage, colon flush or purgation may be used. A respirator may be used, as may a central nervous system stimulant (analeptic agent) given intravenously. Later treatment includes drugs like antibiotics to combat pneumonia.

Chronic opium poisoning is discussed in more detail in Chapter 6, Drug Abuse, since it occurs almost exclusively in the addict. Briefly, the symptoms are weakness and gastrointestinal disturbances such as anorexia, occasional nausea, diarrhea or constipation. The latter two sometimes alternate. The patient is listless and tends to withdraw from his normal social contacts. He becomes careless about his person. The almost continuous constriction of the pupils causes eye strain; consequently he wears dark glasses. There may also be abscesses or sores on the anterior surface of the arms and legs resulting from unsterile and repeated injections. Long sleeves are often worn to conceal the condition.

Interactions. The narcotic drugs potentiate the action of the phenothiazines, sedative-hypnotics, alcohol and the monoamine oxidase inhibitors by additive effect. They are enhanced by the monoamine oxidase inhibitors by microsomal enzyme inhibition.

Contraindications. Morphine and related opium alkaloids, excluding codeine, should be used with caution in cases of lowered respiratory reserve such as occurs in emphysema, kyphoscoliosis, cor pulmonale and even severe obesity. There are few specific contraindications. The opiates are used with caution in head injury because of the danger of increased respiratory depression (below 12 respirations per minute.) Many persons have undesirable reactions following the use of morphine or other opium alkaloids. The nurse may be the first member of the staff to know that a patient cannot tolerate the medication. If the drug has already been ordered, she should withhold it until consulting with the attending physician.

Patient Teaching. The nurse should do all she can to reduce the patient's dependency on opium or other drugs. She should be ready to answer questions freely and accurately. It is essential that the patient realize that as the cause of the pain is removed, he will automatically require less and less of the analgesic. Drug dependency induced by illness is rare and the nurse can assure the patient of this fact. However, it does occur, mainly in patients with painful chronic diseases such as cancer. The physician realizes the danger and he, not the nurse or the patient, has to decide on the proper procedure to adopt.

Other Nursing Problems. The nurse should be aware of the fact that analgesic drugs are not primarily hypnotics. It is true that morphine sulfate and other analgesics will help the patient to sleep, but they do so mainly by indirect action. If the patient is suffering from severe pain he will not sleep. If that pain and the accompanying nervous tension stop, he will sleep. The patient does not feel the sore spots, noise and light are lessened because of reduced sensory perception and, as the senses are dulled and the pain relieved, the patient sleeps. Many times the nurse is faced with a real problem. The nurse may encounter a patient who is not sleeping. He is restless, he has some pain, but it may be minor. There are p.r.n. orders on the chart: one for a narcotic for pain and one for a hypnotic for sleep. The nurse must decide: Will nursing measures such as a back rub or change of position secure the desired result? Will the hypnotic be best? Should the analgesic be given? The nurse must consider all the factors and then proceed as seems best for the patient. Certainly, the nursing measures should be tried, unless the patient is too exhausted to stand further movement. There is no universal answer to such questions. Each patient is a different individual; each presents a new problem. The nurse must be alert to the needs of each individual and do what seems best for him.

The Patient. Opium is one of the few truly addictive drugs. It has been abused for ages and will likely continue to be so in the foreseeable future. However, this does not mean that everything possible should not be done to prevent its occurrence. Many emotionally disturbed patients use drugs as a crutch (V-2), and the euphoria produced by the opiates is a welcome relief from their unpleasant feelings (V-2). However, most people who become dependent upon opium did not start using drugs during illness. This is an assurance the nurse can give the patient who needs a narcotic but is afraid of dependency. To the patient in severe pain, the bringing of relief is all important. That the drug also gives a sense of well being and relaxation is a welcome adjunct. If the patient is to take a narcotic drug at home, the nurse should carefully explain its use and possible side effects. As with all drugs, any untoward reaction should be reported to the physician.

SYNTHETIC ANALGESICS

Several synthetic drugs are effective analgesics. They all act roughly like the opiates and for the same purpose. Most of the discussion of opium applies to these preparations, some of which are nonaddictive and most of which are less addictive than morphine.

MEPERIDINE HYDROCHLORIDE (DEMEROL) AND RELATED DRUGS

THE DRUG. Meperidine is one of several similar drugs which will be discussed together. The others are Alphaprodine hydrochloride (Nisentil), Anileridine (Leritine) and Piminodine (Alvodine).

Physical and Chemical Properties. Meperidine, alphaprodine and anileridine are related phenylpiperidine derivatives. They all form acid salts that are readily soluble. Piminodine is chemically similar.

Action. Meperidine appears to act, as does morphine, by altering the affective reaction to pain. It produces sedation and relaxation and decreases the tidal volume, but not the rate of respiration. In the recumbent patient, no appreciable effect is noted on the cardiovascular system. However, the ambulatory patient may show a drop in blood pressure and an accompanying syncope. Meperidine is not an antispasmodic. It may cause some decrease in gastrointestinal activity, but constipation is not a common side effect. It does not produce miosis.

Therapeutic Uses. These drugs combat moderate to severe pain. They all act in a similar manner, but meperidine is more popular than the others. They are used for pre and postoperative analgesia and for obstetrical analgesia. Anileridine has frequently been used to induce the last condition. These drugs produce less depression than the opiates.

Absorption and Excretion. Meperidine, readily absorbed by all routes of administration, is distributed through the body fluids. Some is bound to the blood proteins. It is demethylated by the liver and excreted by the kidneys.

Preparations and Dosages. See Table 2.

THE NURSE

Mode of Administration. There are no specific methods to be employed. Parenterally they can be given I.M. or I.V. With Anileridine it is important to use the correct form of the drug.

Side Effects, Toxicity and Treatment. Generally they are all similar to the opiates. However, these drugs are less toxic and somewhat less addictive. The main side effects are increased perspiration, dizziness, euphoria, palpitation, syncope and nausea. They are less constipating than the opiates. In acute poisoning they induce less respiratory depression than morphine does. Nalorphine (Nalline) is an effective antidote. Other symptoms are treated as they occur. Acute withdrawal produces symptoms similar to the toxic side effects.

Interactions. When meperidine (Demerol) is given concurrently with atropine there is an additive effect. If given with furazolidone (Furoxone), the action of meperidine is enhanced, but that of furazolidone is inhibited. The same is true with the monoamine oxidase inhibitors; meperidine is enhanced, and the monoamine oxidase inhibitors are inhibited. Phenothiazine tends to increase the sedative effect of meperidine. If promazine (Sparine) is given parenterally simultaneously with meperidine, or within a short period of time after administration, the patient may collapse.

Contraindications. The drugs should not be used with the monoamine oxidase inhibitors or administered to patients sensitive to the drug.

Other Nursing Problems. These drugs will, in most cases, produce some tolerance when given over extended periods of time. Originally they were thought to be nonaddictive, but this belief having proved to be false, the possibility of drug dependency must be kept in mind.

THE PATIENT. Relief of pain is the most important thing to the patient and any drug which will bring it is welcome. In acute conditions this is usually easy to accomplish, but with chronic pain the situation is entirely different. Use of the drug must be weighed against the possibility of dependency. The nurse can do much to aid the patient to adjust his medicines so that as little dependence is produced as circumstances allow.

SOME OTHER SYNTHETIC ANALGESICS

Methadone hydrochloride, U.S.P., B.P. (Adanon, Dolophine, Amidone [C]) may be given orally or subcutaneously. It is a synthetic drug, the structure of which is dissimilar to that of morphine; its action, however, is much like that of morphine. Orally it is more effective than morphine. Readily absorbed from the gastrointestinal tract and partially inactivated by the liver, it is excreted by the kidneys. Dosage is 5 to 10 mg. orally or parenterally. It is effective for three to four hours. Methadone acts more slowly than morphine and its action is cumulative. It is used for the relief of pain, renal colic and severe cough. Methadone is often a substitute for morphine or heroin in the treatment of addiction. It, like morphine, is addictive, but withdrawal symptoms are less severe. Methadone produces respiratory depression, constipation and miosis. It may also cause nausea, vomiting, dry mouth and drowsiness.

Levorphanol tartrate, U.S.P. (Levo-Dromoran; levorphan [C]) is similar to morphine when given parenterally and to methadone when administered orally. It is a white crystalline powder with a bitter taste. It is only moderately soluble in water. Its action is more prolonged and its dosage lower, 2 to 3 mg., than that of morphine. It is used to combat moderate to severe pain. Levorphanol is capable of producing tolerance and addiction, but more slowly than morphine.

Methotrimeprazine (Levoprome), *levomepromazine* (Nozinan [C]) is a synthetic analgesic derived from phenothiazine. It is given intramuscularly in doses of 20 mg. (5 to 10 mg. in the older patient). Since it causes orthostatic hypotension, it is rarely given to patients other than those confined to bed. As with all these drugs, see Table 2 for details.

Phenazocine (Xenagol [C]) is a benzomorphan derivative. More potent than morphine, it has the same side effects, tolerance and addictive properties. It is given intramuscularly in 2 mg. doses as needed.

PENTAZOCINE (TALWIN)

THE DRUG. Pentazocine is a congener of phenazocine but unlike it and others of this group, it is a mild narcotic antagonist with analgesic properties.

Physical and Chemical Properties. Pentazocine is a synthetic drug with a complex chemical structure. It is a benzazocine (or benzomorphan) derivative. Pentazocine is a white crystalline substance which is soluble in acidic aqueous solution.

Action. Pentazocine relieves all types of pain, but the exact mode of action is incompletely understood. A dosage higher than morphine but lower than meperidine is required to secure the same effects, and its antinarcotic activity is much less than that of nalorphine.

Therapeutic Usages. It is used in the relief of acute and chronic pain, especially of moderate or severe degree, as a pre and postoperative medication, in emergencies and during labor.

Preparations and Dosages

Pentazocine lactate, N.F. (Talwin) 20 to 60 mg. orally, 50 to 100 mg. parenterally q 3 to 4 h p.r.n.

THE NURSE

Mode of Administration. The drug is manufactured in tablets, ampules or vials, and may be given orally, subcutaneously, intramuscularly or intravenously. Consult directions on the package before administering the drug.

Side Effects. The usual side effects associated with the narcotic drugs such as constipation and respiratory depression rarely occur with pentazocine. The most frequently reported side effects in decreasing order of frequency are vertigo, dizziness, vomiting and euphoria. Many other side effects have been reported but the number of patients affected by them is very small.

Toxicity and Treatment. Severe toxicity with moderate respiratory depression occurs only with excessive dosage. Nalorphine or levallorphan should not be used for these cases. Instead, naloxone (Narcan) is the drug of choice.

Contraindications. The safety of this drug for children and pregnant women has not been established. It should be used cautiously, if at all, for patients in these catagories. It is contraindicated for patients with increased intracranial pressure.

Other Nursing Considerations. Pentazocine, being a narcotic antagonist, is less prone to produce dependency and does not require reporting as do the usual narcotic drugs.

THE PATIENT. Pentazocine relieves pain, making it very acceptable to the patient, and since drug dependency is not as common as with most analgesics, it is a good drug for long term use. Originally, it was available only for parenteral use, limiting it primarily to the hospitalized patient. Now, however, it is available in tablet form, the preparation most commonly used in the home.

Narcotic Antagonists

(See Current Drug Handbook.)

The narcotic antagonists are, as the name

implies, drugs used to antagonize the action of narcotics. Their main use is to prevent or overcome the respiratory depression caused by the narcotic drugs.

Nalorphine hydrochloride, U.S.P., *nalorphine hydrobromide,* B.P., (Nalline) 5 to 10 mg. given parenterally is used for acute narcotic poisoning. It is also used to test for opium addiction. It is not used to treat chronic opium poisoning. As a test, the drug is given to the person suspected of taking one of the opium alkaloids, usually heroin. If he has been taking the narcotic, withdrawal symptoms will set in. Nalorphine (Nalline) is not effective in barbiturate poisoning.

Naloxone hydrochloride (Narcan) is a narcotic antagonist (a synthetic congener of oxymorphone). Like nalorphine, it is used in the treatment of respiratory depression due to narcotic drugs (natural or synthetic preparations). It is also effective in pentazocine-caused respiratory depression. Like nalorphine, it is used to test for narcotic addiction. Naloxone may be given intramuscularly, intravenously or subcutaneously. The intravenous route is used in emergencies. The usual dose is 0.4 mg. (1 ml.). It may be repeated at 2 or 3-minute intervals. Toxicity is relatively low. Nausea and vomiting have been reported.

Levallorphan tartrate, (Lorfan) N.F., B.P., 0.3 to 1.2 mg. given parenterally is used mainly to lessen respiratory depression occurring from narcotic drugs. It may be combined with the narcotic when respiratory depression is a hazard such as during parturition when the infant might be affected by a narcotic administered to the mother.

Drugs Which Potentiate Analgesics

(See Current Drug Handbook.)

Two of the phenothiazine tranquilizers have been shown to potentiate the action of the narcotic drugs when given at the same time. These drugs permit a lower dosage of the narcotic drug, especially important when long term administration of a narcotic is required. These drugs are:

Promethazine hydrochloride, U.S.P., B.P. (Phenergan) 25 to 50 mg. parenterally;

Propiamazine hydrochloride (Largon) 10 to 30 mg. parenterally.

Various Analgesic Agents Used to Relieve Minor Pain

There are several drugs available for the relief of minor pain that are not of the analgesic-antipyretic group. Their value varies, especially from patient to patient. Usually they are more effectual in combination than when used alone. These include ethoheptazine citrate, N.F. (Zactane) and propoxyphene (Darvon), dextropropoxyphene (Leradol, Proxyphene [C]).

Ethoheptazine is chemically related to meperidine but possesses much less analgesic action. It is usually given with aspirin and appears more effective when so used.

Propoxyphene has been equated with codeine in pain control, but it takes more propoxyphene than codeine to secure the same pain relief. Thus, it would usually take at least 65 mg. of propoxyphene to give the same result as 32 mg. of codeine.

These agents are further covered in Table 2.

Analgesic Antipyretics

This group comprises the synthetic phenol derivatives excluding the salicylates except aspirin. The salicylates are covered with acute rheumatic fever, Chapter 18. Aspirin is acetylsalicylic acid and is used extensively for arthritis. However, aspirin has a much wider use, hence its inclusion here. See Current Drug Handbook and accompanying table.

ASPIRIN

The Drug. Aspirin is one of the most commonly used drugs in the world. One wonders what people did before its discovery to rid themselves of minor aches and pains. Aspirin is universally popular because of the relief it affords for most minor pains.

Physical and Chemical Properties. A white crystalline substance with a bitter taste, it is moderately soluble in water and readily soluble in the digestive juices.

Action. The action of aspirin is largely that of the salicylates which will be discussed with the antiarthritic drugs. Briefly, it affects a number of bodily functions. Its analgesic action is probably due to the blockage of the thalamic pathways, decreasing the perception of pain. Aspirin reduces fever in the febrile patient, but does not change the temperature in the nonfebrile person. It tends to increase respiration, but affects cardiovascular activity very little. Aspirin irritates the gastric mucosa and may cause bleeding. It is used with caution, if at all, for patients on anticoagulant therapy since aspirin has some anticoagulant properties. It may also prompt the recrudescence of a latent ulcer. There is usually an initial respiratory alkalosis followed by prompt renal compensation (the excretion of bicarbonates, sodium and potassium). The electrolyte changes are not pronounced except with heavy dosage. As with the other salicylates, aspirin palliates the arthritic changes in affected joints, but it does not cure arthritis.

Therapeutic Uses. Advertising has long regaled the public with the major uses of the mild analgesics such as aspirin: the relief of cold, headaches, muscular aches and pains. To these might be added relief of dysmenorrhea. Aspirin is used for all minor pain. Except in arthritis, aspirin should not be used for persistent or chronic pain. The cause of such pain should be determined and the proper treatment instituted.

Absorption and Excretion. Readily absorbed from the gastrointestinal tract, aspirin is rapidly transported to all parts of the body and excreted, largely unchanged, by the kidneys. As a buffered preparation it probably reduces gastric acidity.

Preparations and Dosages

Aspirin, U.S.P., Acetylsalicylic acid, B.P., (many trade names). 0.3 to 0.6 Gm. orally q 3 to 4 h. Aspirin is prepared in many forms for adults and for children. In arthritis the dosage may be increased, but no more than 3 Gm. should be taken in any 24 hour period.

Salicylamide, N.F. (Dropsprin, Salamide, Cetamide) 0.3 to 2 Gm. orally q 3 to 4 h is a similar drug used for the same purposes as aspirin.

Aspirin is an ingredient in any number of preparations for the relief of minor pains.

THE NURSE

Mode of Administration. Aspirin is given orally. It comes in many forms: capsular, tablet, effervescent, buffered, gum and so forth. Aspirin is an ingredient in many compound drug preparations such as aspirin, phenacetin and caffeine. Such compounds may include codeine or propoxyphene to combat more severe pain or phenobarbital to induce sleep. All of these preparations are given orally. Some patients find that they have better results and less distress by taking aspirin with a little food.

Side Effects, Toxicity and Treatment. Adverse symptoms are rare due to low dosage. In massive doses, such as might be used in arthritis, salicylate poisoning may occur. This will be discussed with the salicylates later. Small doses of aspirin may, in some patients, cause gastric irritation and skin rashes. Some people are allergic to aspirin, death from edema of the larynx having resulted from a single dose of aspirin. Although such occurrences are rare, the nurse should be alert to the fact that they can happen. If the patient tells the nurse that he cannot take aspirin, this fact should be relayed promptly to the physician and no aspirin or other salicylate should be given until additional orders are received. There are no contraindications to the use of aspirin except what was previously stated. Occasionally children take excessive amounts of aspirin, especially in the candy form of the drug, and become very ill. For information about salicylate poisoning, refer to Rheumatic Fever, Chapter 18.

Interactions. Aspirin, which is acetylsalicylic acid, shares interactions with the other salicylates. These include enhancing the action of the oral anticoagulants, amethopterin (Methotrexate) and para-aminosalicylic acid (PAS). In this latter case, toxicity may occur owing to additive action.

Patient Teaching. In this area the main responsibility of the nurse is not teaching but "unteaching." The patient will doubtless already be aware of the value of aspirin, but he may not know the dangers. In this respect "self-medication" can be dangerous, particularly if the person has other allergies. Aspirin can kill as well as cure, as noted before. The patient may ask about the relative merits of the various forms and brands of aspirin. The forms are merely for the patient's convenience, since one patient may prefer a liquid, another finds a capsule easier to swallow than a tablet, and so forth. Aspirin in gum form is convenient on a trip where fluid or food to take with the tablet may be difficult to obtain. The gum is also effective in the relief of sore throat. Concerning brands, any aspirin marked "Aspirin, U.S.P." is the same as any other aspirin so marked. If asked, the nurse should advise the patient against taking aspirin too often or using it for prolonged pain. The patient may assume that his pain is arthritis whereas actually the etiology may be something quite different. Even aspirin should not be taken without medical advice.

The Patient. Aspirin can easily become a "crutch." How often does one hear the plaint, "I can't sleep without aspirin," or similar remark (V-2)? Aspirin has certainly become a cure all, but it still can relieve only minor pain. Aspirin is made by the ton. Millions of tablets are used each year, but it is safe to guess that a high percentage are used without medical advice and probably most of the aspirin used is not really needed.

Other Analgesic Antipyretics

(See Current Drug Handbook.)

PYRAZOLON DERIVATIVES

Aminopyrine, dipyrone and antipyrine are synthetic derivatives of pyrazolon used for analgesia and antipyresis. They have been largely replaced by more efficient and less toxic drugs. Commonly, antipyrine is used to reduce fevers, and aminopyrine to bring about analgesia, whereas dipyrone, an aminopyrine derivative, is used for both purposes. All three drugs are toxic: aminopyrine and dipyrone have been shown to cause agranulocytosis. They also provoke skin rash, dizziness, depression, tachycardia, cyanosis, diaphoresis and collapse. Aminopyrine was formerly the main ingredient in many headache remedies, but such compounds are now prohibited. All of the pyrazolon derivatives require a prescription and are no longer sold over the counter. They are given in oral dosages as follows:

Aminopyrine (Amidofebrin, Amidopyrine, Pyramidon) 0.3 Gm. q 4 h p.r.n.

Antipyrine, N.F. (Pyrazoline) 0.3 Gm. q 4 h p.r.n.

Dipyrone (Nevaldin, Diprone) 0.3 to 0.6 Gm. t.i.d. or q.i.d.

Dipyrone is also given parenterally 0.5 to 1 Gm. q 3 h p.r.n.

PARA-AMINOPHENOL OR ANILINE DERIVATIVES

Acetaminophen, acetanilid and phenacetin – aniline derivatives – are used for all types of minor pains, such as headache, myalgia, arthralgia, dysmenorrhea and neuralgia; they also have some antipyretic action. They are capable of causing either acute toxic (excessive dosage) or chronic toxic (prolonged use) symptoms. Acute symptoms include weakness, anorexia, dizziness, nausea, numbness of the extremities and palpitation. Acetanilid is regarded as the most toxic, acetaminophen, the least toxic, of the aniline derivatives. Since less toxic and more efficient drugs are available, they are much less frequently used now than they once were. With acetanilid, habituation may occur. Phenacetin has been implicated in some blood dyscrasias. None of the drugs should be taken for extended periods except under direct medical supervision. They are all given orally, are readily absorbed from the gastrointestinal tract and are excreted by the kidneys. Dosages are as follows:

Acetaminophen, N.F. (Amadil, Tempra, Tylenol, Tralgon) 0.3 to 0.6 Gm. p.r.n.

Acetanilid (Acetylaniline, Antifebrin) 0.2 Gm. p.r.n.

Phenacetin, U.S.P. (Acetophenetidin) 0.3 Gm. p.r.n.

The coal tar analgesics (including aspirin) are often given in combinations with each other and with drugs of the sedative-hypnotic groups. There are an almost endless number of these combinations. One of the popular ones is a preparation which combines aspirin, phenacetin and caffeine. The dosage is usually aspirin 210 mg., phenacetin 150 mg. and caffeine 30 mg. It is marketed under a number of names such as: Empirin Compound, Phenacetin Compound, A.P.C., P.C.A., P.A.C., Acetidine and A.S.A. Compound. The caffeine counteracts the depressant action of the analgesics, especially their tendency to depress heart action. It also appears to have synergistic analgesic action in such a combination. Other medications are often combined with these drugs, the two most common being codeine and phenobarbital.

DRUGS USED TO RELIEVE TENSION AND/OR PRODUCE SLEEP

Sedative-Hypnotics

(See Current Drug Handbook.)

Next to the analgesics, the sedative-hypnotic drugs are probably the most universally used. At one time they were dispensed without prescriptions; however, because of the present stricter drug laws, most of them can be secured only by prescription. This greatly reduces the possibility of self-medication. These drugs are very effective therapeutically and have wide usage in medical practice. The drugs used as sedatives and as hypnotics are usually the same. The difference is one of amount rather than kind of medicine.

CHLORAL HYDRATE. *Chloral hydrate*, U.S.P., B.P., is one of the early preparations used as a hypnotic. It is a synthetic medication and a strong central nervous system depressant. Chloral hydrate is called "knockout drops" by the underworld. Therapeutically, it produces sound sleep from which the patient awakes refreshed and without aftereffects. Chloral hydrate is a heart depressant and is not usually given to the cardiac patient. After having had chloral hydrate, the patient, whether or not he is known to have a heart disorder, should be carefully watched for symptoms of cardiac failure. Chloral hydrate, irritating to the gastric mucosa, should be used with caution, if at all, for the patients with peptic ulcers. In the body, chloral hydrate is reduced to trichloroethanol, in which form it is presumed to be effective. The glucuronic acid conjugate is excreted by the kidneys.

Over prolonged periods, chloral hydrate may produce tolerance and dependency. However, it is a relatively safe and effective hypnotic. Its method of action is only partially understood, but it is thought to depress the sensorimotor areas of the cerebral cortex.

Chloral hydrate can be given either orally or rectally. Originally the drug came in liquid form only but since it has a very disagreeable taste was unpleasant to take. It now comes in capsule form and is given in doses of 0.3 to 0.6 Gm. *Chloral betaine* (Beta Chlor) is a similar preparation with the same side effects as chloral hydrate. It is given orally in a dose of 870 mg. to 1.7 Gm. for the same purposes as chloral hydrate.

By increasing the metabolism of the oral anticoagulants, these drugs decrease the effective half-life of the coumarin compounds.

PARALDEHYDE. *Paraldehyde*, U.S.P., B.P., is a liquid with a peculiar odor and a very disagreeable taste. It is a relatively safe, efficient hypnotic and can be administered orally, intramuscularly or rectally. However, the odor lingers; even the next day it is exuded from the patient. This condition is due, at least in part, to the fact that paraldehyde is excreted partially through the respiratory tract regardless of the route of administration. A small amount is excreted by the liver and some is metabolized by the body into carbon dioxide and water. It is the unpleasant odor and taste that have greatly limited the use of the drug. The nurse should be prepared to deal with the odor when the drug is given, as it is most annoying, not only to the patient but to others in the immediate vicinity. Room deodorants will overcome most of the difficulty. At the present time, paraldehyde is used mainly to produce hypnosis in alcoholism, in any stage from simple drunkenness to delirium tremens. It can be given with a small amount of water, fruit juice, wine or liquor. Of course, the physician will indicate if he desires the drug given with an alcoholic beverage. Paraldehyde may also be given in fluid food. The dose is 8 to 15 ml. Occasionally paraldehyde is given to control convulsions.

BROMIDES. The *bromides* are all salts of hydrobromic acid together with some other element. Bromide was in common use before the advent of the barbiturates and other newer sedative-hypnotics. There are many salts of hydrobromic acid, but the most commonly used in medicine are potassium, ammonium and sodium. It is usual to give a combination of the salts rather than one alone. Bromide preparations produce lethargy and sleep, and tend to reduce muscle as well as mental activity. The effects of drugs are cumulative, and repeated use for insomnia can cause severe toxic reactions. The effect of the bromides is unpredictable; some patients get very good results while others experience con-

TABLE 3. COMPARISON OF SOME OF THE IMPORTANT

NAMES	DOSAGE	ONSET OF ACTION	DURATION OF ACTION
Barbital, Barbitone (Veronal, Barbitone)	300 mg.	30 to 60 minutes	8 to 10 hours
Barbital sodium, Barbitone sodium, B.P. (Medinal)	300 mg.	Same	Same
Mephobarbital, N.F. (Mebaral)	30 to 200 mg.	Same	Same
Metharbital, N.F. (Gemonil)	100 mg.	Same	Same
Phenobarbital, U.S.P., Phenobarbitone, B.P., (Luminal)	50 to 100 mg.	Same	Same
Phenobarbital sodium, U.S.P. Phenobarbitone, B.P. (Luminal sodium, Natribarb sodium)	15 to 100 mg.	Same	Same
Amobarbital, U.S.P., Amylobarbitone, B.P. (Amytal, Amobarb)	20 to 100 mg.	45 to 60 minutes	6 to 8 hours
Amobarbital sodium, U.S.P., Amylobarbitone, B.P. (Amytal sodium)	60 to 100 mg. 100 to 200 mg.	Same	Same
Aprobarbital, N.F. (Alurate)	10 to 160 mg.	Same	Same
Aprobarbital sodium (Alurate sodium)	10 mg.	Same	Same
Butabarbital sodium, Butobarbitone, B.P. (Barbital sodium, Butisol sodium)	15 to 100 mg.	Same	Same
Cyclobarbital calcium, (Phanodorn, cyclobarbitone [C])	200 mg.	10 to 15 minutes	2 to 4 hours
Hexobarbital sodium,	260 to 520 mg.	Same	Same
Pentobarbital sodium, U.S.P. Pentabarbitone sodium, B.P. (Nembutal, Hypnotal)	50 to 100 mg.	Same	Same
Secobarbital sodium, U.S.P. Quinalbarbitone, B.P. (Seconal, Secolone [C])	30 to 100 mg.	Same	Same
Talbutal (Lotusate)	30 to 120 mg.	Same	Same
Vinbarbital sodium, N.F. (Delvinal)	100 to 200 mg.	Same	Same

BARBITURATES (All are derivatives of barbituric acid)

MODE OF ADMINISTRATION	THERAPEUTIC USES	TOLERANCE	DEPENDENCY	REMARKS
Oral	Sedative-hypnosis	Not common	Not common	First barbiturate synthesized
Oral	Same	Same	Same	
Oral	Sedation and anticonvulsant	Same	Same	
Oral	Same	Same	Same	
Oral	Same	Same	Same	Most widely used of all barbiturates; also prepared as an elixir for children
Oral or parenteral	Same	Same	Same	
Oral	Sedation and hypnosis	May occur with prolonged use	Dependency develops with prolonged use	
Oral Parenteral	Same	Same	Same	
Oral	Same	Same	Same	
Oral	Same	Same	Same	
Oral	Same	Same	Same	
Oral	Hypnosis	May occur with prolonged use	Dependency develops	
Oral	Same	Same	Dependency may develop	
Oral, parenteral, rectal	Same	Same	Same	One of the commonly "abused" hypnotics
Same	Same	Same	Same	Same
Oral	Same	Same	Dependency occurs only after prolonged use	
Oral or parenteral	Same	Same	Same	

fusion or "nightmares." Side effects, with prolonged use, and toxic symptoms include anorexia, constipation, salty taste, mental depression, drowsiness, slow speech, slow walk, slow pulse and respirations and a characteristic skin rash. Treatment consists of giving sodium or ammonium chloride to counteract the bromide ion. Dosage of the bromides is 0.6 to 1.0 Gm. if two or more are given together. They are given orally.

FLURAZEPAM HYDROCHLORIDE. *Flurazepam Hydrochloride* (Dalmane) is a benzodiazepine derivative hypnotic. It is related to the benzodiazepine tranquilizers but has more sleep-producing potential. It is given orally in doses of 15 to 30 mg. and usually assures six to eight hours of sleep. For the older or debilitated patient, the lower dose should be used. It is relatively safe and side effects do not commonly occur with therapeutic dosage. The use of this drug with other central nervous system depressants or alcohol is not advised. It may be given to a patient receiving the coumarin type anticoagulants, but it is suggested that the prothrombin times should be determined at frequent intervals. Side effects, if they occur, include dizziness, drowsiness, lightheadedness, staggering and ataxia. As with any hypnotic routine, long-term use is not advisable.

BARBITURATES

THE DRUG. Of all the drugs used for sedation and hypnosis, the barbiturates are by far the most popular. They have an ever widening use from simple sedation to general anesthesia. Any number of compounds have been synthesized, but only a small number have proved to be therapeutically effective. The first barbiturate in general use was barbital (Veronal), introduced by Emil Fisher and Joseph van Mehring in 1903. Phenobarbital (Luminal), the second to come into common use, is one of the most widely used today.

Physical and Chemical Properties. These drugs are the salts of barbituric acid which in turn is a synthetic derivative of malonic acid and urea. The salts of barbituric acid are white crystalline compounds with a bitter taste, some of which are only slightly soluble in water, but all of which are soluble in alcohol. The sodium salts are soluble in water.

Action. All of the barbiturates have a depressant effect on the central nervous system, usually starting with the diencephalon. Some preparations affect mainly the motor centers and hence can be used as anticonvulsants. Therapeutic dosages of the barbiturates do not materially affect the visceral organs, but large amounts can cause respiratory and cardiac depression as well as light to severe hypotension. Some can cause tolerance and dependency.

Therapeutic Usages

(See Table 3 and Current Drug Handbook.)

Absorption and Excretion. Most barbiturates are readily absorbed when given either orally or parenterally. The sodium salts, absorbed most rapidly, are the only form used for parenteral administration. Most of the drug is inactivated by the liver and excreted, either in an altered or unaltered form, by the kidney. The slower acting preparations are inactivated at a much slower rate than the quicker acting ones, and it is possible for cumulative action to occur.

Preparations and Dosages

(See Table 3 and Current Drug Handbook.)

THE NURSE

Mode of Administration

(See Table 3 and Current Drug Handbook.)

Side Effects. Some barbiturates in therapeutic doses produce little or no side effects. However, some patients do not react well to certain forms of the drug. They may have a "hangover" after an ordinary dose used as a hypnotic. Depression may be excessive and nausea and emotional disturbances may occur. Other side effects include skin rashes, urticaria, bad dreams, restlessness and even delirium. The barbiturates are not analgesics, and when the patient has severe pain, unless the medication includes an analgesic, he may experience restlessness and confusion instead of sleep. Restlessness, delirium and confusion are most commonly seen in the elderly patient. Side rails should be used as a precaution.

Toxic Effects and Treatment. Acute and chronic poisoning occur and, being different, will be discussed separately.

Acute Poisoning. Most cases of acute poisoning occur after the ingestion of large amounts of the drug either accidentally or with suicidal or homicidal intent. Regardless of why the drug was taken, the nurse's

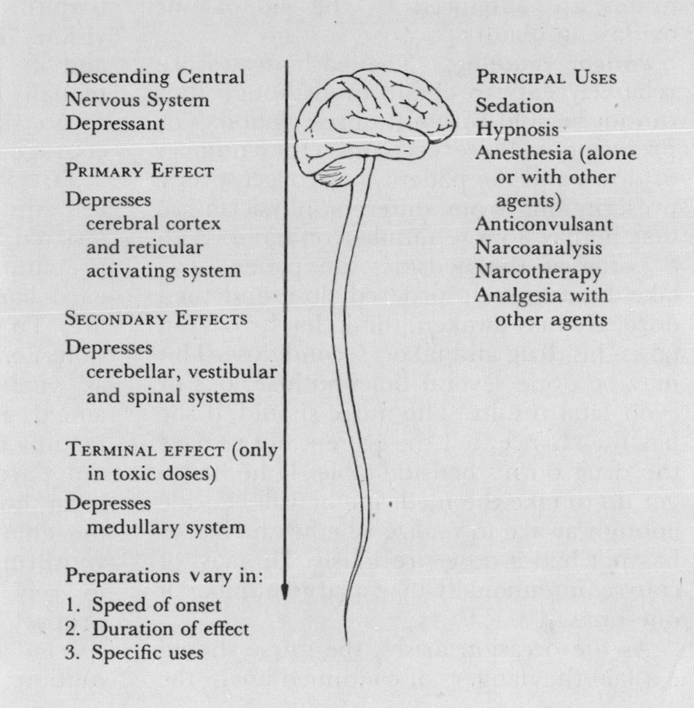

Descending Central
Nervous System
Depressant
PRIMARY EFFECT
Depresses
cerebral cortex
and reticular
activating system
SECONDARY EFFECTS
Depresses
cerebellar, vestibular
and spinal systems
TERMINAL EFFECT (only
in toxic doses)
Depresses
medullary system
Preparations vary in:
1. Speed of onset
2. Duration of effect
3. Specific uses
PRINCIPAL USES
Sedation
Hypnosis
Anesthesia (alone
or with other
agents)
Anticonvulsant
Narcoanalysis
Narcotherapy
Analgesia with
other agents

FIGURE 19. Derivatives of barbituric acid (the barbiturates) as therapeutic agents.

only concern should be for the care of an acutely ill person. However, very accurate records should be kept in case there is legal action later. In acute poisoning, the patient shows mental confusion, often delirium, then drowsiness, lethargy, and finally coma. There is a fall in blood pressure, sterterous breathing, tachycardia, moist skin, respiratory depression with pulmonary edema, lowered body temperature and collapse. Treatment consists of lavage and saline catharsis. The cathartic is instilled after the lavage. Great care must be used in the lavage as respiratory aspiration might prove fatal. The nurse should save the expressed gastric fluid unless told otherwise. Oxygen is given and a respirator used, if indicated. Cardiac stimulants are used. The type and amount will be determined by the patient's condition. Drugs that might be ordered include doxapram (Dopram) or ethamivan (Emivan). Peritoneal dialysis or hemodialysis may be used with or without the drugs.

The seriousness of acute barbiturate poisoning is increased if the patient has also consumed alcohol in any form, since alcohol potentiates the depressive action of the barbiturates.

Chronic Poisoning. Some of the barbiturates easily produce addiction, especially the rapidly acting ones, used as hypnotics, such as secobarbital (Seconal) and pentobarbital (Nembutal). Symptoms of chronic poisoning are headache, weakness, anorexia, anemia, visual disturbances and amnesia. Renal damage or psychoses may occur. Since the withdrawal symptoms are severe and serious, the drug is usually withdrawn slowly. Various nonaddictive sedatives may be substituted for the barbiturate. A stimulant may be ordered. Symptoms are treated as they occur. Additional information on this subject will be found in Chapter 6, The Problem of Drug Abuse.

Interactions. The barbiturate drugs interact with several other drugs. They antagonize, by enzyme induction, the action of such drugs and drug groups as analgesics, anticoagulants (oral), antihistamines, anti-inflammatory agents, diphenylhydantoin (Dilantin), griseofulvin (Fulvicin), hypnotics, steroids and meprobamate (Equanil, Miltown). The barbiturates potentiate other central nervous system depressants by additive effect, so much so, that at times there may be severe toxicity and even death. This is especially true with alcohol. The barbiturates are enhanced by the monoamine oxidase inhibitors.

Patient Teaching. The barbiturates are relatively easy to obtain even though they cannot be sold without a prescription. The prescription, however, is often for a number of doses and the patient may collect several prescriptions from different physicians so that he has a large number on hand. With a bottle at the bedside, the patient may take his regularly ordered dose and then doze. He may awaken, think that he has not taken his drug and take a second dose. This may be done several times with serious or even fatal results. The nurse should, if she has the chance, tell the patient not to have the drug on his bedside table. If he has to get up to take the medicine he will be wide enough awake to realize whether he has or has not had a dose previously. He may, of course, intentionally take a large number at one time.

As the occasion arises, the nurse should explain the dangers of continued use of the barbiturate drugs without medical supervision. Taking a sleeping pill each night and a "pep" pill each morning is a potentially dangerous habit to fall into. The nurse should do all that she can to discourage it.

The Patient. The patient whose restless and disturbed state is effectively alleviated by one of the milder, slower acting preparations like phenobarbital, may regard barbiturates as almost a necessity of life. To the patient susceptible to convulsion, i.e., the epileptic, barbiturates appear as vital. The short acting preparations aimed at inducing anesthesia and hence helping the patient over a trying and fearful time are most welcome preparations. It must, however, be kept clearly in mind that the emotionally disturbed patient and the youthful "experimenter" frequently come to rely upon barbiturates as emotional props. These preparations must be respected and used with the proper degree of caution.

TABLE 4. *SOME OF THE MORE IMPORTANT RESULTS OF STIMULATION BY THE AUTONOMIC NERVOUS SYSTEM*

STRUCTURE INNERVATED	SYMPATHETIC STIMULATION	PARASYMPATHETIC STIMULATION
Eye		
iris	dilated (increased intraocular pressure)	contracted (decreased intraocular pressure)
ciliary muscle	relaxed (far vision)	contracted (near vision)
lacrimal glands	circulatory changes	secretion
Heart		
rate	increased	decreased
stroke volume	increased	decreased
coronary vessels	dilated	usually constricted
Blood Vessels		
skin and mucosa	usually constricted	not usually innervated
abdominal viscera	constricted	dilated
cerebral	constricted	dilated
Lungs		
glands	inhibited	stimulated
muscles	relaxed	constricted
Gastrointestinal Tract		
muscles	decreased tone and motility	increased tone and motility
sphincters	constricted	relaxed
glands	inhibited	increased secretion
Liver	glycogenesis	does not innervate appreciably
Salivary Glands	stimulated – sparse thick secretion	stimulated – profuse watery secretion
Skin		
glands (sweat)	stimulated	does not innervate
pilomotor muscles	contracted	relaxed
Adrenal Medulla	secretion	does not innervate
Uterine Muscle	relaxed	constricted

Reference to Figure 19 will help the student to interpret the action of the barbiturate drugs.

DRUGS ACTING ON THE AUTONOMIC NERVOUS SYSTEM

(See Current Drug Handbook.)

The autonomic nervous system, as its name implies, acts without the intervention of volition. It carries on the activities that are essential to life (Table 4). Functionally, it is divided into two parts, the sympathetic and the parasympathetic (I-4). These divisions act more or less in opposition to each other. Thus, one stimulates and the other depresses the action of any given organ. The parasympathetic is concerned mainly with the maintenance of life (the so-called vegetative state), while the sympathetic is more active in emergencies. (It provides the "second wind" and the great power a person exerts in an emergency.) When each acts properly, a balance is reached and the life processes go on without interruption. Drugs of this classification may act directly upon the nervous tissue or they may, very occasionally, act directly upon the organs innervated by the nervous tissue. Some drugs appear to act in opposite ways upon the two divisions, depressing one and stimulating the other, but this is by no means universally true. Another point to remember is that, though a drug may act in opposite ways upon the two divisions, it may do so in varying degrees. The following brief summary may help to clarify these points (Table 5).

Many of the drugs that act primarily on the autonomic nervous system are not listed here; only representative ones in each group have been given. Since these drugs are usually important for their action on the organ involved, they will be discussed in Section 3. Only those with a variety of uses will be considered here.

Stimulants of the Parasympathetic Nervous System

Drugs in this category are also called cholinergic or parasympathomimetics. They

TABLE 5. *A FEW REPRESENTATIVE AUTONOMIC NERVOUS SYSTEM DRUGS* (Numbers refer to Figure 20)

	GANGLION (3)	PARASYMPATHETIC (2)	SYMPATHETIC (1)
Stimulants		*Cholinergic*	*Adrenergic*
	Acetylcholine	*Simulate acetylcholine*	Epinephrine
	Physostigmine	Methacholine	Ephedrine
	Neostigmine	Carbachol	Amphetamine
		Bethanechol	Phenylephrine
		Pilocarpine	Levarterenol
		Inhibit cholinesterase	
		Physostigmine	
		Neostigmine	
		Pyridostigmin	
		Ambenonium	
		Benzpyrinium	
		Isoflurophate	
		Demecarium	
		Echothiophate	
Depressants	*Ganglion blocking*	*Cholinergic blocking*	*Alpha-adrenergic blocking*
(Blocking)	Acetylcholine (large doses)	Atropine	Ergot and similar drugs
	Tetraethylammonium and similar compounds	Scopolamine	Tolazoline (Priscoline)
		Hyoscyamine	Phenoxybenzamine (Dibenzyline)
		Homatropine and similar atropine-like compounds such as	Phentolamine (Regitine)
		Lescopine	*Beta-adrenergic*
		Propantheline (Pro-Banthine)	Propranolol
		and many others	

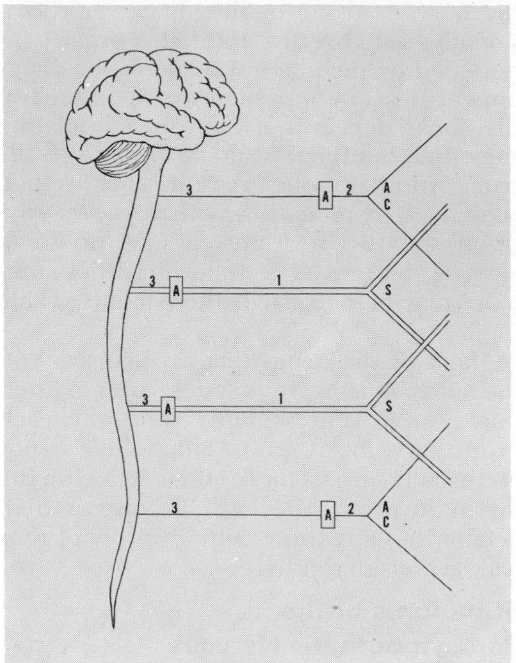

FIGURE 20. The autonomic nervous system. The single lines represent the cranial-sacral (parasympathetic) division. Note that the preganglionic fibers (3) are long and the postganglionic fibers (2) are short. The ganglia are situated in or near the organs which they innervate.

The double lines represent the thoraco-lumbar (sympathetic) division. Note that the preganglionic fibers (3) are short and the postganglionic fibers (1) are long. The ganglia are situated on each side of the spinal column.

The letter (A) represents the area where acetylcholine is formed; (C) where cholinesterase is formed—which counteracts (blocks) the action of acetylcholine; (S) where sympathin is formed. Sympathin consists of epinephrine and norepinephrine.

It should also be noted that the areas of control of the two systems cross, in part. This indicates that most organs receive fibers from both divisions of the autonomic nervous system, but there are exceptions.

act mainly in the following ways: as cholinesterase inhibitors, thus preventing the destruction of endogenous acetylcholine; by increasing the amount of acetylcholine in the body (the choline derivatives); or by simulating the action of acetylcholine. Reference to the diagram and tables will aid in the understanding of their action, and this holds true for all the autonomic nervous system drugs. Those drugs which simulate acetylcholine (the choline derivatives) are used mainly in the treatment of urinary or intestinal retention, including flatulence. The cholinesterase inhibitors are used primarily for two purposes: to constrict the pupils of the eyes in glaucoma and to treat myasthenia gravis. Some of the cholinesterase drugs are used also for retention and flatulence.

The choline derivatives include *methacholine chloride* (Mecholyl chloride; Mecholin [C]) 200 to 500 mg. orally or 10 to 25 mg. subcutaneously, or by ion transfer (iontophoresis) 0.2 to 0.5 per cent solution. *Bethanechol chloride* (Urecholine) 5 to 30 mg. orally or 2.5 to 5.0 mg. subcutaneously. Toxic symptoms include flushing, headache, abdominal cramps, sweating and sometimes asthmatic type attacks and/or hypotension.

The cholinesterase inhibitors include many drugs used for the same purposes as the choline derivatives and also to treat myasthenia gravis and glaucoma. A full discussion of these will be found in Chapters 24 and 32. A simple listing of some of the more important ones will suffice here. *Neostigmine* (Prostigmine; Intrastigmine [C]) is used for urinary retention, flatulence and to treat and diagnose myasthenia gravis. *Benzpyrinium bromide* (Stigmonene) is used for retention, flatulence and delayed menstruation. *Physostigmine* (eserine [C]), an alkaloid of physostigma, has varied actions, but its main use is to counteract atropine poisoning or overdose, or as a miotic. It is also a strong diaphoretic. *Pyridostigmin* (Mestinon) and ambenonium (Mytelase) are used to treat myasthenia gravis. Isoflurophate (Floropryl), demecarium bromide (Humorsol) and echothiophate iodide (Phospholine) are among the more common preparations used to treat glaucoma.

Patients receiving parasympathetic stimulants must be watched for too great a decrease in pulse rate and for respiratory embarrassment. These stimulants must also be used sparingly in bronchial asthma as they increase bronchiole constriction.

Interactions. There have been many reports of possible interaction between the parasympathomimetic drugs with various other medicines, but many of these reports are unsubstantiated. However, a few are well enough documented to warrant discussion. These include neostigmine (Prostigmin), which reduces the neuromuscular blockage of the aminoglycoside antibiotics (streptomycin, neomycin and kanamycin). Neostigmine and edrophonium antagonize the relaxant action of the drugs of the curare type, but they prolong, rather than antagonize, succinylcholine.

Depressants of the Parasympathetic Nervous System

Parasympathetic depressants are also called cholinergic blocking agents or parasympatholytics. Their action simulates that of cholinesterase as it blocks or inactivates acetylcholine.

The parasympathetic depressants will cause thirst when taken in excessive amounts. Even after small doses patients often complain of dryness of the mouth and throat. The nurse must watch for this if the patient is taking any of these drugs for any length of time, even if the dosage is relatively small. Other untoward symptoms include flushed face, dry hot skin, rapid pulse, rise in blood pressure, dilated pupils and rapid shallow respirations. In acute poisoning these symptoms come on suddenly and in chronic poisoning, gradually. In chronic poisoning and in cases of idiosyncrasy the symptoms may all appear but are much less severe than in the acute condition. Stopping the drug is usually sufficient for relief. In acute poisoning, emetics are given or a lavage is done. Tannic acid may be ordered for the lavage. In the home, strong tea may be substituted. Morphine should not be given, for, although atropine is an antidote for morphine, morphine is not an antidote for atropine. The patient will need to be treated for shock. It is well to be prepared for catheterization, as the drug is excreted by the kidneys and the physician may want to prevent any reabsorption. Central nervous system stimulants should be available for use if needed.

These drugs are contraindicated in glaucoma as they increase intraocular pressure. Refer to Chapters 17 and 24.

Atropine, scopolamine and many synthetic compounds that are similar to these are used for a variety of purposes. However, most of these drugs will be dealt with later when the various conditions treated with them are discussed. Only brief mention will be made of them here. All of these drugs are commonly used to decrease secretions of most of the glands. They are used to decrease perspiration and gastric secretions, especially in patients with peptic ulcers. They decrease peristalsis and are, therefore, used in biliary, renal and intestinal colic. They dilate the bronchial tubes and are sometimes added to preparations for the relief of asthma.

Atropine and some of the newer synthetic drugs are used to dilate the pupils of the eyes. This action is directly opposed to that of pilocarpine and eserine. Atropine is a physiologic antidote for morphine and cholinergic drug poisoning. Atropine sulfate is the active principle of belladonna, a drug derived from the plant *Atropa belladonna.* Both act as anodynes and also relax muscle tissue and relieve tension.

Belladonna and *atropine sulfate* are administered in many different ways. Belladonna in the form of a plaster or an ointment is used locally as an anodyne and antispasmodic. Belladonna in the form of the tincture is given orally, usually in 0.3 to 1.0 ml. It is used in this way as an intestinal antispasmodic and to lessen gastric secretions. Atropine sulfate 0.3 to 0.6 mg. may be given either orally or subcutaneously for the same purposes and for many others, such as to decrease secretions during operative procedures. Other uses for this drug will be discussed later (Chapters 15 to 24). Atropine sulfate in a 1/2 to 2 per cent solution is used for instillation in the eyes as a mydriatic. In combination with other drugs, atropine is used in treating many disorders, especially those of the lungs and the gastrointestinal tract.

Scopolamine hydrobromide (hyoscine [C]) is given either orally or subcutaneously in the same dosage as atropine sulfate 0.3 to 0.6 mg. Scopolamine tends to cause more mental relaxation than does atropine. For long continued use it is less desirable, but as a preoperative medication it has the advantage over atropine of reducing mental activity and it produces less tenacious sputum.

Interactions. Most interactions of the parasympatholytic drugs, so far as they are known, are exaggerations of their established pharmaceutical activity. When orphenadrine and propoxyphene (Darvon) are given together, cases of tremors and convulsions have been reported.

Papaverine is often considered with the parasympathetic depressant drugs because of its action on smooth muscle tissue. Papaverine is a non-narcotic alkaloid of opium that does not appear to be habit forming, nor does it usually produce tolerance. It is helpful as an antispasmodic in cases of smooth muscle spasms of the peripheral vascular system, the gastrointestinal tract and, to a lesser degree, the bronchi, coronary vessels and biliary tract. Papaverine is given orally or parenterally in doses of 0.1 Gm. It does not usually cause any toxic symptoms, but liver damage has been reported with long-term usage. There are many drugs in this category. Refer to Current Drug Handbook for further information.

Stimulants of the Sympathetic Nervous System

The sympathetic stimulant drugs are also called sympathomimetic or adrenergic. Many of these substances come from natural sources, plant or animal. In addition, there are a large number of synthetic compounds which have similar actions. All of these drugs have some actions in common but, at the same time, each product displays certain individual effects not necessarily found in the other preparations.

The action of the drugs in the sympathetic stimulant group is similar to those just described. They all tend to decrease muscular tone, dilate the bronchial tubes, dilate the pupils of the eyes, increase cardiac rate and decrease most glandular secretions.

The adrenal medulla secretes powerful hormones called "catecholamines" which mimic the action of the sympathetic nervous system. There are also synthetic preparations which have similar activity. These amines act on peripheral receptor sites known as alpha and beta receptors. (Refer to Chapter 4 for further information on receptor sites.) The alpha receptors are associated with excitatory responses of smooth muscles (contraction). Beta receptors mediate relaxation of smooth muscles, but they also increase the rate and strength of cardiac contraction.

Some specific drugs and their actions on these sites are as follows:

Alpha and beta activation: epinephrine and metaraminol (Aramine).

Alpha blockage: phenoxybenzamine (Dibenzyline) and phentolamine (Regitine).

Alpha activator: norepinephrine.

Beta blockage: propranolol (Inderal).

Beta activation: isoproterenol (Isuprel), phenylephrine (Neo-Synephrine) and methoxamine (Vasoxyl).

Amphetamine sulfate (Benzedrine) and similar preparations have already been considered as central nervous system stimulants. Its action as a sympathetic stimulant is not greatly different. Although amphetamine does stimulate the central nervous system, it also stimulates the sympathetic system as well. It will elicit some or all of the symptoms that have just been mentioned.

Epinephrine hydrochloride (Adrenalin, Suprarenin) is the most important and widely used of all the sympathetic stimulants. Epinephrine has many uses but the most important are: vasoconstriction locally to lessen bleeding and to delay absorption of drugs, such as local anesthetics; vasoconstriction to raise blood pressure; bronchial dilation to relieve the symptoms of bronchial asthma; treatment of other allergies; and as an emergency stimulant in certain cases of heart or respiratory failure. Epinephrine tends to lessen the blood supply to the abdominal area and to increase the blood supply to the skeletal muscles. The body's emergency hormone, it is secreted by the medullary portion of the suprarenal glands. The drug is rendered inert by the digestive juices and cannot be given orally. It is given parenterally in an aqueous solution 1:1000 in strength. The dose is usually from 0.3 to 1.0 ml. Epinephrine also comes in an oil solution 1:500 in strength which is given intramuscularly in doses of 0.2 to 1.0 ml. The aqueous solution is used in a nebulizer for inhalation. Synthetic preparations similar to epinephrine that can be given orally are available, but many physicians feel that they are not so satisfactory.

If the dosage of epinephrine is too great, toxic symptoms may occur but, since it is a normal body secretion, idiosyncrasy is rare. Undesirable symptoms include: rapid irregular pulse, pale blanched skin, throbbing sensation in the head, dilated pupils, tremors and, in severe cases, fibrillation, pulmonary edema and collapse. The patient should be treated for shock and a parasympathetic stimulant administered. The patient receiving epinephrine, especially for the first time, should be closely watched for symptoms of toxic reaction; he should be reassured if any of the untoward symptoms do develop. In most cases, the undesirable reactions are very transitory, the effect wearing off in a few minutes. The drug does not have a prolonged effect at any time. The aqueous solution is often repeated every three or four hours, as often as every hour in severe cases of asthma and it can also be used in a nebulizer. This, of course, is stopped as soon as relief is secured. The time interval is then adjusted to suit the patient's needs.

Ephedrine is the active principle of a plant drug which forms one of the main sympathetic stimulants. However, its use has been largely limited to the treatment of allergies and bronchial asthma, and it will be discussed under that topic.

Levarterenol (Levophed) is the salt of norepinephrine and is used in cases of hypotension, especially the severe type accompanying surgery or emergencies. There are a number of synthetic drugs with similar actions. These are discussed in Chapter 15 and also in the Current Drug Handbook.

Depressants of the Sympathetic Nervous System

None of the drugs listed under this heading will be discussed at this point. Those mentioned at the beginning of the discussion of autonomic nervous system drugs included ergot, which is considered with drugs used in the treatment of patients suffering from gynecologic disorders and in obstetrics (Chapter 28); Pituitrin, which is used in the same ways and also after surgery (Chapter 15); and quinine, which is discussed with drugs used in treating patients with communicable diseases (Chapter 31). Pituitrin is sometimes used for the same purposes as neostigmine, which has been discussed with parasympathomimetics.

Interactions. Azapetine and phenoxybenzamine will reverse the pressor effect of epinephrine, block or diminish the vasoconstrictive effect of levarterenol and prevent epinephrine-induced cardiac arrhythmias after myocardial sensitivity by cyclopropane or chloroform. Methylsergide appears to be potentiated by chlorpromazine.

All the drugs discussed in this chapter will be repeatedly mentioned in the chapters which follow in Section III. As a certain type of patient or condition is discussed, the drugs that deal with that condition will be given. This, of course, necessitates repetition, but in each case the drug will be seen in a different light. It is the intention in every case to consider the individual patient's needs and his possible reactions to the medicines which are given. It may seem logical to say that epinephrine is good for asthma, Mr. Blank has asthma, therefore Mr. Blank should be given epinephrine; but this is not necessarily a valid conclusion. Mr. Blank is an individual person and he may not react to the drug in the usual manner. It is Mr. Blank who is being treated—not just the asthma.

Tranquilizers

Drugs used as tranquilizers may act on the central nervous system, the autonomic nervous system or both, and for some the exact method of action is only partially understood. The tranquilizing properties of the medications were discovered much by accident; most of the drugs, used widely in medical therapy, first were given for conditions other than tranquilization. This fact often decides the best drug to be given to a specific patient. The application of the drugs in various conditions will be covered throughout the clinical section. Here the major groups will be discussed briefly. Refer to Chapter 30 for detailed information. See Current Drug Handbook.

PHENOTHIAZINE DERIVATIVES. The phenothiazine tranquilizers can be classified according to their principal use or their chemical structure. Some are antinauseants and were used for that purpose before their tranquilizing properties were known. Some potentiate other drugs, especially the analgesics, which makes them extremely valuable in conditions requiring long periods of analgesic use (cancer and other chronic painful conditions). In such cases less of the narcotic is needed.

Here follow the main tranquilizers; they are discussed in detail in the areas of their importance.

- Phenothiazine Derivatives
  - Dimethyl amine side chain
    - Chlorpromazine (Thorazine; Elmarine [C])
    - Promazine (Sparine; Atarzine [C])
    - Promethazine (Phenergan)
    - Propiomazine (Largon)
    - Triflupromazine (Vesprin; fluopromazine [C])
    - Trimeprazine (Temaril)
  - Piperidine side chain
    - Pipamazine
    - Thioridazine (Mellaril)
  - Piperazine side chain
    - Acetophenazine (Tindal)
    - Butaperazine (Repoise)
    - Carphenazine (Proketazine)
    - Fluphenazine (Prolixin; Permitil [C])
    - Perphenazine (Trilafon)
    - Prochlorperazine (Compazine; Stemetil [C])
    - Thiopropazate (Dartal)
    - Thiethylperazine (Torecan)
    - Trifluoperazine (Stelazine)
- Thioxanthenes
  - Chlorprothixene (Taractan; Tarasan [C])
  - Thiothixene (Navane)
- Benzodiazepines
  - Clorazepate dipotassium (Tranxene)
  - Chlordiazepoxide (Librium)
  - Diazepam (Valium)
  - Oxazepam (Serax)
- Butyrophenones
  - Haloperidol (Haldol)
  - Droperidol (Inapsine)

THE BENZODIAZEPINES, CHLORDIAZEPOXIDE (LIBRIUM), DIAZEPAM (VALIUM), OXAZEPAM (SERAX)

The Drugs. The benzodiazepine tranquilizers are useful for so many conditions that it seems appropriate to give them more extensive coverage here. These drugs include Clorazepate dipotassium (Tranxene), Chlordiazepoxide (Librium), Diazepam (Valium) and Oxazepam (Serax). Oxazepam has a large number of undesirable side effects and is not extensively used.

Physical and Chemical Properties. These are benzodiazepine derivatives. They are colorless crystalline substances. Chlordiazepoxide is readily soluble in water, diazepam is not.

Action. They have wide action, varying with the dosage. They relax skeletal muscle, decrease tension and anxiety, produce sedation and tranquilize. They act not only on the central nervous system, but on the autonomic and the peripheral nervous systems as well. Their exact mode of action is unknown.

Therapeutic Uses. Chlordiazepoxide (Librium) in small doses is used for tension associated with various disorders of the skin and gastrointestinal, cardiovascular and reproductive systems; anxiety; some types of headaches; menstrual tension and dysmenorrhea; pre- and postoperative apprehension; chronic alcoholism; and behavioral problems in children. In larger doses it is used for severe tension and anxiety. It is also used in some cases of skeletal muscle spasticity and other neuromuscular disorders.

Diazepam (Valium) is used in much the same conditions as with chlordiazepoxide especially when there is concomitant emotional disturbances with the various somatic conditions. It is helpful in the alleviation of muscle spasm associated with cerebral palsy and athetosis. The drug is not effective in the treatment of psychotic anxiety and should not be used in cases of known psychoses.

Absorption and Excretion. The exact fate of these drugs in the body is not known. However, it is known to take several hours to reach the peak blood level. The drug remains in the body in appreciable amounts for 24 to 48 hours and is slowly excreted by the kidneys over several days. Some of the drug is excreted unchanged; some is in the conjugated form.

Preparations and Dosages

Clorazepate dipotassium (Tranxene) 15 to 60 mg. daily, orally in divided doses.

Chlordiazepoxide hydrochloride, N.F. (Librium) 5 to 25 mg. orally t.i.d. or q.i.d. 100 mg. I.M. q 4 to 6 h.

Diazepam (Valium) 2 to 10 mg. orally, I.M. or I.V., b.i.d. to q.i.d.

Oxazepam (Serax) 10 to 30 mg. orally t.i.d. or q.i.d.

THE NURSE

Mode of Administration. There are no special problems in the oral administration of these drugs. However, the amount administered is highly individualized. Parenteral medication should be prepared immediately prior to use and given slowly and deeply, intramuscularly. After parenteral injection it may be wise to have the patient remain recumbent for approximately three hours so that his reactions can be observed.

Side Effects. It is rare to have to discontinue either chlordiazepoxide or diazepam due to side effects although it may be necessary to reduce the dosage in some cases. The main side effect is drowsiness. Other side effects have been reported with chlordiazepoxide including ataxia, constipation, headache, dizziness, muscle tenderness, confusion, syncope, urinary frequency and menorrhagia. With diazepam the most common side effects are, in addition to drowsiness, nausea, dizziness, excitement, disturbances of sleep, hallucinations, diplopia, headache, slurred speech, tremors and incontinence. The side effects of oxazepam are similar to the other two drugs of this group, but as stated previously they occur more often than with either chlordiazepoxide or diazepam.

Toxicity and Treatment. Because the blood level is so slowly reached, acute toxicity is rare. However, with chlordiazepoxide, cumulative effects may occur while maintenance level is being reached, and abrupt withdrawal symptoms may occur if the drug is discontinued rapidly. These symptoms include tremors, nausea and vomiting, insomnia, profuse diaphoresis and abdominal and muscle cramps. Convulsions have been reported to have occurred after the drug was discontinued.

Interactions. The benzodiazepine compounds are enhanced by alcohol, the barbiturates and the monoamine oxidase inhibitors.

Contraindications. These drugs tend to potentiate other psychogenic agents such as the phenothiazines, barbiturates, monoamine oxidase inhibitors and alcohol. They are used with caution, if at all, when these drugs are being given. Chlordiazepoxide is used with caution for individuals known to tend to drug dependency because, in large doses, it has been shown to have addictive tendencies. Diazepam is contraindicated in infants, patients with a history of convulsive disorders and patients with glaucoma. It is used only in low dosage for elderly or debilitated patients. Refer to Current Drug Handbook for contraindications to oxazepam.

Patient Teaching. The nurse should explain to the patient that after the drug, which does not act immediately, takes effect he will feel much better. He should be warned not to drive a car or operate dangerous machinery while taking these drugs, especially at the initiation of treatment or if the dosage is large. If asked or if there is an opportunity, the nurse might tell the patient that these drugs potentiate the action of alcohol and that he will be wise to reduce or discontinue the use of alcoholic beverages while taking the medicine.

THE PATIENT. These drugs by reducing tension, anxiety and emotional disturbances make the patient feel much better. Indirectly, the drug also often helps to improve family relationships. A tense, anxious person can often cause many family disturbances. When this same person becomes less tense the whole family relaxes.

RAUWOLFIA DERIVATIVES. These were first used as hypotensive agents and are still used to reduce blood pressure. However, they are used more often now as tranquilizers. They do not cause sedation nor do they potentiate other medications. There are many rauwolfia preparations, such as reserpine (Serpasil and many other trade names), deserpidine (Harmonyl), rescinnamine (Moderil) and rauwolfia root (Raudixin, Rauserpa, Rauserpin, Rauval).

SKELETAL MUSCLE RELAXANTS. Though weak as tranquilizers, these do cause relaxation, especially when muscle tension is a factor. The more important members of this group include such drugs as carisoprodol (Soma, Rela; isomeprobamate, Caricoma, Sonoma [C]), chlorphenesin (Maolate), chlorzoxazone (Paraflex), mephenesin (several trade names), mephenesin carbamate, metaxalone (Skelaxin), methocarbamol (Robaxin) and phenaglycodol (Ultran, Acalo [C]).

Another drug used as a tranquilizer is hydroxyzine hydrochloride (Atarax, Vistaril; Pas Depress [C]). Refer to the Current Drug Handbook for details. Patients taking these drugs should be extremely careful to avoid hazardous occupations, at least until the body adjusts to the drug. This is an ever-expanding area which is very helpful in the treatment of many conditions, but there are times when tranquilization is not the best therapy. Only the physician can determine this.

Interactions. Carisoprodol decreases the action of meprobamate by enzyme induction. It decreases the effect of barbital, phenobarbital chlorcyclizine and diphenhydramine due to enhanced metabolism. There is increased relaxation by enzyme induction with the concurrent use of the monoamine oxidase inhibitors.

IT IS IMPORTANT TO REMEMBER

1. That any drug acting upon a part of the nervous system will also act upon the organ or organs controlled by that portion of the nervous system.
2. That many "nervous system" drugs are given for their effect upon the organs other than the nervous system; for instance, stimulation of the respiratory center may be the action of the drug, but increase in respiration is the desired result.
3. That most analgesic and hypnotic drugs are habit forming, though they may not cause actual addiction. The nurse should avoid their use whenever other measures can be used safely and effectively.

TOPICS FOR STUDY AND DISCUSSION

1. A child is brought into the emergency department of a hospital. The child is restless and shows involuntary contractions of various skeletal muscles. When the bright overhead light is turned on, the child has a convulsion. The parents state that they do not know what the trouble is, but they think that the child may have eaten some rodent poison.
   a. What might the nurse suspect?
   b. What should she prepare while awaiting the arrival of the physician?
   c. What steps might she take?
   d. What questions might she ask the parents?
2. Owing to emotional shock a friend becomes faint. You have her sit down and put her head between her knees. This does not seem to be sufficient. What else might you do?
3. Give some rules for the prevention of self-medication—especially as it applies to nurses who have minor but regularly recurring pains. (You might prepare a sociogram with some of your classmates to dramatize this.)
4. Why do doctors and nurses frequently acquire the "drug habit"? How can this be avoided?
5. What are some of the things a nurse may do to decrease the need of her patients for strong analgesics? Cite specific instances if you can.
6. Ask among your friends and relatives, or your class- or schoolmates:
   a. Do you have aspirin in your home (room)?
   b. Have you taken any in the last 24 to 48 hours?
   c. Why did you take it?
   d. How much did you take? (One aspirin tablet contains 0.3 Gm., gr. 5.)

   Tabulate the results and bring to the class for general discussion.
7. Morphine sulfate gr. 1/6 is ordered. The nurse finds the stock tablets are gr. 1/4. How should she prepare the desired dose?
8. Chloral hydrate gr. 10 has been ordered. The stock supply marked 1.0 ml. contains 0.3 Gm. of the drug. How much should be used?

BIBLIOGRAPHY

Books and Pamphlets

American Medical Association Council on Drugs, *Drug Evaluations*, Chicago, 1971, American Medical Association.
Bevan, J. A., *Essentials of Pharmacology*, New York, 1969, Harper & Row.
Falconer, M., Patterson, H. R., and Gustafson, E., *Current Drug Handbook 1974–76*, Philadelphia, 1974. W. B. Saunders Co.
Goodman, L. S., and Gilman, A., *Pharmacological Basis of Therapeutics, 4th Ed.*, New York, 1970, The Macmillan Co.
Goth, A., *Medical Pharmacology*, St. Louis, 1970, The C. V. Mosby Co.
Robinson, D. S., and Amidor, E., *Interaction of Benzodiazepines with Warfarin in Man*, Burlington, Vermont, University of Vermont College of Medicine.
Sedlock, S., et al., *Drug Sheet for Coronary Nurses*, reproduced by Santa Clara County (California) Heart Association.

Journal Articles

Boyd, E. M., "The safety and toxicity of aspirin," *Am. J. Nurs.* 71:5:964 (May, 1971).
Fass, G., "Sleep, drugs and dreams," *Am. J. Nurs.* 71:12:2316 (December, 1971).
Gates, M., "Analgesic drugs," *Sci. Am.* 215:131 (November, 1966).
Kirby, C. W., "Biosynthesis of the morphine alkaloids" *Science* 155:170 (January, 1967).
McBride, M. A., "The addiction to the alkaloids," *Am. J. Nurs.* 69:5:974 (May, 1969).
Rodman, M. J., "Drugs for pain problems," *R.N.* 34:4:59 (April, 1971).
Williams, D. H., "Sleep and dreams," *Am. J. Nurs.* 71:12:2321 (December, 1971).

CHAPTER 10

DRUGS USED TO MAINTAIN FLUID AND ELECTROLYTE BALANCE

CORRELATION WITH OTHER SCIENCES

I. ANATOMY AND PHYSIOLOGY

1. The body fluid is about 60 per cent of body weight for men and 50 per cent for women; there is a higher percentage of water in the thin individual and a lower percentage in the fat person since adipose tissue contains less water than muscle tissue does.

2. Body fluids are either extracellular (outside the cells) or intracellular (within the cells). The extracellular fluid is either interstitial (within the tissue spaces) or intravascular (within the blood and lymph vessels).

3. The process of urine formation is divided into two phases: The first is the filtration of the plasma which takes place in the glomerulus. The second phase is a modification of the filtered material by tubular reabsorption and secretion.

4. The glomerular filtrate is largely reabsorbed. This takes place all along the tubules, but the great amount of both water and electrolytes is in the proximal tubules.

5. If the three processes—filtration, reabsorption and secretion—are normal, the plasma remains in a normal condition. Any change can result in a plasma imbalance.

6. The kidney must adjust the amount of sodium and water excreted. This serves as a protective mechanism for the body.

7. There are normally a few substances which are actively secreted by the renal tubular cells. Among these are hydrogen, ammonia, potassium, creatinine and certain dyes and drugs used in renal function tests.

II. CHEMISTRY

1. The hydrogen ion is a standard electrochemical unit.

2. The pH of a solution is determined by its hydrogen ion concentration. A pH of 7.0 is neutral, over 7.0 is basic (alkaline) and below 7.0 is acid.

3. The normal pH of the blood is slightly on the alkaline side of neutrality (7.35 to 7.45).

4. If an excess of acid causes the pH of the blood to drop below 7.2, acidosis exists and an excess of basic (alkaline) ions pH above 7.5 will cause alkalosis.

5. In acidosis the amount of hydrogen excreted by the kidneys is increased by reaction with the urinary buffer system and combination with ammonia. The increased excretion is maintained as long as a favorable pressure gradient is present.

6. The normal pH of the urine is 6, or slightly acid.

7. Colloid is a state of matter composed of single large molecules or aggregates of smaller molecules in stable suspension (dispersed particles 1 to 100 mμ in diameter).

8. Diffusion is the movement of molecules from a region of high to low concentration. (In a closed system, an equilibrium is reached which results in a uniform concentration throughout.)

9. A semipermeable membrane allows diffusion of some types of particles (such as molecules or ions in solution), but not others. An equilibrium is usually reached resulting in an equal osmotic concentration on each side of the membrane.

10. Osmosis is the diffusion of solvent molecules (usually water) across a semipermeable membrane. Osmotic pressure is pressure exerted by this movement in a closed system.

11. An equivalent is the unit of measurement of the chemical activity of a substance. The gram equivalent weight of a substance, estimated by dividing the atomic weight of the ion by its valance, is the number of grams of an element that will combine with 1.008 Gm.

of hydrogen ions or 17.008 Gm. of hydroxyl ions. A milliequivalent (mEq.) is 1/1000 of an equivalent.

12. An electrolyte is a chemical substance which, when dissolved in water, separates into charged particles (ions) capable of conducting an electrical current. A cation is an ion with a positive charge; an anion is an ion carrying a negative charge.

13. A mol (mole) is the molecular weight of a substance expressed in grams. A millimol is 1/1000 of a mol. A molar solution contains 1 Gm. molecular weight of solute in each liter of solution (1 mol per 1000 ml.).

A molal solution contains 1 Gm. molecular weight of solute to 1 kg. of solvent (1 mol to 1000 Gm.).

14. An osmol is a unit of osmotic pressure. A milliosmol is 1/1000 of an osmol.

INTRODUCTION

Fluid balance, though discussed separately here, is to be considered in many diseases and disorders. It is especially important in cardiovascular conditions, endocrine imbalance, surgical procedures, diabetes mellitus, burns and fever. In relation to this, reference should be made to diuretics in Chapter 18 and diuretics and intravenous fluids in the Current Drug Handbook.

The human body is approximately one-half water (I-1). All cells, except those on the surface of the body, are surrounded by fluid and are largely water (I-2). This water is in constant motion. It moves through the vessels of the circulatory and lymphatic systems, diffusing across the membranes of these systems into spaces between the cells where it is recognized as interstitial fluid. The water also crosses the membranes bounding the body's tissue and organ cells and through the membranes within these cells. In these locations it is referred to as intracellular fluid. This is the medium of transport utilized to carry nutrients, hormones and enzymes to their needed locations, and the waste products of cell activity to the site of elimination (II-1, 2, 3).

As shown by Figure 21, intake and output in the healthy individual are usually in a dynamic balance as is the proportion of intravascular, interstitial and intracellular fluid. This ever-changing (dynamic) but steady relationship (balance), is commonly called *"water balance."* A change in either intake or output can upset this balance. Likewise a change in the concentration of particles in solution can alter the osmotic characteristic of one of the components (intravascular, interstitial or intracellular) with consequent alteration of their dynamic relationship. Any disturbance of this ratio can be serious. Vomiting, diarrhea, exudation from denuded surfaces or treatments such as gastric suction can deplete the body of fluids very rapidly. Excessive loss of body fluid results in dehydration. (For further information concerning fluid balance refer to "The Severely Burned Patient" (Chapter 23).

If the proper amount of fluid is not excreted, it is retained and edema will result. Edema may be either local, usually due to infection or trauma, or general, due to diseases or disorders such as congestive heart failure, renal insufficiency (oliguria or anuria) or nephrosis.

In any loss or excessive retention of body fluid, there is a concomitant loss or retention of electrolytes. (An electrolyte is a compound which, dissolved in water, separates into charged particles, ions, capable of conducting electricity [II-12].) Ions with a positive charge are called cations; negatively charged ions are anions. Loss of the electrolytes may be as serious or even more serious than the actual loss of water because of their osmotic influence. The major ions in the body are: sodium, potassium, calcium, magnesium—cations—and chloride, bicarbonate, phosphate and sulfate—anions. See the accompanying table for more details.

An isotonic solution has the same osmotic pressure as the solution to which it is compared. Medicinally, isotonic solutions are those which have the same osmotic pressure as blood plasma. Isotonic saline (0.9 per cent) is such a solution. However, it is incorrect to call this solution "normal," since it is not. It

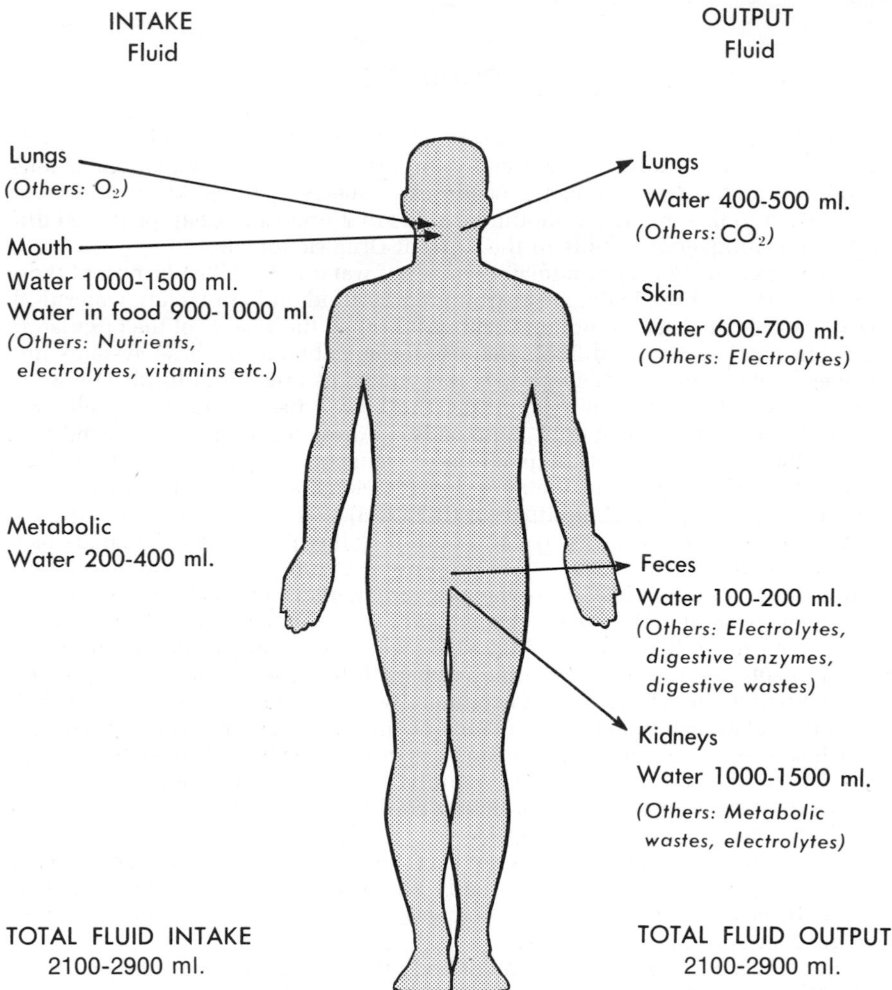

FIGURE 21. Intake and output of the human body.

contains more mEq./L. of both sodium and chloride than does plasma (II-10). It is isotonic in that it neither increases nor decreases the osmotic pressure of the intracellular fluid. Solutions not containing electrolytes may have osmotic pressure. These are usually colloidal solutions (II-7).

It would appear that the medicinal treatment of fluid or electrolyte imbalance would be relatively simple. If there is not enough water, give water, not enough of a specific ion, give a compound containing that ion and so on. Theoretically, this is true, but as is often the case, the practical application may be very involved. Many questions must be answered before treatment is begun, such as: Why is there a deficit? What is the possibility of the patient's absorbing or retaining the replacement? What is the best way to give the required substance? What type of fluid and/or drugs should be used? In some cases, replacement is easy, in some, moderately difficult and very complicated in others.

Because of the nature of this subject, the usual divisions will not be used. Causes of the conditions, major symptoms, laboratory findings and usual treatment will be covered.

FLUID VOLUME DEFICIT

CAUSES. The usual cause of depleted fluid volume is, of course, excessive loss of fluids in such conditions as diarrhea, vomiting, gastric suction, diaphoresis, exudation from denuded surfaces (burns or skin diseases), or polyuria.

There is a great deal of fluid normally present in the gastrointestinal tract both through ingestion and secretion. This is usually reabsorbed in the lower ileum and the colon. However, with vomiting and diarrhea the fluid is not reabsorbed and the loss can be severe. Normal amount of water in the intestines each 24 hours is estimated to be about 8200 ml. divided as follows: saliva 1500 ml., gastric juice 2500 ml., bile 500 ml., pancreatic juice 700 ml., and intestinal juice 3000 ml.

SYMPTOMS. The symptoms of fluid deficit are those of dehydration: dry skin and mucous membranes, longitudinal wrinkling of the tongue, oliguria, acute weight loss (over 5 per cent), lowered body temperature.

LABORATORY FINDINGS. There is an increase in hemoglobin and usually the hematocrit.

TREATMENT. Naturally, the treatment is to supply fluid. If the patient can take fluid by mouth it is usual to give it that way, otherwise the intravenous route is preferred. Of course, there are other routes such as rectal, subcutaneous and intraperitoneal, however, in most cases their disadvantages usually outweigh any advantages.

It must be remembered that there is never only water lost from the body. Replacement must take into consideration the loss of electrolytes and possibly other substances such as proteins. The solution the physician selects for replacement will be one that includes all the things which laboratory studies indicate are needed. If the solution is to be given orally, it must contain more than just water. Of course, the needed electrolytes and colloids may be given as medicines or foods or both, but they must be secured. Water alone is not sufficient.

Of the various constituents that may be lost with water, sodium is perhaps the most important, with potassium ranking second. The reason for this is that the dynamic fluid balance between intracellular and intercellular fluid is maintained by these two substances, potassium being intracellular and sodium, interstitial. They will be discussed further in this chapter.

FLUID VOLUME EXCESS

This condition is generalized edema. It is treated by removing as nearly as possible the cause of the edema. Diuretics may be used according to the condition. Fluid intake may or may not be restricted. See Congestive Heart Failure, Chapter 18.

Acid-Base Ratio

It is not possible to discuss fluid balance without at least touching on the subject of the acid-base ratio of the body fluids. Any change in the normal pH of the blood is serious, whether there has been loss of fluid volume or not. Acidosis and alkalosis are both severe conditions (II-1, 2, 3, 4). Buffers are substances which aid in maintaining the normal pH; they reduce the tendency to change from a stable condition. Carbonic acid (H_2CO_3) allows less basic change, bicarbonate (HCO_3^-) allows less acid change. The presence of these in the plasma is an important factor in maintenance of the normal pH. Acids are hydrogen donors, they give up the hydrogen atom relatively easily; bases are hydrogen acceptors. The acid-base ratio is maintained by the concentration of the hydrogen ions in the extracellular fluid. Carbon dioxide combines with water to form carbonic acid. The cations, sodium, potassium, calcium and magnesium, combine with the anion, bicarbonate, to form a compound which is called a base bicarbonate. The ratio of the base bicarbonates to carbonic acid under normal conditions is one to one. Table 6 gives information on the basic ions.

Acidosis is a condition of reduced alkalinity of the blood. Any pH under 7.35 is considered to be acidosis. Alkalosis is the reverse, occurring when the pH is above 7.45. There are two forms of acidosis and alkalosis. One, caused by a disturbance of metabolism, is called metabolic acidosis or metabolic alkalosis; the other, occurring in respiratory dysfunction, is called respiratory acidosis or respiratory alkalosis.

Refer to Table 7 for comparisons.

Metabolic Acidosis (Primary Base Carbonate Deficit)

CAUSES. Excessive infusion of isotonic saline solution is one cause; others include thyrotoxicosis, starvation, excessive use of certain drugs, such as the salicylates or paraldehyde, or any condition in which fats and proteins are metabolized by the body instead of carbohydrates. An excessive loss of intestinal fluids, which are mostly basic, can cause a rise in the amount of the acidic ions.

BUFFER SYSTEMS. Before clinical symptoms appear, the body will have tried to correct the condition by means of its buffer systems. The three most important of these are the bicarbonate system, which is the ratio of carbonic acid to sodium bicarbonate, the phosphate, or the ratio of disodium phosphate to monosodium phosphate and the protein buffer system, which is probably the most important. The protein molecule, by releasing acid or basic radicals, counteracts the acidic or the basic increase, thus bringing the acid-base ratio into balance. If these buffer systems cannot correct the condition, respiratory changes, the second line of defense, take place.

SYMPTOMS. Shortness of breath appears early with rapid deep respirations in more serious conditions. Other symptoms include weakness, malaise, disorientation, stupor progressing to coma. The respiratory increase is a compensatory action to aid in the lowering of the carbonic acid by excreting carbon dioxide.

LABORATORY FINDINGS. Urine pH is below 6.0 and plasma pH below 7.35. Plasma bicarbonates will be decreased; below 25 mEq./L. (adults) or 20 mEq./L. (children).

TREATMENT. Sodium bicarbonate solution or glucose solution or both is the usual choice. However, any solution that is neutral or basic (alkaline) will usually overcome the difficulty.

Metabolic Alkalosis

CAUSES. The most common cause of alkalosis is the loss of gastric fluid by vomiting, suction or fistula. Alkalosis can also be caused by the intake of large amounts of alkaline drugs such as sodium bicarbonate (baking soda). This is often done without medical supervision and the patient becomes ill without any idea what has caused his illness.

SYMPTOMS. Note buffer systems above. Slow shallow respirations, to conserve carbon dioxide, and therefore carbonic acid, are common. Other symptoms include: irregular pulse, cardiac dilatation or decompensation or both, hypertonic muscles, tetany, convulsions (due to calcium ionization), azotemia, personality changes, disorientation, delirium.

LABORATORY FINDINGS. Urine pH is above 7.0 and plasma pH above 7.45. Plasma bicarbonates are above 29 mEq./L. (adults) and 25 mEq./L. (children). Plasma potassium and sodium normal or below;

TABLE 6. ELECTROLYTES IN THE EXTRACELLULAR AND INTRACELLULAR FLUIDS OF THE BODY (II–10)

NAMES	SYMBOLS	mEq./L. EXTRACELLULAR	mEq./L. INTRACELLULAR	ATOMIC WEIGHT	VALENCE
CATIONS					
Sodium	Na^{+}	142	15	23	1
Potassium	K^{+}	5	150	39	1
Calcium	Ca^{++}	5		40	2
Magnesium	Mg^{++}	3	30	24	2
		155	195		
ANIONS					
Bicarbonate	HCO_3^-	27		64	1
Chlorides	Cl^-	104		35	1
Phosphates	HPO_4^{--}	2	125	96	2
Sulfates	SO_4^{--}	1	10	96	2
Proteinate		16	60		
Organic acid		5			
		155	195		

TABLE 7. CLASSIFICATION OF THE SYMPTOMS OF ACIDOSIS/ALKALOSIS

	RESPIRATORY	METABOLIC
ACIDOSIS	CNS (CO_2 excess) Disorientation Comatose Respirations – labored Pathologic Conditions Emphysema Asthma	CNS (HCO_3 deficit) Disorientation Comatose Respirations – rapid and deep Pathologic Conditions Uremia Diabetic acidosis Diarrhea
ALKALOSIS	CNS (CO_2 deficit) Convulsions Peripheral excitability Tetany – begins in forearms Extreme nervousness Respiratory muscle tetany Respiration – rapid and deep, later stertorous Pathologic Conditions Salicylate poisoning Hyperventilation	CNS (HCO_3 excess) Convulsions Peripheral excitability Tetany – begins in forearms Extreme nervousness Respiratory muscle tetany Respiration – slow and shallow Pathologic Conditions Excessive vomiting Bowel obstruction

plasma chlorides markedly decreased and sodium bicarbonate increased.

TREATMENT. Removal of the cause is the first and most important thing to do. Intravenous solution of ammonium chloride 0.9 per cent may be given. It must be infused *very slowly*. Some physicians feel that it is best to use sodium chloride 0.9 per cent solution since it is less toxic than is the ammonium chloride. Potassium deficit often accompanies metabolic alkalosis and should be treated by giving it in the solutions.

Respiratory Acidosis (Primary Carbonic Acid Excess)

CAUSES. Respiratory acidosis can be caused by anything which interferes with the normal respiratory function (failure to properly excrete carbon dioxide). This occurs in such conditions as pneumonia, emphysema, certain drug poisonings, congestive heart failure, bronchiectasis, pulmonary edema.

SYMPTOMS. The primary symptom is respiratory embarrassment. There may be tachycardia, cyanosis, weakness, disorientation or coma.

LABORATORY FINDINGS. Urine pH is below 6.0 and plasma pH below 7.35. Plasma carbonates are above 29 mEq./L. (adults) or 25 mEq./L. (children). Serum chloride is normal or low with the serum sodium elevated.

TREATMENT. In this condition, the removal or amelioration of the underlying cause is the prime treatment.

Respiratory Alkalosis (Primary Carbonic Acid Deficit)

CAUSES. Deep, rapid breathing is one common cause. It may be deliberate or unconscious. It may follow hysteria or anxiety. Other causes include: fever, salicylate poisoning, central nervous system diseases or trauma, anoxia of high altitudes.

SYMPTOMS. Symptoms of this condition are not always diagnostic, but may include unconsciousness, rapid deep breathing, which tends to become slower and more shallow, and tetany.

LABORATORY FINDINGS. Urine pH is above 7.0 and plasma pH above 7.45. Plasma bicarbonates are below 25 mEq./L. (adult) or 20 mEq./L. (children). Serum chloride is normal or elevated and the serum sodium is normal or decreased.

TREATMENT. Removal of the cause is the first thing to be done; and often it is all that is required.

It will be noted that respiratory acidosis and alkalosis are not primarily disorders of fluid balance. However, they are conditions in which electrolytic imbalance occurs. One important thing to remember is the significance of frequent checking of the patient's respirations, noting changes not only in rate but, more important, in character, depth, and so forth. The decreasing respiration may not mean improvement; in acidosis a decrease is an unfavorable sign.

It is entirely possible to have an imbalance of one of the electrolytes or ions. Imbalance of some ions does not appear to cause serious consequences; but for others, a little too much or not enough can produce severe disorders. The more important imbalance of specific ions follows. The student should remember that these ions are measured in the body by mEq. usually per liter of plasma (II-10).

Sodium (Na) Depletion or Deficit (Hyponatremia)

CAUSES. Hyponatremia can be caused by prolonged vomiting, gastric suction, excessive sweating, electrolyte loss due to adrenal insufficiency, too much infusion of carbohydrates and water. It should be noted that the sodium content of gastric juice is high.

SYMPTOMS. Symptoms include apprehension, abdominal cramps, hypotension, oliguria, cold clammy skin, convulsions, rapid thready pulse and, sometimes, diarrhea.

LABORATORY FINDINGS. Plasma sodium below 137 mEq./L. Specific gravity of the urine below 1.010.

TREATMENT. The usual replacement for sodium deficit is the infusion of isotonic saline solution. Orally, the use of salt tablets is indicated. As with any of the ions, if other ions are also in short supply a combination solution will be used.

Sodium Excess (Hypernatremia)

CAUSES. It may be caused by repeated infusions of isotonic saline solution. Other causes include tracheobronchitis, copious, watery diarrhea, inadequate intake of water.

SYMPTOMS. Symptoms include excitement progressing to mania and convulsions, dry sticky mucous membranes, oliguria, firm tissue turgor.

LABORATORY FINDINGS. Plasma sodium in excess of 147 mEq./L. Specific gravity of urine above 1.030.

TREATMENT. Treatment will depend largely upon the amount of excess sodium. Most of the solutions low in or lacking sodium can be used provided other conditions do not contraindicate their use.

Potassium (K) Deficit (Hypokalemia)

CAUSES. Most common causes are diarrhea, ulcerative colitis, sprue, recovery from diabetic acidosis, severe vomiting, burns, starvation, use of diuretics, low sodium diet and adrenocortical hormone therapy.

SYMPTOMS. Symptoms are anorexia, gaseous distention of the gastrointestinal tract, silent intestinal ileus, soft muscles, tremors and disorientation. In severe cases there may be paresthesia and flaccid paralysis of the extremities, heart block or cardiac arrest or both.

LABORATORY FINDINGS. Plasma potassium below 4 mEq./L. Specific findings with the electrocardiogram.

TREATMENT. The treatment is intravenous infusions of solutions containing potassium, usually potassium chloride, or any potassium medicine orally.

Potassium Excess (Hyperkalemia)

CAUSES. Common causes include burns, crushing injuries, renal disorders, excessive infusion of solutions containing potassium, adrenal insufficiency.

SYMPTOMS. The symptoms are oliguria progressing to anuria, intestinal colic, diarrhea, weakness, bradycardia and lowered blood pressure.

LABORATORY FINDINGS. Plasma potassium above 5.6 mEq./L. Characteristic changes in the electrocardiographic tracings occur in severe conditions.

TREATMENT. Treatment consists of giving calcium gluconate, glucose and insulin intravenously and the use of the artificial kidney.

TABLE 8. *A FEW REPRESENTATIVE INTRAVENOUS SOLUTIONS USED IN THE TREATMENT OF FLUID*

SOLUTIONS	Per cent	Hypotonic	Isotonic	Hyper-tonic	CONTENTS mEq./l. Na$^+$	K$^+$	Ca^{++}	Cl$^-$
Saline	0.45	*			77			77
	0.9		*		154			154
	3.0			*	513			513
Multiple solutions								
Butler's solution			*		42	30		35
Fox's solution			*		140	10	5	103
Talbot's solution		*			40	35		40
Darrow's solution			*		121	35		
Sodium lactate (1/6 molar)	5.00 to 5.75		*		130	4	3	109
Sodium bicarbonate			*		600			600
Ammonium chloride	2.4			*				400
Dextrose or glucose	varies							
Protein replacement and Total alimentation								
Protein hydrolysate T.P.A.–900	5							
Free amine								
Colloidal solution								
Dextran	6 to 12							

Solutions from human sources

Albumin which contains the normal blood protein (Normal human serum).

Plasma which contains all blood factors except cells.

Whole blood which contains all blood factors including cells.

Packed red blood cells which contain extracted red cells from whole blood.

Blood factors which are extracted from blood serum. (There are many of these which are used for specific purposes.)

*See also Current Drug Handbook.

*AND ELECTROLYTE IMBALANCE**

HCO_3^-	$HPO_4^=$	SO_4^{--}	Mg^{++}	Lactate	Acetate	pH	PRINCIPAL USES
						4 to 5.7	With glucose or dextrose is isotonic. Sodium and chlorine replacement and/or meet daily needs.
						4 to 5.7	Sodium, chlorine and volume replacement and/or meet daily needs.
						4 to 5.7	Rapid replacement in severe loss. Given slowly in small amounts (200 to 300 ml.).
25	16		5			7.4	Supply fluid and electrolytes.
55			3				Same as above plus correct sodium deficit.
20	15						Same as above plus general replacement and maintenance.
55		103				6.5 to 7.5	Same as above and correct potassium deficiency.
				28			Supply fluids and electrolytes and correct metabolic acidosis.
600							Treat metabolic or respiratory acidosis (shock, diabetic coma, salicylate or barbiturate intoxication, severe hepatic disease).
			—				400 mEq · NH_4^+. Treat severe metabolic alkalosis. Give required calories. Often used with electrolytic solutions and/or as a vehicle for other substances. Strong solutions are hypertonic and act as diuretics which tend to reduce edema of the central nervous system.
							Intravenous protein replacement for emergencies and short-term use. Contains 900K† calories (dextrose), amino acids furnishing 4.17 grams nitrogen or 26 grams protein equivalent. Used for total alimentation.
							1000 ml. solution contains 850K* calories (dextrose), amino acids (8 essential, 7 non-essential) providing 6.25 grams nitrogen plus 39 grams protein equivalent.
							Temporary expedient to increase blood volume. Half-life 6 to 12 hours. Comes in specific strengths for special purposes. A glucose polymer. Consult brochure before using.
							For replacement of blood loss. Supplies fluid and protein.
							As above.
							As above.
							As above, especially when it is not necessary to increase blood volume appreciably.

†These amounts represent the calories after the addition of 500 ml. of 50 per cent dextrose.

Calcium (Ca) Deficit

CAUSES. The causes include sprue, acute pancreatitis, hypoparathyroidism, excessive infusion of citrated blood, massive subcutaneous infections, generalized peritonitis.

SYMPTOMS. The symptoms are tetany progressing to convulsions, muscle cramps, tingling of the extremities.

LABORATORY FINDINGS. Plasma calcium below 4.5 mEq./L. Characteristic changes in the electrocardiogram are seen. Sulkowitch's test on urine shows no precipitation.

TREATMENT. Solutions of calcium given intravenously are used and various calcium salts are given orally, if possible.

Calcium Excess

CAUSES. The more common causes are tumors or over-activity of the parathyroid gland and excessive intake of vitamin D in the treatment of arthritis and multiple myeloma.

SYMPTOMS. The symptoms include relaxed muscles, flank pain and deep thigh pain.

LABORATORY FINDINGS. Plasma calcium above 5.8 mEq./L. Sulkowitch's test on urine shows increased precipitation. Electrocardiograms reveal characteristic changes.

TREATMENT. This is treated with infusions of sodium sulfate with concentrations of sodium 160-200 mEq./L. Disodium edetate can be used to chelate calcium, and it aids in the excretion of calcium.

Magnesium (Mg) Deficit

CAUSES. The causes of magnesium deficit are chronic alcoholism, prolonged vomiting or gastric suction, diarrhea, impaired intestinal absorption, enterostomy drainage, prolonged maintenance with magnesium-free solutions.

SYMPTOMS. The symptoms of magnesium deficit are disorientation, confusion, hallucinations (usually visual), convulsions, hyperactive deep reflexes, positive therapeutic test (the giving of magnesium to see if it overcomes the symptoms).

LABORATORY FINDINGS. Plasma magnesium below 1.4 mEq./L.

TREATMENT. Solutions which include magnesium are given intravenously or the drug is given orally. As much as 2 mEq./kg. of body weight may be given within the first four hours. The dose is then adjusted to the response of the patient.

Magnesium Excess

CAUSES. The main cause is renal insufficiency.

SYMPTOMS. The symptoms are varied; depression of the central nervous system and diminution in the amplitude of the potential of the neuromuscular end-plate may occur. There may be loss of deep tendon reflexes, and respiratory paralysis.

LABORATORY FINDINGS. Plasma level more than 4 mEq./L. is considered moderate excess; above 10 mEq./L. is severe excess.

TREATMENT. Solutions containing calcium will be effective in controlling the excessive magnesium.

So far the major electrolytes and ions in the body have been briefly outlined as to causes of excess or deficit, symptoms of these disorders, laboratory findings and treatment. Although the picture may appear somewhat disconnected, the chemicals are very much interdependent within the body. Each has a specific function or functions, but none functions entirely alone. An increase or decrease in any one chemical will affect the proper actions of one or more of the others.

The body fluids have been divided into intracellular and extracellular. The latter category was subdivided into interstitial (intercellular) and intravascular. The various electrolytes can be similarly divided. Usually only the placement of the various substances is intracellular and extracellular. It should be understood that when ions are said to be either in or out of a cell, this means that the majority are so placed. The major placement of the various ions is easily determined for the vascular fluids but is more difficult for the intracellular ones. This must be estimated from various data. (See Table 8.)

The disturbance of the amounts of sodium and potassium probably poses the most serious threat to the general health of the individual. The excretion of sodium is in direct relation to that of water. Hence, retention of sodium (its reabsorption over normal amounts) is accompanied by a reabsorption of extra amounts of water, with resultant edema. This accounts for the low-salt diet in cases of edema or potential edema, such as occurs in nephrosis and some cardiac disorders. Excessive sodium excretion results in dehydration, which is less common, but should not be overlooked. This will be discussed in a later chapter.

Most diuretics cause the excretion of sodium, water and potassium by blocking their reabsorption in the renal tubules. Unlike sodium, the excretion of potassium is not associated with that of water, so its loss or retention is harder to evaluate than that of sodium. Excessive amounts of potassium (hyperkalemia), while serious, are less common than is potassium deficit (hypokalemia). (See Potassium Excess and Deficit, this chapter.) Potassium deficit occurs rather frequently, especially with the long-term use of diuretics as in the treatment of hypertension. Such use of diuretics is not uncommon in weight reduction. A diuretic is ordered by the physician to be used only until the "water weight" has been brought down to normal. The diuretic should then be discontinued, but some patients may continue beyond this point. In any case, if the potassium loss exceeds the intake, marked symptoms can occur which the patient will not associate with the diuretic, if one is being used. The most distinctive early symptom is muscle weakness. This may progress, and if the patient has any cardiac disorder, heart block or cardiac arrest could result. The nurse, in her contact with patients and friends, can advise anyone taking diuretics over any extended period of time to include foods rich in potassium in his diet. This will at least partially compensate for the potassium deficit. She can also advise frequent medical examinations to be sure that all is well.

There are diuretics that are potassium sparers. These are often used with the diuretics that tend to cause potassium excretion and this will aid in maintaining a more normal concentration of potassium in the body. (See Chapter 18.)

NUTRITIONAL DEFICIT

In addition to fluid and electrolytes, two other substances are essential for body nutrition. These are protein (amino acids, nitrogen) for tissue maintenance and calories for fuel. Usually, unless the loss is severe, these can be supplied by an increase in the diet. However, there are circumstances in which these must be supplied by parenteral means, usually intravenously. If this will be needed for a short time only, it is relatively easy to supply the calories by giving a solution of glucose or dextrose. The addition of 100 K calories of dextrose or glucose to 1000 ml. of solution will prevent starvation ketosis. See Table 8 for further information.

Protein Deficit

CAUSES. The cause of a protein deficit may be inadequate intake of protein or the better forms of protein (those containing all the essential amino acids). This will be discussed in more detail in Chapter 20. The other causes of protein deficit include trauma, hemorrhage, severe burns, wound, ulcers and/or debilitating diseases.

SYMPTOMS. Symptoms of protein deficiency include anorexia, pallor, easy fatigability, weight loss and loss of muscle tone and mass. In severe illness, these symptoms may be attributed to the disease rather than to the protein loss. The nurse should be alert to this possibility.

LABORATORY FINDINGS. Hemoglobin and erythrocyte count are usually depressed. Total plasma proteins are below 6 Gm. per 100 ml., plasma albumin is below 3.5 mg. per ml.

TREATMENT. If at all possible, the protein is given orally. However, in severe loss, or if the patient cannot take food by mouth, the protein is given by intravenous infusion as an emergency measure. Refer to Table 8 for a list of three solutions that contain protein.

The protein hydrolysate solution does not allow for the exact measurement of the nitrogen being given. This type of intravenous fluid is used for conditions where the protein deficit is not severe or the patient will need treatment by parenteral means for a short time only. This solution can be given into a peripheral vein.

The solutions called "hyperalimentation"

contain amino acids and glucose for more complete nutrition. These solutions are given by means of a catheter introduced into one of the deep veins such as the internal jugular, subclavian or superior vena cava. These solutions are particularly valuable when the need for intravenously administered nutrients may be prolonged. As shown on the table, they are prepared so that the exact amount of nitrogen, total protein or other substances can be estimated for the particular patient being treated. In some conditions, transfusions of plasma, whole blood or packed red cells may be required before the start of the hyperalimentation solutions. This is often done in emergency situations to carry the patient over until other treatments, including nutrition, can be started.

The Nurse. The nurse has many responsibilities in the area of fluid and electrolytic balance and they go far beyond merely checking an intravenous. If the causes of most imbalance have been noted, it can be seen that many patients have the potential for developing an electrolyte or fluid imbalance. Any patient with persistent vomiting, prolonged gastric suction, diarrhea for an extended period of time, diabetes mellitus, or renal or adrenal disorders, is apt to be out of balance for one or more electrolytes and/or fluid.

With these and other factors in view, some of the more important of the nurse's responsibilities are as follows:

1. As has already been mentioned, the respiratory rate and character should be checked frequently, especially in respiratory acidosis or alkalosis. The respiratory function is important in other conditions as well. It is especially valuable to note if the rate is increasing or decreasing and if the depth is getting shallower or deeper. Naturally, all vital signs should be carefully checked. If there is renal dysfunction, it is important to note in oliguria if it is progressing toward anuria. The urinalysis must be watched and any change called to the attention of the doctor.

2. Accurate recording of all fluid intake and output is vital. Daily weights should be taken and recorded. Remember fluids are also lost through wound drainage, hyperventilation and insensible perspiration. Note Figure 21.

3. Keeping a close watch on laboratory findings and reporting promptly any deviation from normal which might indicate actual or impending imbalance. These findings are important even if the patient is already being treated for imbalance since a reversal is possible. An excess can be treated too long and a deficit occur or the reverse may happen.

4. Of course, when intravenous therapy is being used, the nurse must be sure that she gives the right fluid at the right rate and for the specified time or amount. The nurse must know the electrolytes in the solution being given, the normal mEq./L. and the latest laboratory report for the patient being treated. As soon as a normal (or nearly normal) reading is reached, the physician should be notified and his orders concerning continuation of the intravenous be received. She should not discontinue the fluid unless he has ordered this previously.

5. Careful observation and reporting of symptoms—predisposing, precipitating or actual—of either fluid or electrolyte disturbances.

6. In most cases of fluid and electrolyte imbalance, the nurse will need to do a relatively larger share of the care and observation of the patient than in some other conditions. Most ancillary workers are not qualified to properly interpret the changes in the patient's condition.

7. Attempting to prevent imbalance by seeing that the patient, if able to take food and fluids orally, gets sufficient water and various chemicals to prevent or to overcome fluid and electrolyte disturbances.

SOME PROBLEMS WITH INTRAVENOUS THERAPY (INCLUDING BLOOD TRANSFUSIONS)

Only a few of the more common problems relating to intravenous therapy can be mentioned here. Obviously, the first is the instillation of the needle. The bevel of the needle must be free in the vein (see Chapter 3, Figure 5, page 29) and the area surrounding the insertion point (for peripheral veins) must be watched for signs of infiltration such as swelling due to leakage and discoloration due to bleeding. The amount of fluid must be kept at the amount ordered (ml. per min. or per hour).

Blood transfusions can result in many adverse reactions, such as the following.

1. Antigen-antibody reaction characterized by chills and fever. The transfusion should be stopped, but the needle left in the vein for possible infusion of saline or glucose.

2. Acute hemolytic reaction is much more severe and is characterized by destruction of some erythrocytes (hemolysis). This can progress to an anaphylactic shock, early symptoms of which are chills and fever. If the reaction occurs during surgery, the sign is fine oozing of blood in the wound. The transfusion should be stopped, and treatment for shock given. Mannitol may be given I.V.

3. Allergic reactions usually occur later and urticaria is the predominant symptom. This type of reaction tends to increase with repeated transfusions. Antihistamine drugs usually suffice.

4. Much longer reactions (5 to 10 days after the transfusion) are not common, but are similar to 3. and treated with antihistamines.

5. Serum hepatitis, syphilis, malaria or bacteremia may occur with whole blood transfusions, hepatitis being the most common. Blood banks attempt to prevent these infections, but an occasional case (most commonly hepatitis) does occur. These diseases are discussed in other chapters—serum hepatitis in Chapter 19, malaria in Chapter 31 and syphilis in Chapter 26. Bacteremia will be covered later in this chapter.

There are a few other problems that may come up in the course of intravenous therapy such as "circulatory overload." This is more common in infants, small children and the elderly. The symptoms are similar to those of congestive heart failure (see Chapter 18). The infusion should be stopped, at least temporarily, and the patient raised to a sitting position. This may be all that is required.

Air embolism is another rare possibility. This causes chest pain, cough and dyspnea. The patient should be positioned head down on the left side. If the condition is severe, the physician may aspirate the right heart to remove the air.

Septicemia or Bacteremia (Blood Poisoning)

Septicemia or bacteremia, as the name implies, is an infection within the circulating blood stream. There are many possible causes such as extension from an infection elsewhere in the body, infected blood or infusion fluid or contamination as an infusion or transfusion is being given. The former is called an "intrinsic" infection and the latter an "extrinsic" infection. The latter is more common.

Almost any organism may be responsible for blood poisoning (septicemia). To differentiate between intrinsic (fluid infection) or extrinsic (handling contamination) is not always easy, but there are some guidelines. If the intravenous infusion was recent, not of long duration and not related to the patient's illness, fluid contamination should be suspected. The infusion should be stopped, the end of the catheter sealed and the entire apparatus, including any unused fluid, put into a plastic container and sent to the laboratory for examination. If the fluid is found to contain microorganisms, all of the equipment should be segregated and the public health agency and the manufacturer notified. If the equipment is not contaminated, it will be necessary to try to locate the source of the infection elsewhere.

Two blood cultures are taken from the patient, at two different points. These are cultured and a sensitivity test is done to determine the proper anti-infective drug to be used. All equipment and personnel should be tested as possible sources. If the patient has any type of infection other than the blood bacteremia, there should be cultures taken to see if it is caused by the same organism. The search for the source may be a very frustrating and difficult task, but it must be pursued to the end.

Nurses and intravenous therapists must be most scrupulous in their technique. Hospital-induced infections are not common, but they are extremely serious and very hard to explain to the patient and to the public.

IT IS IMPORTANT TO REMEMBER

1. That fluid and electrolytic balance is absolutely essential for health. Any imbalance results in some dysfunction.
2. That an important part of her duty is to watch for the early symptoms of fluid and electrolyte imbalance, in all patients, so that the condition may be corrected before it becomes serious.
3. That certain diseases and disorders tend to fluid and electrolyte imbalance and in these the nurse must be exceptionally careful to report any deviation from normal. These disorders include: burns, fever, oliguria, cardiovascular dysfunction, diabetes mellitus, nephrosis, surgery.

TOPICS FOR STUDY AND DISCUSSION

1. Estimate the mEq. of the following ions:

Ion	Atomic weight	Valence
Magnesium	24	2
Chloride	35	1
Sodium	23	1
Sulfate	96	2

2. In dehydration "hemoconcentration" (increase in concentration of non-water components of the blood) results. Explain how this may be expected to affect interstitial and intracellular fluids.
3. Parents often panic when children hold their breath. What are the ultimate physiological consequences of holding the breath?
4. Discuss the merits and demerits of the "buffered" aspirin preparations.

BIBLIOGRAPHY

Books and Pamphlets

Beeson, P. B., and McDermott, W., *Cecil-Loeb Textbook of Medicine, 13th Ed.*, Philadelphia, 1971, W. B. Saunders Co.

Chatton, M. J., Margen, S., and Brainerd, H., *Handbook of Medical Treatment, 12th Ed.*, Los Altos, California, 1970, Lange Medical Publications.

Conn, H. F., et al., *Current Therapy, 1974*, Philadelphia, 1974, W. B. Saunders Co.

Dutchee, J. E., and Fuilo, S. B., *Water and Electrolytes*, New York, 1967, The Macmillan Co.

Free Amine, Parenteral Hyperalimentation, Bulletin from McGraw Laboratories Division of American Hospital Supply Corporation, Glendale, California, and Milledgeville, Georgia.

Ganong, W., *Review of Medical Physiology, 5th Ed.*, Los Altos, California, 1971, Lange Medical Publications.

Goodman, L. S., and Gilman, A., *Pharmacological Basis of Therapeutics, 4th Ed.*, New York, 1970, The Macmillan Co.

Meltzer, L., Abdellah, F., and Kitchell, J. R., *Concepts and Practices of Intensive Care for Nursing Specialists*, Philadelphia, 1970, The Charles Press.

Meng, H. C., and Sandstead, H. H., *Total Parenteral Alimentation*, Bulletin, Vanderbilt University School of Medicine, Nashville, Tennessee.

Metheny, N. M., and Snively, W. D., *Nurses' Handbook of Fluid Balance*, Philadelphia, 1967, J. B. Lippincott Co.

Reed, G. M., and Sheppard, V. F., *Regulation of Fluid and Electrolyte Balance*, Philadelphia, 1971, W. B. Saunders Co.

Walter, B. L., Asinov, J., and Nicholas, M. K., *Chemistry and Human Health*, New York, 1956, Blakiston Division McGraw-Hill Book Co.

Journal Articles

Anderson, J., "Emergency nursing techniques: venipuncture," *Nurs. Clin. North Am.* 3:1:165 (1968).

Betson, C., and Lends, U., "Central venous pressure," *Am. J. Nurs.* 69:7:1466 (July, 1969).

Donn, R., "Intravenous admixture incompatibility," *Am. J. Nurs.* 71:2:325 (February, 1971).

Donn, R., "Programmed instruction on potassium imbalance." *Am. J. Nurs.* 67:2:343 (February, 1967).

Humphrey, N., Wright, P. S., and Swanson, A. B., "Parenteral hyperalimentation for children," *Am. J. Nurs.* 72:2:286 (February, 1972).

Lennon, E. J., and Lemann, J., "Defense of hydrogen ion concentration in chronic metabolic acidosis," *Ann. Intern. Med.* 65:2:265 (February, 1965).

Mazzara, J. T., and Ayres, S. M., "Fluid, electrolyte and acid-base disturbances in the coronary care unit," *Nurs. Clin. North Am.* 7:3:549 (June, 1972).

Parsa, M., Thorton, B., and Ferrer, J., "Central venous alimentation," *Am. J. Nurs.* 72:11:2042 (November, 1972).

Voda, A., "Body water dynamics—A clinical application," *Am. J. Nurs.* 70:12:2594 (December, 1970).

Wilmore, D. W., "The future of intravenous therapy," *Am. J. Nurs.* 71:12:2334 (December, 1971).

CHAPTER 11

TOXICOLOGY

CORRELATION WITH OTHER SCIENCES

I. ANATOMY AND PHYSIOLOGY

1. Hemoglobin (the red substance in the erythrocytes) is the oxygen carrying medium of the body. It forms an unstable compound with the oxygen in the lungs, oxyhemoglobin. The oxygen is released to the tissues in exchange for carbon dioxide as needed, and the hemoglobin returns it to the lungs where the carbon dioxide is exchanged for more oxygen.
2. The exposed portion of the eye, as framed by the eyelids, is an ellipse. The two ends of this ellipse are called the canthi. The one next to the nose is the inner or medial canthus; the one on the outer end, the outer or lateral canthus.

II. CHEMISTRY

1. An acid and an alkali (base) will react to form a salt. If both are either weak or strong the result will be a neutral salt. If the acid is strong and the alkali weak, the result will be an acid salt, while the reverse will produce a basic salt.

IV. PHYSICS

1. If a solution is diluted (made weaker), it will take longer to pass through a permeable membrane because it is greater in volume.

INTRODUCTION

The nurse plays a most important part, often a vital part, in the care of the accident victim. She must understand not only what she should do in an emergency situation but, also equally important, what she must not do. As far as the nurse is concerned, emergency situations may be divided into three classes: those in which she must act on her own initiative since there is not time to await the arrival of the physician; those in which she should start treatment; and those for which she need give only palliative treatment until the physician arrives. There can be no hard and fast rule. In any specific case, the nurse will need to use her own good judgment, basing her decision for a given situation on what is best for the patient.

Would it be wisest to wait for the doctor? If I give first aid treatment am I sure the patient will be better than if I delayed? If I do start treatment, how far should I go? These are questions that each nurse must ask herself in each case. In the discussion which follows, a few general rules will be given which may aid the nurse in reaching a satisfactory conclusion. The nurse must understand that these are only *general directions*. They cannot possibly apply in every case, probably not even for the majority of situations, but they may help the nurse to answer the questions she must ask herself.

If she feels she is not qualified to treat the patient, and in the majority of cases this is the correct decision, she must know what things the physician is apt to need and see that these are ready for his use. Much valuable time can be saved if the nurse has everything ready when the doctor arrives. It is much better to have things on hand that are not required than to lack what is needed. The nurse is also responsible for giving the physician, by telephone, some indication of the patient's condition. This will allow him to give advance verbal orders and also to determine which drugs or supplies he should bring and which the nurse will be able to secure.

In most emergency situations, the nurse will have not only the patient to care for but also relatives and friends, all eager to help but usually, unfortunately, in the way. Often the nurse can overcome this difficulty by using these people as assistants. She may have one notify the physician or get the doctor on the telephone so that she can talk to him. Others can be sent for needed equipment or drugs. This will aid the nurse, give those wanting to help a feeling of being able to do something useful and relieve the patient from the attention of oversolicitous people.

In almost all emergency cases there is an element of shock. It may be so slight as to cause few symptoms or so profound as to endanger life. In any event, the nurse can at least do something about this. External heat is usually indicated. The patient should be covered with blankets, coats or whatever material may be available. These may be warmed, if heat is available, and if heat seems indicated. Care must be taken that they are not too warm. A child may be wrapped in a warmed, large turkish towel.

Accidents can be classified, as are diseases, into surgical and medical. The latter includes poisoning. Since the various medical and surgical emergencies treated pharmacologically can best be included in the chapters in Section 3 dealing with the specific organ or organ system involved, only poisoning as a specific entity will be discussed here. Toxicology cannot be divorced from the discussion of drugs in general, but excessive action of drugs or the accidental intake of poisons not medicinally used warrants some direct consideration. Toxic symptoms occurring from cumulative action, mild overdosing, idiosyncrasy and such will be given with each drug discussed in Section 3. This chapter will deal with excessive accidental intake of a drug or other poisonous substance.

GENERAL RULES

A word of caution concerning antidotes is necessary. The nurse should remember that it is better not to use any antidote than to use the wrong one. It is impossible for the average person to remember a long list of antidotes. Consequently, aside from a few exceptions, lists of antidotes should not be memorized but used for reference.

The nurse has several sources of antidote listings. Among these are:

1. The label on the package of commercial poisonous substances. The nurse should always ask for and save for the doctor any bottle or box known or thought to have contained the material taken by the patient.

2. Many households have lists of common poisons and antidotes. These are easily available from most drug stores. The nurse is wise to have one for herself.

3. The entire country is separated into areas and in each there is a Poison Control Center. These centers are constantly informed of the latest available information about poisons and antidotes. All commercial materials which might be injurious if taken in sufficient amounts are listed along with the trade names, chemical composition and possible antidotes and treatment of poisoning. The nurse should know where the Poison Control Center is in her community. She will not, in most cases, contact the center herself. The doctor will do this, but if the nurse knows where the center is and has the telephone number for the doctor, valuable time can be saved.

There are a few general rules suitable for any case of poisoning that are important and should be learned.

1. Call a doctor—or arrange to get the patient to the doctor.

2. Remove the poison, or the patient from the poison (dilute—wash out) (IV-1).

3. Counteract the poison (chemically, physically, physiologically) (Usually the doctor's responsibility).

4. Counteract the effect of the poison by

treating for shock and other symptoms as they occur (Partly the nurse's responsibility, partly the physician's).

The order in which these rules are given does not apply in all cases, possibly not even in the majority of cases. The various steps are numbered for clarity and not because of increasing importance. Sometimes the removal of the poison is more essential than calling the doctor, although often these can be done simultaneously, the nurse doing one and some friend or relative doing the other. In most instances it is best for the nurse to remain with the patient while some member of the family gets the physician on the phone. Treatment for shock, listed in number 4, may be the first action that should be taken. In any case, the safety of the patient is of prime importance and must be the deciding factor. To get a physician, or to get the patient to a physician is essential, but it is not always the first thing to be done.

Poisons may enter the body by ingestion, inhalation or direct contact with the skin or mucous membranes. In the last two situations, it is usually most important first to remove the poison and then get the patient to the doctor. Removal of ingested poisons may be difficult and require the services of the physician.

POISONING BY INHALATION

When the poison has been inhaled, the first thing to do is to remove the patient from the contaminated area to some place where there is more oxygen available. If pure oxygen can be secured it should be administered. Commercial oxygen such as is used in welding outfits can be used, provided some means of giving it to the patient can be found. In most cities, firemen maintain inhalator squads for such cases, and they should be called. The most commonly inhaled poison is carbon monoxide gas, either from household gas, the exhaust from an automobile engine or, more rarely, sewer gas. It is odorless, but other gases with which it is often mixed may have a distinct odor. Illuminating gas, especially, has an added ingredient which makes its odor rather unpleasant. The nurse must be careful to get the patient out of the contaminated area quickly, not only for the patient's safety but for her own as well. Artificial respiration may be needed, and treatment for shock should be started at once.

SURFACE POISONING

If the poison is on the skin or any of the exposed mucous membranes, the first procedure is to dilute it and wash it off. This is especially necessary if the poison has gotten into the eyes. The area should be washed with a copious amount of running water. Care must be taken to prevent spreading the poison to another part of the body. Thus, in irrigating the eye, the water should be poured from the inner canthus toward the outer canthus in order to avoid washing the poison over the bridge of the nose into the other eye (I-2).

INGESTED POISONS

Most poisons are ingested (swallowed). They may be taken accidentally or purposely, but to the nurse this is immaterial during emergency care. Later on she might find out whether the poison was taken purposely so that she can help to prevent any recurrence, but her first problem is a patient who needs immediate care. The nurse should arrange for the services of a physician immediately. This may be either getting the patient to a doctor or hospital or calling for a physician to come to the patient. In the latter case the nurse should give the doctor as much detail as she can and receive his emergency orders.

Presuming that the nurse arrives when there is reason to believe that the toxic substance, other than a corrosive poison, is still in the stomach, the first thing she should do is to dilute the poison. This will delay absorption and also aid in emptying the stomach by producing vomiting (IV-1). The patient should be given generous amounts of tepid water. If this does not produce vomiting, it should be induced. There are three ways of inducing vomiting applicable to such cases. Tickling the back of the throat (pharyngeal irritation) with a clean feather, a loose cotton applicator, or similar substance may be sufficient to bring about the desired results. If this fails, a solution of mild soap (not detergent) may be tried. Soap should not be used in alkali poisoning as it will increase the alkalinity of the stomach contents. Be sure the solution is just lukewarm since this temperature is nauseating, whereas hot or cold fluids might aid in the retention of the poison. Some doctors use warm (tepid or lukewarm) milk, three or four glasses, for this purpose, but an order for this must be obtained as in some cases milk is contraindicated. If these procedures are not effective, drugs or a stomach tube may have to be used, but a physician's order must be obtained for these. Drugs used to induce vomiting include syrup of ipecac, apomorphine and mustard. The mustard is used in a very weak solution, possibly 1 teaspoonful per gallon of water. Apomorphine hydrochloride 6 to 8 mg. may be given by hypodermic. If available these drugs should be ready for administration when the physician arrives. Syrup of ipecac 4 to 8 ml. may be ordered. It is usually used for children, in appropriate dosage. Ipecac acts much more slowly than apomorphine, but produces less depression. Other emetics that may be ordered include antimony and potassium tartrate (tartar emetic), copper sulfate or zinc sulfate.

Chemical Antidotes

After dilution and removal of as much of the poison as possible, various antidotes are used to stop the action of any poison remaining in the body. The physician will often combine the use of a chemical antidote with the process of diluting the toxic substances. There are times when this may be done by the nurse. When the patient has taken one of the strong alkalis, such as lye, the nurse may give a weak acid immediately. *Vinegar* or *lemon juice* is suitable and easily secured. The acid will neutralize at least a part of the alkali and render it less harmful. The reverse obviously would be true if a strong acid had been ingested. In this case, a weak alkali should be given. *Sodium bicarbonate* (*baking soda*) or a mild soap is effective and easy to secure (II-1).

Some doctors use the so called "universal antidote" as it is effective in a number of cases. It consists of 1 part magnesium oxide, 1 part tannic acid and 2 parts of activated charcoal. About 15 grams (5 to 6 heaping teaspoonfuls) is dissolved in a glass of water and administered. Of course, the nurse does not use this without direct order from the doctor. The magnesium neutralizes any acid present, the tannic acid forms an insoluble salt with many drugs, especially the alkaloids, and the activated charcoal adsorbs many substances.

Most people know that starch turns blue in the presence of iodine. However, not everyone realizes that this blue product is a relatively inert substance. If the patient has swallowed iodine, any starch can be used to neutralize it, although commercial starch used for starching clothes should not be used if something better is available since it may contain other ingredients which may be injurious to the patient. *Cornstarch* or *flour* in solution will act best. Cooked starches are most effective and may be easily secured in the home.

Some poisons can be counteracted at least in part by giving the appropriate medication. The choice of the drug, its amount and the method of administration is the responsibility of the physician. But, as mentioned earlier, the nurse may need to procure the drug and have it ready when the doctor arrives. Among the drugs which may be used are:

Ascorbic acid in large doses, since it has a detoxifying effect on lead, arsenic and some toxins.

Dimercaprol (British anti-lewisite, B.A.L.) is used mainly in severe arsenic or mercury poisoning.

Edathamil calcium disodium (Calcium disodium versenate; sodium calcium edetate [C]) is used for poisonings due to certain metals such as copper, nickel and lead, especially the latter. Apparently the metal forms a more stable compound than the calcium chelate which it replaces in the molecule.

Penicillamine (Mercaptovaline [C]) also can chelate copper and other metals. However, it is considered less effective than the last two drugs mentioned. It does have one definite advantage in that it appears to be effective when given orally.

Commercial companies manufacturing preparations that are poisonous must always label them as such and, in most cases, give the antidote to be used and other emergency care. Many of the new insecticides contain several poisonous compounds of a highly complex nature. These require special treatment. The companies, through their research divisions, have discovered the best remedies to be used, and these should be used when at all possible. The nurse should ask to see the package if the patient or his relatives know what has been taken. This may be lifesaving.

Physical Antidotes

In many situations no chemical antidote is available or adaptable for use on the human patient. Many things are workable in the chemical laboratory that cannot be used for the human being. If a chemical antidote cannot be given, if it is too late to use it, or after the chemical antidote has been used, use of the physical and/or physiologic antidote is indicated. Usually by the time these are needed a physician is in charge, and the nurse will be following his orders in her usual role. It is extremely rare for the nurse to have to administer either the physical or the physiologic antidote on her own initiative. She should understand why these are given and what will be used in order to be able to have needed materials on hand. The nurse is expected to anticipate the physician's wishes and, thus, to save valuable time for the patient.

Physical antidotes are used to counteract the tissue damage done by the poison. They are most important following the ingestion of irritant and corrosive poisons such as alkalis, acids, phenol, iodine and the salts of heavy metals. These substances and others like them cause extensive damage to the mucous membranes and the skin with which they come into contact. The use of a stomach tube is contraindicated in these cases lest the injured tissue be further damaged. Perforation might even occur. Demulcents and emollients are usually used as physical antidotes, the type used depending upon the circumstances. Usually some bland or mucilaginous substance is effective, such as starches, especially *cooked starches, acacia* and, when not contraindicated, *olive, cottonseed* or *linseed oil.* No oil is used if the poison contained any phosphorus since this aids in its absorption.

Physiologic Antidotes

Physiologic antidotes are given to counteract the effect of the poison on the body. These are most important when the poisonous substance taken is a drug. For example, if the patient has taken an overdose of a depressant drug (an analgesic or hypnotic), a stimulating drug will be given to overcome the depressant action of the medicine taken. The reverse would also be true. If the patient has taken a stimulating drug such as strychnine in excessive amounts, a depressant drug is given to offset the effect of the strychnine. For the depressant drugs, *caffeine* is the effective physiologic antidote and may be given orally, rectally or subcutaneously. *Coffee,* orally or rectally, may be substituted for the drug. There are many depressant drugs that could be used in the case of overstimulation, but the exact drug selected and the amount given will depend upon individual cases.

It should be remembered that although *atropine sulfate* is considered a physiologic antidote for *morphine sulfate,* the reverse is not true. Morphine is not an antidote for atropine. Naloxone Hydrochloride (Narcan) is the drug of choice for opium poisoning. Other narcotic antagonists include *nalorphine hydrochloride* (Nalline) and *levallorphan tartrate* (Lorfan). Atropine sulfate depresses the autonomic nervous (parasympathetic) system so, to counteract overdosing with atropine, one of the parasympathetic stimulants is given. The ones most commonly used are *physostigmine salicylate* (Antilirium), *eserine salicylate* (Isopto-Eserine Salicylate [C]) or *pilocarpine.*

Some poisons destroy constituents of the blood. Carbon monoxide, for example, forms a fixed compound with the hemoglobin called methemoglobin (I-1). This destroys the ability of the hemoglobin to form the unstable compound oxyhemoglobin, and the hemoglobin is then unable to carry oxygen to the body cells. Poisons of this kind require special treatment to overcome the damage to the body's vital fluid—the blood.

Counteracting the Effect of the Poison

Although counteracting the effect of the poison has been placed last, it may be the first thing the nurse will be called upon to do. One effect of most poisoning, as with any emergency, is shock. This should be anticipated and treated even before the first symptoms occur; it is often the very first thing the nurse should do. This is especially true if the nurse does not see the patient until some time after his contact with the poison.

Other systemic effects of poisons are so varied there can be only one rule to follow—treat the symptoms as they occur. Obviously, this includes an almost endless range of conditions. Poisons usually produce damage to the gastrointestinal tract if ingested and to the kidneys because of their function in removing waste materials from the blood. In addition, injuries to liver, blood and/or the nervous system are not uncommon. These conditions are treated as is any disease or disorder of the organs involved.

CAUSES OF POISONING

Causes of poisoning are many and varied, but most of them can be placed in one of two categories, those taken accidentally and those taken or given with suicidal or homicidal intent. The former far outnumber the latter. If the drug is taken intentionally, the patient rarely reaches a nurse early enough for her to do much on her own initiative. She must await the physician's orders. However, in an established emergency or first aid department she will have standing orders for such cases. The nurse must not draw any conclusions about the possible criminal action involved. She should, however, be aware of such a possibility and be especially careful of what she says or does. She must also be exceptionally accurate in recording such cases in detail.

By far, most poisonings are accidental. There are any number of ways in which poisonous substances can be taken unintentionally. A few of the more common ones include:

1. Leaving poisonous substances where children can get them.
2. Taking a poisonous substance instead of a medicine.
3. Taking more than the prescribed dose of a medicine.

The nurse can do a great deal to help to prevent accidental poisoning by spreading information about the dangers involved. A few rules would eliminate most accidental poisonings.

These can be listed briefly as follows:

1. Put ALL poisonous substances where children cannot get them. This includes insecticides, rodent poisons, garden poisons, cleaning supplies, matches and household antiseptics, as well as drugs. Do not leave them, even for a minute, where a small child can reach them. Note the labels of commercial containers to see if emergency treatment is given and be familiar with where this information can be found.
2. Have household medicines in a separate cupboard from cosmetics and bathroom supplies.
3. Have the household medicines so arranged that those for internal and those for external use are on separate shelves or, if possible, in separate cupboards.
4. Never take a drug at night without sufficient light to be able to read the label. (The nurse's old rule—read the label three times—is as good in the home as in the hospital and as good at night as in the daytime.)

If these few rules were consistently followed little accidental poisoning would occur. It is often lack of understanding the seriousness of these things that makes the average layman careless. The nurse has a responsibility to spread information about the potential dangers of poisoning.

FIRST-AID MEASURES FOR POISONING*

Emergency telephone numbers:
PHYSICIAN....................FIRE DEPT....................
HOSPITAL.........(resuscitator)..............................
PHARMACIST....................POLICE....................
RESCUE SQUADS..

The aim of first-aid measures is to help prevent absorption of the poison. SPEED is essential. First-aid measures must be started at once. If possible, one person should begin treatment while another calls a physician. When this is not possible, the nature of the poison will determine whether to call a physician first or begin first-aid measures and then notify a physician. Save the poison container and material itself if any remains. If the poison is not known, save a sample of the vomitus.

Measures to be taken before arrival of physician

I. Swallowed poisons

Many products used in and around the home, although not labeled "Poison," may be dangerous if taken internally. For example, some medications which are beneficial when used correctly may endanger life if used improperly or in excessive amounts.

In all cases, *except those indicated below,* REMOVE POISON FROM PATIENT'S STOMACH IMMEDIATELY by inducing vomiting. This cannot be overemphasized, for it is the essence of the treatment and is often a life-saving procedure. Prevent chilling by wrapping patient in blankets if necessary. Do not give alcohol in any form.

A. Do not induce vomiting if:
   1. Patient is in coma or unconscious.
   2. Patient is in convulsions.
   3. Patient has swallowed petroleum products (kerosene, gasoline, lighter fluid).
   4. Patient has swallowed a corrosive poison (symptoms: severe pain, burning sensation in mouth and throat, vomiting). CALL PHYSICIAN IMMEDIATELY.
      (a) Acid and acid-like corrosives: sodium acid sulfate (toilet bowl cleaners), acetic acid (glacial), sulfuric acid, nitric acid, oxalic acid, hydrofluoric acid (rust removers), iodine, silver nitrate (styptic pencil).
      (b) Alkali corrosives: sodium hydroxide-lye (drain cleaners), sodium carbonate (washing soda), ammonia water, sodium hypochlorite (household bleach).

If the patient can swallow after ingesting a *corrosive poison,* the following substances (and amounts) may be given:

For acids: milk, water, or milk of magnesia (1 tablespoon to 1 cup of water).
For alkalies: milk, water, any fruit juice, or vinegar.
For patient 1-5 years old—1 to 2 cups.
For patient 5 years and older—up to 1 quart.

B. Induce vomiting when non-corrosive substances have been swallowed:
   1. Give milk or water (for patient 1-5 years old—1 to 2 cups; for patient over 5 years—up to 1 quart).
   2. Induce vomiting by placing the blunt end of a spoon or your finger at the back of the patient's throat, or by use of this emetic—2 tablespoons of salt in a glass of warm water.

When retching and vomiting begin, place patient face down with head lower than hips. This prevents vomitus from entering the lungs and causing further damage.

II. Inhaled poisons

1. Carry patient (do not let him walk) to fresh air immediately.
2. Open all doors and windows.
3. Loosen all tight clothing.
4. Apply artificial respiration if breathing has stopped or is irregular.
5. Prevent chilling (wrap patient in blankets).
6. Keep patient as quiet as possible.
7. If patient is convulsing, keep him in bed in a semidark room; avoid jarring or noise.
8. Do not give alcohol in any form.

III. Skin contamination

1. Drench skin with water (shower, hose, faucet).
2. Apply stream of water on skin while removing clothing.
3. Cleanse skin thoroughly with water; rapidity in washing is most important in reducing extent of injury.

IV. Eye contamination

1. Hold eyelids open, wash eyes with gentle stream of running water *immediately.* Delay of few seconds greatly increases extent of injury.
2. Continue washing until physician arrives.
3. *Do not use chemicals;* they may increase extent of injury.

V. Injected poisons (scorpion and snake bites)

1. Make patient lie down as soon as possible.
2. Do not give alcohol in any form.
3. Apply tourniquet above injection site (e.g., between arm or leg and heart). The pulse in vessels below the tourniquet should not disappear, nor should the tourniquet produce a throbbing sensation. Tourniquet should be loosened for 1 minute every 15 minutes.
4. Apply ice-pack to the site of the bite.
5. Carry patient to physician or hospital; DO NOT LET HIM WALK.

*"Recommendations of Committee on Toxicology on First Aid Measures for Poisoning," *J.A.M.A.* 165:686–687 (October, 1957).

VI. Chemical Burns

1. Wash with large quantities of running water (except those burns caused by phosphorus).
2. Immediately cover with loosely applied clean cloth.
3. Avoid use of ointments, greases, powders, and other drugs in first-aid treatment of burns.
4. Treat shock by keeping patient flat, keeping him warm, and reassuring him until arrival of physician.

Measures to prevent poisoning accidents

A. Keep all drugs, poisonous substances, and household chemicals out of the reach of children.
B. Do not store nonedible products on shelves used for storing food.
C. Keep all poisonous substances in their original containers; do not transfer to unlabeled containers or to food containers such as soft drink bottles.
D. When medicines are discarded, destroy them. Do not throw them where they might be reached by children or pets.
E. When giving flavored and/or brightly colored medicine to children, *always* refer to it as medicine—*never* as candy.
F. Do not take or give medicine in the dark.
G. READ LABELS before using chemical products.

IT IS IMPORTANT TO REMEMBER

1. That fear may be more destructive than a poison. The patient or his relatives may seriously hamper treatment by overzealous attention which is the result of fear.
2. That the use of an antidote is often more dangerous and less important than other procedures that the nurse may safely perform.
3. That shock is an important factor in cases of poisoning and may be more deadly than the poison.
4. That prevention is much more important than cure.

TOPICS FOR STUDY AND DISCUSSION

1. Look in the newspapers for reports of accidental poisoning. What types of poisons predominate? What was the general age group or groups represented? In each case, what would the nurse's duties have been?
2. Give some rules for the home in which you live—your own or the dormitory—which will prevent accidental poisoning.
3. What antidotes were mentioned as essential for the nurse to remember? Can you recall all of them? Why are these considered important?
4. Why is an accurate detailed record of any poisoning case necessary? What should be recorded?
5. Locate and visit the Poison Control Center in your area and report to the class on its functions.
6. The doctor wishes to give a lavage of 2 per cent sodium bicarbonate solution. The nurse will need about 2 quarts. How much sodium bicarbonate will be required?
7. Apomorphine hydrochloride 6 mg. is ordered as an emetic. The nurse finds that the apomorphine is in hypodermic tablets marked gr. 1/8. How should she prepare this dose?

BIBLIOGRAPHY*

Books and Pamphlets

A Programmed Learning Course in Toxicology II, Madison, Wisconsin, University of Wisconsin Press.

American Medical Association Council on Drugs, *Drug Evaluations*, Chicago, 1971, American Medical Association.

*See also Chapter 6 bibliography.

Bergersen, B., *Pharmacology in Nursing*, St. Louis, 1973, The C. V. Mosby Co.
Goodman, L. S., and Gilman, A., *Pharmacological Basis of Therapeutics*, 4th Ed., New York, 1970, The Macmillan Co.
Goth, A., *Medical Pharmacology*, St. Louis, 1970, The C. V. Mosby Co.
Haavik, C. O., *Accidental Poisoning, Prevention and Treatment*, Madison, Wisconsin, 1970, University of Wisconsin Press.

Journal Articles

Miller, R. R., and Johnson, S. R., "Poison control—Now and in the future," *Am. J. Nurs.* 66:9:1984 (September, 1966).
Rodman, H. J., "Poisonings and their treatment, *R.N.* 35:11:5272.
Rodman, H. J., "Poisonings and their treatment," *R.N.* 35:12:57.

CHAPTER 12

THE PSYCHOLOGICAL ASPECTS OF DRUG THERAPY

CORRELATION WITH OTHER SCIENCES

V. PSYCHOLOGY

1. People normally want both time to be alone, and time to be with others. Long enforced periods of isolation have a very depressing effect upon most individuals.
2. In this modern age, time has become a most important factor in everyone's life. People are used to planning all their activities by the clock, and any marked deviation produces tensions which disturb the normal functioning of the individual.
3. Most people like attention, but in some this desire is much stronger than in others. If controlled, this is a normal need, but uncontrolled, it can lead a person to use any ruse for securing the attention he desires.
4. People become dependent upon artificial and physical means of bolstering their egos. They must lean on something or somebody to keep their equilibrium.
5. All human beings are alike in many respects, but each one has individual characteristics which make him different from all others.
6. People react to those about them. If the influence is good, the reaction is usually satisfactory; but if the influence is poor, the reaction is apt to be unsatisfactory.

VI. SOCIOLOGY

1. Many families do not include medical and hospital costs in their budgets, or if they do it is in inadequate amounts. A sudden severe illness, especially if it strikes the breadwinner, is a financial catastrophe.
2. Current medical insurance plans vary widely in their provisions. Some pay all or nearly all of the patient's hospital bill; others pay only a very small per cent. Some people are ineligible for medical insurance, yet these are often the people who need the coverage most.
3. Every person regardless of race, creed or nationality deserves the same opportunity for adequate health care.

INTRODUCTION

What is the significance of that little tablet that was just given to Mr. Blank? How many nurses, or doctors for that matter, ever really try to answer that question? In Chapter 6 some of the social aspects of drugs were discussed, but mainly from the angle of self-medication and drug dependency. There it was stressed that drugs should be ordered by a physician and taken only under his direction. But what of those drugs that are given only on the advice of and under the close supervision of the physician? What are the sociologic and psychologic factors which interact to make each patient's experience with his medicine unique? Just what do these white pills, or green capsules or bitter liquid, ordered by the doctor and administered by a nurse or delegated member of the family, represent in the eyes of the patient? A brief exploration of some of these questions might make a routine nursing task a bit more interesting and vastly more purposeful.

Except in rare instances, drugs should always be considered as temporary expedients to be dispensed with at the earliest possible moment. This is not meant to imply that the nurse should start reducing the medications too soon or should deny the patient any needed medication, but it is intended to remind all concerned that drugs are an aid to be used only until the patient can carry on adequately without them. There are, of course, certain exceptions to this—such as the hormones administered in cases of deficiency which must often be used for the entire life of the individual.

MEDICINES FROM THE PATIENT'S VIEWPOINT

When a person is very sick, his medicine, no matter what its composition or form, means a great deal to him. In the first place, it usually means relief from pain or discomfort. It is the first step on the road to recovery and a return to home (if in the hospital), to his family and to his job. It is the starting of the path that will lead to increased activity. To the patient in the hospital, especially the one in a private room, medication time is a diversion, a time when his isolation is broken and he has a chance, if time is allowed, to speak to someone (V-1). It is a very welcome break in the monotony of the day. Most patients know when their drugs are due and they wait eagerly for the nurse to appear, often becoming very upset when she is late (V-2). For instance, if the patient has glaucoma and his eye drops are late in coming, he may become extremely anxious, since he realizes that these drops mean his sight. These are all things that retard recovery but, since their existence may be unrecognized by the patient, the observing nurse must be aware of her patient's need. However, she will also recognize the patient who uses his medication as an attention-getting mechanism or a crutch (V-3, 4). These last few remarks apply mainly to the so-called "p.r.n." drugs—those given whenever, in the opinion of the nurse, the patient needs the drug. The nurse needs a great deal of understanding to evaluate properly the various factors involved.

Some Reasons Why Patients Refuse Medications

Sometimes patients will refuse to take prescribed drugs, and the busy nurse may simply write "refused" on the chart and await the arrival of the physician for further orders. The nurse who is interested in the welfare of the patient, however, may often, with patience and tact, uncover the reason for the refusal. A few of the more common reasons might be considered. These are only examples, for the actual list is unlimited, and the nurse will need to use imagination and understanding in dealing with each individual case.

The reasons for refusal may be very simple, such as unpleasant taste or odor of a fluid drug or difficulty in swallowing a large tablet or capsule. Powders and grainy materials are very unpleasant and often difficult to swallow, and many patients become nauseated by them. This is also true of oily medicines, which often "repeat," thus nauseating the patient or at least making food distasteful. In such cases a simple explanation as to the purpose of the drug, and why that particular form has been ordered, may be all that is needed to secure cooperation. For instance, bitter drugs are often given before meals to stimulate appetite and to increase the secretion of the digestive juices. The bitterness is an essential part of the drug. If the patient understands that the bitterness will aid digestion and thus recovery, he will be more willing to take the drug. Sometimes the physician can be asked if another form of the medicine could be used. Large tablets can be crushed and put into capsules or they can be given with a small amount of food if this is permissible. Oils taken directly after holding ice in the mouth for a few seconds cannot be tasted. Powders and grainy drugs taken with a little food (unless this is contraindicated) or with water are much easier to swallow. The ingenious nurse will think of many ways of getting the patient to take his medicine willingly in such situations.

Parenteral administration may be very painful, and adults as well as children may fear such procedures. To most nurses, many of whom have not had such treatments themselves, the injection of subcutaneous or intramuscular drugs is a very simple thing, but to the patient these may be traumatic, often frightening, experiences. Some people feel that such methods are used only when the patient is in a critical condition and to these patients the sight of a hypodermic means a last attempt to secure help—in other words they experience the "if this doesn't help I'm going to die" feeling. In other cases, an unpleasant past experience may be the cause of the fear. Sometimes the tissues are not in good condition or, if the needle accidentally strikes a small blood vessel, ecchymosis may result. This causes a sore area which increases the patient's discomfort. Some drugs cause a stinging, burning sensation, and even pain, at the point of injection. Although the nurse cannot avoid such situations, if she is careful she can minimize them. A sharp needle of the correct size expertly inserted into the best area will avoid much of the discomfort. To decide what areas are "best," the nurse may be aided by observation of the patient's preferred positions; for instance, if the patient lies most of the time on his right side the left buttock might be the best place for injection if there is nothing to contraindicate this.

Some Fears Patients Have

Medicinal therapy is also affected by many other matters. The patient may be worrying about finances (VI-1). Having heard about the high cost of the "new wonder drugs," he may make excuses to avoid taking the medicine if he fears he cannot pay for it. Although he may not put his fears into words, the nurse can usually get enough hints to suspect the cause of the trouble. The nurse can do much to overcome such worries. She can explain, if such is the case, that the drug in question is not very expensive. If the drug is one of the higher priced ones, she can assure the patient that the hastened recovery and shorter hospital stay will more than recompense for the expense of the drug. The drug, though it costs a great deal, may in the long run be an actual saving for the patient, since with recovery will come regained productiveness.

The nurse should be extremely careful to avoid any waste of the patient's medicines no matter how inexpensive they may be. Each patient's drugs, if the individual drug system is used, must be kept strictly for that patient; and when he goes home, if the drug is not given to him to take home, it should be returned to the pharmacy so that proper credit may be given and the patient will not have to pay for something he did not use. Even one dose might mean a refund of several dollars. Many patients are covered by the governmental insurance plans, Medicare and Medicaid. These pay for the medicines as do some private insurance policies. These facts do not relieve the nurse of the responsibility of not wasting a patient's medicines.

Money is only one of many worries commonly associated with medicines. Probably the most serious ones are those associated with the habit-forming properties of drugs, and in this respect the nurse has a great responsibility (discussed in some detail in previous chapters). It must be remembered that although the nurse should not give a "p.r.n. order" when it is not needed, it is equally important that she not withhold such a drug when the patient really should have it. Some nurses, overzealous in the prevention of drug habituation, do not give medications that are actually best for the patient's speedy recovery or for his comfort. In addition to the responsibility of deciding when a drug is needed, it is important for the nurse to be able to assure the patient that not all drugs are habit forming and that, even with those drugs that can produce habituation, such a result is extremely rare following illness. It is unusual for a patient to continue to want a medicine when the physical need for the drug is past; as soon as the patient has recovered sufficiently, the need and desire for the medicine cease simultaneously.

Patients are often fearful that the treatment given may not be effective. They want to know what can be done if it is not. It is usually sufficient to assure the patient that there are many drugs and many treatments for most disorders and that, if one is not effective, perhaps another will be. Similar to this is the situation, encountered so often, of the patient who has a friend or relative with the same condition who has had this or that treatment or drug, and who wants to know why the doctor does not order the same thing for him? Again it can be explained that there are many drugs and treatments for each disease and that, in general, they are all effective. The physician selects the one which he feels will be best for the individual he is treating. Each person is different from every other, and what is good for one may or may not be good for someone else with the same disease (V-5).

Tolerance is another matter of concern for many patients, especially those with chronic conditions. The drug is extremely helpful, and they fear the time when their systems will no longer tolerate it or when it will cease to be effective. Many drugs do not produce tolerance to any great degree, and the nurse need only assure the patient that this particular drug rarely ever ceases to be effective nor does it produce undesirable symptoms when taken over a long period of time. However, many drugs do tend to become less and less efficient the longer they are taken, making larger and larger doses necessary to secure the same effect. With increasingly large doses the body may react unfavorably, and toxic reactions occur, or the drug may cease entirely to give the desired results without actual toxic action. In these cases the nurse will need to be very tactful, even cautious, in her explanations. Usually there is more than one drug which can be used to treat any specific disorder, and this fact can often be of help in allaying the patient's fears.

SOME POINTS TO BE CONSIDERED

It is important for the nurse to remember that spoken words do not constitute the entire means of communication. Nonverbal communication is equally impressive, often more so. The toss of the head, the shrug of the shoulder, the smile or the lack of one, all tell much. In fact, all the bodily movements may be more expressive than any words spoken. The considerate nurse will be careful to show only concern and understanding for the patient in her acts as well as her conversation. She must not in any way let worries, tiredness or pressure of other duties affect her dealing with the patient at hand.

Patients of all races and creeds are admitted to our hospitals, treated in our outpatient departments and cared for in their homes by nurses and doctors who also are of all races and creeds (VI-3). Every nurse should keep this fact always before her in dealing with patients. Many churches and religions impose restrictions upon their members that may interfere with the regular routine of the hospital. Especially is this true in relation to the kinds of foods the individual may eat and the time he may eat. Although the problem is most important for the dietary department, it may also concern the nurse in her administration of drugs. If the patient is supposed to be fasting, he may feel that oral drugs should not be taken or, if they are taken, that no water or food should be used to aid in swallowing the drug. It is not the nurse's prerogative to announce glibly, "Oh! It's all right for you to break your fast. Medicines don't count. Anyway, patients are exempt from the rules." Although this may well be true, it is not for the nurse to decide. She should have the church representative assure the patient about these matters. If the patient feels that he is violating a religious principle which he considers important, the very violation of the rule may cause a great deal of psychic damage, the result far outweighing any benefit to be gained from the drug.

The sympathetic understanding of the nurse for all her patients and their problems cannot be stressed too much. The nurse should try to place herself in the position of the patient and then apply the golden rule.

If the patient is seriously ill, the nurse should be prepared to receive the spiritual advisor of the patient and should aid in securing such a person if requested by either the patient or his family. If the administration of a drug produces a severe untoward reaction, the minister, priest or rabbi should be notified as well as the physician. It is difficult, almost impossible, to set any rules, but the sympathetic, understanding nurse will find a way to solve these problems if she is thinking always of the patient's welfare.

The nurse should remember that every person responds differently and must be allowed to do so. She should not attempt to reply for him. It is very often easier for an older nurse than a younger one to communicate with an elderly patient. This is not because of any particular skill or knowledge the older nurse has, but because, consciously or not, the patient feels the older nurse has "lived more" and hence has a better idea of life's problems than the younger nurse who may well have a much greater technical knowledge. Each can help the other and both can help the patient by understanding their "long and short points."

One other thing that is often forgotten in dealing with patients, especially in attempting to perform a treatment or give a medication the patient does not want is that "a little praise can be a therapeutic agent."

IT IS IMPORTANT TO REMEMBER

1. That investigations in psychosomatic medicine have proved that the mental and emotional outlook of the patient often spell the difference between sickness and health, regardless of the treatment given.
2. That a cheery word is often worth as much as a medication.
3. That the nurse must understand the emotional problems of her patients and try to find remedies for them.
4. That "haste makes waste," and a persistent hurried air will make patients lose confidence in the nurse.

TOPICS FOR STUDY AND DISCUSSION

1. Secure a list of 25 drugs in common use on the division to which you are assigned. Find the retail price of each and estimate the cost per average dose. What are your conclusions about wasted medicines?
2. Presuming that the medical insurance plan pays $25.00 for medicines, select a patient from your division and figure out how long this will last and what the patient might have to pay. Refer to the information gained under Topic 1.
3. Study various religious tenets that might affect the giving of medicines, and show how each might be dealt with without disturbing the patient's religious practice or the hospital routine. (This might be a project for several students.)

BIBLIOGRAPHY

Books and Pamphlets

Beland, J. L., *Clinical Nursing, 2nd Ed.*, New York, 1970, The Macmillan Co.

Duskin, D. A., et al., *Psychology Today*, Del Mar, California, 1970, Communication Research Machine Co.

Kempf, F. C., and Useem, R. H., *Psychology*, Philadelphia, 1964, W. B. Saunders Co.

Price, A. L., *The Art, Science and Spirit of Nursing, 3rd Ed.*, Philadelphia, 1965, W. B. Saunders Co.

Watson, J. E., *Medical-Surgical Nursing and Related Physiology*, Philadelphia, 1972, W. B. Saunders Co.

Journal Articles

Cooper, S. J., et al., "Symposium on nursing practice—Expectation and reality," *Nurs. Clin. North Am.* 3:68:3.

Domming, J. J., "That certain feeling," *Am. J. Nurs.* 71:11:2156 (November, 1971).

Gage, F., "Suicide in the aged," *Am. J. Nurs.* 71:11:2153 (November, 1971).

Gauld, G. T., et al., "Symposium on compassion and communication in nursing," *Nurs. Clin. North Am.* 4:69:12.

SECTION II

DRUGS USED FOR SPECIFIC AGE GROUPS

CHAPTER 13

CHANGES IN DRUG THERAPY FOR INFANTS AND CHILDREN

CORRELATION WITH OTHER SCIENCES

I. ANATOMY AND PHYSIOLOGY

1. Growth is the process of increasing in size, while development refers to the anatomic and physiologic changes that occur.
2. The greatest postnatal growth period is in infancy; however, there is a second period of rapid growth during preadolescence and adolescence.
3. Physical and emotional growth and development are sequential patterns of normal functioning and children progress through these patterns at different rates.
4. Growth and development of a child depend upon the hereditary background received from each parent as well as various environmental factors.
5. Development is measured by improvement in skill and functional capacity.
6. The onset of menstruation is usually considered as the period when the girl becomes a woman, but it must be remembered that the period of change spans several years, not just one month.
7. Illness threatens physical and emotional growth and development of the child.
8. Illness in children is manifested by the physiological and psychological differences between the immature child and the mature adult.

III. MICROBIOLOGY

1. The infant at birth has antibodies received from his mother. However, he almost immediately begins to form his own immunity. The building of antibodies is rapid during the period of growth and development, so that by the time he reaches adulthood, he has become immune to those communicable diseases with which he has been in contact.

V. PSYCHOLOGY

1. Mother-child relationships are not necessarily dependent upon the amount of time spent together, but rather on the quality of the time spent.
2. Parental reactions to a child's illness or need for hospitalization are reflected in a variety of behaviors specific for that family.
3. Hospitalization may be a psychologically traumatic experience creating anxieties in the child regarding separation from the family.
4. During illness, children may regress in behavior and reflect increased dependency needs.
5. Play is an effective way of dealing with anxiety in children.
6. How a child views death depends upon his degree of maturity and his past experience with death (if any).
7. The nurse must recognize her own feelings and reactions to death in order to interact effectively with and care for a dying child and his family.

VI. SOCIOLOGY

1. The family unit is called the nuclear family and is composed of parents, children and sometimes grandparents.

2. One-parent families are not uncommon. The parent may be lost through death or divorce or the situation may be the result of an out-of-wedlock birth.

3. The home culture or ethnic group, the geographical location (urban, suburban or rural) and the family social class affect the child's growth and development.

4. Parenthood, if it is to be successful, requires the capacity to give unselfish love which finds its satisfaction in the happiness of the children.

INTRODUCTION

People in the medical professions, including nurses, usually think of life as a continuum, beginning with conception and ending with death (I-1). They do not feel that it is possible to set up arbitrary divisions. However, for the purpose of discussion it is essential to make certain distinctions among general age groups. Fortunately, there are some rather definite developmental changes, and these do occur at approximately the same ages in most individuals. It is important to remember that these are rough divisions and that no definite rules can be made. Each person is an individual and must be looked upon as such. Averages are set by taking the mathematical mean of a large number of people, but no one can say that the mean is the normal figure. For instance, the time of the onset of menstruation taken from the mean age of 1000 women might be 14½ years (I-6). Is that the normal age for all women? Or can it be assumed that that is normal even for the group studied? What is normal for one person is not necessarily normal for another. This example is to try to impress upon the reader that the divisions made in this and other chapters are for convenience only and may not suit any specific person.

It is essential to remember that the developmental stage is far more important than the chronologic age of the individual. Age is a rather indefinite factor. In studying a person we arrive at many ages. The child on his sixth birthday (chronologically) may have a mental age of eight, a social age of ten, an emotional age of three and a developmental age of seven. It is the developmental age that is of importance in our present discussions; however, when other information is lacking, the chronologic age must be used.

For purposes of discussion the developmental groups may be given as follows:

1. Infancy—birth to 1 year
2. Toddler—1 to 3 years
3. Preschool—3 to 6 years
4. School age—6 to 12 years
5. Adolescence (Puberty)—12 to 20 years

Changes in drug administration for each age group may include:

1. Dosage
2. Form of the drug
3. Method of administration
4. Kind of medicine

CHANGES FOR INFANTS THROUGH THE PRESCHOOL AGE CHILD

Since the adult dose is considered as the standard, it is necessary to ascertain the child's dose from that of the adult. There are several ways of calculating doses according to weight or age as follows:

Fried's rule: (child less than one year of age)

$$\frac{\text{age in months}}{150} \times \text{adult dose} = \text{infant's dose.}$$

Young's rule: (child two years of age and over)

$$\frac{\text{age in years} \times \text{adult dose}}{\text{age in years} + 12} = \text{child's dose.}$$

Clark's rule: (infant or child)

$$\frac{\text{weight in pounds} \times \text{adult dose}}{150 \text{ (average adult weight)}} = \text{child's dose.}$$

This rule is based upon the assumptions that the average adult weight is 150 pounds and that the child's weight is a good indi-

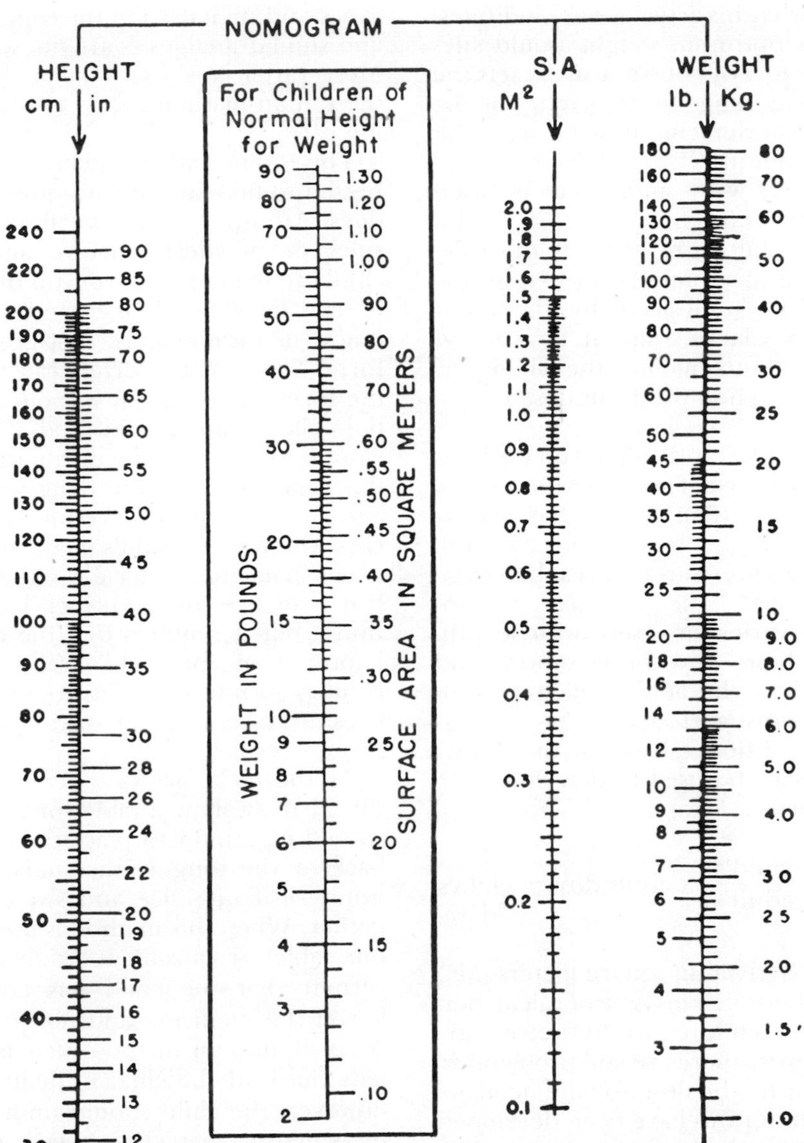

FIGURE 22. West nomogram (for estimation of surface areas). The surface area is indicated where a straight line connecting the height and weight intersects the surface area column or, if the patient is roughly of average size, from the weight alone (enclosed area). Nomogram modified from data of E. Boyd by C. D. West. (From Shirkey, H. C., and Barba, W. P., in Nelson, W. E., *Textbook of Pediatrics, 9th Ed.*, Philadelphia, 1969, W. B. Saunders Co.

cation of his development. However, this may not be so accurate as it seems. Let us consider a 9 pound infant who is six months old. He is underweight. Suppose that the drug ordered is one to improve appetite or to increase the secretion of the digestive juices. It might be better for this infant to receive, not what his actual weight indicates, but what his optimum weight would suggest. The doctor, of course, usually sets the dosage for the drugs to be given, but the nurse should understand how he arrives at the correct amount.

Fried's rule is very similar but is based upon the age relationship between the infant and the adult in months. By this rule, the child's age in months is divided by 150 and the result multiplied by the adult dose, as with Clark's rule. It is assumed that by the 150th month the child has reached a time when the adult dose can be tolerated.

Dosage may also be calculated on the basis of body surface area. The use of the surface area is dependent upon the fact that, in relation to their weight, smaller objects (children) have a greater surface area than large objects (adults). The surface area-to-weight ratio varies inversely with length. Thus, the infant, since he is shorter and weighs less than the adult, will have proportionately more surface area.

In this type of dose calculation the following formula can be used to determine the dose from surface area:

$$\frac{\text{surface area (child's)}}{\text{surface area (adult's)}} \times \text{adult dose} = \text{child's dose.}$$

Surface area is given in square meters (M^2) or fractions thereof. This type of calculation can be used for children up to twelve years of age. However, there are still problems in the estimation of the dose for the neonate.

Several nomograms have been developed for determining body surface area. The Boyd and West nomogram is given as an illustration (see Fig. 22). To use such nomograms, it may be necessary to use any or all of the following formulas:

$$\begin{aligned} \text{pounds} &\div 2.2 = \text{Kg.} \\ \text{grains/pound} &\div 7 = \text{Gm./Kg.} \\ \text{Gm./M}^2 &\div 30 = \text{Gm./Kg.} \\ \text{mg./M}^2 &\div 30 = \text{mg./kg.} \end{aligned}$$

As mentioned in earlier chapters, dosage is only one of the factors to be considered in pediatric drug administration. It is well known that infants tolerate some drugs better than others. For instance, most vitamins can be given in larger doses than the rule would indicate. The same is true for cathartics and digitalis. On the contrary, opiates and similar analgesics are not well received. Most physicians use smaller quantities of these than mathematical calculations would indicate.

The infant and small child cannot be expected to take oral medications as the adult does. An infant cannot swallow tablets, capsules or powdered drugs, and the little child can manage these only if they are small or can be chewed like candy. During infancy, medications are best given in liquid form. Some of the drugs can be added to the formula and given without difficulty. If the child is eating solid food, it may be unwise to disguise the medicine with food lest the child associate the drug with his food and an eating problem result. Most pharmacists will mix the child's medicine with some sweet palatable vehicle so that the child learns to like his medicine. This is a good thing, but it requires that the medicine be kept out of the child's reach. Often the child is so intrigued with the drug that he tries to take it all at once, perhaps with serious results.

As the child grows older he can be induced to swallow a tablet or a capsule. He should be taught to place the tablet on the back of the tongue, then take a drink of water or fruit juice and swallow both together. When this method is used, give only one tablet or capsule at a time and be very certain that the child has actually swallowed the medicine and not just the fluid. A small amount of food such as custard or jelly may aid the child in taking the drug; however, the child should understand that he is getting medicine, since it is unwise to trick him. If the child is unable to swallow the drug, the tablet may be crushed and dissolved in a small amount of water or food; a capsule may be emptied and its contents treated in the same manner. Delayed-release drugs, tablets, capsules or pills should not be crushed or emptied as this may permit the drug to be absorbed too rapidly or in the wrong area of the gastrointestinal tract. If in doubt, the physician should be consulted. It is wise to give the child's medicine at a time when it will not interfere with his regular meals unless, of course, it is a drug to be given with meals.

Special precautions must be observed in giving medications to children by parenteral routes. The needles should be very sharp and of the correct size. As small a caliber should be used as is consistent with the fluid to be injected. The needle should not be too large since there is not so much tissue to penetrate as in the adult; too small a needle may bend or "wobble" when inserted, and this is distressing to the patient. A helper should hold the child lest he move suddenly and break the needle. However, the nurse should not approach the patient as an army about to conquer the enemy. If the child is old enough to understand, she should explain briefly what is to be done. She can make a game of it so that the child will cooperate more willingly (V-5). In the actual administration, she should be quick and efficient. After it is over the child can be praised, or loved, even if uncooperative. He should feel that the nurse appreciates his attempt to "be good" and that she knows that it did hurt. Maybe the next time there will be less resistance.

Other approaches that are useful in helping the older toddler and the preschool child handle a painful intrusive procedure such as an intramuscular injection are: (1) spending time with the child in order for him to become familiar with the nurse; (2) allowing the child some reasonable choices, e.g., determining which side to use for the injection; (3) allowing the child to cry during the procedure or to hold a hand or a toy; (4) permitting him to put on the Band-Aid over the injection site; (5) allowing aggressive behavior after the procedure is complete, e.g., punching a bag and (6) remaining with the child for comforting after the procedure. The nurse will need to be constantly innovative in her approach to children. What works effectively with one child will not necessarily be effective with another. Also, repeated experience with the same child will require modifications in the nursing approach.

It is very important to decide upon the exact area to be used for the injection, being sure that the part selected is right for the particular type of medication used. Intramuscular injections may be given in various areas. The ventrogluteal and the vastus lateralis are sites which are preferred for intramuscular injections on children less than two years of age. The ventrogluteal and the posterior gluteal sites are preferred for children over two years of age. These recommendations are based on the fact that the gluteal muscles are not sufficiently developed until the child has been walking for about one year. If there are several to be given, alternation of the sides and variations in the point of insertion will be necessary. Recording is important—drug, dose, time and site of injection should be charted.

In the giving of medications to children, much can be done to make things easier if the nurse will give some thought to the procedure before attempting to administer the drug. Children react to the attitude of the adult and, if the nurse acts as if she expected the child to take the medicine, she will often secure cooperation without further effort. Small children are afraid of strange things but, as a rule, they have no conditioning against drugs. It is a common thing to see a small child lick the spoon that contained cod liver oil until some adult makes a face or says something like "doesn't that taste terrible." From then on the child refuses the cod liver oil. The nurse should never be guilty of such conditioning. Children like to play games and to be "big." Knowledge of this can be used to persuade the child to take his medicine. Also the child's desire to make his own decisions can be used to secure cooperation. Thus, if the child is to have two medicines, he may be allowed to choose which one he will take first, or he may be allowed to decide the kind of food or drink that is to be given with the medicines if this is allowable. The resourceful nurse will find many ways to get the child to take his medicine willingly.

If the child is old enough, he should be told why the medication is being given in words that he can understand. The nurse should not go into details for these bore the young child, whose attention span is very short. Here it is especially necessary that the nurse know her patients. She should take time to study each child enough to understand his basic problems and needs. If her first approach "falls on

TABLE 9. *APPROXIMATE RELATION OF SURFACE AREA AND WEIGHTS OF INDIVIDUALS OF AVERAGE BODY DIMENSIONS**

KILOGRAMS	POUNDS	SQUARE METERS	PER CENT OF ADULT DOSE
2	4.4	0.12	6
3	6.6	0.20	10
4	8.8	0.23	12
5	11.0	0.25	13
6	13.0	0.29	15
7	15.0	0.33	17
8	18.0	0.36	18
9	20.0	0.40	20
10	22.0	0.44	22
15	33.0	0.62	31
20	44.0	0.79	40
25	55.0	0.93	42
30	66.0	1.07	51
35	77.0	1.20	60
40	88.0	1.32	65
45	99.0	1.43	70
50	110.0	1.53	75
55	121.0	1.62	80
60	132.0	1.70	85
65	143.0	1.78	90
70	154.0	1.84	92
75	165.0	1.95	95
80	176.0	2.00	100

*Adapted from data in Crawford, J. D., Terry, M. E., and Rourke, G. M., "Simplification of Drug Dosage Calculation by Application of the Surface Area Principle." Read in abstract form at the Annual Meeting of the Society for Pediatric Research, Atlantic City, N.J., May 4, 1949. (Received for publication September 12, 1949.)

deaf ears," she should try another. She should not become discouraged or angry since the child will sense her feelings very quickly and will react accordingly. The nurse should try to maintain an even temper at all times when dealing with infants and children. She should be cheerful, resourceful, patient, understanding and truthful, and she should expect cooperation. If, in addition, the nurse genuinely likes children she will have no difficulties.

CHANGES DURING CHILDHOOD

From Preschool Age to Adolescence

As with the infant's, the child's dose must be reduced from that of the adult. There are certain general averages that will be helpful in estimating the doses for various age groups and in checking calculations. When comparing Young's rule to the adult dose, the 12 year old child receives about half the amount; the six year old child, a third; and the four year old child, about a quarter. Since there can be no sharply defined point at which childhood begins, almost everything mentioned under infancy and early childhood applies to the older child.

During infancy and childhood the emphasis is upon the maintenance of adequate health, including proper growth and development, and the prevention of disease. The preponderance of medicinal substances used during childhood are for these purposes.

When the child is sick he receives medicines much as the adult except that the amount is in direct relationship to his age and size. Mode of administration may vary, but the actual drugs used do not. The nearer the child approaches adulthood, the more the adult forms of administration may be used. It is often easier to get the child to take his medicine if he realizes that it is the way "grownups" take theirs.

Gradually, as the child nears the "teen"

years his medicines approach the adult type. The drugs and the modes of administration vary little though the dosage usually remains less.

Each year the child undergoes both physical and psychologic changes. The nurse should be familiar with these changes and use this knowledge to aid her in gaining proper rapport with her charges. The small child is an individualist and, although he may play with other children, he maintains his own sense of values. Later on, the "gang" becomes important, and the sexes tend to play separately. The child then wants to do as the "gang" does and is scornful of anything not approved by his group. This fact can often be used as a means of securing cooperation. If the proper atmosphere is maintained in the children's ward, for instance, each new child can be made to feel one of the group and, as such, will follow the example of the other children in the ward.

It often helps to know something of the child's background. Is he an only child or are there siblings? If the latter, are they older or younger, the same or opposite sex? The child can be made to feel more at home if the nurse knows of his brothers and sisters and can speak of them by name. This information is usually available from the chart or can be obtained from the parents or the child himself. This may be a way of establishing rapport. There are many ways to overcome fear, secure cooperation and get the child to do the things which are essential for recovery.

Preventive medication has been discussed in detail in Chapter 7. It is customary to begin inoculations when the infant is one or two months of age. These are continued at intervals until the desired immunizations have been obtained.

"Booster shots" are often given just before the child enters school to insure production of sufficient quantities of antibodies to prevent the diseases. The sudden association with a large number of his peers greatly increases the possibility of his exposure to the various communicable diseases.

During an epidemic, specific precautions may be used such as "booster shots" or gamma globulin if the child has had no immunization against the specific disease. This product contains the antibodies for most of the common communicable diseases since it is obtained from the blood of a number of adults (III-1).

Vitamins and minerals form a large segment of the drugs used for the infant and child. When these materials can be secured in the diet, additions need not be made; however, if the diet is inadequate, vitamins, especially vitamins A, D and C and minerals such as calcium should be added. Since there is a tendency for the family to add these without a physician's advice, a note of warning is important. Vitamins are essential food products and must be provided in sufficient amounts, but only the physician can determine whether or not a given child is receiving the correct amount. It can be dangerous to give additional vitamins. Avitaminosis (a condition produced by the lack of vitamins) is well advertised, but one hears less of the serious consequences of hypervitaminosis (a condition caused by excessive vitamin intake).

CHANGES DURING ADOLESCENCE

From Preadolescence to Young Adulthood

This period includes preadolescence, adolescence and immediate postadolescence. It spans the age group from approximately 11 or 12 years to about 20 or 21 years of age. It includes the much maligned, grossly misinterpreted and overly emphasized teen ages.

Changes in dosage gradually disappear during this stage. The young person of 18 or 20 years is able to tolerate the regular adult dose of most, if not all, drugs. The child of 12 years receives about half the adult dose, but from this time on the child gradually becomes adult in physical makeup and hence is able to tolerate the same strengths of medicines as the adult.

The form and mode of administration for medications during this period is the same as for the adult; the 12 year old child is usually able to take drugs by the same routes as the adult. In most cases no special persuasion is needed to secure cooperation. Usually all one needs to do is to approach the child as if he were an adult, and he will do what is desired.

Changes in the type of drugs used during this period are not striking. Glandular products may be needed to aid the individual in adjusting to maturity. This is more often true of the girl than it is of the boy. Delayed, early or abnormal rhythm may occur in the menstrual cycle which can often be overcome by estrogen, progesterone or testosterone. One or all three may be used, depending upon the type and cause of the dysfunction. Disturbances of thyroid function are not uncommon during puberty and may require thyroid therapy. Fröhlich's syndrome may first appear during adolescence and requires hormone therapy, usually including both anterior pituitary secretion and/or thyroid hormone.

Adolescence is a period of rapid growth, and the youth often cannot or does not eat enough of the proper foods to maintain this excessive growth and development. Food accessories such as vitamins and minerals are helpful.

During these years, the adolescent is changing from a child to an adult—at one moment he is "grown-up" and at another he is still a dependent child. These factors must be understood and properly evaluated if the nurse is to deal sympathetically with the mood swings and unpredictable actions of these patients. She should never become resentful or sarcastic about the unusual actions of youth. He cannot help these reactions and is often surprised and ashamed of them but will never acknowledge this. The nurse must realize the reasons behind such behavior and aid the young person in making the necessary adjustments to adult life.

PEDIATRIC INTRAVENOUS THERAPY

The intravenous route is definitely preferred for all pediatric parenteral fluid administration. It can be readily carried out by using a scalp vein, arm vein or foot vein. Total parenteral nutrition or hyperalimentation utilizes a silicone catheter in the external or internal jugular vein or the axillary vein. In all instances, careful nursing observations are necessary to prevent circulatory overload and to keep the parenteral system patent.

Accurate records of the type, rate and amount of fluid administered are essential. It is also very important to record the body weight, central venous pressure and the chemical data from the laboratory.

The nurse must be especially cautious in administering intravenous fluid or drugs to infants and small children since they have greater difficulty in handling excessive fluids than do adults. Circulatory overload and subsequent pulmonary edema occur more rapidly in children than in adults. The nurse must also be cautious in using adult-sized equipment, e.g., bottles of fluids. Accidental administration of an additional 500 ml. could prove fatal. A general rule recommended by many health professionals is to never give more than 250 ml. of fluid to a child under 5 years of age or 500 ml. of fluid to any child.

Special pediatric bottles and administration sets should be used. The physician will prescribe the volume of fluid to be given within a designated period of time. By using such data and the drop factor of the equipment, the nurse can accurately determine fluid administration. The flow rate should be checked every 15 minutes and the condition of the patient noted at the same time. Dangerous situations can occur within a short time span when dealing with small children.

IT IS IMPORTANT TO REMEMBER

1. That adjustments in the use of drugs—kinds, preparations, dosage—go on from birth to death, and that there are no "hard and fast" rules to go by. The doctor and the nurse must make each change in the light of the individual patient concerned.
2. That though the average four year old child needs only a quarter of the adult dose of a drug, the child for whom the dose is being estimated may be far

from average and may need an entirely different amount of the particular drug under consideration.

3. That body surface area in relationship to weight is the most accurate means of determining doses for children.

4. That the knowledge of the child's stage of physical and emotional development will assist the nurse in understanding how to cope with the individual child's anxieties.

TOPICS FOR STUDY AND DISCUSSION

1. List some of the things a nurse might do to get a reluctant three year old boy or girl to take his or her medicine.
2. Describe in detail your nursing approach to a small child to give an intramuscular injection.
3. How might you secure the cooperation of a young person who needs glandular treatment but who does not want to be "different" from the "gang"?
4. The recommended adult dose of a drug is 0.5 mg. How much should be given to a six year old child?
5. Calculate the dose of piperazine citrate for pinworms for the following children in the Swiss family: Alfred, weight 21 pounds, Sara, weight 48 pounds, and Ted, weight 80 pounds. Single dose administration is based on 1 gm./M^2 basis. Refer to Boyd and West nomogram.
6. Describe how to give a vastus lateralis intramuscular injection to a child less than two years of age.

BIBLIOGRAPHY

Books and Pamphlets

American Pharmaceutical Association, *Usual Doses for Infants and Children*, Washington, D. C., 1965, American Pharmaceutical Association.

Blake, F., Wright, F., and Waechter, E., *Nursing Care of Children*, Philadelphia, 1970, J. B. Lippincott Co.

Goodman, L. S., and Gilman, A., *Pharmacological Basis of Therapeutics*, New York, 1965, The Macmillan Co.

Marlow, D., *Textbook of Pediatric Nursing, 4th Ed.*, Philadelphia, 1973, W. B. Saunders Co.,

Shirkey, H. C., *Pediatric Therapy, 3rd Ed.*, St. Louis, 1969, The C. V. Mosby Co.

Journal Articles

Brandt, P., Smith, M., Ashburn, S., and Groves, J., "Intramuscular injections in children," *Am. J. Nurs.* 72:8:1402 (August, 1972).

Dittman, L. L., "A child's sense of trust," *Am. J. Nurs.* 68:1251 (1968).

Erickson, F. H., "Helping the sick child maintain behavioral control," *Nurs. Clin. North Am.* 2:695 (1967).

Erickson, F., "When 6- to 12-year olds are ill," *Nurs. Outlook* 13:48 (July, 1965).

Frankenburg, W. K., and Dobbs, J. B., "The Denver developmental screening test," *J. Pediatr.* 71:181 (August, 1967).

Humphrey, N., Wright, P., and Swanson, A., "Parenteral hyperalimentation for children," *Am. J. Nurs.* 72:2:286 (February, 1972).

Kern, M. S., "New ideas about drug systems," *Am. J. Nurs.* 68:1251 (June, 1968).

Leavitt, S. R., Gofman, H., and Harvin, D., "A guide to normal development in the child," *Nurs. Outlook* 13:56 (September, 1965).

Milis, N., "Values, social class, and community health services," *Nurs. Res.* 16:26 (Winter, 1967).

Payne, J., and Kaplan, H., "Alternative techniques for venipuncture," *Am. J. Nurs.* 72:4:702 (1972).

Pitel, M., "The subcutaneous injection," *Am. J. Nurs.* 71:1:76 (1971).

Shaffer, J. H., Sweet, L. C., "Allergic reactions to drugs," *Am. J. Nurs.* 65:100 (1965).

Webb, C., "Nursing support for your young patients' parents," *R.N.* 30:44 (February, 1967).

Webb, C., "Tactics to reduce a child's fear of pain," *Am. J. Nurs.* 66:2698 (1966).

Wu, R., "Explaining treatment to young children," *Am. J. Nurs.* 65:71 (July, 1965).

CHAPTER 14

CHANGES IN DRUG THERAPY FOR THE OLDER PATIENT

CORRELATION WITH OTHER SCIENCES

I. ANATOMY AND PHYSIOLOGY

1. Bodily changes are both progressive and regressive. In the child and the young adult, the progressive changes predominate, but as the person grows older, the regressive changes become more pronounced.
2. As the onset of menstruation can be given as the beginning of sexual maturity in the female, so the cessation of menstruation can be set as the end of that period. Just as the period of adolescence spans several years, so the period of menopause also covers many years. This is the time when the degenerative processes begin, and a woman is no longer able to bear children. Though she may seem to be in better health than she has been previously, certain body processes are gradually becoming less active.
3. The male does not have any abrupt, spectacular change to correspond with the menstrual function of the female; however, the preadolescent male undergoes many developmental changes.
4. The male also experiences a period corresponding to the cessation of menstruation in the female. The male sex organs become less active, and general regressive changes begin. The male climacteric usually occurs later than does the female.
5. The period of senescence is the period when the physical powers wane. The regressive changes may be mental as well as physical. The entire body is undergoing regressive changes, and the process may be relatively rapid or it may be very slow.

III. MICROBIOLOGY

1. The building of antibodies is rapid during the period of rapid growth and development. This carries over into the adult period so that most individuals build up immunity by about 30 years of age to those communicable diseases with which they have been in contact. This will occur even though the person may not have had the disease in a recognizable form. Later in life some of these antibodies may be lost.

IV. PHYSICS

1. Due to cellular changes during senescence there is a decrease in the processes of dialysis, osmosis and diffusion.

V. PSYCHOLOGY

1. People tend to enter into the emotional pattern of those with whom they are associated. A cheerful attitude is likely to gain cooperation, while anger will beget resentment.
2. It is natural to be afraid of what is strange or unusual. Knowledge dispels fear.
3. No person likes to be tricked. The practical joker is unpopular. People respect the simple truth, but they do not like the individual who says one thing but does another.
4. Most people want to make their own decisions. This becomes apparent in early infancy and persists throughout life.
5. Desire to be accepted and liked by one's peers is a normal trait.

VI. SOCIOLOGY

1. The problem of old age is an ever-increasing one since each year life expectancy increases. With increased longevity have come many problems. The older person must be kept productive as long as possible for the good of the over-all economy and also to help him to feel needed.

2. The cost of medicines is very high, and this is an important factor in treating the elderly patient who may be living on a fixed, low income, which usually does not change with the changes in the value of the dollar.

INTRODUCTION

Medical science has done much to lengthen the life span of mankind, especially in the last 50 to 100 years. Thus, many more people are living longer than in previous centuries. However, this has not been an unmixed blessing, since much of these latter years is spent in the grip of chronic (so-called degenerative) diseases. Little is really known of the causes and processes of aging. In this short chapter, some of the known facts, as they affect the administration of medications, will be considered. Much research into the problems of the aged and the aging is being done, and it is hoped that this will provide means of overcoming and/or preventing many of the medical problems of this increasingly large segment of society.

CHANGES DURING THE CLIMACTERIC

From Adulthood to the Postclimacteric Period

The climacteric or menopause begins at different ages in the different sexes and varies widely within the sexes. Most women reach this period at about 45 or 50 years of age while most men do not begin the "change" until about 55 or 60 years of age. However, some women begin as early as the middle thirties, whereas others do not reach it until nearly 60. The climacteric does not occur in a single day or month or year. It is a physiologic change and as such takes place very gradually (I-2, 3, 4). Like adolescence, the climacteric is easier to date in women than in men since the cessation of menstruation can be recognized and its time noted. However, even this may not be too accurate, as irregularity of menstrual flow during this period is apt to occur. In the male, the period of change is hard to recognize, for the symptoms are vague and indefinable, with no dramatic change occurring as in the female. Some people (both men and women) go through the climacteric without showing any disturbing symptoms. Such individuals, however, are in the minority, since most men and women experience some difficulties at this time varying from very slight to very severe symptoms. Many men resent the implication that they are getting old or losing any of their youthful vigor; they will not accept suggestions or help and will often overdo in an attempt to prove that they are "just as strong as ever."

Drug therapy during this period does not include any change in dosage or in the form of the medicines, but it does include some changes in the types of medicines used. Drugs used at this period may fulfill the following needs:

1. Relief of the symptoms of the climacteric
2. Maintenance of good health
3. Prevention of the so-called degenerative diseases which often make their first appearance about this time

The most important drugs used to relieve the symptoms of menopause are the hormones. The sex hormones naturally predominate, and these include the female hormones, estrogen and progesterone, and the male hormone, testosterone. A description of their use will be found in Chapter 27. It is sufficient here to state that these hormones may be given individually or in any combination. The use of estrogen and progesterone is not limited to women, for they are also used in treating certain symptoms in men. The reverse is also true, since testosterone is often used to aid in reducing some of the very disagreeable symptoms of the menopause in women. Hormones are capable of relieving most of the symptoms of this period.

Some patients are bothered by only one or two symptoms and, in these cases, the physician may feel that it is best to treat just these symptoms rather than to use hormones. For instance, the patient may complain of restlessness and insomnia, and a small dose of a sedative or tranquilizer may be all that is required. If insomnia is severe, a stronger acting hypnotic may be needed for one or two nights. Other symptoms may be similarly treated without hormones; however, if the symptoms are severe or multiple, one of the hormones is often ordered with or without the addition of other drugs.

Menopause is an indication of beginning decline in the physical vigor of the individual. This does not mean that activity ends with this stage, for many people feel much better and stronger after the menopause than they did before it began. However, it does indicate that certain physiologic changes are occurring, and these changes are of the regressive type. During the climacteric, it is usually helpful to give some preparation which will, insofar as is possible, delay these changes. Vitamins and certain minerals are the main drugs used for this purpose, but the exact preparations given will depend upon the condition of the individual patient.

Drugs used to reduce the tendency to degenerative diseases will depend upon the conditions which the physician anticipates might occur in the patient. The term "degenerative diseases" is one that is not easily defined. Technically, it includes all diseases in which the pathologic changes are retrogressive. Of course, such changes may occur at any age. However, the term has come to be applied mainly to the diseases associated with the process of aging. These diseases can be grouped into several broad classifications: cardiovascular disorders, neurologic disturbances, arthritic conditions and neoplasms, especially those of a malignant nature.

In most cases, it is more important to advise the patient of a proper regimen than it is to order any specific medication. These people are at the crossroads between the prime of life and its decline. They are reluctant to acknowledge that they cannot do all the things they are accustomed to doing. Many have experienced most of the interesting things they have desired to experience—there are no more "worlds to conquer." They do not have the enthusiasm of youth and yet are not ready to take the quiet seat on the side lines which most older people must take. Many are afraid of "old age"; they worry about financial security; they have not acquired an avocation and often their vocation is one they can no longer follow. All these things and many more complicate the medical problem. As a consequence, the physician must not only be able to aid the patient physically, but he must understand and be able to help with the psychologic problems as well. The nurse has the same obligation.

CHANGES FOLLOWING THE CLIMACTERIC

There is a period following the "change" when the individual feels and acts much as he did before the change occurred. Often, in fact, he is in better health than he was in the immediate preclimacteric period. During this stage no specific type of drug therapy is indicated. As signs develop which indicate that a disease or disorder may be beginning, suitable therapy is instituted as it might be at any age. The early signs of aging should be noted and everything possible done to halt or delay the process. However, it is unwise to try to overlook the fact that the person is getting older; "be your age" is excellent advice.

Changes During Presenescence

With the advent of social security and often with forced retirement at a specific age, many individuals are, as they might express it, "put on the shelf" when they are well and able to continue working. If they have not prepared for this, the results can be almost catastrophic. Some simply give up and wait to die. Others have serious mental and emotional difficulties which are usually depressive in nature. Certainly, no drug is going to correct all the possible ill effects of enforced idleness. However, medical treatment can help with some, especially if it is accompanied by counseling. If the individual has been seeing a physician regularly, the doctor and/or the nurse can suggest the establishment of an avocation before retirement occurs. Many individuals can see no reason for even thinking of the loss of work at age 50 or 55, even though they know that retirement is set for 60 or 65. Ten years seems a long time, but it passes all too soon. For the immediate treatment of "retirement illness," it may be desirable to give an antidepressant or other medication which the patient's condition might indicate.

Changes During Senescence

Old age is inevitable, and in this period many changes in medicinal therapy are essential. Dosage is usually reduced since the elderly individual cannot tolerate so much of most drugs as might be given to a younger person. Of course, if the patient has been receiving the drug over a long period of time he may have developed a tolerance and, therefore, can take more than the average adult dose. Stimulating drugs can usually be tolerated in larger than average doses, but sedative and hypnotic preparations are usually best given in smaller doses; depression from the sedative drugs may be too severe.

Senescence, old age, does not come on at once. It is a very gradual process reached by different individuals at widely varying ages. One person may be senile at 55 while another may show very few symptoms of senility even at 90 (I-5).

MEDICINAL CHANGES DURING SENESCENCE. Drug changes for the older patient include the following alterations.

Morphine sulfate should be used with caution in the elderly patient because of the potential danger of respiratory depression.

Codeine (phosphate or sulfate) may cause retention of bronchial secretions with a resultant possibility of infection, especially in the case of chronic lung disorders. It also tends to cause constipation in many individuals.

Analgesics are generally required less owing to a higher threshold of pain.

Tranquilizers may cause a dangerous fall in blood pressure.

Chlordiazepoxide (Librium) and *diazepam* (Valium, Tridan [C]) should be given in the smallest effective dose to prevent development of ataxia or oversedation. This is true of all of this type of drugs.

Bromides and *barbiturates* can cause confusion. The patient is apt to repeat doses without realizing he has taken the drug before.

Antibiotics are likely to be less effective in treating bronchial disorders owing to increased fibrosis, emphysema and lowered vital capacity. Renal excretion of parenterally administered kanamycin, neomycin or streptomycin may be diminished in the elderly.

Antihypertensive agents such as *reserpine* or *pargyline hydrochloride* (Eutonyl, Eudatin [C]) should be initiated with about one half of the usual adult dose. The antihypertensive drugs may cause a severe drop in blood pressure.

Digitalis preparations may be poorly tolerated, especially in the patient with considerable loss of body mass. *Digitalis leaf, digitoxin* and *digoxin* should be given in one-half to two-thirds the amount given the younger adult. The mean blood half-life of digoxin has been reported to be 73 hours for elderly men, as opposed to 51 hours for young men.

Elderly female patients are particularly susceptible to bleeding episodes following intravenous administration of anticoagulants such as *heparin*. The risk is much greater in women over 60 years of age than in younger women.

All antidepressant drugs should be given to the older patient in doses lower than those for the average adult. Such drugs as *amitriptyline* (Elavil, Laroxyl, Tryptisol [C]) *desipramine hydrochloride* (Norpramin), *imipramine hydrochloride* (Tofranil, Dynapin [C]), *isocarboxazid* (Marplan), *nialamide* (Niamid), *nortriptyline hydrochloride* (Aventyl, Acetexa [C]), *protriptyline hydrochloride* (Vivactil, Triptil [C]), *tranylcypromine sulfate* (Parnate), *phenelzine dihydrogen sulfate* (Nardil, Nardelzine [C]) and *methyldopa* (Aldomet, Sembrina [C]) may cause syncope when given to the older patient with advanced arteriosclerotic vascular disease. This can be avoided by giving a smaller dose of the drug. Having the patient remain seated or lying down for thirty minutes to one hour following the administration of the drug will also help.

Potassium deficiency may occur with the following diuretics—*thiazide* diuretics, *chlorthalidone* (Hygraton, Igroton [C]), *ethacrynic acid* (Edecrin), *furosemide* (Lasix), *quinethazone* (Hydromox, Aquamox [C])—in patients having inadequate or marginal potassium intake and may be complicated by digitalis intoxication. Oral diuretics may precipitate myocardial infarction or cerebral thrombosis when used in patients with advanced arteriosclerosis. In these patients, the usual dose should be cut in half initially and increased only if needed. *Triamterene* (Dyrenium; Jatrepur [C]), since it is a "potassium" sparer, may aid in preventing hypokalemia.

THE NURSE. It is important for the nurse to understand the problems facing the older patient. These problems are economic, social, religious, psychologic and physiologic as well as pathologic. Drug therapy is influenced by all of these factors. The older person is apt to be in difficult financial circumstances. With the steady reduction in the buying power of the dollar, many older people who have small fixed incomes find these incomes wholly inadequate for their needs (V-1). Some are, of course, dependent upon relatives, friends and charity, public or private. Often older people feel that illness makes them an added burden which those upon whom they are dependent can ill afford. If the drugs ordered are expensive, the patient may well feel that he cannot afford such a luxury (V-2). One prescription may be secured but, when the amount of money entailed is known, no renewals are made. This may be true even though the drug is still needed and is definitely beneficial. It may be the nurse who first discovers such a situation, and she can then consult the physician to see if a less expensive drug can be substituted or other financial arrangements made. It may be possible for the nurse to direct the patient to some clinic or organization which will give aid. Many older people do not want to be "charity patients," and great tact is needed to secure their cooperation.

The patient may not want to take the drug if it is given in such a way as to violate some religious rule. This situation also requires great tact, and it is usually best to obtain the physician's permission to administer the drug in such a way as not to interfere with the church edict. Common rules that are apt to cause difficulty include fasting and specific regulations of diet.

There are many other intangible problems that will face the nurse in caring for the elderly patient. Usually the patient will want to know what medications he is getting and for what purpose. He will probably compare his medicines favorably or unfavorably with the drugs given to his friends and relatives. Most people have definite ideas about medicines which have become fixed by the time the individual has reached an advanced age. Some patients want drugs, while others are afraid of them.

SPECIFIC PROBLEMS. Some of the reasons given for not wanting to take prescribed medications are: fear of becoming an addict; fear that the drug may be too strong or too weak to be of value; inability to swallow the pill or capsule; fear that the drug may upset the stomach, and on and on. These are very real problems to the individual and will require tact and patience on the part of the nurse, as well as ingenuity in finding ways of overcoming the patient's objections. Some of these fears are, of course, groundless, but many have a basis in fact. The patient may have had unpleasant experiences with similar medicines. They may have upset his stomach, been difficult to swallow or even have caused severe choking spells. The fear of choking is not confined to medicines, but may include food as well. The nurse should recognize this possibility in all patients, especially the very young and the very old. It is also an ever-present problem with the patient who has cardiac or respiratory trouble and who has difficulty in breathing.

There are many physical conditions which must be considered. The patient may not absorb food and medicines so readily as a younger person, so that drugs given orally may not have the desired effect (III-1). Pills, hard or coated tablets, may pass through the intestinal tract without even being broken down. The nurse should watch for this in the stools, especially if the patient does not seem to be deriving the expected benefit from the medicine. Even with drugs in capsule and liquid form the absorption may be delayed or incomplete. If the patient has trouble in taking the drug it can be given with a little food or drink if this is not contraindicated. This will usually aid in swallowing and will often prevent gastric disturbance.

If the medicine is to be given parenterally, special precautions must be taken. The tissues of the older person tend to lose their elasticity, and tissue fluid is often either increased or decreased. Dehydration or edema may be severe, or it may be so slight as not to be noticeable (III-1). Other tissue changes include either an excess of adipose tissue (obesity), emaciation or a marked reduction in the normal amount of muscle mass. These conditions make parenteral administration difficult.

General Rules

A few general rules may help the nurse to overcome these conditions. The needles used should be very sharp, and a long bevel is usually best. A dull or hooked needle can cause considerable tissue damage, and this should be avoided. The nurse should use a large enough needle so that the fluid can be given quickly and the needle will not "wobble" when it is inserted. When the drug is to be given intramuscularly, the nurse will find it best to use the buttocks unless the patient has dependent edema whereupon other sites must be selected. If several intramuscular injections are to be given, it is necessary to alternate the site of insertion from side to side and to vary from one point to another. The nurse should notice on which side the patient prefers to lie and should use that side least, if possible. Many patients tend to bleed or ooze after a hypodermic is given. This tendency continues even when pressure is used. The Z technique described previously will aid in preventing this, or the opening may be sealed with a circular (spot) adhesive bandage. The rectangular adhesive bandage used for small lacerations is not suitable as it does not give enough pressure.

There are many specific changes in drug therapy in senescence. The older person does not have so much resistance to infection as does the younger individual and, hence, needs more drugs to aid him. This is especially true of persons with respiratory conditions. Since vitamin A may help to prevent respiratory infections, its inclusion in the diet and drug therapy is essential. Vitamin B-complex is needed since it is not stored in the body, and the type of diet the average elderly person eats often is not too well supplied with this vitamin. The physician will usually order one of the general mixed vitamin products.

Sedatives or tranquilizers are often needed to insure rest and to prevent undue worry or excitement. It takes less of the sedative drug to produce the desired effect in the older person. Phenobarbital is one of the preparations that is often used. Bromides are good at intervals or for an occasional dose but they must not be given over long periods since they are apt to cause toxic symptoms. Any one of a number of tranquilizers may be used. Physicians usually try to avoid giving the more habit-forming drug since the elderly patient often needs the drug for an extended period and habituation is likely to result.

Analgesics, like sedatives, are usually given in smaller amounts than would be given to the younger adult. Of course, tolerance must be taken into consideration. Since the drugs are given over many weeks, the patient may gradually build up tolerance so that the drug will have to be given in much greater amounts than when it was started. The severity of the condition will determine what analgesic is to be used. The antipyretic analgesics, with or without codeine, are very popular and give excellent results when the pain is not severe. If these are not sufficient the use of a synthetic analgesic or the opiates will be required. If there is a chronic disease that will require the use of analgesics for a long time, the type will have to be varied to avoid excessive habituation. When the patient is receiving any of the more potent analgesics the nurse must watch carefully for symptoms of respiratory depression.

In the use of any sedative or analgesic there is danger of the patient's sleeping too heavily and not moving enough, which may lead to hypostatic pneumonia or thrombosis (especially of the legs). The nurse should see that the patient turns frequently and that at no time is he in the position to cause undue pressure on any part of the body. An abnormal position can cause deformities such as foot drop, and these must be avoided. The patient may be too drowsy to realize that the position is uncomfortable.

Although diet should be used to regulate bowel activity as much as possible, there are times when a laxative is needed. It cannot be stressed too much that everything possible must be done to avoid having the patient become dependent upon a laxative. The nurse may find that the patient already has an established laxative habit that will need to be broken. In any case, the nurse should understand what laxatives are best to use for the elderly person. Some of the more acceptable ones are mineral oil and agar-agar compounds, the bulk laxatives and the saline laxatives if there is a tendency to edema. Mineral oil should be used with caution since it tends to prevent the absorption of the fat-soluble carotenes which are essential for these patients. Bulk laxatives, too, must be given very carefully. Many of these preparations are in the form of pellets which are very hard when dry. If chewed they may break teeth or dentures, and if swallowed rapidly they are apt to cause choking. Consequently, it is wise to give them in small amounts and follow with ample water. Water is very important and the entire amount ordered with the drug must be given. These drugs will withdraw water from the tissues if enough is not taken with the medicine. This would be beneficial in patients with edema but in other conditions is undesirable. One of the detergent or surface acting laxatives may prove best. Refer to Chapter 17 for details. Of course, the physician will order the laxative to be used, but the nurse must see that it is used judiciously and watch for any signs that it is acting in an adverse manner.

The physician may order a "tonic" or some simple drug whose main purpose is to build the patient's morale. The nurse must make the patient feel that the medicine will be helpful. Many of these patients need something to rely on, and if a simple pill, capsule or a teaspoonful of a fluid once or twice a day will make them feel better, what difference does it make if no scientific basis for the improvement can be found? It is true that an individual is better when he thinks that he is better. No nurse should ever give a patient the least reason to doubt the efficacy of any treatment.

If the patient is to take his own medicine at home, explicit directions for taking it should be given. It is wise to advise the patient not to have the bottle of sedatives or tranquilizers at the bedside, since he might get drowsy, not remember taking one dose and repeat it. This might be very dangerous. If the patient has to get up to get the medicine he will probably be awake enough to remember having already taken the drug. If the patient does not see too well, it may be helpful to mark the medicine bottle with letters larger than those of the regular prescription. Thus, the bottle containing capsules of a hypnotic could have a large *S* (sleep) put on the cap, vitamins could be marked with a *V* and so on. If the bottles and/or the caps are similar, and there is the possibility of the tops' being exchanged, the large letters could also be superimposed on the label, or a piece of tape or extra label put on with the large letter on that. This would have the additional advantage of keeping the tops and the bottles together. Of course, the whole purpose of this is to prevent the patient from taking the wrong medicine. If one medicine is to be taken once at bedtime, and another three times a day with meals, a mix-up might be disastrous. Therefore, the number of doses per day might be added to the large letters. Thus, if the patient is to take a digitalis preparation twice a day, it might be marked "D 2." It is important that the patient understand exactly how the medicines are to be taken and what the letters and numbers mean. Patients having hearing difficulties often fail to hear what is said clearly and they are reluctant to keep asking "What did you say?" They may pretend to know, when in fact they have only a hazy idea of what was said. In speaking to the person who is hard of hearing, three rules will aid greatly in helping the patient to understand what is being said. The nurse should (1) speak slowly, (2) enunciate clearly and (3) face the patient. Many patients with hearing difficulties lip-read unconsciously even if they have never studied lip reading. The resourceful nurse will find many ways to assure that the older patient receives his medications regularly and in the best possible manner for meeting his particular needs.

IT IS IMPORTANT TO REMEMBER

1. That, although the government and industry may set a chronological time for the beginning of "old age," the term is really a relative one and that each person reaches it at a different time.
2. That as an individual grows older he should recognize and heed the fact that he is not able physically to do everything that he could at an earlier age.
3. That most medical therapy for the older age group is palliative and supportive and not curative.
4. That stress, tensions, and fears play an even greater part in the illnesses of older patients than in those of the young adult.
5. That little is really known of the causes and cures for the so-called degenerative diseases.
6. That adjustments in the use of drugs—kinds, preparations, dosage—go on from birth to death, and that there are no "hard and fast" rules to go by. The doctor and the nurse must make each change in the light of the individual patient concerned.
7. That in doing a procedure, the nurse often tends to spend so much time performing it the way she has been taught, getting the work done, that she forgets the real purpose of the nurse—to help people! No nurse should let the *how* of procedures overshadow the *why*. No nurse should let any routine overshadow the patient for whom nursing and nurses exist!

TOPICS FOR STUDY AND DISCUSSION

1. Check the charts for any medical and/or general surgical floor and segregate the patients according to ages and diagnoses. What, if any, conclusion can you draw?
2. With this same list, check medications and doses. Is either age connected?
3. Why is the problem of medicines for the older person more difficult now than it has ever been? How do you think this problem in the United States compares with the same problem in other countries? (You may select a specific country if you wish.) Defend your answer.
4. Make a list of one dozen drugs that might logically be needed by the older patient at home (for regular use). Secure the retail prices of these drugs from a drug store or the hospital pharmacy. How might use of these affect the budget of a retired individual living on a limited income?
5. How might you aid a patient (age 58) who has just been told that he has diabetes mellitus?
6. How could you help an elderly patient in a private room with few if any visitors to pass the time without his withdrawing or becoming seriously depressed?
7. The average adult dose of chloral hydrate is 600 mg. The physician wishes his patient (who is elderly) to have only three-fourths of the usual dose. The nurse should give __________Gm.

BIBLIOGRAPHY

Books and Pamphlets

American Medical Association Council on Drugs, *Drug Evaluations,* Chicago, 1971, American Medical Association.

Conn, H. F., et al., *Current Therapy, 1974,* Philadelphia, 1974, W. B. Saunders Co.

Jaeger, D., and Simmons, L. W., *The Aged Ill,* New York, 1970, Appleton-Century-Crofts.

Newton, K., and Anderson, H., *Geriatric Nursing, 4th Ed.,* St. Louis, 1966, The C. V. Mosby Co.

Physician's Desk Reference, 27th Ed., Oradell, New Jersey, 1973, Charles E. Baker, Jr.

Price, A. L., *Clinical Nursing,* New York, 1965, The Macmillan Co.

Journal Articles

Drummond, E. C., "Communication and comfort for the dying patient," *Nurs. Clin. North Am.* 5:1 (1970).

Ewt, G. A., "Digitoxin Reduction," *Circulation*, 39:449 (1960).

Fond, K., et al., "Dealing with death and dying through family-centered care," *Nurs. Clin. North Am.* 7:4:53 (December, 1972).

Gaspard, N. J., "The family of the patient with long-term illness," *Nurs. Clin. North Am.* 5:1 (January, 1970).

Hansen, J. M., et al., "Geriatric," *Lancet* 1:1170 (1970).

Hansen, K. B., and Bender, A. D., "Changes in serum potassium levels occurring in patients treated with triamterene and a triamterene-hydrochlorothiazide combination," *Clin. Pharmacol. Ther.* 8:392:1967 (May-June, 1967).

Hayflick, L., "Latest findings in the biology of aging," Report of the IX International Congress of Gerontology in Kiev, U.S.S.R., *Geriatric Focus* 11:3:1 (October, 1972).

Knowles, L. N., et al., "Symposium on putting geriatric nursing standards into practice," *Nurs. Clin. North Am.* 7:2 (June, 1972).

Lane, H. C., et al., "Symposium on care of the elderly patient," *Nurs. Clin. North Am.* 3:4 (December, 1968).

Robstein, M., "Health problems of the aged," *R.N.* 32:8:39 (August, 1969).

Todd, R. L., "Early treatment reverses symptoms of senility," *Hosp. Community Psychiatry* 17:1704 (June, 1966).

Tuck, B., "The geriatrics nurse—Pioneer of a new specialty," *R.N.* 35:8:35 (August, 1972).

SECTION III

DRUGS USED IN THE COMMON MEDICAL-SURGICAL AND RELATED CONDITIONS

DRUGS USED IN SURGICAL INTERVENTION

DRUGS USED FOR DISORDERS OF THE RESPIRATORY SYSTEM

DRUGS USED FOR DISORDERS OF THE GASTROINTESTINAL SYSTEM

DRUGS USED FOR DISORDERS OF THE CARDIOVASCULAR SYSTEM

DRUGS USED FOR DISORDERS OF THE BLOOD AND BLOOD FORMING ORGANS

DRUGS USED TO AID IN OVERCOMING NUTRITIONAL DISORDERS

DRUGS USED FOR DISORDERS OF THE MUSCULO-SKELETAL SYSTEM

DRUGS USED FOR DISORDERS OF THE URINARY SYSTEM

DRUGS USED FOR DISORDERS OF THE SKIN

DRUGS USED FOR DISORDERS OF THE EYES AND EARS

DRUGS USED FOR AN ALTERED ANTIGEN-ANTIBODY RESPONSE

CLINICAL PHARMACOLOGY

DRUGS USED FOR DISORDERS OF THE REPRODUCTIVE SYSTEM

DRUGS USED FOR DISORDERS OF THE ENDOCRINE SYSTEM

DRUGS USED DURING PREGNANCY, DELIVERY AND LACTATION

DRUGS USED FOR MALIGNANT CONDITIONS

DRUGS USED FOR PSYCHOGENIC DISORDERS

DRUGS USED FOR COMMUNICABLE DISEASES

DRUGS USED FOR MISCELLANEOUS DISORDERS

INTRODUCTION

If the student has not already done so, before beginning this section she will find it helpful to read the portion of the book entitled "Suggestions for the Use of the Book for Both Teachers and Students."

In the clinical area, drugs are discussed in connection with the conditions for which they are used. A specific pattern has been adopted. However, only rarely will any drug discussion follow this pattern exactly. Naturally, one drug may be used for a number of disorders. This requires considerable repetition, but this is desirable for emphasis and to show the various uses of the drug. In most instances, there is one major use for each drug. The drug will be given full coverage in the discussion of its main use, with sufficient information in other areas to show the reasons for the drug's usage in other conditions.

The following format will be used for all major drugs.

THE DRUG NAME

THE DRUG. Short statement of the drug, source, if important; history, if interesting.

Physical and Chemical Properties. Brief, simple discussion.

Action. What can be expected of this drug.

Therapeutic Uses. One or multiple.

Absorption and Excretion. Fate of the drug in the body.

Preparations and Dosages. Generic names, initials as indicated, major trade names; Canadian names are indicated by the letter [C]. How and when given.

THE NURSE. Mode of Administration: How given, rationale for administration, problems and so forth.

Side Effects (Desirable and Undesirable). These and the next two may be combined.

Toxicity and Treatment. Usually only serious toxicity is given here.

Contraindications. If any.

Interactions. If any.

Patient Teaching. What the nurse should tell the patient about this drug.

Other Nursing Problems. If any.

THE PATIENT. Psychological, socio-economic, ethical or religious aspects as they apply. Teaching aspects will be discussed here.

The student should remember that the last section of the book, the *Current Drug Handbook*, has brief but explicit information for all drugs mentioned in the text as well as many others. Here, too, Canadian drug names have been indicated by the letter [C].

To find a specific drug, the student will need to consult the index for the main portion of the text or for the *Current Drug Handbook.* In the former, the page on which the drug has been discussed in detail will be in boldface type. If the student desires information about drugs used in a specific disease or condition, the table of contents should be used to refer either to the clinical section or to the handbook portion.

CHAPTER 15

DRUGS USED IN SURGICAL INTERVENTION

CORRELATION WITH OTHER SCIENCES

I. ANATOMY AND PHYSIOLOGY

1. Sensation is the conscious realization (awareness) of a stimulus. It requires an active end organ or receptor, a sensory neuron, association neurons and a nerve center in the cerebrum. Any break in the chain will block the impulse and prevent awareness of the stimulus.

2. Peristalsis is the wave-like motion of the smooth muscle tissue especially notable in the intestinal and urinary tracts. Its purpose is to propel the contents of the tubular organs toward the exterior.

V. PSYCHOLOGY

1. Fear of the unknown is an almost universal trait. The emotion of fear is a combined physical and psychologic state which prepares an individual for emergencies.

2. The perception of illness, surgical therapy and probable prognosis all contribute to a decrease in one's receptivity to teaching and learning.

3. Amnesia is the loss of memory. It may be for any length of time from a few seconds to several years or it may even be permanent. It may be complete, leaving the individual without any knowledge of what happened previously, or partial, with some things remembered while others are forgotten.

4. Each person is different from every other person and will react to any situation in a specific manner.

5. Anxiety produces physical tensions and may result in various physiological or psychological disorders.

6. Because of stress and anxiety during surgical intervention, an individual will need repeated reinforcement of concepts being taught.

VI. SOCIOLOGY

1. Tradition is a major factor in the conditioning of the individual and to a great extent forms his attitudes.

2. Length of hospitalization and nature of the disease or disorder may create economic hardships for the individual and his family.

INTRODUCTION

Modern surgery dates back about a century to the work of such men as Lister, Long, Morton, Pasteur and Koch. Since that time it has risen rapidly to become one of the largest segments of medicine today. Certainly it is the most spectacular. Modern hospitals always are prepared to care for the operative patient and, in all except special hospitals, surgery forms a major division. Medical cases often can be cared for in the home, but modern surgical procedures require the equipment and the personnel found only in the hospital.

Each surgical case is unique in that it deals with a different individual, no matter how common the operative procedure may be. However, routines are much the same for all cases. It makes little difference what part of the body is to be incised; the essential steps will follow a general pattern. The medicines used in these routines are discussed in this chapter.

An operation is a landmark in the life of the patient, even though it may be only the most minor event in the day's routine for the nurse and the physician. The nurse must understand how much the procedure means to the patient, for his operation represents not only a physical strain but usually a severe emotional strain as well. Operations are usually serious, and the patient is well aware of this. To people unacquainted with modern surgery, the record of a few generations ago when some operations were fatal is still representative (VI-1). It is the nurse's responsibility to do all she can to relieve the patient's anxiety and to help him overcome his fears of surgery. The nurse in the surgeon's office or the public health nurse (when one is available) can do much to prepare the patient psychologically and emotionally for the surgery to be done.

DRUGS GIVEN BEFORE OPERATION

Medications often are given some time before the patient enters the hospital. Naturally, if the operation is an emergency, only drugs given immediately before the operation can be used. For elective surgery, however, medicines will often be ordered for several days or weeks before the actual time of the operation since the surgeon wants the patient to be in the best possible physical condition before the operation is performed.

The types of drugs used before an operation will depend to a great extent upon the operation to be done and also upon the condition of the patient. If tests show that the patient is anemic, the usual antianemic drugs will be ordered: *iron; vitamin* B_{12}, *B-complex, folic acid* and/or *liver* and *stomach* extracts. Many combinations of these drugs are available. The physician's selection will depend upon his past experiences with the preparations and with the type of anemia.

Physical examination may reveal that, although no true anemia exists, the patient is not generally in so satisfactory a physical state as the surgeon desires. For such cases, one of the general vitamin compounds is usually prescribed. This will aid in two ways: first, by supplying needed vitamins and, second, by stimulating the patient's appetite so he will eat more, thus helping to improve his general health.

If the surgery involves possible excessive blood loss, the surgeon usually makes sure that the patient's blood will clot quickly. If the prothrombin time is found to be deficient, *vitamin K* is ordered and, in some cases, *calcium* in the form of *lactate* or *gluconate* may be given. If vitamin K is ordered for a patient with faulty fat digestion, as in cases of cholecystitis, *dehydrocholic acid* will be given to insure that the fat-soluble vitamin K is absorbed, since its absorption depends upon the presence of bile or its extracts. Dehydrocholic acid is usually given with the meals to the patient with gallbladder disease to insure proper fat digestion, even if the patient is on the usual low fat diet.

Before a thyroidectomy, some form of iodine is usually ordered to reduce the amount of thyroid hormone in the blood stream and thus put the patient in a better condition for surgery. These patients need a great deal of rest, and most physicians give repeated small doses of one of the barbiturates at fairly frequent intervals to insure this. *Phenobarbital,* 30 mg. at 10:00 a.m. and 2:00 p.m. and 90 mg. at bedtime, is one such order.

Some types of surgery, such as those involving digestive or respiratory organs, are apt to open up avenues of infection for "opportunist" microorganisms. In such cases antibiotic drugs are often given prior to the operation to destroy the organisms before they can become pathogenic. The choice of the antibiotic will depend upon the circumstances. If surgery is to be performed on the intestinal tract, one of the non-absorbable anti-infective drugs will probably be used. Otherwise, a broad-spectrum antibiotic is usually given.

Sedation may be ordered for any preoperative patient whose condition warrants it. Rest is essential, and if it cannot be secured without drugs, then drugs must be used. Any of the mild sedatives will suffice to relax the person and let him rest, such as the barbiturates, chloral hydrate and certain antihistamines.

Admission to the hospital is a severe strain on the patient, and the nurse should do all in her power to ease that strain (V-1). Most hospitals have clerks who take care of all the routine details of admission, but this does not relieve the nurse of her part in lessening the anxiety experienced by the patient preparing for surgery (V-5). Patients are often admitted the afternoon preceding surgery and may have orders already awaiting their arrival. As the nurse prepares the patient for surgery, she may alleviate some of his fears by respecting his rights as an individual and his specific needs for modesty. Through an unhurried and solicitous attitude, the nurse may be able to help the patient to understand what to expect and what may be expected of him (V-2).

Drugs which the patient has been taking at home may or may not be desirable after his admission to the hospital. Some patients will bring with them medications used at home. Institutions vary as to procedures in such cases. The rules of the institution and the physician must be followed in such instances.

Drugs ordered the day preceding the operation are, as mentioned above, sedative, supportive or those used for special purposes. As a supportive measure the surgeon may order an intravenous infusion. This may be of any type, but nutrients (*amino acids* and *glucose*), and the *electrolytic* solutions are most commonly used. *Whole blood* or *plasma* may be given if the condition of the patient or the type of surgery to be done warrants it. The nurse should assure the patient that the giving of an intravenous infusion is not an emergency measure and that it does not indicate that the patient is in a precarious condition.

It is essential that the patient have a good rest the night preceding the operation, and the physician or anesthetist usually makes sure that this is the case by ordering some hypnotic drug to be given at bedtime. A barbiturate is very often the drug used, but chloral hydrate or other hypnotics may be given. The drug may be administered orally, parenterally or rectally, but the oral route is most common since it is least disturbing to the patient. *Pentobarbital sodium* (Nembutal) 0.1 to 0.2 Gm., *secobarbital sodium* (Seconal) 0.05 to 0.1 Gm., *amobarbital sodium* (Amytal) 0.05 to 0.1 Gm. or a combination such as *Tuinal,* a combination of amobarbital and secobarbital 0.05 to 0.1 Gm., each may be given. *Chloral hydrate* is given in doses from 0.25 to 0.5 Gm.

It is customary for the anesthetist to order the drugs to be given immediately before the surgery since he is responsible for the patient's condition during the actual operative procedure. Orders will vary according to the condition of the patient, the type of anesthetic to be used and length of the operation. One common routine is to repeat the barbiturate or other hypnotic given at bedtime early in the morning before the operation. This keeps the patient drowsy, if not actually asleep. The dosage may be the same or it may be increased or decreased, depending upon the situation.

About 20 or 30 minutes before the scheduled time for the operation to begin, a hypodermic containing an analgesic and a parasympathetic depressant may be given. The analgesic (discussed in Chapter 9) may be an opiate such as *morphine sulfate* 10 to 15 mg., *Pantopon* 20 mg. or one of the synthetic analgesics such as *meperidine* (Demerol) 50 to 100 mg. The analgesic may be omitted if a deep anesthesia is contemplated, but it is usually given if a local or light general anesthesia is planned. In young children, a simple hypnotic, e.g., chloral hydrate or one of the phenothiazine tranquilizers may be sufficient for preanesthesia medication.

PARASYMPATHETIC DEPRESSANTS

The Drugs. The parasympathetic depressants (parasympatholytics and cholinergic blocking agents) are used in a number of conditions. Some of them are naturally occurring alkaloids, others are semisynthetic and yet a third group is entirely synthetic in origin. These various groups are used for different purposes. See Current Drug Handbook for additional details. The naturally occurring alkaloids are derived from various plants of the solanaceae family. Under these will be discussed atropine from the plant *Atropa belladonna* and scopolamine from the plant *Scopolia atropoides*. Belladonna, the parent drug of atropine, has a long and interesting history. It was early used as a prolonged poison, hence its original name, atropa, for Atropos, the Fate who cut the thread of life. Its subsequent name is derived from its use by Spanish ladies to dilate their pupils, to enhance their beauty (bella = beautiful; donna = lady).

Physical and Chemical Properties. The alkaloids are organic esters, a combination of tropic acid with a complex organic base, either tropine or scopine. Chemically, atropine and scopolamine are closely related, and their salts are readily soluble in water and in body fluids.

Action. All parasympathetic depressants have similar action, but preparations vary in the degree. The actions have variously been termed parasympatholytic, anticholinergic, antispasmodic and antimuscarinic. They inhibit the action of acetylcholine on structures innervated by the postganglionic cholinergic nerves and on smooth muscles that respond to acetylcholine, but do not have cholinergic innervation. Briefly, they dilate the pupils, decrease glandular secretions, relax smooth muscle tissue and increase the rate of the heart beat. Scopolamine has a calming, sedative action on the higher neural centers, producing a partial amnesia.

Therapeutic Uses. The parasympathetic depressants are used to decrease secretions preoperatively, in asthma and in rhinitis; relax smooth muscle tissue in biliary or renal colic and in gastrointestinal hypermotility; dilate the pupils in certain diseases and disorders and for ophthalmological examination; and in the treatment of parkinsonism. In addition, scopolamine is used in the treatment of motion sickness, with an analgesic or a hypnotic in obstetrics. Locally, they act as anodynes, decreasing secretions of the oral, nasal and bronchial mucosae and of the salivary glands, and allowing for a less obstructed airway during surgical procedures. They tend to decrease smooth muscle activity, another valuable measure in surgical procedures. The sedative action of scopolamine is a desirable asset in preanesthetic medication. Some physicians feel that scopolamine produces a less tenacious sputum postoperatively than that of atropine, and this too is helpful.

Absorption and Excretion. Most of these drugs are readily absorbed from the gastrointestinal tract. They are not well absorbed when used topically in the eyes or from the intact skin. They are widely distributed throughout the body. Some of the drug is changed by the body, probably in the liver, but a significant amount is excreted by the kidneys unchanged.

Preparations and Dosages

Atropine sulfate, U.S.P., B.P., 0.3 to 0.6 mg. parenterally.

Scopolamine hydrobromide, U.S.P., Hyoscine hydrobromide, B.P., 0.3 to 0.6 mg. parenterally.

Scopolamine is one of the ingredients in many analgesic and sedative-hypnotic preparations sold without a prescription. Side effects or toxicity can occur without the patient's or the physician's realizing the cause.

THE NURSE

Mode of Administration. These drugs may be given by any method; inhalation, orally, topically, subcutaneously, intramuscularly or intravenously. However, as preoperative medication they are usually given either subcutaneously or intramuscularly. If, as is usual, an analgesic is also given parenterally, the drugs may be given in one injection, unless otherwise ordered or indicated. It is very important that the preoperative medications be given exactly at the time ordered, since they are really a part of the anesthetic process and are timed so as to aid the anesthetist in giving the anesthesia. A calm, quiet, relaxed patient is much better prepared for the anesthesia than one who is not.

Side Effects. All the effects of these drugs will occur regardless of the reason for their use, although the degree of effects will vary with the preparation being used. As a preoperative sedative, the most common side effects encountered are dilated pupils, (which may react very slowly to light), blurred vision, photophobia and dryness of the mouth, nose and throat. Tachycardia and postural hypotension may be seen. The patient should not be allowed out of bed after the preoperative medication has been given.

Toxicity and Treatment. As with most drugs, the toxic symptoms are an exaggeration of those seen with therapeutic dosage. Early symptoms include thirst, dry mouth and throat, dysphagia, flushed face, "atropine fever" (due to inhibition of sweat glands), dilated pupils and loss of visual acuity, urinary retention and constipation. Respiration and heart rate are increased. Later symptoms include shallow, irregular respirations, dizziness, tachycardia and an atropine "jag" (excitement, delirium, hallucinations), disorientation, sometimes delirium and excessive excitement. These symptoms may be followed by unconsciousness, coma and respiratory failure.

Symptoms are treated as they occur, the treatment often including gavage with weak tannic acid solution or strong tea. Respiratory stimulants are used cautiously—oxygen with positive pressure is usually more satisfactory. One of the parasympathetic stimulants such as neostigmine methylsulfate 0.5 to 1.0 mg. may be used. Sedatives—chloral hydrate, paraldehyde or one of the barbiturates—are often valuable.

Interactions. Atropine and meperidine enhance each other by additive action.

Contraindications. The parasympathetic depressants are not commonly used in glaucoma, prostatic hypertrophy, constrictive lesions of the gastrointestinal tract or coronary heart disease.

THE PATIENT. These drugs help the patient over a most distressing time—just before surgery. The nurse should explain to the patient why the premedication is given. If the anesthetist has already talked to the patient, the nurse can continue to reinforce the information he has given. The patient will better endure the thirst and dry mouth that follow surgery if he understands that the medicine is responsible for them. The nurse can explain that the drugs were given to facilitate induction of the anesthesia and to decrease the amount of anesthesia used during surgery. The patient should remain in bed with the side rail up, to prevent his falling due to postural hypotension.

When the administration of preoperative drugs is accurately timed, the patient enters the operating room either asleep or in a relaxed state. In this way the anesthetic can be easily administered. The patient should be encouraged to relax and sleep if possible. Even though all the drugs used as preanesthetic medication have some disadvantages, e.g., morphine causes bronchial constriction, most anesthetists feel that carefully selected preanesthetic medications are essential.

Further information concerning these drugs will be found in the Current Drug Handbook.

DRUGS USED IN THE OPERATING ROOM

Many drugs are used in the operating room, and for many reasons. However, they can all be placed into a few separate divisions: anesthetic agents or drugs to produce unconsciousness or insensitivity to pain; supportive drugs; antiseptics; muscle relaxants; emergency and miscellaneous drugs. Most of the drugs used in the operating room are administered by the anesthetist, but this does not relieve the nurse from the responsibility of knowing all important details concerning them.

General Anesthetics

Anesthetics fall into two main classes—general and local. The general anesthetic is any agent which produces unconsciousness (coma) from which the patient may not be awakened. These may be administered rectally, intravenously or by inhalation, but inhalation is the method used most. Any combination of drugs and means of administration may be used. For example, anesthesia may be started intravenously and, after the patient is asleep, inhalation may be employed. Local anesthetics block pain impulses without producing unconsciousness. The rectal route is rarely used now, since it has proved to be slow and unpredictable owing to irregular absorption.

For some surgical procedures it is advisable to have the patient conscious or at least close enough to consciousness that he may be easily aroused. This may be accomplished by giving intravenously a combination of a tranquilizer and an analgesic. One such combination is Innovar (droperidol and fentanyl citrate [Sublimaze]). This produces a sort of "twilight sleep." A local anesthetic is used to block pain. Morphine may be used in place of fentanyl.

THE DRUGS. The nurse is referred to Table 9, General Anesthetic Agents, for the information usually given under this heading and also for some usually given under the heading, THE NURSE. See also Current Drug Handbook.

THE NURSE. Though the nurse usually does not give the anesthetic, unless she is specially trained, she should be familiar with the stages of general anesthesia and the signs which indicate passage from one stage to another. The nurse also uses this information as general knowledge regarding levels of consciousness. Most general anesthetic drugs produce the same stages, although the length of these stages may vary widely with different agents. This is especially true of the first and second stages which, in some cases, may be so short that they go undetected. (See Figure 23.)

Authorities divide the stages of anesthesia into four divisions, with subdivisions in the third stage. The first stage, or beginning induction, is one of analgesia with some mucous membrane irritation. There is increasing loss of the awareness of pain, a feeling of warmth, some excessive lacrimation, a feeling of asphyxia and various vague and ill-defined sensations. There is usually no change in pulse, respiration or pupil size during this stage, and there may or may not be an amnesia for this first period (V-3).

The second stage of anesthesia is the stage of excitement or delirium. There is loss of consciousness due to depression of the higher cerebral centers, but the lower areas are as yet unaffected, allowing for varied symptoms. The patient is apt to struggle and cry out, and the respirations and often the pulse are irregular. During this stage the pupils are usually normal, but there is movement of the eyeballs. If the proper premedications have been given and the induction is rapid and smooth, this stage may progress so rapidly as to be unobserved. Occasionally, especially in children and emotionally upset

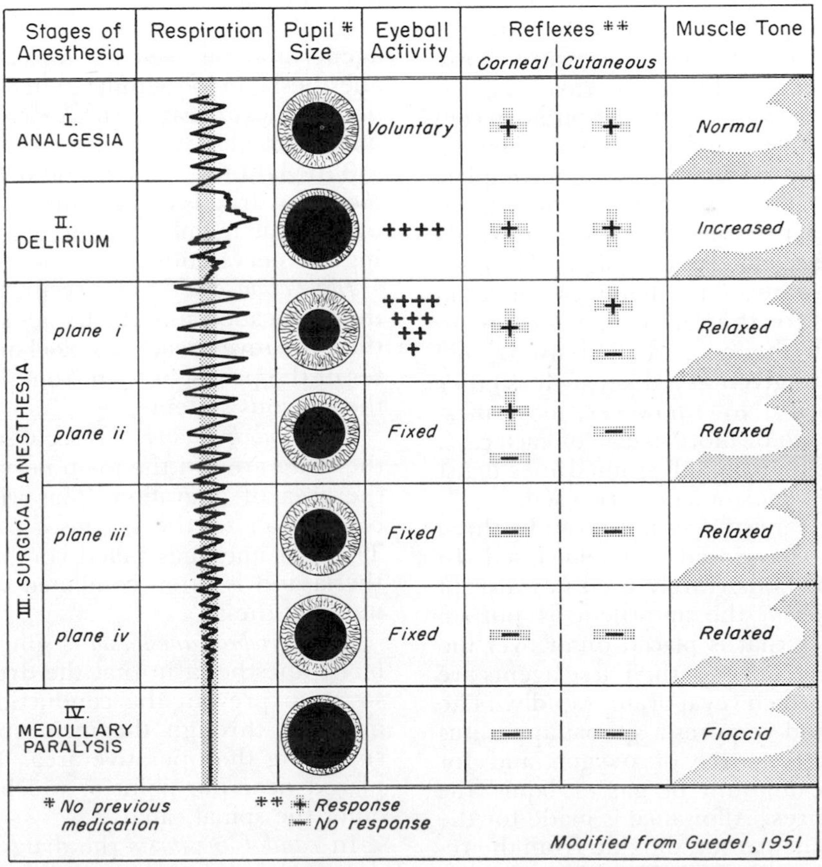

Stages of Anesthesia		Respiration	Pupil * Size	Eyeball Activity	Reflexes ** Corneal	Reflexes ** Cutaneous	Muscle Tone
I. ANALGESIA				*Voluntary*	+	+	*Normal*
II. DELIRIUM				++++	+	+	*Increased*
III. SURGICAL ANESTHESIA	*plane i*			++++ +++ ++ +	+	+ −	*Relaxed*
	plane ii			*Fixed*	+ −	−	*Relaxed*
	plane iii			*Fixed*	−	−	*Relaxed*
	plane iv			*Fixed*	−	−	*Relaxed*
IV. MEDULLARY PARALYSIS					−	−	*Flaccid*

* *No previous medication* ** + *Response* − *No response*

Modified from Guedel, 1951

FIGURE 23. The stages of anesthesia. (From: Brooks, S. M.: Basic Facts of Pharmacology. Philadelphia, W. B. Saunders Co., 1963.)

adults, there may be reflex dilation of the pupils. This also is less likely to occur when induction is smooth and rapid. It should be remembered that pupil size may be controlled by the preoperative medication and, therefore, may not be a reliable indication of the stage of anesthesia.

The third stage, which is often divided into four planes, is the stage of surgical anesthesia. It covers all depths from light anesthesia to an unconsciousness so deep it borders upon respiratory failure. During stage three, when surgical anesthesia without toxic symptoms is maintained, the respirations are deep, regular and slightly increased in rate. Pulse rate is also increased, with the volume and rhythm normal. The eyelid reflexes are lost, but eyeball activity continues. The pupils are normal in size and respond to light, though the response may be less rapid than normal.

As the third stage progresses various adverse symptoms occur. Pupillary reflexes are lost and the pupils are dilated; eyeball activity ceases; respirations are irregular and shallow; the pulse is likely to be thready; with volume low, the blood pressure drops. The onset of the fourth or toxic stage is marked by paralysis of the respiratory center. The pulse may or may not be perceptible, since the patient goes into complete circulatory failure. During the entire anesthetic period, the anesthetist must constantly check and record the vital signs. He must always be aware of the patient's condition and be alert for the various danger signals.

When anesthetics were first used, only one drug was given at a time, such as ether or chloroform. Now, however, most anesthetists use two or more drugs for each case. It takes an expert, highly trained anesthetist to administer most agents now used.

Inhalatory anesthetics are given by three methods: open, closed and semiclosed. In the open methods (rarely used now except in emergencies) the anesthetic is put on a gauze mask that is placed on or over the patient's nose and mouth. These agents are all liquids which evaporate rapidly. The closed method requires a special apparatus to serve as a source of oxygen and for gauging the amount of gas or liquid the patient receives. Allowance is made for the removal of the carbon dioxide from the rebreathed gas. The semiclosed method is similar, but a valve allows the expired air to pass into the atmosphere.

THE PATIENT. The psychological and physiological status of the patient are important factors in his ability to withstand the stress of anesthesia and surgery. Many patients think that surgery is a last resort and that their chances for survival are slim. In many instances, the nurse may be helpful to the patient and his family by allowing them an opportunity to express their fears and worries. The nurse may also serve as facilitator in communications between the physician and the patient and his family so that misconceptions and misinformation can be corrected. The patient will need to feel that all are concerned and interested in his care and welfare.

Local Anesthetics

Drugs included in this category are those that produce insensitivity to pain without loss of consciousness. These anesthetic agents may be used for topical or surface anesthesia, in local infiltration or to produce nerve block, paravertebral, caudal or spinal anesthesia (I-1).

THE DRUGS. For *topical* or *surface anesthesia* the drug is applied directly to the skin or mucous membrane and acts by deadening the nerve endings.

Infiltration anesthesia is secured by putting the medication into the tissues surrounding the operative area, thus blocking the transfer of the pain sensation from the wound to the nervous system.

Nerve block anesthesia is secured by placing the drug around the main nerve supplying the area of operation. This will block the conduction of the impulses to the brain. This is sometimes called conduction anesthesia and is often combined with infiltration anesthesia.

Paravertebral anesthesia is similar to nerve block anesthesia in that the drug is placed so as to prevent the conduction of nerve impulses through the main spinal nerves supplying the operative area. The drug is placed near the point at which the nerves enter the spinal canal.

In *caudal anesthesia* the drug is placed in the caudal or sacral canal and prevents the transfer of impulses from the lower part of the body to the spinal cord. This anesthesia is also similar to the nerve block since it really is directed to the nerves of the cauda equina.

In *spinal anesthesia* the anesthetic drug is introduced into the subdural space. A needle is introduced into the spinal canal in the lumbar region, and a small amount of spinal fluid is withdrawn. The anesthetic is dissolved in this fluid and reinserted into the canal through the same needle. The area thus anesthetized is determined by the amount of the drug and the position of the patient. It is used very rarely for operations above the diaphragm because of the danger of respiratory depression.

Many drugs are used for these types of anesthesia, but the majority are synthetic preparations similar to *cocaine.* These drugs, in dilute solutions – 1 per cent or less – produce insensitivity to pain, loss of temperature sensation and dilation of blood vessels, unless this last is prevented by the addition of *epinephrine hydrochloride* (Adrenalin). Most physicians use epinephrine, especially when giving the agent into the tissues as in infiltration or nerve block anesthesia since it results in vasoconstriction and therefore slows the rate of absorption.

Some local anesthetic drugs are used only topically; these include ethyl chloride (sprayed on) which anesthetizes by freezing, benzyl alcohol and phenol (usually combined in ointments and lotions with other drugs), amolanone hydrochloride (Amethone), which is used directly on skin or mucous membranes, and cocaine hydrochloride, used, as is amolanone hydrochloride, for surface application only. There are many derivatives of cocaine which can be used below the surface. Ethyl chloride is sometimes used to induce general anesthesia and is then given by inhalation.

Cocaine hydrochloride is used only for surface or topical anesthesia as it is too toxic to be introduced into the body tissues. *Procaine hydrochloride* (Novocain) and an entire family of similar synthetics (see Current Drug Handbook) are used extensively for all local anesthesia except surface anesthesia, for which they have proved unsatisfactory. Some of these drugs are relatively nontoxic and are used for spinal anesthesia. Procaine has also been used in very weak solutions intravenously for the relief of pain in such conditions as rheumatic fever, burns, extensive traumatic injuries and severe neuritis. Lidocaine (Xylocaine) has been found useful in correcting ventricular arrhythmias when given by the intravenous route.

Local anesthetics may, and often do, cause severe toxic symptoms. These may occur from giving too much or a too concentrated solution. Idiosyncrasy to these drugs is not uncommon and, where such sensitivity exists, even minute amounts may cause toxic reactions. Toxic symptoms may be mild or severe enough to cause death. The main symptoms are mental confusion, drug delirium, anxiety, choreiform movements, dizziness, palpitation, tachycardia, irregular pulse and respiration, diaphoresis and dilated pupils. The use of one of the barbiturate drugs before the local anesthetic is given will often prevent occurrence of these symptoms; and the use of epinephrine or a similar drug with the anesthetics, by slowing the rate of absorption, will aid in preventing untoward symptoms. Treatment is symptomatic. Spinal anesthetics tend to produce hypotension, and it is for this reason that patients recovering from this anesthetic are usually placed flat or sometimes in shock position. This type of anesthesia sometimes produces postoperative headache. It may be of very short duration or may be intermittent and persist for some time. Better management of the anesthesia has greatly reduced this complication. The nurse should remember that cocaine is habit forming. It is listed in Schedule II of the 1970 Dangerous or Controlled Drug Act. See Chapters 2 and 6 for details.

The student is referred to the Current Drug Handbook for further information on local anesthetic agents.

The local anesthetics pose several problems for the patient. He is unable to move voluntarily, he can hear but often not comprehend what is being said or he may misinterpret the conversation. The patient feels very helpless and alone. Many times there is apparent concern that the anesthetic agent may not prove entirely satisfactory. The nurse can do much by continuing to give emotional and physical support to the patient during the surgical procedure.

TABLE 10. GENERAL ANESTHETIC AGENTS

ANESTHETIC AGENT	CHEMICAL FORMULA	NATURAL STATE, SPECIAL PRECAUTIONS	F—flammable NF—not flammable EX—explosive NEX—not explosive	ADMINISTRATION O—open drop SC—semiclosed C—closed	INDUCTION PERIOD	ANES-THESIA PRODUCED	MUSCULAR RELAXA-TION	TOXICOLOGY, UNDESIRABLE SIDE EFFECTS	MAJOR USES AND REMARKS
Ether, U.S.P., B.P., Ph.I. (dimethyl ether)	$C_2H_5{\cdot}O{\cdot}C_2H_5$	Volatile liquid Do not use after 48 hours in opened can	F Vapor EX in 2% concentration	O, SC, C	Medium to long 10–15 min.	Good	Good	Apt to cause excitement, restlessness, choking during induction and nausea and vomiting after anesthesia	Good emergency and general anesthetic alone or with other anesthetics to give good muscle relaxation
Vinyl ether, N.F., B.P., Ph.I. (Vinethane)	$CH_2{:}CH{\cdot}O{\cdot}CH{:}CH_2$	Volatile liquid Refrigeration necessary Do not use after 48 hours in opened can Has an objectionable odor	F and EX	O usually	Rapid 30–90 seconds	Good	Good	Stimulates respiratory mucus production; respiratory arrest reached quickly; hepatic damage apt to occur if used longer than 30 minutes	Short anesthesias, as in office or clinic and for induction; not used for prolonged anesthesias
Ethyl chloride, N.F., B.P., Ph.I.	$CH_3{\cdot}CH_2Cl$	Highly volatile liquid Do not use in a closed circuit with soda lime	F	O sprayed on mask	Rapid	Good	Good	Toxicity similar to chloroform, which see	Used only for very short anesthesias; more commonly used as a local anesthetic agent; sometimes used for induction
Trichloroethylene, U.S.P., B.P., Ph.I. (Trilene)	$CHCl{:}CCl_2$	Highly volatile liquid Light sensitive	NF	Special inhaler	Rapid	Good	Poor	Toxicity is low in light, short anesthesias	Used only for very short anesthesias and for short-duration but repeated anesthesias; major use is in obstetrics; has been used in tic douloureux
Chloroform, N.F., B.P., Ph.I.	$CHCl_3$	Highly volatile liquid Light sensitive	NF	O very slowly in minute amounts	Rapid 2–3 min.	Good	Good	Immediate—cardiac disorders Delayed—hepatotoxic	Use rare in the United States because of toxicity; used in obstetrics and for surgery elsewhere
Fluroxene, N.F. (Fluoromar)	$CF_3CH_2OCH{:}CH_2$	Volatile liquid	F and EX	O, SC, C Usually not O Special inhaler	Rapid	Good	Medium to poor	May be some excitement during induction; margin of safety is low; should be used only by a skilled anesthetist; heart, respirations and blood pressure may be depressed.	General surgery with muscle relaxants added; epinephrine and levarterenol are contraindicated

Halothane, U.S.P., B.P. (Fluothane)	$CF_3CHBrCl$	Volatile liquid	NF NEX	SC, C Special inhaler	Rapid	Good	Medium	Same as above	General surgery with synthetic muscle relaxants added; epinephrine and levarterenol are contraindicated
Ketamine hydrochloride (Ketaject, Ketatar)		Solid Formulated in slightly (3.5–5.5) acid fluid for injection		I.V.	Rapid (30–60 seconds)	Good	Poor	Relatively low toxicity; too rapid administration may cause respiratory failure, increase blood pressure and, slightly, muscle tone	Short anesthesia when muscle relaxation is not required; induction, to supplement low potency agents
Methoxyflurane, N.F.	$COHCl_2{\cdot}CF_2{\cdot}O{\cdot}CH_3$	Colorless, volatile liquid with fruity odor.	NF NEX	C Special inhaler	Relatively slow	Good	Good	Same as above, but less apt to cause cardiac depression	Same as above
Nitrous oxide, U.S.P., B.P., Ph.I.	N_2O	Gas, always given with oxygen $N_2O-80\%$ } highest safe $O-20\%$ } concentration	NEX NF	SC, C	Medium to short	Fair	Poor	Hypoxia; occurs in higher concentration and even in low concentration in some patients	Obstetrics, dentistry, short surgical procedures and with other agents for longer surgery
Ethylene, N.F.	$CH_2{:}CH_2$	Gas Has an objectionable odor Given with oxygen, not stronger than 80–20 concentration	F EX	SC, C	Rapid	Good	Poor	Relatively nontoxic, but should be given only by a skilled anesthetist	Obstetrics and general surgery
Cyclopropane, U.S.P., B.P., Ph.I.	C_3H_6	Gas, given with oxygen Oxygen 80–90%	F and EX Avoid all sparks	C	Rapid	Good	Good	Toxicity low in the hands of a skilled anesthetist; may cause cardiac arrhythmia	General surgery and obstetrics; especially good for patients with respiratory difficulties
Methohexital sodium, N.F. (Brevital) (methohexitone. Brietal [C])	These are all short acting barbiturates	Solid Hygroscopic powder dissolved in water	NF NEX	I.V. Some can be given rectally	Rapid	Fair	Poor	Respiratory depression and laryngospasm may occur; may cause hypotension and tachycardia; selection of patients for I.V. barbiturates should be very carefully done; these should be given only by a skilled anesthetist; there are many contraindications	As an induction agent in general surgery, in obstetrics and for short surgical procedures
Thiamylal sodium (Surital)	Same as above								
Thiopental sodium, U.S.P., thiopentone sodium, B.P. (Pentothal)	Same as above								

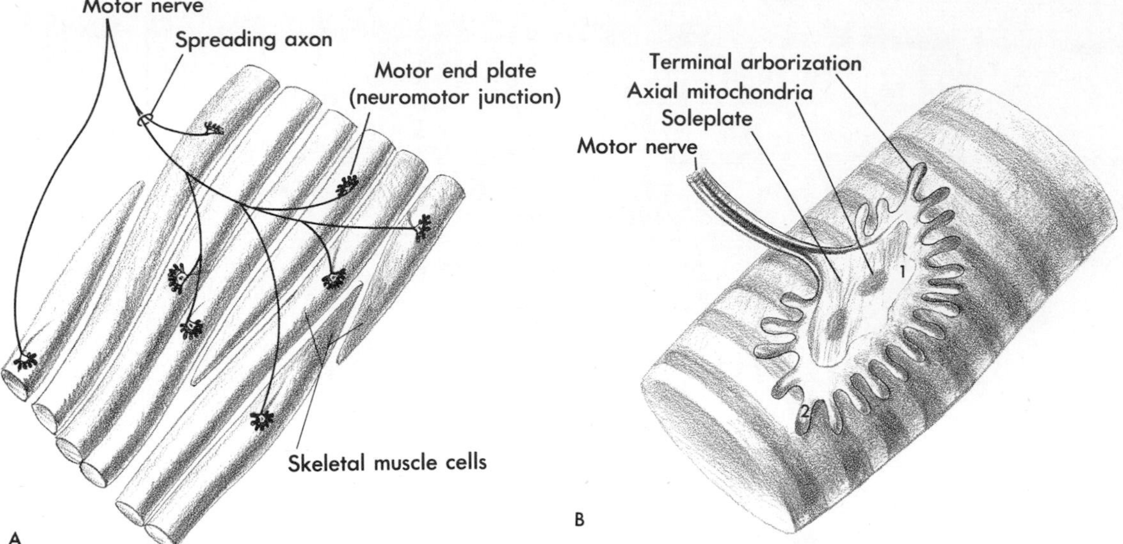

FIGURE 24. *A,* Shows connections between nerve endings and muscle fibers. *B,* Enlargement of motor end plate. Effect of muscle relaxants on muscular contraction. Contraction is initiated by passage of an impulse along the axon. Acetylcholine is liberated at 1. Depolarization increases permeability of cell membrane at 2, followed by initiation of potassium and sodium ion exchange. Muscle excitation and contraction occur.

Curare drugs act on acetylcholine at 1, preventing its action. Succinylcholine decamethonium and neostigmine prolong depolarization, making new contractions impossible.

MUSCLE RELAXANTS

The Drugs. The muscle relaxant drugs have a long and interesting history. They have been used for centuries as an arrowhead poison by the natives of South America, especially those in the upper reaches of the Amazon estuary. The drug paralyzes the game, making capture easy even if the arrow fails to strike a vital spot. Curare is the generic name of the extract obtained from various plants. Muscle relaxants which are secured synthetically will also be considered here.

Physical and Chemical Properties. The curare drugs are the purified alkaloids of various plants. Some have been synthesized and some are semisynthetic. They are mainly quaternary ammonium compounds similar to acetylcholine. The depolarizing agents are entirely synthetic. All these drugs are soluble in water and in body fluids, but they are poorly absorbed from the gastrointestinal tract.

Action. The action of these two types of drugs is antagonistic. However, the final result, muscular relaxation, is the same (Fig. 24). These drugs act in the area of the neuromuscular end plate and not in the central nervous system as other muscular relaxants do. How long the muscle remains inactive depends upon the preparation used and, of course, the kind and amount of other depressant drugs given simultaneously. The curare drugs have a more prolonged action than the depolarizing agents.

Curare and curariform drugs act by blocking the nerve impulse at the motor end plate. They block the transmitter action of acetylcholine. They act on the muscles of the eyes, fingers and toes, continuing until all the skeletal muscles are paralyzed. The respiratory muscles are the last to be affected.

The synthetic, depolarizing relaxants prolong the depolarization interval of the neuromotor end plate delaying muscle contraction.

Therapeutic Uses. The chief application of these drugs is in surgical treatment. They allow for a lighter level of anesthesia since the anesthetic agent is not required for muscle relaxation. They are also used when a strong muscle relaxant is desired such as in tetanus, encephalitis, poliomyelitis and shock therapy, to lessen the convulsion.

Absorption and Excretion. The strong muscle relaxants, poorly absorbed from the gastrointestinal tract, are administered chiefly by the intravenous route, following which they are widely distributed through the body, rapidly inactivated by the liver and excreted through the urinary tract.

Rapid inactivation by the liver and excretion through the urinary tract permits the use of artificial respiration, with a patent airway to be used in respiratory embarrassment. The drug remains active only for a few minutes. The synthetics, particularly succinylcholine, are rapidly deactivated by esterases at the site of activity.

Preparations and Dosages

CURARE GROUP

Tubocurarine chloride, U.S.P., B.P., (d-Tubocurarine, Tubadil, Tubarine) 6 to 9 mg. I.V.

Dimethyl tubocurarine iodide, N.F. (Metubine) 1.5 to 6 mg. I.V.

Gallamine triethiodide, U.S.P., B.P., (Flaxedil) 1 mg./kg. of body weight I.V.

DEPOLARIZING AGENTS

Decamethonium bromide or iodide, B.P. (Syncurine, Eulissin, as the iodide, [C]) 2 to 2.5 mg. I.V.

Succinylcholine chloride, U.S.P., Suxamethonium bromide or chloride, B.P. (Anectine, Sucostrin, Scoline [C]) 10 to 30 mg. I.V. (Refrigerate and protect from light.)

All of these drugs are repeated as indicated by the patient's condition and the progress of the surgical treatment. Although they are short acting drugs, too rapidly repeated dosage can cause adverse symptoms. The duration of the depolarizing group is much shorter than for the curare group, hence they must be repeated more frequently to insure the same results. Succinylcholine is inactivated most quickly of all these drugs.

THE NURSE

Mode of Administration. These drugs are all given intravenously, ordinarily by the anesthetist. However, the nurse will be required to prepare the drug and sometimes to administer it. In most cases the drug is administered by continuous intravenous drip to maintain prolonged relaxation.

Toxicity and Treatment. The curare drugs may cause the release of excessive amounts of histamine with resulting bronchospasm. However, the most serious toxic symptom is respiratory paralysis. Neostigmine methylsulfate 1 or 2 mg. or edrophonium chloride 10 mg. is usually used as an antidote and should be readily available.

Interactions. The action of the curare-type drugs is enhanced by the monoamine oxidase inhibitors, the thiazide diuretics and the antibiotics (neomycin, kanamycin and streptomycin) by the production of hypokalemia. They are inhibited by the anticholinesterases. The action of the depolarizing drugs is enhanced by the anticholinesterases in an additive fashion.

The depolarizing drugs do not cause any release of histamine, hence no bronchospasm. However, respiratory failure can occur. There are no effective antidotes for the depolarizing agents. Neostigmine and edrophonium may actually increase the toxic effects. Mechanical, positive pressure respiration must be continued until the drug has lost its effectiveness and the patient is able to breathe without assistance.

THE PATIENT. Since these drugs are frequently used during surgical treatment, the patient is unconscious; by the time he regains consciousness, their effects have worn off.

Drugs Used in an Emergency

Although every precaution is taken to prevent emergencies in the operating room, such situations do occur and in order to deal with them effectively the necessary drugs and equipment must be readily available. The actual condition of the patient is in the hands of the anesthetist, and he is constantly on the alert to anticipate any untoward change in the patient. Since all patients do not react in the same manner to the same drugs, emergency drugs that might be needed must always be easily available. Not only should the drugs be where they can be quickly secured, but the means of giving them must also be at hand. Usually the anesthetist gives the drug intravenously and, when an intravenous infusion is already in progress, as is often the case, the drug is introduced into the fluid through the tubing. If the nurse gives the medication, she must be very careful to insert the needle into the rubber portion of the tubing. Most intravenous tubes are plastic for the greater portion of their length. This plastic is not self-sealing and must not be punctured. Toward the end of the tubing nearest the patient is a short length of rubber, put there so that drugs may be given while the infusion is in progress.

The most common operative emergencies are shock with circulatory failure, cardiac arrest, respiratory embarrassment or paralysis and hemorrhage. Some of the emergencies can be treated by changing the anesthesia. Increasing the oxygen or carbon dioxide in the gaseous mixture is sometimes effective. If the cause of the emergency is an adverse reaction to a drug that has been given, the proper antidote may be used, for example edrophonium or neostigmine for the curariform drugs. Cardiac arrest is usually treated by manual or electrical stimulation. Respiratory failure may be treated by positive pressure artificial respiration. However, cardiac and/or respiratory difficulties may be treated by giving a central nervous system stimulant. (See Chapter 9.) The predominant symptom of shock, which often accompanies these conditions, is hypotension. A lowering of blood pressure may be the first symptom noted. Shock may be treated by increasing blood volume with an intravenous infusion or transfusion and/or by the use of an antihypotensive drug.

THE ANTIHYPOTENSIVE DRUGS

THE DRUGS. Some of the drugs used for shock, such as epinephrine (Adrenalin) and phenylephrine (Neo-synephrine), find their main use in the treatment of allergy and are discussed under that topic. Refer to Chapter 25 and Current Drug Handbook for further information. The antihypotensive drugs, most of which are prepared synthetically, are sympathomimetics.

Physical and Chemical Properties. The parent compound for the sympathomimetic amines is usually considered to be β-phenylethylamine, consisting of a benzene ring and an aliphatic portion. Substitutions in the ring or side chains vary the action of the drugs. They are all amines and react with an acid to form a salt, the compound used pharmaceutically. The salts are readily soluble in water and body fluids.

Actions. The sympathomimetic drugs all produce, to a greater or lesser degree, mydriasis, decreased tone of the bronchioles, constriction of the blood vessels (other than coronary) and an increased rate and output of the heart. These are all adrenergic agents. The adrenergic receptors have been classified as alpha or beta receptors. The alpha receptors are associated with excitatory responses to smooth muscle tissue. Beta receptors mediate relaxation of smooth muscle tissue, but they also increase the rate and strength of cardiac contractions. Epinephrine strongly affects both alpha and beta receptors. Norepinephrine acts more on the alpha receptors than on the beta receptors, and isoproterenol acts more on the beta receptors than on the alpha receptors.

Therapeutic Uses. There are many uses for the different preparations of the sympathetic stimulants. However, in surgery and emergency they are used to combat hypotension as it occurs in shock, cardiac and respiratory failure and for bronchospasm. Isoproterenol (Isuprel) does not materially raise blood pressure but is of great importance in the relief of bronchospasm or cardiac arrest.

Absorption and Excretion. The sympathetic stimulants used in surgical procedures are introduced directly into the blood stream and are distributed widely. The drugs are inactivated in the body mainly in the liver, but the tissues also aid in their degradation. Their metabolites are excreted by the kidneys.

Preparations and Dosages

Epinephrine hydrochloride, U.S.P., Adrenaline, B.P., (Adrenalin) 0.06 to 1 ml. of a 1:1000 solution parenterally.

Isoproterenol hydrochloride, U.S.P. (Isuprel, isoprenaline, Neo-Ephinine [C]) 0.2 to 1 mg. I.M. or I.V.

Levarterenol bitartrate, U.S.P., Noradrenaline acid tartrate, B.P. (Levophed) 1 to 10 micrograms I.V./minute.

Metaraminol bitartrate, U.S.P. (Aramine) 15 to 100 mg. I.V. usually given in a glucose solution.

Methoxamine hydrochloride, U.S.P. (Vasoxyl) 5 to 20 mg. I.V.

THE NURSE

Mode of Administration. These drugs are given intravenously or intramuscularly, depending upon the drug chosen. They may be added to intravenous infusions, glucose or the electrolytes. The nurse has a grave responsibility to patients who are receiving them. Many specific nursing care implications must be considered according to the drug being used and the pathological condition which has resulted in the severe hypotension. Study Table 11, Antihypotensive Drug/Nursing Care Implications, very thoroughly.

Side Effects, Toxicity and Treatment. Toxic symptoms may include pallor, coldness of the extremities, nervousness, dyspnea, tremors, anxiety, vertigo, diaphoresis, nausea and vomiting and a severe throbbing headache. The patient may complain of palpitation, a slow forceful heart beat, constriction of the chest and a feeling of oppression (fear of dying). Unless the untoward signs and symptoms are alleviated, the patient may progress into ventricular fibrillation, pulmonary edema, or a cerebral vascular accident. Specifically, epinephrine, isoproterenol and levarterenol may cause palpitation, precordial distress and even acute cardiac dilation. Antihypertensive medications are resorted to when rise in blood pressure, owing to peripheral vessel constriction, becomes excessive. The symptoms are treated as conditions indicate, but respiratory and cardiac stimulants are usually ordered. Methoxamine may cause a severe bradycardia.

Contraindications. All antihypotensive drugs must be used with caution when patients demonstrate a history of thyroid or cardiac disease, especially high blood pressure. The incidence of ventricular fibrillation has increased when these drugs are combined with the tranquilizers, monoamine oxidase inhibitors and certain anesthetics such as cyclopropane.

THE PATIENT. In cases that require treatment with these drugs, the patient and the family feel helpless and afraid. They will need repeated instructions and information. Anxiety levels are usually high and often the patient and family are "unable" to tune into them. The nurse can alleviate much of this anxiety by working efficiently, demonstrating patience, reinforcing coping behavior and helping the patient and the family to continue communicating with the physician. Many times she will simply need to listen to the real fears being expressed.

Drugs Used to Overcome Hemorrhage

In surgery, most hemorrhage is controlled by mechanical means. In the discussion of the antihypotensive drugs, it was noted that they constrict peripheral blood vessels. This will help in the control of bleeding.

Plasma, also used for shock, will aid in the stopping of bleeding since it will add extra blood clotting factors to the patient's blood. The same is true of whole blood.

Locally, various substances such as Gelfoam are used to stop bleeding, capillary bleeding in particular since this form of hemorrhage cannot be controlled by ligation. This type of material supplies fibers on which the clot may form more easily. Surface capillary bleeding can be stopped with the common astringent drugs such as silver nitrate, cotarnine biphthalate (Styptol), alum or ferric chloride or antihemorrhagic biological products such as thrombin, thromboplastin and fibrinogen.

Supportive Drugs

Since the maintenance of the patient's general condition is closely related to the occurrence of emergencies, many drugs are useful for both purposes, but custom has restricted the term supportive to materials given intravenously to aid in keeping the patient in good condition during the operation. Many different materials for intravenous injection are available to the anesthetist or the surgeon. Those most commonly used are *whole blood*, especially if there has been excessive blood loss, *plasma*, *glucose* or other *sugar* solution, *saline* and other *electrolyte solutions*. These fluids are used in surgery for the same reasons that they would be used in any disorder: to supply fluid, to maintain blood pressure, to supply needed blood constituents.

Analgesics

It is often advisable to give drugs which will lessen the sensitivity to pain even though the patient is under anesthesia. These medicines allow the anesthetist to

TABLE 11. NURSING CARE IMPLICATIONS OF ANTIHYPOTENSIVE DRUGS

	ANTIHYPOTENSIVE DRUGS				
NURSING CARE IMPLICATIONS	Epinephrine hydrochloride (Adrenalin)	Isoproterenol hydrochloride (Isuprel)	Levarterenol bitartrate (Levophed)	Metaraminol bitartrate (Aramine)	Methoxamine hydrochloride (Vasoxyl)
Rate of flow ordered by doctor is adjusted by nurse to maintain constant blood pressure	*	*	* (Dextrose better than saline)	*	*
Do not leave patient unattended during the infusion	*	*	*	*	*
Observe injection site for subcutaneous extravasation (swelling and/or blanching) leading to tendency to tissue necrosis	*	*	* (May cause severe sloughing)	*	*
Atropine available as antidote to bradycardia			*		*
Drug darkens on exposure to light and air, keep tightly covered in light-resistant container	*	*	*		*
Observe vital signs every five minutes until desired blood pressure is maintained	* (Wide pulse pressure)	*	*	*	*
Closely observe the patient—electrocardiograph, urinary output, peripheral perfusion (skin color) and central venous pressure	*	*	*	*	*
Change intravenous sites every 12 hours	*	* (Not given with epinephrine; wait twelve hours to alternate)	*	*	*
Be alert for changes in blood pressure even after drug has been discontinued	* (Never used with tranquilizers, may cause return of hypotension due to additive action)	*	* (Gradually lessen amount of drug to prevent sharp drop in blood pressure)	* (Repeated injections may result in overdosage when circulation returns to normal)	*

use much less of the anesthetic. The drugs used are the same as those used preoperatively, the opiates or the synthetic analgesics, such as pentazocine (Talwin) or meperidine (Demerol) (pethidine [C]). Many anesthetists use analgesics in conjunction with local anesthetics. This keeps the patient comfortable and eliminates the hazards of general anesthesia. Of course, such routines can be used only in selected cases. See Chapter 9.

Antiseptics

Many chemicals are used for antiseptics in the operating room. Some are used for utensils and instruments while others are used to clean the skin of the patient, the surgeons and the nurses. These drugs do not differ materially from antiseptics and disinfectants used for other purposes. See Chapter 7.

DRUGS USED IMMEDIATELY AFTER OPERATION

The postoperative period begins as soon as the surgeon has completed the actual surgical procedure, even though the patient may not have returned to his room. Many hospitals maintain recovery rooms in which the patient remains until after he has regained consciousness and his condition is such that he may be left alone, at least temporarily. Many of the drugs used at this time are the same as those used in the operating room. This is especially true of analgesic and supportive drugs.

Analgesics

Pain is almost inevitable following an operation. During a surgical procedure many nerve endings are disturbed or severed, and sometimes whole nerves must be cut, thus causing pain—light, moderate or severe, according to the amount of trauma and the normal pain threshold of the individual patient. People vary widely in their ability to withstand pain, and this makes it necessary to vary the type of drug and the dosage (V-4). If the patient has been in pain for a long time, he may have built up a tolerance for one or more of the analgesic drugs. This will necessitate either a different drug or a larger dose of the same drug. Needless to say, the nurse should make sure that the patient is as comfortable as possible before giving any pain-relieving medication. The immediate postoperative period is not the time to withhold narcotic drugs or to try to get the patient to do without such medications. The length of time the patient will need pain-relieving medications will, of course, depend upon the nature of the operation. The analgesic drugs used in the postoperative period are the same as those used to relieve pain from other causes. They have been discussed previously. See Chapter 9.

Supportive Drugs

It is not uncommon for the patient to return from surgery with an intravenous infusion in process. This may be whole blood or any of the usual intravenous solutions. If the patient is unable to retain sufficient fluids or food, the intravenous solutions may be continued for several days. When surgery has been performed on the gastrointestinal tract (such as a gastric resection) the surgeon may wish the organs to remain at rest, and the necessary nutrient materials are given through the veins for the length of time desired. In addition to the intravenous solutions mentioned before, various compounds containing the essential *amino acids* (such as *protein hydrolysate*) and/or *vitamin B-complex* may be given.

Vitamins, especially *vitamins B* and *C*, are also given orally to aid the patient to recover more rapidly. Preparations containing amino acids and the essential vitamins are available and are often given to the postoperative patient when he is able to retain such drugs. Of course, these are food accessories and are not given until the patient is able to accept at least a soft diet.

POSTOPERATIVE DISORDERS AND DRUGS USED TO TREAT THEM

Abdominal Distention

After all laparotomies there is the possibility of abdominal distention. The very fact that the intestines must be disturbed often causes a lessening of the normal peristaltic waves, and this will result in the accumulation of gases in the intestines (I-2). Drugs, especially the opiates, also tend to produce the same effect, and there are other factors which may add to this tendency such as the lack of food materials for the intestinal juices to work upon. When distention does occur it may be slight, causing only mild discomfort, or so severe that it causes respiratory distress. Enemas, rectal tubes and similar treatments may be effective in the more severe cases, or drugs that increase peristalsis may be needed. The most common drug used for this purpose is *neostigmine* (Prostigmin) 1.0 ml. of a 1:2000 solution by hypodermic. This will increase the tone of the intestinal muscles, with a resulting increase in peristalsis, passage of flatus and relief of distention. The use of a rectal tube in conjunction with this drug is often an aid to more rapid relief.

Urinary Retention

Urinary retention is a not uncommon result of anesthesia. It is a condition which usually is more uncomfortable than serious. The patient has the desire to urinate but is unable to do so. This upsets the patient, and the emotional disturbance increases his tension, making voiding even more difficult (V-5). The nurse can reassure the patient that many different nursing measures will be used to help him facilitate a voiding response. No serious harm will result if the urinary retention is neither severe nor of long duration. If it is decided that medical treatment is needed, *neostigmine* (Prostigmin) is usually ordered. This drug increases urinary as well as intestinal peristalsis and is often given to relieve abdominal distention as well as urinary retention. Certain other drugs of the parasympathetic stimulant group (parasympathomimetic) are used for this purpose, such as *benzpyrinium bromide* (Stigmonene), *bethanechol chloride* (Urecholine). All except Stigmonene may be given orally or subcutaneously; usually the latter route is used. Stigmonene is administered intramuscularly. Dosages are as follows: Stigmonene 2 mg.; Urecholine 2.5 to 5.0 mg. subcutaneously, 10 to 30 mg. orally.

Cyanosis

Cyanosis (blueness of the skin) is often encountered in the hours immediately following general anesthesia. It is caused by improper oxygenation of the blood, and the obvious treatment is to remedy the cause by the administration of oxygen. If, at the same time, respirations appear inadequate (shallow or irregular) *carbogen* (a combination of *oxygen* 95 per cent and *carbon dioxide* 5 per cent) is sometimes ordered. The physician's orders as to the amount of carbogen to be used should be very strictly observed, since excessive amounts of carbogen can be toxic.

Singultus

Singultus (hiccup) is an annoying and sometimes serious postoperative complication. It may be due to any one of a number of causes, such as abdominal distention and disturbance of the respiratory center. Obviously, the removal of the cause is the best possible cure. If distention is the reason for the hiccups, *neostigmine* will usually afford relief or, if the distention is in the stomach, *carbonated drinks*, if allowed, or any of the antacid drugs may be effective. If the cause of the hiccups is a disturbance of the respiratory center, *carbogen* is often sufficient to relieve the condition. *Hoffman's anodyne* (spirits of nitrous ether) orally has proved valuable in some persistent cases. Some physicians order sedative, hypnotic or tranquilizing drugs for hiccups. In most cases these give little permanent relief, but they do afford temporary relief and thus give the patient needed rest. *Chlorpromazine hydrochloride* (Thorazine), *promazine* (Sparine) and *prochlorperazine* (Compazine) have been used successfully in the treatment of persistent hiccups. Thorazine can be given either orally or intramuscularly. The usual dose is 25 mg. Sparine is usually given intramuscularly in the same dosage. Compazine may be administered rectally, orally or parenterally, dosage varying from 10 to 75 mg. Any one of a number of tranquilizing drugs may be used. Refer to Chapter 30 for further details.

Acidosis

Acidosis is not uncommon following certain types of surgery and can be easily overcome by the use of *sodium bicarbonate*. It can be given orally or intravenously, whichever is best under the specific circumstances. Many drugs are antacid in action in the stomach, but most of them do not aid in the relief of systemic acidosis as sodium bicarbonate does.

DRUGS USED IN THE LATE POSTOPERATIVE PERIOD

Drugs used during the late postoperative and convalescent periods vary widely according to the character of the surgery and the condition of the patient at the time of the operation. Most of the drugs pertinent to this heading are discussed in other areas which relate to specific conditions. However, for most patients doctors order some type of tranquilizing drug to aid the patient in his adjustment during the often difficult period of convalescence. Also, many feel that vitamin supplements are advantageous, at least until the individual is on an adequate diet and is feeling much improved.

Recovery from surgical procedures at the present time is so rapid and easy there is little need for drugs after the immediate postoperative period. The patients are up and around, often able to resume most activities in a few days, even after major surgery. This should not blind the nurse to the fact that these patients have been really sick and that often the quick recovery may be more apparent than real. She should be ready to explain to the patient why he cannot immediately do all the things he has been accustomed to doing. Some patients need encouragement to do things; others need to be discouraged from doing too much. It takes tact and understanding to judge whether encouragement or discouragement is needed and how much is necessary. Even months after apparent recovery from major surgery, the patient may find that he is unable to do all that he feels he should be doing. It takes time for nature to complete the work that the surgeon started.

IT IS IMPORTANT TO REMEMBER

1. That no matter how simple or routine the surgery may be for the nurse, it is a "once in a lifetime" experience for the patient.
2. That many patients, both younger and older people, are extremely fearful of surgery. They have known others who did not survive such procedures or who have been invalids following an operation. These people need reassurance.
3. That though the patient may be out of bed early, he is nevertheless weak and ill and needs to be encouraged to do what he is able to do, but discouraged from overdoing.
4. That the correct timing of medications given preoperatively may spell the difference between an effective and a relatively difficult anesthesia.
5. That drugs given postoperatively are extremely important, and every care should be taken to give them on time and as ordered. Of course, this is true of all medications. The nurse must be especially observant of the untoward action of these drugs, since the patient may think that the adverse symptoms are the result of the surgery rather than the drugs.
6. That the patient's physiological and psychological status will often determine how effectively he will be able to cope with the stress of anesthesia and surgery.

TOPICS FOR STUDY AND DISCUSSION

1. Prepare a skit to show "good" and "poor" approaches to a newly admitted patient. Presume the patient is to be prepared for an exploratory laparotomy.
2. Check the charts of the patients on the surgical division for preoperative, operative and postoperative drugs. List, compare and explain their uses.
3. Plan means of quieting an emotional patient who is resisting medication and who is averse to having needed surgery done.
4. What analgesics are used in the operating room? Are these all narcotics? Explain your answer. Are these reportable under the federal narcotic act?
5. The preoperative order is for Pantopon 20 mg. and scopolamine 0.4 mg. The nurse finds the floor supply of these drugs to be hypodermic tablets. The Pantopon is gr. 1/3 and the scopolamine gr. 1/100 each tablet. Explain, in detail, what should be done.
6. The local anesthetic ordered is procaine 0.5 per cent solution. There are to be 10 ml. prepared. To this epinephrine (Adrenalin) 1 ml. of a 1:1000 solution is to be added. The nurse finds that the procaine is in a stock solution of 5 per cent strength. How should she proceed?
7. Write a dialogue between you and a family member who is having difficulty speaking with the physician about the use of a general anesthetic for her elderly father (anticipating removal of a part of the pancreas).

BIBLIOGRAPHY

Books and Pamphlets

American Medical Association Council on Drugs, *Drug Evaluations*, Chicago, 1971, American Medical Association.

American Medical Association Council on Drugs, *Evaluations of Drug Interactions*, Chicago, 1971, American Medical Association.

Beeson, P. B., and McDermott, W., *Cecil-Loeb Textbook of Medicine*, Philadelphia, 1971, W. B. Saunders Co.

Beland, I. L., *Clinical Nursing*, New York, 1965, The Macmillan Co.

Bergersen, B. S., King, E. E., and Goth, A., *Pharmacology in Nursing, 12th Ed.*, St. Louis, 1973, The C. V. Mosby Co.

Conn, H. F., et al., *Current Therapy*, Philadelphia, 1972, W. B. Saunders Co.

Goodman, L. S., and Gilman, A., *Pharmacological Basis of Therapeutics, 4th Ed.*, New York, 1970, The Macmillan Co.

Hartshorn, E. A., *Handbook of Drug Interactions*, Cincinnati, 1970, University of Cincinnati Press.

Meltzer, L., Abdellah, F., and Kitchell, J. R., *Concepts and Practices of Intensive Care for Nurse Specialists*, Philadelphia, 1970, The Charles Press.

Moidel, H., Sorensen, G., Giblin, E., Kaufmann, M., *Nursing Care of the Patient with Medical-Surgical Disorders*, New York, 1971, McGraw-Hill Book Co.

Moore, C., and Rose, M., "Working with children and their families to help them through a long-anticipated surgical experience," *in* Bergersen, B., et al., (Eds.) *Current Concepts in Clinical Nursing*, St. Louis, 1967, The C. V. Mosby Co.

Rodman, M. J., and Smith, D. W., *Pharmacology and Drug Therapy in Nursing*, Philadelphia, 1968, J. B. Lippincott Co.

Shafer, K. M., et al., *Medical-Surgical Nursing, 5th Ed.*, St. Louis, 1971, The C. V. Mosby Co.

Watson, J. E., *Medical-Surgical Nursing and Related Physiology*, Philadelphia, 1972, W. B. Saunders Co.

Journal Articles

Bergstrom, N., "Ice applications to induce voiding?" *Am. J. Nurs.* 68:1:62 (January, 1968).

Carnevali, D., "Preoperative anxiety," *Am. J. Nurs.* 66:7:1536 (July, 1966).

Carroll, J., et al., "Symposium on the patient with trauma," *Nurs. Clin. North Am.* 5:4 (December, 1971).

Chandler, J. G., "The physiology and treatment of shock," *R.N.* 34:6 (June, 1971).

DeVeber, G., "Fluid and electrolyte problems in the postoperative period," *Nurs. Clin. North Am.* 1:6:275 (January, 1966).

DiPalma, J. R., "The why and how of drug interactions," *R.N.* 33:3:63 (March, 1970).

DiPalma, J. R., "The why and how of drug interactions," *R.N.* 33:4:67 (April, 1970).

DiPalma, J. R., "The why and how of drug interactions," *R.N.* 33:5:69 (May, 1970).

Healy, K., "Does pre-operative instruction make a difference?" *Am. J. Nurs.* 68:1:62 (January, 1968).

Luessenhop, A., "Care of the unconscious patient," *Nurs. Forum* 4:3:6 (1965).

Quint, J., "Communications problems affecting patient care in the hospital," *J.A.M.A.* 195:36 (January, 1966).

Williams, J., et al., "Symposium on care of the surgical patient," *Nurs. Clin. North Am.* 3:3:489 (September, 1968).

Woss, T., "Nursing the patient after heart surgery," *Can. Nurse* 65:1:35 (January, 1969).

CHAPTER 16

DRUGS USED FOR DISORDERS OF THE RESPIRATORY SYSTEM

CORRELATION WITH OTHER SCIENCES

I. ANATOMY AND PHYSIOLOGY

1. Internally, the nose is divided into a right and a left cavity by the septum and is lined with ciliated mucous membrane.
2. The paranasal sinuses are eight in number, of which the maxillary, the sphenoid, the ethmoid and the frontal sinuses are probably the most important.
3. The pharynx, reaching from the posterior limit of the nose to the esophagus and larynx, is divided into the nasopharynx, the oropharynx and the laryngopharynx.
4. The larynx is made up of three main parts: the thyroid, the cricoid and the arythenoid cartilages.
5. The lungs are composed of an elastic compressible material which is inflated and deflated with each respiration.
6. The lungs perform the essential function of providing needed oxygen to the body and transporting carbon dioxide to the outside air.
7. The bronchi and bronchioles lengthen and widen in inspiration and shorten and narrow in expiration. Drainage is facilitated by these rhythmic contractions, by the normal ciliary action of the epithelium of the tracheobronchial tree, and by the expulsive force of the elastic recoil of the lungs and the piston-like action of the diaphragm.
8. The respiratory center is located in the lower part of the medulla.
9. To have effective pulmonary ventilation, the airways must be patent; the lung and tracheobronchial tree must be elastic and expansile; there must be an adequate musculoskeletal apparatus of the chest wall of related structures; and there must be a normal relation between the amount of air inspired per breath and the amount within the lungs.

III. MICROBIOLOGY

1. Microorganisms which may cause diseases of the respiratory tract include viruses, fusiform bacilli and a spirochete, *Streptococcus, Staphylococcus, Pneumococcus, Haemophilus influenzae, Mycobacterium tuberculosis* and others.
2. Viruses do not contain ribosomes and are dependent on other living cells (host cells) for replication, hence they are called "intracellular parasites."
3. The *Mycobacterium tuberculosis* is an aerobic organism which causes tuberculosis in man. Owing to the high lipid content of the cell wall, this pathogen is highly resistant to many disinfectants and can survive in dust for several months.

IV. PHYSICS

1. The maximal breathing capacity or maximal minute ventilation is the maximal volume of air that can be breathed by voluntary effort per minute.
2. Vital capacity is the maximal volume of air that can be exhaled after a maximal respiration.
3. Tidal air is the actual volume of a single breath—about 500 ml. (cc.). Of the 500 ml. of tidal air inhaled at each breath, about 350 ml. (cc.) (effective tidal air) is well distributed in normal persons throughout the pulmonary alveolar spaces.
4. Normally, pressure within the pleura is always below that of the atmosphere. As the volume of the thoracic cage increases on inspiration, due to lowering of the diaphragm and

expansion of the chest wall, the pressure of the air in the lung decreases. As a result, air from the outside, which is at a higher pressure, enters. On expiration, the diaphragm rises and the volume of the thorax decreases. This is accompanied by an increase in the pressure in the lungs and, because this pressure is now greater than the outside air, air passes out of the lung.

V. PSYCHOLOGY

1. Treatment of some diseases of the respiratory tract is often long, and some diseases tend to recur. This is often discouraging to the patient.
2. The restriction of breathing often present in lung conditions very frequently causes great apprehension on the part of the patient.
3. Many patients feel that because they have a lung disease they have tuberculosis, but this is probably not true.
4. The realization that one has a serious illness that is communicable and apt to be prolonged, such as tuberculosis, may be a severe emotional shock to the patient.
5. Chronic illness may develop with some respiratory diseases. This may result in depression and feelings of helplessness and hopelessness.

VI. SOCIOLOGY

1. The cost of prolonged treatment may become a burden to patients with respiratory diseases. They should be assisted by every means possible to continue treatment.
2. Social stigma is a potent factor in the life of everyone, since people desire the approval of their peers. Certain types of diseases carry a stigma, especially in some segments of society. This may cause the patient, if he fears he has such a condition, to postpone seeking medical help, and this delay may result in a much worse condition than would otherwise have occurred.

INTRODUCTION

Any condition that interferes with the proper exchange of air and carbon dioxide may be of very serious consequence to the patient for, in order to maintain life, there must be this exchange of air at frequent intervals (I-6; IV-1, 2, 3, 4). Some few of the diseases that affect the respiratory tract are relatively minor, but the majority require long-continued treatment and often cannot be permanently corrected without surgery. However, in some cases drug therapy is the only form of treatment possible.

The mucous membrane lining the respiratory tract and the gastrointestinal system is continuous, hence any infection in one area can affect other areas by direct extension. For instance, pharyngitis (sore throat) may travel upward, causing rhinitis, sinusitis or even otitis media via the eustachian tube. It may go downward, causing laryngitis, tracheitis, bronchitis or pneumonia.

DISEASES OF THE NOSE, THROAT AND SINUSES

Acute Rhinitis (Acute Coryza, the Common Cold)

DEFINITION. Occurring the world over, acute rhinitis—the common cold—is in its uncomplicated form a mild disease, but complications occur so frequently that they are almost a part of the disease itself. Though the actual cause is unknown, it is well established that the responsible agent is a virus (III-1).

MAJOR SYMPTOMS. The onset is usually rather abrupt with a feeling of dryness and soreness in the nasal passages and pharynx. Rapidly, nasal congestion develops with a watery nasal discharge, sneezing, lacrimation, headache, a nonproductive cough and occasionally a low-grade fever. The patient also complains of malaise, aching in the back and limbs, chilly sensations and weariness.

DRUG THERAPY. All drug therapy is purely symptomatic, for no medication has been found to ward off the disease or to cure it.

ANALGESIC-ANTIPYRETIC DRUGS. *Aspirin* or *acetaminophen* (Tylenol) in average doses 0.3 to 0.6 Gm. will often relieve the headache and muscular pain and reduce the temperature. These drugs have been discussed in detail in Chapter 9. Some physicians believe that aspirin, phenacetin and a small amount of caffeine (A.P.C., many trade names) may be even more effective than one drug alone.

ANTIHISTAMINES. On some occasions, the use of an antihistamine during the first day of the disease will provide some symptomatic relief. It has no curative action. Coricidin, one of a number of similar preparations, is a combination of *chlorpheniramine maleate* (Chlor-Trimeton) (an antihistamine), *aspirin, phenacetin and caffeine*, and provides an effective antihistaminic action plus an analgesic and antipyretic action. If this drug is taken early in the disease, it definitely lessens discharges and the patient is more comfortable. The usual initial dose is two tablets, followed by one tablet every four hours for three days. This drug may cause drowsiness in some patients.

NASAL DECONGESTANTS. One of the vasoconstrictor drugs administered as nose drops or spray or by inhalation may sometimes be used to relieve nasal congestion. Some physicians believe that the closure of the nose during the acute stage may be a protective mechanism and that the use of nose drops may cause the infection to spread. Some of the more commonly used preparations include: *ephedrine* 1 per cent; *naphazoline hydrochloride* (Privine) 0.05 per cent, *tetrahydrozoline hydrochloride* (Tyzine) 0.05 per cent, *xylometrazoline hydrochloride* (Otivin) 0.05 and 0.1 per cent, *racephedrine hydrochloride* 0.5 to 2 per cent; *oxymetazoline* (Afrin) 0.05 per cent. They may be used in from one to three drops in the nose every four to six hours or longer or by using the plastic squeeze bottle in which most of these drugs are now marketed. All of these are generally contraindicated in hypertension, hyperthyroidism, insomnia, arteriosclerosis, nephritis, coronary disease or glaucoma.

There are several good inhalers available which will also produce constriction of the nasal mucosa.

Chemotherapeutic agents and antibiotics are of no value in acute rhinitis. Occasionally they may be ordered to prevent secondary infections, but they have no effect on the disease itself.

THE NURSE. The proper administration of nose drops is as important as giving the medication when needed (I-1, 2). There are several accepted methods of administration that the nurse may wish to review before giving nose drops. She also will need to instruct the patient in self-administration. This procedure may be uncomfortable for some patients, especially children.

THE PATIENT. While nasal decongestants do have value, as a general rule there is a great tendency to overuse this type of medication. If used as directed with long enough intervals between doses, they will provide fairly good relief. When used too frequently, they tend to cause rebound congestion or continuous swelling of the nasal mucosa, resulting in delayed recovery. The patient may need reinforcement to understand how often to use nasal drops and how much solution is required for each administration.

Acute Sinusitis

DEFINITION. An acute infection of the mucosa of any or all of the paranasal sinuses (I-2), acute sinusitis is caused most commonly by hemolytic streptococci, staphylococci, pneumococci or *Haemophilus influenzae* (III-1, 2, 3). It is probable that the viruses of the common cold and influenza are involved as well.

MAJOR SYMPTOMS. Starting most frequently with a catarrhal stage of acute rhinitis, the symptoms become more pronounced as the rhinitis subsides. Mucus or mucopus is discharged from the anterior and posterior nares. There is an associated sore throat, with irritation of the larynx and trachea and a productive cough. Headache over the affected sinus is usually present and often there is tenderness on pressure over the affected bone. Nasal congestion is to be expected, and fever, malaise and anorexia are frequently present.

DRUG THERAPY. ANALGESIC-ANTIPYRETICS. To relieve the pain associated with sinusitis, one of the simpler analgesic-antipyretic drugs such as *aspirin* or *acetaminophen* (Tylenol) is usually effective. In more severe forms, codeine may be required, alone or in one of a number of combinations.

In severe cases, especially if there is mucopurulent drainage, one of the broad-spectrum antibiotics may be used until culture and sensitivity test disclose which specific drug will be most effective. Occasionally, one of the sulfonamide preparations may be indicated.

Many people say they have "sinus." This of course is a misuse of the term. Actually few people have an infection in the sinuses. The patient with acute sinusitis well realizes the difference (III-2). As in acute rhinitis, the patient must understand the value of the correct use of nasal decongestants and must not overuse them since overdosage will aggravate the condition (V-1).

NASAL DECONGESTANTS. Some physicians feel that the restricted use of a nasal decongestant is indicated to assist in keeping the nasal passages open to facilitate drainage. (See Acute Rhinitis.)

Acute Pharyngitis and Tonsillitis

DEFINITION. These conditions are acute inflammations of the lymphoid tissues of the pharynx (I-3), caused by a number of organisms (III-1) but more commonly by group A hemolytic streptococci. Throat cultures should be taken to determine the actual organism.

MAJOR SYMPTOMS. The onset is usually abrupt with a sore throat soon causing severe pain on swallowing. A chill often follows, with a rapid rise in the temperature and marked malaise, and the anterior cervical lymph nodes at the angle of the jaw become swollen and tender. This infrequently may develop into a peritonsillar abscess (quinsy sore throat).

DRUG THERAPY. ANALGESIC-ANTIPYRETICS. Beside rest in bed and other such measures, the use of one of the more common analgesic-antipyretic drugs—*aspirin* or *acetaminophen* (Tylenol)—is helpful in relieving the pain and fever accompanying these conditions. Some physicians feel that gargling powdered aspirin (five 0.325 mg. [5 gr.]) tablets dissolved in one-half glass of hot water) is often helpful. Hot saline or 5 to 10 per cent glucose throat irrigations every two to three hours provide some relief. Anesthetic throat lozenges relieve some of the soreness.

ANTIBIOTICS. *Penicillin* is the drug of choice if it is not contraindicated. The dosage and times will depend upon the age of the patient and the seriousness of the condition. If penicillin cannot be used, *erythromycin, tetracycline,* or another suitable antibiotic may be given.

ATELECTASIS

DEFINITION. Atelectasis is a collapse of the alveoli of the lungs and may be simple or massive in character. Simple atelectasis may be caused by shock, embolus, foreign bodies, trauma or pneumonia (I-5, 7). The cause of massive atelectasis is uncertain, but most cases follow anesthesia and surgical operations on the abdomen or may follow some physical injury.

MAJOR SYMPTOMS. In simple atelectasis there may be no symptoms or only a dyspnea, tachypnea, some cyanosis and tachycardia. The symptoms that appear in massive atelectasis appear in no other disease and are, therefore, pathognomonic of the condition. About 24 to 48 hours postoperatively the patient suddenly has dyspnea, tachypnea, cyanosis, tachycardia and pain (usually in the lower part of the thorax). The temperature, pulse and respirations rise and the chest wall on the affected side looks flat, with respiratory movements diminished or absent. The patient is very apprehensive (V-2). The condition may be rapidly fatal or may spontaneously subside in a week or ten days.

DRUG THERAPY. The medical treatment is by no means curative but purely for the relief of symptoms. The cause, if possible, should be removed by bronchoscopy. Expectorants such as *syrup of hydriodic acid* 1 to 2 teaspoonfuls three times daily or *potassium iodide* 0.3 to 0.4 Gm. four times daily may be used. To relieve the bronchospasm present, an aminophylline preparation is often used.

Intermittent administration by positive pressure of aerosols such as Bronkosol (isoetharine hydrochloride 1.0 per cent, phenylephrine hydrochloride 0.25 per cent, in a buffered solution or *isoproterenol hydrochloride,* U.S.P. (Isuprel; isoprenaline [C]), in a 1:200 solution (see Bronchitis). The use of postural drainage after bronchodilation may help. Pneumonia almost always develops in 24 hours so it is common to give antibiotics early. *Penicillin,* 600,000 units q 6 h., and *streptomycin,* 0.5 Gm. b.i.d. or 1.0 Gm. daily, intramuscularly for seven days usually are sufficient. For those allergic to penicillin, *tetracycline,* 250 mg. four times a day for seven days, may be substituted.

The best treatment is prevention and this can be done by changing the position of the patient, encouraging deep breathing and mechanically aspirating mucus from the throat.

INFLUENZA

DEFINITION. Influenza is an acute, self-limited, specific, infectious disease of man caused by a virus of the influenza group (A, B and C). It is often epidemic in proportions.

MAJOR SYMPTOMS. The onset is usually abrupt, with chilliness or a frank chill, fever, headache, malaise, lassitude, anorexia and muscular pains. Symptoms referable to the respiratory tract are not marked. The temperature may be elevated to 101 to 103° F.

DRUG THERAPY. There is no specific treatment for influenza but some measures can be taken to relieve the symptoms. Bed rest is recommended and fluids should be taken very freely. *Aspirin,* U.S.P., 0.3 to 0.6 Gm. two to four times daily, helps relieve the headache, malaise and myalgia. Some physicians prescribe, early in the disease, a combination of *codeine sulfate,* 16 mg., and *aspirin,* 0.3 Gm., with or without caffeine, 30 mg., two to four times a day to provide relief for the irritability, cough and substernal pain. For the cough which may be present, any of the many preparations of codeine or dihydrocodeinone may be used. If the cough is not too severe, one containing dextromethorphan may be effective. Continuous steam inhalations are helpful but the value of tincture of benzoin added to this is questionable.

No effective antimicrobial therapy against this viral infection has been found. Secondary infections due to bacterial invasion are so rare that most physicians do not feel it advisable to administer an antibiotic.

Many people advocate the use of large doses of vitamin C for prophylaxis, treatment or both. Scientifically controlled evidence available at present fails to support such use.

There are vaccines available to prevent influenza that will provide protection for 6 to 12 months. There are monovalent vaccines and bivalent vaccines available; the latter are preferable. They are considered to be about 70 per cent effective provided they are given two weeks or more before exposure and that the vaccine contains the same strain of virus prevalent in the community. The difficulty here is that there are many different strains, especially of type A, and each strain does not appear every year in every area. The U.S. Public Health Service regulates the production of this vaccine on a yearly basis, trying to predict which type will appear in different regions of the United States. Usually 1 ml. (cc.) is given subcutaneously in the September to November period and repeated in six to eight weeks.

The vaccine is prepared as a killed suspension from the embryonated chicken egg; therefore this vaccine should not be given to those with a history of sensitivity to eggs, chicken and chicken feathers. The vaccine should be readily available to those who are essential to the conduct of community life (policemen, doctors, nurses, military personnel), those who live in groups (boarding schools, military camps and so forth) and to those who are particularly vulnerable to infections—older persons, those with chronic diseases such as diabetes and those with cardiac, renal or pulmonary disorders.

BRONCHITIS

DEFINITION. An inflammation of the tracheobronchial tree, bronchitis may be caused by a chemical or physical agent or one of the common pathogenic species of *Streptococcus, Staphylococcus, Diplococcus, Hae-*

mophilus or viruses (I-5, 6, 7) (III-1, 2). The disease may be acute or chronic. The acute form is a self-limited disease. The chronic state is one of long standing and there are definite fibrotic, inflammatory and atrophic changes in the bronchial structure.

MAJOR SYMPTOMS. In acute bronchitis the onset is most frequently that of an acute upper respiratory infection with chilliness, malaise, aches and pains, headache, a dry scratchy throat and mild fever, with a corresponding rise in pulse and respiratory rates. Cough may not appear for several days. The cough is at first dry, irritative and nonproductive. After a few days, the patient brings up a scanty viscid sputum which gradually progresses to a looser cough with more abundant and mucopurulent sputum. Though the fever and malaise usually subside in four or five days, the cough and sputum often continue for two or three weeks (V-5).

Chronic bronchitis is an inflammation which recurs from year to year; with each successive attack the sputum and cough are more troublesome.

DRUG THERAPY

ANTIBIOTIC THERAPY. In acute bacterial bronchitis, the administration of one of the antibiotics in average doses may shorten the course of the disease and serves to prevent chronic problems.

EXPECTORANTS AND ANTITUSSIVE AGENTS

THE DRUGS. The term expectorants has led to considerable confusion in classification, arising largely from the use of the terms sedative and stimulant. Since neither means what it appears to mean, no attempt will be made here to classify expectorants into any particular class. With the advent of the new antitussive agents, the classification of expectorants has become less important. Expectorants here are considered to be substances which aid in expectoration, whereas antitussive agents inhibit the cough reflex through the cough center in the central nervous system. Both expectorants and antitussic agents are used in the treatment of bronchitis.

To help in the liquefaction of mucus, the simplest effective method is by using *saturated solution of potassium iodide*, N.F., 10 to 30 drops (in juice) four times daily, or a preparation containing glycerol guaiacolate in doses from 100 to 300 mg. q 4 h may be substituted.

Provision for additional moisture to the inspired air by means of aerosol therapy helps to prevent drying of the bronchial secretions. If wheezing is present, the doctor may order one of a number of drugs that can be used by nebulization. *Isoproterenol hydrochloride*, U.S.P. (Isuprel, isoprenaline [C]) is supplied as a "Mistometer," the sulfate comes as the "Medihaler." *Acetylcysteine* (Mucomyst), a derivative of the amino acid cysteine, reduces the viscosity of the secretions when administered by inhalation. Alevaire, an aqueous solution of 0.125 per cent tyloxapol, 5.0 per cent glycerin and 2.0 per cent sodium bicarbonate, acts as a detergent on the mucous membrane of the bronchial tubes. The package insert should be consulted before using these preparations. These drugs relieve bronchospasm, shrink swollen mucous membranes and reduce the secretion of mucus. They exert a mild expectorant action by liquefying tenacious mucus. These drugs should not be given with epinephrine though they may be used alternately. They are frequently given by means of the intermittent positive pressure apparatus (I.P.P.B.) or with a hand nebulizer. Many institutions now employ inhalation therapists (or specialists) who administer the drugs for loosening and removal of the mucus and who give oxygen and other gases. This does not entirely relieve the nurse of responsibility, since she may be called upon to watch the patient after the therapist leaves and/or give the treatment when the therapist is not available.

Although coughing is a protective mechanism, if it is overdone it may compound the irritation on a mechanical basis. Nonproductive coughing should be discouraged. *Codeine sulfate* in small doses every three or four hours may be used but is addicting.

The newer antitussive agents are usually more effective. All the presently known antitussives act either by raising the threshold of central neurons to sensory impulses or by reducing the number of afferent impulses going toward the medullary cough regulating mechanism (I-8). Some have a central depressant action and also possess secondary peripheral effects. Some of the centrally acting drugs are used mainly for relief of pain and depress the respiration and the associated cough reflex. Others with a varied chemical structure have relatively specific depressant action on the cough mechanism with little, if any, analgesic action or effect on respiration.

Benzonatate, N.F. (Tessalon), is believed to exert its antitussive action by a combination of peripheral and central effects. This drug is a chemical congener of the local anesthetic tetracaine and acts on the vagal stretch receptors. This results in fewer impulses being transmitted centrally. It is believed also that this drug may act centrally to depress polysynaptic spinal reflexes producing a reduction of the transmission of tussal impulses to the cough center. Some physicians use this drug before passing a nasogastric tube. They believe that it suppresses the gag reflex, making the passage of the tube easier for the patient. Benzonatate is given orally in doses of 100 mg. three to six times a day and acts rapidly (within 15 to 20 minutes). Its action lasts from 3 to 8 hours.

Another of the effective antitussives is *dextromethorphan hydrobromide,* N.F. (Romilar), which is related to levorphanol, a synthetic analgesic. It, however, does not possess analgesic action or addicting properties. The drug is usually given orally to adults in doses of 10 to 20 mg. one to four times a day. For children over four years, the dose is reduced to one-half, and to one-fourth for children under four years.

Dimethoxanate hydrochloride (Cothera), a phenothiazine derivative, possesses antitussive, local anesthetic and mild antispasmodic properties. It is believed that this drug acts centrally to depress the cough reflex and is as effective as codeine with a duration of action which is shorter than that of codeine. If slight drowsiness occurs, the patient should neither drive a car nor operate machinery. The usual dose is 15 to 30 mg. three or four times daily.

Still another effective antitussive agent is *carbetapentane citrate,* N.F. (Toclase), which is a phenyl cycloalkane carboxylic acid ester. It seems to have atropine-like and local anesthetic properties and is believed to act selectively on the medullary center suppressing the cough reflex. Given orally, the usual dose for adults is 15 to 30 mg. three to four times a day. For children, the dosage is reduced proportionately.

Many other antitussive agents are available; refer to the Current Drug Handbook.

Almost all of these drugs have some drying action but this is not excessive and does not increase the viscosity of mucus in the respiratory tract.

Cough syrups may be helpful for they tend to reduce afferent impulses arising in the respiratory tract by decreasing the local irritation. There are too many cough syrups to mention them all individually. Many of them contain glycerol guaiacolate with various other ingredients. Elixir of terpin hydrate with or without codeine is still used by some physicians. Most of these drugs are given in 5 ml. doses every three or four hours. The various preparations may contain codeine, dextromethorphan, a sympathomimetic, an antihistamine or other ingredients. Those containing antihistamines are more valuable in asthmatic bronchitis patients. In asthmatic bronchitis, other treatment includes the drugs used for asthma (epinephrine, ephedrine and aminophylline), which are discussed under Asthma (Chapter 25).

The Nurse. The nurse must dilute liquid iodides with either milk, water or fruit juice as they are very bitter and salty. Also, they are given in such small doses that they would be lost in administration unless this is done.

Whenever any iodine preparation is used, the nurse must be constantly alert for symptoms of iodism, which include a brassy taste, a burning sensation in the mouth, sneezing and irritation of the eyes. The patient often complains of severe headache. Skin lesions resembling acne may be present. Gastric disturbances and fever are common. Should any of these appear, the nurse should report them immediately to the physician and stop the medication until further orders are received.

If a cough syrup is used, it may be left at the patient's bedside (unlike other medications) so that he may sip it at frequent intervals as needed. No water should be taken with or for a short time after taking a cough syrup, for this defeats its purpose.

An apprehensive patient is made more anxious by tickling or irritation in the throat or chest. The alert nurse will see that the needed medication is readily available to relieve this condition. She should observe and report the results of these drugs, for if one does not relieve the coughing, another drug may.

Aerosol therapy may be given in the hospital with an I.P.P.B. machine (see Bronchiectasis) or by the use of the small hand nebulizer. The nurse must know how these operate and keep them scrupulously clean.

Side effects from the antitussives (rare) include drowsiness, dizziness, headache and gastric intolerance. If dimethoxanate hydrochloride (Cothera) is used, it is well for the nurse to remember that this is a phenothiazine derivative and is subject to the same untoward effects. Refer to Chapter 30 for further details.

The nurse will encourage the patient to get as much rest as possible and to limit the amount of exposure to others. Additional nursing measures would include forcing fluids and an adequate diet. Additional methods (other than drugs) may be instituted to relieve nonproductive coughing. These might include tea with lemon, sips of honey, and carbonated beverages.

THE PATIENT. Patients who are receiving iodides for any appreciable period should be alerted to contact their physician should any of the symptoms of iodism appear.

If benzonatate (Tessalon) is used, the patient should be instructed not to chew the capsule or allow it to dissolve in the mouth for it exerts a local anesthetic effect on the mucosa that is disagreeable.

The nurse will need to encourage the patient to suppress as much of the irritating nonproductive coughing as possible. Frequently the coughing will interfere with sleep and cause the patient to be further irritated. When the cough becomes productive, it may be more comfortable to be in a sitting position to cough. This phase of illness is most uncomfortable and the patient will require a lot of assurance and encouragement.

MISCELLANEOUS DRUGS. In acute bronchitis, to relieve the malaise and lessen the fever, *aspirin,* 0.3 Gm., every four to eight hours is often used. Steam inhalations may also be helpful, especially in the acute stages.

BRONCHIECTASIS

DEFINITION. A pathologic state of the lungs characterized by dilatation of the bronchi, bronchiectasis more commonly follows some other pulmonary disease such as

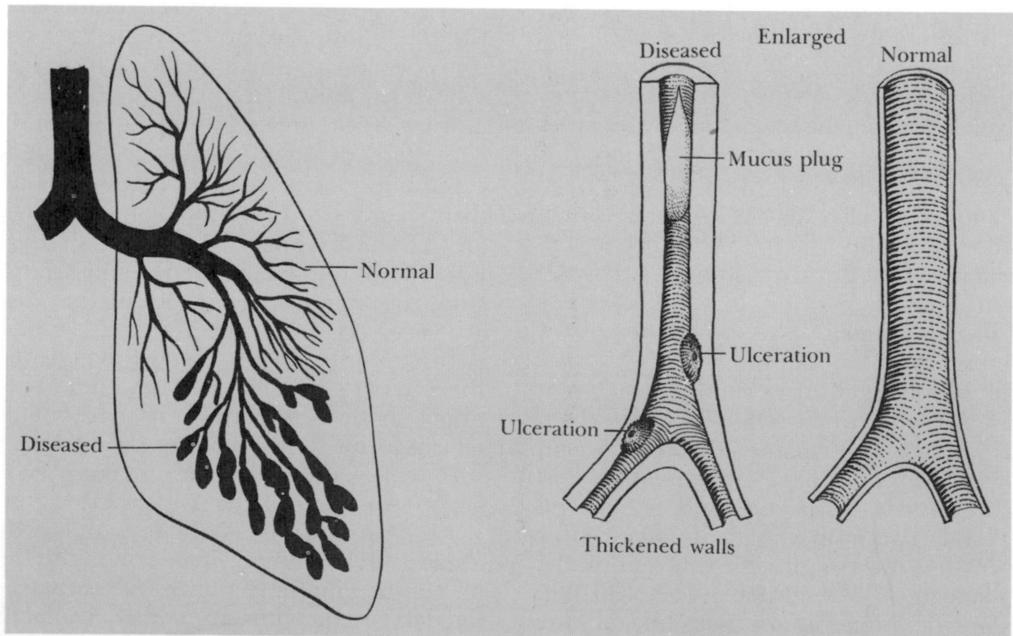

FIGURE 25. Bronchiectasis. Proteolytic enzymes liquefy plug (especially layer next to wall) freeing plug which can then be coughed up (expectorated). Used in various respiratory conditions. Bronchodilators also aid in the removal of plugs.

bronchopneumonia or lung abscess (I-5, 7; III-1). The anatomic changes which appear are permanent.

MAJOR SYMPTOMS. A chronic productive cough is often the first sign of the existence of bronchiectasis. The quantity of sputum is often copious in amount and is usually yellowish or light greenish in color. The sputum often has a fetid odor and hemoptysis is common. Pain in the chest is present only if there is a complicating pleurisy or empyema. Positive diagnosis is made after an x-ray using iodized oil or after bronchoscopic examination.

DRUG THERAPY. Although the only cure for bronchiectasis is resection of the diseased portion of the lung, medical treatment is very helpful in providing for the general comfort of the patient and in preparing him for surgery. Medical treatment usually includes, besides the drug therapy, the use of postural drainage (Fig. 25).

COUGH MEDICATIONS. Medications for the alleviation of the cough in bronchiectasis are generally of little value. Some authorities believe it is undesirable to suppress the cough except when it is exhausting or painful. Although expectorants may not be totally effective, cough syrups containing glycerol guaiacolate may aid in loosening the tenacious secretions. *Codeine* in 15 to 30 mg. doses may be used during acute exacerbations, most frequently with terpin hydrate as a vehicle. These drugs have been discussed in detail under Bronchitis.

Hemoptysis is often alarming to the patient (V-2, 3) and medication may be needed. Along with complete bed rest and reassurance, some mild sedative may be ordered. Morphine is seldom used because of its property of depression of the respirations and cough center.

ANTIMICROBIAL DRUGS. Antibiotic treatment is used mainly for those acutely ill who have purulent sputum. The tetracyclines are effective in doses of 250 mg. four times a day given with food to minimize gastrointestinal upsets. Both penicillin and streptomycin are effective against specific organisms, but this is often difficult to determine for it is often a mixed infection. Sulfonamides are less effective than the other antimicrobials.

Some physicians believe that cyclic therapy is best, using one of the antibiotics for five to seven days each month or three to six days every two weeks. The drugs may be alternated to help reduce the possibility of the development of resistant strains.

INHALATION THERAPY

THE DRUGS. The use of intermittent positive pressure breathing (I.P.P.B.) is often recommended for those patients who have severe impairment of pulmonary function with marked hypoxemia and retention of carbon dioxide. There are several kinds of apparatus available (Fig. 26) which will administer oxygen and drugs in this manner. They are all designed to assist breathing by inflating the lungs more completely during inspiration under safe, controlled oxygen pressure and to permit free unrestricted passive exhalation without pressure. This mechanism helps the oxygen and drugs to penetrate farther into the pulmonary tree than would be accomplished by normal breathing. The addition of bronchodilator drugs also promotes better bronchial drainage. At the beginning of an expiration, there is a rapid release of the inspiratory pressure (because of a "flow-sensitive" valve) and this results in a high velocity of expiration. Thus, obstructions due to mucus plugs are reduced or eliminated. This "flow-sensitive" valve permits complete patient control of the breathing rhythm—in fact, the patient's rate of breathing sets the pace of the machine. As the oxygen is forced through the nebulizer with the prescribed drugs, the medications are blown into the lungs.

Oxygen alone may be used, but more frequently drugs are added. *Isoproterenol* (Isuprel), a bronchodilator, or *bronkosol* may be used in the nebulizer. (See Atelectasis.) The systemic antibiotic therapy may be supplemented by the addition of either penicillin or streptomycin to the nebulization. The choice of medications and dosages is strictly individualized for each patient. The patient usually has his treatments ordered for one to two or more times a day and it takes from 10 to 20 minutes to nebulize the medications prepared for him.

THE NURSE. The intermittent positive pressure breathing (I.P.P.B.) apparatus is arranged so that, after the nurse has prepared the proper medication and placed it in the attached nebulizer (Fig. 26), the patient is instructed to breathe slowly and deeply at his own rate of respiration. The nurse should be sure that the mask fits

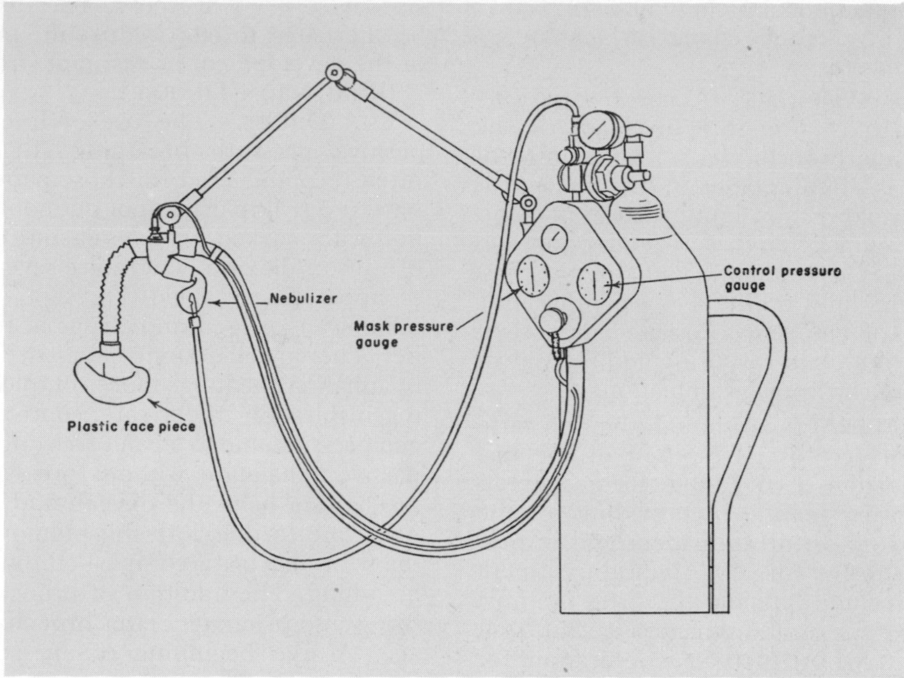

FIGURE 26. The Bennett Valve. One of the several types of intermittent positive pressure breathing apparatus available. The plastic face mask must be cleaned thoroughly after each use. The nebulizer is detachable and the ordered medication is placed therein. The control pressure gauge is set at the prescribed pressure (normally between 12 and 20 cm.). The mask pressure gauge fluctuates with each respiration of the patient, registering the volume of each breath.

snugly over the mouth and nose, for any mask leakage will make inhalation difficult.

This machine is very delicate and the nurse must acquaint herself thoroughly with its operation before attempting to use it. After each patient has had his treatment, she must clean the nebulizer by rinsing in clear, warm water and remove and wash carefully those parts that came in contact with the patient. In addition, the nurse must be sure that the pressure control gauge is set at the prescribed control pressure. If the large size oxygen cylinder is used, it should give between 15 and 20 treatments of 20 minute duration.

To many patients this type of treatment may at first be alarming, and the nurse must reassure the patient that it is a perfectly painless operation and easy for him to do (V-1, 2, 3). She may demonstrate the machine on herself first.

If the patient cannot use the intermittent positive pressure (I.P.P.B.) apparatus or the respirations are seriously affected, a direct positive pressure respirator may be required. In many areas this latter type of apparatus has largely replaced the intermittent type. Again, the inhalation therapist may perform this treatment.

The Patient. When the nurse has fitted the mask to the patient's face, she will find that he usually prefers to hold it himself though it may be strapped to his face. He must understand that deep breathing is essential but should not be carried to the point of fatigue. He sets his own pace of breathing. He should understand, also, that inhalation should not be difficult and if it is, he should tell the therapist or the nurse so that proper adjustments can be made (IV-4). The patient should understand that this type of treatment is not curative but will probably give him considerable relief (I-5, 6, 7; V-1, 5; VI-1). The patient must be taught how to do postural drainage and its purpose.

EMPHYSEMA

DEFINITION. Emphysema is a condition of the lungs in which the alveoli are abnormally dilated and there is often a rupture of the alveolar walls. Prolonged hyperinflation of the lungs may be a cause and the condition is often found in chronic asthma (IV-3; V-1). Chronic bronchitis often accompanies this condition.

MAJOR SYMPTOMS. Usually insidious in onset, the patient suffers from gradually increasing dyspnea on exertion, a cough, cyanosis and asthmatic attacks. When the condition has been present for years, the patient presents a typical picture of what is often called a "barrel shaped" chest. Deep breathing causes wheezing and the movement of the chest is chiefly upper costal in character (IV-2). These patients seem very prone to develop upper respiratory infections.

DRUG THERAPY. Though drug therapy does not cure the condition, much can be done for the symptomatic relief of the patient by improving pulmonary ventilatory function and preventing recurring respiratory infections (I-6, 9; III-1; IV-1). Sedatives and narcotics should be avoided as they depress ventilation.

ANTIMICROBIAL DRUGS. During the periods of an acute exacerbation of the accompanying tracheobronchitis, one of the antibiotics is usually prescribed. It is advisable to do a culture of the sputum to determine the specific microbes present so that the proper drug may be given. Intramuscular *penicillin* in doses of one to two million units a day may be given or one of the *tetracyclines,* 1 to 2 Gm. daily, may be used. These drugs may be used in aerosol therapy also. There is some disagreement among clinicians, but some believe that continuous or intermittent antimicrobial therapy is indicated, especially during the winter months. A tetracycline is usually given in this instance.

EXPECTORANTS. Because of the persistent and tenacious sputum produced by the patient, *potassium iodide* may be used. It is given most frequently as the saturated solution in doses of from 10 to 15 drops three to four times daily. This tends to liquefy the sputum and make it easier to expectorate. The usual precautions whenever iodides are administered apply here. (See Bronchitis.) The conventional cough remedies are not usually given but should the cough be severe, one of the drugs with codeine may be used.

BRONCHODILATORS

THE DRUGS. This group of drugs has probably proved more effective than any other in relieving the symptoms of the disease for, by causing bronchodilation, they make breathing easier for the patient (I-9; V-2, 3). The antihistamines have been tried but, as a rule, are not too effective.

Ephedrine orally in 25 mg. doses every four hours may be effective or may be used in combination with *aminophylline* or *phenobarbital,* U.S.P., 15 mg. *Aminophylline,* U.S.P., is sometimes used alone in 0.2 Gm. doses orally. If the bronchial spasm is especially severe, aminophylline may be administered intravenously but the use of this drug does not produce a uniform response.

Isoproterenol, U.S.P. (Isuprel), is an adrenergic agent that has almost pure beta effects. Its main therapeutic action in the respiratory system occurs in the bronchi by relieving bronchospasm, shrinking swollen mucous membranes and reducing secretion of mucus. It is used alone in doses of 0.25 to 0.5 Gm. orally or rectally. After inhalation, the drug tends to liquefy tenacious mucus, thus producing a mild expectorant action. By aerosol therapy not more than 0.5 ml. (cc.) of a 1:200 solution or 0.1 to 0.3 ml. (cc.) of a 1:100 solution should be used for each dose. Bronkosol, mentioned earlier, or racemic epinephrine in a strength of 2.25 per cent may also be used.

THE NURSE. The nurse will need to allow this type of patient adequate time for rest in order to conserve energy, especially as the emphysema becomes progressively worse. To facilitate the air flow, varying positions may be suggested to the patient. Orthopnea is not uncommon and these patients do better sitting up. Breathing exercises aid in ventilating the lungs, and the nurse will need to teach and supervise the patient doing these exercises. It may also be necessary to decrease the number of respiratory irritants such as smoking.

The nurse must become acquainted with the operation of various nebulizers, including the hand nebulizer so that she may assist the patient in any way possible.

Isoproterenol should not be given at the

same time as epinephrine but the two drugs may be used alternately.

Often the appetite is very poor but the expenditure of energy is high. Therefore, a well balanced diet plus increased amounts of fluids are vital. Added nutrients supply the required energy, and the hydrated condition results in thinner secretions.

Coughing will remain a problem. The nurse can help by supporting the chest and teaching adequate coughing techniques. She may also do tapping, cupping, vibrating and clapping to aid with postural drainage.

Vital signs are constantly monitored. Any indication of increase in heart rate, blood pressure, or pallor (cyanosis is a late sign) should be promptly reported. These, in addition to restlessness, may indicate pulmonary obstruction.

If the patient is to use the I.P.P.B. machine, the nurse should observe him carefully during the treatment. This procedure should not fatigue the patient, and the period of assisted ventilation that can be tolerated is limited.

The Patient. Emphysema is a chronic disease and the patient must understand that he will continue to have some adverse symptoms. He should be warned that smoking, respiratory infections (such as colds) or any inhalatory irritant will increase his difficulties. There will be "good days and bad days."

He must learn to use various equipment such as the inhalator and intermittent positive pressure machine and to supervise postural drainage and administer oxygen by mask or nasal catheter. It is extremely frightening to experience the inability to obtain sufficient oxygen. If he relies too much on drugs or mechanical equipment he may become overly dependent on his family or the health care personnel. Reassurance and confidence are difficult to convey when every breath is an effort.

These patients are often restless and their appetite is poor. However, they must be encouraged to eat a well balanced diet. Several small meals are much better than three large ones. Exercises should be undertaken in a limited amount at first but increasing as much as possible without fatigue as time goes on. Rest periods during the day are beneficial.

The patient will need the assistance of the nurse, his family and any community resources available to help him to readjust his life in view of his limitations and to prevent further disability.

CORTICOSTEROIDS. Physicians do not agree on the advisability of using the corticosteroids in emphysema. It is felt by some that any value for long-term administration is outweighed by the potential complications of their use. (See Corticosteroids, Chapter 27.) They are sometimes effective when bronchospasm is a major complication. One method is to give orally a very high initial dose (40 mg. or more) of *prednisone* or its equivalent. Very soon it can be determined whether this drug will be effective. If it is, the aim is to reduce the daily dose gradually to a minimum of 5 mg. of the drug, if possible. The better way seems to be to give the drug by the aerosol method, three to four times daily. An intermittent positive pressure breathing (I.P.P.B.) apparatus is often used in conjunction with the hand inhalers. (See Bronchiectasis.)

Oxygen Therapy. This type of therapy is used cautiously, for with the decreased ventilation of the patient with emphysema, there is a build up of carbon dioxide tension in the arterial blood. The administration of oxygen injudiciously removes the hypoxic stimulus to ventilation and so further increases carbon dioxide tension. Current methods indicate that if oxygen is to be used, it should be started through a nasal catheter at 1 to 2 liters flow rate. The patient is watched closely for increased somnolence or apnea. If no serious effects appear, the rate may be increased in gradual increments under careful observation.

PULMONARY EDEMA

DEFINITION. As the term implies, pulmonary edema means a grossly abnormal amount of fluids in the lungs. This is actually the case, for there is an escape of serous fluids from the capillaries into the lung tissues, alveoli, bronchioles and often even into the bronchi. Most often it is a factor in general systemic collapse and may be acute or chronic and is often associated with cardiocirculatory collapse or pneumonia. The whole or part of one lung or both lungs may be involved.

MAJOR SYMPTOMS. The onset may be gradual or sudden, with the patient complaining of a feeling of oppression or pain in the chest. The breathing is rapid, with dyspnea or orthopnea, and the patient is bothered with an incessant short cough. Apprehension is marked. He expectorates a copious frothy sputum, sometimes blood tinged, which seems to gush from the mouth and nose. The patient presents a typical picture of shock and, unless adequate measures are taken promptly, the prognosis is poor.

DRUG THERAPY. Mild attacks may pass by themselves, but severe and progressive forms necessitate vigorous treatment, which is often lifesaving.

If the edema is caused by a cardiocirculatory collapse, sedation in the form of *morphine sulfate,* 15 mg., or sometimes *meperidine,* 50 to 200 mg. may be used. *Oxygen* under positive pressure is a definite aid in clearing the respiratory passages if the patient is not in acute shock. (See Fig. 26.) The increased pressure of the oxygen pushes the fluid out of the lungs back into the venous end of the pulmonary capillaries, thus increasing the oxygen intake of the blood (I-5, 6, 7, 8; IV-3, 4). Rapid digitalization may be indicated in frank heart failure. (See Chapter 18.) Intravenous aminophylline, 0.25 to 0.5 Gm. given slowly, may be of real help by decreasing fluid in the lungs and promoting diuresis.

When the pulmonary edema is due to pneumonia, sedation may be used but the cough reflex must be protected; hence, morphine may be contraindicated. Oxygen is undoubtedly useful for the cyanosis and dyspnea, but the use of the I.P.P.B. machine is more effective in asthma and emphysema than in pneumonia. Bronchodilators may be used if the bronchospasm is severe. (See Bronchiectasis.) Vigorous antibiotic therapy is given as indicated.

THE NURSE. This type of emergency involves expert nursing care and observation. Vital signs should be monitored almost continuously. In particular, respiration should be monitored for rate, type, audible sounds, character of secretions, and cyanosis. Any mental change, agitation or restlessness may indicate a decreased blood flow and lowered oxygen uptake. Fluid intake and output should be carefully recorded.

The nurse will need to explain to the patient the various procedures used, such as monitoring of central nervous pressure, and what they are expected to do. During the acute stage, the patient should not be left unattended.

THE PATIENT. Pulmonary edema is a very frightening experience. If the patient survives, the convalescence may be long, and if the edema was the result of a chronic cardiac disorder such as congestive heart failure, there may be only partial recovery, since there will still be the heart condition to treat. (See Chapter 18.)

No matter what the cause, limitation of activities will be necessary to conserve body energies. When ambulation begins, assistance must be provided. Exercise should be increased very gradually, and frequent undisturbed rest periods must be provided. Often, these patients are more comfortable in a semi-Fowler's position in bed or sitting in an easy chair than lying down. The "air chairs" are especially good.

Dietary restrictions may be difficult, but often these patients have previously been on a restricted diet. If sodium is to be avoided, other flavorings do help. There are salt substitutes available and lemon juice or spices may make the unsalted food more palatable.

If the patient indicates in any way that he is harboring fears of dying, he should be not only allowed but encouraged to express these fears. "Talking them out" to a sincerely concerned and interested listener is often a great relief.

During the acute stage, the family also will probably need reassurance and help. They should be allowed to express their fears (away from the patient) and, insofar as is possible, at least one member of the family might stay with the patient most of the time. This may interfere with the hospital rules, but there are times when rules should be set aside.

PULMONARY INFARCTION (PULMONARY EMBOLISM)

DEFINITION. Pulmonary infarction is caused by an embolus or thrombus in the pulmonary artery, or one of its branches, with a resultant mass of airless lung tissue infiltrated with blood. As would be expected, the interruption in the blood supply severely damages the affected area (I-6, 9). It may be rapidly fatal.

MAJOR SYMPTOMS. Too often pulmonary infarction occurs without warning and the patient dies before anything can be done. The patient may complain of a sudden piercing pleural pain which radiates to the shoulder and which may or may not be accompanied by dyspnea. There is an irritating cough with hemorrhagic sputum and the temperature, pulse and respiration rates rise. Signs of collapse are soon present (V-2).

DRUG THERAPY. The object of treatment here is to prevent the formation of more emboli and to treat symptomatically. The patient should be at bed rest in a sitting position and all sudden effort avoided.

GENERAL THERAPY

THE DRUGS. The alleviation of symptoms is one of the first considerations in the therapy of pulmonary infarction. *Morphine sulfate*, or *meperidine*, U.S.P. (Demerol), in the usual doses by hypodermic are often given for the dyspnea, pain and apprehension. The drug may have to be repeated in 15 to 30 minutes and it may be given even in the presence of cyanosis or collapse. Oxygen therapy by tent is helpful in relieving the dyspnea and cyanosis (see Fig. 29). To reduce bronchial spasms and secretions, some physicians may use the intravenous administration of *atropine sulfate*, 0.6 to 1.0 mg., or *papaverine* 30 to 60 mg., but their value is highly controversial. *Aminophylline*, U.S.P., 250 to 500 mg. by either suppository, intramuscular or slow intravenous method, is often helpful when dyspnea is prominent or pulmonary edema is present. (See Chapter 27.) Antitussive agents are used for cough (see Bronchitis). Prophylactic doses of an antibiotic are usually indicated to prevent bacterial invasion of the lungs. *Procaine penicillin*, 600,000 units one to two times daily, or one of the broad-spectrum antibiotics may be used.

Levarterenol bitartrate, U.S.P. (norepinephrine bitartrate; Levophed), 4 to 8 mg. per 100 ml. or *metaraminol bitartrate*, N.F. (Aramine), 50 to 100 mg. in 500 or 1000 mg. isotonic saline or 5 per cent dextrose, by slow intravenous infusion may sustain the arterial blood pressure through the critical period. Metaraminol bitartrate has a more gradual onset, a more prolonged duration and a smoother action than some of the other drugs. Other drugs which may be used to help maintain the blood pressure include *methoxamine hydrochloride*, U.S.P. (Vasoxyl), in doses of 10 to 15 mg. intramuscularly. In emergencies, the drug may be given slowly intravenously in doses of 5 to 10 mg.

THE NURSE. When the nurse observes the signs of impending pulmonary infarction, she should call the doctor immediately and then collect the drugs and equipment which may be needed in emergency treatment for possible complications such as shock, pulmonary edema or cardiac arrhythmias. The patient should never be left alone in this situation.

Even if the condition is not life threatening, the nurse must continue to observe carefully for dyspnea, tachycardia, pleuritic chest pain, apprehension or agitation.

The nurse will need to prepare the patient for the various therapeutic techniques which may be used, such as chest x-ray, lung scanning, electrocardiograms, continuous monitoring, anticoagulant therapy, or pulmonary artery embolectomy.

It will be the responsibility of the nurse to frequently check the blood pressure and adjust the rate of flow of the infusion to maintain the pressure. The prolonged duration of action of metaraminol bitartrate (Aramine) may result in a cumulative effect. In view of this, at least ten minutes should elapse before the dosage (rate of flow) is increased. If methoxamine hydrochloride (Vasoxyl) is being given by slow intravenous drip, the usual rate of flow is one drop every 20 seconds.

THE PATIENT. The patient may be extremely alarmed over his condition. The nurse will then need to direct the entire health team to become sensitive to the patient's feelings and requirements.

The patient who has sustained a massive embolism will often develop complications such as cerebral vascular accident, myocardial infarction, gastrointestinal infarction or acute renal failure. Such a setback is apt to cause considerable depression. Working through the feelings may take some time.

The patient will need help in observing other limitations placed on his mode of living. First passive, and then active, exercises will aid in maintaining and regaining his strength. Larger doses of drugs will be ordered to prevent recurrence of the embolism and the nurse can teach the patient what these drugs are and how to follow a new regimen which includes oral anticoagulants, unhurried activities, regular rest periods and ample fluids to prevent hemoconcentration. The patient must understand that he is not to take any form of aspirin without the doctor's permission, since aspirin and the anticoagulant drugs enhance each other. Special emphasis should be placed on avoiding cuts and bruises while taking anticoagulant drugs to avoid bleeding that might become serious.

Anticoagulant Therapy. Anticoagulants should be started immediately to lessen the danger of recurrent and frequently fatal embolic accident. It is not universally agreed as to the best approach, for some clinicians prefer *heparin*; others, a combination of *heparin and coumarin*; and still others, *coumarin* alone. Heparin does have the advantage of rapid action and more potent antithrombotic effects but it must be given parenterally. These drugs are discussed in detail under Myocardial Infarction (Chapter 18). The usual precautions in their use prevail here. If hemorrhagic complications develop during the administration of heparin, protamine sulfate is used. The dose is determined by the amount of heparin that has been given. For the coumarin type anticoagulants, *vitamin* K_1 *oxide* is given if bleeding occurs. Both protamine sulfate and vitamin K_1 oxide are administered parenterally.

PNEUMOCOCCAL PNEUMONIA

DEFINITION. Pneumococcal pneumonia is an acute bacterial infection of the lungs characterized by its abrupt onset with chills and fever, chest pain, cough and bloody sputum. It is caused by pneumococcus (III-1), a gram-positive diplococcus. There are many types of this organism.

MAJOR SYMPTOMS. The onset is usually sudden, with a severe chill and chest pain which is stabbing in character. The temperature rises rapidly to 103 to 106° F., and the patient is extremely ill. Cough may be absent at first but soon becomes prominent, with the patient raising a bloody or "rusty" sputum. Respirations are limited by pain and each inspiration is often accompanied by a grunting sound.

DRUG THERAPY

Antibiotics. Prompt use of antimicrobial therapy usually brings the disease to a dramatic halt. At the present time, *penicillin* is the drug of choice. This is usually given intramuscularly in aqueous penicillin G, 600,000 to 1,000,000 units four times a day for the first 24 hours. The dose may then be changed to 600,000 to 1,200,000 units of aqueous procaine penicillin every 12 hours. The oral route is seldom used as it requires larger doses and is much slower to act. The pneumococcus does not seem to develop resistance to penicillin.

The *tetracyclines* and *erythromycin* may be used, particularly when a diagnosis has not been clearly established. The usual dose is 0.5 to 1.0 Gm. by mouth every six hours. It must be remembered that when the broad-spectrum antibiotics are used, there is always the danger of developing a staphylococcus enteritis. Erythromycin has been shown to be about as effective as penicillin or the tetracyclines. Treatment should be continued until the patient has been afebrile for 48 to 72 hours.

Alertness for side and untoward effects of the drug must be ever in the nurse's thoughts. If oral penicillin is used, it should not be given just preceding or immediately following a meal. The presence of food further reduces the amount of the drug absorbed and delays the attainment of adequate blood levels.

The patient should understand that the drug cannot be discontinued too early or there may be a relapse or complications.

Analgesics. For pleural pain, the physician may order *codeine*, U.S.P., 30 to 60 mg. orally. If the pain is especially severe, *morphine sulfate*, 10 to 15 mg., or an equivalent analgesic such as *methadone hydrochloride*, U.S.P. (Dolophine, Amidone), 5 to 10 mg. subcutaneously or orally, may have to be used.

Oxygen. *Oxygen* is given to help relieve the dyspnea and cyanosis. If the tent is used, the concentration should be 40 to 60 per cent oxygen; if the nasal catheter is used it is recommended to be at 35 to 50 per cent at 4 to 7 liters per minute.

Supportive Therapy. Fluids and electrolytes are usually given because of the loss of essential body fluids due to the high body temperature.

ATYPICAL (VIRAL) PNEUMONIA

DEFINITION. Primary atypical pneumonia is an acute infectious disease in which there is a varying degree of pulmonary infiltration.

MAJOR SYMPTOMS. In most cases the onset is gradual. The patient suffers from headache, malaise, chilly sensations, sore throat and photophobia. Cough is an outstanding feature and its absence makes the diagnosis questionable. At first, the cough is dry and paroxysmal; later, it becomes productive and mucoid or mucopurulent in character. Frequently the sputum may be blood streaked. The patient complains of a pain in his chest, which is usually substernal in location and aggravated by cough. Anorexia is prominent; in some cases, there may even be nausea and vomiting. The patient is acutely but not seriously ill. The temperature usually ranges from 102 to 104° F. In about 50 per cent of the cases, there is a relative bradycardia present which is of some diagnostic value.

DRUG THERAPY. There is some disagreement over whether or not the use of antimicrobial therapy is warranted. However, some physicians feel it wisest to use one of the *tetracyclines* in about 0.5 Gm. doses every six hours until the temperature falls to normal. The dose is then usually reduced to 0.5 Gm. twice daily and continued for another three days. If side reactions such as nausea, vomiting and diarrhea occur, it may be necessary to reduce the amount of the drug or discontinue therapy.

To help control the cough, *codeine,* 15 to 60 mg., is usually ordered. This will also be useful to relieve the headache and malaise. One of the new antitussive agents may be used (see Bronchitis).

Steam inhalations are very helpful to relieve the soreness and dryness of the upper respiratory passages.

The Nurse. These patients should be kept at bed rest and a limited (respiratory) isolation maintained. Even though there is often rather severe chest pain, the nurse must assist the patient to deep breathe every hour. As soon as there is sputum, the patient is also encouraged to cough and expectorate every hour. The tissue used is deposited promptly in a throwaway paper bag. The nurse will obtain a specimen of the sputum for culture and sensitivity testing. Vital signs are especially important. Any dyspnea or increased pulse or respiratory rate may indicate a further extension of the disease. Oxygen should be available for use. Rales may be heard on auscultation. The areas where they are heard should be noted and any extension recorded and reported. X-rays are usually taken frequently to note the extent of lung consolidation and effect of therapy.

The Patient. The patient may resist enforced bed rest, even limited isolation and decreased activities. He will be more cooperative if he understands that these measures are intended to hasten his recovery and to prevent others from contracting his illness.

Anorexia and halitosis are not uncommon symptoms. Frequent oral care and the preparation of appetizing small meals will aid in overcoming these conditions. The patient is encouraged to take ample fluids, but these need not be limited to water. Fruit juices, "soft drinks" and the like are usually more acceptable.

Coughing may be persistent and annoying. This is taxing and tiring for the patient. Therefore, remedies other than cough syrups may be used, such as limiting talking and smoking, sucking on hard candy and use of environmental humidifiers.

EMPYEMA

DEFINITION. Empyema is often a result or extension of the pneumococcic process, indicating the presence of pus of inflammatory origin in the pleural cavity (III-1). The pus is thick and purulent in character. This condition may be acute or chronic.

MAJOR SYMPTOMS. Usually it appears before another lung disease has subsided. The patient complains of dyspnea, a productive cough with a purulent sputum and unilateral pain and discomfort in the chest. The fever is intermittent in character and profuse diaphoresis is common. On observing the patient, it is noticed that there is a limited respiratory movement on the affected side. X-ray examination usually confirms the presence of pus in the pleural cavity (V-3).

DRUG THERAPY

Antibiotic Therapy. Against gram-positive cocci (pneumococcus, hemolytic streptococcus and the staphylococcus), the intrapleural injection of *penicillin* is often very useful. Though penicillin may be given, and often is, by the intramuscular route in these infections, the concentration of the drug is not sufficient in the pleural fluid to be very helpful. In empyema, from 50,000 to 200,000 units of aqueous penicillin may be injected into the lesion on alternate days, followed by aspiration of this area after 24 hours. If the causative organism becomes resistant to penicillin, some other antibiotic may be used effectively. Suggested substitutes for penicillin include methicillin sodium (Staphcillin) (meticillin, Synticillin [C]) 1.0 to 2.0 Gm. q 6 h.; nafcillin sodium (Unipen) 1.0 Gm. q 4 to 6 h; oxacillin sodium (Prostaphlin) 1.0 Gm. q 4 to 6 h; and clindamycin hydrochloride hydrate (Cleocin, Dalacin C [C]) 150 mg. q 6 h.

LUNG ABSCESS

DEFINITION. Lung abscess is caused by a variety of microorganisms (III-1). There is a localized area of suppuration in the lung tissue and cavitation may be present. If the extent of necrosis is massive, it is usually referred to as gangrene of the lung.

MAJOR SYMPTOMS. Lung abscess may at first simulate bronchitis or pneumonia, but by the end of the second week the patient is coughing up pus which often has a foul odor. There is some pain in the chest which is worse on deep breathing, and a high fever is usually present (V-1, 2, 3).

DRUG THERAPY. Some beneficial effects may result from drug therapy, though surgical excavation of the abscess is the usual treatment. The choice of the antibiotic depends upon the organism present. For pneumococci, streptococci, spirochetes and fusiform bacilli, systemic *penicillin* in very large doses is usually used. If nonspecific bacteria are present, a combination of *penicillin* and *streptomycin* may be used. One of the broad-spectrum tetracyclines in doses of 0.5 Gm. orally every 6 hours is frequently effective.

To help in the evacuation of accumulated secretions, an expectorant such as *ammonium chloride* or *glycerol guaiacolate* can be used in conjunction with postural drainage.

Aerosol therapy often supplements other treatment. Sometimes *isoproterenol hydrochloride* (Isuprel) or *phenylephrine hydrochloride* (Neo-Synephrine) is used to help shrink the inflamed mucosa. (See Emphysema.) Another substance that may help is the mucolytic agent *acetylcysteine* (Mucomyst) 10 to 20 per cent every 4 to 6 hours. It tends to loosen tenacious sputum.

Supportive therapy should include bed rest, high fluid intake, highly nutritious diet, vitamin supplements and even blood transfusions as indicated.

The Nurse. When trypsin is used, the patient should rinse his mouth with water after the aerolization. This is to prevent soreness of the mouth from the medication. Bronchospasm may occur during the nebulization of these drugs, and the patient should be watched carefully and reassured.

If ammonium chloride is used, it should be given before meals and at bedtime, followed by a glass of hot water to aid in the evacuation of the secretions.

The nurse must be alert for a possible vitamin K deficiency if there is prolonged administration of one of the broad-spectrum antibiotics.

TUBERCULOSIS

DEFINITION. Tuberculosis is an infectious disease caused by *Mycobacterium tuberculosis* (III-3). The organism may attack any organ in the body, but by far the majority of cases are pulmonary. Tuberculosis is still one of the most widespread of all diseases; it occurs in almost every climate and in every race. It can and does affect all age groups.

MAJOR SYMPTOMS. The symptoms of tuberculosis will vary with the part of the body affected but there are a few symptoms which occur in all cases: loss of weight, fever especially in the afternoon, fatigue and a general feeling of debility. In pulmonary tuberculosis, cough may be a factor.

DRUG THERAPY. A vaccine against tuberculosis, the BCG (bacille Calmette Guérin), has been used in some other countries for several years. The vaccine was not always successful, but recent refinements have made it much better and its use is being expanded.

CHEMOTHERAPY. Present-day chemotherapy for tuberculosis is not entirely encouraging. Patients often have to take drugs for years and, in some instances, still are not cured (V-1, 4, 5; VI-1, 2). After drug treatment, the incidence of regression is alarmingly high. Best results seem to be achieved by a combination of drugs, surgery and inactivity. The tuberculostatic agents exert their action by preventing the susceptible organism from reproducing at the usual rate as long as it is exposed to effective quantities of the given drug. At the present time, it is believed that chemotherapy merely holds the infection effectively in abeyance, allowing nature to take its course unhindered. When the body's natural defenses are poor or entirely lacking, even the most potent drugs are of little effect. The bacterium very rapidly becomes resistant to chemotherapeutic agents.

Most physicians treating tuberculosis patients use two or three drugs concurrently, since this practice seems to be more effective than one drug given alone. Resistant strains of the organisms develop more slowly. Whenever possible, a bacterial culture and a sensitivity test are done and the starting drugs are selected on this basis. Often, one injectable and two oral drugs are given. One such combination includes isoniazid, streptomycin and ethambutol.

ISONIAZID

THE DRUG. Isoniazid is a synthetic drug which is considered to be one of the better chemotherapeutic agents in the control of tuberculosis.

Physical and Chemical Properties. Isoniazid, the hydrazide of isonicotinic acid, is a white crystalline powder that is freely soluble in water. The pH of a 1 per cent solution is between 5.5 and 6.5.

Action. The exact action of this drug is not known. It is believed to be both bacteriostatic and bactericidal. Resistant strains develop—in some patients faster than in others.

Therapeutic Uses. Isoniazid is used primarily for tuberculosis. It is also used for the newly converted positive tuberculin patient to prevent the development of the active disease.

Absorption and Excretion. Isoniazid is readily absorbed from either the oral or the parenteral route. After oral administration, peak blood levels are reached in one to two hours. The drug has a half life of about six hours and in some patients tuberculostatic amounts of the drug can be detected for as long as 24 hours. Simultaneous use of another antituberculosis drug tends to hold the blood level higher than when isoniazid is used alone. Isoniazid diffuses readily into all body fluids and cells. From 50 to 70 per cent of the drug is excreted in the urine within 24 hours, some unchanged, some as products of degradation. The amounts differ with different individual patients.

Preparations and Dosages

Isoniazid, U.S.P., B.P. (isonicotinic acid hydrazide, Niconyl, Rimifon, Nydrazid, and others). 50 to 200 mg. (not to exceed 10 mg. per kg. or 600 mg. per day). The drug is preferably given orally once daily, but the dose may be divided, with the doctor's permission, into two or three smaller ones if better tolerated by the patient.

THE NURSE

Mode of Administration. Isoniazid is usually given in tablet form and presents no real problem. It is also prepared as a syrup which is valuable for use with children.

Side Effects, Toxicity and Treatment. Untoward side effects and toxicity, directly related to dosage level, are rare if the dose is kept within the limits mentioned earlier. The concomitant administration of pyridoxine 50 mg. greatly diminishes the toxic effects, especially those related to the nervous system.

Isoniazid may produce fever and skin rashes as symptoms of hypersensitivity. Its most serious and common toxic effect is on the nervous system—peripheral neuritis. Other undesirable side effects, which reducing dosage and alkalinizing the patient help to counteract, include pruritus, constipation, dysuria, postural hypotension, dizziness, drowsiness, headache and anemia.

Contraindications. Isoniazid should not be given if the patient is taking adrenergic drugs. It should be used cautiously, if at all, in patients who are elderly or who have renal impairment.

Patient Teaching. As with all antitubercular drugs, isoniazid is usually given for an extended period of time at home. The nurse should not only explain to the patient—or his family—how and when the drug is to be given, but also impress him with the importance of reporting *any adverse* symptoms to the physician at once.

THE PATIENT. What is said here applies as well to all of the antitubercular drugs. Tuberculosis presents a deep emotional shock to the patient (V-1, 4). One thing the nurse can do is dispel some of the fiction and misconception surrounding the disease.

The essence of patient teaching involves developing an attitude that will allow for physical and mental rest. The patient will need to learn how the disease process may be arrested and how to control his life so as to prevent a recurrence. The nurse can aid him in setting up a regimen which would include adequate rest, a nutritious diet, mild exercise and a continuance of the medical therapy. He will need to avoid stressful situations and fatiguing exercise.

The patient with limited means faces a real financial crisis (VI-1). Again, the nurse can help by directing him to agencies whose purpose it is to offer assistance—financial and otherwise.

Patience and understanding are very important to the isolated patient. He may feel rejected by his loved ones and by the health personnel as well. Special effort will be necessary on the part of all concerned to help the patient feel accepted and not neglected.

If the patient is to be cared for at home, the nurse will need to instruct him and the family in various isolation techniques which will be required to prevent the spread of the organisms. Susceptibility is usually highest in children under three years of age and in those who are undernourished. Other family teaching will relate to diet, restful environment, regular daily schedules and the need for some quiet recreation.

The patient must realize that, although treatment is protracted, recovery is the rule, not the exception. Departure from previous living conditions will be radical, with modification of occupation and leisure activities necessary. The nurse can do much to help the patient and the family begin these critical adjustments. Referral may be made to the public health nurse for continuity of care.

STREPTOMYCIN. For the tubercular patient, streptomycin is given parenterally in doses not exceeding 1.0 Gm. daily. If streptomycin is given alone, resistance by the organism develops rapidly. However, when given with other antitubercular drugs, resistance is considerably delayed. Some nurses and other personnel who handle streptomycin, especially over an extended period, develop hypersensitivity to it. This can be avoided in most cases by wearing rubber gloves during preparation and administration of the drug. Streptomycin is never without danger. Damage to the eighth cranial nerve resulting in hearing loss is the most serious toxic effect. For additional details refer to Chapter 7 and Current Drug Handbook.

ETHAMBUTOL HYDROCHLORIDE

THE DRUG. Ethambutol is a synthetic compound first developed in 1961. It was found to be effective against tuberculosis in mice. Later, its use in human tuberculosis was demonstrated.

Physical and Chemical Properties. Ethambutol is an odorless, white crystalline compound. It is water soluble and heat stable. There are several chemically related forms of the drug, but the D-isomer is the only one used in the treatment of human tuberculosis.

Action. The exact action of the drug is not known. It is thought to interfere with the production of metabolites essential for the replication of the mycobacteria. Resistant strains develop slowly when ethambutol is given with other antituberculosis drugs.

Therapeutic Uses. Ethambutol is used in the treatment of tuberculosis both as a primary and a secondary drug, according to circumstances.

Absorption and Excretion. Of the orally administered drug, about 75 to 80 per cent is absorbed. Plasma levels reach a maximum in 2 to 4 hours. About 50 per cent of the peak level concentration is present at 8 hours, less than 10 per cent in 24 hours. Ethambutol enters the red blood cells readily and this may account for the length of time the drug remains in the body; a small amount is released as plasma levels fall. The drug is excreted in the urine and feces almost unchanged, but some is in the form of metabolites, an intermediary aldehyde and a terminal butyric acid derivative.

Preparations and Dosages

Ethambutol hydrochloride (Myambutol) 15 mg. per kg. as a single dose, orally, initially. For retreatment, 25 mg. per kg. as a single dose, orally. After 60 days reduce to 15 mg. per kg.

THE NURSE

Mode of Administration. Ethambutol is given orally, one dose daily in the morning.

Side Effects, Toxicity and Treatment. Ethambutol appears to be relatively nontoxic. However, a reversible diminishing loss of visual acuity and color discrimination may occur. Before beginning therapy, an ophthalmological examination should be done, including testing of color vision. This should be repeated at intervals during therapy. In a few instances the visual loss did not clear up when the drug was discontinued, but in most cases a reduction of the dose usually suffices. The higher the dose, the greater the possibility of the vision's being involved. The seeing of green as gray or white is the type of color distortion that occurs. There are a number of side effects. See Current Drug Handbook for details.

Patient Teaching. (See Isoniazid.)

THE PATIENT. (See Isoniazid.)

OTHER DRUGS USED IN TREATMENT OF TUBERCULOSIS. It was stated previously that whenever possible a culture and sensitivity test were done to determine the best drugs to use for the particular patient being treated. The three drugs so far considered may or may not be the best ones for a specific patient. When retreatment is required for a patient whose symptoms subside, but who is again showing signs of the disease, other drugs usually are needed. It is often found that the organisms are resistant to the original medicines. There are several other drugs that may be substituted. Some of these include the following.

DRUGS GIVEN ORALLY

Ethionamide (Trecator, Trescatyl [C]) is a synthetic derivative of isonicotinic acid which is effective in varying degrees in pulmonary tuberculosis. It should be given in conjunction only with other antituberculosis drugs since, if it is used alone, bacterial resistance rapidly develops. Ethionamide may cause various side effects such as anorexia, nausea, vomiting, postural hypotension, depression, drowsiness and asthenia. It is advisable that, during therapy, urine and hepatic functions be checked frequently. Ethionamide is given orally, 250 to 1000 mg. daily, usually in divided doses. It is common to start with a small dose and increase it each day until the maximum is being given.

Pyrazinamide (Aldinamide) is a synthetic antitubercular agent of moderate potency. Like other drugs of similar use, it is more effective when combined with other preparations. When given alone, bacterial resistance develops within a few weeks. Pyrazinamide is likely to be hepatotoxic; consequently, it is ordinarily reserved for the severely ill patient who either does not respond to or cannot tolerate the less toxic preparations. Untoward symptoms include arthralgia, anorexia, nausea, vomiting, dysuria, malaise and fever. Pyrazinamide is given orally, 25 to 35 mg. per kg. either three or four times daily, and no more than 3 Gm. should be given in any 24 hours.

Rifampin (Rifadin) is a synthetic drug used for the treatment of tuberculosis. Like pyrazinamide, it may be hepatotoxic, possibly to a lesser degree. It is used with caution in patients with known liver damage. Rifampin is believed to inhibit DNA-dependent RNA polymerase activity in susceptible bacterial cells. It is given orally. The dosage is usually 600 mg. once daily. As with other drugs of this kind, the dose may be divided if better tolerated by the patient. It is usually given with at least one other antituberculosis drug. Patients should be warned that this drug colors the urine orange.

Aminosalicylic acid, U.S.P. (PAS and many other trade names) has been used as an antituberculosis agent for a long time. However, it is now used less, since newer preparations are equally or more effective and better tolerated by the patient. Aminosalicylic acid, to be of maximum value, must be given in large doses (as much as 12 to 16 Gm. a day) either in one dose, or divided into two, three, four or five portions in 24 hours. The exact mode of action is not known. It is relatively nontoxic but gastrointestinal symptoms such as anorexia, nausea, vomiting, abdominal distress and diarrhea may occur. Because of the large size of the dose and the gastrointestinal discomfort, it is difficult for the patient to continue taking the drug long enough for it to be effective. It is usually given with other antituberculosis drugs to delay the development of resistant strains.

Cycloserine, U.S.P., B.P. (Seromycin) is an antibiotic derived from *Streptomyces orchidaceous* which is active against gram-positive, gram-negative and acid-fast bacteria. However, its use is restricted to the treatment of tuberculosis. It can be given orally or parenterally, but the former is the preferred route. Parenteral use is reserved for the seriously ill patient. This drug is neurotoxic, causing mental confusion and convulsions in some patients. If these occur, the dose should be reduced or another drug substituted. It is contraindicated in epilepsy. It is presumed to act by competing with D-alanine as a cell wall precursor. As with most antituberculosis drugs, it is rarely, if ever, given alone. The dosage is 0.25 to 0.5 Gm. t.i.d. orally. Other side effects include somnolence, headache, tremors, vertigo and paresis.

DRUGS GIVEN PARENTERALLY

Viomycin (Vinactane, Viocin), *kanamycin* (Kantrex) and *capreomycin* (Capastat) are all given parenterally and share ototoxicity with *streptomycin*, to a greater or lesser extent. They are used interchangeably with streptomycin and each other as the patient's reactions and organism susceptibility dictate.

Viomycin sulfate (Vinectane, Viocin), produced by *Streptomyces puniceus* or *floridae*, is commonly used for patients who cannot take streptomycin or in whom resistant strains have developed. Viomycin is given parenterally in doses of 0.5 to 1.0 Gm. b.i.d., often only every third day. If the drug is administered intramuscularly, a fresh injection site should be used each time, and the drug introduced slowly. Viomycin in dry form can be stored at room temperature indefinitely. If the drug is in solution, the unused portion should be kept refrigerated, under which conditions it will keep for about one week. Viomycin is relatively toxic and can trigger allergic reactions, signs of renal damage, labyrinthine or hearing disorders and electrolyte imbalance.

Kanamycin (Kantrex), another antitubercular agent, is usually given by intramuscular injection in doses of 10 to 15 mg. per kg. Total daily dose should not exceed 1.5 Gm. It is similar to streptomycin in toxicity since it is liable to cause damage to the eighth cranial nerve with resultant loss of hearing and disturbances in equilibrium. Regular audiograms and blood urea nitrogen tests should be carried out routinely during therapy. Any difficulty in hearing should be reported promptly to the physician. Carbenicillin should not be mixed in the same intravenous fluid as kanamycin, since both drugs will be inactivated.

Another of the injectable antituberculosis agents is *capreomycin sulfate* (Capastat). Capreomycin is a polypeptide antibiotic isolated from *Streptomyces capreolus*. As with most antituberculosis drugs, it is used concurrently with at least one other antituberculosis drug. Capreomycin is given intramuscularly 1.0 Gm. daily. Peak blood level is reached in 1 to 2 hours and there is a low serum residue at the end of 24 hours. However, a build-up of the drug does not usually occur. Some cross resistance has been noted between capreomycin and viomycin and to a lesser degree with kanamycin and neomycin. None has been observed with isoniazid, ethambutol, streptomycin, cycloserine, ethionamide or aminosalicylic acid. Capreomycin shares with the other parenteral antituberculosis agents the possible side effects of ototoxicity and nephrotoxicity.

ANTITUSSIVE AGENTS. It is best for the patient to suppress the cough if at all possible and to expectorate by a gentle clearing of the throat. For a distressing cough in those who may have developed a bronchitis, steam inhalations, perhaps with the addition of some medication such as *creosote* or *tincture of benzoin*, may be helpful. If the cough cannot be controlled otherwise, it may even be necessary to give *codeine*, 30 mg., at three to four hour intervals or longer. This will usually permit the patient to get sufficient needed rest.

MISCELLANEOUS DRUGS. Should significant hemoptysis occur, the patient should have rest in bed and be reassured justifiably by the nurse that the bleeding will subside. Some physicians feel that it is best at this time to give the patient 30 to 60 mg. of *codeine* by hypodermic. Morphine is very seldom used as it depresses reflexes unduly and may permit the retention of clots in the bronchi.

IT IS IMPORTANT TO REMEMBER

1. That restriction of breathing can be very alarming to the patient; but with a calm and understanding attitude, the nurse can do much to allay this apprehension.
2. That the nurse should have thorough knowledge of the operation and care of the intermittent positive pressure machine before attempting to assist the patient with its use.
3. That cough remedies are usually given without water.
4. That pulmonary infarction (pulmonary embolism) and edema are medical emergencies that require prompt treatment. The nurse should be prepared to meet such emergencies and should watch for any premonitory symptoms which might indicate an oncoming attack.
5. That there are no medications which are specific in the treatment of acute rhinitis (the common cold).
6. That health teaching is one of the most important duties of every nurse, and at no time does she have a better opportunity than when she is caring for the patient with a respiratory disorder.

TOPICS FOR STUDY AND DISCUSSION

1. Describe the patient with a pulmonary infarction and explain what means are taken to combat this.
2. With the assistance of the instructor and several members of the class, demonstrate how the intermittent positive pressure machine is used in your hospital.
3. Your patient shows signs of pulmonary edema. What type of therapy will the doctor order? How might this condition have been prevented?
4. How and for what reasons are the iodides used in respiratory diseases? For what conditions are they probably best?
5. The capsules of chlortetracycline contain 250 mg. The order is for 4 Gm. a day in divided doses. How many capsules must you give at each time to divide it into four equal parts?
6. In the hospital ward, find a patient who is receiving intermittent positive pressure breathing. Find out what medications are ordered for his use on the machine and figure out how you would prepare these.
7. Demonstrate how you would teach a patient to give himself nose drops.
8. What percent is the solution formed when five, gr. 5 tablets of aspirin are dissolved in 200 ml. of water (for a gargle)?
9. Why are antituberculosis drugs usually given in combinations?
10. Describe the possible toxic effects of long-term therapy with streptomycin or kanamycin.
11. What nursing measures might you institute to relieve a tickly, nonproductive cough?

BIBLIOGRAPHY

Books and Pamphlets

American Medical Association, Council on Drugs, *Drug Evaluations*, Chicago, 1971, American Medical Association.
Asperheim, M. K., *The Pharmacologic Basis of Patient Care, 2nd Ed.*, Philadelphia, 1973, W. B. Saunders Co.
Beeson, P. B., and McDermott, W., *Cecil-Loeb Textbook of Medicine, 13th Ed.*, Philadelphia, 1971, W. B. Saunders Co.
Beland, I. L., *Clinical Nursing, 2nd Ed.*, New York, 1970, The Macmillan Co.
Bergersen, B. S., *Pharmacology in Nursing, 12th Ed.*, St. Louis, 1973, The C. V. Mosby Co.
Bevan, J. A., *Essentials of Pharmacology*, New York, 1969, Harper and Row.
Chatton, M. J., Margen, S., and Brainerd, H., *Handbook of Medical Treatment, 12th Ed.*, Los Altos, California, 1970, Lange Medical Publications.
Conn, H. F., et al., *Current Therapy, 1974*, Philadelphia, 1974, W. B. Saunders Co.

Gangong, W., *Review of Medical Physiology*, Los Altos, California, 1969, Lange Medical Publications.
Goodman, L. S., and Gilman, A., *Pharmacological Basis of Therapeutics, 4th Ed.*, New York, 1970, The Macmillan Co.
Govani, L., and Hayes, J., *Drugs and Nursing Implications*, New York, 1971, Appleton-Century-Crofts.
Hartshorn, E. A., *Handbook of Drug Interactions*, Cincinnati, 1970, University of Cincinnati Press.
Kalan, K. T., and Weinstein, L., *Antimicrobial Therapy*, Philadelphia, 1970, W. B. Saunders Co.
Passmore, R., and Robson, J. S., (Eds.), *A Companion to Medical Studies, Vol. II*, Oxford and Edinburgh, 1970, Blackwell Scientific Publications.
Shafer, K. M., et al., *Medical-Surgical Nursing, 5th Ed.*, St. Louis, 1971, The C. V. Mosby Co.
Watson, J. E., *Medical-Surgical Nursing and Related Physiology*, Philadelphia, 1972, W. B. Saunders Co.

Journal Articles

Block, V. C., "Helping the patients to ventilate," *N.O.* 17:31 (October, 1969).
DiPalma, J. R., "Drugs for tuberculosis," *R.N.* 29:53 (July, 1966).
DiPalma, J. R., "Oxygen as drug therapy," *R.N.* 34:8:49 (1971).
DiPalma, J. R., "Enzymes used as drugs," *R.N.* 35:1:53 (1972).
DiPalma, J. R., "The why and how of drug interactions," *R.N.* 33:3:63 (March, 1970).
DiPalma, J. R., "The why and how of drug interactions," *R.N.* 33:4:67 (April, 1970).
DiPalma, J. R., "The why and how of drug interactions," *R.N.* 33:5:69 (May, 1970).
Foley, M. F., "Pulmonary function testing," *Am. J. Nurs.* 71:6:1134 (June, 1971).
Gaul, A. L., Thompson, R. E., and Hart, G. B., "Hyperbaric oxygen therapy," *Am. J. Nurs.* 72:5:892 (May, 1972).
Helming, M. G., et al., "Symposium on nursing in respiratory diseases," *Nurs. Clin. North Am.* 68:4 (September, 1968).
Itkin, I., "The pros and cons of exercise for the person with asthma," *Am. J. Nurs.* 66:7: 1584 (July, 1966).
Lamy, P. P., and Rotkowitz, I. I., "The common cold and its management," *J. Am. Pharm. Assoc.* NS 12:11:582 (November, 1972).
Mushlin, I., and Nayer, H. R., "Big city approach to tuberculosis control," *Am. J. Nurs.* 71:12:2342 (December, 1971).
Nut, L. M., and Thomas, P., "Acute respiratory failure," *Am. J. Nurs.* 67:9:1847 (September, 1967).
Nut, L. M., and Thomas, P., "Why emphysema patients are the way they are," *Am. J. Nurs.* 70:6:1251 (June, 1970).
Nut, L. M., and Thomas, P., "Pulmonary care unit," *Am. J. Nurs.* 70:6:1247 (June, 1970).
Rodman, M. J., "Drugs used for respiratory tract infections," *R.N.* 34:9:55 (September, 1971).
Rodman, M. J., "Drugs for bacterial pneumonias," *R.N.* 34:11:55 (November, 1971).
Schwaid, M., "The impact of emphysema," *Am. J. Nurs.* 70:6:1247 (June, 1970).
Sedlock, S., "Detection of chronic pulmonary disease," *Am. J. Nurs.* 72:8:1407 (August, 1972).
Soni, M., and Jacob, I., "Use of cuffed tracheostomy tube," *Am. J. Nurs.* 67:6:1854 (June, 1967).
Tatro, D. S., "Current therapeutic concepts—Tuberculosis," *J. Am. Pharm. Assoc.*, NS 12:2:76 (February, 1972).
Totman, L., and Lehman, R., "Tracheostomy care," *Am. J. Nurs.* 64:3:96 (March, 1964).
Vaughan, V. C., III, "The place of drug therapy in childhood asthma," *Am. J. Nurs.* 66:5: 1049 (May, 1966).
Weg, J. G., "Tuberculosis and the generation gap," *Am. J. Nurs.* 71:3:53 (March, 1971).

CHAPTER 17

DRUGS USED FOR DISORDERS OF THE GASTROINTESTINAL SYSTEM

CORRELATION WITH OTHER SCIENCES

I. ANATOMY AND PHYSIOLOGY

1. The walls of the stomach have four coats and the inner or mucosal layer contains the small glands which secrete the gastric juices.
2. The stomach has very slow rhythmic contractions upon which are superimposed from time to time strong peristaltic waves which open the pyloric sphincter and cause the stomach to eject some of the stomach mixture into the duodenum.
3. The secretion of gastric juice is stimulated by both reflex and hormonal mechanisms.
4. Liquids leave the stomach rapidly, but a fatty meal will delay the emptying time.
5. The vomiting center is in the medulla. Vomiting is a complex reflex involving contraction of the muscles of the stomach, the diaphragm and the abdomen.
6. Peristalsis is the movement of the intestines which propels the food along and is composed of alternate longitudinal and horizontal contractions and relaxations of the intestinal musculature.
7. The liver is the largest gland in the body and secretes bile essential in the digestive process. This bile is being formed continuously by the liver and drained into the gallbladder where it is temporarily stored.
8. Besides processing certain foods for general body use, the liver acts upon waste and toxic materials before they are excreted from the body.

II. CHEMISTRY

1. The gastric juice, which is a clear fluid, contains normally about 99 per cent water and 0.2 to 0.5 per cent hydrochloric acid as well as mucus and the important enzymes pepsin and rennin.
2. The pancreas secretes a fluid which is important to proper digestion. This fluid is clear and alkaline in reaction and it also contains several enzymes—trypsinogen, amylase and lipase.
3. Although some digestion does take place in the stomach, the major portion occurs in the intestines.

III. MICROBIOLOGY

1. Bacteria are classified in several ways; by shape—bacilli (rods), cocci (spheres), spirilli (spiral); by staining reaction—gram-negative, gram-positive, and acid-fast; by spore formation—form spores, do not form spores; by oxygen requirement—aerobic (require oxygen), anaerobic (do not require oxygen), facultative (can adapt to either), obligate (must have or not have oxygen).
2. The Gram stain is a general stain used to separate bacteria into two main groups. Those that are gram-positive retain the dark stain and appear bluish-black under the microscope. Those that take the counter stain, appearing pink or reddish under the light microscope, are called gram-negative.
3. Spirochetes are slender, flexible, coiled organisms that resemble both protozoa and the true spiral bacteria.

4. Fusiform bacilli are spindle-shaped organisms with pointed ends.
5. Bacteria occurring in chains have the prefix "strepto," those in bunches, "staphylo," and those in pairs, "diplo."
6. Microorganisms which may cause an infection in the intestinal tract include bacteria such as *Salmonella, Shigella, Staphylococcus, Streptococcus* and *Pneumococcus*, protozoa such as *Entameba histolytica*, and fungi such as *Candida*.

IV. PHYSICS

1. Absorption is the penetration of the molecules of a substance into the body of another substance.

V. PSYCHOLOGY

1. Emotions are believed to be involved in the development of some gastrointestinal disorders.
2. It is especially important in peptic ulcer and ulcerative colitis for the patient to exercise self-control and wise judgment in the choice of foods and activities.
3. Many people falsely believe they are suffering from constipation and, as a result, resort to the over-use of various laxatives. Proper health habits and good mental hygiene can do much to correct this.
4. The unwise use of alcoholic beverages may lead to serious disturbances of the gastrointestinal tract or its associated organs, such as the liver.
5. Most people experience an almost instinctive repulsion at the sight of a worm. This is probably due to attitudes passed from parents to children.

VI. SOCIOLOGY

1. The therapy required in some of the diseases of the intestinal tract is not infrequently of long duration and may well constitute a drain on the family finances.
2. Sociologic elements combined with emotions are sometimes a factor to be considered in the development of some of the diseases of the intestinal tract.
3. Fear of social ostracism is a potent factor in the life of everyone. Everyone desires to be liked by his peers.
4. Crowded living and working conditions are conducive to the spread of some microorganisms and other agents that can infect the gastrointestinal tract.

INTRODUCTION

Diseases and disorders of the gastrointestinal system form a large segment of man's ailments. Since the body is an integrated whole, disturbances in one area will affect, to a greater or lesser degree, all other parts of the body. This is especially true of the digestive system, since it supplies the whole body with the "fuel" to maintain heat and provide energy. If the gastrointestinal tract or its accessory organs do not function properly, digestion is impaired. The food may not be prepared sufficiently for absorption, or the process of absorption may be delayed or blocked.

Some gastrointestinal disorders can be treated by improvement of the diet, many are treated surgically, but drugs play a part in the majority of cases. Exclusive of the communicable diseases, many of the disorders are more or less chronic. This necessitates treatment over extended periods of time, which can be most discouraging to the patient. The nurse will need all her powers of persuasion to help the patient adjust to the situation and continue treatment even if the results are not immediately discernible.

A number of the disorders of the gastrointestinal system appear to have a psychosomatic background. Many are long-term (chronic) illnesses.

Diseases and Disturbances of the Gastrointestinal Tract

DISEASES AND DISORDERS OF THE MOUTH AND ESOPHAGUS

Although oral diseases (glossitis, stomatitis, pyorrhea) are relatively common, medical therapy is limited. Many of these conditions are the result of disorders outside the gastrointestinal tract, and as soon as the underlying cause is removed, the mouth condition improves. A number of others are due to dental disorders. Improvement in dental care may be the treatment needed. Mouthwashes of various types are helpful as are antiseptic-anesthetic lozenges. If there is ulceration, the physician or dentist may treat it by direct application of an astringent or an anti-infective to the ulcer.

Exclusive of peptic ulceration (discussed with gastric and duodenal ulcers) disorders of the esophagus are usually treated by surgical means or by altering the patient's diet and living habits. Hiatal hernia is a disorder of this type. In this condition, the patient is advised not to lie down directly after taking any food and to refrain from eating for two to four hours before retiring.

DISORDERS OF THE STOMACH AND THE INTESTINES

Acute Gastritis

DEFINITION. Acute gastritis is an acute inflammation of the membrane lining the stomach. It may appear by itself, or as is frequently seen, accompanied by a generalized gastroenteritis. There are any number of causative agents such as dietary indiscretions, alcohol and bacterial or viral infection.

MAJOR SYMPTOMS. Symptoms include anorexia, nausea, vomiting, epigastric fullness, tenderness and pain. There may be hematemesis, diarrhea, abdominal cramps and generalized aches and pains.

DRUG THERAPY. Treatment is largely symptomatic and supportive. Fluids and electrolytes may need to be replaced. Antinauseants such as prochlorperazine (Compazine) 5 to 10 mg. t.i.d. or 15 mg. once daily, trimethobenzamide (Tigran) 250 mg. t.i.d. or q.i.d. orally or 200 mg. b.i.d. or t.i.d. parenterally are often given. Any of the aluminum or magnesium antacids will aid in overcoming heartburn and epigastric distress. During the first acute stage, usually during the first 24 hours or until vomiting has stopped, nothing is given by mouth. Then clear liquids are allowed and the diet gradually progresses through bland to soft to regular foods, as circumstances permit.

Chronic gastritis is usually secondary to some other disorder and treatment is aimed at eliminating the underlying cause.

Peptic Ulcer Syndrome

DEFINITION. Peptic ulcer is a condition in which there is a sharply circumscribed loss of tissue in the intestinal tract. It may occur in the lower part of the esophagus, in the stomach or in the duodenum. Though many factors are probably involved in the development of peptic ulcer, the ulcer itself is actually caused by the digestive action of the acid gastric juice (I-1, 3; II-3; VI-1). Contributing factors include excessive adrenal cortical activity, the administration of steroids (especially prolonged heavy dosage), vascular congestion, emotional stress and tension, certain types of burns, and diseases or surgery of the brain. Peptic ulcers are more common in men than in women.

MAJOR SYMPTOMS. Although pain is the outstanding symptom of peptic ulcer, it has definite characteristics. It is chronic in nature, periodic in occurrence, almost invariably gnawing, aching or burning in character and rhythmic in its relation to the digestive cycle. Nausea is not common nor is emesis usual unless there is an obstruction (I-2). Constipation is frequent, but there is no particular disturbance in appetite nor weight loss. The presence of an ulcer is confirmed by x-ray examination, gastroscopy or the finding of a high acid content in the stomach (II-1).

DRUG THERAPY. Though there is little unanimity of opinion about the treatment of peptic ulcer, therapy is essentially medical; surgery is resorted to when medical therapy has failed. Actually, the administration of drugs simply creates conditions under which it is possible for the ulcer to heal. In addition to drug therapy, rest, diet and psychotherapy are also important.

SEDATIVES. Sedation of some kind is often necessary to help the patient achieve the kind of rest prescribed. Phenobarbital in small doses (15 mg. orally) two to four times a day may be used. The dose may be 30 to 60 mg. at bedtime to insure sleep. The dose is individually adjusted to prevent excessive daytime sedation. One of the tranquilizer (ataractic) drugs, such as *prochlorperazine* (Compazine), 5 mg., *chlordiazepoxide hydrochloride* (Librium), 5 to 10 mg., or *meprobamate* (Equanil, et al.) 400 mg. three to four times a day, may be substituted. (See Chapter 30).

ANTACIDS USED IN TREATMENT OF PEPTIC ULCER SYNDROME. Besides neutralizing the strongly acid gastric contents to aid healing, antacids provide symptomatic relief. They do not influence the secretory mechanism. There is considerable controversy over their use, but the fact remains that they are widely used. The ideal preparation, yet to be found, would not produce a systemic alkalosis, would not cause a "rebound" stimulation of acid secretion, would not cause diarrhea or constipation, would not interfere with the digestive process and would not release carbon dioxide on reacting with the hydrochloric acid in the stomach.

THE DRUGS. There are any number of drugs that may be used as antacids in the treatment of peptic ulcers. Sodium bicarbonate (baking soda) is the fastest-acting drug and is the antacid used most often in the home (usually without medical supervision). Its use is limited, since it is readily absorbed from the gastrointestinal tract and can cause a systemic alkalosis. The three most commonly used antacids are aluminum hydroxide, magnesium (hydroxide, oxide or carbonate) and calcium carbonate. Most physicians use a combination either of any two, or, more frequently, of all three.

Physical and Chemical Properties. The names of the drugs indicate their chemical constituents. All, except sodium bicarbonate, are relatively insoluble and thus pass through the digestive tract without entering the systemic circulation.

Action. These drugs act mainly by forming a coating over the ulcer, thus preventing further irritant action by the hydrochloric acid in the gastric juice. Aluminum hydroxide, when mixed with hydrochloric acid, forms aluminum chloride, which is astringent. This also adds protection for the denuded mucosa. These drugs delay the gastric emptying time and do not cause an acid rebound as the faster-acting sodium bicarbonate may do.

Therapeutic Uses. These drugs are used almost exclusively for various forms of gastric irritation, particularly peptic ulcer. Magnesium preparations are laxative in action and are used alone for this purpose.

Preparations and Dosages

The number of antacid preparations is almost limitless. The Current Drug Handbook gives the major drugs as single drugs. Refer to it for additional information.

Aluminum hydroxide gel, 300 to 600 mg. tablets or suspension 5 to 40 ml. q.i.d. with water orally.

Calcium carbonate 1 to 4 Gm. tablets q.i.d. orally.

Magnesium hydroxide (Milk of Magnesia) 300 to 600 mg. tablets, 5 ml. suspension q.i.d. orally.

THE NURSE

Mode of Administration. If the tablet form of the drug is ordered, the patient is instructed to chew it well and follow with a few ounces of water or milk. The suspension form, which is usually one part drug to two or three parts water, may be given either orally or by continuous drip through a Levin tube. About 1500 ml. is the average amount given each 24 hour period. Sometimes, especially in the beginning of therapy, the drugs may be given every one or two hours, alternating with half-and-half (half milk and half cream) or with skimmed milk. The medication is given on the hour and the half-and-half on the half hour, or each is given on the hour with the medicine on the even numbered hours and the milk on the odd numbered hours. This regimen may be ordered continuously, 24 hours a day, or some of the night-time medicine and milk may be omitted to allow for sleep. This is a modification of the "Sippy" diet used for a number of years, the main difference being that sodium bicarbonate was a constituent of that diet.

Side Effects. Aluminum and calcium preparations tend to cause constipation, but the magnesium is a laxative, as noted under Action. This is one reason for using a combination of drugs or an alternating schedule. The aluminum ion interferes with the enzymatic action of pepsin and the absorption of phosphorus. However, the "ulcer diet" is usually high enough in phosphorus to overcome this.

Interactions. Dairy products and preparations containing aluminum, calcium and/or magnesium should not be given concurrently with any of the tetracycline antibiotics, since they will delay or prevent entirely the absorption of the antibiotics.

Patient Teaching. One of the most important and difficult teaching problems the nurse will face is encouraging the patient to continue following the regimen set by the physician. These schedules are often very trying and it is difficult for the patient to accept them. The importance of the treatment must be continuously reinforced. The peptic ulcer regimen is very difficult, especially if it is the half hour schedule, night and day, and it naturally increases the patient's feeling of stress and tension. The nurse will need to be accepting and understanding and have almost unlimited patience. She must do all in her power to insure rest and comfort for the patient by eliminating as many environmental stresses as possible and yet maintain the therapy program.

The continuous drip method, if used, may be very alarming to the patient. The nurse must thoroughly explain to the patient what is done and why this method is used. The patient should understand that this keeps the medication continuously in the stomach rather than intermittently as with the oral route. It also allows the medicine to be given at night without disturbing the patient's sleep. One reason for the night schedule is that the secretion of hydrochloric acid usually is increased at night.

Other Nursing Problems. Peptic ulcer patients receiving antacid drugs which contain alkali and any form of milk in their treatment programs must be carefully watched for signs of the "milk-alkali syndrome." This can be extremely serious, and deaths have occurred from a lack of early treatment. The symptoms of this syndrome include distaste for food, headache, weakness, nausea and vomiting. The laboratory findings are hypercalcemia without hypercalciuria, hypophosphaturia, normal or slightly elevated alkaline phosphatase and renal insufficiency without azotemia. There may be milk alkalosis, conjunctivitis and bad breath.

THE PATIENT. The nurse will need to be quite conscientious about giving medications on time. This is important not only because of the physiological effects, but also because this practice is the beginning of habit establishment for the patient. The patient must be instructed about the importance of a regular therapy regimen, even after he returns home for convalescence. Since ulcers recur as easily as they heal, the therapy is extremely important and the patient must understand why each phase of therapy is necessary. To begin this teaching process, the nurse may leave the medicines at the bedside and supervise the patient's taking his own medicines.

The nurse will also need to establish a relationship with the patient to teach the importance of the peptic ulcer diet. Often it is necessary to coordinate diet teaching plans between the patient and his family. The patient will need a lot of emotional support to change dietary habits, and especially to change those events in his life that create turmoil and tension. If the public health nurse is included in the planning, she may be able to provide the continuity link when the patient returns to his home and community.

ANTICHOLINERGIC DRUGS

THE DRUGS. There are many preparations covered by the anticholinergic (antimuscarine) classification. Some of these, such as *atropine* and *scopolamine*, are natural plant alkaloids. These have already been discussed in detail in Chapter 15. In recent years, many synthetic preparations have been developed. They are similar, and the multiplicity of these drugs has somewhat complicated the task of selecting the "right" one. However this has an advantage. If one preparation does not work, the doctor can prescribe another.

Physical and Chemical Properties. The chemical structure of these drugs varies with their source and preparation. The natural ones are alkaloids or salts of these alkaloids. There are semisynthetic ones made from the original alkaloids. Some are quaternary ammonium derivatives of the plant alkaloids. Of those that are entirely synthetic, most are quaternary ammonium compounds, but some have other structural forms such as tertiary nitrogen compounds.

These drugs are readily soluble in water and body fluids.

Action. As indicated by the name, these drugs inhibit the action of acetylcholine. The value of these drugs in the treatment of peptic ulcer lies in their effect on the gastrointestinal tract in decreasing motility, delaying the emptying time of the stomach and decreasing gastric secretion. These drugs also depress the gastrocolic reflex. The extent of the activity of these drugs varies not only with each preparation, but also with dosage and mode of administration. The quickest and best action takes place with parenteral use. The anticholinergic drugs do not markedly affect the secretion of bile, or pancreatic or intestinal juices.

Therapeutic Uses. The anticholinergic drugs are used for a wide variety of conditions, as preoperative medication, as mydriatics, as antispasmodics and as treatment for various gastrointestinal disturbances, including peptic ulcer.

Preparations and Dosages. There are so many anticholinergic drugs it is suggested that the student refer to the Current Drug Handbook for details. A few representative ones are:

Atropine sulfate, U.S.P., B.P., 0.25 to 0.5 mg. orally or parenterally.
Belladonna tincture, U.S.P., B.P., (Taladonna) 0.3 to 0.6 ml. orally.
Glycopyrrolate, N.F. (Robanul [C]) 4.0 mg., oral.
Hexocyclium methylsulfate (Tral) 25 to 50 mg., orally (available in a sustained release tablet).
Methscopolamine bromide (Pamine) 2.5 to 5.0 mg. orally or parenterally.
Oxyphencyclimine hydrochloride, N.F. (Daricon) 10 mg. orally.
Poldine methylsulfate (Nacton) 4 mg. oral.
Propantheline bromide, U.S.P., B.P., (Pro-Banthine) (Propanthel [C]) 15 mg. orally or 30 mg. I.M. or I.V.
Tricyclamol chloride (Elorine) 200 mg. oral.
Tridihexethyl chloride, N.F. (Pathilon) 5 to 25 mg. orally or parenterally.

All doses are individually adjusted. These drugs are usually given three times a day before meals and also at bedtime. The last dose is usually two to four times the daily dose.

The Nurse

Mode of Administration. Most of these drugs are given orally one-half hour before meals and at bedtime. With the hospitalized patient, the parenteral route may be used. If tincture of belladonna is ordered the nurse should dilute the liquid with water as the dosage is too small to be given directly. This is a very bitter substance and the patient should be given something to take the taste out of his mouth—a cracker or cookie, if allowed, or a mouthwash. Since the tablets also have a very unpleasant taste, it may be suggested that the drug be placed in a gelatin capsule for easier and more pleasant administration.

Side Effects. All the anticholinergic drugs share the same side effects, but with some of the drugs they are more pronounced. Side effects include dryness of the mouth, blurring of vision (due to mydriasis), headache, palpitation, flushing of the skin, difficulty in urination and often constipation. Use of the anticholinergic drugs is limited or contraindicated in patients with prostatic hypertrophy. The nurse must also remember that these drugs should *never* be given to patients with *glaucoma.* Should the drug be given by the parenteral route, physostigmine should be available for immediate emergency use. This antidote will counteract serious untoward side effects such as tachycardia or an anaphylactoid reaction.

Interactions. The anticholinergic drugs are enhanced by the antihistamines and the phenothiazine tranquilizers. Orphenadrine and propoxyphene potentiate each other and may cause tremors and convulsions; concomitant therapy is contraindicated.

The Patient. The patient should learn to take his own medications and be taught the proper time and method of administration. He should be cautioned as to the possible side effects of these drugs and instructed to notify his physician when any of these occur. See The Patient, under Antacids.

Other Drugs. The patient with a peptic ulcer may require others drugs as would any person with a long term illness. One medicine often required is a sedative. It may be necessary to give a tranquilizer and a hypnotic in the early stages, and a mild sedative, such as phenobarbital, or a mild tranquilizer as the condition improves. These drugs are used here as they would be in other diseases.

Some preparations combine several drugs such as an antacid, an anticholinergic and a sedative or tranquilizer.

There are some medications that increase or aggravate peptic ulcers. These may cause perforation, hemorrhage or both. Included are corticotropin, adrenocorticol steroids, rauwolfia preparations, phenylbutazone and the salicylates in large doses.

Regional Enteritis (Ileitis)

DEFINITION. Regional ileitis is a nonspecific inflammation of the small intestine with the formation of an ulcerating mass. This mass grows and forms scars which, in turn, cause fistulae to form from the ileum to the abdominal wall or to other viscera. Its cause is unknown but some authorities believe it is probably of infectious origin.

MAJOR SYMPTOMS. More commonly seen in youth, regional ileitis is usually chronic in nature with a prolonged onset of symptoms. The patient usually gives a history of long periods of diarrhea, abdominal pain and loss of weight. The bowel movements are characterized by generalized abdominal cramps and the stools contain mucus, pus and, occasionally, blood. Anemia is usually present and fistula formation is common. Examination of the patient frequently shows a mass in the right lower quadrant. Some of these patients, if untreated, progress to partial or complete obstruction of the bowel. The clinical picture is sometimes dominated by emotional disturbances—anxiety, tension, irritability, and so forth.

DRUG THERAPY. Although medical treatment is not very satisfactory in clearing the condition, treatment is directed toward allaying symptoms and assisting in building up the general state of the patient before surgery is done. A diet high in calories, high in proteins and with adequate fats is usually ordered. Excessive roughage should be avoided.

SEDATIVES AND ANALGESICS. Some form of a mild sedative several times a day helps foster the needed rest some of these patients find difficult to achieve alone. Phenobarbital in small doses or one of the tranquilizers is usually sufficient. (See Chapter 30.) Opiates should be used only to alleviate severe colic or diarrhea for short periods. Codeine is usually the drug of choice.

ANTIMICROBIAL THERAPY. Although the role of secondary bacterial infection is uncertain, many physicians recommend that an attempt be made to "sterilize" the bowel before surgery. Oral *kanamycin* (Kantrex) in doses of 6 to 8 Gm. per day in divided doses is often used for this purpose. Very little of the drug is absorbed, and not many of the gastrointestinal organisms are resistant to it. Some use the tetracyclines with good results.

Neomycin is also very effective because it is so poorly absorbed by the oral route. It rarely produces systemic action or toxic effects when administered orally. The patient is first placed on a low-residue diet and immediately after the administration of a cathartic (unless contraindicated) is given an oral dose of 1 Gm. every hour for four doses followed by 1 Gm. every four hours for 24 to 72 hours before surgery. This amount usually produces four to eight bowel movements. It is recommended that this drug not be given for longer than 72 hours.

ANTICHOLINERGIC DRUGS. Some physicians feel that the use of an anticholinergic drug is indicated to relieve the intestinal spasms. *Tincture of belladonna* is sometimes adequate or one of the synthetic drugs such as *propantheline* may be ordered (see Peptic Ulcer in this chapter).

STEROID THERAPY. In those patients in whom more conservative medical treatment has failed or in whom surgery is not indicated, some physicians have been able to produce striking but temporary improvement with the use of one of these drugs. They may use *prednisolone* in divided doses totaling 60 to 80 mg. the first day followed by 20 mg. daily for three weeks. The drug is then gradually withdrawn. Refer to rheumatoid arthritis in Chapter 21 for details of the administration of this drug.

GENERAL THERAPY. Iron deficiency anemia is present in most of these patients and is treated with the usual antianemic drugs. (See Chapter 19.) In some cases, psychotherapy aids in helping the patient to adjust to his altered life routine, especially after surgery. This should be done when the acute illness is past.

The Patient. (See Ulcerative Colitis.)

Ulcerative Colitis

DEFINITION. Ulcerative colitis is the term used to describe varying degrees of irritation in the colon. The mucous lining is hyperemic and contains small bleeding points and some ulceration. In some cases, the mucosa of the colon may be extensively denuded. The cause of ulcerative colitis is not well understood. Several possible etiological factors have been suggested such as infection (bacterial or viral), allergy (especially food allergies), psychosomatic (there appears to be an "ulcerative colitis personality") and autoimmune reaction. It is possible that a combination of causes may be required to produce the disease.

MAJOR SYMPTOMS. Ulcerative colitis is a chronic disease characterized by acute exacerbations and remissions. Symptoms include diarrhea, rectal bleeding and abdominal distress with pain during the acute stage. There is usually some anorexia, and nausea and vomiting may occur. Fever is present in the more severe cases. Death may occur from exhaustion or from perforation of the colon, with generalized peritonitis. The less severe cases tend to recur, and anemia, perianal abscesses and stricture formation may be complications, especially in cases of long duration.

DRUG THERAPY. Rest and a nonirritating diet are perhaps the most important factors in the treatment of this disease. There is little unanimity of opinion regarding therapy and most of it is on an empiric basis to give symptomatic relief.

Anti-infectives. Despite the fact the results of anti-infective treatment have been questionable, it is still used frequently. *Azulfidine,* 4 to 8 Gm. every 24 hours in divided doses is often used because it can usually be given over long periods without serious side effects. It seems to produce the most consistent results of the sulfa drugs.

The administration of sufficient fluids is important here as it is when any sulfonamide is given.

Azulfidine will cause an alkaline urine to become orange yellow in color and the patient should be warned of this when he takes the drug. The course of this disease is long and drawn out, and this is often very discouraging to the patient. He should be reassured whenever possible (V-2; VI-1, 2).

The use of antibiotics has not proven to be very satisfactory and there is danger of microbial overgrowth. Neomycin orally has been used to aid in reducing the bacterial count before surgery. Kanamycin is used as discussed under Regional Enteritis.

Corticosteroid Therapy. It is rather generally agreed now that the best use of the corticosteroids in ulcerative colitis is in the acutely ill patient, though they are occasionally used in others who have failed to respond to other therapy.

The dosage of the corticosteroids must be individually adjusted to suit the patient's condition and his response to therapy. In severe cases, corticotropin may be given 10 to 20 units in 500 ml. of a glucose solution by intravenous drip every 12 hours. As the patient's condition improves, the long-acting intramuscular gel may be substituted for the intravenous drip. With further improvement, hydrocortisone, usually starting with 200 mg. per day, or prednisone, 40 to 80 mg. per day, may be given. The dose is reduced until a maintenance dose is established. The same precautions are to be observed in these cases as when these steroids are given for any other reason. See Chapter 27 for further details.

To Control the Diarrhea. It is essential to reduce the number of bowel movements as well as the amount of fluid lost. Diarrhea can be treated by reducing intestinal motility with drugs such as camphorated tincture of opium (Paregoric) 4 to 8 ml., codeine 15 to 30 mg. (usually given after every two or three loose stools), diphenoxylate hydrochloride (Lomotil) 2.5 mg. or propantheline (Pro-Banthine) 7.5 to 15 mg. Increasing the bulk of the stools with bulk laxatives is another method of treatment, or a combination of methods may be used. Refer to Diarrhea later in this chapter.

Sedation. Most physicians give either small doses of phenobarbital or one of the milder tranquilizers to reduce the stress and tension which appear to be a part of the disease. It is not unusual to increase the dose at bedtime or, if required, to give a hypnotic for sleep. Rest is an essential part of the treatment of these patients, and it is essential to see that it is secured not only during the acute stage, but also during remission, to aid in preventing recurrence of severe symptoms.

MISCELLANEOUS THERAPY. The fluid and electrolyte balance should be monitored carefully during the acute phase and any deficiency remedied. The physician's attention should be called to any change in reports. Antianemic therapy is usually required and should be maintained during remission unless laboratory reports indicate sufficient amounts of red cells and hemoglobin and no occult blood in the stools. (See Chapter 19.) Hypoproteinemia may require transfusion with whole blood, blood plasma or human serum albumin. The diet is usually high in protein, high in calories and low in residue. Some physicians give an anabolic drug to aid in improving the patient's general health. Surgical intervention may be required and often produces marked improvement. Psychotherapy may be required, but it should only be given during remission. Therapy should be given by a psychiatrist, although experience has shown that psychoanalysis does not produce the desired results.

THE NURSE. The nurse will find that caring for patients with ulcerative colitis is extremely taxing. Patience, patience and more patience is needed. The nursing staff will also need assistance in coping with their feelings of frustration. Inadvertently, the staff could easily "withdraw" attention from the patient and, unintentionally, appear to "punish" the patient for unacceptable behavior. Therefore, the nurse will need to carefully chart the specific behaviors observed and note those symptoms about which the patient complains. Through doing this, the nurse and others may be able to identify constructive ways of modifying behavior into acceptable patterns.

The course of ulcerative colitis is long and drawn out and is subject to many remissions and exacerbations. This is extremely discouraging and depressing to the patient, and he will need much help in coping with all the aspects of his illness.

Careful observations must be made to prevent drug interactions or side effects, especially with cortisone therapy. (See Chapter 27.) Daily recording of fluid intake, fluid output, weight and blood pressure is essential. The nurse must be alert to the signs and symptoms of ulcerative colitis as distinguished from those caused by drug interactions.

Due to debilitated body conditions, these patients are also extremely susceptible to infection. A clean environment must be provided—perhaps reverse isolation—in the acute stages of the illness. Visitors must also be screened for colds or infections. Daily skin care is necessary with careful attention to irritated areas such as the elbow and anal area. Stomatitis and glossitis are common problems which may be prevented by regular oral care.

Dietary problems are often difficult to manage. The dietitian, family members, nurse and patient must work together to develop an acceptable diet that includes high protein and high vitamin content. It may be helpful to begin dietary instruction by emphasizing foods that are acceptable rather than those that are to be avoided.

THE PATIENT. The patient with ulcerative colitis is difficult to describe without resorting to stereotypes. The nurse and other staff will need to use *all* available resources to help the patient adjust to his condition. Long-term drug therapy is expensive and slow in showing results. Both of these factors lead to feelings of frustration and anger which must be expressed. Environmental stresses also must be decreased as much as possible.

Due to lengthy therapy, the public health nurse or visiting nurse may be consulted for predischarge planning. Encouraging a relationship with a community liaison individual may become extremely beneficial. In this way, continuity of drug and diet therapy, rest regimen and other aspects of nursing care can be provided.

Irritable Colon (Spastic Constipation)

DEFINITION. Sometimes referred to as spastic constipation, the term irritable colon is used to describe a condition of disturbed intestinal motility. There is hyperirritability and hypersensitivity of the colon. This condition has also been referred to as mucous colitis, spastic colitis and hypertonic constipation. This disease is associated with emotional tension and may account for as much as 50 per cent of all gastrointestinal diseases. It is believed by many clinicians to rank with the common cold as a major cause of recurrent minor illness.

MAJOR SYMPTOMS. The patient usually complains of a feeling of fullness and discomfort following the ingestion of food or drink and may even suffer from severe, cramp-like abdominal pain. This pain is generalized in the abdomen and, as a rule, defecation or the expulsion of flatus affords only temporary relief. Nausea is frequently present. True constipation may or may not be present. Various other symptoms such as headache and fatigue may be noticed.

DRUG THERAPY. In contrast to atonic constipation, spastic constipation is best treated by rest. The diet should be adjusted to suit the irritability of the bowel.

Tincture of belladonna in doses of 10 to 15 drops in water before meals may provide sufficient relaxation to assist in correcting this condition. *Atropine sulfate*, 0.4 to 0.5 mg. orally three to four times daily may help. *Phenobarbital,* 15 to 30 mg. three to four times daily, is often a helpful adjunct to the atropine-belladonna group because of its sedative action. One of the tranquilizers may be more effective.

The use of the anticholinergic or antispasmodic drugs may assist in the therapy. *Propantheline* (Pro-Banthine), in doses of 15 to 30 mg. daily may be given. *Diphenoxylate hydrochloride* (Lomotil) 5 mg. three or four times a day may also be helpful. (See discussion of these drugs elsewhere in this chapter.)

If the physician feels it is necessary and feasible, the patient may be referred for psychiatric therapy since the simple reassurance that "nothing is wrong" may not be sufficient.

THE NURSE. (See Ulcerative Colitis.)

THE PATIENT. (See Ulcerative Colitis.)

Diverticulosis

DEFINITION. Diverticulosis is a condition of the gastrointestinal tract characterized by numerous outpouchings of the bowel. Although any portion of the tract may be affected, the sigmoidal portion of the colon is most apt to be involved. The next most common site is the ileo-cecocolic junction.

MAJOR SYMPTOMS. This condition may elicit many symptoms or none. The most common symptoms are pain and tenderness over the affected area. There may be diarrhea, constipation or the alternation of these. However, diarrhea seems to be the more common. If inflammation occurs there may be severe pain, fever, increased pulse rate and bloody or mucus passage or both with or without a stool. Diverticulosis can cause obstruction, perforation or both, conditions which require surgical intervention.

DRUG THERAPY. Drug therapy is entirely symptomatic and palliative. Diverticulitis, inflammation of the diverticula, is treated as any intestinal infection, with the nonabsorbable sulfonamides and the broad-spectrum antibiotics. (Refer to Current Drug Handbook and this chapter for further details.)

Constipation is usually treated with fruit juices and, if required, the bulk laxatives. Strong cathartics are to be avoided since they may cause hemorrhage or perforation.

Diarrhea is treated with *camphorated tincture of opium* often combined with an antacid or a demulcent such as kaolin. *Diphenoxylate hydrochloride* (Lomotil) also may be used.

THE NURSE. The nurse must help the patient live with his disability. Most diverticula do not cause serious symptoms. Many people have lived with the condition for years, unaware of the diverticula until a routine physical examination shows their existence. After becoming aware of his diagnosis, the patient will need to adjust some of his health patterns. His illness is not usually serious. However, serious complications, such as perforation, obstruction or hemorrhage, can occur. These are usually the result of frequent recurrence of constipation or dietary indiscretions. The patient should understand his illness, but undue fears should not be implanted in his mind.

A diet low in roughage is usually ordered during any acute episode, and some patients find that they must continuously limit their intake of the types of food they cannot tolerate. During acute attacks, with pain, tenderness, and diarrhea, the patient should see his physician. As with any chronic disease, the patient should be encouraged to have regular medical check-ups so as to forestall, if possible, serious complications. These patients should be warned, as in the case of abdominal pain, never to take a laxative if there is pain or any indication of intestinal infection.

THE PATIENT. Refer to Ulcerative Colitis.

Generalized Peritonitis

DEFINITION. A generalized inflammation of the peritoneum, peritonitis is almost always secondary to some other disease. The causative bacteria are more frequently of the colon group because of the more frequent association with diseases of the intestinal tract (III-6).

MAJOR SYMPTOMS. The symptoms which occur usually merge with or follow the primary disease responsible, and it is important to recognize the difference between the original symptoms of the disease and those of peritonitis. Pain is an important symptom and, as the disease progresses, usually becomes more intense. Tenderness is present in the abdomen over the involved area; the abdominal muscles are rigid, most markedly over the site of origin. Nausea and vomiting are early and common signs. Fever is present and the pulse rate is usually elevated out of proportion to the temperature. A marked leukocytosis is present.

DRUG THERAPY

ANTI-INFECTIVES. Peritonitis is usually treated with one of the broad-spectrum antibiotics such as ampicillin or one of the cephalosporins. The dosage may be 500 mg. every four hours until the temperature reaches normal. Then it usually is reduced to 250 mg. every four hours for a week. If these drugs do not prove effective, tetracycline may be given. In very severe, persistent cases, chloramphenicol may be tried. If a Miller-Abbott tube is in place, the doctor may wish the drug given by that route. The nurse may then be permitted to clamp the tube off for one half hour after the drug is given. The drug also may be given intravenously in a 5 per cent glucose in water or an isotonic sodium chloride solution in doses of 500 mg. to 1 gm. every 6 hours.

FLUID THERAPY. The use of intravenous fluids is almost always indicated in this disease. Solutions of *glucose* 5 to 10 per cent and the *balanced electrolyte solutions* assist greatly in maintaining the patient through this critical period.

SYMPTOM COMPLEXES ASSOCIATED WITH THE GASTROINTESTINAL TRACT

Diarrhea

DEFINITION. An acute or chronic state in which there is the evacuation of watery or unformed stools, diarrhea may be a symptom of some other disease or it may be a primary disorder. In the latter case, the cause may be an enteric infection, food sensitization or some other condition (III-1).

MAJOR SYMPTOMS. Although the symptoms will vary a great deal, nausea, vomiting, abdominal cramps accompanied by tenesmus and frequent watery stools are common to almost all cases. The attack may last from one to three days, with a varying number of stools a day (3 to 15 or 20). Severe or prolonged cases may result in dehydration, prostration and collapse.

DRUG THERAPY

FLUIDS. Rest is important and should include rest in bed and rest from food for at least the first 24 hours. If the dehydration has been severe, intravenous fluids may be used to advantage and these usually include 5 per cent *glucose* and one of the *balanced electrolyte solutions.* The latter are preparations that contain sodium chloride, calcium and magnesium similar to that of normal human blood plasma, with the potassium and bicarbonate equivalent to twice that of normal plasma. When the balanced electrolyte solutions are given, they should be administered slowly at the rate of 1 liter in two to three hours. The use of these solutions helps to restore the normal electrolyte balance of the body.

ANTISPASMODICS. *Atropine sulfate* by hypodermic in full doses – 0.6 to 1 mg. – is often given every four to six hours and may be effective in relaxing the spasms of the intestinal tract.

Diphenoxylate hydrochloride N.F. (Lomotil), 2.5 mg. with atropine sulfate, U.S.P., 0.025

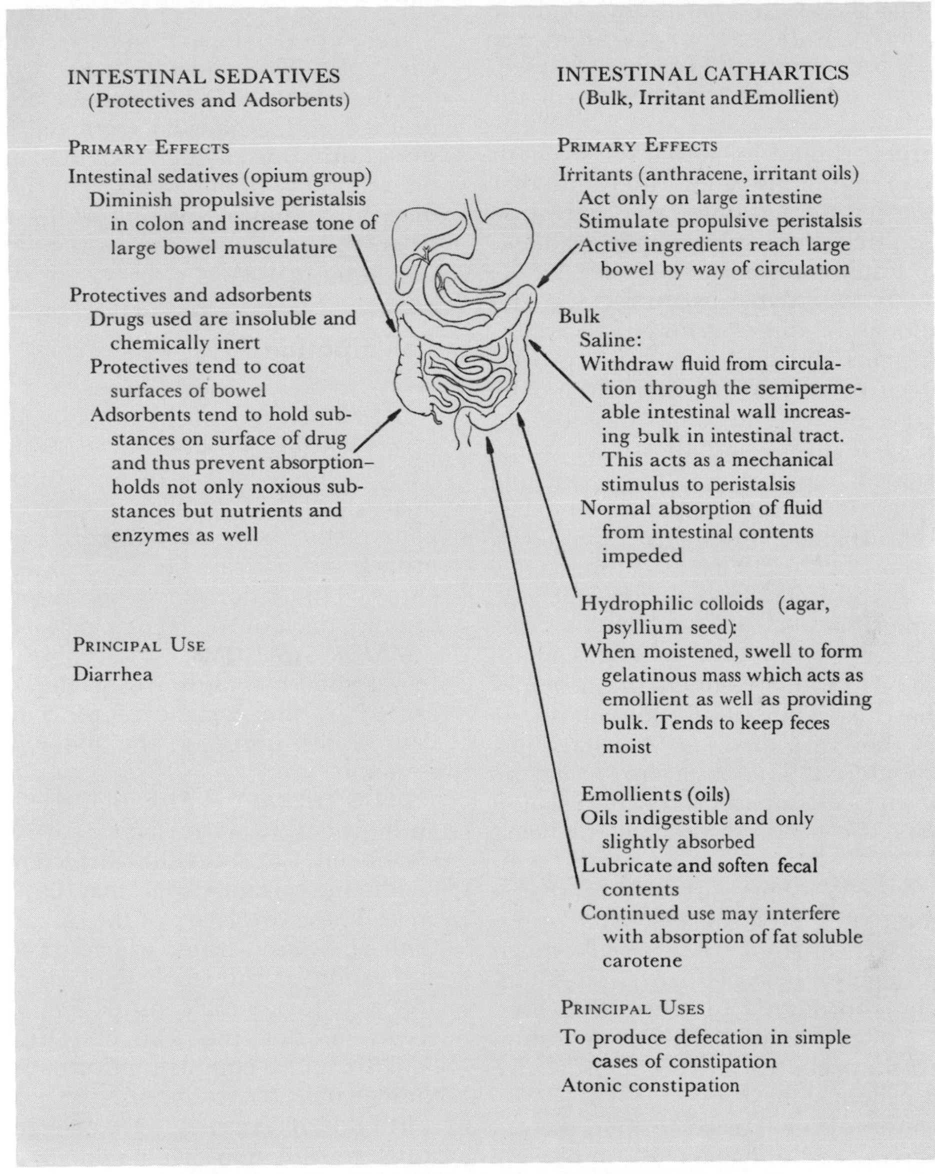

INTESTINAL SEDATIVES
(Protectives and Adsorbents)
PRIMARY EFFECTS
Intestinal sedatives (opium group)
Diminish propulsive peristalsis in colon and increase tone of large bowel musculature
Protectives and adsorbents
Drugs used are insoluble and chemically inert
Protectives tend to coat surfaces of bowel
Adsorbents tend to hold substances on surface of drug and thus prevent absorption–holds not only noxious substances but nutrients and enzymes as well
PRINCIPAL USE
Diarrhea
INTESTINAL CATHARTICS
(Bulk, Irritant and Emollient)
PRIMARY EFFECTS
Irritants (anthracene, irritant oils)
Act only on large intestine
Stimulate propulsive peristalsis
Active ingredients reach large bowel by way of circulation
Bulk
Saline:
Withdraw fluid from circulation through the semipermeable intestinal wall increasing bulk in intestinal tract. This acts as a mechanical stimulus to peristalsis
Normal absorption of fluid from intestinal contents impeded
Hydrophilic colloids (agar, psyllium seed):
When moistened, swell to form gelatinous mass which acts as emollient as well as providing bulk. Tends to keep feces moist
Emollients (oils)
Oils indigestible and only slightly absorbed
Lubricate and soften fecal contents
Continued use may interfere with absorption of fat soluble carotene
PRINCIPAL USES
To produce defecation in simple cases of constipation
Atonic constipation

FIGURE 27. Comparison of intestinal sedatives and cathartics.

mg. (each tablet), 5 to 10 mg. (2 to 4 tablets) four times daily, before meals and at bedtime, is an effective drug in the treatment of diarrhea, whatever the cause. Chemically related to the opiates, this drug has been shown to markedly decrease peristalsis without analgesia. It has not shown addictive tendencies, but may be habit forming.

Many combination drugs are used for this and similar conditions. Most contain antispasmodics, materials having a soothing (emollient or demulcent) action and, sometimes, a small dose of a sedative.

INTESTINAL SEDATIVES. Two members of the opium group of narcotics are sometimes helpful in correcting diarrhea by their action of checking and slowing down peristalsis (I-6). *Camphorated tincture of opium* (paregoric) contains 0.4 per cent opium and is given in 4 ml. doses after each bowel movement. It is equivalent to approximately 1.6 mg. morphine. Codeine phosphate 16 to 60 mg. may be used. See Figure 27 for a comparison of intestinal sedatives and cathartics. A discussion of the latter follows.

The nurse should know that the strength of these preparations varies widely and that they are given diluted with water. Paregoric is brown in color but when water is added, it forms a milky white liquid.

Protectives and Adsorbents. The conventional binding agents such as bismuth, pectins and kaolin have not proved very effective but may be tried if the diarrhea is not severe. The nonlaxative antacid drugs may be given, since they tend to coat the irritated membranes. These include such drugs as calcium carbonate and bismuth subcarbonate. *Aluminum hydroxide gel* in large doses 20 to 40 ml. four times a day is often helpful (IV-1). (See Peptic Ulcer, this chapter.)

There are any number of combination preparations for the treatment of uncomplicated diarrhea. They usually contain two or three of the types of drugs that have just been considered. The physician selects the drug on the basis of its content in relation to the specific needs of the patient being treated.

The Nurse. The nurse will base the nursing care needed on the origin and number of diarrheal stools. Skin irritation can become severe. Perianal irritation is relieved by thorough cleansing after each stool, use of soft tissue, and the application of petroleum jelly to provide a protective water-repellent shield.

The nurse also will need to help the patient keep up his fluid intake to compensate for water lost in the stools. Iced drinks, coffee and fruit juices should be avoided, since these tend to be laxative in action. Tea, taken without milk or sugar, may be used as much as desired. A bland diet should be encouraged. Dry toast and well ripened bananas seem to help reduce the watery content of the stools. Plain yogurt and buttermilk may be taken, since they encourage the normal intestinal flora to reestablish residence.

The nurse must carefully chart the characteristics of the stools—frequency, color, odor, consistency, presence of blood, mucus, flatulence and the like. The presence or absence of tenesmus should be noted. The effect of the drug therapy on controlling the diarrhea also will need to be recorded concurrently.

The Patient. The patient often feels drained and exhausted from the frequent stools with consequent loss of fluid and from interruptions of his sleep. The nurse can help to minimize discomfort by allowing frequent restful naps during the day and by providing privacy.

Constipation

DEFINITION. Constipation is said to be present when the stools are hard and dry. This is due to a lack of tone in the intestinal tract (V-3). Constipation may accompany or be a part of many diseases or disorders, or it may be a separate clinical entity. This latter form has been termed "atonic" (lack of tone) constipation.

MAJOR SYMPTOMS. There are relatively few symptoms aside from the difficulty caused by the passage of the hard stool. Pain or discomfort in the abdomen is not common.

DRUG THERAPY. Although diet, exercise and proper habit formation are the best treatments to use in the correction of this condition, certain drugs may be of assistance. These drugs are of the cathartic class. Cathartics are drugs which increase the evacuation of the stools. Not all cathartics are used for atonic constipation, as will be discussed later. (See Current Drug Handbook for more complete information about these drugs.)

Bulk Cathartics. In many instances, atonic constipation may be due to the overuse of cathartic drugs, yet certain drugs classed as cathartics may be helpful in correcting this condition by increasing the bulk in the intestinal tract.

Agar U.S.P. (agar-agar) is rich in indigestible hemicellulose and, when moistened, swells to form a gelatinous mass which acts as a demulcent and softens the intestinal contents. In addition, this substance adds to bulk and keeps the feces moist by absorbing water from the intestinal tract. This drug is available as a coarse powder or in shredded form and is often eaten as a cereal substitute or added to other foods. The usual dose is 10 Gm. but up to 40 Gm. may be taken before the desired effect is obtained. *Methylcellulose*, U.S.P. (many trade names), is similar to agar and used in the same way. The usual dose is 1.5 Gm. as needed. Preparations made from psyllium seed are also valuable as bulk cathartics. Similar to agar, they swell in the bowel to form a demulcent, indigestible mass. The preparation Psyllium hydrophilic mucilloid (*Metamucil*) is probably the most widely used and is given in 4 to 7 Gm. doses one to three times daily.

In administering agar, the nurse must dissolve the drug in boiling water and allow it to gel before it is taken. Psyllium hydrophilic mucilloid (Metamucil) comes in two forms, plain and effervescent. The effervescent form contains a significant amount of sodium and should not be used for patients on sodium-restricted diets. The plain type may be stirred into water, fruit juice or milk at the bedside immediately before administration. It is best followed by another glass of liquid. For the effervescent form, the directions on the label should be followed.

The nurse can be very helpful in teaching the patient who is accustomed to the use of cathartics to institute the proper rules of hygiene to overcome this tendency. The proper bulk foods can be recommended and the value of establishing regular habits should be explained to the patient.

Lubricants. *Liquid petrolatum*, U.S.P., liquid paraffin, B.P. (mineral oil) is an indigestible oil and has only a slight absorption from the intestinal tract. It lubricates and softens the fecal contents. Both light and heavy grades are available and there is little if any difference in their action. The dose is 15 to 45 ml. (cc.). Though a relatively safe laxative, this drug absorbs fat-soluble substances such as certain vitamins and, in so doing, may deplete the body of these other needed substances. Its continued use over a long period is to be discouraged.

Mineral oil should not be given with meals as it will delay emptying of the stomach (I-4). Although tasteless, the drug may be obnoxious to many because of its oiliness and consistency. This may be overcome by chilling the oil and encouraging the patient to place it on the back of tongue in order to keep the drug from coming in contact with the lips. It may be followed by a slice of orange to cut the oily sensation, or the drug may be mixed with a fruit juice. Repeated use of mineral oil may result in its seepage from the rectum, soiling clothes and causing embarrassment. In the child and the very ill or debilitated patient, there is danger of some of the oil's being aspirated and possibly causing serious respiratory complications.

Many preparations of mineral oil are on the market but the best to use is the cheapest one bearing the U.S.P. label.

Irritant Cathartics. Irritant cathartics increase the propulsive peristaltic activity by irritating the mucosa or by directly stimulating the smooth muscle of the intestine. Of this group, *cascara sagrada* U.S.P., B.P. may be used occasionally in atonic constipation. Its action is mild and not accompanied by discomfort or griping and no tolerance develops. It may be given in decreasing doses so as to wean the patient from the drug. The most effective and palatable form is aromatic cascara sagrada fluid extract in doses of 2 to 4 ml. at bedtime.

Several older drugs such as rhubarb, aloe and jalap are seldom used now but occasionally are found as constituents of proprietary cathartics. Each of these is rather strong in action and is not without toxic manifestations. Aloe, for example, is commonly found in various "liver pills" on the market but it is not a cholagogue as is often claimed.

Castor oil (oleum ricini) is an irritant cathartic which owes its rapid action to this property. It is a fatty substance and retards gastric emptying time. The adult dose is 15 to 30 ml. Larger doses are not more effective. The child's dose is 4 ml. The consistency and taste of the oil are objectionable. Castor oil is prepared in allegedly flavored and tasteless forms. However, it is still disagreeable. One of the simplest ways of avoiding the "bad" taste is to have the patient hold an ice cube in his mouth for a minute or two directly before taking the drug. If allowed, it can be followed by a cracker or bland cookie which will remove any oil from the mouth. Fruit juice may be helpful in changing the taste. The use of castor oil is confined almost exclusively to special purposes such as preparation for x-rays of the large bowel. It is rarely, if ever, used for simple constipation.

Saline Cathartics. This group of drugs promote evacuation by binding water and providing liquid bulk in the stool. *Milk of magnesia,* 15 to 45 ml., may be used in gradually decreasing doses. Most of the drugs in this group are not useful in correcting atonic constipation but do help if edema is present. These include magnesium sulfate, magnesium citrate and magnesium carbonate and some of the potassium salts. (See Current Drug Handbook for others.)

SUPPOSITORIES. *Glycerin* rectal suppositories may be helpful and may be used frequently. Patients should be encouraged to wean themselves from the use of any drugs.

MISCELLANEOUS CATHARTICS. Another group of drugs which act as wetting agents or as contact laxatives are gaining popularity because of their gentle action. *Dioctyl sodium sulfosuccinate,* N.F. (Colace, Doxinate) acts internally as a wetting agent, permitting water and fatty material to penetrate and to mix better with the fecal material. This results in a softer stool. The usual dose is 60 to 300 mg. one to five times daily for adults; children may be given 10 to 20 mg. daily. Dioctyl sodium sulfosuccinate is often combined with other compounds such as carboxymethylcellulose and cascara derivatives.

Bisacodyl N.F. (Dulcolax) is a drug that is classed as a contact laxative. It acts by stimulating nerve endings in the mucosa of the colon, thereby initiating reflex peristalsis. It is given in an oral dose of 5 to 15 mg. in the evening or before breakfast. This method usually produces evacuation within six hours. After the rectal suppository form is used, a response usually occurs within 15 to 60 minutes. The tablets should not be crushed or chewed nor should they be used within one hour after taking antacids since the presence of the drug in the stomach without its enteric coating may cause vomiting. Very occasionally a patient may complain of slight cramping several hours after the drug is ingested but it is one of the gentlest laxatives available.

Phenolphthalein is one of the older group of cathartics which is more commonly found in proprietary medications. It will cause alkaline urine to appear red and may do the same with the stool if it is alkaline. This should not be mistaken for blood. In average doses this drug is not too potent. There are a few hypersensitive people who react violently to it, with severe skin rashes or excessive purgation and collapse. These individuals should be cautioned never to take the drug again in any form. This substance is a frequent constituent of certain chewing gum and chocolate laxatives, and it is these that children sometimes ingest in large amounts. This is not necessarily poisonous and should be treated simply by the replacement of fluids lost in the purgation. However, a physician should always be contacted as there may be shock or other adverse symptoms. These are highly advertised laxatives which claim to be "safe, gentle and effective." They often are not nearly as safe, etc., as they are said to be.

THE NURSE. These patients should be encouraged to set up proper habits of eating food high in bulk but not high in roughage, exercise and establishing regular habits of defecation to overcome constipation but some have become so accustomed to the use of cathartics that this will not be an easy task. It would be wise to say a few words here regarding cathartics in general. It is well known that cathartics are often overused and misused. The public should be educated as to their proper use. It is good practice never to give a cathartic of any kind without the specific order of the physician when there is an undiagnosed abdominal pain. Many cases of ruptured appendix result from this. Many people, too, become so habituated to the use of cathartics they feel that they cannot do without them. This often results in atonic constipation or other serious illness.

THE PATIENT. The patient may need to relearn how to respond to previously ignored defecation stimuli. Establishing a regular time of the day—often after a meal—will begin a pattern of behavior. With instruction and encouragement, this habit reestablishment can occur, but it is difficult and takes time. Many people think that there must be a stool each day. However, it is not unusual or abnormal for some individuals to have a stool every second or third day and for others to have one two or three times every day.

DISORDERS OF THE LIVER, GALLBLADDER AND PANCREAS

Portal Cirrhosis

DEFINITION. Portal cirrhosis is a chronic degenerative and inflammatory disease of the liver characterized by a recurring degeneration and regeneration of the parenchyma of the liver (I-7, 8). This process eventually results in fibrosis in and about the interlobar and portal spaces leading eventually to an obstruction of the portal circulation. It is a slowly progressing disease and its cause is not always known but it is probable that several factors contribute to its beginning. One possible factor is nutritional deficiency. This is also called Laennec's cirrhosis or hypertrophic cirrhosis.

MAJOR SYMPTOMS. The onset is insidious, with considerable weight loss over a long period, anorexia, nausea and vomiting. After a few months, the patient notices an increased abdominal fullness (first due to flatulence, later to ascites). The patient is weak and mentally dull, suffers from thirst and abdominal discomfort or pain. The skin is dry and inelastic and the venules over the face become prominent. The breathing is shallow because of the elevated diaphragm. The pulse is rapid. Edema of the legs may be present. A low-grade fever is present for a long period of time. Bleeding, especially epistaxis, is frequently seen. The icterus is seldom conspicuous.

DRUG THERAPY. There is no specific treatment for cirrhosis and often therapy is of little or no avail. Bed rest is indicated and an adequate diet is essential.

VITAMINS. The use of vitamins and liver extract is usual but there is seldom little if any result. The *vitamin B-complex, thiamine chloride* and *folic acid* especially, is recommended. Because of a defect in fat absorption, oral supplements of the fat-soluble vitamins—A, D, E and K—are usually added.

DIURETICS. In an attempt to relieve the ascites and edema when present, sodium intake is restricted to 1 to 3 Gm. daily. Diuretics may be used but results are often disappointing. *Ammonium chloride,* 6 Gm. daily in divided doses may be used. *Spironolactone* (Aldactone) is an orally effective agent that blocks the sodium-retaining effects of aldosterone on the distal convoluted renal tubule producing diuresis. Although moderately effective alone, it works better when one of the thiazide diuretics is used. Spironolactone potentiates the thiazide diuretic and counteracts the excessive potassium excretion occurring in thiazide therapy. The dose is from 50 to 200 mg. daily in divided doses and will usually produce diuresis by the fifth day. Side effects include headache, confusion, dermatitis, ataxia and abdominal pain. Other diuretics which may be used are *mercaptomerin* (Thiomerin), *chlorothiazide* (Diuril), *furosemide* (Lasix) or *ethycrynic acid* (Edecrin). But, potassium levels must be maintained when the last two drugs are used. These are discussed in more detail in Chapter 18.

CHOLINE. Choline, a lipotropic substance, may be used in the treatment of cirrhosis of the liver and may produce some improvement. Choline is an essential for the normal transport of fat in the body and when it is absent, fat accumulates in the liver. It is on this basis then that choline is administered to patients with cirrhosis. This drug is absorbed readily from the gastrointestinal tract and so it is always given orally. Precise dosage is not definitely determined as yet but may range from 1.5 to 3 Gm. daily. Preparations available are *choline chloride* and *choline dihydrogen citrate.*

METHIONINE. *Methionine,* N.F. (Meonine, Metione), is a sulfur-containing amino acid which is considered an indispensable dietary component. It is a helpful adjunct in early liver disease, especially in those patients who cannot take an adequate diet. There is evidence, however, that in those with severe liver damage, large doses may be harmful. Usually given by mouth as a supplement to a high protein diet, 3 to 6 Gm. is given daily.

CONCENTRATED NORMAL HUMAN SERUM ALBUMIN. *Normal human serum albumin* may be used in an attempt to reduce edema and raise the serum protein level but, like the other drugs, may not prove too effective. This drug is a sterile solution of the serum albumin component of blood from healthy donors prepared by a fractionation process. It is given intravenously in doses of approximately 2.2 ml. per kilogram of body weight at a given rate not greater than 2 ml. per minute with physiologic salt solution or 5 per cent glucose. This solution is a moderately viscous, clear, brownish liquid. If any change in it is noted, it should not be used.

SEDATIVES. As the disease progresses, it becomes more difficult for the patient to rest so that the use of some mild sedative is often indicated. Probably *paraldehyde* or *chloral hydrate* in their usual dosages are best.

Corticosteroid Therapy. The use of steroids is questionable except in some few cases in which the bilirubin level is excessively high or when vomiting cannot be controlled (I-5).

Acute Cholecystitis

DEFINITION. Inflammation of the gallbladder (cholecystitis) may be caused by infection, cholelithiasis or unknown agents. Infection is most commonly caused by organisms of the colon-typhoid group. Staphylococci, streptococci or pneumococci are seen less frequently (III-1). The causative organism may reach the gallbladder by way of the blood stream or by ascent from the duodenum. Frequently, however, no demonstrable organism can be found in an acute inflammation. A large number of cases of cholecystitis are associated with cholelithiasis.

MAJOR SYMPTOMS. The symptoms vary from a mild form of indigestion with moderate pain and tenderness in the right upper quadrant to the more severe forms in which pain and tenderness are pronounced and muscle spasm is present. Abdominal distention is common and icterus may soon be obvious. The urine often is dark in color because of increased amounts of urobilinogen. The attack may last from several hours to several days and there is the possibility of perforation or rupture of the inflamed gallbladder.

DRUG THERAPY. Although conservative measures may bring about improvement in a few days, this is not always true and surgery may be indicated. The medical treatment is purely symptomatic and palliative and should include diet regulation as well.

Analgesics and Antispasmodics. *Sodium phenobarbital* given subcutaneously, 50 to 100 mg., may relieve the discomfort. In other cases, stronger analgesics may be indicated. *Meperidine* (Demerol, pethidine [C]) is often used intramuscularly in 50 to 100 mg. doses. Morphine sulfate is not usually prescribed because of its tendency to constrict the sphincter of Oddi. *Nitroglycerin,* 0.6 mg., may be given sublingually or an amyl nitrate pearl may be used simultaneously to help relax the smooth muscles of the cystic duct. *Papaverine* 30 to 100 mg., may be given intravenously. Since it relaxes smooth muscle tissue, it will tend to relax the sphincter.

Fluid Therapy. Intravenous infusions of 5 per cent *glucose* in saline or water are often given to help maintain the patient.

Antibiotics. If the inflammation is due to a bacterial agent, antibiotics are certainly indicated. Until the responsible organism is identified, one of the broad-spectrum antibiotics should be given. When the organism is identified, the appropriate drug to which it is sensitive is then prescribed.

Miscellaneous. *Magnesium sulfate* is sometimes beneficial because it has a relaxing effect on the sphincter of Oddi.

Nasogastric suction may be needed for relieving abdominal distention and vomiting (I-5).

Cholelithiasis

DEFINITION. The formation of stones in the gallbladder is known as cholelithiasis. There are probably several causes. It is known that these stones are composed chiefly of cholesterol and some are caused by a precipitation of calcium carbonate. The stasis of bile in the gallbladder is important to consider as is the cholesterol content of that bile. Infections and the bilirubin concentration of the bile may play a part in stone formation (III-6).

MAJOR SYMPTOMS. The size and location of the stones in the gallbladder greatly influence the severity of the symptoms. When the stone is in the gallbladder, the patient may have vague sensations of fullness and dull distress in the epigastrium, especially immediately after eating, and he often complains of pyrosis and flatulence. When a stone obstructs one of the ducts (cystic or common), biliary colic is present and the onset is abrupt, occurring usually several hours after a heavy meal. The pain is very great and is probably one of the most severe felt by man. Profound diaphoresis accompanies the pain, which is located in the right upper quadrant somewhat near the midline. It often radiates through to the back beneath the right scapula. Vomiting is common and usually affords the patient some temporary relief. The pain is caused by smooth muscle spasm or stretching of either the gallbladder or ducts. Itching is common and jaundice usually appears in about 24 hours after biliary colic. The attack may last several hours.

DRUG THERAPY. The choice of treatment — medical or surgical — will depend upon the condition of the patient. Medical therapy, though it may not remove the stone, may at least make the patient more comfortable. Diet is of prime importance.

ANALGESICS AND ANTISPASMODICS. Because of the intensity of the pain, one of the stronger analgesics is usually needed. *Morphine sulfate* is often the drug chosen even if it does increase spasm of the sphincter choledochus. This action may be counteracted by the simultaneous administration of *nitroglycerin,* an antispasmodic, 0.6 mg. sublingually. Atropine in doses of 0.3 to 0.4 mg. may also be used for acute pain or spasm. Morphine may be given in doses of 10 mg. to 20 mg. hypodermically or even 30 mg. may have to be given within a half hour period. Even better and faster relief is obtained when the morphine is given intravenously in 10 to 15 mg. doses. *Meperidine* (Demerol; pethidine [C]) may be used in place of morphine. It is given intramuscularly in 50 to 100 mg. doses. *Papaverine hydrochloride,* 60 to 120 mg. intravenously, may be given with the inhalation of an *amyl nitrite* pearl or with *nitroglycerin,* 0.6 mg. sublingually. *Aminophylline* may also be used to advantage for its spasmolytic effect. The use of a rectal suppository (0.5 Gm.) helps to minimize for several hours the spasmogenic activity of opiates or meperidine. Some physicians feel that the use of an anticholinergic drug such as *pantheline* (Banthine) or *propantheline* (Pro-Banthine) parenterally helps to diminish ductal and duodenal spasms.

BILE SALTS. The use of bile salts is highly controversial. It is argued by some that because there is not a normal deposition of bile in the intestines, so important for proper digestion and absorption of foods, a bile salt is beneficial (II-3; IV-1). These cannot be used if there is complete obstruction of the common bile duct. *Dehydrocholic acid* (Decholin) is perhaps the most commonly used. It is given orally in doses of 25 to 50 mg. three times a day. Others that may be used are *desiccated whole bile* (Desicol) and *ox bile extract.*

Bile salts are not without their toxic properties and this is especially true if the drug is given parenterally. Following intravenous administration, there may be a marked fall in the blood pressure with a bradycardia. The bile salts may cause muscular twitching and spasm and a decrease in the threshold of nerve impulses. Vitamin K may be given preoperatively, postoperatively or at both times. This vitamin is concerned with the biosynthesis of prothrombin by the liver, hence it aids in blood clotting and preventing excessive blood loss. (Refer to Chapters 19 and 20, and the Current Drug Handbook for further information.)

THE NURSE. Signs of abdominal distention and distress must be carefully recorded by the nurse. Anorexia, nausea and vomiting will be common indications of this distress. All abdominal discomforts are usually preceded by extremely severe pain. The nurse will need to evaluate the patient very carefully and give the pain medication before the pain becomes too severe. Otherwise, larger doses of analgesics will be needed to achieve relief.

The nurse also will need to provide for relief from pruritus, which is another form of pain. This symptom may be relieved by limiting the use of soap, using bath oils or emollients and applying soothing lotions such as calamine to the skin.

Another observation of importance is the characteristic color or change in color of the urine and feces. With gallbladder blockage, the urine is apt to become very dark, and the feces take on a light (clay) color.

THE PATIENT. Unspoken fears of surgery and possible cancer are always underlying the anxiety expressed by many patients. The patient will need to be able to voice these fears without embarrassment. The nurse can do much to create an open atmosphere for discussion. If the disease is to be treated medically, the patient also will need to be taught the specific components of his diet and medical regimen.

Viral Hepatitis

DEFINITION. Two clinical and epidemiologically distinct entities are recognized and are believed to be caused by different agents. One, commonly called "infectious hepatitis" (infectious jaundice) has a relatively short incubation period (20 to 40 days) and is thought to be transmitted by the fecal-oral route or poor sanitary conditions. The disease referred to as "serum hepatitis" is characterized by a long incubation period (60 to 120 days) and may be transmitted by blood or plasma transfusions or by contaminated instruments that have not been adequately sterilized. Cases have been reported in laboratory personnel, suggesting that the virus may be able to gain access through the skin. Therefore, blood specimens from suspected patients should be handled with this possibility in mind.

MAJOR SYMPTOMS. The prodromal (preicteric) stage may be abrupt or gradual. Fever and prostration are more noticeable in the infectious type than in serum hepatitis. Other symptoms include a transient skin rash, arthralgia, lymph node enlargement, anorexia, malaise, distaste for tobacco, fatigability, headache, chilly sensations, nausea and vomiting. The patient may complain of abdominal distress, pruritus, dark urine, light stools, constipation or diarrhea. With the onset of the icterus, the symptoms may abate promptly.

DRUG THERAPY. Bed rest is extremely important for these patients. Drug therapy is merely supportive and symptomatic.

If vomiting is a problem, slow infusions of 10 per cent *glucose,* 3000 to 4000 ml. daily are used (I-5). Human *plasma* or *blood* transfusions are indicated in toxic cases. *Diphenhydramine hydrochloride,* U.S.P. (Benadryl) and *dimenhydrinate,* U.S.P. (Dramamine) may be used to combat the nausea and restlessness. No phenothiazine drugs should be given because they are often hepatotoxic.

Opiates and barbiturates are not well tolerated, for opiates have hepatotoxic properties and barbiturates are excreted by way of the liver. If a sedative is essential, *chloral hydrate* is the agent of choice.

Most physicians feel that there is insufficient evidence of the efficacy of vitamins, but occasionally the intramuscular administration of the *B-complex* may stimulate a lagging appetite. *Vitamin K* is given only when the prothrombin level is low.

When other measures fail after about six weeks of treatment, some physicians feel that it is worth trying a corticosteroid preparation. This may produce a very temporary remission but there is no evidence that their use improves the prognosis.

Blood and stools are regarded as infectious. Disposable needles and syringes should be used.

Immune globulin given to contacts in a dose of 0.01 to 0.02 ml. intramuscularly per pound of body weight will be effective for about four to five weeks in protecting the person from the disease.

THE NURSE. The nurse's first responsibility is prevention. She must explain the methods and modes of transmission to prevent reinfection or exposure of others to the disease. The nurse can easily do this teaching when the patient is being prepared for reverse isolation (intestinal isolation) to protect others from contamination. Isolation of virus-infected feces is accomplished by special handling of linens and using the bedpan hopper.

The nurse also can encourage the patient to increase his dietary intake. A high protein, high carbohydrate diet, plus supplementary vitamins is the usual order for these patients.

THE PATIENT. The patient is often quite distressed about contracting hepatitis. His being placed in isolation almost immediately can also be upsetting. Much of the therapy seems primitive, even though it is intended to protect. Extended bed rest is still necessary and becomes quite a task to achieve. The nurse needs to show patience and understanding without reflections of censure or punishment. When the patient is well enough, some form of quiet, nonactive entertainment can be suggested and provided.

Pancreatitis

DEFINITION. An acute inflammatory process in the pancreas, pancreatitis may develop from one of several causes. It may be due to a bacterial invasion or to an escape of the enzymes of pancreatic juice through the acinar cells because of an obstruction. It may also be caused by a rupture of a large vessel with a sudden hemorrhage into the organ (II-2, III-6). It may be acute or chronic.

MAJOR SYMPTOMS. In the acute type, the onset is abrupt, with a sudden, acute excruciating pain in the epigastrium or upper abdomen which often radiates to the back. Tenderness is present over the upper abdomen. Vomiting is usually severe. When caused by interstitial hemorrhage and necrosis of vessels, shock is produced. In these cases, the patient may die within a few hours, sometimes in spite of treatment. In chronic pancreatitis, the onset is more gradual. There is loss of weight, and the patient has foul, bulky, fatty or greasy, yellow or grayish stools. He complains of epigastric discomfort or pain. Jaundice may be present.

DRUG THERAPY. Actually little may be done for these patients in the way of drug therapy. Therapy is symptomatic and palliative only.

FLUID THERAPY. Circulatory collapse is often present in the severe stages and its immediate correction is important. The blood volume may be restored by *whole blood* or *serum albumin* or *plasma*. Other intravenous fluids which may be used include 5 per cent *dextrose* in water, saline or lactated *Ringer's solution* with added potassium and calcium salts. Vitamin supplements, particularly the *B-complex* and *ascorbic acid*, are also often added to the fluids. The amount given daily (from 3000 to 6000 ml.) is estimated by determinations of blood volume, hematocrit, urine volume and specific gravity and the amount of perspiration.

ANALGESICS AND ANTISPASMODICS. The pain is often very severe and the choice of a drug for its alleviation is argued. *Meperidine* (pethidine [C]), 100 to 150 mg. intramuscularly every three to four hours, is often preferred. The property of opiates (morphine) to increase pancreatic intraductal pressure by causing a spasm of the sphincter of Oddi limits their use, though they may have to be given.

The stimulation of pancreatic secretion may be further minimized by nothing per mouth and a continuous aspiration of the stomach contents. To add further assistance, the subcutaneous administration of *atropine sulfate*, 0.6 mg. as often as every three hours, will block the parasympathetic innervation of the pancreas. One of the anticholinergic drugs may be used with caution to lessen the motility of the intestines during the first 48 to 72 hours. (See Peptic Ulcer in this chapter.)

ANTIBIOTICS. Broad-spectrum antibiotics are given as prophylactic agents against the potential septic complications of abscess formation and peritonitis. *Penicillin* and *streptomycin* are also effective.

CORTICOSTEROIDS. These drugs are contraindicated unless used as a lifesaving measure in an acute fulminating condition.

THE NURSE. As indicated, there is little that can be done other than palliative therapy. Control of pain is accomplished by means of medications and nursing comfort measures. By controlling pain, the patient can rest more comfortably and adequately, thereby allowing nature a better chance to reduce the inflammation.

Dietary restrictions may be helpful. Often a low fat, high carbohydrate diet is ordered and is divided into several small meals. It is felt that these measures will result in decreased pancreatic secretions. This will reduce the incidence of pain. Alcohol in any form should be avoided.

THE PATIENT. Patients suffering from pancreatitis are often very nonreceptive to changes in life style patterns, especially in decreasing or completely abstaining from alcohol ingestion. The pain is so severe that it serves as a strong warning signal. The patient may be frightened at the thought of possible surgery and have strong unspoken fears of cancer. Pain increases these fears, requiring much compassion and caring on the part of the nurse. By her understanding attitude the nurse can do much to comfort and help the patient over these stressful times.

INFECTIOUS DISEASES OF THE GASTROINTESTINAL TRACT

Vincent's Infection

DEFINITION. Vincent's infection (Vincent's angina, trench mouth) is an ulceromembranous inflammation of the gums and/or tonsils in which an anaerobic spirochete and a fusiform bacillus live in symbiotic relationship. Unless other organisms (III–3, 4) are involved, the destruction of either of the main organisms will eliminate the condition.

MAJOR SYMPTOMS. There is a gradual onset of dryness, soreness, pain on swallowing, otalgia and often a few swollen cervical glands. The lesions are seen as a sloughing ulcer with a soft purple-red surrounding zone of swollen tissue and a gray membrane formation. Fetor is common.

DRUG THERAPY. This condition is usually treated locally and systemically. Mouth washes of saline or, more commonly, of hydrogen peroxide, at frequent intervals are soothing and help remove necrotic tissue and organisms mechanically. The hydrogen peroxide will aid in destroying the spirochetes since it liberates oxygen. Sodium perborate also may be used in dilute form as a mouth wash, since, like hydrogen peroxide, it liberates oxygen. If the condition is not severe and is discovered early, the local treatment may suffice. However, most cases require systemic treatment as well. *Procaine penicillin G* 600,000 units intramuscularly daily, usually is given first. *Potassium phenoxymethyl penicillin* (Penicillin V) 250 mg. every six hours orally for one week, may be used. If the patient cannot take penicillin or it proves ineffective, *tetracycline* is given. For very severe cases, if all other therapy fails, *chloramphenicol* may be resorted to.

Mild analgesics may be needed for the pain as well as *vitamins C* and *K* for bleeding and for the general improvement of the patient. Vincent's infection is chronic and relapses are extremely common so the patient should be encouraged to continue treatment even after apparent recovery.

Sometimes the condition is so painful that the patient cannot eat properly or chew his food as it should be chewed. The nurse must see that the patient obtains ample nourishment. Bland foods that are easily swallowed are most acceptable.

Vincent's infection does not usually require bed rest and often the patient will be able to continue with his usual occupation. The nurse must explain to the patient the contagiousness of the disease and the precautions he must observe to prevent others from contracting the disease. Kissing is a potent means of transmitting the disease, as is careless disinfection of eating utensils and other contaminated articles. It is imperative that the patient's dishes and silverware be boiled after use.

Staphylococcal Food Poisoning

DEFINITION. Staphylococcal food poisoning is usually caused by the ingestion of food contaminated by the toxin produced by some strain of *staphylococcus aureus.*

MAJOR SYMPTOMS. The symptoms usually appear within about three hours after the ingestion of the contaminated food. These include salivation, nausea, vomiting, retching, abdominal cramps, prostration and diarrhea. If the infection is severe, blood and mucus may be seen in both vomitus and stool.

DRUG THERAPY. To combat the nausea and vomiting, rectal suppositories of an antiemetic may be useful. It may be *prochlorperazine* (Compazine), 25 mg., *chlorpromazine* (Thorazine), 25 to 100 mg., *promethazine hydrochloride* (Phenergan), 25 mg.; or even *sodium pentobarbital* (Nembutal), 60 to 200 mg. After the nausea and vomiting have subsided, it is wise to use carbonated beverages, clear broths, tea, gelatin and tap water by mouth. Fruit juices, milk, milk products and ice cold food and drink should be avoided.

If the diarrhea is not too severe and it can be tolerated, an oral mixture of equal parts of *milk of bismuth* and *paregoric* may be used. This is best given immediately after every loose stool. Should the diarrhea and vomiting be severe, it is not necessary to use purgation or gastric lavage.

The fluid loss may be extreme in some cases and this may be combated with the use of 5 per cent glucose in isotonic saline intravenously, 2000 to 4000 ml. in 24 hours.

For severe abdominal pain and cramps, it may be necessary to use *meperidine* (Demerol, pethidine [C]), 50 to 100 mg. every three to four hours, *codeine sulfate*, 30 to 60 mg., or *morphine sulfate*, 15 mg., with *atropine sulfate*, 0.4 mg.

When shock is present, it may be combated with the use of the pressor amines. These include *levarterenol bitartrate* (Levophed), 4 ml. in 1000 ml. of diluent at the rate of 0.5 to 1 ml. per minute, or metaraminol bitartrate (Aramine) U.S.P. 2–10 mg. subcutaneously or intramuscularly, p.r.n.; 15–100 mg., usually given in dextrose, intravenously, p.r.n. to maintain the blood pressure. In extreme cases, the intravenous administration of blood or plasma with a cortisone preparation may be required.

No other specific therapy is usually given. Antibiotics are used only if there are complications, since it is the toxins which cause the poisoning. The correct choice is difficult because many of these staphylococcal organisms change their susceptibility to the antimicrobial therapy rapidly.

The Nurse. The Patient. The nurse will need to teach the patient and his family how to avoid food poisoning situations. Staphylococcal food poisoning occurs most frequently during the summer months when large groups of people are gathering for fun. Foods that are easily contaminated with soluble exotoxins are ham, seafoods, potato salad, sausage, stuffing, custard and whipped cream. Especially when large crowds are served, these foods may be left standing without adequate refrigeration. This allows the organisms to grow and to produce the toxin. Therefore, public education is needed. The public health agencies can be encouraged in establishing an instructional program for the community.

Botulism

DEFINITION. Botulism is a type of food poisoning caused by the ingestion of the toxins produced by *Clostridium botulinum.*

MAJOR SYMPTOMS. Botulism is characterized by increasing fatigue, muscle incoordination, various gastrointestinal symptoms and descending central nervous system paralysis.

DRUG THERAPY. There is a vaccine available for botulism but it is not in common use except for laboratory workers or others who might come in contact with the organism or its toxins. The antitoxic serum is sometimes used to produce a passive immunity. The only specific treatment for botulism is the administration of the polyvalent antitoxin which is available through the local health department in the United States and in Canada from Connaught Laboratories, Willowdale, Ontario. General treatment includes the use of artificial respiration, since respiratory failure is the most serious symptom. Sedatives, hypnotics and most analgesics are avoided because of their effect on respiration. Hyperbaric oxygen has proved successful in some cases. Guanethidine has been tried investigationally. It is given orally, by naso-gastric tube if required, and it appears to delay the progress of the paralysis. If the case is diagnosed early, evacuants are given and also a gastric lavage with *sodium bicarbonate.* Supportive drugs may be used such as *oxygen,* intravenous *glucose* for fluid and nutritional needs, *digitalis* for cardiac complications and *neostigmine* (Prostigmin) or similar drug to aid in maintaining muscle tone.

Botulism occurs most frequently in home canned products, especially those of low acidity, such as beans, peas and meat products. It also occurs with foods cooked in a barbecue pit, especially beans. Since the toxin is destroyed by heat (100° C.), the precaution of boiling these foods for five minutes eliminates the potential hazard.

Colon-Typhoid Diseases

The diseases in this group vary from a mild type of "food poisoning" to serious, often fatal, typhoid fever, but they have several things in common. All are caused by gram-negative rods, many of them are motile, all are intestinal diseases and most cause gastrointestinal distress, anorexia, nausea and vomiting and usually diarrhea and systemic symptoms of toxemia and dehydration. The diseases included in this group are typhoid fever, paratyphoid fever (III-6) A and B, shigellosis and salmonellosis.

Since they are all treated with much the same drugs, the discussion of these diseases will be combined.

Prevention can be approached by improvement of general sanitation—these diseases are extremely rare where sanitary controls are adequate—and by vaccination. The latter is available for typhoid and should be used wherever sanitation is inadequate or where contact is apt to occur. It is not uncommon for an individual who has recovered from typhoid to harbor the organisms even though he is asymptomatic. These individuals are known as "typhoid carriers" and are capable of transmitting the disease to others, especially if they do not observe clean, hygienic habits.

Typhoid fever responds well to the administration of 2 to 3 Gm. of *chloramphenicol* daily for the first few days until the temperature is normal. Then a total daily dose of 1.0 to 1.5 Gm. has been found to be adequate. The daily dose is divided into two or four parts and given at 12 or 6 hour intervals. There is often no change for the first two days; then, on the third day, dramatic improvement is noted—the temperature subsides and symptoms abate. Relapses are prevented by continuing the medication at 1 Gm. doses daily for three or four weeks. Even more dramatic improvement is evidenced when *hydrocortisone* 200 mg. daily for four or five days is given in conjunction with the chloramphenicol. *Ampicillin* may be given in place of chloramphenicol, but it is usually less effective. Carriers are not treated with chloramphenicol. *Penicillin*, ten million units daily for ten days, usually helps some, though surgery to remove an infected gallbladder is more apt to ensure a cure since it removes the organisms from the carrier.

Salmonellosis (enteric fever, acute gastroenteritis) should be treated promptly with intravenous fluids to correct the dehydration and electrolyte imbalance frequently present. *Chloramphenicol* is the drug of choice and is given in divided doses of 50 mg. per kilogram body weight per day for at least two weeks. It may have to be continued for as long as four to six weeks for complete eradication of the organism. If the organism is sensitive in vitro to it, *Neomycin* in 0.5 Gm. tablets every six hours for five days may be used, though its effectiveness has not been universal. *Kanamycin sulfate* (Kantrex), is also effective against the salmonella organism. It is given in a total daily dosage ranging from 15 to 30 mg. per kilogram body weight per day. *Furazolidone* (Furoxone), a nitrofuran derivative, is useful when given orally in doses of 100 mg. four times a day. An antispasmodic such as *tincture of belladonna* or *atropine* in the usual doses may be advisable for severe cramps. *Bismuth subcarbonate* and/or *paregoric* may be given for the diarrhea.

Shigellosis (bacillary dysentery) should not be treated with paregoric or other opiates because they cause an artificial intestinal stasis which is not desirable. Dehydration and electrolyte imbalance are treated with intravenous fluids. Of the broad-spectrum antibiotics, the *tetracyclines* and *chloramphenicol* are the most effective. One of the tetracyclines is usually the drug of choice and is given in a dosage schedule of 2 Gm. initially followed by 1 Gm. every 12 hours. The therapy should be continued for 48 to 72 hours after the acute diarrheal symptoms have subsided.

Amebiasis

DEFINITION. Amebiasis (amebic dysentery) is an invasion of the mucosa of the large bowel by *Entamoeba histolytica*. It is usually transmitted through contaminated drinking water or raw foods, especially those which grow close to the ground.

MAJOR SYMPTOMS. The majority of patients with amebic infections do not have dysentery. Symptoms vary from slight digestive upsets to severe dysentery and constitutional manifestations. Diarrhea is a common but by no means a constant symptom.

DRUG THERAPY. In severe amebiasis, the course of treatment usually starts with *emetine hydrochloride*, 1.0 mg. per kilogram body weight (maximum 65 mg.) daily deep intramuscularly. It is divided in two doses so that any idiosyncrasy may be detected. This is evidenced by a change in pulse rate and quality, loss of muscle tone and vomiting. This form of therapy is not continued for longer than five days to avoid serious toxic effects on the heart. *Emetine hydrochloride* is used with caution, if at all, in patients known to have cardiac disorders. *Metronidazole* (Flagyl, Trikamon [C]) may be used in amebiasis, 400 to 800 mg. three times a day for five days.

Antibiotics are not directly amebicidal; they act by changing the intestinal flora so that organisms necessary for the survival of the ameba are reduced. The *tetracyclines* are most commonly used and the usual dosages apply. Other antibiotics that may be given are *erythromycin* (Erythrocin, Ilotycin) and *paromomycin* (Humatin).

Many other drugs have been and are still being used in amebiasis, among them *diiodohydroxyquin* (Dioquin, Diiodohydroxyquinoline, Direxide [C]), *carbasone* (Ameban), *fumagillin* (Fumidil), *iodochlorhydroxyquin* (Vioform, iodochlorohydroxyquinoline, Domeform. Quinambicide [C]) and *glycobiasol* (Milibis, Bismuth glycolylarsanilate [C]). Some of these drugs are relatively toxic. The hydroxyquinoline derivatives are hepatotoxic; however, they are poorly absorbed; the arsenicals have wide toxicity. (For specific details consult the Current Drug Handbook.)

Cases of acute amebic liver abscess or acute amebic hepatitis are treated with *chloroquine phosphate* (Aralen). The dose is 0.25 Gm. three times a day for two weeks. *Chloroquine phosphate* is often given with emetine. This appears to enhance the effectiveness of both drugs. Visual disturbances are common when this drug is used but they are not serious. If marked nausea, dizziness or severe insomnia develops, the dose is reduced to 0.25 Gm. twice a day and treatment prolonged so that the total dosage is still 10 to 11 Gm.

INFESTATION WITH HIGHER ORGANISMS

Helminthic Infestations

Helminths (worms) infest the body in several ways, but by far the largest number locate in the intestinal tract. There are some that infest the blood, muscles and various other parts of the body. Not all of these conditions are correctly called helminthic, but they are diseases caused by animal organisms that are more complex than the protozoa. For most of these conditions there is specific, effective treatment but, as with all communicable diseases, prevention is the best possible cure, and good sanitation will eliminate the largest number of these diseases.

ANCYLOSTOMIASIS (HOOKWORMS)

DEFINITION. The hookworm is an intestinal parasite that reaches the intestines by a rather devious route from its entrance as a larva through the skin. It attaches itself to the intestinal wall and feeds upon the blood of the victim.

MAJOR SYMPTOMS. At the point of entrance, the larva of the hookworm causes a skin irritation commonly called "ground itch." Later there are symptoms of abdominal distress and, still later, abdominal distention, lethargy, loss of energy, loss of weight, anemia and various symptoms associated with depletion of the blood supply.

DRUG THERAPY. *Bephenium hydroxynaphthoate* (Alcopara, Alcopar) is used in the treatment of hookworms. It is given orally in one dose of 2 to 5 Gm. Very little of the drug is absorbed, hence side effects are rare. Purgation is not required. Other drugs which may be used are *tetrachloroethylene* or *hexylresorcinol* (Caprokol, Crystoids).

The loss of blood from the parasite's feeding activity causes an iron deficiency anemia, treated with large doses of iron as in any such condition. Any of the iron products may be used. Refer to Chapter 19 for details of their administration, dosage and so on. A diet rich in iron and vitamins also helps the patient to recover.

THE NURSE. The nurse should bear in mind the usual precautions when giving iron compounds. (See Anemia.) If hexylresorcinol is used, it is important that the capsule not be chewed as it will burn the mucosa of the mouth.

THE PATIENT. The treatment of patients with intestinal worms is similar in all cases. Drugs form the main therapy and it is very important that the directions for the administration of the medications be followed carefully. Although the orders surrounding the actual administration of these drugs may be very detailed and exacting, they are absolutely essential for the safety of the patient and the effectiveness of the treatment. These rules apply to any of the therapeutic regimens used against intestinal worms, not just to the treatment of hookworms.

Patients usually feel ashamed and even repulsed by the fact that they have worms, and the nurse must allay this feeling as much as she possibly can (V-5). No one can help having a cold or any other disease, and the nurse should reassure the patient that he is in no way to blame for his condition. He is the innocent victim of the disease. The patient may also rebel against the treatments which are often rather harsh, and here again the nurse must be reassuring, explaining to the patient the reason for each order.

ASCARIASIS (ROUNDWORMS)

Ascariasis is treated effectively with piperazine preparations which paralyze the roundworms. Fasting and purgation are not required. Prepared in a syrup and tablet, a maximal dose of 3 to 4 Gm. for the adult on two consecutive days is usually adequate for roundworms. Dosages for children are 2 to 3 Gm. for those weighing more than 60 pounds, 2.5 Gm. for those weighing from 30 to 60 pounds and 1.5 Gm. for those weighing from 15 to 30 pounds. If the infection persists, there should be a week's rest before the second course. Side effects in ordinary doses include urticaria and other sensitivity reactions but when large doses are given, vomiting, headache, blurred vision, muscular weakness, vertigo, tremor, incoordination and impairment of memory have been reported. Preparations available are: *piperazine calcium edetate* (Perin); *piperazine citrate*, U.S.P. (Antepar, Multifuge, Parazine, Pipizan); *piperazine phosphate* (Antepar) and *piperazine tartrate* (Piperat).

Of the many other anthelmintic drugs that may be used probably the best alternate drug for ascariasis is *thiabendazole* (Mintezol) given 20 to 25 mg./kg. twice daily for two days.

ENTEROBIASIS (OXYURIASIS, PIN OR THREADWORMS)

Treatment of one person for pinworms is ineffective if the remainder of the family remains untreated, for there is then continual reinfection. The drugs of choice are the piperazine compounds. The daily dose is calculated on the basis of 50 mg. per kilogram body weight and is limited to not more than 2 Gm. daily per patient. The drug may be given as a single dose or in two equal doses morning and evening for seven days. If the infection persists, there should be a week's rest before the second course of seven days. (See Ascariasis for preparations available and side effects.)

Gentian violet in enteric-coated tablets is effective and is relatively well tolerated. It is given for ten consecutive days, in an adult dose of 65 mg. three times a day before meals; children take 10 mg. per year of age but never more than the adult dose.

Pyrvinium pamoate (Povan; viprynium, Pamovin [C]) is useful in enterobiasis but not in ascariasis. The drug is given orally in a single dose of 5 mg. per kilogram body weight. This is often sufficient to eradicate the worms, but one or two subsequent doses may be needed at intervals of two to three weeks. Side effects are minimal but it may cause some nausea, cramping and vomiting. This drug is a dye and it stains the stools bright red.

TAENIASIS (TAPEWORMS, CESTODIASIS)

DEFINITION. A rather large percentage of the worms infesting the human patient are tapeworms. They are usually transmitted from animal to man rather than from man to man, as is true of many helminthic infestations. The more common tapeworms are the *Taenia solium* (pork), *Taenia saginata* (beef) and *Diphyllobothrium latum* (fish). As the name implies, the worms are shaped like a tape. Some are segmented.

MAJOR SYMPTOMS. Tapeworms produce many symptoms that are similar to those of hookworm: anemia, lethargy, fatigue, emaciation and, in addition, a ravenous appetite.

DRUG THERAPY. *Quinacrine hydrochloride*, U.S.P. (Atabrine, Mepacrine [C]), is the best drug to use in the treatment of tapeworm. A prescribed routine must be followed in order to achieve the optimal results. For two days before treatment is to be started, the patient should be on a low-residue or liquid diet. In the evening, a soapsuds enema is given and a saline purgative taken. The following morning, breakfast is omitted and the drug administered. For adults, the dose is 0.8 Gm.; children's doses are calculated on the basis of weight. To prevent vomiting, the total dose may be divided in two to four portions and given with 15 to 30 minute intervals. One to two hours after the drug is taken, a saline cathartic is given to flush out the worm. If the worm is not brought out by purgation, a soapsuds enema should be given. All stools must be saved for laboratory examination because if the head of the worm remains (is not found in the stool), the tapeworm will grow again. To reduce nausea, sodium bicarbonate may be given with the drug. Some physicians give a mild sedative throughout the treatment.

THE NURSE. The therapeutic regimens used in the treatment of intestinal worms are often harsh and difficult for the patient to accept. However, the rules are required to destroy the organisms effectively and at the same time, protect the patient. Some drugs used in these conditions become toxic if mixed with other substances such as alcohol or fats. The nurse will need tact and patience in dealing with the patient. Many patients, especially adults, are horrified at the very thought of "worms" and when given a lengthy set of "do's and don't's," tend to rebel. Fortunately, most of the newer helminthic drugs do not require regimens as strenuous as those used in the past, but some do have set rules to be followed.

One set of rules, a therapeutic regimen for pinworms in the adult or child, might be noted.

1. Careful handwashing after toileting and before eating.
2. Keeping fingernails clipped short.
3. Changing bed linen daily and handling carefully; folding linen inward to prevent eggs from flying about in the air.
4. Vacuuming the bedroom (and the bathroom, if carpeted) daily to pick up any eggs dropped from the clothing. Otherwise, wet mopping of tile surfaces daily.
5. Showering immediately upon arising in the morning to cleanse the rectal area of eggs deposited during the night. Putting on clean underwear.
6. Disinfecting the toilet seat after each use.
7. Treating the entire family, even if only one member is known to be infected, since the others are apt to harbor the organisms or eggs, is advised by most public health authorities.

This program helps to establish habits of standard cleanliness, especially in younger children. Most schoolchildren in the United States have been exposed to pinworms and thereby have become capable of transmitting the worms to other members of the family. The public health agencies and the school authorities may, at times, initiate a program aimed at the eradication of the worms, but only if the situation is extreme.

THE PATIENT. Refer to The Patient under Ancylostomiasis Hookworms.

IT IS IMPORTANT TO REMEMBER

1. That peptic ulcer may often be controlled by the proper use of drug therapy and the nurse can teach the patient how to live with his illness.
2. That many people have become habituated to cathartics and the nurse can teach these people about proper habits of eating and personal hygiene.
3. That ulcerative colitis is not easily cured in most cases and this may prove very discouraging to the patient and his family.
4. That peritonitis in many instances could have been prevented by early medical attention. The rule about never giving (or taking) a cathartic in the presence of abdominal pain, unless so ordered by the physician, should always be kept in mind.
5. That curative measures have not as yet been found for cirrhosis of the liver and the prognosis is not good.
6. That an anticholinergic should never be given to a patient with glaucoma or prostatic hypertrophy.
7. That patients with some of the gastrointestinal diseases such as ulcerative colitis are often very demanding and hostile. The nurse must be able to tolerate this behavior and allow the patient an opportunity to identify and express his frustrations.
8. That some patients with gastrointestinal disorders such as peptic ulcer, regional ileitis, ulcerative colitis or irritable colon have rather deep-seated emotional problems. These patients often can be helped with behavioral modification techniques.
9. That pinworms are common in a large number of children and adults in the United States.
10. That treatment for chronic constipation often requires that the person relearn to experience (and react to) sensory stimuli that identify with defecation.

TOPICS FOR STUDY AND DISCUSSION

1. Describe the continuous-drip administration of aluminum hydroxide gel. For what condition is it given and what is its action? At what rate is it given?
2. From a peptic ulcer patient's chart, list the medications he has received. How do they compare with those listed in this chapter?
3. What drugs may be used in the treatment of spastic constipation?
4. What are the real names for laudanum and paregoric? From what are they derived? What is their action in the intestinal tract? What is the usual dose? How do they differ?
5. What is dehydrocholic acid and why is it used?
6. Banthine comes in 50 mg. tablets and the patient receives one tablet before each meal and 100 mg. at bedtime. How many grains is this as a total for the day?
7. Sodium phenobarbital is prepared in 0.2 Gm. hypodermic tablets. The dose ordered is 0.12 Gm. How would you prepare this?
8. You must prepare an intravenous 1000 ml. solution of 3 per cent dextrose and all you have available is a 5 per cent solution. How would you prepare this?
9. Identify how the habitual use of alcohol is presumed to effect cirrhosis of the liver.
10. Explain how you would teach a young mother to care for a five year old child with diarrhea.
11. What precautions would you take with food when going on an all-day picnic?
12. Describe the psychological components related to the etiology of ulcerative colitis. What medications are used in this aspect of the therapy?

BIBLIOGRAPHY

Books and Pamphlets

American Medical Association Council on Drugs, *Drug Evaluations*, Chicago, 1971, American Medical Association.

American Medical Association Council on Drugs, *Evaluations of Drug Interactions*, Chicago, 1971, American Medical Association.

Asperheim, M. K., *The Pharmacologic Basis of Patient Care, 2nd Ed.*, Philadelphia, 1973, W. B. Saunders Co.

Beeson, P. B., and McDermott, W., *Cecil-Loeb Textbook of Medicine, 13th Ed.*, Philadelphia, 1971, W. B. Saunders Co.

Beland, I. L., *Clinical Nursing, 2nd Ed.*, New York, 1970, The Macmillan Co.

Bergersen, B. S., *Pharmacology in Nursing, 12th Ed.*, St. Louis, 1973, The C. V. Mosby Co.

Bevan, J. A., *Essentials of Pharmacology*, New York, 1969, Harper and Row.

Conn, H. F., et al., *Current Therapy, 1974*, Philadelphia, 1974, W. B. Saunders Co.

Falconer, M., Patterson, H. R., and Gustafson, E., *Current Drug Handbook, 1974–76*, Philadelphia, 1974, W. B. Saunders Co.

Gangong, W., *Review of Medical Physiology*, Los Altos, California, 1969, Lange Medical Publications.

Goodman, L. S., and Gilman, A., *Pharmacological Basis of Therapeutics, 4th Ed.*, New York, 1970, The Macmillan Co.

Govani, L., and Hayes, J., *Drugs and Nursing Implications*, New York, 1971, Appleton-Century-Crofts.

Hartshorn, E. A., *Handbook of Drug Interactions*, Cincinnati, 1970, University of Cincinnati Press.

Passmore, R., and Robson, J. S., Editors-in-Chief, *A Companion to Medical Studies, Vol. II*, Oxford and Edinburgh, 1970, Blackwell Scientific Publications.

Rodman, M. J., and Smith, D. W., *Pharmacology and Drug Therapy in Nursing*, Philadelphia, 1968, J. B. Lippincott Co.

Shafer, K. M., et al., *Medical-Surgical Nursing, 5th Ed.*, St. Louis, 1971, The C. V. Mosby Co.

Watson, J. E., *Medical-Surgical Nursing and Related Physiology*, Philadelphia, 1972, W. B. Saunders Co.

Journal Articles

Cupit, G. C., Garnet, W. R., and Powell, J. R., "Antacids," *Am. J. Nurs.* 72:12:2210 (December, 1972).

DeLuca, J., "The ulcerative colitis personality," *Nurs. Clin. North Am.* 5:1:35 (1970).

Dericks, V., "Rehabilitation of patients with ileostomy," *Am. J. Nurs.* 61:5:48 (May, 1961).
DiPalma, J. R., "The why and how of drug interactions," *R.N.* 33:3:63 (March, 1970).
DiPalma, J. R., "The why and how of drug interactions," *R.N.* 33:4:67 (April, 1970).
DiPalma, J. R., "The why and how of drug interactions," *R.N.* 33:5:69 (May, 1970).
Downs, H., "The control of vomiting," *Am. J. Nurs.* 66:1:76 (January, 1966).
Farmer, R. G., "Anemia: gastrointestinal causes," *Postgrad. Med.* 52:4:95 (1972).
Henderson, L. M., "Nursing care in acute cholecystitis," *Am. J. Nurs.* 64:93 (May, 1964).
Hirschman, J. L., and Herfindel, E. T., "Current therapy concepts—Peptic ulcer," *J. Am. Pharm. Assoc.* NS 11:8:445 (1971).
Horowitz, C., "Profiles in o.p.d. nursing: a rectal and colon service," *Am. J. Nurs.* 71:1:114 (January, 1971).
Jackson, B., "Ulcerative colitis from an etiological perspective," *Am. J. Nurs.* 73:2:258 (February, 1973).
Kretzer, M., and Engley, F., "Preventing food poisoning," *R.N.* 33:6:50 (June, 1970).
McKittrick, J., and Shatkin, J., "Ulcerative colitis," *Am. J. Nurs.* 62:8:60 (August, 1962).
Most, H., "Treatment of the more common worm infections," *J.A.M.A.* 185:874 (September, 1963).
Putt, A., "One experiment in nursing adults with peptic ulcers," *Nurs. Res.* 19:6:484 (1970).
Reif, L., "Managing life with chronic illness (ulcerative colitis)," *Am. J. Nurs.* 73:2:258 (February, 1973).
Secor, S., "Colostomy rehabilitation," *Am. J. Nurs.* 70:11:2400 (November, 1970).
Simmons, S., and Given, B., "Acute pancreatitis," *Am. J. Nurs.* 71:5:934 (May, 1971).
Stitcher, J. E., and Roth, J. L., "The aerophagic patient," *Am. J. Nurs.* 66:5:1014 (May, 1966).
Williams, L., Jr., "An acute abdomen," *Am. J. Nurs.* 71:2:299 (February, 1971).
Wood, C., "Medications for vertigo and motion sickness," *Am. J. Nurs.*, 66:8:1764 (August, 1966).

CHAPTER 18

DRUGS USED FOR DISORDERS OF THE CARDIOVASCULAR SYSTEM

CORRELATION WITH OTHER SCIENCES

I. ANATOMY AND PHYSIOLOGY

1. The heart serves as a pump to propel the blood through the arteries to the various organs of the body.
2. An inherent property of the myocardium is its ability to contract rhythmically independent of the nerve supply.
3. The sino-atrial node is the pacemaker of the heart.
4. The vagus nerve is the cardiac inhibitor and the sympathetic nerves function as a cardiac accelerator.

III. MICROBIOLOGY

1. Several diseases of the heart and blood are caused by microorganisms, some of which are known and recognized; others are still to be identified. Some of the more common are the *Streptococcus, Staphylococcus, Treponema pallidum* and *Mycobacterium tuberculosis.*

IV. PHYSICS

1. Work is done only when a force (the heart in this case) moves an object (the blood) through a distance (the blood vessels) in the direction of the force.
2. Work (of the heart) is measured by the product of the force (the rate of heart beat) and the distance through which the force acts.
3. Energy is the capacity for doing work.
4. Power is the rate at which work is done.
5. The heart transmits the energy of its motion to the blood. If resistance is present (such as is found in arteriosclerosis), the wave of motion is slowed and finally stopped.
6. The electrocardiogram is a recording of the waves produced by electric currents of active heart muscle.

V. PSYCHOLOGY

1. The majority of patients with heart disease will need help to develop the proper mental attitude toward their disease.
2. Cardiac patients should not be permitted to become psychic cripples. This can often be prevented by the patient's understanding of his condition and his limitations.
3. Severe emotional stress can become a factor in several heart conditions by putting an added burden on the cardiac apparatus.
4. The patient with cardiac disease must learn to accept some responsibility for his recovery.

VI. SOCIOLOGY

1. The intelligent cooperation of the family must be gained in order to help cardiac patients.
2. A diagnosis of heart disease need not mean impending death but, with adequate medical and nursing care, may well make the patient's life longer than otherwise.
3. The family should not transmit their fears to the patient.
4. The patient will need love, approval and understanding from his family and friends.
5. The long-range therapy needed in many cases may prove expensive for the family. They should seek adequate help through social service agencies and through the local heart association to make satisfactory plans for this long-term care.
6. Rehabilitation of the patient may be needed, and the local heart association may assist by helping the family find the facilities for this education.

INTRODUCTION

Although the body is an integrated whole, everyone is aware of the importance of certain specific organs: the brain, which controls our every action, the liver, which is our chemical laboratory, the stomach and intestines, which supply our fuel and building materials and the vascular system, which is our transport system carrying, among other things, the waste products to the kidneys for removal and excretion. However, the one organ that probably has attracted the most attention throughout the ages is the heart. In different eras, it was thought to be the center of the being (the soul) and the center of love (leading to the heart-shaped valentine).

Any disorder of the heart affects every part of the body. This is one reason so much attention is given to heart diseases and disorders. The other is the fact that heart disease is the number one killer in our country today. It is also a fact that deaths from heart disorders often occur in what might be called the prime of life. Of course, deaths from heart disorders can occur at any age, from infancy through senility.

Despite all of this, there is hope for the cardiac patient. Many individuals live for years with a known heart disorder. Although surgery and various manipulative procedures play an important part in some types of heart disorders, by far the majority of cardiac diseases are treated medically.

DISEASES OF THE HEART—DISORDERS OF CARDIAC RHYTHM

There are many different forms of cardiac arrhythmias. Drug therapy is similar in most of them. Only two, one atrial and one ventricular, are discussed here in detail.

Atrial Fibrillation

DEFINITION. Atrial fibrillation is perhaps the most common of all the heart arrhythmias and may or may not be associated with cardiac failure. The sino-atrial node has entirely lost control of the heart rhythm (I-1, 3) with the result that the auricles beat so rapidly (400 or more a minute) that not all of the impulses reach the ventricles. Only about one of every three or four atrial beats reaches the ventricles but even so there is a rise in the ventricular beat. Other similar conditions include atrial flutter and paroxysmal atrial tachycardia. In all of these there is increased atrial rate with decreased effectiveness. Treatment is comparable.

MAJOR SYMPTOMS. This disease usually results in what is known as a pulse deficit—with the radial pulse considerably less than the apical beat. If allowed to continue, this may rapidly exhaust the heart (I-3, 4). The ventricular rate may be one and a half times the pulse rate with irregular force, rate and rhythm. The patient with this disturbance usually complains of palpitation, sometimes pain, breathlessness, pallor, vertigo and nausea. He soon finds that exercise definitely aggravates these symptoms (IV-1, 2).

DRUG THERAPY. The urgency of treatment requires that the heart be slowed as soon as possible so that the heart muscle is not exhausted (I-2, 3, 4). The correct drug will depend upon two factors: the duration of the arrhythmia and the cause of the arrhythmia (e.g., cardiac failure, hyperthyroidism). Arrhythmias of recent origin respond better than those of long standing. The best drug at the present time is thought to be digitalis.

DIGITALIS. Digitalis reduces the ventricular rate by decreasing conduction through the atrioventricular node (I-3). Administration of digitalis intravenously is the most rapid and satisfactory approach. *Deslanoside* (Cedilanid-D) may be given in doses from 1.2 to 1.6 mg., either in one injection or divided into two separate doses of 0.6 to 0.8 mg. several hours apart. *Digoxin* (Lanoxin) may be substituted for the deslanoside. During early therapy for atrial fibrillation continuous monitoring of the electrocardiogram is done, circumstances permitting. If this is impossible, the apical and radial pulse rates should be taken frequently. In some patients, it is possible to use the oral route to begin treatment and with all patients it is used for maintenance. The preferred preparation is digoxin. It may be given in doses of 0.25 mg. three times a day for two days. For maintenance the dose is 0.25 to 0.5 mg. once a day. Digitalis is discussed in detail under Congestive Heart Failure later in this chapter.

If digitalization of the patient does not relieve the fibrillation, propranolol hydrochloride (Inderal) may be ordered; so may quinidine.

PROPRANOLOL HYDROCHLORIDE

THE DRUG. Propranolol hydrochloride is a synthetic preparation used as a beta adrenergic blocking agent in the management of certain cardiac arrhythmias.

Physical and Chemical Properties. Propranolol is a naphthoxyl substituted propanol. It is a stable, colorless crystalline solid readily soluble in water and in ethanol.

Action. As just noted, propranolol blocks the beta adrenergic reflexes, but not the alpha receptors. (See Chapter 9 for further information.) Propranolol reduces the rate of heart beat, cardiac output, resting stroke volume and oxygen consumption but increases ventricular end-diastolic pressure. Propranolol blocks the adrenergic stimulation of catecholamines like isoproterenol, epinephrine and norepinephrine.

Therapeutic Uses. Propranolol is used as a myocardial depressant in various cardiac arrhythmias. It is also used in the treatment of hypertrophic subaortic stenosis, pheochromocytoma and angina pectoris.

Absorption and Excretion. Oral absorption is good, if the drug is given on an empty stomach. It is widely distributed throughout the body with the highest concentration in lungs, spleen and kidneys. After intravenous injection, the metabolic half-life of the drug is about one hour, but considerable effect can still be noted for as long as six hours.

Preparations and Dosages

Propranolol hydrochloride (Inderal) for cardiac arrhythmias:

- 10 to 30 mg. t.i.d. or q.i.d. orally, 1 to 3 mg. I.V. (Not more than 1 ml. [1 mg.] per minute.)
- 20 to 40 mg. t.i.d. or q.i.d. orally for hypertrophic subaortic stenosis.
- 60 mg. orally daily in divided doses for three days preoperatively for pheochromocytoma together with an alpha adrenergic blocking agent.
- 30 mg. orally daily for inoperable pheochromocytoma.

THE NURSE

Mode of Administration. Oral doses of propranolol should be given a.c. and q.i.d.; the fourth dose is given h.s. In intravenous administration, the drug must not be given too rapidly. As soon as normal rhythm is established, the drug should be stopped. If arrhythmia starts anew, the drug may be continued, but usually administration can be given orally. Take the apical and radial pulse, and note and record the pulse deficit before giving each dose. This will aid the physician in the determination of dosage. This is not necessary when continuous monitoring of an electrocardiogram is being done.

Side Effects. The several side effects of the drug are nausea, vomiting, diarrhea, lightheadedness, constipation, lassitude, weakness and fatigue. Skin rash, paresthesia of the hands, drug fever, sore throat and visual disturbances have also been reported.

Toxicity and Treatment. Excessive cardiac depression is the most serious toxic effect of this drug. If excessive bradycardia does occur, 0.5 to 1.0 mg. atropine is usually given intravenously.

Interactions. Propranolol antagonizes the action of isoproterenol. Propranolol inhibits the glycogenolytic action of epinephrine and norepinephrine. With digitalis it may cause bradycardia, and with quinidine it promotes sinus rhythm. Propranolol is potentiated by diphenylhydantoin. With tobacco smoking it causes increased blood pressure, and it enhances the action of the sulfonylurea oral antihyperglycemic agents (Diabinese, Dymelor, Orinase, Tolinase).

Contraindications. Contraindications include bronchial asthma and allergic rhinitis, especially during hay fever season. The drug is not given in patients with sinus bradycardia, heart block, cardiogenic shock, right ventricular failure secondary to pulmonary hypertension or in congestive heart failure, unless the failure is secondary to tachyarrhythmia. Propranolol is also contraindicated in patients receiving heart depressing anesthetics such as ether and chloroform or certain adrenergic augmenting psychotropic drugs including the monoamine oxidase inhibitors or within two weeks after discontinuance of such drugs. Safety during pregnancy has not been established.

Precautions. When propranolol is given intravenously, cardiac monitoring is essential. Intravenous administration of propranolol may be considered hazardous, resulting in cardiac standstill or severe hypotension. The drug is used with caution in patients with diabetes mellitus or hypoglycemia, those receiving catecholamine depleting drugs like reserpine or those with known renal or hepatic dysfunctions.

Patient Teaching. If the fibrillation is acute and the patient seriously ill, the nurse can do little but reassure the patient and his family that the medication usually controls the emergency in a short time. However, if the patient must continue taking the drug after he goes home, he should be told to take the drug before—and not after—meals, because it is more effective that way. The tablet should not be chewed but should be swallowed immediately. The patient should be assured that the drug usually helps; however, he should report to the doctor immediately if dryness of the mouth or other adverse symptoms recur.

Palpitation and other symptoms of cardiac arrhythmias are very distressing and alarming. The nurse should assure the patient that these symptoms will soon be relieved by the drug.

THE PATIENT. The patient with acute, severe atrial fibrillation is very apprehensive; this would be true even if the condition were not acute. It is terrifying to feel as if the heart were "running away" or, as some patients have expressed it, "jumping out of the chest." By allowing the patient to express his fears, the nurse may be better able to reassure him. The frequency and the severity of the palpitation and arrhythmias will be the major factor in his anxieties. The nurse can help him to learn to cope with his illness. If the disorder is such as to cause a major reduction in his capacity to function as he previously did, the stress will be very great.

The patient will need to be instructed about monitoring (if he is so placed). The nurse can briefly explain that the device picks up the electrical impulses of the heart and records them in the nurses' station and that the nurse can see immediately if any change in therapy will be required. Most patients have already had electrocardiograms taken. If the patient has not had an electrocardiogram before, the procedure should be explained to him. The nurse will need to create an atmosphere of dependability and help the patient develop confidence in the treatment he is being given. (VI-1, 2, 3, 4).

QUINIDINE

THE DRUG. Quinidine is an alkaloid derived from the bark of the cinchona tree and as such is similar to quinine.

Physical and Chemical Properties. Quinidine, the d-isomer of quinine, is an alkaloid not readily soluble in water, although its salts are.

Action. Quinidine and quinine have similar actions, although quinine is more effective against malaria, whereas quinidine acts better as a cardiac depressant. Quinidine shares with quinine, but to a lower degree, antimicrobial, antipyretic and oxytoxic actions.

DIGITALIS

PRIMARY EFFECTS

Increases force of systolic contraction by acting on myocardium
Slows cardiac rate by stimulating vagus nerve
Decreases diastolic size of heart
Cardiac output increased
Slows A-V conduction
Shortens functional refractory period of ventricle
Blood pressure affected only by action on heart muscle-not remarkable

PRINCIPAL USES

Congestive heart failure
Atrial fibrillation and flutter if accompanied by heart failure
Certain cases of paroxysmal tachycardia

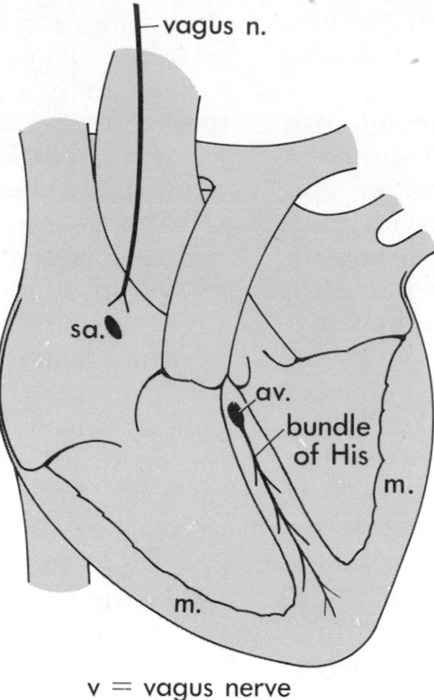

v = vagus nerve
sa = sinoauricular node
av = atrioventricular node
m = myocardium

QUINIDINE

PRIMARY EFFECTS

Depresses cardiac vagal receptor mechanism
Some hypotension caused mainly by peripheral vasodilation
Depresses myocardial excitability
Prolongs conduction time through the bundle of His
Prolongs effective refractory period of cardiac muscle

PRINCIPAL USES

Atrial fibrillation and flutter
Ventricular tachycardia
Certain cases of paroxysmal tachycardia
Premature systoles
In certain cases of coronary thrombosis with serious arrhythmias

FIGURE 28. A comparison between the effects of digitalis and quinidine on the heart.

Quinidine is used almost exclusively in the treatment of cardiac arrhythmias, especially atrial tachycardia and fibrillation. It increases the refractory period of the heart which, in turn, decreases myocardial excitability. As a result, heart rate is altered and the conduction of impulses in the heart muscle is slowed. Quinidine is most effective in the treatment of atrial fibrillation of recent origin. It is much less useful in those patients who have had the syndrome for some time. However, if the patient with a chronic atrial disturbance does not respond favorably to digitalis, quinidine may be ordered.

Therapeutic Uses. As has been stated, the primary use of quinidine is in atrial fibrillation. However, it is also used for other cardiac arrhythmias such as atrial flutter, premature beats, paroxysmal supraventricular tachycardia and ventricular tachycardia.

Absorption and Excretion. Quinidine is almost completely absorbed from the gastrointestinal tract. After oral dose, it reaches a peak effect in one to three hours and persists for six to eight hours. If doses are given at two to four hour intervals, a cumulative effect, often desirable, occurs. Following intramuscular injection, maximum effect is seen in 30 to 90 minutes. Even with intravenous injection, effect is not immediate. Quinidine is rapidly bound to plasma albumin to the extent of about 60 per cent. Some quinidine is metabolized by the body, and from 10 to 50 per cent is excreted unchanged by the kidneys, which also excrete the metabolites.

Preparations and Dosages

Quinidine sulfate, U.S.P., B.P. (Asarum, Quinicardine, Quinidate, Quinidox). 200 to 400 mg. orally. Time schedules vary, but the drug is usually administered every 6 hours.
Quinidine gluconate, U.S.P., (Quinaglute, Quinate [C]) 300 to 500 mg. I.M. or I.V. p.r.n. 200 to 400 mg. orally q 12 h.
Quinidine hydrochloride, U.S.P. 200 to 400 mg. p.r.n., orally, I.M. or I.V.
Quinidine polygalacturonate (Cardioquin) 275 mg. b.i.d. or t.i.d., orally.

THE NURSE

Mode of Administration. Quinidine is administered orally, intramuscularly and intravenously, and all of the methods are aimed at building a blood level which will convert atrial fibrillation into normal sinus rhythm. Ideally, the patient should be hospitalized so that close medical supervision and continuous cardiac monitoring can be carried out (VI-6). If the dysfunction is not critical, a day or two of bed rest with mild sedation is helpful before beginning treatment.

If continuous monitoring is not being done, and before administering each dose, the nurse should check the apical and radial pulse, noting and recording the pulse deficit. A more accurate measurement is made after simultaneously counting both the apical and radial pulses for a full minute. Frequent checking of the pulse rate, quality and rhythm assists in developing a baseline parameter. Any variation would indicate that the physician should be notified. Daily blood pressure recordings are also vital. It is common to give one dose of quinidine as a test dose. If no adverse reactions are produced, the drug is continued for as long as it is effective and devoid of toxic effects.

Schedules of administering quinidine vary. If given orally, quinidine sulfate is used. The patient should be instructed not to let the tablet dissolve in the mouth since quinidine, like quinine, is very bitter. If the tablet is given with food, some of the untoward gastrointestinal symptoms may be eliminated. One schedule for oral administration is to give quinidine 400 mg. every two to four hours. The dosage is adjusted to suit the individual. Improvement is indicated by a gradual decrease in the pulse rate and a diminution of the pulse deficit (Fig. 28). If continuous monitoring is not possible, repeated electrocardiograms should be made (IV-6). Usually, if there is no sign of improvement in three or four days, the drug is discontinued since it probably will not be effective.

For intravenous therapy, quinidine gluconate or hydrochloride is used. The drug is usually dissolved in a 5 per cent glucose solution and injected *very slowly*. The patient should be closely watched for signs of hypotension.

If and when normal rhythm is established, most physicians continue quinidine for three or four weeks and then gradually reduce the dosage. The length of time the drug is given depends upon the patient's response.

Side Effects. The side effects of quinidine are similar to those of quinine, i.e., nausea, vomiting, headache, diarrhea and ringing in the ears, which are usually relieved by reduction of dosage.

Toxicity and Treatment. Serious cardiac symptoms such as paradoxical ventricular tachycardia and even ventricular fibrillation have occurred. This is one reason for continuous monitoring when quinidine is given, especially intravenously. Such conditions are best treated in the premonitory period rather than after the actual occurrence. Hypotension during intravenous administration has been reported, making constant observation of blood pressure essential. Petechial hemorrhages may occur due to thrombocytopenic purpura. Frequent inspection of mucous membranes (especially oral) will need to be made. If these hemorrhagic areas are noted, the drug should be stopped immediately. Treatment of all these conditions is symptomatic.

Interactions. Oral anticoagulants are enhanced by quinidine. Quinidine is inhibited by urinary acidifiers through increased excretion in acid urine.

Patient Teaching. (See Propranolol.)

THE PATIENT. (See Propranolol.)

OTHER DRUG THERAPY. In patients with atrial fibrillation of short duration, a normal sinus rhythm may be restored by the use of procainamide (Pronestyl). The total daily oral dose ranges from 1 to 5 Gm. given in three or four divided doses. If normal rhythm is established, a maintenance dose of 500 to 1000 mg. every three to six hours may be used. This drug is discussed in more detail under Ventricular Tachycardia.

Ventricular Tachycardia

DEFINITION. Ventricular tachycardia is a condition of the heart caused by an irritable focus in one of the ventricles (I-3, 4). The ventricular beat often is 150 to 200 beats per minute and this may persist for several minutes, hours or many days. It may be resistant to treatment. It is usually found in connection with organic heart disease.

MAJOR SYMPTOMS. The patient is usually aware of the disturbed rhythm and complains of a fluttering of the heart starting suddenly. In addition, there is a rapid heart beat and a throbbing or fullness of the neck vessels. There may be apprehension and nervousness. Nausea, vomiting, dizziness, fainting and loss of consciousness may be experienced and the patient appears very ill.

DRUG THERAPY. Patients with ventricular tachycardia should be hospitalized, if possible, so that continuous monitoring can be performed. An external pacemaker and defibrillator should be at hand. If actual ventricular fibrillation occurs, closed chest resuscitation and electrical defibrillation are necessary.

If digitalis intoxication is the cause of paroxysmal ventricular tachycardia, potassium, either citrate or chloride, is usually given. Dosage depends upon the condition of the patient, but orally as much as 4 Gm. may be given, best administered in fruit juice. If given intravenously, the chloride salt is used. Three grams are added to 500 ml. of a 5 per cent glucose solution and instilled about three to six milliters per minute.

Other drugs that are used are procainamide hydrochloride (Pronestyl) and Quinidine. Use of the latter, discussed under Atrial Fibrillation, is not markedly different here. The dosage is the same and as with atrial fibrillation it is individually adjusted according to the patient's response. Procainamide hydrochloride is usually the drug of choice for paroxysmal ventricular tachycardia.

PROCAINAMIDE HYDROCHLORIDE

THE DRUG. Procainamide hydrochloride is a synthetic drug which has been found to be effective in cardiac arrhythmias, especially those of the ventricles.

Physical and Chemical Properties. As the name indicates, procainamide hydrochloride is the hydrochloride salt of the amide derived from procaine. It is a white to tan, odorless, crystalline salt, readily soluble in water.

Action. The action of procainamide is similar to that of quinidine, as well as to that of the parent drug, procaine. However, it has more cardiac action and less central nervous system effect than procaine. Procainamide depresses the excitability of the myocardium and slows the conduction impulses from the atria to the ventricles. Cardiac output is decreased. When given intravenously, especially if the injection is rapid, procainamide may cause hypotension, the systole being more affected than the diastole.

Therapeutic Uses. Procainamide hydrochloride is used almost exclusively in the treatment of cardiac arrhythmias, especially paroxysmal ventricular tachycardia.

Absorption and Excretion. Procainamide is rapidly and completely absorbed from the gastrointestinal tract. By the oral route, peak blood levels are reached in about one hour. If given intravenously this may occur in 15 to 60 minutes. The drug is slowly hydrolyzed by plasma esterases. About 15 per cent of the procainamide is bound to non-diffusible blood constituents. The remainder is widely distributed throughout the body. A considerable amount is found in the tissues, especially the brain. The drug is mainly excreted by the kidneys. 2-10 per cent of a given dose is excreted as free or conjugated p-aminobenzoic acid. Patients with congestive heart failure or renal impairment excrete the drug slowly so that cumulative effects can occur.

Preparations and Dosages

Procainamide hydrochloride, U.S.P., B.P. (Pronestyl, Novocamide [C]), 250 to 750 mg. q ½ to 2 h orally, 250 to 750 mg. q 6 h I.M., 25 to 100 mg. per minute I.V. to a total of not more than 1.0 Gm. (I.V.).

Dosage regulated by the response and condition of the patient. Often the first dose is relatively large with subsequent doses at or near the minimum. Refer to Current Drug Handbook for other uses.

THE NURSE

Mode of Administration. Whenever practicable, the patient receiving procainamide should have continuous monitoring. If this cannot be done, the pulse and the blood pressure should be checked frequently, especially if the drug is given intravenously. Because of the danger of hypotension, norepinephrine or phenylephrine should be ready and orders established as to when and how to give them. Intravenous administration requires that the drugs be added to an intravenous infusion so that dosage can be regulated more easily.

Side Effects. Procainamide is usually well tolerated, but side effects have been re-ing, flushing, a bitter taste, diarrhea, weakness, mental depression and giddiness, as well as hypersensitive reactions (chills, fever, arthralgia, skin rash, urticaria and malaise). Symptoms are treated as they occur. Reduction of dosage may be sufficient to overcome the side effects. Allergic reactions may necessitate the use of another drug.

Toxicity and Treatment. As was previously mentioned, hypotension is a serious hazard when procainamide is given by the intravenous route, and may result in cardiovascular collapse, convulsions or coronary insufficiency. These untoward effects can be minimized by introducing the intravenous drug very slowly. The blood pressure and pulse should be taken prior to and frequently during administration so that sudden changes can be readily noted. If the blood pressure drops 15 mm. Hg during the infusion, the drug should be discontinued. A continuing fall in blood pressure is treated with norepinephrine or other antihypotensive agents.

Agranulocytosis has been reported during chronic procainamide therapy. Frequent blood counts should be taken when the drug is used for extended periods of time.

Interactions. Procainamide has a blocking effect on some antibiotics. It enhances the neuromuscular effect of the muscle relaxant drugs and the anticholinergic agents. The cholinergic drugs are antagonized by procainamide. The thiazide diuretics potentiate the hypotensive effects of procainamide.

Patient Teaching. (See Propranolol.)

THE PATIENT. (See Propranolol.)

Another drug used mainly in postoperative arrhythmias and arrhythmias of acute onset with severe symptoms is Lidocaine, U.S.P., Lignocaine hydrochloride, B.P. (Xylocaine). It is given by slow intravenous injection at about 0.3 to 2 mg./kg. The most serious toxic effect of lidocaine is convulsive seizures.

Congestive Heart Failure

DEFINITION. The heart serves as a pump to propel the blood through the arteries to the various organs and is endowed with the unique property of undergoing continuous activity (I-1, 2, 3, 4). When for some reason it has been overworked, heart failure ensues (IV-2, 3, 4). The ventricles of the heart are unable to empty themselves properly, while the auricles empty the usual amount of blood into the ventricles. Because the ventricles do not empty adequately, the blood backs up in the auricles and this, in turn, leaves most organs congested with blood that is dammed back (IV-5). The ventricles, in an effort to do the extra work required of them, hypertrophy. This condition is referred to also as cardiac decompensation or failure or myocardial insufficiency.

MAJOR SYMPTOMS. Patients with cardiac failure usually suffer from dyspnea of varying degrees, edema (largely dependent edema), cyanosis, cough and expectoration, anorexia, nausea and vomiting. In addition, there is usually headache and oliguria. The dyspnea is worse on exertion of almost any kind and before long results in orthopnea. These symptoms usually produce a state of anxiety in the patient.

DRUG THERAPY. Patients with cardiac failure are usually put to bed so that the strain on the heart will be decreased by the lessened activity. If at all possible, the patient with congestive heart failure should be in a hospital where continuous monitoring is available.

Many drugs are used for the patient with congestive heart failure, including two groups that are commonly used in all cases: some preparation of the digitalis group (including strophanthus) and diuretics (any one of a number of drugs). Other medicines are used as indicated by the symptoms and reactions of the individual patient, such as sedatives and hypnotics for restlessness and insomnia, alkalinizers for acidosis, electrolytes as required and so on. The primary use of digitalis is in the treatment of congestive heart failure.

DIGITALIS

THE DRUG. (See Current Drug Handbook.) Digitalis is derived from the *Digitalis purpurea* or *lanata* (purple or white foxglove). It has been used for "dropsy" and similar conditions for centuries. Its medical importance was first noted by William Withering, a British physician, in 1785. There are several other plants with actions similar to digitalis. The more important ones are strophanthus and squill. Strophanthus was first introduced into medicine in 1890 by Sir Thomas Frazer,

TABLE 12. DIGITALIS AND RELATED COMPOUNDS **(There are any number of digitalis drugs. Only a sample is given below. However, the drugs most commonly used are included. Refer to Current Drug Handbook for others.)**

DRUG NAME	INITIAL OR DIGITALIZING DOSE		MAINTENANCE DOSE	AFTER ORAL DOSE	
	Oral	Intravenous	Oral	Onset of Action	Duration of Action
Powdered digitalis, U.S.P., B.P. (Digicortin, Digitora, Digifortis [C])	1.5 Gm.		100 to 200 mg.	3 to 4 hours	14 to 21 days
Digitalis tincture, N.F.	10 to 15 ml.		1 ml.	3 to 4 hours	14 to 21 days
*Digitoxin, U.S.P. (Crystodigin, Glucodigin, Purodigin, Digitoxoside [C])	1.0 to 1.5 mg.	1.0 to 1.5 mg.	0.05 to 0.2 mg.	3 to 4 hours oral ½ to 2 hours I.V.	14 to 21 days
Acetyldigitoxin (Acylanid)	1.0 to 2.0 mg.		0.1 to 0.2 mg.	8 to 10 hours	9 to 12 days
*Digoxin, U.S.P., B.P. (Lanoxin, Natigoxin. Nativelle, Raugoxin [C])	2.0 to 4.0 mg.	0.75 to 1.0 mg.	0.25 to 0.75 mg.	1 hour oral 5 to 10 minutes I.V.	3 days
*Deslanoside, N.F. (Cedilanid D)		1.2 to 1.6 mg.		5 to 10 minutes	2 to 3 days
Gitalin (Gitaligin)	4.0 to 8.0 mg.		0.25 to 1.0 mg.	2 to 4 hours	7 to 20 days
*Lanatoside C, N.F. (Cedilanid C)	8.0 mg.		1.0 mg.	variable	2 to 3 days
Ouabain, U.S.P.		up to 0.5 mg.		3 to 10 minutes	1 to 3 days
Strophanthin K		up to 0.5 mg.		3 to 10 minutes	1 to 3 days

*Digitalis products most commonly used.

but it had been used as an herb and arrow poison for many years. Squill was mentioned in the Egyptian Eber's Papyrus (ca. 1500 B.C.) and has been used more or less continuously ever since. Since strophanthus and squill are used for the same purposes as digitalis and usually only when the patient cannot tolerate digitalis, they will be discussed together. Squill is rarely used, but is included here since it may be used for the patient who does not respond to or cannot take either digitalis or strophanthus, and also for its historical interest.

Physical and Chemical Properties. All of the active principles of digitalis and the related plant drugs are glycosides (Table 12). Although there may be several glycosides in the various plants, the ones used medicinally in this country are: from *Digitalis purpurea:* digitoxin, gitoxin, gitalin; from *Digitalis lanata:* digitoxin, gitoxin, digoxin; from *Strophanthus kombe* (seed): strophanthin (K-strophanthin beta), cymarin, from *Strophanthus gratus* (seed): ouabain (g-strophanthin); from *Urginea maritima* from India (squill, bulb): proscillaridin. These glycosides are combinations of an aglycone (genin) and from one to four molecules of a sugar. The aglycone portion is made up of a steroid—similar to the hormonal steroids—and a lactone.

There are several semisynthetic preparations. Some of the glycosides are readily soluble in water; others much less so.

Action. Digitalis stimulates the vagus nerve and the ventricular myocardium. Simultaneously it inhibits transmission of the impulse from the atria to the ventricles, resulting in a slower cardiac beat, a stronger systolic contraction and an increased cardiac output, and effecting a more complete emptying of the ventricles. Backflow to the atria is reduced, the reduction gradually decreasing the size of the heart and providing all the body organs with improved blood supply. The net result is decreased dyspnea, edema and other symptoms associated with cardiac failure. Although not a diuretic, digitalis increases urinary output because more blood passes through the kidneys.

Therapeutic Uses. Digitalis is used primarily in congestive heart failure, but also for many other cardiac disorders. Specific preparations are selected on the basis of severity of the condition, type of cardiac involvement, preferred method of administration and so on. Preparations from *Digitalis purpurea* have slower and more prolonged action and are therapeutically usually preferred for maintenance. Preparations from *Digitalis lanata* and from strophanthus have more rapid action. The former is used in emergencies as well as for maintenance. The strophanthus glycosides are used principally for the patient who cannot tolerate digitalis or for the maintenance of the patient with cumulative digitalis poisoning.

Absorption and Excretion. Absorption of the digitalis products from the gastrointestinal tract is usually adequate. The glycosides from strophanthus and squill are poorly and irregularly absorbed by this route so that their use is much less than digitalis. Ouabain, from strophanthus, must be given parenterally. Absorption of these drugs from subcutaneous or intramuscular sites is also irregular and undependable. Since these products are irritating to the tissues, the only parenteral route in common use is intravenous. Rectal absorption of the digitalis drugs is adequate, but not often used.

Digitoxin and some of the other glycosides are bound to plasma protein to a considerable degree. Lanatoside C is much less bound; ouabain not at all. The drugs are widely distributed, and are found especially in the heart, skeletal muscles and kidneys. Metabolic degradation of digitalis occurs mainly in the liver. Some products are almost completely metabolized, whereas others like digoxin and lanatoside C are excreted largely unchanged.

Excretion by way of the kidneys varies widely from one of these drugs to another. The half-life of digitoxin is about nine days, that of digoxin about 46 hours. However, excretion is rapid for all types during the first 48 hours and then gradually decreases.

Preparations and Dosages. (See accompanying table and Current Drug Handbook.)

Powdered digitalis and the tincture were used extensively, but since the introduction of the purified glycosides, they are now rarely given. Strophanthin and ouabain are used when immediate action is required, since they act more quickly than the digitalis preparations in digitalis intoxication to sustain the patient until the excess digitalis is excreted, and in the patient who cannot tolerate digitalis. Usually, the physician does not use the strophanthus glycosides within a few days of the last dose of digitalis because of the likelihood of toxic reactions.

Digitalization. Digitalization involves two problems: (1) determination of the amount needed to obtain therapeutic effects (initial digitalization) and (2) determination of the amount needed to maintain these effects (maintenance dose). The doctor must consider that it is the total accumulated dosage that is more important than the single dose, that practically no therapeutic effect is produced until the total dosage approaches the toxic and that the dosage must be reduced when the desired action has been obtained. There are two approaches to digitalization (the term used to describe the process of reaching the desired therapeutic effects). The rapid (intensive) method consists of giving large doses initially, followed by gradually diminishing doses until the maximal effects are reached. The patient is then placed on a maintenance dose. This is usual in treating seriously ill patients. In the cumulative or gradual method, small doses are given regularly until the maximal effects are reached, and the patient is then placed on a maintenance dose.

The total amount of digitalis to be given in a short period of time usually depends upon the immediate previous use of the drug by the patient. Most physicians now prefer the purified forms as they give a more uniform result.

THE NURSE

Mode of Administration. Before administering any digitalis preparation, unless the patient is on a maintenance dose, the nurse must take (for one full minute) and record the apical and radial pulse and the pulse deficit; this, of course, unless continuous monitoring is being done. If the apical rate is 60 or less, the physician should be notified before the dose is given, unless he has left orders covering such a contingency. Because of the slowing action of digitalis on the heart, there is danger with continued administration of producing heart block which could prove very serious.

Digitalis is usually given orally at meal time to minimize any possible irritating effects upon the gastric mucosa. If the drug is ordered intramuscularly, it is important that it be given deep intramuscularly. Digitalis products are irritating to the tissues and this route is therefore seldom used. Rectal instillation of digitalis preparations may be used, especially if the patient is vomiting. A cleansing enema is given and the digitalis in one of the acceptable water soluble, parenteral forms is instilled through a small rectal tube or the drug may be given in the form of a suppository. When digitalis is given intravenously it must be injected *very slowly*. The nurse should thoroughly understand the differences among the various preparations, when and how each is used, different levels of toxicity and the like. Refer to Current Drug Handbook if needed.

The nurse must watch the patient for clinical signs of improvement, as well as for signs of toxicity. Generally good signs include a gradual slowing and strengthening of the pulse, a gradual decrease in edema, an improved color, diminishing orthopnea and dyspnea and a general improvement in condition. Patients in cardiac failure should be weighed daily, preferably before breakfast, and the weight recorded. This is often a guide to the rate of diminution of edema. The fluid intake and urinary output should also be recorded accurately. Salt intake is usually limited.

Side Effects, Toxicity and Treatment. There is a narrow margin of safety between side effects and toxicity with digitalis. Numerous side effects of digitalis include anorexia, nausea and vomiting. Anorexia usually precedes by a day or two the development of nausea and vomiting. It was formerly believed that the nausea and vomiting following digitalis administration were due to gastric irritation, but this has been practically disproved by the fact that even parenteral administration of digitalis may cause it. The nausea often occurs in "waves." This drug is irritating to the mucous membranes and subcutaneous tissues but the nausea and vomiting which may occur are due to systemic action after absorption and are toxic symptoms. This emesis is secondary to selective stimulation of the chemoreceptor trigger zone for emesis in the medulla. Salivation is frequent and may be copious.

Diarrhea is occasionally noted but rarely occurs alone. Abdominal discomfort or pain often accompanies the other gastrointestinal symptoms. Headache, fatigue, malaise, drowsiness and neuralgic pain commonly appear soon after administration of the drug. Disorientation, confusion, aphasia and even delirium and hallucinations may also occur. Vision may be blurred, and the patient may complain of white borders or halos on dark objects. Disorientation and visual disturbances are more likely to develop in elderly arteriosclerotic patients.

Symptoms of cardiac toxicity may be manifested as a very slow radial pulse due to partial heart block or any one of a number of arrhythmias. Ectopic beats may indicate the beginning of ventricular tachycardia. In some cases excessive amounts of digitalis may tend to increase the coagulability of the blood; heparin seems to reduce this tendency.

Mild digitalis toxicity can usually be prevented by lowering the dosage. Some physicians stop the drug until the undesirable side effects disappear and then start the drug at a lower dosage level.

More serious cardiac toxicity involves, in addition to stopping the digitalis, administration of potassium salts either orally, intravenously or both, since hypokalemia has been demonstrated as a factor in digitalis poisoning. This is probably due to the fact that diuretics are usually administered at the same time the patient receives the digitalis. Other symptoms are treated as they occur.

Hypokalemia may also result from the administration of corticosteroids, gastrointestinal suction, vomiting, diarrhea, or kidney disease with greater than normal potassium loss. See Chapter 10 for signs and symptoms. These unexpected results may cause the patient to seek additional medical attention for potassium deficiency rather than cardiac supervision.

Interactions. The action of digitalis, even to the point of toxicity, can occur with the concurrent use of diuretics such as the thiazides, mercurial, ethacrynic acid (Edecrin) or furosemide (Lasix) because of potassium loss. The alternate or concurrent use of either spironolactone (Aldactone) or triamterene (Dyrenium) preparations will tend to decrease the loss of potassium and aid in overcoming this problem. Reserpine and the digitalis glycosides potentiate each other by additive action.

Patient Teaching. Probably the most important point for the nurse to emphasize is the need for the patient to "live within his physical capacities." For a person who has led an active life to be told that he must curtail all or most of his physical activities is a very difficult idea to accept. It is no easy matter to readjust a lifetime of deeply entrenched habits and patterns. Frequently, the adjustment requires changing a job and even leisure activities.

Often, the patient fears that he will be a burden to his family or, if he is the breadwinner, that he may be unable to care for them (V-1, 2, 3, 4; VI-5, 6). The nurse cannot solve these problems, but she can help the patient adjust to them, suggesting agencies that can aid him. Teaching the patient how to live with his physical limitations is an important function of the nurse.

The nurse can also help to educate the patient's family and friends to become aware of the situation. The patient needs their support and, although they may be fearful of the outcome, each family member and friend must be helped to cope with and acknowledge these fears in a healthy way. This does not mean that the family should not have concern for the patient, but it does mean that they should not increase the patient's anxiety by showing undue fear.

THE PATIENT. The person with cardiac failure usually has much to learn about his condition (V-1, 2, 3, 4). The fact that he is first put on strict bed rest and is totally dependent upon others is usually upsetting to an active person. He must learn that both physical and mental rest are important to him. Mental rest is usually more difficult to achieve, frequently because the patient is in the habit of expending large amounts of emotional energy in his daily activities and frequently because the illness itself has caused severe life-threatening stress and fear for his own survival. All resources, including help from the community and church, should be used if needed to help the patient (VI-1, 2, 3, 4, 5, 6).

The patient will need instruction about the other areas of treatment, including beginning limited activity, pain medications, routines concerning vital signs or monitoring, necessary laboratory procedures, intravenous and oral anticoagulant therapy, dietary restrictions and the reason and need for fecal softeners. This amount of data cannot be learned rapidly or all at once. The nurse and other personnel will need to develop a teaching plan incorporating small elements of the information to be learned, giving preference to those things that either come first or are apt to be most misinterpreted. Reinforcement and encouragement are vital for successful learning and cooperation.

The patient under digitalis therapy should be seen routinely by his doctor who will determine his progress and perhaps readjust his dosage. In some instances, it might be advisable to teach the patient or some member of his family to take the usual precaution of noting the radial pulse before administering the drug. The nurse can also emphasize the need for lifetime supervision. However, the patient should be encouraged to be as active as the physician will allow and to gradually, as he gains strength, resume more and more of his normal activities and life patterns.

DIURETICS

The use of diuretics in cardiac decompensation is aimed at reducing the fluid accumulation (edema) and thus aiding the ailing heart. Normally, the control of the volume and composition of body fluids is governed by the kidneys. In some conditions, such as those of the heart and kidneys, this control is no longer maintained and there is a retention of salts and water resulting in edema. Diuretics may be classified by the mechanism of action or by their chemical composition. The reduction of edema will help to relieve the patient with cardiac failure; there are several methods by which this may be accomplished. (See Current Drug Handbook for additional information.)

Thiazides and Sulfamyl Diuretics. These drugs block the tubular reabsorption, mainly in the distal tubules, of both sodium and potassium, with a lesser change in the rate of excretion of bicarbonate than some of the other drugs. *Chlorothiazide,* U.S.P. (Diuril), has some properties of the carbonic anhydrase inhibitors as well. It is rapidly and uniformly absorbed from the gastrointestinal tract, its onset of action is rapid (within two hours) and its action persists for 6 to 12 hours. Few serious side ef-

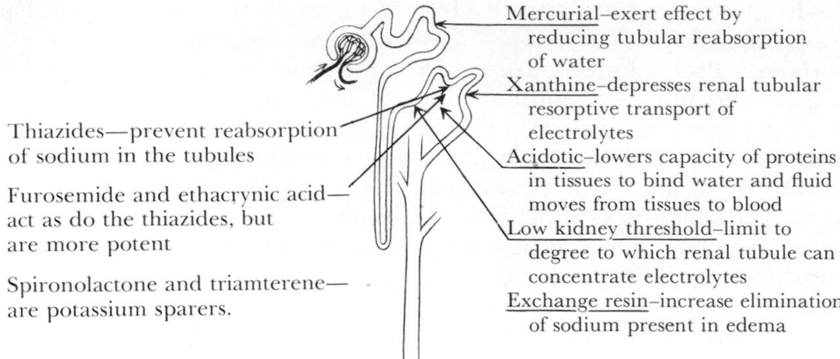
Mercurial–exert effect by reducing tubular reabsorption of water
Xanthine–depresses renal tubular resorptive transport of electrolytes
Thiazides—prevent reabsorption of sodium in the tubules
Acidotic–lowers capacity of proteins in tissues to bind water and fluid moves from tissues to blood
Furosemide and ethacrynic acid—act as do the thiazides, but are more potent
Low kidney threshold–limit to degree to which renal tubule can concentrate electrolytes
Spironolactone and triamterene—are potassium sparers.
Exchange resin–increase elimination of sodium present in edema

fects have been noted, but it should be borne in mind that its influence on fluid and electrolyte excretion is potent. An electrolyte imbalance may occur.

Although doses are highly individualized, the usual oral dose ranges from 0.5 to 1.0 Gm. one or two times a day. *Chlorothiazide sodium* (Lyovac Diuril) is the preparation for intravenous use. *Hydrochlorothiazide,* U.S.P. (Esidrix, Hydrodiuril, Oretic; dihydrochlorothiazide, Aquarius [C]), is effective in doses only one-tenth as great as that required for chlorothiazide. Promptly effective by oral administration, its maximal effect occurs within a few hours, and some residual effects may persist for as long as 12 hours or more. The patient should be watched closely for electrolyte depletion—weakness, lethargy, thirst, xerostomia, nausea, vomiting, muscle cramps, oliguria and hypotension. The total daily dosage should not exceed 200 mg. and should be given early in the morning. Daily administration of a banana or citrus juice may help to prevent potassium depletion. This drug, like chlorothiazide, has some properties of the carbonic anhydrase inhibitors. Others in this group include: *bendroflumethiazide* (Naturetin), *benzthiazide* (NaClex), *cyclothiazide* (Anhydron), *methyclothiazide* (Enduron; Duretic [C]), *polythiazide* (Renese) and *trichlormethiazide* (Naqua). The related sulfamyl compounds are *chlorthalidone* (Hygroton; chlorphthalidone [C]) and *quinethazone* (Hydromox; Aquamox [C]).

Interactions. The thiazides potentiate the action of digitalis, the muscle relaxant agents, the antihypertensive drugs and the monoamine oxidase inhibitors by additive effect. They potentiate the sulfonylureas by displacement at the binding sites. They are potentiated by the monoamine oxidase inhibitors by additive hypotensive effect. The thiazides inhibit the hypertensive action of norepinephrine and, if they are given with the phenothiazine drugs, shock may result. With the uricosuric agents, both drugs are inhibited. For this and all of the diuretics, refer to the Current Drug Handbook for additional information and additional drugs.

With the use of diuretics which excrete large amounts of sodium and potassium, the chlorides are also excreted. There is a decrease in the excretion of the citrates and bicarbonates. This results in a lowered urinary pH (more acidic) and an increase in the pH of the blood (systemic alkalosis). This is sometimes called hypochloremic alkalosis.

Stronger Acting Diuretics

Ethacrynic acid (Edecrin) is a rapid acting potent diuretic. It is believed to act upon both the proximal and distal tubules and the ascending loop of Henle. Dosage varies with the condition of the patient, but is usually from 2 to 4 mg./kg. given orally or 0.5 to 1.0 mg./kg. intravenously once a day. The dosage is initiated at a low level and increased as indicated by the diuresis effected and the number and severity of the side effects. As with many of these drugs, electrolytic imbalance may occur, for evidence of which the patient should be tested frequently. Ethacrynic acid initially causes substantial loss of sodium and larger amounts of chloride. With prolonged use, there usually is a decrease in the chloride excretion and an increase in the potassium loss. If used alone for a prolonged period, potassium supplements are advisable through either special diet or by giving potassium. This is true of most diuretics. Ethacrynic acid has little or no effect on glomerular filtration, and it does not decrease renal blood flow. It enhances the action of digitalis and the antihypertensive agents. It inhibits the uricosuric agents.

Furosemide (Lasix) is also a very effective diuretic which acts quickly. As with ethacrynic acid, furosemide acts upon both the proximal and distal tubules and the loop of Henle. It can be administered orally, I.M. or I.V. Parenteral injections are reserved for the seriously ill patient when oral administration is impractical. The onset of action following oral administration is about one hour. Its diuretic action lasts for six to eight hours. Furosemide appears to have only a few side effects and its toxicity is relatively low. However, excessive diuresis with dehydration and electrolytic imbalance can be severe if dosage is excessive. The commercial brochure should be consulted for all the side effects, warnings, and so on. Dosage is 20 to 600 daily mg. I.M. or I.V. (intravenous injection should be given very slowly), 40 to 600 mg. orally daily. Usually after the initial dose, the dosage is individually adjusted.

The reason that ethacrynic acid and furosemide have given results in the treatment of refractory edemas may be that they increase the renal blood flow, whereas the thiazides and the mercurials reduce renal blood flow.

Furosemide and ethacrynic acid are contraindicated for use in children, in pregnancy, anuria, severe renal disorders and in certain hepatic diseases.

The selection of the best diuretic to use depends upon many factors such as the patient's condition, the presence or absence of renal or hepatic disorders and so on. Most physicians try the thiazide diuretics first. If they do not prove to be effective, either furosemide or ethacrynic acid is tried. If these fail, the doctor then tries one of the mercurial diuretics.

Mercurial diuretics. Historically, mercury in the form of calomel (mild mercurous chloride) was used by Paracelsus in the eleventh century. It was an ingredient in Guy's Hospital Pill (calomel, squill, digitalis) to which it contributed a share of effectiveness by its diuretic action. However, because of its laxative action and the introduction of the organic mercury compounds, calomel is no longer used as a diuretic.

Even the organic mercury compounds are being used less and less, owing to the availability of newer, more effective and less toxic drugs. However, for the severely ill, edematous patient, they are sometimes life saving.

There are any number of organic mercurial compounds. A few of the representative ones follow. Refer to Current Drug Handbook for further information on these and other compounds.

Mercurophyllin (a combination of an organic mercurial and theophylline) (Mercupurin) 0.2 Gm. daily, orally.

Mercaptomerin sodium (Thiomerin) 0.5–2.0 ml. subcutaneously, daily. (Should not be given I.M.)

If the urine is alkaline, ammonium chloride—1.0 Gm. four times a day—is usually given with these drugs, since they act best in an acid urine. The mercurial diuretics are enhanced by acidifiers and the chloride ion. They are inhibited by the alkalinizing agents.

Diuretics which Act as Potassium Sparers

Spironolactone (Aldactone) is a different type of diuretic which acts by antagonizing the action of the adrenocortical hormone, aldosterone, inhibiting the reabsorption of sodium and producing diuresis. It increases the urinary excretion of sodium and chloride, reduces excretion of potassium and ammonium and decreases the acidity of the urine. Since spironolactone blocks the excretion of potassium, if it is given with a diuretic that causes excretion of both sodium and potassium, it will aid in maintaining electrolyte balance. When given alone, it can cause an electrolytic imbalance. Spironolactone enhances the action of digitalis and the antihypertensive agents. With the thiazides there is increased diuresis. Spironolactone should not be used in patients with severe renal insufficiency. It is given orally in an initial dose of 100 mg. per day in four divided doses and continued for at least five days in order to evaluate the response properly. Adjustments in dosage may then have to be made.

Triamterene (Dyrenium) is a diuretic with effects resembling those of spironolactone, but its action is different. It causes an excretion of sodium and chloride, but not potassium. It is used in edema caused by congestive heart failure, cirrhosis of the liver and the nephrotic syndrome. Best results are obtained when it is given with one of the thiazide diuretics. Side effects are usually mild. Some of these are nausea, vomiting, mild diarrhea, and headache. Adverse effects are minimized by giving the drug after meals. The usual dose is 100 mg. orally, twice daily to begin with and gradually decreasing until 100 mg. daily or every other day is sufficient for maintenance. In giving triamterine with a thiazide, the action of each is enhanced, so the dose of each drug should be decreased. As with all diuretics, frequent checks of blood serum electrolytes should be done. Like spironolactone, triamterine preserves the potassium so that if given with a drug which normally excretes both sodium and potassium, potassium supplements should not be given. If it is given alone, it may cause an electrolyte imbalance with excess potassium.

Carbonic Anhydrase Inhibitors. There are several drugs in this group, each having slightly different actions but proving to be valuable.

Acetazolamide, U.S.P., B.P. (Diamox), depresses the tubular reabsorption of bicarbonate—both sodium and potassium—promoting the excretion of bicarbonate ion rather than chloride ion and producing diuresis, alkalinization of the urine and a mild degree of metabolic acidosis. After oral administration the drug is active for about 8 to 12 hours but its action is not so dramatic as the mercurials. Acetazolamide and mercurials may be given on alternate days. Undesirable side effects, though rather frequent, are usually not serious and are rapidly reversible. The most common complaints are drowsiness, paresthesias over the face and extremities, fatigue, excitement, gastrointestinal upsets and polydipsia. The dose for patients with cardiac failure is 250 to 375 mg. daily in the morning. *Acetazolamide sodium* (Diamox Sodium) is the preparation for either the intramuscular or intravenous routes and is given only when oral administration is impractical.

Ethoxzolamide (Cardrase) is similar to acetazolamide in actions and uses. Usually well tolerated, there are few side effects. These may include nausea, dizziness, and numbness and paresthesias of the fingers and toes. Given orally either alone or in combination with mercurial diuretics, a single dose of 62.5 to 125.0 mg. is given in the morning before breakfast for three consecutive days of each week or it may be given on alternate days. Other drugs of this group include dichlorphenamide (Daranide) and Methazolamide (Neptazane).

The carbonic anhydrase inhibitors are inhibited by acidifiers.

Xanthine Diuretics. Refer to the discussion of caffeine, Chapter 9 and aminophylline, Chapter 25 for more information about the xanthine drugs. This group of drugs is used mainly to supplement digitalis and mercurials. The diuresis is proportional to the cardiac effusion, sets in promptly and ceases when the drugs are withdrawn. They are especially helpful for two or three days at the beginning of the more slowly acting digitalis therapy.

The three main drugs—caffeine, theophylline and theobromine—are not equally potent as diuretics. *Caffeine* is seldom used as a diuretic because its stimulant action on the central nervous system is more potent than its diuretic action. *Theophylline* has the strongest diuretic action (this is not marked) and is given in 300 mg. doses three to five times a day for a few days. *Theobromine* is slightly less potent but longer acting and may be given in doses of 600 mg. three to five times a day for several days. This group of drugs has little use in the absence of edema and is of no value if there is renal impairment. Side effects are mild and not serious—gastric distress, nausea and vomiting. These drugs are best given after meals to minimize the possibility of gastric irritation or may be given in enteric-coated tablets.

The Acidotic Diuretics. Salts which produce acidosis are powerful diuretics and are used in treatment of heart disease with accompanying edema. The reduction of the alkaline reserve lowers the capacity of proteins in the tissues to bind water, and fluid moves from the tissues to the blood, producing diuresis. This group may be used alone or to intensify the action of mercurial diuretics. In the latter case, it is recommended that the acidifying salt be administered in full doses for at least 48 hours before the use of the mercurial diuretic.

The most widely used are *ammonium chloride, ammonium nitrate* and *calcium chloride*. All of these are given orally. The best forms are enteric-coated tablets or capsules.

They are given in amounts from 8 to 12 Gm.

Because there is a strong possibility that these drugs will produce gastric distress, it is important that the nurse bear in mind that they should be given in divided doses at mealtime. She must be alert to notice any signs of this distress, such as nausea and vomiting. Ammonium nitrate produces the fewest gastrointestinal disturbances but may occasionally cause methemoglobinemia. These are bitter drugs and the tablet or capsule should not be allowed to dissolve in the mouth. Sufficient water should be given so that it may be swallowed easily.

Miscellaneous Diuretics. *Aminometradine* (Mincard; mictine [C]) is a synthetic uracil derivative and is believed to inhibit reabsorption of sodium ions by the renal tubule. It does not affect carbonic anhydrase nor does it cause significant changes in the systemic acid-base balance. It is sometimes effective when organic mercurials fail. Minor side effects (nausea and vomiting) are common but rarely necessitate discontinuance of therapy or reduction of dosage. Aminometradine is given orally, the dosage depending on the severity of the edema. The range is from 200 to 800 mg. daily and to minimize gastric disturbances it is best given on an interrupted schedule. This may be done either by giving the dosage every other day in divided doses during meals or by giving the amount in divided doses during meals for three consecutive days and then omitting for four days.

Amisometradine (Rolicton), is related to aminometradine and is similar in its actions and uses. This drug has less incidence of gastrointestinal upsets and is equally as potent as the parent drug. Given orally, the dosage is dependent on the severity of the edema. Generally, 400 mg. may be given four times daily with meals on the first day and then twice daily thereafter.

Oxygen Therapy. The administration of oxygen is usually very helpful to these patients. Because the heart muscle is incapable of pumping the blood as it should, oxygenation is inadequate and there is a resulting anoxia. The patient must then be supplied with the needed oxygen. The methods of administration are discussed under Myocardial Infarction.

The Nurse. When the nurse administers a diuretic intramuscularly, especially a mercurial, the drug should be given deep into the gluteal muscle, carefully aspirating to avoid blood vessels. The nurse should give a brief, vigorous massage at the site of injection. The sites of injection should be rotated regularly.

Whenever diuretics are used, an accurate account of the fluid intake and urinary output should be kept. The output in edematous individuals may be very markedly increased following the administration of a diuretic; as much as ten liters in 24 hours is not unusual. The nurse should see that the necessary toilet facilities are easily accessible. The patient should be weighed once daily (preferably before breakfast) to help ascertain the amount of fluid lost. An accurate and detailed account of the decrease (if any) of the visible edema should be kept in the nurse's notes. The nurse may check for pitting edema of the lower extremities in ambulatory patients and recumbent edema for patients on bed rest.*

With the loss of large amounts of body fluids, the patient must be carefully observed for signs of electrolyte imbalance. A diet rich in potassium or a potassium supplement may be necessary to prevent hypokalemia, unless a potassium sparing diuretic such as spironolactone or triamterene is given with or alternated with the main drug such as a thiazide, mercurial, ethacrynic acid, furosemide or any diuretic in which both sodium and potassium are excreted. Dehydration is another side effect that could easily result and create increased hemoconcentration and intravascular clotting. Since all diuretics place increased burden on the kidneys, careful monitoring of kidney function will become invaluable. (For individual drug side effects, toxicity and treatment as such, refer to the Current Drug Handbook.)

The Patient. It is essential that the patient understand that not too long after he has had the drug he will be voiding more than previously and that the necessary facilities are close at hand. If this is not fully understood, the patient may be unduly

*It should be noted that edema of the lower extremities in the elderly patient may not be of the ankle, but rather of the back of the leg, just below the heavy muscles (the soleus and gastrocnemius).

alarmed over frequent, excessive urinary output.

The patient will need to learn how he can maximize his diuretic therapy. If he has returned home, he can maintain a record of daily weight and abdominal girth measurements, avoid obviously salty foods (ham, potato chips, olives) and carefully report any signs or symptoms of electrolyte imbalance. Assisting in collecting data on his therapy may provide a useful tool in helping the patient feel "in control" and not so completely dependent.

Body image is greatly affected during acute phases of edema. Often the patient is unable to wear shoes or even dress appropriately due to increase in body size. Edema and obesity are factors contributing to the changes in body image. Depression and anger result in withdrawn or hostile behavior. Many times it may appear that the patient is uncooperative. These are difficult periods and the patient will need a great deal of understanding and help in coping with the changes in body size.

Angina Pectoris

DEFINITION. Angina pectoris is a disease of the coronary arteries caused by a periodic spasticity of the coronary vessels resulting in cardiac hypoxia.

MAJOR SYMPTOMS. The onset is usually sudden and may strike without warning. After his first attack, however, the patient often has some premonition of an attack. The patient is suddenly struck with a severe pain—usually substernal or precordial, which may remain localized or radiate to the shoulders and inner aspects of the arms or to the jaw, neck or back. Of importance, too, are the attendant circumstances which bring on the attack. It most frequently follows exertion, strong emotion or eating. However, this is by no means universal. Some patients have most of their attacks early in the morning after an apparently good night's sleep. The pain is excruciating and lasts about three to five minutes, during which time the patient is forced to rest. He often has a sense of impending death. With proper treatment, some patients may survive for many years (V-1, 2, 3, 4; VI-1, 2, 3, 4, 5, 6).

DRUG THERAPY. Before drug therapy can be really effective, the patient must reorganize his life so that he is exposed to a minimum of exciting situations (VI-5, 6). The drugs of choice are the organic nitrites and the nitrate, nitroglycerin.

THE ORGANIC NITRITES AND NITRATES

(See Current Drug Handbook.)

THE DRUGS. There are a large number of drugs in this group. Two of these, glyceryl trinitrate (nitroglycerin) and amyl nitrite, have been used as vasodilators for more than 100 years. All the nitrite and nitrate preparations have similar properties.

Physical and Chemical Properties. Both the organic and the inorganic nitrite ions are active. However, only the organic nitrate is active. The inorganic nitrate is pharmaceutically inert. Physically, all except amyl nitrite are solids and most of them are readily soluble in water. Amyl nitrite is a volatile liquid.

Action. The pharmaceutical action of the nitrites is relaxation of smooth muscle tissue. All noted results of these drugs are due primarily to their effect upon the smooth muscles. They tend to reduce blood pressure, dilate small blood vessels and the coronary arteries and relax the bronchial, biliary and urinary tubes.

All of this group of drugs have similar actions on the blood vessels, their differences being in methods of administration and the rapidity of action. Although the nitrites exert no direct action on the myocardium, they produce a dilation of the blood vessels, especially the fine vessels of the heart. They act on the musculature of the vessels directly, irrespective of their autonomic innervation.

Therapeutic Uses. The main therapeutic use of the nitrites is in relief of angina pectoris. The long acting forms can be used to help prevent anginal attacks. The nitrites are also used in other conditions (such as biliary or renal colic) in which relaxation of smooth muscle tissue is desirable.

Absorption and Excretion. Most of these drugs are readily absorbed through the mucous membranes. Sites of optimum absorption vary with the preparation. Amyl nitrite, for example, is maximally absorbed through the lungs, nitroglycerin and some others through the buccal mucosa and pentaerythritol tetranitrate and others through the gastrointestinal tract. Some, such as nitroglycerin, can be absorbed through the skin. The nitrates and the nitrites disappear rapidly from the blood stream. About two-thirds of absorbed nitrite ions disappear in the body, probably by conversion to ammonia and the remainder is voided with the urine. The fate of the nitrates in the body is not known.

Preparations and Dosages

Amyl nitrite, N.F., Isoamyl nitrite, 0.2 ml. (one pearl) by inhalation.

Nitroglycerin, U.S.P., Glyceryl trinitrate, B.P., 0.3 to 0.6 mg. sublingually (several trade names).

Erythrityl tetranitrate, N.F. (Cardilate, erythrol tetranitrate [C]) 5 to 15 mg., sublingually, 5 to 30 mg., orally.

Isosorbide dinitrate (Isordil, Sorbitrate, Sorbid Nitrate, Coronex [C]) 2.5 to 10 mg. every 4 hours or whenever necessary, orally or sublingually.

Pentaerythritol tetranitrate, N.F., B.P. (Peritrate, PETN [C]) 5 to 20 mg. p.r.n. for attacks; orally t.i.d. or q.i.d. for prevention.

Mannitol hexanitrate (Nitranitol) 15 to 60 mg. q 4–6h, orally, for prevention.

THE NURSE

Mode of Administration

Nitroglycerin, U.S.P. (glyceryl trinitrate, trinitrin), remains the most effective agent for the relief of attacks of angina pectoris and is administered in the form of a readily soluble tablet placed under the tongue. Though it is not decomposed by the gastric juice, it is absorbed more effectively by the sublingual method. The drug may be given hypodermically, but it is not often used in this manner. The usual dose is from 0.1 mg. to 0.6 mg. and the effects are noted, as a rule, within two to three minutes. In most instances, this affords prompt relief. If a single dose is not effective, the patient may be instructed to take an additional one, two or even three doses at intervals of five minutes. Tolerance to nitroglycerin may be delayed a little by using the smallest effective dose at the beginning of therapy and increasing the dose as needed.

The patient should be warned that nitroglycerin (and in fact all of these products) causes a fall in blood pressure due to dilatation of the blood vessels. He should not get up quickly (from bed or chair) after taking the drug, since fainting may result.

Nitroglycerin and alcohol interact to cause a severe drop in blood pressure. Cardiovascular collapse may occur when both are used at the same time.

Amyl nitrite is a clear, yellow, volatile and inflammable liquid with a fruity odor. It is available in small glass ampules (called pearls), each of which contains a therapeutic dose of 0.2 ml. The pearl is crushed and the vapor inhaled. For this reason the glass ampule is enclosed in a heavy fabric in order to minimize the possibility of cutting one's fingers while breaking the glass. Relief of the attack is usually prompt, occurring as a rule within one minute. The pearls may be used as needed.

Isosorbide dinitrate (Isordil, Sorbide Nitrate, Coronex [C]) is a nitrate which is prepared both for emergency and preventive use. The sublingual form is used for those patients who do not react well to nitroglycerin, and the oral preparation is used as a substitute for pentaerythritol tetranitrate (Peritrate).

Pentaerythritol tetranitrate (Peritrate Tetranitrate; PETN, Tetranite [C]) has the same properties as other slow-acting vasodilator organic nitrate compounds. The action of this drug is not immediate; hence, it is not intended to replace nitroglycerin in the relief of an anginal attack. It is believed to release small amounts of its active constituents over long periods of time and to thus aid in preventing acute attacks. There is little effect on the heart rate but it does increase moderately the rate of respiration. There is little evidence that tolerance to pentaerythritol tetranitrate (Peritrate) develops, and significant toxic manifestations have not been observed. Transient headache and nausea, which are seen occasionally, disappear after four or five days of medication and seldom call for a cessation of the drug. Peritrate is administered orally in doses of 10 to 20 mg. three to four times daily as needed for maximal effect. In some patients, a regular dose of not less than 10 mg. three or four times daily may reduce the number of anginal attacks or lessen the severity of those which are not prevented.

Erythrityl tetranitrate (Cardilate; erythrol tetranitrate [C]) is another of the nitrates and is used both for immediate and for preventive therapy. It is given orally in doses of 15 to 30 mg. every four to six hours.

Side Effects, Toxicity, Contraindications. Some of the side effects have already been included. In addition, while administering nitroglycerin sublingually, it is extremely important for the nurse to gain the complete cooperation of the patient. He should be instructed to place the tablet under his tongue at the first premonitory sign. He should allow the tablet to dissolve completely in the mouth and retain the saliva containing the nitroglycerin for at least a brief interval before swallowing. The patient should be warned of the possibility of dizziness, flushing and cranial throbbing (due to drop in blood pressure) and be reassured that these are harmless though unpleasant side effects. When these symptoms appear he should, if at all possible, lie down. Even if these signs do not appear, the patient should be instructed to rest for at least a brief period after using the drug. It is important to have fresh tablets as those older than six months lose much of their potency.

It is usually the duty of the nurse to instruct the patient in the use of pearls of amyl nitrite. She should teach the patient, at the earliest sign of an attack, to place a pearl in a handkerchief and crush it. The handkerchief should then be held near the nostrils and the vapor inhaled. Generally, the crushing of the ampule is accompanied by a noise owing to the escape of vapors which may be alarming to the uninstructed patient. The vapor of amyl nitrite is disagreeable and may cause a feeling of vertigo and faintness, but this is transitory and the patient should be taught that this is the expected pattern. It is wise to caution the patient that this is an inflammable drug and should not be used where it may be ignited.

The longer-acting nitrites may cause a severe headache, and nitrite syncope may occur after the administration of any of these drugs. Nitrite syncope may be evidenced by nausea, vomiting, weakness, restlessness, pallor, cold sweat, collapse and involuntary passing of urine and feces. The patient usually recovers within an hour. The head-low posture, deep breathing and movements of the extremities assist in recovery.

The Patient. Those patients for whom nitroglycerin tablets have been prescribed should carry a sufficient number at all times in a labeled container. The patient must learn to place the tablet under his tongue at the earliest sign of an impending attack and thus, many times, may relieve the pain before it really takes hold.

Those for whom amyl nitrite is ordered should always carry with them a sufficient supply of the pearls in a noncrushable, well-labeled container. The patient should use them when indicated as he has been instructed. Amyl nitrite pearls are the most costly of the preparations of nitrites.

While the patient is hospitalized, he will need to be instructed and supervised in taking his nitroglycerin. In the hospital a small dark glass container with a specific number of tablets may be left at the bedside. The patient should be told to use a tablet as needed, but to close the container immediately after taking it. At home, he will have a larger number of tablets in the container, since the pharmacist may not open the bottle, but must dispense the unopened bottle as it came from the manufacturer. The bottle may contain as many as 100 tablets. Whatever the number, the patient is instructed to take out only one tablet at a time and to close the container immediately afterwards. The reason for this is the fact that the drug quickly loses its strength when exposed to the air. The fresh drug is much more effective. The bottle is small, even if it does contain 100 tablets, and the patient should keep it with him at all times. Most physicians allow the patient to take from one to four tablets if necessary at about 5 to 15 minute intervals. Should these not be effective, the patient should contact the doctor before taking any more than he has been told to take. Since nitroglycerin is relatively inexpensive, the patient may find that it is convenient to have more than one bottle on hand.

Occasionally, attacks occur with, or immediately following, a meal, especially if it has been a large one. If this occurs many times, the patient may need to adjust to eating several small meals rather than the usual three large ones each day.

Smoking is not advisable, owing to its tendency to increase vasoconstriction. This is a very difficult habit to stop and sometimes the patient will not succeed. However, every attempt should be made by the patient, his family and friends to aid him in breaking the smoking habit.

In addition to modifying its life style, the family must learn how best to assist the patient during an attack (VI–1, 3, 4, 5). Everyone should know where the medicine is and how it is given. The family members will need to learn not to become overly excited when an attack occurs. Their calm attitude may be reassuring to the patient.

Other Drugs Used for Angina Pec-

TORIS. The wise use of sedative and analgesic drugs may be of great value in the routine care of angina pectoris. They are often helpful in allaying apprehension and making possible the acceptance of a more moderate daily routine.

Drugs that are often used are *codeine phosphate* in 8 mg. doses orally four times a day as an analgesic and *phenobarbital*, 32 mg. three to four times daily by mouth. Should insomnia be a factor, one of the shorter-acting barbiturates may be used before retiring. *Pentobarbital sodium* (Nembutal) or *secobarbital sodium* (Seconal) in 100 mg. doses may be used orally. These have been discussed elsewhere (see Chapter 9). Some of the tranquilizing drugs may be helpful in calming the patient (see Chapter 30).

The beta adrenergic blocking agent *propranolol* (Inderal) has been used successfully in some cases. This drug has been discussed elsewhere in this chapter.

Acute Myocardial Infarction

DEFINITION. In acute myocardial infarction, sometimes called coronary occlusion or coronary thrombosis, a branch of a coronary artery is suddenly and completely closed. This may be caused by an embolus or thrombus. As a result, the area of the heart beyond the occlusion is deprived of blood and the tissues die. Most attacks cannot be related to any special event.

MAJOR SYMPTOMS. The onset is often preceded by an abrupt appearance of a severe persistent pain, most commonly in the upper or middle third of the sternum. This pain grows more severe and may radiate to the left and at times to the right arm. In contrast to the relative immobility caused by the angina pain, these patients become restless and may even pace the floor. The patient becomes cyanotic, pale or ashen gray; his skin is clammy with a cold sweat on the brow. He cannot seem to get his breath, is extremely apprehensive and often has a strong feeling of impending death. Nausea and vomiting are often present. The pulse may not be detectable radially and the blood pressure may be at shock level. Collapse, coma or quick death often ensues. The person ordinarily survives the first attack, but subsequent attacks eventually prove fatal.

DRUG THERAPY. Although the basic treatment is rest for the heart for a prolonged period (often six weeks or longer), there are some drugs which have proved to be helpful adjuncts in prolonging life. For the relief of the initial pain some strong analgesic is usually needed.

THE NARCOTIC ANALGESICS. The opium alkaloids, of which morphine sulfate is one, have no rivals for the relief of pain. Though the action of morphine is mainly upon the cerebral centers, it does mildly dilate the coronary arteries. Here, however, the drug is used primarily to relieve the acute pain accompanying myocardial infarction. *Morphine sulfate*, 15 mg., may be given subcutaneously at one-half hour intervals during the acute attack until the desired effects are obtained, but the total dose should not exceed 60 mg. It should be noted here that larger doses than are usually recommended are given in these cases.

Meperidine hydrochloride (Demerol) may be used in place of morphine but if relief is not afforded by a dose of 200 mg., larger amounts will not be effective. *Methadone* may be substituted in doses of 5 to 15 mg. by mouth or subcutaneously, as may pentazocine (Talwin) in 30 or 60 mg. dose, I.M.

Keeping in mind the severity of the pain the patient is suffering, the administration of larger doses of narcotics than is usual may be left to the discretion of the nurse on the doctor's specific order. The effect of each dose should be carefully evaluated before administering the next dose, but the nurse must not withhold the drug when the patient actually needs it.

Patients suffering the excruciating pain of coronary occlusion are very restless and apprehensive so that much reassurance must be given by the nurse. The patient should be assisted to assume the most comfortable position possible.

Often patients' families become a problem at this time. They are naturally much concerned over the patient, but many times their presence is disturbing to the acutely ill patient. No visitors are usually allowed for several days—at least until the acute phase of the attack is over. Family members permitted to visit should be instructed to limit their visits to a few minutes and to avoid disturbing conversation with the patient (V-1, 2, 3, 4; VI-1, 2, 3, 4, 5, 6).

OXYGEN THERAPY. Oxygen therapy is indicated in almost all cases of coronary in-

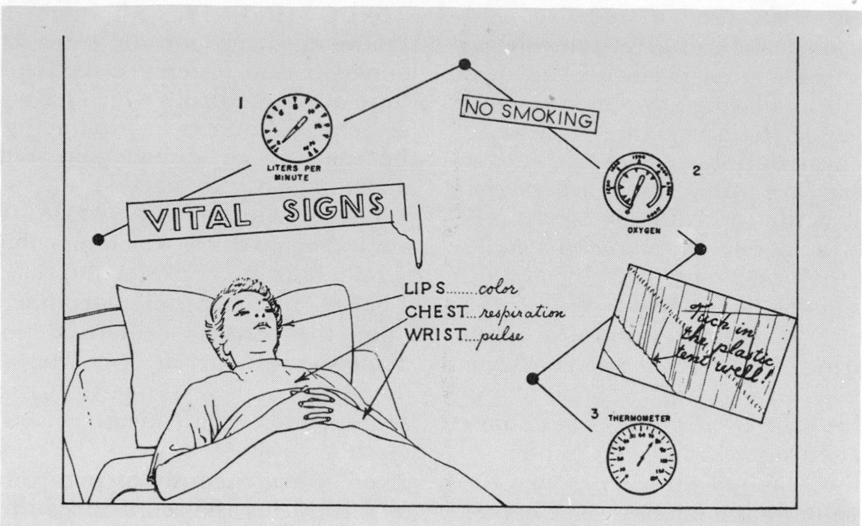

FIGURE 29. Oxygen therapy. The gauge showing liters of oxygen delivered per minute (1) should be kept at the prescribed rate of flow. When the valve (2) showing the amount of oxygen remaining in the tank goes below 500 it is wise to have another tank ready to exchange. The thermometer (3) showing the temperature inside the tent is kept at the prescribed temperature (usually cool). It is extremely important that the tent be tucked in securely all around the head of the bed and across the bed. The patient's color, respirations and pulse are good indications of response. Precautionary signs should always be prominently displayed.

farction and especially whenever cyanosis is present (Fig. 29). This is essential because a vicious circle of events has occurred: due to the occlusion, there is impaired cardiac function; the resulting passive congestion may lead to pulmonary edema; this, in turn, results in poor absorption of oxygen and incomplete aeration of the blood in the lungs; as a result, anoxia is increased. When oxygen is used, dyspnea is relieved, pain is lessened and the heart rate is slowed. This often enables the patient to lapse into the needed sleep.

High concentrations of oxygen should be used – 80 to 100 per cent. The use of the oxygen tent is probably best as it allows for some freedom of movement for the restless patient; however, a nasal catheter may be used to advantage. The use of the oxygen mask is probably not advisable because of the patient's restlessness.

As in all oxygen therapy, the nurse must set up and apply the equipment and see that the supply is maintained at the proper level. She must note the progress of the patient while under this type of therapy. It is advisable to check the mechanism of operation of the oxygen tents available.

In some institutions, specially trained personnel known as "inhalation specialists" or "inhalation therapists" assume these duties. However, the nurse will need to check the oxygen intake between visits of the therapist.

Whatever method of administration is employed in oxygen therapy, the patient should be told of the reasons for its use, and the nurse should try to gain his cooperation insofar as possible. He should be assured that this will help him over the acute stage and that before too long it will be removed. Though the usual precautions in administering oxygen are carried out (no smoking signs posted and so forth) visitors should be instructed to be careful when in the room, especially with matches.

Anticoagulant Therapy. It is almost standard practice to use one of the anticoagulant drugs in the treatment of coronary occlusion. The theory behind their use is that these drugs may prevent extension of the blood clot and also prevent the formation of other emboli or thrombi. The prolonged period of inactivity of the patient always carries with it the possibility of thrombophlebitis or pulmonary embolism and for this reason, also, these drugs are often employed.

The two best known anticoagulants – *heparin* and *coumarin* derivatives – complement each other in their uses. Heparin is used when rapid anticoagulant action is required and followed by a coumarin drug for more prolonged effect. Neither drug should be used indiscriminately, and each patient receiving these drugs should be under very close medical supervision.

HEPARIN

THE DRUG. Heparin is a refined tissue extract made principally from beef lung or intestines. Heparin is a normal constituent of the human body.

Physical and Chemical Properties. Heparin is a mucopolysaccharide compound of sulfated d-glucosamine and d-glucuronic acid, soluble in water and body fluids.

Action. Heparin inhibits the clotting of blood. It is believed to inhibit the conversion of prothrombin to thrombin and fibrinogen to fibrin. Heparin does not dissolve the clot but it does tend to prevent its extension. This means that it does not produce excessive bleeding after small lacerations.

Therapeutic Uses. Heparin is used to prolong clotting time and to treat coronary thrombosis, thrombophlebitis, pulmonary embolism or any disorder in which there is excessive or undesirable blood clotting.

Absorption and Excretion. Heparin is ineffective after oral administration because it is destroyed by the digestive process. It is well absorbed from parenteral sites and is widely distributed in the body. Heparin is found in the blood plasma, but not in blood cells. The rate of removal from plasma is directly related to dosage. Thus, the half-lives of 100, 200 and 400 units per kilogram of body weight, injected intravenously are 56, 96 and 152 minutes respectively. The exact fate of heparin in the body is not well understood. Some of it is metabolized by the liver. From a very large dose, as much as 50 per cent may be excreted unchanged by the kidneys. One degradation product, erroheparin, is excreted by the liver.

Preparations and Dosages

Heparin sodium, U.S.P., B.P., (Lipo-Hepin, Liquaemin, Pan heparin; Hepalean [C]) 5,000 to 30,000 units I.V.

Depo-heparin, U.S.P. 20,000 to 40,000 units I.M.

THE NURSE

Mode of Administration

In preparing heparin for intravenous use, the nurse must be extremely accurate in her technique and in figuring the doses. The continuous-drip method requires almost constant attendance by the nurse to maintain the flow at the prescribed amount per minute—milliliters (or fractions thereof) or minims. Drops are less accurate and usually not recommended for this type of therapy. Before starting a continuous drip for extracorporeal hemodialysis for post-myocardial infarction, the nurse should make the patient as comfortable as possible, since the therapy will be in progress for a long period of time. Should a chill develop or any spontaneous bleeding occur, the drug must be stopped immediately and the physician notified. In these cases, a transfusion of fresh whole blood may be needed. Protamine sulfate (1%) also may be administered via a slow intravenous route for 1 to 3 minutes to counteract the anticoagulant action of the heparin. If intravenous administration is too rapid, the patient should be observed for sudden drop in blood pressure, bradycardia, flushing and a feeling of warmth. Shock may occur.

Heparin may also be given via the subcutaneous route, using a tuberculin syringe. The following procedure may be used to avoid as many complications as possible.

1. Repository heparin often comes in individual packages. The nurse should consult the accompanying literature *before* attempting to administer the drug.
2. Since heparin may be ordered in units versus milligrams, the nurse must carefully check the dosage. The daily coagulation time should also be noted.
3. Heparin should be drawn in a tuberculin syringe (its finer calibration facilitates measurement of the dose). A #25 or #26 gauge, 1/2″ to 5/8″ length, needle is used. A small amount of air may be placed at the plunger end of the syringe (1/10 ml.) to facilitate clearing the needle of the drug and preventing its drag through the tissues while the needle is being withdrawn.
4. Select an iliac or abdominal site and make a small roll. Sponge area with alcohol; let dry before inserting the needle. Wipe needle with a dry sterile sponge to free it of heparin.
5. Insert needle in elevated fatty tissue roll (see Fig. 30). Release skin and administer the heparin slowly. It is *not* necessary to withdraw the plunger and check for capillary insertion.
6. Withdraw needle quickly. Press firmly

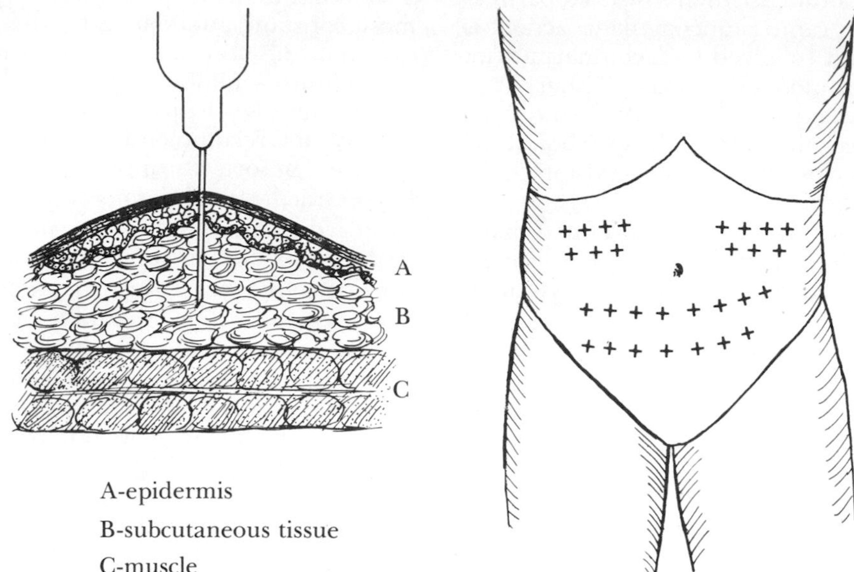

FIGURE 30. Heparin injection. Drug must be given subcutaneously, not intramuscularly. Note short needle with short bevel. Area is pinched and held up to avoid penetrating the muscle.
Injections should not be given closer than two inches apart. Avoid getting close to any bony places (iliac crest, pubic arch, etc.). The points below the umbilicus are the preferred points, but those above may be used if required.

with sponge for a few seconds. DO NOT MASSAGE.

7. Separate charts should be kept in the patient's record on the results of daily coagulation time, amount of drug given and location of each injection.

Intramuscular injections have been reported to result in a high incidence of hematoma formation at the injection site. Hence, the preferred route of administration is subcutaneous.

Side Effects, Toxicity, Treatment. Although not common, hemorrhage may occur during heparin therapy. It may be either one large or several small bleeding points. Protamine sulfate may be ordered. Heparin is, of course, stopped immediately. In an acute situation, a blood transfusion may be administered (see Table 13).

It is generally recommended that heparin be discontinued slowly, for the abrupt withdrawal may cause the production of more thrombi or emboli. It is usual to start a coumarin drug before the doses of heparin are reduced, gradually and finally discontinuing it and letting the coumarin take over the anticoagulant action.

The size of the dose will vary from patient to patient and from injection to injection. The effects of heparin wear off quickly, so the nurse must always be alert and observe for new clot formation or enlargement of old ones. Doses, however, will be dependent on blood coagulation times – the Lee-White method. The normal Lee-White coagulation times are 9 to 12 minutes. Under heparinization, the therapeutic regimen usually attempts to maintain the blood coagulation time at two to three times the normal.

BISHYDROXYCOUMARIN AND RELATED COMPOUNDS

The Drugs. The anticoagulant qualities of the coumarin products were first demonstrated in the early 1920's when a bleeding disease broke out in cattle that had been fed improperly cured (spoiled) sweet clover hay. Some of these products are still derived from spoiled sweet clover and some are produced synthetically. There are two groups, the coumarin and the phenindione drugs.

Physical and Chemical Properties. These drugs are all derivatives either of 4-hydroxy-

TABLE 13. BISHYDROXYCOUMARIN AND RELATED COMPOUNDS

DRUG NAME	PEAK EFFECT (HOURS)	DURATION OF EFFECT (DAYS)	MAINTENANCE DOSE	SIDE EFFECTS
Bishydroxycoumarin, U.S.P., Dicoumarol, (Dicumarol, Dicoumarin, Dufalone [C])	36 to 48	5 to 6	25 to 150 mg.	Rare, but gastrointestinal disturbances may occur; hemorrhage, one large or several small, are possible; cumulative action can happen; for hemorrhage, vitamin K is usually ordered
Acenocoumarol (Sintron, Acnocoumarin, Nicoumaline [C])	36 to 48	1½ to 2	4 to 16 mg.	As above
Cyclocumarol (Cymopyran, cyclocoumarol [C])	36 to 60	6 to 8	25 mg.	As above
Ethyl biscoumacetate, N.F. (Tromexan)	18 to 30	2 to 3	150 to 300 mg.	As above, plus erythema and alopecia
Phenprocouman, N.F. (Liquamar, Marcumar)	48 to 72	7 to 14	0.75 to 4.5 mg.	See bishydroxycoumarin
Warfarin sodium, U.S.P., B.P. (Coumadin, Panwarfin, Warfilone, Warnerin [C])	36 to 72	4 to 5	2 to 25 mg.	Side effects are not common but are similar to those of heparin when they occur
Anisindione, N.F. (Maradon, Uridone [C])	24 to 72	1½ to 3	25 to 50 mg.	As above, plus orange-red urine
Diphenadione, N.F. (Dipaxin)	24 to 48	15 to 20	3 to 5 mg.	Nausea; see warfarin sodium
Phenindione, B.P. (Danilone, Hedulin, Indon)	24 to 48	1 to 4	25 to 300 mg.	See warfarin sodium; can cause more serious symptoms such as blood dyscrasias, hepatitis and so on

coumarin or indan-1-3-dione. The solubility varies from one product to another.

Action. The exact mechanism of action is unknown, but it is believed that they inhibit the production of prothrombin from vitamin K by the liver. Their action is much slower and more prolonged than that of heparin.

Therapeutic Uses. These are the same as for heparin—the treatment of diseases and disorders in which there is a tendency to clot formation. The coumarin drugs act slowly and are thus used for long-term therapy. They are not useful in acute conditions.

Absorption and Excretion. The absorption of these drugs from the gastrointestinal tract is slow and—with some of them—erratic. Most are completely absorbed. The variation in absorption rate not only varies with the different products, but from patient to patient for the same product. Peak plasma levels are not usually seen for several hours after oral use. Most bishydroxycoumarin is bound to plasma proteins. It is distributed widely, but concentration varies in the different tissues. It is found in lung, liver, spleen and kidneys in rather high concentration. Little or none is found in the brain. It does cross the placental barrier and is excreted in the milk. The exact fate of these drugs in the body is unknown. Less than 1 per cent of bishydroxycoumarin is recovered in the urine.

Preparations and Dosages. (See Table 13.)

THE NURSE

Mode of Administration

Bishydroxycoumarin, probably the best known of the coumarins, is given by mouth but requires from 12 to 72 hours before its maximal effects are noted. For this reason it is not valuable as an emergency drug. It more often follows the initial use of heparin. Its action continues for 24 to 96 hours after the drug is discontinued. Some clinicians believe that in myocardial infarction bishydroxycoumarin (Dicumarol) should be given for a minimum of 30 days unless toxic reactions or contraindications occur. Though toxic reactions are not common, the patient should be under very close medical observation since there is the possibility, as in heparin administration, of hemorrhage.

The dose varies from day to day, depending upon the results of daily prothrombin tests. It is absolutely imperative if the drug is to be administered safely that when it is used a reliable laboratory technician perform the prothrombin test each morning. Normal prothrombin time is 12 to 15 seconds. Therapy usually attempts to depress the prothrombin activity 15 to 20 per cent of normal. The nurse should *always* report a prothrombin time over 30 seconds *before* administering the oral anticoagulant. The usual first dose is from 200 to 300 mg.; subsequent daily maintenance doses vary from 25 to 100 mg. depending upon the laboratory reports.

The anticoagulant action persists for several days after the drug is withdrawn. Should bleeding of any kind occur, the drug should be stopped and large doses of a suitable vitamin K preparation (K_1) given immediately intravenously. This drug counteracts the hypoprothrombinemia (I-7). Because of the fact that the effect of vitamin K is somewhat delayed, a transfusion of whole blood or fresh plasma may be advisable to control the immediate bleeding. (Stored plasma should not be used.)

Long-term anticoagulant therapy with a drug of the coumarin group is possible. These drugs are strikingly free of serious side effects. They have been given to patients, under their physician's direction and care, for long periods of time—5 to 15 years. They are not indicated in all patients but do improve the prognosis for those patients who use them. The dose is highly individualized. (See Table 13.)

Side Effects, Toxicity, Treatment. In both types of therapy, it is important that the nurse be sure that the proper laboratory work is done promptly at the specified times. In all anticoagulant therapy, the dosage is dependent on coagulation or bleeding times, and the drug should never be given without a specific order for each dose.

In administering both heparin and the coumarin drugs, there is danger of hemorrhage. The nurse caring for patients on any anticoagulant therapy must be alert to specific signs and symptoms related to the actions of the drugs. These might include epistaxis, bleeding from the gums, tarry stools, dark red or coffee-colored urine (not the orange color with indandione therapy), petechiae, ecchymosis, and hematomas—particularly from parenteral injections. Emergency measures were specifically outlined previously in this chapter. Hemorrhage may become fatal due to internal hemorrhage, cerebral hemorrhage, or intrapericardial hemorrhage (cardiac tamponade).

Interactions. The oral anticoagulant preparations have a large number of interactions. They are enhanced by phenylbutazone, sulfonamides, and clofibrate, probably by displacement at the binding sites. They are also enhanced by the anabolic agents and phenyramidol, probably by enzyme inhibition, by quinidine because of additive effect and by the salicylates by additive action on coenzyme systems. Their action is also enhanced by d-thyroxine, the bromelains, and papain. The method of action is not well known in these interactions. The oral anticoagulants potentiate the sulfonamides and diphenylhydantoin owing to enzyme induction. They are inhibited by sedatives, haloperidol and griseofulvin by enzyme inhibition.

Patient Teaching. Since many patients take these drugs for extended periods, the nurse should give the patient detailed information as to when to take the drug and the possible side effects. A routine may be established for taking the medication. This measure may help to prevent overdoses and forgetfulness. A public health nurse may be able to continue to give additional care within the home. She may be able to follow up on the routine scheduling and caution the family to keep these medications out of the reach of children. The patient should be instructed to keep in touch with his physician and to notify him immediately if any adverse symptoms develop. Routine physical examinations to check progress and to aid in maintaining health are advised. The patient should be warned not to take aspirin or any salicylate drug without specific orders from his physician, since salicylates also tend to depress blood clotting.

The Patient. These drugs, often taken for extended periods, help to prevent further attacks of coronary occlusion of this type. In order to alert others to the patient's physical condition and drug therapy regimen, the patient is often advised to carry an identification card specifying this information. This card may also contain the physician's name and telephone number in case of an accident.

The patient and his family will need help in understanding that anticoagulant therapy may be a long-term drug treatment. They must be taught how to observe for small bleeding tendencies, e.g., cuts from shaving that continue to bleed, or bruising more easily than usual.

Patients receiving heparin are usually very ill and need continuous reassurance. The nurse should do all in her power to allay the patient's fears, but she should not be overly optimistic if conditions do not warrant it. This is also true for the patient's relatives and friends. They may be overly solicitous, but they should be warned not to add their own fears to the patient's anxiety. If the patient is the head of the house, as is often the case, there may be serious financial considerations. Although the nurse cannot solve these problems, she can suggest agencies or places where help can be obtained for the patient and his family. The nurse should do everything within her jurisdiction to help the patient secure the rest he needs. Later, after the acute stage is over, she may be able to help him adjust to a new routine of life. As with most cardiac patients, these patients must learn an entirely new mode of living, often including a change of avocation as well as vocation.

Miscellaneous Drugs. *Quinidine sulfate* is extremely valuable in those cases of myocardial infarction in which an arrhythmia develops. It is given orally in 200 to 400 mg. doses four times daily. This drug has been discussed in more detail elsewhere in this chapter.

Papaverine has been used fairly effectively for the severe pain of coronary occlusion. The relief is produced by the increased blood flow through the collateral vessels. This drug is antispasmodic to smooth muscles.

Atropine sulfate is sometimes used in an attempt to block adverse vagal reflexes, but recent evidence shows that there is no significant coronary vasodilation produced. There is grave danger, too, of causing an elevated heart rate.

Digitalis may be employed if there is evidence of congestive failure or a rapid ventricular rate due to atrial fibrillation or flutter. In the absence of these definite indications, digitalis is not used.

Drugs Used to Combat Bleeding Caused by Anticoagulant Therapy

Phytonadione, U.S.P., *phytomenadione,* B.P. (Vitamin K_1, Aquamephyton, Konakion, Mephyton). Phytonadione is prepared both for oral and, in a colloidal solution, for parenteral use. Phytonadione is indicated in the treatment of anticoagulant induced prothrombin deficiency (as with the coumarin type drugs), prophylaxis and treatment of hemorrhagic diseases of the newborn, some hepatic disorders and any disorder attended by hypoprothrombinemia. Dosage and mode of administration depend upon the gravity of the condition. Intravenous use is reserved for the most serious, intramuscular or subcutaneous for those situations in which time is a factor of secondary importance. The oral route is used for those patients who are not so acutely ill. The oral dose is usually 5 mg., the parenteral dose, 2 to 100 mg. If after 12 to 24 hours oral dose or 6 to 8 hours after parenteral dose, the prothrombin time has not reached a satisfactory level, the dose may be repeated. If given intravenously, the injection should be made very slowly. The prothrombin time should be checked frequently during therapy. If the drug is introduced too rapidly intravenously toxic reactions can occur such as flushing, dizziness, rapid pulse, weak pulse, sweating, brief hypotension, dyspnea and cyanosis. With subcutaneous or intramuscular injection there may be pain at the penetration site. Too much phytonadione in the treatment of excessive anticoagulant dosage may cause a recurrence of the clot formation.

Protamine sulfate, U.S.P., is used as a heparin antagonist and is effective for combating bleeding from an overdose of heparin. This is somewhat paradoxical, for protamine itself is an anticoagulant and will cause prolongation of the clotting time. However, when protamine is given in the presence of heparin, the attraction of the two substances for each other is much greater than their individual attraction to the blood elements, and they tend to neutralize the anticoagulant activity of each other. Protamine is effective in direct ratio to heparin—1 mg. of protamine to 78 to 95 units of heparin. Protamine is given intravenously in heparin overdosage as a 1 per cent solution injected slowly—over one to three minutes. The dosage can be calculated on the basis of the amount of heparin given over the previous three or four hours. The dosage should not exceed 50 mg. at any one time.

Drugs That Reduce the Size of Intravascular Thrombi

Fibrinolysin (Actase, Hydrolysin, Thrombolysin) is the naturally derived fraction of human plasma. It tends to cause the lysis (dissolution) of blood clots intravascularly. It has been most successful in the treatment of thrombophlebitis, phlebothrombosis and pulmonary embolism. It is given intravenously, comes in vials of 50,000 MID units and is reconstituted by adding 25 ml. of sterile water or glucose 5 per cent solution. Saline solution should not be used. The reconstituted drug is added to an intravenous infusion of 5 per cent glucose. Dosage varies with the reaction of the patient but is usually 50,000 to 100,000 units per hour for one to six hours per day. The reconstituted drug should be promptly used since its strength is lost upon standing. Dosage is higher when the clot is arterial than when it is in the vein. Fibrinolysin is contraindicated in hemorrhage disorders, fibrinogen deficiency or major liver dysfunction. The side effects include febrile reaction, chills, nausea, vomiting, dizziness, headache, muscle pain, backache, tachycardia and hypotension.

Complications and other symptoms of coronary disease are treated as they occur. In cardiac arrest the treatment is usually not medicinal but external or internal massage, artificial respiration and/or defibrillation; for shock, the usual antihypotensive agents, continuous monitoring and administration of glucosteroids may help.

Rheumatic Fever and Rheumatic Heart Disease

DEFINITION. Though not interchangeable, the terms rheumatic fever and rheumatic heart disease go hand in hand. Rheumatic heart disease is one of the most common and serious complications of rheumatic fever (III-1). Rheumatic fever gets its name because of the rheumatic symptoms, pain and swelling in the joints, associated with it. Although predominantly a disease of childhood and early adult life, it may appear later in life. But the fact remains that those who have rheumatic fever very frequently develop a heart lesion of some sort.

MAJOR SYMPTOMS. The prodromata of rheumatic fever are usually those associated with any streptococcal infection. The general symptoms of anorexia, loss of weight, weakness and fatigability are almost always present. The actual onset may be gradual or acute, often precipitated by overexertion or chilling. The temperature may rise to 102 to 104° F. A rapid pulse, profuse perspiration, severe prostration and polyarthritis are other symptoms. The arthritis is of migratory character, with involvement of new joints in rapid succession. It is characterized by pain, tenderness, swelling, heat and local redness. Rashes of varying degrees may be noticed. There are frequently subcutaneous nodules present as well.

Cardiac involvement is a common feature and may be of the obvious type or more subtle in character. Carditis, valvulitis, pericarditis, myocarditis or congestive heart failure may be present, each with its own variations in symptoms. The development of signs of cardiac insufficiency terminating eventually in congestive heart failure may not develop for several months or even years following an acute attack of rheumatic fever. Life expectancy is shortened by rheumatic fever and rheumatic heart disease (VI-2, 3, 4, 5, 6).

DRUG THERAPY. As yet no specific prevention or cure has been found for rheumatic fever. The relative merits of the various suggested forms of therapy are still under investigation and there is no general agreement as to which is best.

THE SALICYLATES

The Drugs. The salicylate drugs were originally obtained from plants, but are now produced synthetically. Their use as antipyretics and analgesics and probably in the treatment of other conditions was well known to ancient civilizations. However it was not until the 19th century that the active principle was isolated.

Physical and Chemical Properties. As the name shows, salicylates are either salicylic acid or its derivatives. These derivatives may be esters of salicylic acid, salicylic esters of organic acids, direct salts of salicylic acid or others such as salicylamide, which is the cogener of salicylic acid and strictly speaking not a salicylate. It is included because it has many of the actions of the salicylates. The degree of solubility varies with the preparation.

Action. The primary action of the salicylates are analgesia and antipyresis. The antipyretic action is thought to be due to the effect of the drug on the heat regulating center in the hypothalamus. The drugs seem to "reset" the "thermostat" to a lower level. The peripheral blood vessels are dilated, there is more heat loss and with no change in heat production and the temperature is lowered. These drugs do not affect the temperature if it is within normal range.

The actual mechanism of action of the salicylates which causes analgesia is not completely understood. However, it is believed to be selective depression of the central nervous system.

The salicylates tend to stimulate respiration and change the acid-base ratio and electrolyte balance in the blood; they may cause epigastric irritation and increase the output of uric acid. Except in toxic dosage, none of these actions causes serious difficulties.

The direct action of the salicylates in rheumatic fever is due to its primary actions, antipyresis and analgesia. These drugs do not alter the progress of the disease.

Salicylic acid is irritating to the skin and mucous membranes as are some of its derivatives. This is discussed further under "Mode of Administration."

Therapeutic Uses. The uses of the salicylates are almost unlimited, but they all revolve around the primary actions of antipyresis and analgesia. In addition to rheumatic fever they may be used for arthritis, headache, dysmenorrhea, fever (from almost any cause), the "common cold," muscular aches and pains and backache.

Absorption and Excretion. Orally ingested preparations are rapidly absorbed from the gastrointestinal tract. Within 30 minutes appreciable amounts appear in the blood. Peak levels are reached in about two hours, then gradually decline. They are widely distributed throughout the body in all tissues and fluids. They cross the blood-brain barrier and in pregnant patients the placental barrier and appear in the milk. They are also found in synovial and peritoneal fluids, but not in gastric juice after absorption. The salicylates are excreted mainly by the kidneys in both unchanged and metabolite forms. They may lend a green-brown color to the urine.

Preparations and Dosages

Salicylic acid, U.S.P. *Topical use only.*

Methyl salicylate, U.S.P., B.P. (oil of wintergreen). *Topical use only.*

Aspirin, U.S.P., acetylsalicylic acid, B.P., (many trade names), 0.3 to 0.6 Gm. orally.

Sodium salicylate, U.S.P., B.P., 0.3 to 1.0 Gm., orally.

Salicylamide, N.F. (many trade names), 0.3 to 2.0 Gm. q 3 to 4 h p.r.n. (not more than 3 Gm. in 24 hours).

Aspirin and salicylamide are constituents of many combination preparations used mainly for the relief of "minor aches and pains."

THE NURSE

Mode of Administration. Salicylic acid and methyl salicylate are used only for external application. Methyl salicylate (oil of wintergreen) is the product most commonly used. It is a liquid with a characteristic odor and taste. It is used as a counterirritant solely for its local action. Although it can be used full strength, it is generally recommended that it be diluted with two parts olive oil or incorporated in an ointment. It is applied directly to the joint and the part is then wrapped in cotton or soft lint to help preserve the warmth generated by the medication. Salicylic acid is incorporated into ointments, plaster and solutions. Concentration varies with the different products.

The oral drugs, aspirin, sodium salicylate or salicylamide, have about the same use in rheumatic fever. There does not appear to be much difference in their effects. Aspirin is probably the most commonly used, but it does not seem to have any advantage over the others. Of course, if the patient cannot tolerate one drug, another is substituted for it. The total daily dose is usually divided into four parts which are given as nearly q 6 h as circumstances permit or, if the patient is sleeping, as soon as he awakens. The last dose of the day is given at bedtime. Sodium bicarbonate should not be given with these drugs because it accelerates urinary excretion of the salicylates and reduces the efficiency of their absorption. If the patient complains of gastric distress after taking the medicine, the physician should be consulted. He may order one of the "buffered" preparations. These are usually more expensive and are recommended only if the patient cannot tolerate the "unbuffered" forms. It is always a good idea to give the salicylate drugs after meals, or with milk and cookies so as to minimize gastric irritation.

During the first three or four days of therapy, the patient may complain of anorexia, nausea or tinnitus. Usually this does not warrant stopping the drug, although the doctor should be aware of these symptoms. Common practice in rheumatic fever is to give full doses until the patient has been asymptomatic for at least two weeks and all evidence of acute infection is gone. Then the drug is decreased gradually over several days and finally discontinued.

Side Effects. Untoward side effects are uncommon, except when large doses are used for a patient who has not previously had much of the drug. In addition to those mentioned previously, side effects include headache, confusion, excessive perspiration, thirst and skin manifestations. Vomiting, other gastrointestinal disorders, lassitude and apathy have also been reported. Change of dosage or preparation is usually all the treatment that is required.

Idiosyncrasy to the salicylates is not uncommon, usually causing skin rashes or anaphylactic phenomena. Most patients reacting unfavorably have a history of allergy, a type of reaction that may occur with the first dose. However, even if the drug has been taken previously without ill effects, this is no guarantee against the occurrence of an untoward reaction with later doses.

Toxicity and Treatment. Severe salicylate poisoning is rare, and ordinarily involves the small child who ingests too many of the sugar-coated children's aspirin tablets. Mental excitation—"salicylate jag"—may be the first symptom, followed by mental depression, stupor or coma. Other symptoms include heart depression, polyuria, impairment of hearing and vision, skin eruptions and acidosis. Treatment is symptomatic.

Interactions. The salicylates potentiate penicillin, methotrexate, sulfonylurea and para-aminosalicylic acid by displacement from binding sites. Salicylates should not be given concurrently with probenecid or sulfinpyrazone, since they counteract the uricosuric effect of probenecid and sulfinpyrazone. The salicylates are enhanced by phenobarbital due to enzyme induction. The concurrent use of the salicylates with the oral anticoagulants should be avoided or closely monitored due to the additive effect seen when these drugs are given at the same time.

Patient Teaching. Probably the most important thing for the nurse to tell the patient or, if he is a child, his parents, is that just because a "little is good" does not mean that "a lot is better." Often, the patient gets some relief from the dose ordered, but he feels that if he took more he would receive more relief and this goes on until a toxic dose has been taken. The dosage schedule and the advisability of giving some food at the same time should be stressed.

If the topical preparations are to be used, the nurse should give detailed information on how to use the drug.

THE PATIENT. The patient with rheumatic fever must be kept in bed and as quiet as possible. Since the patient is usually a child, keeping him in bed and even moderately quiet can be a problem. Family and friends can often help by supplying reading material and quiet games that can be played by the patient lying in bed (VI-5, 6). The prognosis of rheumatic fever is always guarded for it is not possible to know immediately the extent of the cardiac involvement.

The patient needs an untold amount of patience and understanding. However, especially with a child, care should be taken not to make him a dependent, insecure individual (V-2; VI-1, 3, 4). He should be encouraged to face his problem and not develop a defeatist attitude. All this is difficult, but essential. The nurse can do much to assist the patient, his family and friends in coping with the limitations required.

Other areas for instruction relate to avoiding individuals with upper respiratory infections, maintaining fluid and nutrition balance during fever episodes, keeping a rigid schedule for taking prescribed drugs, and protective handling of body joints—slow and deliberate movements. Salicylates may be given approximately 30 minutes prior to activity in order to reduce the incidence of painful stimuli. Through these efforts, the patient's goals and medical therapy goals may coincide.

Antimicrobial Therapy. When rheumatic fever is first diagnosed, the physician usually prescribes a course of penicillin to help to eliminate completely any hemolytic streptococci in the body.

One routine calls for 1.2 million units of benzathine penicillin G (Bicillin) intramuscularly or 1.2 million units of oral penicillin daily for ten days. If the patient cannot take penicillin, erythromycin is given, 250 mg. four times a day for ten days.

Since recurrence of the disease is not uncommon and streptococcal infections which usually trigger it often go undetected, most physicians feel that any person who has had rheumatic fever should have prophylactic treatment for the prevention of streptococcal infections. The duration of prophylaxis depends upon the severity of the original attack and the presence or absence of cardiac involvement. Prophylactic treatment may be benzathine penicillin (Bicillin) 1.2 million units intramuscularly monthly, or oral penicillin 200,000 to 400,000 units daily.

Corticosteroids. The use of the steroids is a controversial subject among clinicians. Some feel they should be reserved for lifesaving measures or when other drugs cannot be used. Others believe they should be given early in the disease. Yet a third group feels that it should be used in rheumatic heart disease with symptoms of congestive heart failure. They do produce a response similar to the salicylates in about the same time—relief of symptoms. The dangers attendant with the administration of the steroids must be considered. (See Chapter 27.) Ideal dosage schedules have not yet been determined. Some feel that if *cortisone* is used, the initial dose (orally) is 2 to 4 mg. per pound per day in divided doses. If *prednisone* is used, a suppressive dose is usually 40 to 80 mg. a day in divided doses. It is generally agreed, however, that before the steroids are discontinued, salicylates should be started to help ease the shock to the body with the withdrawal of the suppressive dose of the steroid.

Rheumatic fever may cause a variety of cardiac disorders. These are treated as they occur. There is no standard procedure either for prevention (except as noted previously) or for treatment. Each case must be considered individually.

Bacterial Endocarditis

DEFINITION. Endocarditis is an inflammation of the endocardium (lining of the heart) with involvement of the heart valves. It is often classified as nonbacterial and bacterial endocarditis and it is with the latter that we are concerned here (III-1).

In bacterial endocarditis the bacteria circulate in the blood stream and lodge in some portion of the heart—frequently a damaged valve. The typical vegetations produced impair valve function further. Almost every known pathogenic bacterium has been found to cause this disease at one time or another, but the nonhemolytic streptococcus accounts for about 90 per cent of all cases (III-1). Bacterial endocarditis is classified as acute or subacute, based on the rapidity of progress of the untreated disease.

MAJOR SYMPTOMS. The onset of subacute endocarditis is usually insidious. The patient complains of having the "grippe" for a long period of time, weakness, easy fatigability, anorexia, fever, malaise, chills, sweating and arthralgia. Petechiae are frequently seen on the conjunctiva. Significant heart murmurs are almost always present but may not be prominent at first. In acute endocarditis, the onset is rapid as is the course of the disease and, if untreated, proves fatal in a few months.

DRUG THERAPY

Antibiotic Therapy. Antibiotic therapy is considered best, the choice of a specific drug depending upon the sensitivity of the offending organism to the antibiotic.

Penicillin is probably the antibiotic most commonly used. In bacterial endocarditis, it is extremely important to attain and maintain a high blood level of the drug for a relatively long period of time. It is recommended that from 600,000 to 2.4 million units q 6 h intramuscularly or intravenously be given for at least six weeks or more. It

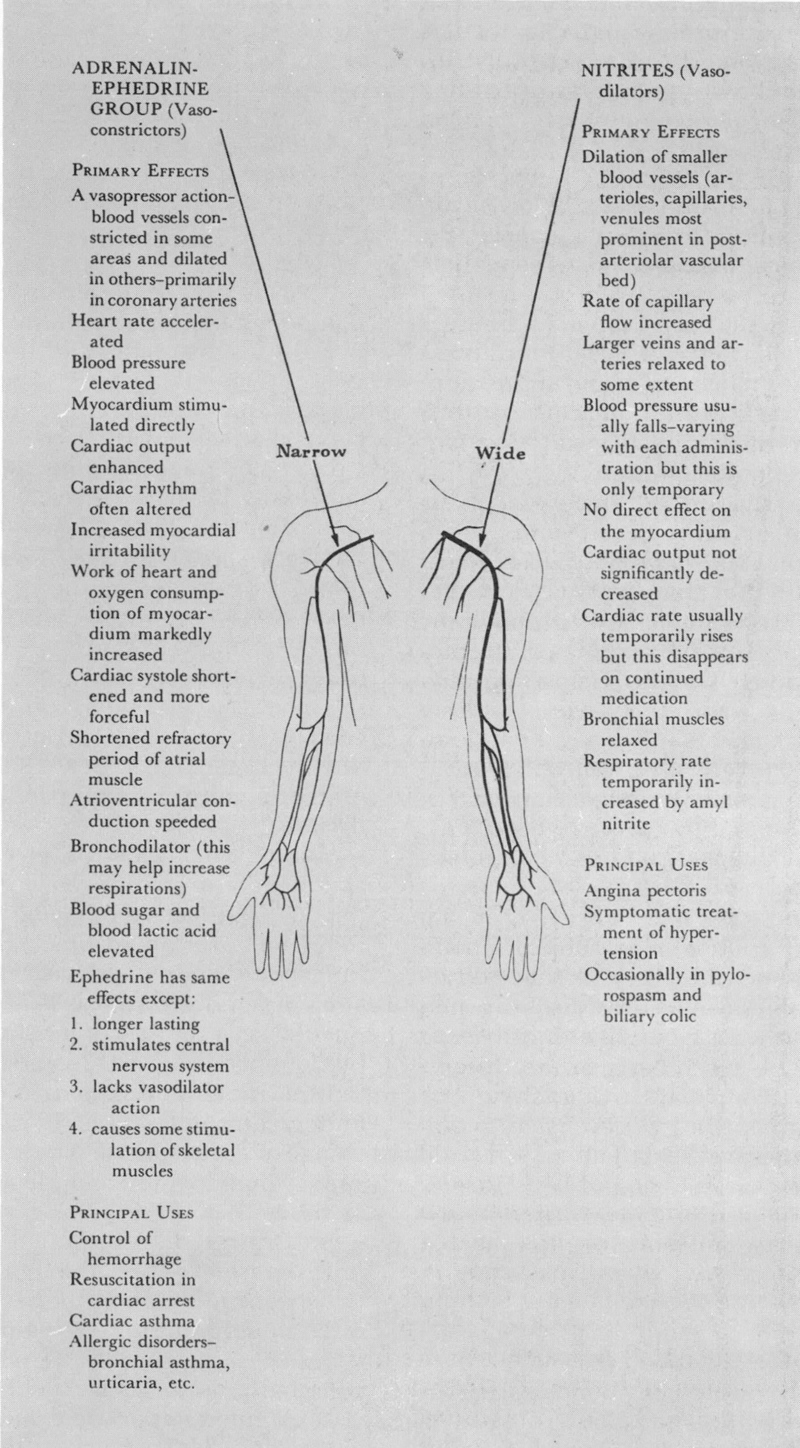

ADRENALIN-
EPHEDRINE
GROUP (Vaso-
constrictors)
PRIMARY EFFECTS
A vasopressor action–
blood vessels constricted in some areas and dilated in others–primarily in coronary arteries
Heart rate accelerated
Blood pressure elevated
Myocardium stimulated directly
Cardiac output enhanced
Cardiac rhythm often altered
Increased myocardial irritability
Work of heart and oxygen consumption of myocardium markedly increased
Cardiac systole shortened and more forceful
Shortened refractory period of atrial muscle
Atrioventricular conduction speeded
Bronchodilator (this may help increase respirations)
Blood sugar and blood lactic acid elevated
Ephedrine has same effects except:
1. longer lasting
2. stimulates central nervous system
3. lacks vasodilator action
4. causes some stimulation of skeletal muscles
PRINCIPAL USES
Control of hemorrhage
Resuscitation in cardiac arrest
Cardiac asthma
Allergic disorders–bronchial asthma, urticaria, etc.
Narrow
Wide
NITRITES (Vaso-
dilators)
PRIMARY EFFECTS
Dilation of smaller blood vessels (arterioles, capillaries, venules most prominent in postarteriolar vascular bed)
Rate of capillary flow increased
Larger veins and arteries relaxed to some extent
Blood pressure usually falls–varying with each administration but this is only temporary
No direct effect on the myocardium
Cardiac output not significantly decreased
Cardiac rate usually temporarily rises but this disappears on continued medication
Bronchial muscles relaxed
Respiratory rate temporarily increased by amyl nitrite
PRINCIPAL USES
Angina pectoris
Symptomatic treatment of hypertension
Occasionally in pylorospasm and biliary colic

FIGURE 31. Comparison of vasoconstrictors and vasodilators.

may also be given by continuous intravenous drip. The long-acting preparations should not be used since they do not provide sufficiently high and consistent blood levels. Good results may be obtained in some cases by using penicillin together with streptomycin for two weeks. Relapses are treated promptly with larger doses and a longer course of the drug. Large doses may be used prophylactically in patients with a past history of endocarditis should any surgical procedure have to be done.

If the patient is allergic to penicillin, vancomycin is regarded as the next best.

Because such large doses of penicillin are given daily, it is wise to divide the daily dosage into equal portions and give it intramuscularly every three hours day and night. It is extremely important that the medication be given promptly at the designated times to maintain the high blood level necessary. The site of injection should be varied each time and the best of techniques should be used to make the injections as painless as possible.

DISORDERS OF BLOOD PRESSURE

Vascular Hypertension

DEFINITION. Hypertension is usually defined as a pathologic elevation of the blood pressure. However, there is no universal agreement on where normotension ends and hypertension begins. Hypertension is a physical sign reflecting a disturbance of the heart, the blood vessels or both. There is no single known cause for hypertension, but there are several predisposing factors such as renal disorders, adrenal tumors, and the like. Most cases of hypertension are classified as "idiopathic." Whatever the cause, there is a definite narrowing of the arterioles. The heart tries to pump the blood through this narrowing vascular bed but this provides an increasing resistance to the flow of blood (IV-5).

MAJOR SYMPTOMS. Although headaches and a sensation of pressure in the head may be noted by some patients, often this condition will remain undetected for some time until picked up by accident, such as during a physical examination. The symptoms are few and often vague at first.

DRUG THERAPY. The treatment of hypertension presents one of the major challenges in the medical field today. The very term is often in dispute. Some patients maintain a consistently elevated pressure, but others, for unexplained reasons, have a spontaneous return from elevation to a normal level for a few weeks or months. Then, without any apparent cause, the blood pressure rises to its former high level. The importance of diet in relation to this disease has long been controversial. There are no drugs now available which can be depended upon to consistently lower blood pressure for long periods of time, but some of the newer preparations offer at least a hope for the future. See Figure 31 throughout this discussion for the action of the vasodilators and vasoconstrictors.

ANTIHYPERTENSIVE AGENTS

THE DRUGS. A large number of drugs which cause vasodilation and reduction of blood pressure are available. Because their uses are similar, they will be discussed together, but the usual divisions will be omitted. Each drug will be discussed briefly, then the place of the nurse and the patient will be given for all the drugs together.

RAUWOLFIA ALKALOIDS

(See Current Drug Handbook.)

Extracts from the root of the Rauwolfia serpentina (a climbing shrub of India and surrounding countries) have been used for centuries and are still used in the treatment of psychoses and hypertension.

These alkaloids are readily absorbed from the gastrointestinal tract and are widely distributed throughout the body. They cross the blood-brain barrier. The exact metabolism is not known. Although the whole root product is available, the refined alkaloids are more commonly used.

In the management of hypertension, the alkaloids are usually reserved for mild hypertension, especially if it is accompanied by anxiety and emotional factors. They produce slight lowering of blood pressure and a tranquilizing effect.

Undesirable side effects of the Rauwolfia derivatives are not uncommon, but usually are relieved by a change in dosage. Side effects include sedation, nasal congestion, gain in weight, various gastrointestinal disturbances and orthostatic hypotension.

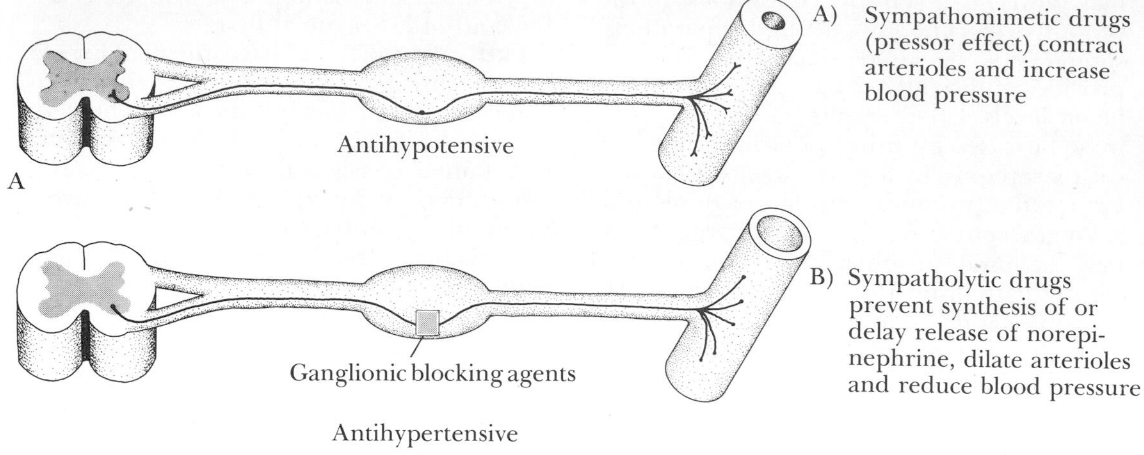

FIGURE 32. A) Sympathomimetic drugs (pressor effect) contract arterioles and increase blood pressure. B) Sympatholytic drugs prevent synthesis of or delay release of norepinephrine, dilate arterioles and reduce blood pressure.

Preparations and Dosages

Doses given here are maintenance ones. In beginning digitalization or crisis situations, doses may be much higher.

Reserpine, U.S.P., B.P. (many trade names), 0.1 to 0.5 mg. daily, orally or parenterally.

Rescinnamine, N.F. (Moderil) 0.25 to 0.5 mg. two to four times a day, orally.

Deserpidine (Harmonyl) 0.1 to 1.0 mg. as above.

Alseroxylon (several trade names), 2.0 mg., as above.

Syrosingopine, N.F. (Singoserp) 0.5 to 1.0 mg. two to three times a day, orally. (This is a synthetic product.)

Interactions. In patients who have been on long-term reserpine therapy there can be a decreased cardiovascular response to normal doses of ephedrine or metaraminol. This can be overcome by use of a direct acting agent such as norepinephrine or phenylephrine, since the musculature in reserpine-treated patients is often hypersensitive to the pressor action of the direct acting drugs. Reserpine should be used with caution in patients taking tricyclic antidepressants, since it has been known to cause "reserpine reversal." Reserpine's hypotensive effect may be enhanced by the phenothiazines, quinidine, the thiazide diuretics and procainamide. With alcohol, both drugs are potentiated because of additive action.

HYDRALAZINE HYDROCHLORIDE

(See Current Drug Handbook.)

Hydralazine is a synthetic derivative of phthalazine. It is used to reduce blood pressure and in the treatment of peripheral vascular diseases. The exact method of action is incompletely understood, but it produces peripheral vasodilation, which in turn reduces blood pressure. This same action aids in reducing symptoms of the peripheral vascular diseases. Hydralazine is believed to act mainly on the midbrain. The effects of hydralazine are delayed, even after intravenous injection. It is readily absorbed from the gastrointestinal tract and from parenteral sites. Peak blood levels are reached in three to four hours and some drug remains for as long as 24 hours. Little is known of the fate of hydralazine in the body. Side effects occur frequently, the most common ones being headache, palpitation, anorexia, nausea, vomiting and diarrhea. Cases have been reported of conditions resembling lupus erythematosus and rheumatoid arthritis which usually subside when the drug is withdrawn. Preparations and dosages: hydralazine hydrochloride, N.F. (hydrallazine, B.P.) (Apresoline) 10 to 100 mg. orally, 20 mg. I.M. or I.V. Dosage is individually adjusted.

METHYLDOPA

(See Current Drug Handbook.)

Methyldopa, a synthetic preparation

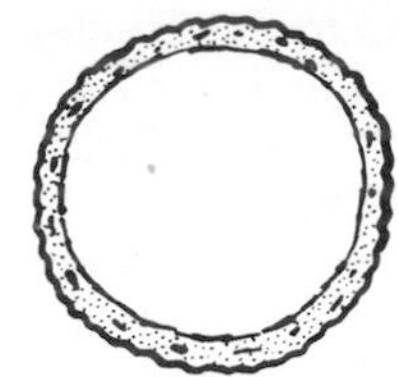
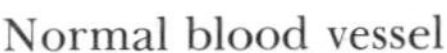

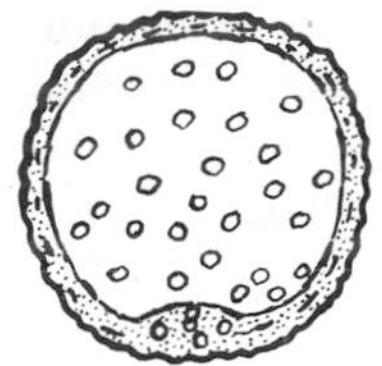

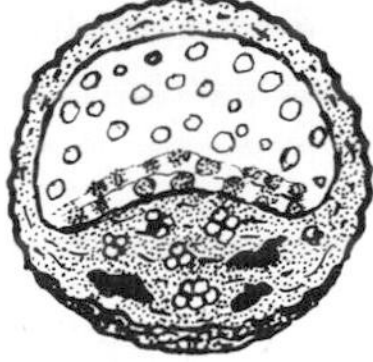

FIGURE 33. One cause of hypertension is the narrowing of the lumen of the blood vessels due to atherosclerotic or arteriosclerotic plaques.

which effectively lowers blood pressure, reduces serotonin in the brain and norepinephrine in peripheral tissues, inhibits dopa carboxylase and reduces blood pressure more in the hypertensive person than in the normotensive individual. Its exact fate in the body is not known. Absorbed from the gastrointestinal tract, a single dose reaches peak blood level in four to six hours and persists for 24 hours. Side effects include sedation, postural hypotension, anxiety, dizziness and apprehension. Psychic depression, reversible drug fever and impairment of the liver may also develop. Preparation and dosage: Methyldopa (Aldomet) 0.5 to 1.0 Gm. orally or 250 to 500 mg. q 6 h intravenously. Dosage individually adjusted.

Interactions. Methyldopa is enhanced by anesthetic agents and inhibited by the sympathomimetics. It potentiates levarterenol.

GUANETHIDINE SULFATE

(See Current Drug Handbook.)

Guanethidine is a synthetic drug whose main use is to reduce blood pressure in relatively severe hypertension. Its exact method of action is not known, but it is believed to interfere with the release of norepinephrine at the sympathetic neuroeffector junction. Guanethidine is preferred by some physicians over the ganglion blocking agents since its action is postganglionic. It does not produce parasympathetic blockage and is slow acting. After oral dose, which is well absorbed, it begins to produce hypotension in 36 to 48 hours. With continued medication, a maximum effect is reached in 72 hours. Postural hypotension is the most common and persistent side effect. Persons taking the drug should be warned to avoid strenuous exercise because of the danger of syncope from hypotension. Guanethidine may also inhibit sexual ejaculation. It is contraindicated in pheochromocytoma and in pregnancy. Other side effects are similar to others of this group and are usually controlled by dosage adjustment. Preparation and dosage: Guanethidine hydrochloride, U.S.P., B.P. (Ismelin) 10 to 25 mg. orally. Dosage individually adjusted.

Interactions. The hypotensive effect of guanethidine is enhanced by the thiazide diuretics and the phenothiazines. It is antagonized by the tricyclic antidepressants and inhibited by amphetamines which block the uptake of guanethidine. Guanethidine potentiates levarterenol, since it prevents the uptake of pressor onto inactive sites.

GANGLIONIC BLOCKING AGENTS

(See Current Drug Handbook.)

The ganglionic blocking agents, which are mainly quaternary ammonium compounds, inhibit the transmission of impulses through the autonomic ganglia, both the sympathetic and the parasympathetic. They produce symptoms of both sympatholytic and parasympatholytic drugs. All of these preparations lower blood pressure and are usually more effective in severe than in mild hypertension. The lowering of the blood pressure is due to the blocking of the sympathetic stimuli which tend to constrict the peripheral blood vessels. Thus there is vasodilation which is more pronounced in the upright than in the reclining position. The side effects are the same as for other drugs causing vasodilation, with postural hypotension being relatively common. Since these drugs also block the parasympathetic system, additional side effects often occur such as constipation, blurring of vision, dryness of the mouth and difficulty with micturition. The absorption of these drugs from the gastrointestinal tract is incomplete and unpredictable, and larger doses are required than for the parenteral route. The drugs are mainly found in the intracellular fluids and are not present to any great extent in the brain. Mecamylamine is completely absorbed after oral administration. It also is not confined to the extracellular spaces and does cross the blood-brain and the placental barriers. These drugs are all excreted by the kidneys and cumulative effects may occur in the patient with renal impairment.

Preparations and Dosages

All doses are individually adjusted.

Hexamethonium chloride (Bistrium, Methium) 125 to 250 mg. orally usually started q.i.d.

Mecamylamine hydrochloride, U.S.P., B.P. (Inversine) 2.5 to 10 mg. orally. (Not a quaternary ammonium product.)

Pentolinium tartrate, B.P. (Ansolysen, pentolonium [C]) 20 to 200 mg. usually started q 8 h orally, subcutaneously or I.M. Not given I.V.

Trimethaphan camphosulfonate, U.S.P., B.P. (Arfonad) usually given I.V. in a 5 per cent glucose or saline solution 1 to 4 mg./min. until blood pressure has reached desired level.

Trimethidium methosulfate, N.F. 20 mg. usually started twice a day, orally. Best given in fasting or near fasting stage.

Veratrum Viride Alkaloids

(See Current Drug Handbook.)

The veratrum viride products are derived from green hellbore and have been used medicinally for many years. Their use as antihypertensive agents has been irregular. Their hypotensive response is due to action on the central nervous system and is variable. It reduces both systolic and diastolic pressure and usually causes a bradycardia. Recent use of these drugs has been confined to parenteral use in emergencies when reduction of blood pressure is essential. In such cases as toxemia of pregnancy, acute glomerulonephritis and hypertensive encephalopathy, the veratrum alkaloids may be life saving. Side effects include weight gain, epigastric burning sensation, anorexia, nausea and vomiting. In acute poisoning, cardiovascular collapse may occur. Epinephrine or similar medication is usually ordered to counteract the effects of veratrum. All preparations of veratrum are combinations of alkaloids and, as with most of these drugs, the dosages are individually adjusted.

Preparations and Dosages

Alkavervir (Veriloid) 3 to 5 mg. usually started q 6 to 8 h (t.i.d.) orally.

Cryptenamine acetate (Unitensin acetate) 1 to 2 mg. q 1 to 2 h I.V. until desired pressure is reached.

Cryptenamine tannate (Unitensin tannate, unitensyl [C]) 1 to 2 mg. b.i.d. or t.i.d. orally.

Protoveratrine A and B Maleate (Veralba) 0.1 to 0.5 mg. b.i.d. or t.i.d. orally. 0.1 to 0.5 mg. q 1 to 3 h I.V. until desired pressure is reached.

Pargyline

(See Current Drug Handbook.)

Pargyline hydrochloride is a synthetic preparation. It is a monamine oxidase inhibitor and is used as an antihypertensive agent and an antidepressant. It is not recommended for labile hypertension or for patients amenable to treatment with mild sedation and the thiazide diuretics. The exact mechanism of action of pargyline in hypertension is incompletely understood. Its side effects are similar to other antihypertensive drugs and also to those of the antidepressant group. Side effects include insomnia, euphoria, impotence, gain in weight, edema, postural hypotension and various gastrointestinal symptoms. The drug has cumulative effects so dosage is usually started at a low level and increased gradually until desired pressure level is reached. The preparation is Pargyline hydrochloride, N.F. (Eutonyl) 10 to 50 mg. daily, usually in one dose, orally.

Interactions. Pargyline enhances the central nervous depression when given with anesthetic agents. With narcotics it may produce hypotension. Pargyline given with the sympathomimetic amines and foods containing tyramine causes hypertension because of decreased metabolism of the catecholamines.

The Nurse. Method of administration and side effects have been discussed with each drug, but some remarks will bear repeating.

Because of the frequent occurrence of postural hypotension when any antihypertensive agent is given, the patient receiving these drugs parenterally should continue in a recumbent position for two to three hours following the initial dose. Upon arising, not suddenly, the patient should be instructed to lie down at the first feeling of faintness.

Any marked deviation of the systolic or diastolic pressure should be recorded and reported. If the patient is also taking digitalis, both drugs will exert a bradycardiac effect.

The nurse should take and record the blood pressure at frequent intervals (at least every five to 15 minutes for the first hour following parenteral administration). Most of these drugs when given orally are given with meals. However, some such as trimethidium are given in the fasting state.

In most cases, in the diet of patients on antihypertensive therapy, especially with the ganglionic blocking agents, salt is not restricted. The physician's recommendations in this matter should be followed.

Constipation which is not uncommon with the blocking agents can usually be controlled by diet or a mild laxative.

Daily weight measurements are also valuable to determine evidence of loss (edema) through the more efficiently functioning kidneys. Records of routine output and intake are helpful in determining the significance of weight loss (amount of diuresis). If severe diarrhea is noted, reduction in the dose may be indicated.

The nurse should be familiar with and watch for the side effects of each hypotensive drug administered. If the patient is to take the drug at home, the nurse should provide the patient or some member of the family with explicit directions on how to give the medication and what adverse symptoms may occur. They should be advised of the need for frequent medical consultation. Many patients continue to take a drug once it is prescribed for long periods without seeing the doctor. This is bad practice with any drug, but is especially so for the antihypertensive medicines.

The Patient. It is very important that the patient understand the possibility that postural hypotension may develop during therapy with these drugs. He should be reassured and know what to expect and what to do should it occur. He should be warned not to attempt strenuous exercise until he has adjusted to the new blood pressure level; there is danger of syncope and possible injury.

If the patient is receiving one of the ganglionic blocking agents, he should be advised to stop the drug immediately and contact his physician if abdominal distention or other signs of intestinal stasis develop.

The patient should understand that when these drugs are given orally, the blood pressure lowers gradually which is desirable (V-2, 4).

MISCELLANEOUS DRUGS USED IN THE TREATMENT OF VASCULAR HYPERTENSION

Sedatives. Sedatives or tranquilizers are usually used to good advantage in hypertension. By lessening nervous excitability, they decrease the tension of the whole body and thus assist in lowering the blood pressure.

Phenobarbital (Luminal; phenobarbitone, Bartol [C]) in doses of 15 to 60 mg. or elixir of phenobarbital in appropriate doses may be used several times a day. Elixir of phenobarbital contains 16 mg. of phenobarbital per 4 ml. (fdr. 1). *Chloral hydrate,* 300 mg. two or three times a day, is also effective. Some sedation may be expected if the rauwolfia drugs are used.

Diuretics. Various diuretic drugs are used in the management of hypertension with or without other antihypertensive agents. However, they are usually used in conjunction with one of the medicines just discussed. Diuretics have been discussed in some detail under acute cardiac decompensation earlier in this chapter. The preparations most often used for reduction of blood pressure include the thiazide derivatives such as bendroflumethiazide, chlorothiazide and hydrochlorthiazide, the zolamide drugs such as acetazolamide, dichlorphenamide and ethoxzolamide and the aldosterone blocking agent spironolactone. For long term use of these drugs, except spironolactone, development of electrolyte imbalance may occur, especially a lowering of potassium. The concomitant administration of potassium is sometimes used. The nurse can advise the patient of foods rich in potassium which may be included in the diet. These are mainly the fruits and vegetables.

DISORDERS OF THE BLOOD VESSELS—PERIPHERAL VASCULAR DISORDERS

Chronic Occlusive (Peripheral) Arterial Disease

DEFINITION. Chronic peripheral arterial disease is characterized by the partial or complete occlusion of the arteries of the extremities (usually the legs) by atherosclerosis or atherosclerotic plaques. There may be small sacculations with or without the plaques.

MAJOR SYMPTOMS. The most noticeable symptom is difficulty in walking. There is need to stop often to let the legs rest. Other symptoms include pain, coldness and pallor in the extremities. Since this is usually a complication of atherosclerosis or arteriosclerosis, there are usually systemic symptoms as well as local ones.

DRUG THERAPY. The drugs used for this condition are almost legion, but they are only palliative at best. They may help to prevent or at least slow the progress of the disease, but they do not overcome the damage already done. The drugs employed are mainly those used for hypertension, which usually accompanies peripheral arterial disease, plus the direct vascular antispasmodics. Hormones, especially estrogen in the female patient, often help.

The direct antispasmodics which act on the peripheral blood vessels include *cyclandelate* (Cyclospasmol) 200 mg. and *nicotinyl tartrate* (Roniacol) 50 to 150 mg. These drugs may cause dizziness and flushing as with the coronary dilator nitroglycerin. Other drugs used include the adrenergic blocking agents, ganglionic blocking agents, sympathetic amines, drugs used to reduce cholesterol, antibiotics if ulcers occur, direct antihypertensive agents and, in some cases, heparin or dextrothyroxine. These drugs are discussed in more detail in other areas (see Hypertension).

THE NURSE. In this condition, the nurse has many responsibilities, not the least of which is to aid in early diagnosis. Often among her friends and relatives or in a public health or other nonhospital nursing field, she may well be the first to notice that there is real trouble. Often this condition goes untreated until very little can be done. The first time the physician sees the patient is when there is an ulcer or even beginning gangrene. The observant nurse would have noted the patient's difficulty in walking, his complaints of coldness, muscle aches and pains and so on. Patients often attribute these discomforts to "getting old."

When the diagnosis is made, the nurse will be called upon to explain to the patient the therapeutic regimen he is to follow. She should inform him that he may not see much improvement but should continue his medication, since it will prevent any worsening of the condition. She will also aid him in adjusting to any change in life style which the physician orders. It is customary to prohibit smoking, start a program of controlled exercises and reduce the intake of saturated fats. Alcohol in moderation is usually encouraged, since it tends to relax the blood vessel muscles.

THE PATIENT. This condition is chronic and usually progressive in spite of medications which slow the process but rarely halt it. This may require that the patient change his occupation, avocations and usual life routines. Since this is most commonly a disease of the older age group, change is difficult. It is important that the family, as well as the patient, understand the situation. The nurse, the family and the intimate friends will need patience and forbearance in dealing with the patient.

Raynaud's Disease

DEFINITION. Raynaud's disease or syndrome is a primary disorder characterized by paroxysmal bilateral symmetrical cyanosis of the digits either with or without local gangrene. The cause is unknown and it is usually brought on by cold or emotion and relieved by heat. The paroxysmal cyanosis is due to a constriction of the digital, palmar or plantar arteries causing a complete interruption of the local blood flow. Later, the digital capillaries become markedly dilated but the cyanotic blood remains there for a while, leaving the skin cold. After the disease has been present for some time, the intima of the blood vessels is thickened and the muscular coat of the arteries becomes hypertrophied. Eventually, there is thrombosis of small arteries leading to small points of gangrene. It is more often confined to the hands alone but the feet, nose, cheeks, ears and chin may be affected.

MAJOR SYMPTOMS. Beginning gradually, the attacks soon become bilateral—one to four digits (thumb often excepted) on each hand become deeply blue or first white, then blue. The fingers are cold, more or less numb and occasionally are covered with perspiration. These attacks usually end spontaneously or are terminated by immersing the hands in warm water or on entering a warm room. If the cyanosis is prolonged, there is often pain and awkwardness in fine movements. As the circulation returns, the digits become brilliantly red and there is tingling, throbbing or a slight swelling present. If allowed to continue, trophic changes are noticed—the skin becomes smooth and shiny, less mobile and eventually tightly stretched.

DRUG THERAPY. General health measures must be followed, including the elimination of smoking as this produces vasoconstriction and aggravates the disease. The vasodilator drugs of long action may help to relieve the frequency and intensity of the attacks. Beverages containing ethyl alcohol (dose 0.5 ml. per kg. body weight) produce some vasodilation for as long as four hours, but their long-term effect is questionable.

PHENTOLAMINE HYDROCHLORIDE, N.F. (REGITINE HYDROCHLORIDE; ROGITINE [C]). More commonly known as *Regitine*, this chemical compound is a potent adrenergic blocking agent, producing adrenolytic and sympatholytic effects. Although it is relatively nontoxic, it may produce untoward side effects such as tachycardia, orthostatic hypotension, nasal stuffiness and gastrointestinal disturbances such as nausea, vomiting and diarrhea. Most patients do not tolerate the dosage for sustained therapy because of the tachycardia.

The usual oral adult dose is 50 mg. four to six times daily but larger doses (up to 100 mg. four to six times daily) may be necessary in severe cases of peripheral vascular disease. Phentolamine methanesulfonate is a preparation which may be used for parenteral administration.

PHENOXYBENZAMINE HYDROCHLORIDE (DIBENZYLINE). This drug and its closely related congener dibenzyl-β-chlorethylamine (Dibenamine) act directly and specifically on adrenergic receptor cells so that the receptiveness to adrenergic (sympathomimetic) stimuli is decreased or abolished. The effects are largely those of peripheral vasodilation, which increases the peripheral blood flow and skin temperature and lowers the blood pressure. After a single full dose the action persists for three to four days or longer.

Most of the side effects are extensions of its therapeutic actions. These include nasal congestion, miosis, tachycardia and postural hypotension and tend to decrease with continued therapy. *Phenoxybenzamine hydrochloride* is given orally in an initial dose of 10 to 20 mg. once daily for four days. Then the dose may be increased by 10 mg. increments until satisfactory response is obtained. At least two weeks or more are required before maximal results are obtained.

MISCELLANEOUS DRUGS. *Nylidrin hydrochloride,* N.F. (Arlidin), acts as a peripheral vasodilator and appears to have an almost selective action upon the small arteries and arterioles of skeletal muscles. Minor side effects may occur such as nervousness or palpitation, but these are usually transient and disappear on continued therapy or reduction of dosage. This drug may be administered orally or parenterally (subcutaneously or intramuscularly). The suggested initial oral dose is 6 mg. three times a day and increased to four to six times a day as indicated.

Azapetine phosphate (Ilidar) is a potent adrenergic blocking agent which blocks the vasoconstrictive response of smooth muscle to circulating or injected epinephrine and exerts a direct vasodilating effect on the wall of small blood vessels. Occasionally drug fever occurs but serious untoward effects are rather rare. Nausea, vomiting, lightheadedness, weakness, malaise, syncope and postural hypotension may complicate therapy. The drug is given orally in an initial test dose of 25 mg. three times a day for seven days to screen out the occasional patient who cannot tolerate the drug. If it is used, the usual adult dose is about 50 to 75 mg. three times a day.

Nicotinyl alcohol (Roniacol), related to nicotinic acid, produces cutaneous vasodilation. Side effects include flushing of the face and neck. This flushing may be necessary to obtain the required amount of vasodilation. The drug is given orally in doses of 50 to 100 mg. three times a day.

Some physicians prefer the rauwolfia products in the treatment of Raynaud's disease. These have been discussed under Vascular Hypertension in this chapter. Other drugs used include the ganglionic blocking agents also discussed under Hypertension.

If the drugs which dilate the peripheral blood vessels do not help, or as an addition to them, thyroid or androgenic hormones may be given. These drugs are discussed in Chapter 27.

THE NURSE. The nurse will need to watch for signs and symptoms related to each drug used in treatment for peripheral vascular disease. In addition, she will need to monitor the blood pressure and peripheral pulses about every 4 hours. Through careful observations of intermittent claudication, skin temperature, postural color changes and arterial pulsations, the patient may develop minimal arterial impairment. All of this is done in an effort to prevent surgical amputation.

THE PATIENT. The patient will need a great deal of teaching in order for him to preserve his skin and tissue integrity. All of his efforts should be geared toward preventing gangrene and amputation. Instruction for prevention of further injury will include avoidance of mechanical, thermal or chemical trauma (contusions to feet, extremely hot water or corn cures), optimum warmth for extremities (socks in bed), alternate vasoconstriction and vasodilatation (exercise) and avoidance of *smoking*. By concentrating on teaching the above, as well as cogent aspects of drug and diet therapy, the nurse can assist the patient in maintaining his health status.

Cerebrovascular Accident (Cerebral Hemorrhage, Apoplexy, Stroke)

DEFINITION. A cerebrovascular accident is the rupturing of a blood vessel within the cranial cavity with resulting damage to the brain. It is a relatively common occurrence and is familiar to most people.

MAJOR SYMPTOMS. Cerebral hemorrhage may produce any number of symptoms, depending on its location and severity. One of the more common locations is in the internal capsule. In this location bleeding gives rise to paralysis of the side of the body opposite to the hemorrhage because of the desiccation of the fibers of the pyramidal motor tracts. In most cases restlessness is an early symptom.

The patient who has had a cerebrovascular accident may present a picture of profound coma, or the hemorrhage may have been so slight that only nominal reduction of the usual activities results.

DRUG THERAPY. The medicines used in the treatment of these patients will depend upon the severity of the condition. If the patient is conscious and there is only mild functional disturbance, drugs will form only a minor part of the treatment.

MILD CONDITION. Sedative drugs, usually the barbiturates, are used early and in fairly moderate dosage to insure adequate rest. *Phenobarbital* (phenobarbitone [C]), 60 mg. twice during the day and 90 mg. at bedtime, is not an unusual order.

Restlessness may also be controlled by a drug like *chlorpromazine* (Thorazine) 25 to 50 mg. (This drug is discussed in Chapter 30.)

Various preparations are used to augment the diet, which may be limited for a time. The diet is usually low residue and such things as glucose, high nitrogen products and vitamins may be added to it.

The combination of sedative medications, bed rest and the decrease in muscular activity resulting from the disorder often produces mild or severe constipation, so that most physicians order a mild laxative as a preventive measure. Straining at stool may increase the bleeding or start it again after it has stopped, since such straining causes an increase in intracranial pressure. This is another reason for the use of a cathartic.

Aspirin compound with or without codeine or *propoxyphene* (Darvon) orally or codeine 30 mg. parenterally may be given for pain.

If convulsive seizures occur, *diphenylhydantoin* (Dilantin) 250 mg. I.M. q 4 h is often ordered.

THE NURSE. The administration of these drugs will depend upon the exact condition of the patient. If the patient is conscious and there is no involvement of the deglutitive muscles, the oral route is used. If the patient cannot take the medications orally, they must be given parenterally or rectally.

The patient tends to be restless, and every effort must be made to reduce this since the extra movement may increase the hemorrhage. If the amount of the sedative ordered is insufficient to insure adequate rest, the physician should be notified.

THE PATIENT. The nurse must help the patient to turn frequently but, even with this help, the patient remains longer in one position than would be the case if he were not ill. This inactivity is one of the reasons that laxatives are needed. If the laxative cannot be taken orally, enemas or suppositories may be required until the patient is able to swallow a drug.

With elderly patients, in whom this condition is more common, this inactivity may produce any number of adverse symptoms, perhaps the most serious of which is pneumonia. It is essential that the mucus be removed from the lungs and bronchial tubes, by aspiration, if the patient cannot do it himself. If he is able to swallow easily and safely, an expectorant may be ordered to ensure that there is no retention of the mucus.

It is essential that these patients take sufficient nourishment and fluids and, if these cannot be taken orally, intravenous infusions or rectal instillations may be needed.

The patient with a cerebral hemorrhage is very restless and apprehensive and needs constant assurance and reassurance to aid him to obtain sufficient rest to prevent further damage. All therapy, in the early stages, is directed to that end. Later, drugs will be used to aid healing and to repair, insofar as is possible, any damage that has occurred.

SEVERE CONDITION—THE UNCONSCIOUS PATIENT. If the cerebral hemorrhage has been severe enough to produce unconsciousness, the nurse's responsibilities become vastly increased and the medical treatment much more important. The types of drugs used do not vary materially, but the route of administration does. Care of an unconscious patient is a nursing challenge of the first magnitude, whatever the cause of the unconsciousness may be. The vital functions of the patient must be maintained, which means that essential oxygen, fluid and nourishment must be supplied, excretion of wastes continued and the skin and musculature kept in as good condition as possible under the existing circumstances. Most of these things are the responsibility of the nurse, under the guidance of the physician.

To reduce the cerebral edema, the physician may order *mannitol* injection (Cystosal) (Osmitrol [C]). It is administered as an intravenous infusion. The usual adult dose ranges from 50 to 200 gm. in 24 hours. However, the actual amount given any individual patient varies widely according to the patient's condition and response to the drug. A urine flow of at least 30 to 50 ml. per hour is desirable. Another drug given for the same purpose is *dexamethasone sodium phosphate* (Decadron, Hexadrol Phosphate). The initial dose is 10 mg. given intravenously. This is followed by 4 mg. intramuscularly, every 6 hours until maximum response has been obtained. Oral dosage is started as soon as possible, 1 to 3 mg., three times a day, tapered off over a period of 5 to 7 days. Some patients may require more continuous use to remain edema free. The smallest possible dose should be used for maintenance.

Oxygen may be needed if cyanosis is encountered. The amount will depend upon the needs of the patient and will vary from time to time.

In order to allay restlessness, some mild sedative may have to be administered. Laxatives and enemas may have to be employed to ensure proper functioning of the intestinal tract. *Neostigmine methylsulfate* (Prostigmin), 0.5 to 1.0 mg. or *bethanechol* (Urecholine) 2.5 to 5 mg., may be ordered for flatulence and retention. These drugs will help to increase peristalsis in both the urinary and intestinal tract and will aid the patient to expel flatus and to void urine. It may not cause passage of the stool, but it is far more important in the early stages to rid the intestines of gaseous accumulation than it is to eliminate the solid excreta. Gas in any appreciable amount may interfere with the proper functioning of the heart and lungs, and this may be a serious complication.

Fluid and electrolyte balance must be maintained for the unconscious patient, especially if he is perspiring freely. Various electrolyte solutions are usually ordered either intravenoulsy or by hypodermoclysis. If the latter route is used, *hyaluronidase* (Alidase, Wydase), 1 ml., may be added to aid in the absorption of the fluid. *Glucose,* 10 to 25 ml. of a 50 per cent solution, may be given intravenously in the first few days to decrease intracranial pressure. Additional fluid and nutrients may be given by adding *amino acids* or *vitamins* or both to the solutions. Total parenteral nutrition may be used.

Stimulants are contraindicated in the early stages of cerebral hemorrhage lest they increase the bleeding. However, these may be used later when this danger is considered past.

Many of the drugs used for the unconscious patient are no different from those used for the patient who is conscious, though the dosage may vary somewhat in certain instances.

Oxygen can be administered by any method, but the unconscious patient must be watched very closely to see that an adequate supply is being delivered at all times, especially if a closed circuit is used. Since it may be necessary to leave the unconscious patient, nasal catheters are often used as these do not interfere with the normal intake of air.

The unconscious patient should be kept in such a position that he is able to breathe easily, but no one position should be maintained for more than a short time lest hypostatic pneumonia, decubitus ulcers or other undesirable conditions result. Frequent turning and the use of alcohol or skin lotion will aid in keeping the skin in good condition and help to prevent its breakdown. It is important for the nurse to watch heart and respiratory action since these may be difficult or weak. The unconscious patient is immobilized in spite of all the nurse may try to do to prevent this.

Since the unconscious patient cannot speak for himself, the nurse will need to be very alert to any change in his condition. Observation and recording of all symptoms becomes vitally important since only in this way can the physician be kept aware of the patient's progress. The physician needs the nurse's record to judge the effectiveness of the drugs and the treatments used and to plan for further treatment.

For the unconscious patient the nurse must do the things that he would ordinarily be doing for himself. The nurse will have to decide when the patient needs drugs ordered p.r.n. since he is not able to request them. She must be ever alert to make the patient as comfortable as possible, but at the same time she must avoid giving sedatives when they are not needed.

Staying in one position for a long time, even though every effort is made to change the patient's position frequently, may give rise to circulatory or respiratory involvement. With the latter, there may be need for an anti-infective drug. Some physicians routinely order an antibiotic as a preventive measure. The type and amount of the drug will depend upon circumstances. The use of the antibiotic in such a case may need to be explained to the patient's relatives or friends. They will wonder why such a drug is used when there is no apparent infection.

The paralysis which accompanies this type of condition should be given immediate attention by the use of passive exercises. There is no medical treatment for this, but if massage and passive exercises are begun early and done routinely, much of the common residual contractures and/or loss of muscle function can be avoided.

If relatives request religious aid this should be given first preference. It is the duty of the nurse to give all help possible in securing the proper religious advisor and providing him with anything he may need.

IT IS IMPORTANT TO REMEMBER

1. That digitalis is not given if the heart rate is below 60 per minute unless there is a specific order from the physician to do so.
2. That overdoses of salicylates may produce salicylism which may mean potential danger to the patient.
3. That during diuretic therapy, keeping an accurate daily weight and intake and output record is important.
4. That when giving antiarrhythmic drugs, one should count the apical and radial pulse for one minute and then calculate the pulse deficit.
5. That nitroglycerin tablets should be available at the bedside or carried in the patient's pocket.
6. That antihypertensive ganglionic blocking agents may cause orthostatic hypotension.

TOPICS FOR STUDY AND DISCUSSION

1. Why is it important to take the heart rate (preferably apically) before administering digitalis preparations?
2. What are the actions of digitalis on the heart and the rest of the body?
3. Describe the signs and symptoms of hypokalemia.
4. For what disease are the salicylates of great value? What is salicylism?
5. Identify the extracardiac toxicity reactions that may occur when quinidine is used as an antiarrhythmic agent.
6. The order reads: digitoxin 0.1 mg. How many grains is this?
7. The ordered dose of morphine sulfate is 15 mg. All that is on hand is 10 mg. How would you give this?
8. Differentiate between digitalization and maintenance doses. Why does this difference exist?
9. Describe how the nurse would instruct a patient in taking Digoxin so as to decrease the probable incidence of side effects.

BIBLIOGRAPHY

Books and Pamphlets

American Medical Association Council on Drugs, *Current Medical Terminology*, Chicago, 1966, American Medical Association.

American Medical Association Council on Drugs, *Drug Evaluations*, Chicago, 1971, American Medical Association.

American Medical Association Council on Drugs, *Evaluations of Drug Interactions*, Chicago, 1971, American Medical Association.

Beeson, P. B., and McDermott, W., *Cecil-Loeb Textbook of Medicine, 13th Ed.*, Philadelphia, 1971, W. B. Saunders Co.

Beland, I. L., *Clinical Nursing, 2nd Ed.*, New York, 1970, The Macmillan Co.

Bergersen, B. S., King, E. E., and Goth, A., *Pharmacology in Nursing, 12th Ed.*, St. Louis, 1973, The C. V. Mosby Co.

Chatton, M. J., Morgen, S., and Brainerd, H., *Handbook of Medical Treatment, 12th Ed.*, Los Altos, California, 1970, Lange Medical Publications.

Conn, H. F., et al., *Current Therapy, 1974*, Philadelphia, 1974, W. B. Saunders Co.

Goodman, L. S., and Gilman, A., *Pharmacological Basis of Therapeutics, 4th Ed.*, New York, 1970, The Macmillan Co.

Hartshorn, E. A., *Handbook of Drug Interactions*, Cincinnati, 1970, University of Cincinnati Press.

Miller, B. J., and Keane, C. B., *Encyclopedia and Dictionary of Medicine and Nursing*, Philadelphia, 1972, W. B. Saunders Co.

Rodman, M. J., and Smith, D. W., *Pharmacology and Drug Therapy in Nursing*, Philadelphia, 1968, J. B. Lippincott Co.

Shafer, K. M., et al., *Medical-Surgical Nursing, 5th Ed.*, St. Louis, 1971, The C. V. Mosby Co.

Watson, J. E., *Medical-Surgical Nursing and Related Physiology*, Philadelphia, 1972, W. B. Saunders Co.

Journal Articles

Aagaard, J. N., "Treatment of hypertension," *Am. J. Nurs.* 73:4:620 (April, 1973).
Adolph, E. F., "The heart's pacemaker," *Sci. Am.* 216:3:32 (March, 1967).
Anderson, L. C., et al., "Symposium on nursing challenges in cardiovascular and metabolic diseases," *Nurs. Clin. North Am.* 4:1 (1969).
Andreoli, C. K., "The cardiac monitor," *Am. J. Nurs.* 69:6:1238 (June, 1969).
Cafruny, E. J., "Ethacrynic acid and furosemide," *Ann. Rev. Pharmacol.* 8:131 (1968).
Coleman, D., "Surgical alleviation of coronary artery disease," *Am. J. Nurs.* 68:4:763 (April, 1968).
DiPalma, J. R., "Oxygen as drug therapy," *R.N.* 34:8:49 (1971).
DiPalma, J. R., "Precautions with the anticoagulants," *R.N.* 34:10:57 (1971).
DiPalma, J. R., "Enzymes used as drugs," *R.N.* 35:1:53 (1972).
DiPalma, J. R., "The why and how of drug interactions," *R.N.* 33:3:63 (March, 1970).
DiPalma, J. R., "The why and how of drug interactions," *R.N.* 33:4:67 (April, 1970).
DiPalma, J. R., "The why and how of drug interactions," *R.N.* 33:5:69 (May, 1970).
Elwood, E., "Nursing the patient with a cerebrovascular accident," *Nurs. Clin. North Am.* 5:1:47 (1970).
Freeman, E., and McCarty, M., "Rheumatic fever," *Sci. Am.* 229:3:66 (September, 1973).
Frohman, I. P., "Digitalis and its derivatives," *Am. J. Nurs.* 57:2:172 (February, 1957).
Fulcher, A., "The nurse and the patient with peripheral vascular disease," *Nurs. Clin. North Am.* 1:47 (March, 1966).
Gibbs, D., "Nursing assessment of circulatory function," *Nurs. Clin. North Am.* 3:53 (1968).
Griep, A., and DePaul, Sister, "Angina pectoris," *Am. J. Nurs.* 65:72 (June, 1965).
Griffith, E. W., and Madera, B., "Primary hypertension—patient's learning needs," *Am. J. Nurs.* 73:4:624 (April, 1973).
Hirschman, J. L., and Herfindal, E. T., "Current therapy concepts—essential hypertension," *J. Am. Pharm. Assoc.* NS 11:10:555 (1971).
Jackson, B. S., "Chronic peripheral arterial disease," *Am. J. Nurs.* 72:5:928 (May, 1972).
Jacobansky, A. M., "Stroke," *Am. J. Nurs.* 72:7:1260 (July, 1972).
Jenkins, A. C., et al., "Symposium on the care of the cardiac patient," *Nurs. Clin. North Am.* 4:4 (December, 1969).
Kerr, R. A., "Current therapy concepts—angina pectoris," *J. Am. Pharm. Assoc.* NS 12:4:178 (1972).
Lehman, Sister Janet, "Auscultation of heart sounds," *Am. J. Nurs.* 72:7:1243 (July, 1972).
Mayer, G. G., and Kaelin, P. B., "Arrhythmias and cardiac output," *Am. J. Nurs.* 72:9:1597 (September, 1972).
Pidgeon, V., "The infant with congenital heart disease," *Am. J. Nurs.* 67:2:290 (February, 1967).
Pinneo, R., et al., "Symposium on concepts in cardiac nursing," *Nurs. Clin. North Am.* 7:3 (1972).
Rodman, M. J., "Drugs used in cardiovascular diseases," *R.N.* 36:4:41 (1973).
Ross, E. J., "Hypochloremic alkalosis," *Clin. Pharmacol. Therapy* 8:131 (1968).
Smith, A. M., Theirer, J. A., and Huang, S. H., "Serum enzymes in myocardial infarction," *Am. J. Nurs.* 73:2:277 (February, 1973).
Smith, B., "Congestive heart failure," *Am. J. Nurs.* 69:2:278 (February, 1969).
Sobel, D., "Personalization in the coronary care unit," *Am. J. Nurs.* 69:7:1439 (July, 1969).
Spencer, R., "Problems of drug therapy in congestive heart failure," *R.N.* 35:8:46 (1972).
Wiecken, D. E. L., et al., "Reserpine's effect on structure of heart muscle," *Science* 157:3794:1332 (September, 1967).

CHAPTER 19

DRUGS USED FOR DISORDERS OF THE BLOOD AND THE BLOOD-FORMING ORGANS

CORRELATION WITH OTHER SCIENCES

I. ANATOMY AND PHYSIOLOGY

1. The blood is remarkably constant in composition, both chemically and in the number and proportion of the various types of cells.
2. Circulating blood is the main vehicle for the transport of nutrients, regulating substances, waste products and defense elements (leukocytes, antibodies) throughout the body.
3. The functions of the leukocytes (white blood cells) are defense against invading organisms and the mediation of the antibody response.
4. The total white cell count varies considerably from time to time, but most authorities place the normal limits at about 5000 to 10,000 per cu. mm. of blood.
5. The normal number of red blood cells (erythrocytes) is between 4,500,000 and 5,000,000 per cu. mm. of blood. The absolute average (normal) per cent of hemoglobin is 100 per cent, though most authorities consider 85 to 100 per cent or 14 to 16 Gm. per 100 ml. of blood within normal limits.
6. The primary function of the erythrocytes (red blood cells) is to act as containers for hemoglobin which carries oxygen from the lungs to the metabolizing tissues and carbon dioxide back to the lungs for discharge.
7. The site of erythrocyte production is the red bone marrow where cells undergo a recognizable series of maturation stages resulting in the mature red blood cell which is released to the circulating blood. Immature forms are normally not observed in the circulation.
8. Leukocytes and thrombocytes (platelets) undergo maturation stages in a manner somewhat similar to that of the erythrocytes. Some types of leukocytes are produced in the red bone marrow and others are produced primarily in lymphoid tissue. Like the red blood cells, usually only the mature forms appear in the circulating blood.
9. The genes that control hemoglobin (an iron-protein complex contained in the erythrocytes) production have undergone a variety of stable mutations and are present in a small proportion of the population. Inheritance of such "abnormal" genes may result in deficiency of normal hemoglobin production and/or oxygen-carrying abilities. These are referred to as hemoglobinopathies.

II. CHEMISTRY

1. The protein and electrolyte content of the plasma maintains a constant osmotic pressure relationship between it and the intercellular fluids.
2. Relatively simple laboratory tests can be used to distinguish various molecular differences of the hemoglobin molecule.

III. MICROBIOLOGY

1. Several diseases of the vascular system are caused by microorganisms, some of which are known and recognized; others are still to be identified. Some of the more common ones are the *Streptococcus, Staphylococcus, Treponema pallidum* and the *Mycobacterium tuberculosis*.

V. PSYCHOLOGY

1. The patient, when first told that he has pernicious anemia and will require injections for the remainder of his life, usually suffers a severe emotional shock.
2. It is very difficult for anyone, especially those in the older age groups, to revise lifelong habits and routines.
3. Individuals with genetically inherited diseases or traits must learn to adapt to their limitations.

VI. SOCIOLOGY

1. Pernicious anemia may pose a financial burden, especially if the family breadwinner is affected. Referral to the proper social agency is important.
2. Genetic counseling is of the utmost importance for any person known to have a genetic defect or trait. This is especially important if marriage is contemplated. The couple should be given all the important facts and understand the possibilities of spontaneous abortions or the birth of a child with the defect.

INTRODUCTION

The body is dependent on the circulating blood for its nourishment, in the form of nutrients and oxygen, and for carrying waste products to the kidneys and the lungs for excretion. It is also dependent on the blood for carrying agents of defense to the site of need in case of invasion or infection. Deficiencies of erythrocytes or hemoglobin result in a lowered oxygen-carrying capacity to the tissues, and interference with leukocyte function results in deficient defensive capacity.

Anemias are deficiencies in the oxygen-carrying capacity of the blood due to diminished or faulty production of erythrocytes (red blood cells) and their precursors or of hemoglobin in the bone marrow (I-7, 8). Anemias may result from a primary physiological deficiency such as the inability to absorb essential nutrients as in pernicious anemia, or they may be secondary to predisposing conditions such as nutritional deficiency, chronic or acute hemorrhage, infection with intestinal parasites or intestinal surgery. A third group results from inherited characteristics related to the synthesis of the hemoglobin molecule (I-8). Decreased cell production can also be caused by chemical agents or drugs that interfere with normal function of the bone marrow.

The anemias are frequently classified as macrocytic, normocytic, microcytic or hypochromic, depending on whether the erythrocytes are larger than normal, normal in size, smaller than normal, or deficient in their amount of hemoglobin.

ANEMIAS DUE TO NUTRITIONAL DEFICIENCY AND/OR BLOOD LOSS

Iron Deficiency Anemias

DEFINITION. Iron deficiency anemias are described as microcytic (erythrocytes smaller than normal) and hypochromic (erythrocytes pale in color owing to less-than-normal amount of hemoglobin).

Iron is normally obtained from foods rich in iron such as liver, heart and other meats, egg yolks, dried beans and peas, dried fruits and dark leafy vegetables. Normally, there is a large reserve of iron stored in the liver, spleen and other tissues. There is considered to be only limited normal excretion of iron. There are several circumstances which may lead to an iron deficiency anemia. First, there may be an insufficient amount of iron in the diet, but this is rarely seen except in infants on a strict milk diet. Impaired absorption of iron may be another causative factor, but this is not common. Increased requirements such as are necessary for growth are also possible and not too infrequent. Probably the most common cause is chronic blood loss, which includes infection with intestinal parasites that use the host's blood for their nutrition.

MAJOR SYMPTOMS. There are a variety of vague symptoms, many relating to the gastrointestinal tract. Anorexia, heartburn, sore tongue and mouth, dysphagia, palpitation, dyspnea, edema, achlorhydria, neuralgic pains, vasomotor disturbances and numbness and tingling may be found. The patient usually presents a tired, lifeless appearance with pallor, inelastic and often dry and wrinkled skin, dry, scanty hair and nails that break easily.

Examination of the blood shows a red blood cell count normal or nearly so or even greater than normal with small, thin, pale erythrocytes poorly filled with hemoglobin. The white blood cell count is normal or slightly reduced (Fig. 26).

DRUG THERAPY. IRON PREPARATIONS

THE DRUGS. Iron is required for the production of hemoglobin. As a medicine iron is of value only in iron deficiency anemia. However, this may be anything from a mild, almost asymptomatic condition to one so severe as to be life threatening. Iron has been used for anemia since ancient times. The use of blacksmith's water (in which iron had been cooled) to treat "pallor" was common for many years.

The cure for iron deficiency anemia depends on finding the cause for excess loss or impaired intake and treating that cause. The patient's intake is usually supplemented initially, and the supplement is continued until elimination of the cause is accomplished and the body's reserve is replenished.

Physical and Chemical Properties. Elemental iron is insoluble, unlike most of its salts.

Action. Iron given as a drug acts first to replenish the deficiency in red blood cells and then, when this has been accomplished, restores the body reserve (Fig. 34).

Therapeutic Uses. The only proven value of iron is in the treatment of iron deficiency anemia.

Absorption and Excretion. Absorption of iron is dependent on "acceptors" in the mucosa of the intestines and a "transport protein" in the plasma. The iron is thought to be bound to the acceptor which passes it to the plasma transport protein. This process is most active in the duodenum. Conservation of body iron is quite effective and only about 0.5 mg. is lost via feces and urine each day.

Preparations and Dosages. There are many iron preparations, each with advantages and disadvantages. The following are the forms most commonly used in the treatment of anemia:

Ferrous sulfate, U.S.P., B.P. (several trade names) 60 to 320 mg. t.i.d. a.c. or with meals, orally.

Ferrous gluconate, N.F., B.P. 300 mg. t.i.d. a.c. or with meals, orally.

Ferrous fumarate, U.S.P. 200 mg. t.i.d. a.c. or with meals, orally.

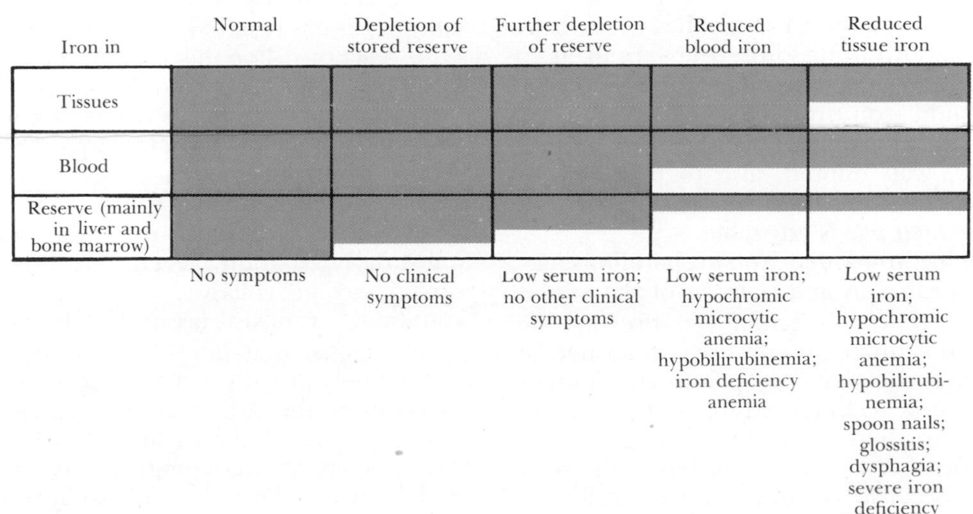

Iron in
Normal
Depletion of stored reserve
Further depletion of reserve
Reduced blood iron
Reduced tissue iron
Tissues
Blood
Reserve (mainly in liver and bone marrow)
No symptoms
No clinical symptoms
Low serum iron; no other clinical symptoms
Low serum iron; hypochromic microcytic anemia; hypobilirubinemia; iron deficiency anemia
Low serum iron; hypochromic microcytic anemia; hypobilirubinemia; spoon nails; glossitis; dysphagia; severe iron deficiency anemia

FIGURE 34. Iron deficiency anemia. (Adapted from Coleman, Stevens and Finch in Beckman.)

Because of the side effects, iron therapy is usually started slowly. One routine calls for one dose daily and addition of doses gradually until the desired dosage is reached. If the patient's condition is critical, or if the oral route cannot be used, parenteral preparations are available. These include:

Iron dextran injection, U.S.P. (Imferon) 50 to 250 mg. I.M., or 100 mg. I.V., daily. Dosages individually adjusted.

Dextriferron, N.F. (Astrofer) 20 to 100 mg. I.V., dosage started low and increased gradually. Must be injected slowly. Avoid infiltration. Must not be given into the tissues.

The Nurse

Mode of Administration. The dosage of all iron compounds is based upon the hemoglobin response in the patient. However, the drug is not discontinued when the hemoglobin reaches the desired level, since only after this is the stored reserve replenished. However, in building up the hemoglobin or hematocrit, the dosage is varied to suit the patient's response.

Iron therapy should not be prolonged indefinitely. The patient should be advised to consult with his doctor at frequent intervals during nonhospital use of any iron product.

It has been shown that oral iron preparations are absorbed best when taken on an empty stomach. However, many patients cannot tolerate this, so most physicians order the oral iron taken with meals. Ferrous sulfate should not be given with milk because it forms a heavy coagulum. Iron tablets should not be chewed or kept in the mouth to dissolve—they are likely to stain the teeth and cause feelings of nausea. If a liquid iron product is ordered for oral administration, it should be given through a tube, well diluted, also to prevent discoloration of the teeth. A mouth wash following such use is advisable.

The intramuscular iron preparations may cause local pain and staining of the skin at the site of the injection. To prevent the latter, the nurse should use a long needle and give the drug deep into the muscle, using the Z technique (refer to Chapter 3). Not more than 5 ml. should be given into any one site. If more is ordered, the dose should be divided and given in two different areas.

When administered intravenously, iron should be given very slowly, not more than 5 ml. in two minutes. The patient should remain recumbent for a short while after the injection to prevent postural hypotension.

Accurate recording is essential—amount, time, site, etc. It is wise to consult the package insert before giving any iron preparation either I.M. or I.V.

Overloading with parenteral iron may cause excess storage of iron with the possibility of exogenous hemosiderosis. This is most apt to occur in patients with hemoglobinopathies erroneously diagnosed as iron deficiency anemia.

Even with oral iron, overloading is possible, e.g., patients taking multivitamin-plus-minerals preparations without medical supervision. An adequate diet usually supplies all the iron an individual requires.

Side Effects. The side effects of iron therapy occur chiefly with oral administration and relate primarily to the gastrointestinal tract. All of the oral preparations cause black and pasty stools. The patient should be advised to include in his diet foods which are laxative in nature such as fruits and fruit juices. Other side effects include gastric distress, colicky pains, diarrhea or, more commonly, constipation. There may also be a feeling of fullness in the head, insomnia, tachycardia and skin eruptions. These latter symptoms are most likely to occur after a single large dose has been administered.

Toxicity and Treatment. Serious toxicity is rare with the oral administration of iron. However, the parenteral use of the iron complexes has resulted in fatal anaphylactic-type reactions. For this reason, these preparations should be used only in serious iron deficiency that cannot be controlled by oral iron therapy. The accidental ingestion of a large amount of iron medicine, usually by small children, can have serious or even fatal results. The symptoms are severe gastrointestinal irritation, even necrosis and cardiovascular collapse. There is nausea, vomiting, cyanosis, lassitude, drowsiness, hematemesis, diarrhea of green and later tarry stools. Death may occur within six hours after the drug has been taken, or it may be delayed for as long as 24 hours. Treat by inducing vomiting, giving milk and eggs and lavaging with sodium bicarbonate if seen early. Phosphate salts tend to bind both ferrous and ferric ions into complexes which are poorly absorbed and are used in the early treatment of iron poisoning. Since the Fleet enema is composed of sodium diphosphate and sodium phosphate, it may be diluted by one half with water and used. Do not lavage late because of the danger of gastric necrosis and possible perforation. An iron chelating agent such as desferoxamine mesylate (Desferal) may be given 1 to 2 Gm. in 5 per cent glucose solution intravenously by slow drip over a 24 hour period. Another chelating drug which may be ordered is calcium disodium acetate (EDTA). Dimercaprol (BAL) should not be used because it combines with iron to form a toxic compound.

Patient Teaching. Most of the instructions to the patient have already been given: how to take the drug, when to take it, the relationship to diet, possible side effects that may occur and how to cope with them and the need for medical supervision. There is one more important point the nurse should make—the proper diet the patient should follow to insure that iron requirements are met during and after iron therapy. The main foods rich in iron are meats, especially liver and heart, poultry, fish and egg yolk. Iron in lesser amounts is also present in some grains, fruits and vegetables. Milk and milk products are poor sources of iron.

THE PATIENT. Iron deficiency anemia tends to be a chronic condition. The patient must be encouraged to continue treatment even if it does not seem to help. If he understands that it takes weeks or even months for the body to absorb sufficient iron to restore depleted supplies, he will be more willing to continue therapy. If it is necessary to use parenteral iron preparations, the cost and discomfort may be factors that will need to be dealt with in accepting long-term therapy. The nurse can often aid the patient who is financially burdened by suggesting an agency which can help to subsidize part or all of the treatment. It is important that treatment and medical supervision be continued for as long as six months.

Pernicious Anemia

DEFINITION. Often called Addisonian anemia, this disease is a symptom complex characterized by a macrocytic anemia, central nervous system involvement and a deficiency in gastric secretions. There is a primary physiologic deficiency in the ability to absorb cyanocobalamin which is required for normal production and maturation of the erythrocytes.

It is generally believed that the characteristic lack of gastric secretion deprives the patient of a thermolabile substance (intrinsic factor) apparently specifically needed for the efficient absorption of vitamin B_{12} (extrinsic factor) from foods. Binding of the vitamin by the intrinsic factor is essential, but the mechanism is not yet completely understood. The substance which is normally formed by this binding is called the antianemia principle. This substance is stored in the liver and probably the liver elaborates this principle. When this antianemia principle is released from the liver, it enables the bone marrow to produce normally matured red blood cells. The patient with pernicious anemia is incapable of producing adequate quantities of the antianemia principle.

MAJOR SYMPTOMS. There are often insufficient characteristic symptoms to permit a diagnosis. The onset of the disease is insidious and the most common early complaint is that of chronic fatigue. Glossitis is frequent and early, but the tongue is seldom coated. Soon anorexia, nausea, vomiting and diarrhea occur. Symmetrical paresthesias of the hands and feet may occur as the spinal cord becomes involved. A yellow tinge to the skin is often noticed.

The blood picture shows evidence of abnormal bone marrow activity. The red cell count is usually below two million and the corpuscular constant is increased; the white blood count and platelets are reduced in number and a large proportion of the red blood cells are immature.

DRUG THERAPY. Therapy in pernicious anemia is directed toward replacement—that is, supplying the cyanocobalamin that the patient is unable to absorb from his diet and making up for the lack of acid in the stomach. Without adequate treatment, the patient rapidly declines; with treatment, life can be prolonged to its normal span and the patient may lead a normal life.

CYANOCOBALAMIN (VITAMIN B_{12}; COBALAMIN)

(See Current Drug Handbook.)

THE DRUG. Historically, pernicious anemia has been recognized clinically for more than 100 years. In 1926, Minot and Murphy demonstrated the value of liver in the treatment of this condition. At first, the patient was instructed to eat one-half to one pound of liver each day. This was an almost impossible task. Then an extract of liver was produced and used in the treatment of pernicious anemia. Still later, folic acid (pteroyl monoglutamic acid) and vitamin B_{12} (cyanocobalamin) were discovered. Both of these drugs appeared to be effective in the treatment of pernicious anemia. It was soon found that folic acid relieved only the hematologic aspect of the disease without affecting the neurological symptoms. This allowed the neurological damage to persist. Cyanocobalamin is now established as the main treatment for pernicious anemia. Folic acid alone is dangerous as it may mask the disease until serious neurological impairment has occurred.

Physical and Chemical Properties. Vitamin B_{12} is a very complex organic compound. It has been called the "red vitamin" since solutions of cyanocobalamin are a pinkish red in color. Cyanocobalamin is a crystalline substance that is readily soluble in water.

Action. Cobalamin, the shortened form of the word often used, appears to be concerned with most metabolic processes in man. It is essential for normal growth and nutrition, for normal hematopoiesis, normal production of epithelial cells (mucous and cutaneous) and for the maintenance of myelin throughout the nervous system.

Therapeutic Uses. Cobalamin is used primarily for the treatment of vitamin B_{12} deficiency, including pernicious anemia, nutritional macrocytic anemia, tropical and nontropical sprue. It has been used with questionable success in any number of conditions such as multiple sclerosis, trigeminal neuralgia, infectious hepatitis, anorexia, aging and various forms of malnutrition.

Absorption and Excretion. Absorption from parenteral sites is rapid and complete. Absorption from the gastrointestinal tract is erratic and unpredictable. When the latter route is used high doses of the drug must be given. Cobalamin is distributed throughout the body. The drug is metabolized in the body and excreted as its various components. Small amounts, about 1 to 2 micrograms daily, are excreted mainly through the feces. With oral administration this is markedly increased since much of a given oral dose is not absorbed.

Preparations and Dosages

Cyanocobalamin, 25 to 30 mcg. (micrograms), orally.

Cyanocobalamin injection, U.S.P., B.P. (Vitamin B_{12}) (many trade names), 10 mcg. to 1 mg. I.M.

Hydroxocobalamin (Vitamin B_{12a}), B.P. 10 mcg. to 1 mg. I.M. (This is said to have a more prolonged action, hence dosage intervals may be further apart.)

The oral drug is given daily. Parenteral preparations are given every day to once a month. In pernicious anemia, the drugs are given for life at intervals determined by the response of the individual patient.

THE NURSE

Mode of Administration. Though the drug is occasionally given orally in mild conditions, by far the most common method is intramuscular injection. Cobalamin is not irritant to the tissues and poses no problem in its administration. Since it is usually given regularly for indefinite periods, it is wise to rotate the site of injection.

Side Effects, Toxicity and Treatment. There is practically no adverse reaction to the use of cyanocobalamin.

Patient Teaching. It may be necessary for the nurse to teach some member of the patient's family how to give the intramuscular injections. However, some physicians want the patient to come to the office for the injections. In this way the doctor has more complete control of the administration and it also allows for frequent medical checking of the condition of the patient. The patient may not want this expense and the nurse may need to explain why the doctor prefers the drug given in the office.

THE PATIENT. The patient with pernicious anemia faces a real problem which he is often emotionally incapable of handling easily. It is not a simple matter for him to realize that he has a condition which will require injections regularly for the remainder of his life. It will mean, in most cases, a restructuring of his life patterns. At this time, the patient is a person who is usually tired, depressed and feeling generally below par. The nurse can often aid the patient by just being a good listener. Patients want to express their feelings and the nurse who will take the time to allow the patient to do so may be doing him as much or more good than many treatments. In this type of condition, it may be the nurse who can explain in "layman's language" what the trouble really is and emphasize the importance of the medicine being given.

DILUTED HYDROCHLORIC ACID. Most clinicians now feel that the administration of diluted hydrochloric acid is not necessary, especially if vitamin B_{12} is used. If the acid is used, it must be well diluted with water and taken during or immediately after meals. It should be taken through a glass straw to avoid injury to the teeth. A capsule form of glutamic acid hydrochloride (Acidulin) may be used; it is easier to take than the solution.

Vitamin B_{12} or Folic Acid Deficiency Anemias

DEFINITION. These are macrocytic anemias in which the blood picture is identical to that of pernicious anemia. In the vitamin B_{12} deficiency state, clinical symptoms are identical also. However, the cause of the anemia is not related to the primary physiologic deficiency in ability to absorb this essential vitamin.

Simple dietary deficiency of vitamin B_{12} is rare in the United States, but it does occur in individuals on prolonged strict vegetarian diets. In developing countries where diets contain little animal protein, dietary deficiencies are more common. Patients with gastrectomy, gastric carcinoma or resection of the ileum require supplemental, parenteral B_{12}, as do those with steatorrhea or infections of the intestinal tract resulting in prolonged diarrhea and impaired absorption. In areas where fish tapeworm is a frequent parasite, an anemia may develop, owing to successful competition of the parasite for the available vitamin in the intestines.

The major cause of folic acid deficiency in the United States is of dietary origin, in contrast to the rarity of this cause in the case of vitamin B_{12} deficiency. Folic acid deficiency is also frequently associated with alcoholism. Other causes include impaired absorption due to tropical and nontropical sprue, surgical alteration of the intestinal tract and infections resulting in prolonged diarrhea.

DRUG THERAPY. CYANOCOBALAMIN (VITAMIN B_{12}). (See pernicious anemia for details.) The drug may be given orally in cases of nutritional deficiency. However, it is usually given parenterally in cases of impaired absorption.

FOLIC ACID PREPARATIONS. Several preparations of folic acid are available. *Calcium leucovorin*, U.S.P. (leucovorin), is given intramuscularly and the usual dose is 3 to 6 mg. per day. *Folic acid*, U.S.P. (Folvite), is given orally in doses of 1 to 5 mg. daily. It may be given intramuscularly but ordinarily this has no advantage over the oral route. *Sodium folate* (Sodium Folvite) is the drug preferred when parenteral therapy is indicated.

Hemoglobinopathies

INTRODUCTION

Hemoglobin is a complex protein made up of two pairs of polypeptide chains, each having a "heme" group which is responsible for combination with oxygen and carbon dioxide.

The chemical makeup of the earlier-described polypeptides is quite constant and is such that small changes in amino acid content and sequence can noticeably alter physicochemical characteristics of the protein and, in some cases, its affinity for oxygen and carbon dioxide.

During the first three months of fetal life, the hemoglobin is made up of pairs of alpha (α) and epsilon (ϵ) chains. Production then shifts to a variety called "fetal hemoglobin" or HbF which is composed of pairs of alpha (α) and gamma (γ) chains. At birth, the production of the gamma (γ) chains is suppressed and adult hemoglobin (HbA) composed of alpha (α) and beta (β) chains becomes the predominant variety, accompanied by 2 to 3 per cent of HbA_2 having pairs of alpha (α) and delta (δ) polypeptide chains.

HEMOGLOBIN VARIANTS AND RESULTING DISORDERS

Over one hundred mutations involving alteration of amino acids in the alpha (α) and beta (β) chains have been noted, some of which result in anemias. Inherited impaired ability to synthesize alpha (α) and beta (β) chains also results in clinical anemia.

About 1948, Linus Pauling and his associate Harvey Itano published their observations of the physicochemical characteristics of hemoglobin from patients with sickle cell anemia, sickle cell trait (abnormal hemoglobin variants to be discussed later) and from normal individuals. They noted that the hemoglobin from patients with the anemia was less soluble than normal hemoglobin (HbA), and that it demonstrated different electrophoretic properties. They also noted that patients with the trait had equal amounts of HbA and the less soluble hemoglobin, which they termed hemoglobin S (HbS). It was later determined that the difference between HbA and HbS results from the substitution of an amino acid (valine for glutamic acid) at one position in each of the beta (β) chains of HbA. Because patients with the trait showed nearly equal parts of HbA and HbS, and those with the anemia had practically all HbS, Pauling suggested that this resulted from the presence of a mutant gene for the production of hemglobin and that it was evidence of a molecular disease. This then resulted in a chemically and physically different end product from the usual one. The anemias, he proposed, result from homozygous SS condition, and the trait represents the heterozygous SA state. Family studies for the most part have supported this theory of the molecular expression of gene mutation with resultant molecular disease.

Sickle Cell Anemia

DEFINITION. Sickle cell anemia is a genetically determined defect causing an abnormal hemoglobin (HbS). It is an autosomal recessive and the primary form appears almost exclusively in the black race. Sickle cell trait occurs in many apparently healthy individuals. However, if both partners in marriage carry the trait, the chance of their having a child with the disease is one in four (25 per cent). Two

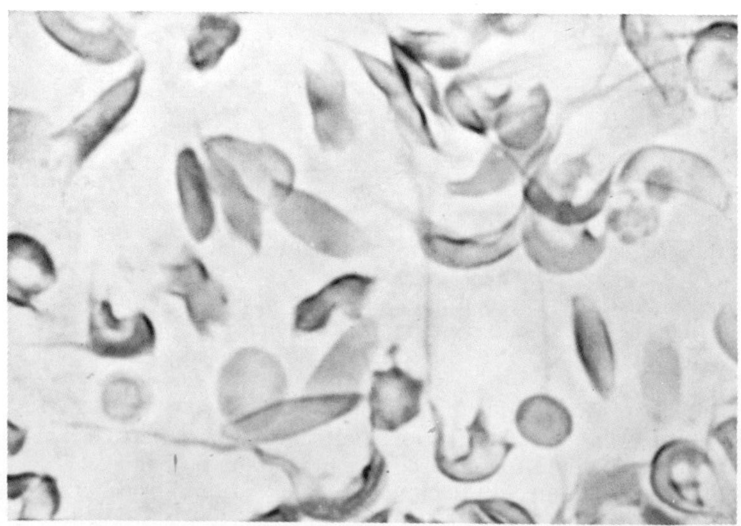

FIGURE 35. Sickle cell preparation with sodium metabisulfite. (From Leavell and Thorup, *Fundamentals of Clinical Hematology, 3rd Ed.,* Philadelphia, 1971, W. B. Saunders Co.)

similar conditions which occasionally occur in the United States are sickle cell-hemoglobin C (HbC) disease and sickle cell-thalassemia (Mediterranean) disease.

Sickle cell anemia is characterized by a tendency of the erythrocytes to become deformed into rod-like or sickle-shaped cells (whence the disease gets its name) or other irregular forms. These abnormally shaped cells cause occlusion and infarction of the spleen, liver, kidneys, brain and lungs. The misshapen cells are destroyed (hemolyzed) at a rapid rate with accompanying jaundice. The condition has long been recognized in two forms: as a disease of youngsters with spontaneous sickling and a high mortality rate (terminal sickle cell anemia), and as a milder form (sickle cell trait) in both youngsters and adults in which sickling crises are precipitated only infrequently, by exposure to high altitudes or other situations resulting in hypoxia.

MAJOR SYMPTOMS. Babies born with "sickling tendencies" usually appear normal at birth. From age six months to two years they begin to have difficulties. The condition is characterized by remissions (chronic or silent stage) and exacerbations (crisis stage). These children tend to develop slowly, have difficulty walking, are fretful and trying to care for. They are often thought to be mentally retarded. During crises, there is pain in the area affected, fever, anorexia and sometimes nausea and vomiting. Abdominal pain and rigidity are not uncommon. Splenomegaly may be noted as may hepatomegaly. Symptoms vary with the area involved. The erythrocytes containing HbS look and act as the normal hemoglobin (HbA) does until, for some reason, they become deoxygenated. This causes the hemoglobin molecules to become bound to each other. The cells then become misshapen, brittle, fragile and rigid. These cells break down easily. They tend to aggregate and plug the small blood vessels. This naturally stops the circulation at that point which causes an infarct. These infarcts may be minute or massive. If they are very small, there may be no symptoms. However, even small infarcts in a vital area may prove serious. If the infarct is in the brain, it may cause convulsions or death. However, most patients survive many crises. These crises are brought on by hypoxia. The attacks can develop from being at a high altitude (over 4,000 feet) without either extra oxygen or a pressurized chamber such as those in the larger airliners. Other causes include infections (especially those of the respiratory system), excessive exercise (resulting in severe fatigue), stressful situations or trauma (physical or emotional). As the patient grows older, the attacks of sickling crises diminish. However, there may be continuance of some infarction with resulting pathology, especially splenic or renal. The renal involvement may be serious, especially after 50 years of age.

Individuals with sickle cell trait are usually asymptomatic. However, under severe stress conditions or when going into a high altitude area, they may develop some of the symptoms of sickling crisis.

DRUG THERAPY. There is no direct cure for sickle cell anemia. However, recently the molecular cause has been determined and, it is hoped that a drug may be found to overcome this defect. In the meantime, much can be done to help these patients. Hyperbaric oxygen during crisis has been beneficial for some patients, but this treatment is not available for the majority. Infections should be prevented as much as possible and should be treated early and vigorously. Immunizations are important. Although the anemia is often marked, the usual antianemic drugs (iron and B_{12}) are rarely effective. Iron may be contraindicated, since these patients usually have ample reserves of iron. Folic acid (Folvite) has been successfully used for some patients. The dose is highly individualized, but the average is 0.25 to 1.0 mg. orally, once each day. It is used mainly during crisis, but may be continued intermittently during the "quiescent stage." As with all the present drug therapy, this is experimental, but it has proved valuable for some patients.

Transfusions are given as indicated by the hematocrit and the hemoglobin. Some physicians give small repeated transfusions in an effort to keep enough normal hemoglobin to prevent the sickling crisis. One routine is to give 350 ml. of whole blood every three or four months after withdrawal of 500 ml. of the patient's blood. This reduces the number of cells containing HbS and increases the number of cells containing HbA.

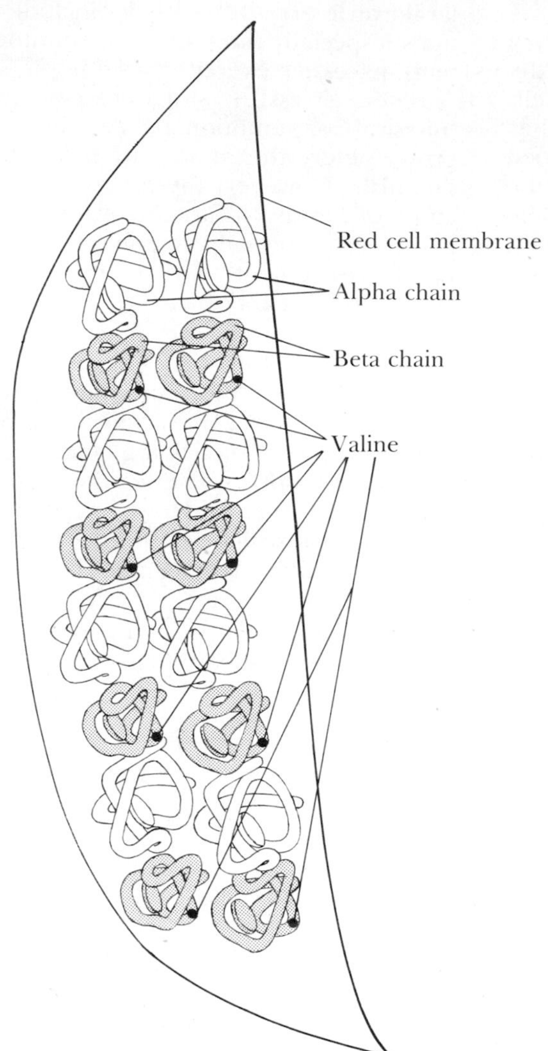

FIGURE 36. Substitution of valine for glutamic acid in the beta chain of hemoglobin. (Adapted from Foster, S., "Sickle cell anemia: Closing the gap between theory and therapy," *Am. J. Nurs.* 71:10:1953 [October, 1971].)

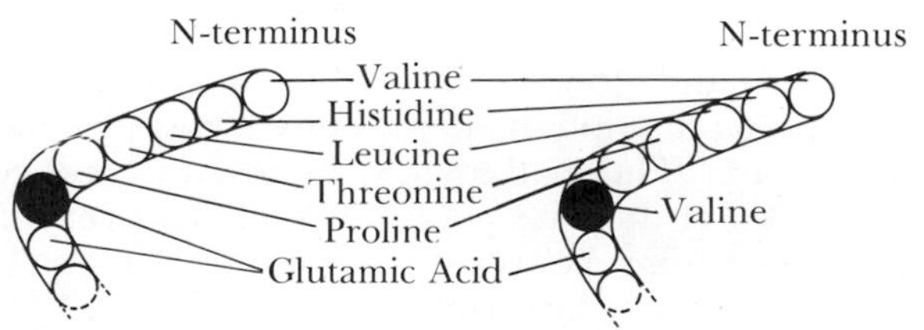

Urea and potassium cyanate are being investigated for use in the prevention and treatment of sickle cell anemia and the crises it produces. Reports so far vary as to routines being employed as well as to the effectiveness of the therapy.

The Nurse. The course of sickle cell anemia varies considerably owing to whether or not there is early diagnosis and early institution of supportive therapy. This means that the nurse will need to be specifically skilled in teaching about the illness, supporting the parents, being helpful in community endeavors to raise funds and begin diagnostic clinics and being able to understand and interpret aspects of genetic counseling to those involved.

During acute phases of the illness, the nurse will need to observe the patient carefully for infections—a critical secondary problem—and respiratory difficulties—largely due to infarcts resulting from stress situations. Periodic blood transfusions, prophylactic antibiotics and experimental drugs (urea and potassium cyanate) may be used in therapy.

The nurse must be alert to any reaction that may occur, especially from the transfusions these children usually receive. If experimental drugs are used, the results should be carefully noted and reported.

The blood pH is carefully observed, since it is known that acidity promotes sickling. Dehydration is to be avoided, and adequate fluid intake, particularly of orange juice, is encouraged. Acid compounds such as aspirin are also to be avoided. Analgesics may be ordered to alleviate joint, back and abdominal pain.

The nurse, especially the public health nurse, will need to observe and record carefully the child's growth rate and progress and continue screening him for dental and eye problems. Often follow-up is needed with school personnel to help the child with sickle cell anemia cope with the stresses of school and for the school personnel to understand the specific requirements of these children. The public health nurse can also aid the family to cope with and understand the enuresis which occurs from the inability to concentrate urine—and help the parents not to feel the need to punish the child for this behavior.

Regardless of all the supportive care given, the nurse must be alert to and prepared to deal with the concept of death. The fear of death is most prevalent among the affected children—and rightfully so. However, most of these children succumb from infection rather than from the disease itself. In these situations, the nurse will need to understand and deal with cultural and racial backgrounds—perhaps different from her own—which may encompass many different views of death and dying.

The Patient. The nurse will need to be especially skillful in helping the patient and family members understand the genetic mechanism of the disease. She will need to help them accept their feelings of guilt and blame for producing offspring with sickle cell anemia. Much is being done with research and new supportive therapies so that hope is valuable for all to retain.

Parent education is vitally important—especially since more than one child in the family may be affected. After approximately five years of age, the survival rate is quite high. Although the chronic illness continues to exist, the patient can become a productive member of society. Additional teaching and follow-up are always needed in addition to supportive emotional assistance through the various stages of life. Teaching continues to revolve around protection of the individual from his environment to insure that warmth, avoidance of trauma and precautions against infections are provided. In addition, if high altitude transportation is necessary and infarctions have been previously noted, special arrangements, such as having extra oxygen available, will need to be made.

The Thalassemias

Another group of syndromes with deficient hemoglobin production is characterized by inherited deficiency in production of either the alpha (α) or beta (β) polypeptide chain of normal hemoglobin. These abnormal genes have the greatest prevalence in the geographic regions bordering the Mediterranean Sea, through countries of the Middle East and in Southeast Asia. They are likewise found in the United States among concentrations of the population whose ethnic origins are in these regions. The name Mediterranean anemia was once applied because of the high incidence of the disease in those areas.

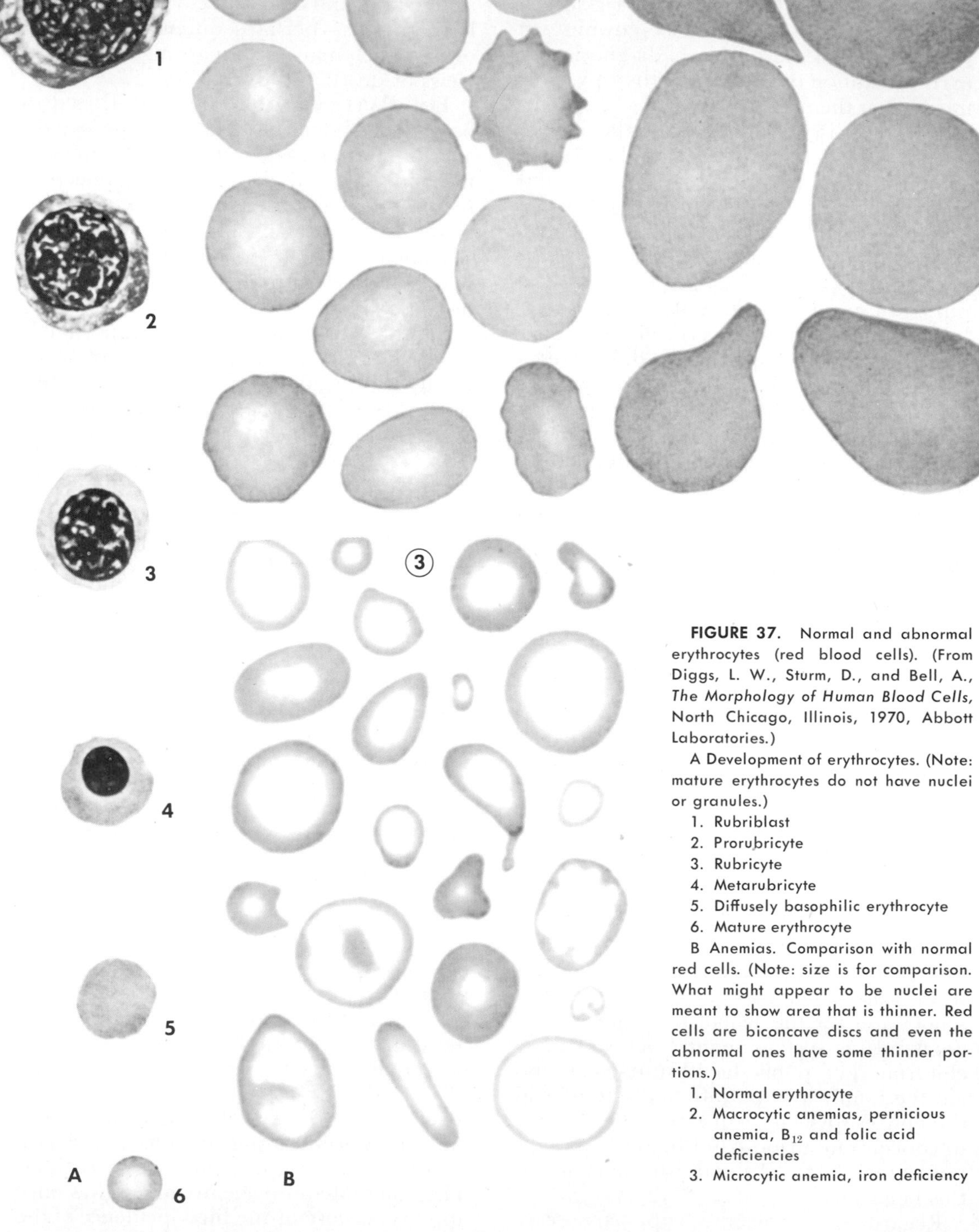

FIGURE 37. Normal and abnormal erythrocytes (red blood cells). (From Diggs, L. W., Sturm, D., and Bell, A., *The Morphology of Human Blood Cells,* North Chicago, Illinois, 1970, Abbott Laboratories.)

A Development of erythrocytes. (Note: mature erythrocytes do not have nuclei or granules.)

1. Rubriblast
2. Prorubricyte
3. Rubricyte
4. Metarubricyte
5. Diffusely basophilic erythrocyte
6. Mature erythrocyte

B Anemias. Comparison with normal red cells. (Note: size is for comparison. What might appear to be nuclei are meant to show area that is thinner. Red cells are biconcave discs and even the abnormal ones have some thinner portions.)

1. Normal erythrocyte
2. Macrocytic anemias, pernicious anemia, B_{12} and folic acid deficiencies
3. Microcytic anemia, iron deficiency

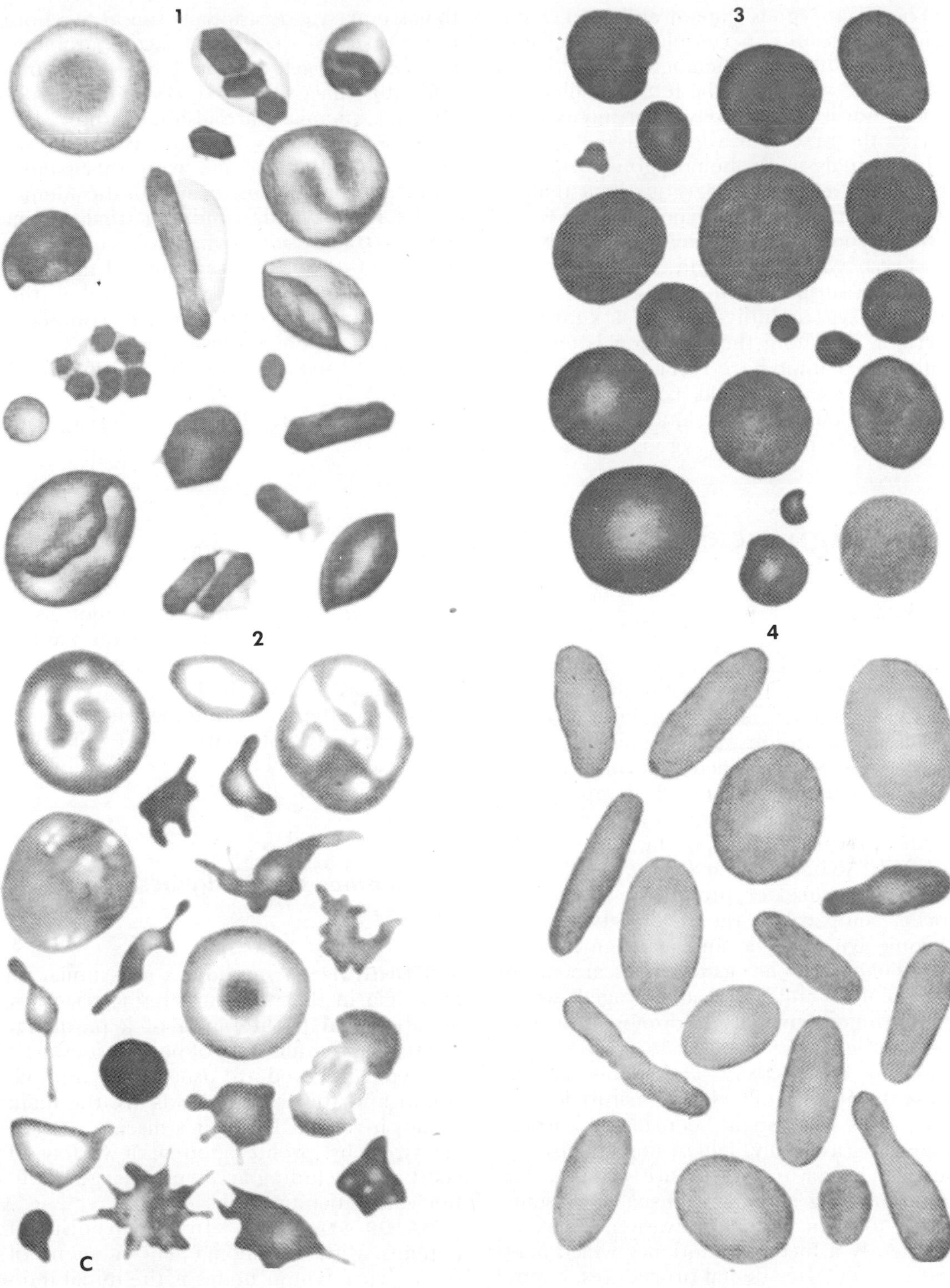

C Hemoglobinopathies.
1. Sickle cell anemia
2. Thalassemia major
3. Homozygous C disease
4. Sickle cell-hemoglobin C disease

The homozygous state of alpha (α) chain deficiency results in complete suppression of the production of hemoglobin and is incompatible with life. The fetus usually dies in utero or is prematurely born and expires during the first hour after birth.

Individuals with homozygous beta (β) chain deficiency (homozygous beta thalassemia or thalassemia major) suffer from severe hypochromic anemia and usually do not live beyond the second or third decade, even with supportive therapy.

Heterozygous individuals, also known as carriers, in whom the condition is termed thalassemia minor are rarely symptomatic. They may exhibit a mild hypochromic anemia and a characteristic blood picture.

Patients with heterozygous sickle cell-thalassemia are occasionally found in whom the severity of the disease is comparable to that of sickle cell anemia. HbC-thalassemia and HbD-thalassemia—relatively mild hypochromic anemias—are also encountered.

DRUG THERAPY. Therapy is rarely required for the carriers with thalassemia minor. Because of the severity of the anemia in the homozygous condition (thalassemia major) transfusions of whole blood or packed erythrocytes are required to maintain the oxygen-carrying capacity of the blood. Supportive therapy for complications of the anemia is also required.

THE NURSE. (Refer to Sickle Cell Anemia.)

THE PATIENT. (Refer to Sickle Cell Anemia.)

Malignancies

Leukemias

DEFINITION. Leukemias are conditions arising from abnormal proliferation of one of the leukocyte series and its immature forms and invasion of the tissues by these cells. They are classified according to the type of leukocyte involved (lymphocytic, myelogenous, monocytic) and the maturity of the predominant type, the more immature disease being termed acute and the disease with a greater proportion of mature forms being called the chronic type as in chronic lymphocytic and acute myelogenous leukemia. The acute forms are more prevalent in children and the aged, while the chronic forms are predominant during the middle years.

MAJOR SYMPTOMS. The blood picture presents large numbers of immature leukocyte forms not usually seen in the normal blood. Occasionally, leukocytosis is absent, but the immature forms are present. An accompanying anemia is usually present, owing to bone marrow invasion. There is frequently a bleeding tendency which may first be seen after dental procedures, minor surgery or trauma.

DRUG THERAPY. With the introduction of chemotherapeutic agents and their application to malignant diseases, the survival time for patients with acute leukemia has been extended from three to six months to two years or more, and that for the patient with chronic leukemia has been extended to six or more years. These drugs are represented by the alkylating agents, antimetabolites, corticosteroids, plant alkaloids and antibiotics. (See Table 14 and Current Drug Handbook for details.)

Lymphomas and Hodgkin's Disease

DEFINITION. Lymphomas are similar to leukemia in that they are characterized by an abnormal proliferation of a particular cell type and infiltration of body tissues. The cell types involved are usually of lymphoid origin and the lymph glands are the main tissues involved. Hodgkin's disease is characterized by proliferation of a variety of cell types including an atypical large multinucleate reticulum cell.

MAJOR SYMPTOMS. In the majority of patients with lymphoma, enlargement of the cervical lymph nodes is the initial indication of the disease. Progression is by extension of the process (dissemination) to involve other nodes and, eventually, other tissue.

Anemia and infections are secondary

complications resulting from invasion of the bone marrow. Immune deficiency, probably resulting from interference with lymphoid tissue, is responsible for the patient's increased susceptibility to infection.

DRUG THERAPY. Therapy for lymphoma (lymphosarcoma) includes irradiation of the affected nodes and chemotherapy. As with other malignancies, early detection and therapy provide the best prognosis. Early adequate radiotherapy may result in a cure in approximately 50 per cent of these patients. The usual life span for patients with Hodgkin's disease is four years. However, remissions are obtained with the judicious use of chemotherapeutic agents. These drugs are represented by alkylating agents, antimetabolites, corticosteroids, plant alkaloids and antibiotics. (See Table 14 and Current Drug Handbook for details.)

THE NURSE. In caring for these patients, the nurse has a very challenging problem or set of problems. The various chemotherapeutic agents exhibit many untoward side effects which must be known and watched for. The nurse must be able to differentiate between the symptoms of the disease and the side effects of the drugs. Physically, the patient must be shielded from infections which might prove very serious. Most of the drugs produce, at least in the initial use, anorexia (if not actual nausea and vomiting), yet food is all important. Strict oral hygiene is essential, as is skin care, since the skin and the mucous membranes tend to be more "fragile" than normal. If the drugs are given intramuscularly, rotation of sites is imperative.

However, with these patients (as with most patients) the physical care is just about half of the fulfillment of "good nursing care." The psychosocial problems of the patient and his family are much more difficult to resolve. The nurse must be able to give support to these people. She must be able to counsel when it is requested (not just verbally, but subtly by implication). In most cases there are remissions of months or even years and in some cases, cures. The nurse can plan with the patient and his family for home care during remissions.

THE PATIENT. The adult patient with leukemia or lymphoma usually understands the situation, but it is still a severe emotional shock to be told of his condition. He may react with anger, denial, resentment, resignation or even depression bordering on psychosis. He may consider suicide as an alternative to long treatment with no assurance of success. The nurse must realize that the "difficult" patient may actually be expressing his inner fears. He must be given an opportunity to express his feelings. He needs support and encouragement. Often, especially in the hospital, these patients feel very much alone. The nurse can do much to overcome this if she will take time for frequent visits, even if only for a minute. Many patients do not like to call for a nurse unless it is absolutely necessary and they may be left alone for hours before the busy nurse realizes it. The frequent visits mean that "someone does care."

With the sick child, this is equally true. It is important to make such children feel that someone is always near and ready to help. The family of the sick child will need help in planning for home care. If there are other children, their place in the scheme may be very important. Often the mother is so busy with the sick child that she appears to neglect the well children. However, if the well children are given a chance to help, even if it is ever so little, they will feel more "important" and will not consider that they are being neglected.

When the patient (adult or child) goes home, the public health nurse can give continuity of care if the hospital personnel plan with her and the family for the patient's needs.

Aplastic Anemia

DEFINITION. Aplastic anemia is a term used to describe a condition characterized by failure of the bone marrow to produce, or rarely, to release, cells to the circulating blood. The condition shows a profound reduction in those cells normally produced by the bone marrow. It is a relatively rare condition and is known to have been caused by a variety of drugs, chemicals and ionizing radiation as x-rays. The blood picture of these patients shows a normocytic anemia with some oddly shaped cells.

Treatment of the condition involves removal of the drug or chemical causing the suppression of the bone marrow and supportive care.

TABLE 14. *SPECIFIC AGENTS USED IN CANCER CHEMOTHERAPY*

AGENTS	ADMINISTRATION AND DOSAGE	USES	ACTION AND FATE	UNTOWARD REACTIONS	COMMENTS
Mechlorethamine hydrochloride, U.S.P. Other names: Nitrogen mustards (HN_2) Mustargen Mustine injection (B) Chlormethine [C]	I.V.: 0.1–0.4 mg./kg. body weight daily for 4 successive days On occasion, may be given by intra-arterial, intrapleural and intrapericardial injection	1. Chronic leukemia 2. Cancer of lung, ovary, breast 3. Hodgkin's disease 4. Lymphosarcoma 5. Lymphoblastoma of skin and mycosis fungoides Can be used in alternating courses with x-ray Not used in terminal cases	1. Cytotoxic to all cells with special affinity for intestinal and corneal epithelium, germinal tissues, lymphatic and hematopoietic systems and rapidly proliferating cells of certain neoplastic growths 2. Subsequent courses usually not so effective as preceding course 3. May cause temporary remission of varying duration 4. Also affects normal tissue, causing toxic reactions 5. Shrinks tumor masses in 12 to 24 hrs.	1. Nausea and vomiting usually within 1 to 3 hrs. after administration; emesis may disappear in first 8 hrs. but nausea can persist for 24 hrs. or more 2. Anorexia, weakness, diarrhea 3. Occasional skin rash 4. Amenorrhea 5. Depression of hematopoietic system – leukopenia, thrombocytopenia – may last up to 50 days after starting therapy 6. Thrombophlebitis and thrombosis may result from direct contact with intima of injected veins 7. Because of excessive cell destruction, may cause multiple hemorrhages in various parts of body	1. Prepare fresh solution before each use 2. Best given in divided doses on four successive days 3. Margin of safety extremely narrow 4. Extravasation of drug into subcutaneous tissues results in painful inflammation with induration and sloughing; may be minimized by infiltration of 0.16 molar sol. sodium thiosulfate with ice compresses to part 5. Preliminary blood picture necessary 6. Vesicant – may cause blistering of skin – those handling drug should use rubber gloves; if there is contact with skin, wash with large amounts of water immediately 7. One of antiemetics helps control nausea and vomiting
Triethylenemelamine, N.F. Other names: TEM Tetramine Triethanomelamine [C] Tretamine [C]	I.V.: 5–20 mg. over several days Orally: 2.5–5 mg. on 2 successive mornings	1. Hodgkin's disease 2. Lymphosarcoma 3. Chronic leukemia 4. Polycythemia vera 5. Mycosis fungoides 6. Cancer of lung Usually used as adjunct to x-ray	1. Depresses mitosis (I-5) especially of lymphoid tissue and bone marrow 2. Inhibits growth of neoplasms, especially lymphomas 3. Acts like nitrogen mustards 4. Relieves anorexia, weakness and pruritus and diminishes size of tumor	1. Gastric irritation – nausea and vomiting less frequent than in nitrogen mustards 2. Bone marrow depression (similar to nitrogen mustards) which may not be noted until 14 to 21 days after last dose	1. Given before breakfast with sodium bicarbonate in water to favor absorption of drug, and food withheld for 1 to 2 hrs. 2. Slow onset – results may not be noted for 7 to 10 days 3. Prolonged effect may be continued as long as subjective improvement continues without excessive bone marrow depression 4. Periodic check of hemoglobin, total white blood cells and platelets 5. Therapy discontinued when white blood count falls rapidly or is below 4000

Triethylenethiophosphoramide, U.S.P. Other names: Thio-TEPA TESPA TSPA	I.M. I.V.: 30 mg. once a week or less as determined by white blood count Intra-arterial Intraserosal Intratumor Orally: 60 mg. once a week	1. Similar to nitrogen mustards 2. Metastatic cancer of ovary and breast 3. Chronic granulocytic and lymphatic leukemias 4. Hodgkin's disease 5. Carcinoma of lungs, gastrointestinal, genito-urinary tracts and central nervous system	1. Markedly depresses blood cell formation 2. Slow onset of action; results may not be noted for several weeks 3. Results variable	1. Nausea and vomiting minimal 2. Effects on bone marrow unpredictable 3. Anorexia, headache 4. Occasional febrile and allergic reactions 5. Amenorrhea in female; diminished spermatogenesis in male	1. Not used as initial treatment of choice 2. Frequent blood studies during and for some time after therapy – depression of blood cells may occur as late as 30 days after drug stopped 3. Powdered sterile preparations stored in refrigerator; study literature accompanying vial for correct method of diluting. Reconstituted solution may be kept 5 days in refrigerator; if precipitate present at any time, discard
Busulfan, U.S.P. Other names: Myleran Busulphan [C]	Orally Initial dose: 2–6 mg. daily until maximal hematologic and clinical improvement attained; then reduce to maintenance dose of 1–3 mg. daily	1. Chronic myeloid (myelogenous) leukemia 2. Not in acute or terminal stages	1. Produces remission for a few weeks to months 2. Depresses bone marrow function and may cause depression of platelets and erythrocytes 3. Lymphoid tissue not affected 4. Does not affect germinal tissues or lymphatic or intestinal epithelium	Hemorrhagic symptoms because of extreme thrombocytopenia which may not be apparent for 4 to 6 months	1. Complete blood count including thrombocyte levels at least once a week 2. If untoward signs do not appear, continue administration until clinical improvement noted – 3 weeks to several months
Chlorambucil, U.S.P. Other names: Leukeran Leukran [C]	Orally Initial dose: 4–10 mg. Maintenance dose: 2–4 mg. daily	1. Chronic lymphocytic leukemia 2. Lymphosarcoma 3. Hodgkin's disease	1. Cytotoxic – often produces remission of variable duration 2. Relief of pain and pruritus, regression of nodes, weight gain 3. Rapid reduction in total leukocyte count	1. Bone marrow depression may be irreversible if dosage not reduced or discontinued with remission 2. Anorexia, nausea and vomiting minimal, except with large doses.	1. Complete blood count mandatory at least once a week 2. Thrombocyte count at regular intervals 3. This drug potentiated by other cytotoxic drugs and radiation therapy. Not given for at least four weeks after other agents discontinued
Cyclophosphamide Other names: Cytoxan Procytox [C] Endoxan [C]	I.V.: 3–5 mg./kg. body weight twice weekly Orally: 100–250 mg. daily I.M. Intrapleurally Intraperitoneally If indicated, infiltration of tumor	1. Hodgkin's disease 2. Multiple myeloma 3. Chronic lymphocytic and granulocytic leukemias 4. Monocytic leukemia 5. Carcinoma of breast and ovaries, neuroblastoma and mycosis fungoides	Drug transported to malignant cells and there transformed to active agent	1. Serious bone marrow depression 2. Anorexia, nausea, vomiting, diarrhea 3. Weight loss 4. Dizziness, blurred vision 5. Mental changes 6. Alopecia 7. Cystitis	1. Watch hematologic picture closely – weekly blood counts 2. Use usually reserved for those with widely disseminated disease 3. Increase water intake if possible

Table continues

TABLE 14. *SPECIFIC AGENTS USED IN CANCER CHEMOTHERAPY (Continued)*

AGENTS	ADMINISTRATION AND DOSAGE	USES	ACTION AND FATE	UNTOWARD REACTIONS	COMMENTS
Melphalan Other names: Alkeran L-Sacolysin Compound CB 3025	Orally: 6 mg. daily Discontinue after 2 or 3 weeks for about 4 weeks Another course may be given when white blood count and platelet count rise with maintenance dose of 2 mg. daily	Multiple myeloma	Depresses bone marrow production	1. Usually well tolerated 2. Single large doses may cause nausea and vomiting 3. Avoid serious or irreversible bone marrow depression	1. Not given if similar agents or radiation have been used in recent past 2. Frequent white blood counts and platelet counts 3. Repeated courses should be given for improvement may be slow
Methotrexate, U.S.P. Other name: Amethopterin	Orally: 5–10 mg. 3 times a week I.M. I.V. Intra-arterial Intratumor	1. Metastatic choriocarcinoma 2. Acute lymphoblastic leukemia 3. Acute monocytic and myelocytic leukemia 4. Lymphosarcoma in children	Interferes with action of folinic acid in nucleic acid synthesis; disrupts mitotic process	1. Nausea, vomiting, diarrhea 2. Hematologic depression 3. Oral and digestive tract ulcerations	1. Blood counts daily for first month then 3 times a week 2. Bone marrow examination weekly to monthly 3. Absorbed readily from G.I. tract and excreted via urine 4. Sodium (parenteral form of drug) reconstituted only with sterile water; if precipitate forms, discard; may be stored at room temperature for 2 weeks; caution in using in conjunction with salicylates and sulfa drugs
6-Mercaptopurine, U.S.P., B.P. Other names: Purinethol 6-M.P.	Orally Initial dose: 2.5 mg./kg. body weight daily Doubled if no clinical response after 4 weeks	1. Primarily in acute leukemia 2. Possibly of help in chronic myeloid (myelogenous) leukemia	1. Believed to interfere with nucleic acid biosynthesis 2. Provides temporary remission and prolongation of life 3. Depresses bone marrow	1. Bone marrow depression 5 to 10 days after initiation of therapy 2. Nausea and vomiting means excessive dose 3. Ulceration of intestinal epithelium	1. Frequent blood counts mandatory 2. Drug withdrawn temporarily at first evidence of abnormally large fall in white blood count
5-Fluorouracil Other name: 5-F.U.	I.V. Dosage strictly individualized but daily dose must not exceed 1 Gm.; discontinued after twelfth day of therapy Locally	1. Cancer of breast, colon and rectum All patients *very* carefully selected 2. Solar keratosis	Apparently blocks synthesis of deoxyribonucleic acid (DNA) and inhibits formation of ribonucleic acid (RNA)	1. Leukopenia, thrombocytopenia 2. Stomatitis, diarrhea, gastrointestinal ulceration and hemorrhage	1. Contraindicated in those with poor nutritional state and with previous bone marrow depression 2. Not given to those with recent surgery 3. Absolutely *must* be in hospital for first course of treatment 4. Consult package insert for details of administration 5. Narrow margin of safety

Hormone Therapy (I-4) *Androgens* Testosterone Methyltestosterone Fluoxymesterone	I.M. Orally Dosage individualized	Cancer of breast	1. Changes environment of gland, interfering with neoplastic process 2. Causes regression of soft tissue masses 3. Subjective improvement—relief of pain and increased sense of well-being, increased appetite, weight gain	1. Masculinization in female 2. Fluid retention 3. Marked hypercalcemia 4. Mild gastrointestinal disturbances occasionally	1. One of safest forms of cancer therapy 2. Mammary cancer in postmenopausal women responds better to estrogens
Estrogens Diethylstilbestrol Ethynylestradiol Estradiol benzoate Oestradiol monobenzoate [C]	I.M. Orally Dosage individualized	Cancer of prostate and breast (mainly in those over 60 yrs.)	1. Changes environment of gland, interfering with neoplastic process 2. Relieves pain 3. Heals bone lesions 4. Prolongs life	1. Nausea 2. Fluid retention 3. Feminization in male 4. Uterine bleeding 5. Marked hypercalcemia	1. Safe form of therapy 2. May be used indefinitely, as long as therapeutic benefits continue
Corticosteroids Prednisone Prednisolone	I.M. Orally Dosage strictly individualized	1. Acute childhood leukemia 2. Hodgkin's disease 3. Lymphosarcoma 4. Multiple myeloma 5. Chronic lymphatic leukemia	Method of action not clear but often helpful in early stages	See Chapter 27	1. Most helpful in acute leukemia when followed by other antineoplastic agents 2. In other conditions, variable results
Plant Alkaloids and Antibiotics *Vinblastine sulfate* Other names: Velban Velbe [C]	0.1 to 0.2 mg./kg. body weight for 1 or 2 weeks I.V.	1. Hodgkin's disease 2. Other lymphomas 3. Solid cancers	Not well understood but may arrest mitotic division at metaphase	1. Nausea and vomiting 2. Stomatitis 3. Alopecia 4. Loss of reflexes 5. Local irritation	
Vincristine sulfate Other name: Oncovin	0.01 to 0.03 mg./kg. body weight weekly I.V.	1. Acute lymphocytic leukemia 2. Hodgkin's disease 3. Other lymphomas 4. Solid cancers	As above	1. Local irritation 2. Peripheral neuritis 3. Paralytic ileus 4. Mild bone marrow depression 5. Areflexia	
Dactinomycin Other names: Actinomycin D Cosmegen	0.015 to 0.05 mg./kg. body weight weekly for 3 to 5 weeks I.V.; wait for bone marrow recovery (3 to 4 weeks); then repeat	1. Wilms' tumor 2. Testicular cancer 3. Rhabdomyosarcoma 4. Ewing's sarcoma 5. Osteogenic sarcoma 6. Other solid cancers	Exact mechanism unknown	1. Local irritation 2. Nausea and vomiting 3. Stomatitis 4. Oral ulcers 5. Alopecia 6. Mental depression 7. Bone marrow suppression 8. Diarrhea	

TABLE 14. SPECIFIC AGENTS USED IN CANCER CHEMOTHERAPY (Continued)

AGENTS	ADMINISTRATION AND DOSAGE	USES	ACTION AND FATE	UNTOWARD REACTIONS	COMMENTS
Mithramycin Other name: Mithracin	0.025 to 0.05 mg./kg. body weight, q 2 days for up to 8 doses I.V.	1. Testicular carcinoma 2. Trophoblastic neoplasms	Believed to act by inhibiting cellular ribonucleic acid and enzyme synthesis	1. Nausea and vomiting 2. Bone marrow depression 3. Hepatotoxicity 4. Hypocalcemia	Can be used in treatment of hypercalcemia and hypercalciuria associated with a variety of advanced neoplasms
Other Agents					
Hydroxyurea Other name: Hydrea	80 mg./kg. body weight orally q 3 days or 20 to 30 mg./kg. body weight daily orally	Chronic granulocytic leukemia	Possible interference with DNA synthesis by inhibition of formation of deoxyribonucleotides	1. Depression of leukocytes 2. Depression of platelets 3. Buccal ulceration 4. Nausea and vomiting	
Procarbazine hydrochloride Other names: Matulane Natulan [C]	Start 1 to 2 mg./kg. body weight daily, orally. Increase over one week to 3 mg./kg. Maintain for 3 weeks, then reduce to 2 mg./kg. daily until toxicity appears	1. Hodgkin's disease 2. Non-Hodgkin's lymphomas 3. Bronchogenic carcinoma	Inhibition of DNA and RNA synthesis, but exact mechanism unknown	1. Nausea and vomiting 2. Bone marrow depression 3. Central nervous system depression	
Investigational Drugs (July, 1973)					
Adriamycin	60 to 90 mg./M^2, I.V. single dose or over 3 days, repeated q 3 weeks	1. Soft tissue, osteogenic and miscellaneous sarcomas 2. Hodgkin's disease 3. Non-Hodgkin's lymphomas 4. Bronchogenic carcinoma 5. Breast carcinoma	See Daunorubicin	1. Nausea 2. Red urine (not hematuria) 3. Bone marrow depression 4. Cardiotoxicity 5. Alopecia 6. Stomatitis	Differs from Daunorubicin only in having a hydroxyl group in place of a hydrogen
Bleomycin Other name: Blenoxane	10 to 15 mg./M^2 weekly or twice weekly I.V. or I.M. to total dose of 200 to 300 mg.	1. Hodgkin's disease 2. Non-Hodgkin's lymphomas 3. Squamous cell carcinoma 4. Testicular carcinoma 5. Some renal carcinomas 6. Some soft tissue sarcomas	Interferes with DNA synthesis	1. Nausea and vomiting 2. Fever 3. Edema of hands 4. Pulmonary fibrosis 5. Alopecia 6. Stomatitis	An antibiotic isolated from cultures of *Streptomyces verticillus*

Daunorubicin Other names: Daunomycin Rubidomycin Cerubusine	30 to 60 mg./M²/days 3 or 30 to 60 mg./M² weekly I.V.	Acute lymphocytic and acute granulocytic anemias	Inhibits both DNA dependent DNA synthesis and DNA dependent RNA synthesis	1. Nausea 2. Red urine (not hematuria) 3. Bone marrow suppression 4. Cardiotoxicity 5. Alopecia	Antibiotic isolated from *Streptomyces peucetius* and *caeruborubidus*
Carmustine BCNU Other name: Bischlorethyl nitrosourea	100 mg./M²/day times 2; not to be repeated for 6 weeks	1. Primary and secondary central nervous system neoplasms 2. Hodgkin's disease 3. Non-Hodgkin's lymphomas 4. Multiple myeloma 5. Gastrointestinal adenocarcinomas 6. Burkitt's tumor	An alkylating agent that interferes with DNA and RNA synthesis	1. Nausea and vomiting 2. Hepatotoxicity 3. Leukopenia 4. Thrombocytopenia	
Lomustine CCNU	130 mg./M² single dose orally; repeated at 6 week intervals	1. Hodgkin's disease 2. Central nervous system neoplasms (primary and secondary) 3. Gastrointestinal adenocarcinomas 4. Bronchogenic carcinoma 5. Renal cell neoplasms	See Carmustine	1. Nausea and vomiting 2. Hepatotoxicity 3. Leukopenia 4. Thrombocytopenia	

DRUG THERAPY. Transfusions with whole blood or packed erythrocytes may be necessary to maintain the oxygen-carrying capacity of the blood.

Infection as a result of reduced leukocytes is probable and must be detected and treated promptly with the appropriate anti-infective agents.

Androgenic hormones appear to stimulate bone marrow response. However, prolonged therapy of four to six months is required. The following may be used: fluoxymesterone 10 to 20 mg. daily, orally, testosterone enanthate 300 to 600 mg. every one to three weeks intramuscularly and oxymetholone 2 to 4 mg. per kg. of body weight daily, orally.

Agranulocytosis (Agranulocytic Angina)

DEFINITION. This disease is fairly rare and is thought to result from causes similar to those involved in aplastic anemia. The bone marrow suppression results in a severe deficiency of granulocytes and platelets with a high probability of spontaneous bleeding and infection. The disease is an acute, fulminating and often fatal condition with sudden onset, high fever, headache, malaise and sore throat. The red blood count is normal or slightly depressed in contrast to the white count which shows a severe leukopenia.

Successful treatment depends on identification and removal of the offending agent or stimulation of the myeloid marrow and supportive therapy as in aplastic anemia.

THE NURSE. The patient with either aplastic anemia or agranulocytosis is suddenly an extremely ill person. Often he has no idea why. The first thing for the nurse to do is to reassure the patient. Try to ease the shock. Explain repeatedly, if need be, what is being done, and what it is expected to do. Infection is an ever-present danger and hospital contamination could be fatal. Reverse isolation may be required, and this will certainly need to be interpreted so that it will not increase the patient's anxiety. The earliest sign of infection must be noted and reported.

Transfusions are usually given to these patients, and it is necessary to watch for signs of adverse reactions. If the patient is unable to retain food, total parenteral nutrition may be needed after the initial transfusion. This is also a frightening experience which the nurse will have to explain to the patient. As with leukemia, oral hygiene is extremely important.

Drug therapy is begun as soon as the acute stage begins to subside, and it is prolonged for weeks or months as with leukemia. Plans for home care are important, especially the precautions against infection, its early detection if it does occur and the fact that the least sign of infection should be reported to the physician.

THE PATIENT. The nurse, by adroit questioning or just by getting the patient to talk, may be able to discover the possible cause of the condition. This knowledge will facilitate the treatment of the case by the physician. Removal of the offending drug or chemical is "half the battle won."

These patients, like any very ill patients, need a great deal of reassurance and support. They need help in planning for the future, for until the blood picture reaches, or at least approaches, normal, there is always potential trouble.

IT IS IMPORTANT TO REMEMBER

1. That the treatment of iron deficiency anemia must be continued until the body's reserve has been replenished (usually three to six months).
2. That the patient on oral iron therapy needs to be advised to include ample amounts of fruits and vegetables in his diet to aid in overcoming the constipating effect of the iron.
3. That patients with pernicious anemia, or vitamin B_{12} deficiency anemia (unless due to dietary deficiency) will usually require parenteral vitamin B_{12} for the remainder of their lives.
4. That sickle cell anemia and other hemoglobinopathies are inherited condi-

tions and that the patients and any relatives who carry the trait will need genetic counseling.

5. That although there is no "sure cure" at this time for malignancies associated with the blood and the blood-forming organs, chemotherapy in many cases can prolong the "useful" lifetime by months and often years.

TOPICS FOR STUDY AND DISCUSSION

1. Describe a diet you might suggest for a patient on iron therapy. What dietary advice would you give when the therapy has been completed?

2. A patient with pernicious anemia has a friend who has diabetes mellitus. The friend gives herself insulin injections. The patient with pernicious anemia asks why the doctor insists that she come to his office for her "shots." What would be your reply?

3. Sickle cell anemia defect is a Mendelian recessive gene. How would you explain these terms and the effect of the disease to a person who has just been told that he has sickle cell trait?

4. A white patient, upon being told that he has thalassemia minor (which is similar to sickle cell anemia trait), asks how it is possible for him to have this type of disease, since he had thought it only affected black people. What would your reply be?

5. Many new drugs and treatments for various cancers (including those of the blood) are being tried. Check the available literature (medical, nursing, scientific) for the last year and see what the newest therapy is. (This might be a project for several students.)

BIBLIOGRAPHY

Books and Pamphlets

American Medical Association Council on Drugs, *Drug Evaluations*, Chicago, 1971, American Medical Association.

Beeson, P. B., and McDermott, W., *Cecil-Loeb Textbook of Medicine, 13th Ed.*, Philadelphia, 1971, W. B. Saunders Co.

Bergersen, B., *Pharmacology in Nursing, 12th Ed.*, St. Louis, 1973, The C. V. Mosby Co.

Conn, H. F., *Current Therapy, 1974*, Philadelphia, 1974, W. B. Saunders Co.

Diggs, L. W., Sturm, D., and Bell, A., *The Morphology of Human Blood Cells*, North Chicago, Illinois, 1970, Abbott Laboratories.

Goodman, L. S., and Gilman, A., *Pharmacological Basis of Therapeutics, 4th Ed.*, New York, 1970, The Macmillan Co.

Gothe, A., *Medical Pharmacology*, St. Louis, 1970, The C. V. Mosby Co.

Meltzer, L., Abdellah, F., and Kitchell, J. R., *Concepts and Practices of Intensive Care for Nurse Specialists*, Philadelphia, 1970, The Charles Press.

Rodman, N. T., and Smith, D. W., *Pharmacology and Drug Therapy in Nursing*, Philadelphia, 1968, J. B. Lippincott.

Shafer, K. M., et al., *Medical-Surgical Nursing*, St. Louis, 1971, The C. V. Mosby Co.

Watson, J. E., *Medical-Surgical Nursing and Related Physiology*, Philadelphia, 1972, W. B. Saunders Co.

Journal Articles

Brady, C. M., "The lymphomas, concepts and current therapies," *Nurs. Clin. North Am.* 7:4:763 (March, 1972).

Christian, D. G., Cornelis, W. A., and Fortner, C. L., "The acute leukemias," *Am. J. Nurs.* 72:9:473 (September, 1972).

Cornelis, W. A., Christian, D. G., and Fortner, C. L., "Hodgkin's disease," *J. Am. Pharm. Assoc.* NS 13:3:147 (March, 1973).

Cunningham, J. J., et al., "Cancer—A clinical trial of i.v. and intracavitary bleomycin," *J. Am. Pharm. Assoc.* 222:29:1413 (1971).

Farmer, R. G., "Anemia—gastrointestinal causes," *Postgrad. Med.* 52:4:95 (1973).

Fewer, D., et al., "Chemotherapy of brain tumors," *J.A.M.A.* 222:5 (1972).

Fischer, D. S., et al., "Acute iron poisoning in children—The problem of appropriate therapy," *J.A.M.A.* 218:8:1179 (1971).

Foster, S., "Sickle cell anemia—Closing the gap between theory and therapy," *Am. J. Nurs.* 71:10:1952 (October, 1971).
Grant, J. A., "The nurse's role in parenteral hyperalimentation," *R.N.* 36:7:27 (July, 1973).
Hussar, D. A., "Drug interactions, the pharmacist's opportunities and limitations," *J. Am. Pharm. Assoc.* NS 12:9:467 (1972).
Isler, C., "Blood—The age of components," *R.N.* 36:6:31 (June, 1973).
Jackson, D., "Sickle cell disease—Meeting a need," *Nurs. Clin. North Am.* 7:4:727 (December, 1972).
Jerne, N. J., "The immune system," *Sci. Am.* 229:1:52 (July, 1973).
Lerner, R. A., and Dixon, F. J., "The lymphocyte as an experimental animal," *Sci. Am.* 228:6:82 (June, 1973).
Levin, R. H., "Current therapeutic concepts—Iron deficiency anemia in the pediatric patient," *J. Am. Pharm. Assoc.* NS 11:12:670 (December, 1971).
Patterson, P. C., Shuman, D., et al., "Symposium on patients with blood disorders," *Nurs. Clin. North Am.* 7:4:743 (December, 1972).
Pochedly, C., "Sickle cell anemia," *Am. J. Nurs.* 71:10:1948 (October, 1971).
Rodman, M. J., "Drugs for treating nutritional anemia," *R.N.* 35:6:61 (June, 1972).
Silverstein, M. J., and Morton, D. L., "Cancer immunotherapy," *Am. J. Nurs.* 73:7:1178 (July, 1973).
Wilson, P., "Iron deficiency anemia," *Am. J. Nurs.* 72:3:502 (March, 1972).
Wong, F. T., et al., "Cancer—Adriomycin," *J.A.M.A.* 221:28:837 (1972).

CHAPTER 20

DRUGS USED TO AID IN OVERCOMING NUTRITIONAL DISORDERS

CORRELATION WITH OTHER SCIENCES

I. ANATOMY AND PHYSIOLOGY

1. Metabolism is the term used to denote the sum total of the chemical processes of the body cells. It is divided into two processes: anabolism, the building of tissue, and catabolism, the breaking down of tissue. Anabolism builds and repairs the body cells. Catabolism supplies heat and energy.
2. When total food intake is in excess of the body needs, the extra material is laid down as adipose (fatty) tissue.
3. When total food intake is below body requirements, the fat stored in the body is used to supply the body requirements for heat and energy.
4. Calcium and phosphorus form a large proportion of the mineral content of bones and teeth.
5. Calcium salts are essential for the proper clotting of blood.
6. The body is made up of a number of elements, four or five forming the major portion. Many elements are found in very minute quantities and are called trace elements.
7. Vitamin K plays an essential part in the mechanism of blood clotting. It is needed for proper prothrombin activity.

II. CHEMISTRY

1. A solution is a combination of a solute dissolved in a solvent. There are various solvents, such as water, oil, ether, benzene and other materials. The solute may be another liquid, a gas or a solid.

V. PSYCHOLOGY

1. Many people need emotional aids to meet the more severe trials of life. They cannot make themselves do the appointed tasks without help from others.
2. Individuals differ greatly in their likes and dislikes. These preferences are often difficult to change.
3. What an individual believes to be important is important to him. Each person has his own standard of values.

VI. SOCIOLOGY

1. Social effectiveness is the relationship of the individual to those with whom he lives —how well he serves society and, conversely, how well society serves him.

INTRODUCTION

The principal treatment of the nutritional disorders is obviously dietary rather than medicinal, but medicines may be used to aid in a more rapid and satisfactory recovery. These disorders often present definite psychologic, as well as physical, problems. The overly stout individual or the person with a pellagrous dermatitis is most unattractive, and the knowledge of this unattractiveness may produce serious emotional trauma. This is especially true of certain age groups. The correction of the disorder may give the person an entirely new outlook on life and greatly enhance his social effectiveness (VI-1).

Disorders resulting from poor nutrition may be either quantitative—the result of either too much or too little food—or qualitative—the result of an unbalanced diet, with some foods deficient and others in excessive amounts.

Nutritional disorders, especially deficiencies, may damage vital organs, particularly if they are of long duration. The conditions produced may require extensive medical as well as dietary treatment. Most of these conditions are discussed under the systems mainly concerned; thus, malfunction of the liver may be caused by lack of proper vitamins or other food substances such as protein. This disorder, even if it is of dietary origin, will be discussed with other diseases of the liver.

DISORDERS CAUSED BY ABNORMAL QUANTITATIVE FOOD INTAKE

Obesity

DEFINITION. Obesity, a condition in which excessive fat is stored in the body, is one of the foremost nutritional problems of our day. It appears almost natural for the individual in the middle years of life to put on extra weight, but this is a time when he can least afford it. However, even children and young adults frequently are burdened with many more pounds than is consistent with the best health.

If there is one continuous national food fad, it is "dieting." That the overweight person should eat less is, of course, true. Weight is the direct result of caloric intake in proportion to metabolic needs. Most overweight is caused by eating more than the body requires (I-1, 2). Certain disorders, mainly of endocrine origin, do produce a tendency to an increase in weight, but these are not numerous and cannot be blamed for most obesity.

TREATMENT OF OBESITY WITHOUT DRUGS. The best way to avoid obesity is to limit the food intake to the amount needed to maintain adequate nutrition. To overcome the condition it is necessary to reduce the intake somewhat below the actual requirements so that stored fats will be utilized for the maintenance of body heat and energy (I-3). The food reduction must be continued as long as there is excessive weight. After the desired weight has been reached, the diet is standardized so as to maintain the normal body weight level. It sounds simple, but many find it very difficult to avoid overeating.

Any person needing weight reduction should first find out how much he should lose and estimate a possible time schedule for that reduction. Let us assume the individual is a man of medium build—five feet 10 inches in height, weighing 210 pounds. The scale for that build and height is 146 to 160 pounds. Therefore, he should lose at least 50 pounds. Most physicians advise a relatively slow steady loss of 1 to 3 pounds per week. If the midpoint is taken at 2 pounds per week, it will take 25 weeks or about six months to lose 50 pounds. It has been found that diet alone is a very slow process, but if increased exercise is added, reduction will be much more rapid and the person will feel and look better, since muscle tissue will be gradually built up to replace the fatty tissue lost.

DRUG THERAPY. To aid the patient in keeping to the prescribed diet, some drug is often ordered. The medicine serves two purposes: the physical value and the psychologic effect. The drug acts as a sort of crutch, for most patients feel that the diet alone is too difficult to maintain (V-1). However, if the patient feels that the drug will help him, he is more willing to continue with the prescribed routine.

Drugs for obesity are always used as an adjunct to the dietary regimen. Several drugs may be employed. Sometimes a simple sedative, such as phenobarbital or a tranquilizer will suffice. Other drugs which may aid include thyroid products, which increase metabolism, methylcellulose, which decreases feelings of hunger and diuretics, which decrease the amount of fluid in the body and also increase waste disposal. A short discussion of these follows.

THYROID HORMONE. The *thyroid hormone,* either the extract or the active principle, is used only in patients who have a low basal metabolic rate. These are in the minority and are treated as any hypothyroid case. When used for reducing purposes, thyroid extract is usually given orally once or twice daily, the total dosage ranging from 15 to 200 mg. The active principle, thyroxin, is usually given each morning. Dosage is 0.2 mg. It is also given orally.

When the drug is being used for weight reduction, the nurse must impress the patient with the need to keep the caloric intake at or below the previous level or the drug will be of no avail. Patients receiving the thyroid hormone for obesity must be watched for symptoms of hyperthyroidism, nervousness, irritability, palpitation, tachycardia and sometimes dyspnea.

When obesity is caused at least in part by endocrine imbalance, it is of real psychological help to the overweight individual to realize that his excess weight is not caused entirely by overeating and that there is a drug that can help him to reduce without a severely limited diet.

A more complete discussion of this drug will be found in Chapter 27.

METHYLCELLULOSE. *Methylcellulose,* prepared from the indigestible portion of vegetables, is used mainly as a cathartic and is discussed in detail under that topic. Since it is hydrophilic, it absorbs water and forms a soft bulky mass. As an anorexic agent, it is prepared as "cookies" or "crackers" to be eaten 20 to 30 minutes before meals. They should be taken with a glass of water. This fills the stomach and the patient then needs much less food to satisfy his appetite.

DIURETICS. Some physicians give synthetic oral diuretics to aid in weight reduction. These are most effective when there is a tendency to fluid retention, however slight it may be. They are also best with patients who have elevated blood pressure. Any of the oral diuretics may be used such as *acetazolamide* (Diamox), *chlorothiazide* (Diuril), *ethoxzolamide* (Cardrase) or *hydrochlorothiazide* (Esidrix). These have been discussed previously. Drugs used in the past to reduce appetite have been given for weight reduction. Their use appeared to be more psychological than physical. These drugs were primarily central nervous system stimulants (the amphetamines and related compounds). They are no longer used in programs for weight reduction in the United States. See Chapter 9 for further details.

THE NURSE. It is important for patients on a reducing diet to limit their intake, but the nurse should discourage any reduction beyond that ordered by the physician. Some patients tend to starve themselves, especially at the beginning of the treatment. Such a procedure is not wise and, if the patient is taking drugs to increase the effectiveness of the diet at the same time, may actually be dangerous. These things should be explained to the patient and his cooperation secured, if possible, so that the diet and the drugs may be of utmost value. Some physicians may also wish the nurse to assist with concurrent behavior modification programs in order to develop more helpful eating patterns.

Some physicians start the patient out with an extremely low caloric intake. A 24 to 48 hour liquid diet may be the doctor's choice. The duration the patient adheres to a liquid diet or to a limited caloric diet will depend upon the patient's weight and physical condition. He may be hospitalized temporarily when severe caloric restrictions are being instituted, allowing for closer medical supervision than is available in the home.

Most reducing diets are carefully planned to include all essential food principles, and any variation from that prescribed may reduce necessary elements, especially vitamins, below the requirements of the patient. Sometimes the diet may be lacking in one or more vitamins, and if such is the case, these will be added in the form of drugs.

THE PATIENT. The overweight adult has often been so since childhood and has received many adverse remarks about his condition. "Fatty" or "fatso" may have been a nickname which he hated. In his frustration, he either fought back or retired within himself. Many obese patients use the alibi, "My whole family is heavy. It's heredity." However, no genetic grounds have been found to substantiate this. The probable explanation is "an excellent cook and good appetites all around." These people need support and understanding from the nurse. She must not be judgmental but must try to aid the patient in recognizing his condition and in helping him "rebuild" his eating habits.

Undernutrition

DEFINITION. Undernutrition may be any grade from a simple temporary disorder to actual starvation (I-3). Extra food intake should correct the condition, but often the patient has been on an inadequate diet for so long a time that food has become distasteful, and some means of stimulating the appetite must be found. If the condition is severe, it may be necessary to add foods gradually. The selection should be made carefully. Drugs will be needed to aid the patient to digest his food properly.

DRUG THERAPY. This problem is approached medicinally in two ways. The flow of the digestive juices may be increased by giving bitters before meals or by giving a drug which will increase the body's need for food. The patient then will be more willing to eat, since he feels the need of food. One of these methods is usually sufficient to develop the patient's natural desire for food.

BITTERS. *Gentian*, in various preparations, or drugs such as *iron, quinine* and *strychnine elixir* (elixir of I. Q. & S.) may be used. Most bitters are given as fluids 5.0 ml. in a small amount of water about 20 minutes before meals.

Excessive amounts of water should be avoided, as should any attempt to disguise the taste, since it is the bitterness which creates the beneficial effect. There are two reasons for avoiding extra fluid intake: first, it will decrease the bitter taste and, second, it will fill the stomach with water and the patient will not feel the need for food. The nurse will need to encourage the patient to take the medicine, which certainly does not taste "good." She should explain, briefly, that the very bitter taste is a desirable attribute.

The increase of the digestive juices stimulated by the bitter drugs will increase the patient's appetite and, as a consequence, he will want to eat more. The increased output of digestive juices also increases the amount of food prepared for absorption. Thus, more nutrient enters the system. Other factors conducive to increasing the appetite (quiet comfortable surroundings; rest before the meals; attractive, well-cooked meals and any other factors which will induce a happy emotional outlook) will help to make the drug more effective.

INSULIN. *Insulin* is often given to cause a mild hypoglycemia (lowered blood sugar). The dose is varied to suit the individual patient's needs, but is often units 4 or 5. It is given three times a day, 20 minutes before meals.

Insulin is given subcutaneously, and the nurse may need to teach a member of the patient's family how to administer the drug. The family should also be advised of the symptoms of severe hypoglycemia and what to do should this occur. In such an event the patient must be given sugar (or orange juice) at once. (Insulin and its administration are discussed in some detail in Chapter 27.)

OTHER THERAPY FOR SEVERE UNDERNUTRITION. In more severe undernutrition, amino acids may be added to the diet. These come in powder or granule form and are dissolved, usually in milk, before being given to the patient. If the condition is extremely severe, the patient may be hospitalized and total alimentation given intravenously. This has been discussed in Chapter 10.

THE NURSE. The nurse will need to explain the regimen to the patient or a member of his family and instruct him in the care of the patient and to notify the doctor if any problems arise.

She must try to instill in the patient a desire to eat more and usually to eat a better selection of foods. An estimation of the caloric intake previous to treatment, what weight would be considered adequate for the patient's age and general physique (not using his underweight as a major factor) and how many calories over this amount would be needed to increase his weight should all be spelled out to the patient. When the desired weight gain has been accomplished, a maintenance diet should be established. The nurse should stress not only caloric intake, but also types of food, so that the diet is a balanced one. She will also need to make sure the patient actually eats the foods offered. Personal preferences should be noted and followed as much as possible.

THE PATIENT. Like the obese person, the undernourished individual has often been the victim of taunts such as "Skinny" or "Slim Jim." He is often as frustrated as is the fat individual. Similarly, he may blame heredity, since many members of his family are thin. As with the obese individual, the condition is more apt to stem from improper eating habits than from a "bad gene."

DISORDERS CAUSED BY ABNORMAL QUALITATIVE FOOD INTAKE

Malnutrition

The food requirements of the body are many, and the elimination of any one essential item from the diet for a period of time will produce qualitative malnutrition. Some substances can be substituted for others, but there are certain essentials that must be secured in adequate amounts to maintain health. Though any item may be lacking, the ones most commonly in short supply are the vitamins and the minerals. Lack of essential vitamins produces specific syndromes, and a lack of vitamins in general produces an indefinite state of ill health. Need of a specific vitamin is treated by giving that vitamin, and when this is done the patient is restored to health.

Vitamins are essential substances found in natural foods. They are needed in minute quantities to maintain health. Some vitamins are not synthesized or stored by the body in large enough amounts to fulfill the daily needs and, hence, must be replenished regularly through outside sources. Vitamins are not foods in the strictest sense of the word but rather food adjuncts that are essential for the proper functioning of the body. They are substances that help to regulate the physiologic processes.

The first vitamin to be isolated was vitamin B. It was found that rice polishings contained a substance that would prevent beriberi, and this substance was called a "vital amine" or "vitamine." Later research showed that all the vitamins were not "amines," so the "e" was dropped. Vitamin C, which prevents scurvy, was known long before it was isolated and named. A British sailor is still called a "limey" because for years each sailor was required to eat a lime each day to prevent his getting scurvy. Later it was found that vitamin C, the deficiency of which produces scurvy, is a constituent of most citrus fruits, and other fruits and vegetables.

Vitamins are administered for many reasons, the more important ones being:

1. To overcome specific deficiencies
2. To maintain health
3. To restore health
4. To aid in overcoming the damaging effects of some diseases and disorders
5. As an accessory treatment of certain diseases

The consistent low intake of any vitamin will produce a specific syndrome. This syndrome can be overcome, unless irreparable damage has been done, by the intake of a sufficient amount of the needed vitamin.

Vitamins were originally given letters for names, possibly because their actual nature was not known, but it was soon found that this means of designation was inadequate. It seemed that there would not be enough letters to go around. It also became apparent that what had been thought to be one vitamin was, in fact, several different substances with quite different properties. The next step then in the naming process was to add subnumerals, so B_1, B_2, B_6, etc., made their appearance. Later with the synthesis of some of the vitamins and the analysis of others, specific names were given. This is now the main means of designation.

All vitamins may be divided into two main groups—those that are soluble in water and those that are soluble in fat (II-1). (See Current Drug Handbook.)

THE FAT SOLUBLE VITAMINS

Vitamin A—the preformed vitamins A are secured from animal sources. The precursors, carotenes (alpha, beta, gamma) and cryptoxanthin, are derived from yellow and dark green vegetables. Vitamin A is needed for proper maintenance of the epithelial cells and proper visual functioning.

Vitamin D – the precursors are ergosterol and 7-dehydrocholesterol. Vitamin D is needed for proper calcium and phosphorus metabolism.

Vitamin E – the precursors are the tocopherols (alpha, beta, gamma, delta). The beta tocopherol is the most important. Vitamin E has not been shown to be associated with any specific syndrome in the human, but it appears to be essential to health. The exact mechanism has not been established.

Vitamin K – this vitamin is known to have two divisions, vitamin K_1 and K_2. Menadione (which must be metabolized by the body before it is useful as vitamin K) and mephyton (K_1) are preparations similar to, if not exactly the same as, vitamin K. Vitamin K is required for the proper production by the liver of prothrombin and, thus, for the proper clotting of blood.

THE WATER SOLUBLE VITAMINS

Vitamin B – this vitamin has been divided and subdivided many times. All the factors have specific functions, though many of them have not been demonstrated as essential in human nutrition. The uses of the various members of the group are numerous. Included is the maintenance of a healthy condition of such organs as the nerves, skin and blood. The following is a list of the more important fractions of the B-complex:

Thiamine (B_1)
Riboflavin (B_2) (Also called vitamin G)
Pyridoxine (B_6)
Cobalamin (B_{12})
Nicotinic acid or *nicotinic acid amide* and *niacin* or *niacinamide*
Pteroylglutamic acid (folic acid)
Pantothenic acid
Choline
Para-aminobenzoic acid

Vitamin C – (*cevitamic acid, ascorbic acid*) – this vitamin is used to prevent and to treat scurvy and similar conditions.

Many of the water soluble vitamins have important functions in cell metabolism as coenzymes or essential parts of coenzymes.

GENERAL VITAMIN PREPARATIONS AND THEIR USES

There are many reasons for multiple vitamin deficiency and also for the use of multiple vitamin products. A brief discussion will suffice to acquaint the nurse with the reasons such preparations are so often included in the medications ordered for the patient.

An adequate diet will include all the essential vitamins that are known, and probably many that are not known as well. However, how can an individual be sure he is receiving an adequate diet? This is a question that is extremely difficult to answer. Most well-balanced diets do contain sufficient vitamins for the average adult, and most people do not need to worry about the vitamin content of the foods they eat. However, even if the diet appears adequate it may be deficient in vitamins, since the vitamin content of food is often changed by its production, storage and cooking.

Although a general or specific vitamin deficiency may occur in the presence of an apparently adequate diet, it is much more apt to occur because the individual simply does not eat the proper foods. A meal may contain all the essential food elements, but if a person consistently eats only a part of the foods served, he may readily become deficient in needed vitamins. People are prone to food fads. "I never eat so and so" is heard over and over again. Often the foods not eaten are the very ones that are high in vitamin content, such as fruits and vegetables.

Some age groups are more prone to vitamin deficiencies than others. The very young, because of their rapid growth, need more vitamins than do adults, yet they may not be able to eat sufficient foods to fulfill their needs. The aged person may also be unable to eat enough of the right kinds of

UNITED STATES RECOMMENDED DAILY ALLOWANCES (US-RDA)*

	UNIT	INFANTS (0–12 MO.)	CHILDREN UNDER 4 YRS.	ADULTS AND CHILDREN 4 OR MORE YRS.	PREGNANT OR LACTATING WOMEN
Vitamin A	IU	1500	2500	5000	8000
Vitamin D	IU	400	400	400	400
Vitamin E	IU	5	10	30	30
Vitamin C	mg	35	40	60	60
Folic Acid	mg	0.1	0.2	0.4	0.8
Thiamine (B_1)	mg	0.5	0.7	1.5	1.7
Riboflavin (B_2)	mg	0.6	0.8	1.7	2.0
Niacin	mg	8	9	20	20
Vitamin B_6	mg	0.4	0.7	2	2.5
Vitamin B_{12}	mcg	2	3	6	8
Biotin	mg	0.05	0.15	0.3	0.3
Pantothenic acid	mg	3	5	10	10
Calcium	g	0.6	0.8	1.0	1.3
Phosphorus	g	0.5	0.8	1.0	1.3
Iodine	mcg	45	70	150	150
Iron	mg	15	10	18	18
Magnesium	mg	70	200	400	450
Copper	mg	0.6	1.0	2.0	2.0
Zinc	mg	5	8	15	15

*From Food and Drug Administration, "New regulations on vitamins and minerals," *FDA Drug Bulletin*, (December, 1973).

foods to secure needed vitamins and other food principles. Often with older individuals there is a combination of conditions which produces vitamin deficiency. They may have definite food likes and dislikes, and it is often useless to try to reason with them (V-2). They "never have been able to eat such and such a food"—and that is that. They may lack teeth or have false teeth which makes chewing difficult, and this removes from their diet many foods that are rich in vitamins. In addition, the elderly person often has gastrointestinal difficulties. Not only will this limit his diet but it may also result in incomplete digestion of the foods taken and inhibit complete absorption. All these and many other factors may combine to make the vitamin intake of the elderly patient inadequate.

Certain pathologic or borderline pathologic conditions are apt to produce a general avitaminosis. Patients on restricted diets may not secure enough vitamins for their needs. This may be specific (lack of a single vitamin) or general (lack of several vitamins). An example of the former would be the reduction in the intake of fat-soluble vitamins in a patient on a fat free diet. A nonresidue diet may be overloaded with concentrated carbohydrates, and this may cause a lack of essential vitamins. It should be pointed out that in the hospital where special diets are under the supervision of a competent dietitian, vitamin shortages are not apt to occur because provision for the inclusion of all essential food substances is made. However, in the home where knowledge of nutrition is not so complete, the restricted diet often lacks some of the necessary foods. Another point to remember is that unless the food is eaten by the patient, its inclusion in the diet is valueless. Fevers of long duration may reduce the individual's normal food intake and be the cause of a vitamin shortage. The alcoholic and the drug addict often suffer as much from the lack of proper food essentials as from the toxic effects of the drugs. They are too busy getting enough of the drug to eat the proper foods, often to eat at all.

VITAMIN PREPARATIONS

In the preceding paragraphs an attempt has been made to show some of the factors which produce general avitaminoses. The term "general vitamins" has been used several times. It is employed here to cover any preparation which will give the patient several different vitamins at the same time. Few if any products give all the known vitamins. (How many unknown vitamins there are is a question which few would even try to answer.) This is one reason why supplementary vitamins must always remain just that—supplementary. They are additions to the adequate diet. Until our knowledge of these food adjuncts is much greater, no pill, capsule, or fluid—however well advertised—will take the place of a well-rounded diet.

The various multiple vitamin products each contain certain specific vitamins in definite amounts. The amount often is listed in relation to the known minimum daily requirements. The label on the product will state that it contains the minimum requirement, or a percentage of that amount. If the minimum daily requirement has not been established, the amount given is what the producer, through research, finds the most desirable. The number of multiple vitamin preparations on the market is legion. It would take an entire volume to discuss them all, and by the time the volume was printed it would be out of date. However, these preparations fall into a few general categories:

1. Those containing just those vitamins whose minimum daily requirements are known
2. Those containing the above plus one or two other vitamins
3. Those containing the above (1 and 2) plus other essential substances such as minerals
4. Those whose contents are the same as 1 and 2, but include certain essential amino acids in addition to or in place of the minerals or the extra vitamins
5. Those that disregard the known minimum daily requirements, listing the vitamins contained in the preparation and their amounts without regard to minimum daily requirements
6. Those that follow the form of number 5 with additional minerals, or amino acids, or both

Since, where there is a gross vitamin deficiency there may also exist a mineral and/or a protein deficiency, those products containing the minerals or proteins (amino acids) are often very valuable. The exact product to be used in a specific case and the amount must be decided by the physician.

There are several other reasons for giving various multiple vitamin products. Sometimes vitamins are given as a sort of placebo; that is, for their psychologic effect upon the patient. This is not to say that the patient is psychotic or even neurotic. Many people feel that unless they are "taking medicine" they cannot get well (V-3). The physician may order various other treatments to help, but if there is nothing to "take" the patient feels that he is being neglected and, in fact, he may even seek another doctor who will "give me something to help me get well." In cases of this kind the physician may order supplementary vitamins.

Additional vitamins are often ordered where a subclinical avitaminosis exists. This is a condition in which, though the patient does not show definite symptoms of a lack of vitamins, such a deficiency really exists. The deficiency may be of one or several vitamins but most commonly is the latter. These patients feel much improved when their vitamin requirement is replenished.

Supplementary vitamins may be given prior to surgery. This is especially true when the patient is an older person, but it is also important when the patient has been ill for a long time. The vitamin preparation is given for several days or even for some weeks preceding surgery, if the time of operation is known far enough in advance. Though a mixed vitamin product is usually used, vitamin K is almost always included because of its action in aiding blood coagulation (I-7). In the same way, a vitamin preparation is used to aid in convalescence following surgery or during convalescence from any disease.

Patients often need vitamins in excess of the minimum daily requirements. The minimum daily requirement is estimated on the amounts needed to maintain health but this is usually inadequate to restore health. It is necessary, therefore, to give supplementary vitamins to many patients during illness and during convalescence.

Not all vitamins are needed in equal amounts even when a number are to be given. Some are more important in one age group or in one condition than in another. Though the physician will decide the vitamins to be used in each individual case, the nurse should have some knowledge of the more important needs in order to be able to care for her patients intelligently. She will often be called upon to answer questions concerning the relative value of the different vitamins and to tell why one patient receives one preparation while another patient receives some other product.

The patient needing supplementary vitamins usually needs vitamins of the B group, since various fractions of the B group are not stored in the body and hence need to be given regularly. If there is a tendency to excessive bleeding, vitamins C and K will probably be ordered. For patients with an excessive susceptibility to infections, especially of the upper respiratory tract, vitamin A may be ordered. A common combination is vitamins A, D, C and several factors of the B group. This gives the patient a general feeling of well-being, reduces the likelihood of infections, aids in the maintenance of good bones and teeth and helps to prevent bleeding (interstitial or external).

Vitamins are administered in many ways but, by far, the major route is oral. They are prepared in tablets, capsules (plain or enteric-coated) and fluids. The fluid form is the form most commonly used for infants and children. There are vitamin preparations for children which can be eaten like candy. These are easily given, but the bottle must be kept away from the child lest he eat many of them with possible serious results. Tablets and capsules usually are given to the adult. Since some of the vitamins, especially the fat-soluble ones, are apt to cause belching and an aftertaste that is very disagreeable, they are best given at mealtime, and not when the stomach is empty.

Some vitamins, mainly those in the B group, are occasionally given intravenously. They come in solutions ready for intravenous administration or are added to other intravenous solutions being given to the patient.

Specific Vitamin Deficiencies

VITAMIN A

CONDITIONS PRODUCED BY DEFICIENCY. Xerophthalmia, an eye disease, keratosis, a skin condition, nyctalopia (night blindness) and hemeralopia (glare blindness) may result from vitamin A deficiency. Nyctalopia and hemeralopia occur in the early stages of deficiency. Insufficient amounts of this vitamin also tend to decrease the resistance to infections, especially of the respiratory and the genitourinary tracts.

MAJOR SYMPTOMS. Xerophthalmia, if unchecked, may continue until corneal ulceration, scarring and impairment of vision occur. If the cornea has become scarred over the pupillary area, visual acuity will be decreased in direct proportion to the amount of scarring. The skin condition keratosis is relatively common since vitamin A appears to be necessary for the proper functioning of epithelial tissue.

DRUG THERAPY. The recommended daily allowance of *vitamin A* is 3000 to 5000 international units. Dietary vitamin A is divided into the preformed vitamin A, secured directly or indirectly from animal sources such as fish and fish liver oils, liver, milk fat and egg yolk, and the precursor vitamin A, secured from vegetable sources. It is necessary for the body to convert the precursor vitamin into the form that can be used by the body, but the preformed vitamin can be used without change as it has already been formed by the animal from the original vegetable sources. The vegetable source for the human is mainly in the form of the carotenes (alpha, beta, gamma) derived from yellow and dark green vegetables. Therapeutic vitamin A is usually given as the concentrate from these oils, dosage 25,000 to 50,000 units per capsule. If it is to be given in the form of drops, the dosage is indicated on the commercial package or bottle. As much as 75,000 units may be required for short periods of time in cases of severe deficiency. A water-soluble form of vitamin A may be given parenterally in such a situation.

THE NURSE. Vitamin A is usually administered orally and is best given with or after meals. If given before meals when the stomach is empty, it may produce eructation or flatulence. If the fluid form of the drug is given it can be added to the food or, if allowable, a little salt can be added which makes the oil more palatable.

The patient should be told which foods are rich in vitamin A so that these may be added to the diet, especially after the drug has been discontinued. This will aid in the prevention of a recurrence of the disorder for which the extra vitamin intake was required. Overdosing with vitamin A can produce toxic symptoms, but these occur only when the vitamin is taken in doses greatly in excess of requirements.

The Patient. The patient with a severe vitamin A deficiency may be very emotionally disturbed by his condition. This is especially true when xerophthalmia is present. The nurse should try to reassure the patient but she must not build up false hopes. If corneal ulceration has occurred, there will be some loss of visual acuity, which only the physician can determine. The nurse may aid the patient to understand the value of the drug without being overconfident.

Keratosis usually clears completely with the use of the vitamin, and the nurse can be more reassuring in this case. Keratosis is often rather disfiguring, and the patient will welcome the assurance that this will not be permanent.

The nurse can often aid an individual to avoid serious deficiency by recognizing the early signs and advising the person to consult a physician.

VITAMIN D

CONDITIONS PRODUCED BY DEFICIENCY. If vitamin D is insufficient for the needs of a child, rickets may occur. If the vitamin is lacking in an adult, a condition known as osteomalacia may result.

MAJOR SYMPTOMS. Rickets is manifested by symptoms of improper bone and tooth development. Severe deformities may result if the condition is allowed to progress unchecked. Enlargement of the epiphyses of the long bones, bowing of the legs and protrusion (bossing) of the frontal bones are some of the deformities which often result. If tetany accompanies the deficiency of the vitamin, muscle spasms occur, producing a peculiar claw-like position of the hands and a similar position of the feet. These are called carpopedal spasms.

DRUG THERAPY. *Vitamin D* comes from many of the same sources as does the preformed vitamin A, and the two vitamins are often administered together. Vitamin D is also derived from sunshine and has been called the "sunshine" vitamin. Vitamin D_2 is activated ergosterol (calciferol, viosterol) and vitamin D_3 is activated 7-dehydrocholesterol. These are the important forms of vitamin D. Vitamin D is required for the proper metabolism of calcium and phosphorus. It aids in the maintenance of the proper level of blood calcium and in the functioning of the parathyroid glands.

Vitamin D, in the form of cod or other fish liver oil or in a concentrated preparation, is used both to prevent and to cure the deficiency. As a prophylactic, 400 international units daily is considered advisable for the infant. This same amount is recommended during pregnancy. A lesser amount is needed for the adult. The dosage in cases of actual deficiency is greatly increased and will depend upon the age and the condition of the patient. Dihydrotachysterol is often used therapeutically in vitamin D deficiency. It is similar to vitamin D_2. The drug is prepared in a solution, 1 ml. containing 1.25 mg. of the crystalline drug. It also comes in capsules containing 0.625 mg. each. The amount given will depend upon conditions but as many as 3 to 10 ml. or 6 to 20 capsules may be used. They are given orally each day with meals. It is usual to include plenty of milk in the diet or to give calcium gluconate or lactate to insure adequate amounts of calcium.

The Nurse. Vitamin D is administered in the same manner as is vitamin A. For prevention, sunshine and a well balanced diet are usually sufficient, with the possible exception of the infant and the small child. Once the patient has developed symptoms of shortage, it is necessary to supply the vitamin in medicinal form. Dietary control is usually inadequate to supply enough of the vitamin in a short enough space of time to prevent deformities.

Excessive amounts of vitamin D can cause toxic symptoms. These must be watched for and reported to the physician if they occur. Early symptoms include anorexia, nausea, vomiting, diarrhea, drowsiness and headache. Later symptoms include calcium deposits in the kidneys and nephritis. Circulatory collapse may occur because of the increased viscosity of the blood from hypercalcemia.

The Patient. Recovery from vitamin deficiencies is usually prompt, but the completeness of that recovery will depend upon the amount of damage that has occurred. No amount of vitamins will completely change severe deformities that have resulted from rickets.

It is much better to prevent this condition. The nurse can do much to aid by "spreading the word" that the small child needs to receive this vitamin in some way. Playing outdoors as much as possible helps. Milk, enriched with vitamins, is good for the small child. However, this same milk may be inadvisable for the adult since excessive amounts of vitamin D can cause toxic symptoms (noted earlier) especially after growth has been completed.

VITAMIN C

CONDITIONS PRODUCED BY DEFICIENCY. The result of the lack of vitamin C is scurvy. Scurvy was perhaps the first disease definitely to be associated with vitamin deficiency. Severe scurvy is rare in most countries now, but subclinical conditions caused by restricted diets and inability to secure sufficient foods rich in the vitamin are not uncommon.

The lack of vitamin C may produce associated conditions such as defective bones and teeth, especially in the infant or small child.

MAJOR SYMPTOMS. Scurvy is a condition in which the intercellular ground substance and collagen are deficient. There is a tendency to bleed, especially subperiosteally and from the mucous membranes of the mouth and the intestinal tract. The gums tend to ulcerate. Vitamin C is essential for the proper maintenance of capillary tonus. It is used medicinally for any bleeding in which there is increased capillary fragility. Ascorbic acid is used also in the treatment of extensive burns, multiple fractures and certain blood dyscrasias.

DRUG THERAPY. *Vitamin C,* a water-soluble vitamin also called *ascorbic acid* or *cevitamic acid,* is found in all citrus fruits, tomatoes, raw cabbage and many other foods. For both prevention and cure of deficiency, the vitamin is given in drug and food form. The recommended daily allowance is about 10 to 50 mg. for the child, 50 to 70 mg. for the adult. In cases of severe deficiency, as with any of the vitamins, the dose may be greatly increased. As much as 500 mg. may be given orally per day for children and 400 to 600 mg. for adults. Initially, the drug may be given by slow intravenous infusion.

THE NURSE. Giving foods rich in vitamin C alone is often too slow and uncertain for therapeutic purposes. The vitamin may be given either orally or parenterally as may be deemed best by the physician. The nurse should be prepared to advise the patient or his family as to the foods rich in this vitamin and to help them to decide which foods are best under any given set of circumstances, such as the condition of the patient and availability and expense of food items.

Vitamin C is given for a wide variety of conditions, and the patient receiving this drug may not have any severe condition such as scurvy. The vitamin is helpful in any disorder in which there is a tendency to bleed, either externally, internally or interstitially.

THE PATIENT. The patient who tends to bleed or bruise easily can often overcome this by adding fresh citrus fruit or fruit juices to the daily menu. Though no substantiated research has proved it to be true, many people feel that vitamin C aids in the prevention of respiratory infections. Though excessive amounts of vitamin C usually do not cause serious side effects, long continued use should be discouraged. Research has implicated this excess in the production of urinary calculi. Even though the body does not store this vitamin, the average diet includes, in most instances, a sufficient amount for the minimum requirement.

VITAMIN K

Vitamin K, like vitamin C, is used to treat conditions in which bleeding is a symptom. The lack of this vitamin has not been associated with any specific disease; however, petechial hemorrhage and ecchymosis will occur when it is in short supply. It is used in the treatment of any condition in which a delayed prothrombin time is a factor. It is especially important in disorders of the liver, since this organ elaborates many of the blood factors, including those connected with blood clotting.

Vitamin K is not only obtained from dietary sources but is also elaborated by bacterial activity in the intestines. Gastrointestinal disorders such as diarrhea and malabsorption can cause a deficiency in the face of adequate dietary intake. This is of particular importance in extended spells of diarrhea in infants and adults. It may also be of importance in patients on coumarin type anticoagulants.

Therapeutically, vitamin K is used mainly to counteract the action of the oral anticoagulant drugs. Vitamin K is valueless in the treatment of heparin-induced bleeding. It is also used in lesser dosage in the treatment of certain disorders of blood clotting.

There are several preparations of vitamin K used medicinally. These include *Phytonadione*, U.S.P. (Mephyton, Konakion; *phytomenadione*, Aqua Mephyton [C]) or *vitamin* K_1, which may be given orally, subcutaneously, intramuscularly or intravenously. When given by the latter route it is usually given with an intravenous infusion and not more than 5 mg. of the drug is given per minute. For nonemergency therapy, the dosage is 1 to 25 mg.; in emergency situations as much as 10 to 50 mg. may be given slowly.

Other preparations of vitamin K include the following. *Sodium menadiol diphosphate* (Synkayvite), a water-soluble vitamin K analogue which does not require bile salts for absorption. Its usual dose is 3 to 6 mg. daily. It can be given orally or parenterally. Doses as high as 75 mg. may be ordered in an emergency. *Sodium menadione bisulfite* (Hykinone) is also water soluble but relatively more toxic than others of this group. The nonemergency dose is 0.5 to 2.0 mg., orally. In emergencies, 50 to 100 mg. may be given by slow intravenous drip. *Vitamin* K_5 (Synkamin) is also water soluble. The usual dose is 1 to 5 mg. daily.

The Nurse. In the administration of these preparations, it is important that the prothrombin time be checked frequently as with the anticoagulant drugs. If the reports indicate any substantial change, the physician should be notified immediately. With intravenous administration, care must be exercised that the solution be given very slowly and that the amount given per minute be accurately timed and estimated. This is especially important with phytonadione, which if given too rapidly can cause various adverse symptoms such as flushing, sweating, cyanosis, a feeling of constriction in the chest and peripheral vascular collapse. If any such symptoms occur, the administration should be stopped immediately and the physician notified.

The Patient. When the vitamin K preparations are given in emergencies, the patient is usually too ill to need much except reassurance and emotional support. He should be made to feel that the drug is given to make him more comfortable and better. In nonemergencies, the nurse should explain the method and amount of the drug to be taken and the importance of constant medical supervision.

VITAMIN E

The term vitamin E refers to a group of fat-soluble substances—alpha, beta, gamma and delta tocopherol. The alpha tocopherol is the most active and also the most commonly used of these substances. No exact deficiency or use has been shown in man. But in experimental animals, disturbances such as abortion, muscular dystrophy, cardiac disorders and hemolysis have been demonstrated. It has been established as an essential nutrient in man, but the exact mechanism of action is not known. It aids in the metabolism of unsaturated fats, and the more unsaturated fats in the diet, the more this vitamin should be included. Untoward symptoms which occur only with overdosing include muscular weakness, gastrointestinal disturbances, and reproductive disorders. The dose is alpha tocopherol 30 to 400 international units daily.

VITAMIN B

Vitamin B was the first to be isolated as a distinct substance. It was observed that a diet of polished rice produced beriberi, whereas unpolished rice did not. It has since been found that vitamin B is a highly complex substance with many components. For a time each new fraction was given a subnumber, such as B_1, B_2, B_6 and so on. Still later many of these substances were isolated, synthesized and given names. In the process of separation the various parts of vitamin B were found to be essential factors in many diseases. The complete story of vitamin B probably has not yet been revealed.

The various fractions of the vitamin B are discussed separately, but it should be pointed out that clinical evidence of the lack of one factor often is accompanied by subclinical deficiency of other factors. Therefore, many physicians routinely give the entire vitamin B-complex in any case showing symptoms of the lack of one factor.

VITAMIN B_1 (THIAMINE HYDROCHLORIDE)

CONDITIONS PRODUCED BY DEFICIENCY. Deficiency of thiamine hydrochloride will produce beriberi, certain gastrointestinal phenomena, visual phenomena, polyneuritis (especially that associated with alcoholism), arrested growth in children and, when other fractions of the B-complex are deficient, pellagra.

MAJOR SYMPTOMS. The symptoms of a thiamine hydrochloride deficiency include a tendency to edema, especially of the legs, neuritis, neuralgia, visual disturbances, gastrointestinal disorders, muscular weakness and many other minor symptoms.

NONDRUG THERAPY. The diet of the average citizen of the United States contains sufficient amounts of thiamine hydrochloride so that actual deficiency is rare. However, when the diet is limited for any reason, a mild deficiency may occur. The foods rich in vitamin B_1 include yeast, liver, egg, whole grain, meat, legumes, various vegetables and rice polishings. These should be added, if possible, to the diet of a patient showing any symptoms of a lack of the vitamin.

DRUG THERAPY. The recommended daily allowance of *thiamine hydrochloride* has been estimated to be 1 to 2.5 mg. for the adult and 0.03 mg. per 100 calories of food for the child. Thiamine hydrochloride is rarely given alone but rather in conjunction with other fractions of the vitamin B-complex. Treatment dosage as high as 50 to 100 mg. may be used. In emergencies 30 to 50 mg. may be given intramuscularly.

Since this vitamin is not often entirely lacking in the average diet in this country, beriberi rarely occurs in the United States. However, some of the early symptoms may occur when the diet is limited, and the nurse should be alert to note these symptoms and to report the fact to the doctor. She should also be ready to advise the patient to add, unless contraindicated, foods rich in thiamine to his diet. Thiamine hydrochloride may be administered either orally or parenterally.

As mentioned earlier, thiamine is rarely given alone. There is some indication that it may actually be harmful if taken alone over an extended period of time. Lack of the vitamin produces, even very early, a feeling of depression and an excessive tiredness. The patient should be reassured that this is temporary and that it will soon disappear when the vitamin is supplied in sufficient quantity.

NICOTINIC ACID AND NIACINAMIDE

CONDITION PRODUCED BY DEFICIENCY. Pellagra is produced when *nicotinic acid* or *niacinamide* (a derivative of nicotinic acid) is taken in insufficient amounts. A deficiency of this vitamin may also play a part in other conditions, especially where other vitamins of the B-complex are concerned. Nicotinic acid was one of the first fractions of vitamin B to be discovered. Its relation to pellagra was demonstrated in the United States early in this century, first by experiments on animals and later on man. Pellagra had been a serious, fairly common disease in the southeastern portion of the country, since the diet there was often deficient in protein, especially of animal origin.

MAJOR SYMPTOMS. The symptoms of pellagra are an intestinal disturbance, with spells of diarrhea; a dermatitis, especially of the exposed areas of the skin; and dementia. This syndrome has been referred to as the three "D's"—diarrhea, dermatitis and dementia.

NONDRUG THERAPY. Pellagra is now a relatively rare condition, since more care is taken to see that the diet contains sufficient proteins—the main source of vitamin B. If the disease occurs in a severe form, dietary treatment is insufficient; but if treated early it can be cured by an adequate diet. The foods richest in nicotinic acid are yeast, liver, wheat germ, fish, organs and muscles of animals, egg yolk and most vegetables.

DRUG THERAPY. The recommended daily allowance of *nicotinic acid* for the adult is 10 to 20 mg. When deficiency exists the dosage may be greatly increased. As much as 50 to 100 mg. may be given either orally or intravenously two or three times a day. Like other fractions of the vitamin B-complex, it is usually given with other factors of vitamin B since it is felt that when there is a demonstrable deficiency of one fraction there is a subclinical deficiency of others. *Niacinamide* is often employed in place of nicotinic acid since it does not have as many adverse side effects as nicotinic acid. Patients with pellagra sometimes suffer with anemia, usually of the hypochromic or macrocytic type. The usual treatment for these anemias is followed, i.e., iron for hypochromic anemia and folic acid for the macrocytic form.

THE NURSE. The nurse is faced with many problems in the care of patients with pellagra, since mental and emotional deviations may exist as a result of the disease. Attempting to secure the patient's cooperation in taking the prescribed diet and medication may tax the patience and ingenuity of the nurse. The nurse must use tact and patience but, at the same time, firmness in dealing with these patients. The very life of the patient depends upon his taking the drugs and the diet as ordered.

When nicotinic acid is given, the nurse must watch for undesirable side effects such as flushing (superficial vasodilation). Sometimes the physician may desire this vasodilation, especially if the patient has an elevation of the blood pressure. The nurse should explain to the patient what he may expect and assure him that this is more beneficial than harmful. This does not occur when niacinamide is used.

THE PATIENT. The patient suffering from pellagra is often very difficult to understand. The reason for the condition is a deficient diet, but even though this is explained to him over and over again, he still does not want to eat those foods which will aid him. He may also refuse needed medications. The patient may need to change his entire eating habits, and this may be very hard to do, especially for an older patient.

There are other things to be considered, too. The diet used for pellagra is relatively expensive, and this may be one factor in the patient's apparently unreasonable attitude. It is often necessary to aid the patient to work out his finances in order to provide the foods and drugs ordered by the doctor. During the acute stage, whatever preparation is ordered by the physician must be obtained; but later, to prevent a recurrence, a cheaper product may be allowed. Brewer's yeast, for instance, contains the entire vitamin B-complex and is quite inexpensive. The nurse can also explain the possibilities of using cheaper cuts of meats in place of the more expensive ones.

The nurse must remember that an emotional disturbance is one of the major symptoms of pellagra. She will need to use every method possible to help the patient to understand his own condition and to aid him to overcome the disease.

VITAMIN B_2 (RIBOFLAVIN)

When riboflavin is in short supply, vascularization of the cornea, glossitis, cheilosis, weight loss and a general rundown condition may result. With the addition of adequate amounts of riboflavin these symptoms disappear, and the patient experiences a feeling of well-being. Often this vitamin is given to aid the general recovery of a patient who is convalescing from other diseases, since it does give the patient such an uplift.

When symptoms of riboflavin deficiency exist, symptoms of the lack of other B-complex fractions usually occur; therefore, like others of the B-complex, it is rarely given alone. The dosage varies with the condition of the patient and the purpose for which the drug is being administered. The estimated daily allowance for the adult is 1.5 mg. and 1.0 to 2.5 mg. for the child. *Methylol riboflavin* (Hyflavin) is a preparation which can be given parenterally. The dosage is 2 to 10 mg. usually given daily.

VITAMIN B_6 (PYRIDOXINE)

No specific disease has been associated with the lack of pyridoxine, but it is presumed to be a necessary dietary constituent and its use often aids in recovery from such conditions as pellagra. Infants given diets low in this vitamin develop dermatitis and epileptiform convulsions. With adults, the lack produces skin and oral lesions. Most diets contain adequate amounts of pyridoxine. It has been used to treat persistent and pernicious vomiting, irradiation sickness and various neuromuscular conditions. The dosage is regulated to suit the individual needs of the patient but is usually from 10 to 50 mg. for the adult patient. The drug may be administered either orally or parenterally. When used in treating vomiting, it is often added to the intravenous solutions which are being given to the patient at the same time. Pyridoxine in doses exceeding 5 mg. daily may reduce or negate the effect of levodopa in parkinsonism.

VITAMIN B_{12} (COBALAMIN)

Cobalamin, U.S.P. (cyanocobalamin, many trade names) is considered to be the antianemic factor of the liver and is required for the proper formation of the red blood cells. Deficiency of this factor results in macrocytic anemia. It is used to treat this condition. The drug is very potent and 1 microgram (mcg., one thousandth of a milligram) is considered to be the recommended daily allowance for adults. In conditions of deficiency it is usually given parenterally in doses of 15 to 30 mcg. twice weekly until symptoms subside and then a maintenance dose is established, often 15 mcg. every other week. There are several oral preparations of cobalamin but these are not as satisfactory as the parenteral drugs since absorption from the intestinal tract is varied and irregular. No adverse symptoms have been reported from the use of this vitamin. A more complete discussion will be found in Chapter 19 under Pernicious Anemia.

OTHER FRACTIONS OF THE B-COMPLEX

Folic acid (pteroylglutamic acid) is also used in the treatment of various macrocytic anemias. Alone it does not control the neurological symptoms of pernicious anemia. It is effective in sprue and some of the other anemias. It is also used as an antidote in over-dosing with the folic acid antagonist drugs which are used in the leukemias and similar conditions. Folic acid (Folvite) may be given orally or parenterally. Therapeutic dosage is usually 0.25 to 1.0 mg. (regardless of age) and the maintenance dose is usually 0.1 to 0.25 mg. daily. Close medical supervision is essential. Doses above those recommended may cause hematologic remission of pernicious anemia but mask the neurological manifestations, so that the disorders progress until irreparable damage is done. Folic acid is considered in more detail in Chapter 19.

Pantothenic acid (a part of coenzyme A), biotin, inositol, para-aminobenzoic acid and choline: these and others appear to be essential for the proper metabolic processes of the body, probably in relation to the cell enzyme systems. However, specific deficiencies have not been demonstrated in man. No recommended daily allowance has been established, and drug therapy is limited. Most diets include ample amounts of these fractions and the B-complex preparations contain these and other fractions.

DEFICIENCIES OF MINERALS AND OTHER ELEMENTS

Deficiency of the various minerals and elements produces a number of adverse symptoms which are treated more fully under the specific conditions they are associated with. Thus calcium and phosphorus are essential in the proper development and maintenance of bones, teeth and to a lesser degree muscle and general body cell activity; iron is most important in iron deficiency anemia, iodine in the proper functioning of the thyroid gland and so on.

In the great majority of cases there is sufficient supply of these elements in the diet and there is no need for supplementary use. However, they are used in specific conditions and will be discussed with these conditions.

Some elements are required in minute amounts called "trace elements." Included are copper, manganese, cobalt, zinc, and nickel. These too are usually secured in the average diet although occasionally the physician will include them in a vitamin-mineral preparation.

IT IS IMPORTANT TO REMEMBER

1. That the known vitamins probably are only a fraction of the "vital" compounds secured in the diet.
2. That though vitamins are essential to the proper maintenance of health, they may or may not be needed in excess of those obtained in the diet.
3. That supplemental vitamins are useful in a number of conditions, but the physician is the only person qualified to decide when they are needed, what kinds are best and how they should be administered.
4. That vitamins may be given to aid the patient psychologically as well as physically, and that one reason may be as important as the other.
5. That nutritional disorders are often difficult to recognize and treat.
6. That, if the patient has an adequate diet, drug therapy will usually not be required. However, it is necessary for the individual to eat all of the foods presented if the diet is to be adequate for him.
7. That though drugs have a very important place in the treatment of nutritional disorders, they are always secondary to the dietary regime.
8. That nutritional disorders are always relative and are rarely singular. For instance, a deficiency in one vitamin is usually accompanied by deficiencies in other vitamins, some to a greater degree than others.
9. That emotional disturbance may occur in many deficiency conditions, but it is one of the major symptoms of pellagra.

TOPICS FOR STUDY AND DISCUSSION

1. Make a list of vitamin products you see advertised. What vitamins are contained in these preparations? What claims are made by the producers? Do these claims appear justified?
2. Go to a drugstore and see how many different vitamin products are displayed. What kinds are there? Are special claims made? Do these claims seem justified?
3. What are some of the reasons (in addition to those given in the text) for the fact that an apparently adequate diet may not contain all the vitamins needed to maintain health?
4. What specific vitamins might be ordered before a patient is to have surgery done? Why do you think these would be helpful?
5. What vitamins might be added to the diet of the patient who is convalescing from a long illness? Justify your answer.
6. Discuss the psychologic reasons for which vitamins may be used. Do you feel these are justified?
7. Have you ever taken supplementary vitamins? What was the reason for this? Was it on doctor's orders? Did they help? (A census of the class on this point might be interesting.)
8. Suggest means of inducing a patient with pellagra to take needed food and drugs when he insists, "I've never taken such stuff, and I don't see why I should do it now."
9. What are the main problems in weight reduction? How can the nurse aid the patient?
10. What factors tend to induce qualitative nutritional disorders? How might these be overcome? What are the pharmaceutical implications?
11. The physician has ordered the patient to have 200 micrograms of vitamin B_{12} intramuscularly every other day for three doses, then weekly. The nurse finds a 10 ml. (cc.) vial marked 1 ml. contains 100 micrograms of the vitamin. She should give ________ minims each dose. The vial will last ________.
12. Thyroxin gr. 1/240 is ordered to be given orally twice daily to a patient on a reducing diet. The nurse finds the drug is in scored tablets 0.5 mg. each. She should give ________. What would be the best times of the day to give the thyroxin?

BIBLIOGRAPHY

Books and Pamphlets

American Medical Association Council on Drugs, *Drug Evaluations*, Chicago, 1971, American Medical Association.

Bogert, L. J., Briggs, G. M., and Calloway, D. H., *Nutrition and Physical Fitness, 9th Ed.*, Philadelphia, 1973, W. B. Saunders Co.
Canadian Pharmaceutical Association, *Compendium of Pharmaceutical Specialties, 7th Ed.*, Toronto, 1972, Canadian Pharmaceutical Association.
Conn, H. F., *Current Therapy, 1974*, Philadelphia, 1974, W. B. Saunders Co.
Cooper, L. F., et al., *Nutrition in Health and Disease, 13th Ed.*, Philadelphia, 1971, J. B. Lippincott Co.
Goodman, L. S., and Gilman, A., *Pharmacological Basis of Therapeutics, 4th Ed.*, New York, 1970, The Macmillan Co,
Howe, P. S., *Basic Nutrition in Health and Disease*, Philadelphia, 1971, W. B. Saunders Co.
Krause, M. V., and Hunscher, M. A., *Food, Nutrition and Diet Therapy, 5th Ed.*, Philadelphia, 1972, W. B. Saunders Co.
Lehner, E., and Lehner, J., *Folklore and Odysseys of Food and Medicinal Plants*, New York, 1961, Tudor Publishing Co.
Robinson, C. H., *Normal and Therapeutic Nutrition, 14th Ed.*, New York, 1972, The Macmillan Co.

Journal Articles

Mayer, J., "Obesity control," *Am. J. Nurs.* 65:6:112 (June, 1965).
Mushlin, H. R., "Drugs and food for the disaster shelter," *Am. J. Nurs.* 64:10:116 (October, 1964).
Naeye, R. L., et al., "Urban poverty: Effects on prenatal nutrition," *Science* 166:3908:1026 (November 21, 1969).
Peper, G. M., "Nutrition services in home health agencies," *J. Am. Diet. Assoc.* 50:23 (January, 1967).
Sebrell, W. H., Jr., "Clinical nutrition in the United States," *Am. J. Public Health* 58:2035 (November, 1968).
Schachter, S., "Obesity and eating," *Science* 161:3843:751 (August 23, 1968).
Schaefer, A. E., and Johnson, O. C., "Are we well fed? The search for the answer," *Nutr. Today* 4:2 (Spring, 1969).
Schaumburg, H. H., et al., "Monosodium L-glutamate: Its pharmacology and role in the Chinese restaurant syndrome," *Science* 163:3869:826 (February 21, 1969).
Wann, E., and Miesem, M. L., "Care of adolescents with anorexia nervosa," *Am. J. Nurs.* 67:11:2356 (November, 1967).
Zitnik, R., "First you take a grapefruit," *Am. J. Nurs.* 68:6:1285 (June, 1968).

CHAPTER 21

DRUGS USED FOR DISORDERS OF THE MUSCULO-SKELETAL SYSTEM

CORRELATION WITH OTHER SCIENCES

I. ANATOMY AND PHYSIOLOGY

1. The growth of bone is controlled by a secretion of hormones from the pituitary, thyroid, adrenal cortex, parathyroids and male and female sex glands.
2. Vitamins also play a large part in bone growth: vitamin A promotes endochondral growth; nicotinic acid of the vitamin B-complex stimulates and accelerates callus formation in fractures; vitamin C stimulates osteoblastic activity; and vitamin D promotes absorption of calcium from the alimentary tract.
3. The adrenocorticotropic hormone (ACTH) (corticotropin) is composed of a mixture of proteins and polypeptides which apparently carry the activating substance. This acts by stimulating the endogenous production of cortisone. The biologically active substances of the adrenal cortex are classed as corticosteroids. Both elements are essential for the metabolism of carbohydrates, protein and fat and exert a profound effect on neuromuscular metabolism.
4. Adult human bone consists of a mass of protein tissue in which is deposited a calcium-phosphate-carbonate salt.
5. Bone formation and bone resorption are going on at the same time.
6. The nervous system is made up of the brain, spinal cord, ganglia and peripheral nerves.
7. The basal portion of the brain contains various centers, collectively called the basal ganglia. These centers control many bodily functions which are largely uncontrolled by conscious effort.
8. The point at which the nerve fibrils reach the muscle cell is called the myoneural junction. At this point the impulse may be blocked or intensified by action of enzymes or drugs.

II. CHEMISTRY

1. The inorganic matter of bone consists chiefly of calcium, phosphate and carbonates.
2. Purines are simple organic nitrogenous bases derived from the breakdown of nucleoproteins.
3. Uric acid is an end product of purine metabolism and has a renal threshold largely dependent on the blood level of the substance.
4. Calcium and phosphorus are constantly being released from bone in a normal ratio but this release is accelerated by an increase in the acidity of body fluids and probably to a slight extent by the direct action of the parathyroid hormone. This release is retarded by an increase in the alkalinity of body fluids.

III. MICROBIOLOGY

1. The pyogenic organisms—*Staphylococcus aureus, Streptococcus viridans* and *Streptococcus pyogenes*—are the main causes of muscle, bone and joint infections.

IV. PHYSICS

1. The nerve impulse is a combination of physical-chemical-electrical change.

V. PSYCHOLOGY

1. Patients with muscle and joint diseases must understand that these are generally long, protracted conditions.
2. Patience, though often difficult to develop, is an absolute essential for the patient with rheumatoid arthritis.
3. Emotional factors play an important role in rheumatoid arthritis.
4. Chronic illness or long enforced idleness produces adverse emotional reactions.

VI. SOCIOLOGY

1. Many of the patients who have muscle or joint disorders will need rehabilitation.
2. The chronic arthritic patient will require long-continued therapy. The drugs used may be expensive and this, combined with the cost of medical attention, is often a heavy burden to the patient and his family. All means possible should be investigated to continue treatment.
3. Fear of being unable to compete with the average person produces an unfavorable reaction in the individual, especially if he is the breadwinner of the family.

INTRODUCTION

There are many conditions which restrict the normal muscular activity. Some of these are due to neurological disturbances such as parkinsonism and myasthenia gravis, some to infections such as osteomyelitis, and some to injuries. With many conditions the real cause is not known, as with most forms of arthritis. Not many of these disorders respond to medical therapy. However, drugs, in the majority of cases, do aid the patient by lessening adverse symptoms.

Most arthritic conditions are chronic, long-term illnesses that are crippling to a greater or lesser degree. Even the traumatic injuries of the bones, joints and muscles tend to be longer in healing than are the soft tissues such as the skin. These and many other factors make the patient with a musculo-skeletal disorder very discouraged and often difficult to care for. The nurse needs a great deal of patience and understanding in dealing with him.

BONE AND JOINT DISEASES

Acute Osteomyelitis

DEFINITION. Acute osteomyelitis is an infection of the bone, most frequently caused by the hemolytic *Staphylococcus aureus* and the hemolytic *Streptococcus* (III-1). The organism is usually transmitted to the bone by the blood stream from some focus of acute infection elsewhere in the body. The resulting inflammatory reaction causes necrosis of the bone.

MAJOR SYMPTOMS. The disease is often sudden in onset with fever, chills and, commonly, nausea and vomiting. There is usually pain and tenderness over the involved bone, with surrounding muscle spasm. As it progresses, redness and swelling occur at the site of the infection, and the patient runs a very high temperature and is critically ill.

DRUG THERAPY. The use of antibiotics has greatly improved the outlook for the patient with acute osteomyelitis. *Penicillin* is the antibiotic of choice and should be given at the earliest possible moment. The dosage, 1,000,000 or more units intramuscularly every three to four hours, will vary with the severity of the disease. If severe, some physicians prefer to administer the penicillin by continuous intravenous infusion with the total dosage remaining the same. Sometimes penicillin is injected directly into the site of inflammation after it has been aspirated.

Every effort is usually made to isolate the causative organism and to administer the antibiotic to which it is most susceptible. The appropriate antibiotic therapy should be continued for several weeks or until the temperature of the patient has been normal and the local lesion quiescent for a week or more.

During an acute septicemia, small repeated *blood* transfusions may be useful. Intravenous infusions of 5 per cent *glucose* or isotonic *sodium chloride* are often used to help to maintain a high fluid intake. The composition of the fluid will vary with the electrolyte content of the patient's blood serum.

Chronic Osteomyelitis

Chronic osteomyelitis often follows an acute attack. It is characterized by remissions and relapses. During remission the patient is usually asymptomatic and medicinal treatment is not used; during relapse, the patient is treated as during the original acute phase. This condition may be treated surgically. It is very discouraging to the patient (V-4, VI-3).

Osteomalacia

DEFINITION. Osteomalacia is a condition marked by a decrease in calcified bone tissue because of inadequate bone formation (I-1, 2, 4, 5, II-1) resulting from insufficient saturation of body fluids with calcium and phosphorus (II-4). The disease is sometimes referred to as adult rickets and results from one of three causes: (1) decreased intestinal absorption of calcium; (2) increased urinary excretion of calcium; or (3) abnormally rapid deposition of calcium and phosphorus in the skeleton (usually after the surgical removal of a parathyroid adenoma).

MAJOR SYMPTOMS. These patients complain of anorexia, loss of weight, muscular weakness and pain in the bones. The pain is aching in character and the bones are tender to pressure. Because of the softness of the bones, the long, weight-bearing bones have a tendency to bend, causing deformity. Tetany is almost always present. Frequently, urinary complications in the form of calculi result because of the excretion of large amounts of calcium.

DRUG THERAPY. The therapy is directed at the cause. In those patients in whom there is insufficient absorption of calcium, it is recommended that the calcium intake be greatly increased. In addition to one to three glasses of milk a day, *calcium* as the *lactate* or *gluconate* by mouth in doses of from 5 to 30 Gm. a day with *vitamin D*, 50,000 units daily, are given. If the condition is the result of vitamin D resistance, this dose of vitamin D may be as high as 1,000,000 units a day. Following the removal of a parathyroid adenoma, the calcium may be given intravenously, 10 to 30 ml. of 10 per cent calcium gluconate.

Osteoporosis

DEFINITION. Osteoporosis is a condition in which there is a deficiency of bone matrix formation. This results from deficient osteoblastic activity or from a lack of or inability to retain the essential nitrogenous components of which matrix is composed. The most common form is postmenopausal.

MAJOR SYMPTOMS. The skin of these patients is thin; they complain of weakness, anorexia and pain in the bones, particularly the back. There are frequent fractures, particularly of the spine and pelvis, and these result in deformity.

DRUG THERAPY. The treatment is directed toward the cause. If it is due to an estrogen lack, replacement therapy with *diethylstilbestrol* or another estrogenic compound, 1 to 3 mg. daily by mouth, produces symptomatic relief. This may be discontinued for five to seven days each month. When there is an androgen lack, testosterone therapy (usually with *methyltestosterone*) 10 mg. a day by linguet is used (IV-1).

If the diagnosis is "senile" osteoporosis, a combination of *estrogens* and *androgens* is the therapy of choice. In women, it is recommended that the dose of *testosterone* be reduced after the first 40 days to avoid masculinization.

The Nurse. The nurse will need to be cognizant of some of the etiologies of the disease processes, such as immobilization, infection or decreased plasma levels of calcium. If pathology is related to infection, the nurse must quickly encourage nose, throat, blood and drainage cultures and sensitivities to drugs to determine the antimicrobial therapy of choice. If surgical intervention is eventually required, the nurse and her staff will be responsible for preventing the spread of the infection by giving special attention to contaminated wound packing and drainage. Any new signs and symptoms of fever, pain, bone tenderness or general malaise may alert the nurse to further complications.

All patients suffering with bone diseases need sufficient amounts of rest and adequate limb support to prevent possible contractures. Although rest is vitally important, too much bed rest—which can occur because the patient fears the pain of moving—can be extremely detrimental. The nurse will need to encourage movement and mobility as much as possible and to be able to cope with negative responses from the patients. If mobility is not achieved, the patient may actually suffer from decubitus ulcers, respiratory complications and further depletion of bone calcium resulting in decreased bone strength. Passive exercises may help a patient to later move on his own initiative. Such exercises should be slow and gentle. The physical therapist may be responsible for this.

Through efforts to increase patient mobility, the nurse will be required to teach proper wearing of braces (skin care, padding) and crutch-walking techniques. A walker may also be used within the home if crutches seem too cumbersome. Regardless of the type of ambulation assistance used, the nurse will need to help the patient develop specific muscle groups to command the power to move the body efficiently. The nurse can facilitate the work of the physical therapist by providing continuity of the rehabilitation and retraining process. Encouragement by all the health care workers allows for reinforcement of small accomplishments as quickly as they occur.

In addition to these measures, the nurse may need to assist the patient in adjusting to some dietary modifications. This can include high caloric intake to offset the high energy expenditure of the increased work required for mobility and increased protein to combat tissue destruction and to aid in its regeneration. Avoidance of additional weight gain will also become a necessity if decreased body mass is essential to facilitate movement.

The Patient. The patient will find the limitation of movement very distressing. If possible, a public health nurse should be secured to supervise home care after the patient leaves the hospital. The nurse can critically evaluate the home and the work environments to determine hazards and to teach the patient how he can avoid them. This may require the addition of handrails in bathrooms, removal of throw rugs and the putting away of unnecessary stumbling hazards such as magazine racks and hassocks. Waxing the linoleum in the home may need to be discontinued.

If infection was the instituting factor in the bone disease, any presence of boils or acne in the teenager must be carefully reported and closely observed to determine if it might represent a focus of infection.

Levels and amounts of mobility will also need to be carefully watched. Contractures can develop very quickly and the patient should be instructed that the best and sometimes the only treatment is prevention.

Gout and Gouty Arthritis

DEFINITION. Gout is an undefined error of metabolism shown by hyperuricemia, recurrent attacks of arthritis and most often by eventual tophaceous deposits of urates in joints and an increased level of serum uric acid (II-3). It is more frequent in middle life and occurs in males more often than in females and in patients on diets rich in proteins more often than in those on less protein-rich diets.

MAJOR SYMPTOMS. Gout often appears abruptly as a fulminating arthritis of a peripheral joint, most often involving the feet. Characteristically, the metatarsophalangeal joint of the great toe is affected but it may be the ankle, instep or heel. Usually the initial attack is monarticular. The affected joint exhibits all the local manifestations of acute inflammation: swelling, redness, heat and exquisite tenderness. The blood picture shows an elevated serum uric acid, white blood count and erythrocyte sedimentation rate. The disease is subject to remissions followed by exacerbations and, as the frequency of the attacks increases, there is a characteristic deformity (V-1). There is always some renal impairment. Gout cannot be cured but it can be minimized in most cases with medicines.

DRUG THERAPY. Drug therapy is especially helpful in gout. Medicines are used during an acute attack and to prevent or minimize subsequent attacks. Sometimes the same drugs are used, the dosage and times being different. During an acute attack, in addition to administering various medicines, it is usual to immobilize the affected joint. The application of cold is more beneficial than heat. Early ambulation is encouraged as soon as the acute attack has subsided.

The physician may aspirate the affected joint. This is of value in making a differential diagnosis. He may then instill one of the corticosteroids. This will provide a swift anti-inflammatory effect. *Hydrocortisone acetate* or a similar preparation may be used. For a large joint such as the knee 20 to 40 mg. is usually sufficient; 10 to 20 mg. for the elbow or shoulder and lesser amounts for the smaller joints.

Analgesics are used as required but, since this is a chronic condition, narcotics are avoided.

COLCHICINE

THE DRUG. Colchicine is an alkaloid derived from the plant *Colchicum autumnale* (meadow saffron), which has been used for the treatment of joint pain for centuries. The alkaloid was isolated in 1820.

Physical and Chemical Properties. Colchicine, a pale yellow powder which is soluble in water and body fluids, is an alkaloid with a rather complex chemical structure.

Action. The exact action of colchicine in the body is not known, but it is believed to decrease the reaction of the joint to excessive uric acid in the body fluids. It is not uricosuric, and it reduces cell division. Colchicine is analgesic only in gout. Even in gout it may be the reduction of the inflammation which causes the apparent analgesic effect.

Therapeutic Uses. At present, the only use of colchicine is in the treatment of gout and gouty arthritis.

Absorption and Excretion. Colchicine, given orally, enters the bloodstream from the intestinal tract; it then goes to the liver. A considerable amount of colchicine is returned to the intestines by the bile. Some is reabsorbed. When the drug is given intravenously, most passes rapidly from the bloodstream into the tissue spaces, and is found in the liver, kidneys, spleen and the intestinal tract. There is little or none found in the heart, skeletal muscles or brain. Some of the drug is degraded by the liver. Colchicine is excreted as free colchicine and various metabolites via the urine and the feces.

Preparations and Dosages. All doses and times of administration of colchicine are individually adjusted. To prevent recurrent attacks of gout, colchicine may be given 0.5 mg. orally one to four times a day.

Colchicine, U.S.P., B.P. (Colchineos [C]) 0.5 mg., orally or intravenously.

THE NURSE

Mode of Administration. Colchicine, in an acute attack, may be given orally 0.5 mg. every one to two hours until there is some relief or until toxic symptoms appear. The early toxic symptoms are related to the gastrointestinal tract. It is not advised to give more than 15 mg. over a 72-hour period.

If the drug is given intravenously, 2 mg. in 20 ml. of isotonic saline solution is infused slowly (over at least five minutes), followed by 1 mg. every eight to 12 hours, not to exceed 4 mg. in 24 hours. Great care must be exerted to avoid infiltration as the drug is very irritating to the tissues.

Side Effects. Side effects from colchicine are mainly related to the gastrointestinal tract—nausea, vomiting, diarrhea. In order to continue the therapy to prevent the development of a severe attack of gout, paregoric may be ordered to control the diarrhea. It often takes some time to establish the maximum dose the patient can take without the appearance of side effects. Intravenous use of the drug rarely produces undesirable side effects.

Tolerance to colchicine apparently does not occur. Some physicians may prefer to increase the fluid intake to 3000 to 4000 ml. per day for prevention of urate precipitation in the kidneys. These precautions will necessitate careful recording of daily intake and output.

Toxicity. Severe toxic symptoms include intestinal bleeding, scanty or bloody urine or both and weak pulse. Therefore, the nurse must be constantly alert to evidence of hidden bleeding through the stools or urine. Death occurs from cardiorespiratory failure. Prolonged use may cause agranulocytosis, neuritis or anemia. Treatment is symptomatic after withdrawal of the drug.

Patient Teaching. Patient teaching includes not only the usage (times, doses, etc.) of the drug, but its possible toxic effects. The patient must know all the side effects of the drug, to stop the drug immediately if any appear and to consult his physician before resuming the use of the drug.

In some instances, the nurse may be responsible for dietary instructions. In order to decrease dietary purines (which break down to uric acid in the body), the following foods should be eliminated or avoided: liver, heart, shellfish, sardines and meat extracts (II-2). Other modifications of the diet might include abstaining from alcohol, reduction in total calories (if overweight), decrease in protein and fat intake and increasing foods higher in alkaline ash (most fruits and vegetables except corn, lentils, plums and prunes).

Any patient on long-term therapy with colchicine should have frequent physical examinations including complete blood count, hemoglobin and serum uric acid determination, urinalysis and occult blood and pH determination, since there is marked acidity in gout.

The Patient. The patient who suffers repeated attacks of gout should carry colchicine with him at all times (in a labeled container) so that at the earliest warning of the onset of an attack, he may take the medicine. In this way, he may partially abort an acute attack. Many patients are advised by their physician regarding dosage. Patients should be instructed as to the early signs of toxicity, how to test their own urine pH and told to stop the drug when adverse symptoms occur. Some patients are able to regulate themselves fairly well (V-1).

OTHER DRUGS WHICH MAY BE USED. **Phenylbutazone (Butazolidin).** This chemical compound is a pyrazolone derivative related to aminopyrine and possessing potent anti-inflammatory action. The best use of phenylbutazone, U.S.P., B.P. (Butazolidin; Butaphen [C]) is in those with acute gout who fail to respond to colchicine. The untoward and toxic effects are very frequent and often severe and the use of this drug requires that the patient be under constant medical supervision. When it is used, an initial oral dose of 400 mg. is followed by doses of 100 mg. every four hours until articular inflammation subsides. At this dosage schedule, it should not be given longer than four days before the dose is reduced.

Oxyphenbutazone, N.F. (Tandearil), (Iridil, Tanderil [C]), a derivative of phenylbutazone, has the same antipyretic and analgesic properties of the parent drug. It also shares the same dosage and the same precautions, as well as all the properties of phenylbutazone except that it produces slightly less gastrointestinal distress. Usual dose is 100 mg. three times a day (300 to 600 mg. per day).

Frequently phenylbutazone causes nausea, epigastric pain, stomatitis and gastrointestinal bleeding, especially in patients with a history of peptic ulcer. It is contraindicated when edema is present and in those with hypertension or cardiac decompensation because it tends to cause retention of salt and water. Phenylbutazone may also cause leukopenia, agranulocytosis, thrombocytopenia, anemia and various other blood dyscrasias. The drug should be immediately discontinued and the doctor notified if any of the following symptoms occurs, sore throat, stomatitis or glossitis, fever, marked weight gain, or if the stools become black and tarry.

Because of the possibility of causing gastric irritation, this drug should be administered in conjunction with meals or with milk.

Those receiving phenylbutazone or oxyphenbutazone must be under close medical supervision. This should include frequent blood examinations (red blood and white blood count determinations) and a restriction of dietary electrolytes if indicated. The patient should be instructed in the proper time and method of administration and that he is to stop the drug and notify the physician at the first unusual sign.

Either of these drugs may be given in conjunction with a non-sodium antacid and/or an antispasmodic. This allows for lower dosage.

Phenylbutazone enhances the action of the oral anticoagulants and the sulfonamide compounds. Reduction in the dose of these medications is usually indicated when phenylbutazone or oxyphenbutazone is given at the same time.

INDOMETHACIN. Indomethacin, N.F. (Indocin) (Amuno, Indomed [C]) may be used in place of or with either colchicine or phenylbutazone. Usual starting dose is about 150 mg. This is followed by 50 to 75 mg. every four hours. It markedly diminishes symptoms within 24 hours. Once a satisfactory response has been achieved, daily dosage may be decreased until the maintenance dose is established or the episode is arrested.

Side effects of indomethacin include gastric irritation, headache, vague sensations of drunkenness or unreality. More severe reactions may occur, especially with long term use. This drug is contraindicated for children and for patients with gastric ulcer or ulcerative colitis. Renal tests should be done regularly with prolonged use.

Indomethacin increases the action of the oral anticoagulant drugs. Dosage is usually adjusted to prevent bleeding when they are given at the same time.

CORTICOTROPIN OR CORTICOSTEROIDS. Most physicians use these only as a last resort. Corticotropin has appeared to be more effective than the corticosteroids. The gel is given intramuscularly 40 to 80 units every six to 12 hours for one to three days. Rebound acute inflammation may result when the drug is stopped. However, one of the corticosteroids, as mentioned earlier, may be injected intra-articularly with good results in many cases.

DRUGS USED TO PREVENT ATTACKS OF GOUT. PROBENECID. Probenecid, U.S.P., B.P. (Benemid) (Uricosid [C]) is chemically related to benzoic acid and the sulfonamides. It is known to promote the elimination of urates by depressing their renal tubular resorption. This increases the urinary excretion of the urates and reduces the serum level of uric acid. Probenecid is of no value for acute attacks and should be given only after the acute attack has subsided. During the first few weeks of administration of this drug, an acute flare-up of joint pain may occur. Should this happen, colchicine should be given without discontinuing probenecid.

Absorbed rapidly into the blood stream after oral administration, in chronic gout probenecid in doses of 250 to 500 mg. daily for one week is recommended. The blood uric acid level is then determined and the dose increased if blood level has not been reduced to normal. Usually an adequate maintenance dose is 1.0 Gm. daily in two divided doses. Gradual increases may be made as determined by uric acid plasma levels. The maximum dose is 3 Gm. daily in two divided doses. When this drug is given, it is extremely important to maintain an alkaline (to litmus) urine. This is necessary because it is possible that the drug favors the formation of uric acid stones when the urine is acid. The alkalinization of the urine may be done effectively by the daily administration of sodium bicarbonate, 3.0 to 7.5 Gm. (gr. 45 to 120), or with the use of potassium citrate, 1.0 Gm. The patient's acid-base balance should be checked regularly to avoid systemic alkalosis. Serious side effects are rare.

Probenecid interacts with several other drugs. It delays the excretion of penicillin, para-aminohippuric acid, the sulfonamide compounds and possibly of other drugs. This increases their blood level and lengthens their effective action. Probenecid inhibits the therapeutic action of the thiazide diuretics and ethacrynic acid.

Salicylates should not be administered when probenecid is used as these two drugs are antagonistic in therapeutic action.

It will become the duty of the nurse to test the urine of the patient routinely with indicator paper to determine its alkalinity. Should the urine be acid, it should be reported to the physician immediately.

Although side effects are not too frequent, nausea may appear and if it does, the physician should be notified. He will probably then reduce the daily dosage. Very rarely skin rashes, gastrointestinal disturbances or headache may occur, and if they do, the drug should be stopped and the physician notified. The nurse should advise the patient of the possible side effects and instruct him to notify his physician if they occur when he is not in the hospital.

When the patient takes probenecid, he should be instructed in how to test his urine at home for alkalinity and the reasons for this testing. The patient must understand that the drug should be taken regularly, not intermittently, if it is to help to prevent attacks. The patient should be advised not to take aspirin, any compound containing it or any salicylate without the express order from his physician.

SULFINPYRAZONE (ANTURANE). Chemically related to phenylbutazone, sulfinpyrazone (sulphinpyrazone, Anturan [C]) is a potent uricosuric agent found useful in chronic gout. Its best use is in the prevention rather than in the treatment of attacks of acute gouty arthritis. It may be used in patients who are refractory to other uricosuric agents.

This drug, like probenecid, produces its uricosuric effect by preventing tubular reabsorption of uric acid without altering the rate of glomerular filtration. Suppression of new tophi, a reduction of the size of old tophaceous deposits and alleviation of joint pain and stiffness are usually attained only after several weeks or months of treatment. Most patients require concomitant administration of colchicine or other drugs for adequate symptomatic relief because sulfinpyrazone has weak analgesic and anti-inflammatory actions.

The marked increase in urate excretion induced by the drug may provoke urolithiasis and renal colic. All urinary tract infections should be cleared up before the drug is given. Sufficient fluid intake and the maintenance of an alkaline urine are indicated.

The initial dose is often 50 to 100 mg. four times a day orally. This is gradually increased over a period of a week until a total daily dosage of 400 to 600 mg. in divided doses is reached. When a satisfactory reduction of serum urates is attained, the dose is adjusted for adequate maintenance. Thereafter the medication is continued without interruption even if an acute exacerbation of gouty arthritis occurs, when colchicine or phenylbutazone may be added.

Sulfinpyrazone and probenecid may be given together to achieve more effective uricosuric action in refractory cases. The severity and frequency of attacks is reduced by the long-term administration of sulfinpyrazone, probably because of its ability to promote renal excretion of uric acid.

The nurse should see that a high fluid intake (3 liters) is maintained and should record the intake and output daily. She will probably be required to test the urine routinely for alkalinity. In order to minimize the possibility of gastric distress (a common side effect), this medication should be given either with meals or with milk. It is important that the nurse observe and record accurately the patient's response to the drug and its periodic increases so that the proper maintenance dose can be determined.

Many pyrazolone derivatives, of which this is one, are known to depress hematopoietic function. For this reason, patients who receive sulfinpyrazone should have blood cell counts done at regular intervals. Because of its action, this drug should not be given to patients with active or latent gastric ulcers.

Those receiving this drug must keep their fluid intake high. They must also know that blood cell counts must be done at regular intervals and why. In addition, they should understand that there may be acute exacerbations early in the administration of the drug but that with time these usually subside.

ALLOPURINOL. Allopurinol, U.S.P. (Zyloprim) is an analogue of hypoxanthine and a potent competitive inhibitor of xanthine oxidase. Xanthine oxidase is the enzyme that oxidizes hypoxanthine to xanthine and xanthine to uric acid. It therefore reduces uric acid formation. Allopurinol also acts on purine catabolism without disrupting the biosynthesis of the purines. See Current Drug Handbook for further details.

Allopurinol is usually started with 300 to 600 mg. orally, daily in divided doses. More than 800 mg. in any 24-hour period is not recommended. The drug should be given with meals or food. For best results the urine should be alkaline.

Side effects include skin rashes, gastrointestinal disorders and, very occasionally, chills, fever and/or blood dyscrasias. Safety for use during pregnancy or lactation has not been established.

Allopurinol enhances the action of several drugs. By inhibiting their metabolism, it enhances the action of azathioprine. Allopurinol and probenecid enhance each other, increasing the excretion of uric acid. The action of the xanthine diuretics is inhibited by allopurinol.

MISCELLANEOUS ANALGESICS. Because of the severe pain associated with gout, analgesics are indeed helpful adjuncts. *Aspirin* (acetylsalicylic acid) orally, 2 to 5 Gm. a day in divided doses, or sodium salicylate 0.3 to 1.0 Gm. is often satisfactory and, in addition to producing a mild analgesia, helps promote the excretion of uric acid. As mentioned before, salicylates cannot be given when probenecid is given as the two drugs are antagonistic. If the pain is very severe, *codeine* in 30 to 60 mg. doses or *propoxyphene hydrochloride* (Darvon; Doloxene [C]) 65 to 130 mg. by mouth may be used. Narcotics are usually avoided because the condition is chronic, and addiction can be a real problem.

Rheumatoid Arthritis

DEFINITION. Also known as atrophic or chronic proliferative arthritis, this is a systemic disease with inflammatory changes in the articular and periarticular structures. The causes are not clearly understood. It is a chronic disease with spontaneous remissions and exacerbations and is often classed as a collagen disease. It occurs chiefly in young adults, in women more than men, and is more common in the white race.

MAJOR SYMPTOMS. Characteristically, the disease has a gradual onset, often with vague aches and pains in various muscles and joints. The patient is aware of stiffness in a joint at the end of the day and is subject to easy fatigability. This frequently goes on for some time before joint swelling, tenderness and pain on motion are noted. Although the skin over the joint is warm, it is seldom reddened. Gradually this leads to deformity of the part, the hands and feet being the usual place of affliction (V-1, 2, 3; VI-1, 2). Eventually rheumatoid arthritis tends to involve several joints.

DRUG THERAPY. Treatment must of necessity be directed to the patient as a whole, for this is a systemic condition. There is no specific cure, but some drugs are helpful (VI-2).

ANALGESICS. These drugs have been discussed in detail in Chapter 9. See also Current Drug Handbook. To relieve pain and discomfort, the best drugs found yet are the salicylates. Sodium salicylate may be used but it is more common to use *aspirin* (acetylsalicylic acid) in doses of 0.6 Gm. three to four times a day to as high as 0.9 to 1.2 Gm. every four hours while awake. Patients suffer less gastric irritation if the aspirin is given with an antacid. Enteric-coated tablets are fairly satisfactory but the gastrointestinal absorption is incomplete. There are many combinations of medicines containing aspirin and one of them may be more effective than aspirin or sodium salicylate alone. However, many contain such drugs as phenacetin or aminopyrine which have been known to cause blood dyscrasias. If these drugs are used for long periods of time, frequent blood tests should be done. Only occasionally should a stronger analgesic be needed. Opiates should be avoided because of the chronicity of the disease and the danger of addiction. If it becomes necessary to use a stronger analgesic, *propoxyphene* (Darvon) is preferred over codeine as it is less apt to cause dependency and it does not have as many side effects.

Phenylbutazone (Butazolidin, Butaphen [C]) is sometimes used but its effects are not superior to the salicylates and it has a higher incidence of toxic reactions. Recurrence of symptoms occurs when the drug is stopped. If used, it may be given orally in doses of 100 mg. two to four times a day. This drug is discussed in more detail under Gout and Gouty Arthritis.

GOLD SALTS

THE DRUGS. Gold salts were first used in the treatment of syphilis and tuberculosis, but the results were disappointing. Subsequently they were employed in the treatment of rheumatoid arthritis and lupus erythematosus with considerable success. Their use is still considered empirical and not curative, and in recent years has decreased as newer, less toxic, drugs have become available.

Physical and Chemical Properties. The therapeutically effective gold salts are all aureus salts attached to sulfur. The gold is bound to sulfhydryl sulfur. The thio compounds are more stable with less tendency to decompose to elemental gold. The compounds used in medicine all contain hydrophilic groups in addition to the thioaure group.

Action. The exact action of the gold salts in rheumatoid arthritis is not known. It has been demonstrated that such salts have antibacterial action in certain laboratory animals, but their effect in man has not been shown.

Therapeutic Uses. The gold salts are used almost exclusively in the treatment of rheumatoid arthritis and lupus erythematosus.

Absorption and Excretion. Water soluble salts of gold are rapidly absorbed from intramuscular sites. Their absorption from the gastrointestinal tract is erratic and incomplete. These salts are largely bound to plasma proteins. Their distribution is irregular. The highest concentration is in the kidneys with lesser amounts in the liver and spleen. Pathological joints contain more of the compound than non-affected ones. The gold salts are very slowly excreted by the kidneys. Excretion may not keep up with the intake and hence there may be a gradual build-up of the drug in the body. This may result in cumulative poisoning.

Preparations and Dosages. All gold salts are given intramuscularly. The usual dose is 25 to 50 mg. weekly. The initial dose may be as small as 10 mg. This is given to test sensitivity and possible effects of the drug. After the drug regimen has been established, it is continued until 1.0 Gm. has been given. Then the drug is given only every two to four weeks.

Aurothioglucose, U.S.P. (Gold thioglucose, Solganal)

Gold sodium thiomalate, sodium aurothiomalate, B.P. (Myochrysine)

THE NURSE

Mode of Administration. As stated above, all these drugs are given intramuscularly. The injection area should be selected on a rotation system so as to avoid local irritation.

Side Effects and Toxicity. All the gold salts are potentially toxic. The most common, undesirable side effects are: urticaria, dermatoses, transient albuminuria, gastrointestinal disturbances and more serious agranulocytosis. Because of this last, frequent blood counts should be done during therapy. If acutely severe toxic symptoms occur, dimercaprol (BAL) is usually given. Though this drug is less effective in gold poisoning than in arsenic poisoning, it does aid in chelating and eliminating gold. Gold salts may also prove toxic to the kidneys; hence, regular urinalysis should be done.

THE PATIENT. Since these drugs are given intramuscularly, the patient, in most cases, must go to the physician's office on a regular weekly schedule for four to six months. This gives the doctor a chance to see the patient and determine his condition.

In the early stages of therapy the patient is usually hospitalized. When he goes home, he should understand the possible dangers of the drug and the necessity of immediately reporting to his doctor any untoward symptoms, however insignificant they may seem.

Many patients cannot tolerate these drugs, but for others they are extremely helpful.

ADRENAL CORTICOSTEROID THERAPY. The enthusiasm with which this group of drugs was greeted in 1949 has now faded to careful utilization. They did not fulfill their promise of being a "cure without toxicity." They are now used only with great discretion and in selected cases. The corticosteroids are discussed in more detail in Chapter 27. (See also Current Drug Handbook for further information.) Only their use in rheumatoid arthritis will be considered here.

These drugs do relieve the symptoms of arthritis, but they do not retard or cure the disease. Used intra-articularly, they may delay the disease process. This seems to be their most important use.

When these drugs are used for arthritis, they are started with a very low dosage which is gradually increased until optimum effect is obtained. The initial response shows a decrease in subjective stiffness, diminution in articular tenderness and a decrease of pain on motion, followed by a reduction in joint swelling. All this makes the patient feel better and there is usually an increase in appetite. This initial response is not always maintained even though the drug is continued. Many patients, particularly those with active disease, show exacerbations after a period of a month or two, though not so severe as before. Discontinuance of the therapy very frequently leads to a prompt return of the signs and symptoms (I-3, 4).

Not only is this a serious physical mishap, but it is extremely depressing to the patient. The corticosteroids tend to give a feeling of euphoria, and sudden stoppage can cause the reverse—depression. The preparations most commonly used are listed below with their comparative dose values:

Cortisone acetate	25 mg.
Hydrocortisone	20 mg.
Prednisone	5 mg.
Methylprednisolone	4 mg.
Triamcinolone	4 mg.
Paramethasone	2 mg.
Dexamethasone	0.75 mg.
Betamethasone	0.6 mg.

The best results are obtained when the corticosteroid is given in very small doses with a salicylate. The dose for older persons should be less than that for the younger individual.

The Nurse. These drugs have untoward and toxic effects which may, in some cases, be cause for discontinuance of the medication. They are capable of upsetting the normal physiologic processes of the body with sometimes serious results. Cortisone and hydrocortisone, as noted previously, promote sodium retention with resulting edema (water-logging) and potassium loss and for these reasons are not used very often in rheumatoid arthritis at this time. Prednisone, prednisolone and dexamethasone have these properties to a somewhat lesser degree than the parent drug, but sodium may still be withheld from patients receiving them. Triamcinolone is relatively free of these properties and salt need not be restricted.

It is important for the nurse to remember when she is preparing any of these preparations for parenteral injection that sodium chloride is not used as the diluent. Intramuscular injections of cortisone should be given deep into the gluteus muscle (never into the deltoid). Complications from extended use may occur and include sterile abscesses, subcutaneous atrophy or change in the pigmentation over the injection area.

Potassium loss is seldom serious unless the dietary intake is below normal. The nurse should watch the patient's food intake to insure that it is adequate. Fruit juices are especially valuable for natural potassium replacement. Sometimes the physician may order additional dietary requirements such as salt restriction, high protein intake and supplementary oral potassium. It is recommended that oral medications be given with a snack or at mealtime to avoid gastric irritation. If this does occur, an antacid or an anticholinergic may be given concurrently.

The observations of the nurse must include detailed information about the effects of the drugs (relief of pain, deformity and so forth), for through this the doctor may be in a better position to judge the effectiveness of medication. Routine laboratory studies are important tests for monitoring safe cortisone maintenance. These studies should include urinalysis, chest x-ray, blood electrolytes, complete blood count and two-hour postprandial blood sugar.

Other signs for which the nurse must be alert include acne, hyperpigmentation of the skin, hirsutism, muscular weakness, nervousness and insomnia. The patient may at first be euphoric, partly from relief of pain and partly as a side effect of the drug. Mental depression with suicidal tendencies has been known to develop. A gain in weight may be noted; this may be due to both fluid retention and accumulation of fat. This accumulation often produces a "moon face." These drugs may also cause a reactivation of a gastric ulcer with hemorrhage. Demineralization of the bones may occur, resulting in osteoporosis with the potential danger of pathologic fractures.

Withdrawal symptoms are common when the drug is discontinued and this is understandable when one considers what has happened in the body while the drug was being given. The glucocorticoids suppress adrenocortical function and also suppress the corticotropic activity of the pituitary gland. As a result, there is an inhibition of all the corticotropic-adrenocortical function while the drugs are given. It may be several days after the drug is stopped before the endogenous secretion of the adrenal cortex is adequate, and hypocortism may develop. The patient complains of headache, nausea, vomiting, loss of appetite, malaise, papilledema and muscular weakness. For these reasons, the drug should be withdrawn gradually. Sudden withdrawal is extremely dangerous.

The Patient. Though the relief provided is great, it is necessary to maintain continuous therapy. This may be discouraging to the patient and his family (V-1, 2, 3). They will need to understand that when the drug is withdrawn, symptoms even more severe than before may occur. This can be very discouraging.

The patient should wear a "Medic-Alert" tag and have information available so that in an emergency those caring for him will understand his condition and problems. The family also should be able to give any required information.

The patient and his family should be taught to carefully observe for subtle signs and symptoms of "hidden" mycotic or bacterial infection due to an anti-inflammatory response to the cortisone therapy. Such infections might easily be overlooked. Warning signs include sore throat, anorexia, fever or malaise.

MISCELLANEOUS DRUGS. Antimalarial therapy is still occasionally resorted to and does have a slight ameliorating effect. Its mode of action and true value are not clear. Either *chloroquine* (Aralen) or *hydroxychloroquine phosphate* (Plaquenil) may be used. Results are not usually noted for one to three months after treatment is started, and there is considerable danger from side reactions with the higher dosages. For further information refer to Malaria in Chapter 31.

Phenylbutazone (Butazolidin), *oxyphenbutazone* (Tandearil) or *indomethacin* (Indocin), discussed previously in this chapter, are sometimes used, but they are much less effective in rheumatoid arthritis than in gout and gouty arthritis.

Osteoarthritis

DEFINITION. Osteoarthritis is a degenerative disease of the joints, unknown in origin, which affects older persons much more than those of a younger age. It has been called the "arthritis of the aged."

MAJOR SYMPTOMS. Osteoarthritis is subdivided into two groups: primary, characterized by the formation of Heberden's nodules; and secondary, a post-traumatic reaction. Osteoarthritis is a painful condition, especially when the joint is first affected. It is a progressing condition with gradual loss of the articular cartilage. Joints may or may not ankylose. Function is reduced in relation to the extent of the damage to the joint. It is also related to the amount of use the patient makes of the joint. Excessive use in the acute stage is not advisable, but complete immobilization of the joint tends to produce ankylosing.

DRUG THERAPY. The salicylates are the drugs of choice in the treatment of this condition. If the pain is severe, it may be necessary to employ other analgesics, but the opiates should not be used because of the chronicity of the condition. *Acetaminophen* (Tylenol), *ethoheptazine* (Zactane) or *propoxyphene* (Darvon) may be given. These have been discussed in Chapter 9.

Indomethacin (Indocin) or *phenylbutazone* (Butazolidin) may be used and, for some patients, afford considerable relief. Their use in this condition is the same as discussed earlier in the chapter.

The adrenal corticosteroids are not used for this condition except for intra-articular injections. This may be very beneficial and may allow for much more and easier use of the joints.

These patients need to be encouraged to do as much as they can without undue pain. Often, they tend to become depressed as they see one after another of their joints becoming involved. They need patient and sympathetic nursing without the nurse being too optimistic. Many patients live happy and relatively comfortable lives for years with this disease.

IT IS IMPORTANT TO REMEMBER

1. That the fluid intake of patients receiving sulfinpyrazone should be kept at adequate levels.
2. That though the adrenal corticosteroids are often helpful, much has yet to be learned about them and their actions. Untoward effects are common and are not usually mild.
3. That the patient with gout should always have colchicine available and should take it at the first sign of an attack.
4. That probenecid is useful in the treatment of gout as an adjunct to other therapy, but it should not be given with the salicylates as these two are antagonistic.

5. That patients who are receiving any of the adrenal corticosteroids should routinely have their fluid intake and output and daily blood pressures recorded and should be weighed daily.

6. That if one of the glucocorticoids is to be used for parenteral injection, sodium chloride is *not* used as the diluent.

TOPICS FOR STUDY AND DISCUSSION

1. How are the adrenal corticosteroids given?
2. Go to the pharmacy and find out the cost of these drugs and calculate the cost of each dose.
3. For which diseases of the musculoskeletal system are adrenal corticosteroids effective?
4. List all the diseases you have encountered so far in which adrenal corticosteroids are used.
5. For which disease of the musculoskeletal system are the sex hormones used and why?
6. Describe the nursing care measures you would utilize when caring for chronically ill individuals with restricted motion. Be specific.
7. If a patient receives 0.5 mg. of colchicine q 2 h (day only—8:00 A.M. to 10:00 P.M.) and the doctor wishes the patient to have a total of 12 mg. on this schedule, how long would this take?
8. What signs and symptoms would the nurse identify when inquiring about "hidden" infection for patients on cortisone therapy? Explain why this may occur.

BIBLIOGRAPHY

Books and Pamphlets

American Medical Association Council on Drugs, *Drug Evaluations*, Chicago, 1971, American Medical Association.

Beeson, P. B., and McDermott, W., *Cecil-Loeb Textbook of Medicine, 13th Ed.*, Philadelphia, 1971, W. B. Saunders Co.

Beland, I. L., *Clinical Nursing, 2nd Ed.*, New York, 1970, The Macmillan Co.

Bergersen, B. S., and Goth, A., *Pharmacology in Nursing, 12th Ed.*, St. Louis, 1973, The C. V. Mosby Co.

Conn, H. F., et al., *Current Therapy, 1974*, Philadelphia, 1974, W. B. Saunders Co.

Gagong, W., *Review of Medical Physiology*, Los Altos, California, 1969, Lange Medical Publications.

Goodman, L. S., and Gilman, A., *Pharmacological Basis of Therapeutics, 4th Ed.*, New York, 1970, The Macmillan Co.

Govani, L., and Hayes, J., *Drugs and Nursing Implications*, New York, 1971, Appleton-Century-Crofts.

Watson, J. E., *Medical-Surgical Nursing and Related Physiology*, Philadelphia, 1972, W. B. Saunders Co.

Journal Articles

Cowell, H. R., "Genetic aspects of orthopedic disease," *Am. J. Nurs.*, 70:4:763 (April, 1970).

Decker, J. L., et al., "Prostaglandins," *Sci. News* 103:12:181 (1973).

DiPalma, J. P., "Recent development in bone disease treatment," *R.N.* 36:1:72 (January, 1973).

Herman, I., and Smith, R., "Gout and gouty arthritis," *Am. J. Nurs.* 164:12:111 (December, 1964).

Jowsey, J., Riggs, B. L., and Kelley, P. J., "New concepts in the treatment of osteoporosis," *Postgrad. Med.* 52:4 (1973).

Katcher, B. S., "Rheumatoid arthritis," *J. Am. Pharm. Assoc.* NS 12:7:383 (July, 1972).

Keely, M., "Exercises for the bedrest patient," *Am. J. Nurs.* 66:10:2209 (October, 1966).

Kelley, W., and Beardmore, T., "Allopurinol: alteration in pyrimidine metabolism in man," *Science* 169:3943:388 (1970).

Kraicer, J., Milligan, J. V., et al., "Potassium, corticosterone and adrenocorticotropic hormone release *in vitro*," *Science* 164:3878:426 (1969).

Loomis, W. F., "Rickets," *Sci. Am.* 223:6:76 (December, 1970).

Mendell, J. R., Engel, W. K., and Derrer, E. C., "Duchenne muscular dystrophy: functional ischemia reproduces its characteristic lesions," *Science*, 172:3988:1143 (1971).

Olsen, E., and Edmond, R., "The hazards of immobility: effect on motor function," *Am. J. Nurs.* 67:4:788 (April, 1967).

Potter, T. A., and Nalebuff, E. A., (Eds.), "Symposium of the surgical management of rheumatoid arthritis," *Nurs. Clin. North Am.* 49:4.

Walike, B. C., et al., "Rheumatoid arthritis," *Am. J. Nurs.* 67:7:1420 (July, 1967).

Walike, B. C., et al., "Rheumatoid arthritis—Personality factors," *Am. J. Nurs.* 67:7:1427 (July, 1967).

CHAPTER 22

DRUGS USED FOR DISORDERS OF THE URINARY SYSTEM

CORRELATION WITH OTHER SCIENCES

I. ANATOMY AND PHYSIOLOGY

1. The kidneys must adjust the amount of sodium and water excreted. This serves as a protective mechanism for the body.
2. There are normally a few substances which are actively secreted by the cells of the renal tubules. Among these are hydrogen, ammonia, creatinine and certain dyes and drugs used in kidney function tests.
3. The ureters are capable of wave-like contractions which propel the urine down from the kidneys into the bladder.
4. The urinary bladder is a contractile sac composed of smooth muscle and serving as a storehouse of urine for its periodic discharge.
5. The normal daily urine volume is 1 to 2 liters.

II. CHEMISTRY

1. A semipermeable membrane allows diffusion of some types of particles (such as molecules and ions in solution) but not others. An equilibrium is usually reached, resulting in an equal concentration on each side of the membrane.

III. MICROBIOLOGY

1. The most frequently encountered organisms causing infections of the urinary system are those common to the intestinal tract—the so-called "colon group" and the gonococcus. Streptococci and staphylococci may also cause infection.

IV. PHYSICS

1. Urine flowing out of the collecting tubules into the pelvis of the kidney collects until the pelvis is full. The muscles then contract, forcing part of the urine into the ureter. The pressure is normally low here.
2. Owing to the wave-like contractions of the ureter, the pressure in the ureters is considerably greater than in the kidneys.
3. As the urine collects in the urinary bladder of normal individuals, the pressure increases. The walls of the bladder automatically relax, however, to keep the pressure low. The bladder is capable of adjusting to increasing volumes of urine with only a slight rise in intravesical pressure until urination occurs, when the pressure rises rapidly to high levels.
4. The specific gravity of normal urine is considered to be around 1.010 to 1.020.
5. The interchange of water between blood and tissue spaces depends on the concentration of the plasma proteins. A decrease, especially in albumin, will cause water to flow from the blood into the tissues, resulting in edema.

V. PSYCHOLOGY

1. A diagnosis of a chronic disease can be a severe emotional shock. The patient will need understanding to aid him in adjusting to a new life style.
2. The patient with a chronic disease must develop a "healthy mental attitude" toward the disease and the limitations it puts on his activities.

VI. SOCIOLOGY

1. The intelligent cooperation of the family must be gained to help the chronic patient pattern a new life routine.
2. The expenses of chronic illness are sometimes very heavy. Social agencies should be consulted to find what resources there are to help with the costs of treatment.

DRUGS USED FOR PATIENTS WITH URINARY DISORDERS

INTRODUCTION. Diseases of the urinary tract may be divided into three classifications: those that are peculiar to men, those that affect only the women, and those that affect the sexes alike. The majority belong in the last category.

Urinary disorders vary from a simple, relatively easily treated infection to a life-threatening renal failure. Some disorders respond to medical therapy, but drugs are of little value in others. Urinary infections may be primary, occurring first in that system, or secondary, as a complication of another disease elsewhere in the body. These diseases may be direct extensions from nearby organs or brought to the urinary system by way of the blood or lymph streams. In turn, renal or cystic disorders may infect other organs.

Those urinary diseases that are a complication of another disorder will be considered with the primary disease.

Urinary Tract Infections

URETHRITIS—MALE, FEMALE AND CHILD

DEFINITION. Urethritis is usually classified as gonorrheal or nongonorrheal. Gonorrhea will be discussed in Chapter 26 under Venereal Diseases. Nongonorrheal urethritis is an infection that may be caused by a variety of organisms such as bacteria, viruses or protozoa (*Trichomonas*). The common bacterial invaders, in addition to the gonococcus, include pyogenic cocci and bacteria of the coliform group. Because of structural differences in the female, the infection may be an extension of an infection in adjacent organs. Urethritis may result from trauma, strictures, calculi or unhygienic habits.

MAJOR SYMPTOMS. Regardless of the cause, the symptoms include purulent discharge, dysuria, burning on urination, low backache, low abdominal pain and if the infection is severe, fever, anorexia and malaise. With the small child, restlessness, fretfulness, enuresis and possibly crying on urination may be the only symptoms. In any urinary disorder, the child may react in an entirely different manner from the adult, with such symptoms as vomiting, diarrhea, fever or convulsions.

DRUG THERAPY. The choice of an anti-infective drug depends upon the identity and the sensitivity of the organism. The list of possible drugs is very long, but a few that may be used include *penicillin, kanamycin, gentamicin, colistimethate, tetracycline, nitrofurantoin* (Furadantin) or the sulfonamides. (See Chapter 7 and the Current Drug Handbook for further information.) Locally, *neomycin* may be applied.

Symptoms are treated as they occur. Mild analgesics are usually required. In some cases antispasmodics may be employed to make voiding less traumatic, since they relieve the spasms that often accompany this condition.

Prostatitis

DEFINITION. Prostatitis is an inflammation of the prostate gland which may result from invasion by any of the pyogenic organisms with about one-half of the cases due to the gonococcus (III-1). The gland may be infected either by direct ascent up the urethra or by way of the blood stream from a distant focus of infection.

MAJOR SYMPTOMS. There may be difficult urination or urine retention, malaise, headache, fever and a sacral backache. The gland is often swollen and tender. In gonorrheal infections, there is usually a profuse urethral discharge.

DRUG THERAPY. Antibiotics are used, the choice depending upon the responsible organism and the severity of the infection. If the type of organism is not known, the drug most commonly used is *ampicillin,* 500 mg. Other drugs that can be given orally include *penicillin G* 250 mg. and *cephalexin* (Keflex) 250 mg. q.i.d. Other drugs include: *cephalothin* 0.5-1.0 Gm. q 6 h, *kanamycin* 0.5 Gm. b.i.d. or *polymyxin B* 2.5 mg./kg. daily in divided doses parenterally. If the infection is very severe *chloramphenicol* 250 to 500 mg. q.i.d. may be used. Prophylactic therapy to prevent recurrence may be: *sulfamethoxazole* (Gantanol) 1.0 Gm. b.i.d., *nitrofurantoin* (Furadantin) 50 mg. q.i.d., *nalidixic acid* (NegGram) 500 mg. q.i.d. or *methenamine hippurate* (Hiprex) 1.0 Gm. b.i.d. Also see Current Drug Handbook.

Interactions. Nitrofurantoin is inhibited by antacid compounds. When given with probenecid or sulfinpyrazone the excretion of nitrofurantoin is decreased, and toxic side effects may occur. Nalidixic acid is also inhibited by antacids.

Cystitis

DEFINITION. Cystitis is an inflammation of the bladder which is very common in both sexes at all ages. Its cause may be nonbacterial, nonspecific or some specific organism or parasite. Mixed infections are common, but the most frequent responsible organism is the colon bacillus (III-1). It may be a descending infection from the upper urinary tract or it may be ascending, from the urethra. A persistent or significant infection rarely occurs in the bladder unless there is a stasis of urine or trauma is present.

MAJOR SYMPTOMS. The patient usually complains of pain on urinating, frequency, low back pain, fever and malaise (IV-3). Urinalysis reveals the presence of pus.

DRUG THERAPY

URINARY ANTISEPTICS

THE DRUGS. Many drugs are used for the elimination of bacteria from the urinary tract. Most of these are the general anti-infective drugs used for many conditions. They were discussed in detail in Chapter 7. Here will be discussed those antiseptics used primarily or exclusively for urinary tract infections. These are mandelic acid and methenamine. They are not the same drug, but the combination of these, methenamine mandelate, is used extensively.

Physical and Chemical Properties. Mandelic acid is also known as alpha hydroxy phenylacetic acid. Methenamine is a combination product of formaldehyde and ammonia. Both drugs are readily soluble in water and in body fluids.

Action. Mandelic acid and methenamine are antiseptic in acid urine.

Therapeutic Uses. These drugs are used almost exclusively for urinary tract infections.

Absorption and Excretion. Both drugs are readily absorbed from the gastrointestinal tract and are rapidly excreted in the urine. Usually, these medicines are entirely eliminated within 12 to 24 hours.

Preparations and Dosages. See the Current Drug Handbook for further information.

Mandelic acid, 2-3 Gm. q.i.d. orally.

Methenamine, N.F. (Urotropin), 0.5-1.5 Gm. q.i.d. orally.

Methenamine hippurate (Hiprex), 1.0 Gm. b.i.d. or t.i.d. orally.

Methenamine mandelate, U.S.P. (Mandelamine), 0.25-1.5 Gm. q.i.d. orally. This is the drug most commonly used.

THE NURSE

Mode of Administration. These drugs are given orally. When mandelamine is administered, it may be helpful to give it with at least a half glass of water to reduce gastric irritation from the formaldehyde released in the stomach. The main precaution for the nurse is to make certain that the urine is acid all the time during therapy. Alkaline ash foods should be avoided. Many doctors routinely order an acidifying agent with these drugs, such as ascorbic acid, ammonium nitrate or sodium acid phosphate. Most physicians wish the patient to have adequate fluids. However, some physicians limit the intake to about 1200 ml. each 24 hours when mandelic acid is given alone.

Side Effects and Toxicity. Side effects or toxic symptoms are not common with therapeutic doses. Mandelamine in combination with a sulfonamide may result in turbid urine. This sign is not clinically important (it results from precipitation of formaldehyde with the sulfonamide), but it may cause the patient some concern unless he is aware of this possibility. However, mandelic acid may cause gastrointestinal disturbances, lessened auditory acuity and ringing in the ears. If these occur, the drug should be stopped, fluids given freely and the symptoms treated as they occur. Methenamine rarely causes adverse symptoms, but dysuria, hematuria and albuminuria have been reported in a few cases. Reactions are treated as are those to mandelic acid.

Patient Teaching. If the patient is to take these drugs at home, the nurse should be sure the patient understands the importance of proper fluid intake (usually 1500 to 2000 ml. per day), drug administration and adequate diet containing elements to facilitate the maintenance of urine acidity at a pH of 5.5 or below. Cranberry juice will aid in this. The doctor also may order ascorbic acid tablets. The patient should be instructed to contact the doctor if any undesirable symptoms occur. The nurse may need to teach the patient how to test the urine for acidity.

THE PATIENT. Urinary tract infections are usually very uncomfortable and disturbing to the patient. This type of infection is apt to be prolonged (up to six to eighteen months), and this is discouraging. The nurse can do much to make the patient understand the nature of the condition and what the medicines are expected to do. She can also assure the patient that if one drug does not help, the physician has many others he can use.

Except when receiving mandelic acid, patients with cystitis usually should be encouraged to keep up their fluid intake since this will help maintain normal kidney function.

ANTI-INFECTIVES. The choice of a chemotherapeutic agent depends upon the sensitivity of the organism to the drug. The

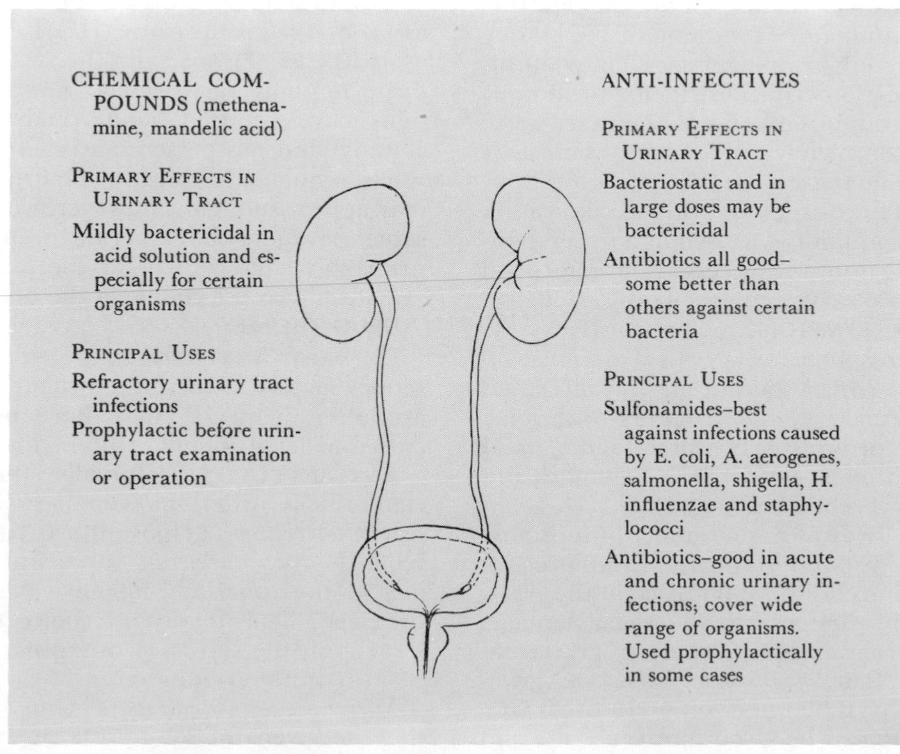

FIGURE 38. Comparison of urinary antiseptics.

aim is to achieve a bactericidal effect not only in the tissues but also in the urine.

The drugs are usually the same as those given for urethritis. When the culture and sensitivity test disclose the preferred medicine, unless the patient is known to be allergic to it, it is given in the usual doses. Unless otherwise ordered, fluid intake is kept high. For information concerning a specific drug, refer to Chapter 7 and the Current Drug Handbook.

Miscellaneous Drugs. Bladder spasms are frequent and may be very painful. Antispasmodics for smooth muscle, such as *tincture of belladonna,* may be ordered in doses of 0.6 ml. For severe pain with any urinary tract infection, *opium and belladonna suppositories* often help, since they contain an analgesic and an antispasmodic.

Irrigation of the bladder is seldom done during the acute stages but often is helpful later. Solutions often used include *physiologic saline, acetic acid* 0.25 per cent or Neosporin Genito-Urinary Irrigant.

ACUTE GLOMERULONEPHRITIS

DEFINITION. Acute glomerulonephritis is an inflammatory condition of the kidney characterized by a plugging of a large number of the glomeruli, obstructing the flow of blood through the kidney. The exact cause is not completely understood, but it is known that there is no direct bacterial invasion. There is good evidence indicating that the condition is caused by a hypersensitivity reaction to successive streptococcal infections elsewhere in the body.

MAJOR SYMPTOMS. The earliest signs are a gross hematuria with a decrease in the total urinary output and an increased specific gravity of the urine (IV-4). Edema becomes progressively worse, and a mild hypertension is noted. If it continues unchecked, cerebral edema occurs.

DRUG THERAPY. Glomerulonephritis does not respond to the usual anti-infective drugs. Diuretics have no place in the treatment, for they add to the renal damage. When cerebral edema is present, it is recommended that *magnesium sulfate* be given orally (if possible) in doses of 15 to 30 Gm. This drug can be given intravenously, and 25 ml. of a 10 per cent solution is introduced *slowly.* The drug is given to aid in the removal of fluid and tends to prevent convulsive seizures. A *hypertonic glucose* (50 per cent) may also be given intravenously to aid in withdrawing fluid from the central nervous system. Anti-infectives may be used to prevent infection. Diet and rest are important.

Heparin may be given to decrease fibrin formation. The oral anticoagulants do not help. Symptoms are treated as they occur. If the condition persists for more than six weeks, many physicians give one of the antimetabolite agents. *Azathioprine,* used with organ transplants, is used by some doctors, but it is investigational. For information on the antimetabolite drugs, refer to the Current Drug Handbook and Chapter 29. For azathioprine, refer to Chapter 25.

Much of the treatment of glomerulonephritis is palliative and symptomatic.

PYELONEPHRITIS

DEFINITION. An infection involving both the pelvis and the medulla of the kidney, pyelonephritis may be either of hematogenous or of ascending origin. Very commonly, *Escherichia coli* is the cause (III-1).

MAJOR SYMPTOMS. In the acute stage, the symptoms vary widely. Few outward signs may be noticed, but a urinalysis shows albumin and pus present and there may be some frequency, or burning on urination. It may appear suddenly, however, with a chill, some elevation of temperature, headache, prostration and a pain in the loin which radiates down the course of the ureter.

DRUG THERAPY

Urinary Antiseptics. Urinary antiseptics may be used in the usual doses and are often helpful. These have been discussed in detail under Cystitis in this chapter.

Anti-infectives. Initially, the physician usually orders *sulfisoxazole* (Gantrisin) or *sulfamethizole* (Thiosulfil) 0.5-1.0 Gm. b.i.d. If these are not successful, almost any of the usual anti-infective drugs may be given. The physician's choice depends largely on the causative organism and the severity of the condition.

Methenamine mandelate 1 Gm. q 4-6 h may be given for low grade or recurring infections. Very severe conditions may be treated with *chloramphenicol*. These drugs are discussed in Chapter 7 and the Current Drug Handbook.

The fluid intake must be maintained so that the total urine volume is not less than 1000 ml. daily (I-5). An intake and output record should be kept on these patients. Symptoms are treated as required—analgesics, sedatives, hypnotics, and so forth. Dysuria may be controlled by the use of *phenazopyridine* (Pyridium) 100-200 mg. q.i.d. The use of antispasmodic drugs may relieve the ureteral and bladder spasms which often accompany this condition.

THE NEPHROTIC SYNDROME

DEFINITION. The nephrotic syndrome (nephrosis) is primarily the result of an injury to the glomerulus, increasing its permeability to plasma proteins. There is no unanimity of opinion about the cause.

MAJOR SYMPTOMS. The condition is insidious in onset and may be present for many years before it is evidenced to any great extent. Then it may be shown by anorexia, nausea and diarrhea, and a gradual development of edema. This, if allowed to continue, progresses from a generalized edema to anasarca, with fluid in the serous cavities (IV-5). The urine contains large amounts of albumin and an increased number of casts. The blood shows a low total serum protein with a reduced serum albumin and a high blood cholesterol.

DRUG THERAPY. Drugs usually ordered include *prednisone* 60 mg. per M. of body surface, daily. This is continued until one week after the urine is protein free. Then it is given every other day for about six months. The dose for a child should not exceed 60 mg. in any one day. One of the thiazide diuretics with *spironolactone* (Aldactone) in the usual doses may be given. These are continued until the patient is edema free. With severe edema, it may be necessary to use either *furosemide* or *ethacrynic acid* for a short time and then change to the thiazide. With severe hypoalbuminemia, albumin may be given intravenously together with a diuretic. These drugs are discussed in more detail in the Current Drug Handbook. The diuretics are covered in Chapter 18, and prednisone is discussed in Chapter 27.

NEPHROLITHIASIS

DEFINITION. The formation of concretions of crystalline urinary constituents in the calices or pelvis of the kidney is known as nephrolithiasis, or kidney stones. The cause is usually unknown.

MAJOR SYMPTOMS. The symptoms will vary with the size, shape and position of the stone. Some are passed unnoticed and others may remain in the kidney for years without outward signs. The most common symptom is dull pain of intermittent character in the flank or back which is more acute on movement. Renal colic occurs when a stone enters the ureter and obstructs it (I-4; IV-2). The pain is excruciating and is often accompanied by nausea, vomiting, profuse diaphoresis, faintness and even shock. There is usually frequency and urgency present but only a small amount of urine is passed (IV-1, 3). The pain may persist for many hours.

DRUG THERAPY. The treatment of urinary calculi depends upon factors such as size and location of the stone, the presence of infection, and the possibility of obstruction to the flow of urine. Infection is treated as has been discussed earlier in this chapter. If there is a stone in one of the ureters, pain may be very severe, and it may require a strong analgesic to control it. Anticholinergic preparations such as *propantheline* (Pro-Banthine) may aid in relaxing the ureter and thus facilitate the passage of the stone. Nausea and vomiting often accompany this condition, and they are treated with an antinauseant such as *prochlorperazine* (Compazine) 10 mg. intramuscularly. Surgery may be required, especially if the stone is large and if there is an obstruction that is not rapidly overcome. Fluids are usually restricted in renal colic, since they increase the tendency to nausea and vomiting.

ACUTE RENAL FAILURE (ACUTE UREMIA)

DEFINITION. Acute renal failure is a sudden failure of the kidneys to function properly. There is retention in the blood of substances usually removed by the kidneys. This explains the second name, "uremia."

MAJOR SYMPTOMS. The principal early symptom is a rapidly progressive oliguria. The patient is "uncomfortable." Later, headache, nausea and vomiting are common. If the condition is not corrected, it may progress to anuria with a "uremic" (ammonia) breath, convulsions and/or coma.

DRUG THERAPY. Acute renal failure is usually a complication of another disease or due to poisoning. The first treatment is the removal of the cause, if possible. Fluid intake is usually restricted. Balancing of the serum electrolytes is imperative. This is generally done by intravenous infusions as long as nausea and vomiting persist. The oral route is used as soon as circumstances permit. Symptoms are treated as they occur. Antiemetic-type tranquilizers are often very helpful. Sedation may be required. It is important that the drugs selected be those that are not nephrotoxic. If medicinal and intravenous treatments are not successful, hemodialysis or peritoneal dialysis may be employed. The process of dialysis is further discussed under chronic renal failure, which follows. Most cases of acute renal failure do respond to treatment and the patient recovers in one to six weeks. There may be some residual kidney damage.

THE NURSE. (See Chronic Renal Failure.)

THE PATIENT. (See Chronic Renal Failure.)

CHRONIC RENAL FAILURE (CHRONIC UREMIA)

DEFINITION. Chronic renal failure is a persistent failure of the kidneys to function properly. It may be caused by repeated infections, nephrolithiasis (kidney stones) – especially if obstructive – or other renal disorders, or it may be the result of diseases not directly related to the kidneys, such as diabetes mellitus, collagen disorders and so forth.

MAJOR SYMPTOMS. The onset is insidious. There is a gradual decrease in urinary output. Occasionally, there may be an increase in fluid output but not in the solutes usually excreted. There is a build-up in the blood of substances normally removed by the kidneys. General symptoms also come on gradually. They include lassitude, anorexia, possible nausea and vomiting, edema, hypertension, diminution in visual acuity due to retinal hemorrhages and a gradual physical deterioration. If unchecked, this leads to stupor, coma and death.

DRUG THERAPY. There is no curative drug therapy for renal failure. Symptoms are treated as they occur.

If it is deemed advisable, considering all factors – age, general physical condition, finances – dialysis may be started. It may be done in one of two ways – hemodialysis or peritoneal dialysis. The latter is done by perfusing the peritoneal cavity with the dialyzing solution, leaving it for a specific time and then withdrawing the fluid. With hemodialysis, an arterial-venal shunt is installed. This is connected to the dialyzing machine and the blood is pumped through the dialyzing fluid with a partially porous (semipermeable) plastic membrane to protect the cells. The dialysis is usually done three times a week for 8 hours each time, but this may vary to from two to four times and from 4 to 14 hours each time, depending upon circumstances. Permanent dialysis is extremely expensive, but it is life saving. For acute uremia, only one or a few treatments may be needed. Also, peritoneal dialysis is more apt to be used for the acute form than for the chronic form of the disease.

With chronic renal failure, if the patient is to be placed on permanent dialysis, the first few treatments are given in a hospital. If home treatment is not anticipated, the patient returns to the hospital or clinic for the treatments. However, if he is to be treated at home, he or some member of his family is taught the entire procedure. A dialyzing machine is installed in the home and the patient is "on his own." Of course he is still under very close medical supervision for the remainder of his life. It is customary for a public health nurse, a technician or both to visit the home regularly to check on the patient's progress, the condition of the machine and other circumstances which might need to be clarified with the patient or his family.

A comparison of the dialyzing solution and the normal blood plasma concentrations follows. (All values are in mEq/L unless otherwise marked.)

NORMAL BLOOD PLASMA ELECTROLYTES		STANDARD DIALYZING SOLUTION
Sodium	142.0	134.0
Potassium	5.0	2.6
Calcium	5.0	2.5
Magnesium	2.0	1.5
Chloride	105.0	104.0

Bicarbonate	24.0	
Phosphate	2.0	
Organic acid	6.0	(Not necessarily mEq.)
Proteinate	16.0	(Not necessarily mEq.)

Sodium acetate	36.6	(Not necessarily mEq.)
Anhydrous glucose	2.0	(Not necessarily mEq.)

The dialyzing solution is varied to suit the needs of the patient and for specific purposes (such as the removal of a poison). Variations are usually in sodium, potassium or calcium.

In hemodialysis, the pump is primed with saline solution. *Heparin*, 4500 μ. of the aqueous solution, is added to the first blood, and 1000 μ. per hour of the solution is added thereafter. *Protamine* is usually added when the treatment is terminated to inactivate the heparin. The dose is, as usual, based upon the amount of heparin given.

THE NURSE. Maintenance of fluid and electrolyte balance is the goal of the medical therapy. The fluid intake must be watched carefully, because there is great danger of overloading the circulatory system. The patient should be weighed each morning before breakfast to note any weight changes. Precise recording of intake and output (including the dialyzing fluid) should be made each day. Temporary and sometimes long-term improvement may be obtained by dialysis.

Dialysis is based upon the physical laws of fluid movement through a semipermeable membrane from a region of higher to one of lower concentration until an equilibrium is established (II-1). Through this procedure, the end products of protein metabolism (urea, creatinine) are removed, and a more normal plasma electrolyte concentration is maintained.

Diet is an important nursing concern. Intravenous replacements are used until the patient can tolerate oral administration of food and fluids. Thirst—a common complaint due to the increased urea levels—may be partially relieved by giving ice chips made with 20 to 50 per cent glucose solution.

After oral foods and fluids are allowed, the diet is often very restricted. This is temporary for acute renal failure, but it may be more or less permanent for the chronic case, depending upon circumstances. One such diet includes 20 to 40 grams of protein, 500 mg. of sodium (very restricted), foods low in potassium, 500 ml. of fluids and a high intake of carbohydrates and fats. The latter two are to decrease the endogenous metabolism of proteins. This is a very restricted diet and the patient will need a lot of encouragement to continue on it.

A vital area of nursing care is the elimination of all possible respiratory infections. Reverse isolation may be needed, especially for the acute case and in the beginning of treatment for the chronic form. Pneumonia is not uncommon because of the fluid differential which makes the mucus very thick and tenacious. The cough reflex is apt to be depressed because of the acidosis which affects the central nervous system. Early ambulation, frequent turning, tracheal suction and positive pressure therapy are all beneficial. Oral care is important in helping to prevent infection and in decreasing odor.

THE PATIENT. The patient suffering from chronic uremia is often very depressed and has a feeling of impending death. However, his prognosis may be better than he anticipates. With dialysis, it is now possible to prolong life for years beyond what was previously possible. Even with dialysis, the patient must accept the fact that other measures, such as a restrictive diet, low fluid intake and usually a change in life style must be taken. Becoming so completely dependent upon a "machine" for his life is depressing and demoralizing to the extent that some patients are unable to face it. Everyone connected with the case must do all in his power to help the patient adjust to his condition in a mentally healthy way.

The patient with chronic uremia undergoes personality changes due to the uremia and the depression which accompanies long-term illness. The patient, his family and his friends will all need help in learning to cope with the changes the disease imposes.

It may be necessary for the patient to change his vocation and his avocations, and he will need the help of various social agencies to make the required changes. The expense of dialysis is very great and may be entirely beyond the financial resources of the patient. These same agencies can often aid in this area as well.

IT IS IMPORTANT TO REMEMBER

1. That urinary antiseptics are extremely helpful in infections of the urinary tract.
2. That when methenamine and mandelic acid preparations are used, it is usually essential to acidify the urine with another drug to obtain the best results.
3. That the only condition of the urinary system in which the use of diuretics is indicated is nephrosis.
4. That the fluid intake and output should be measured for all patients with diseases of the urinary tract.

TOPICS FOR STUDY AND DISCUSSION

1. Discuss the merits and demerits of the "buffered" aspirin preparations.
2. What is the action of corticotropin and the adrenocortical steroids in nephrosis?
3. What precautions are necessary when methenamine and mandelic acid preparations are used? Why?
4. For what reason is potassium citrate administered in nephrolithiasis?
5. In what conditions of the urinary system are diuretics used?
6. List the medications shown on the chart of a patient with one of the urinary tract diseases and compare them with those listed in this chapter.
7. An ampule contains 50 ml. of 50 per cent glucose solution. How much sterile distilled water would you add to this to make a 10 per cent solution?

BIBLIOGRAPHY

Books and Pamphlets

American Medical Association Council on Drugs, *Current Medical Terminology, 3rd Ed.*, Chicago, 1966, American Medical Association.

American Medical Association Council on Drugs, *Drug Evaluations*, Chicago, 1971, American Medical Association.

Beeson, P. B., and McDermott, W., *Cecil-Loeb Textbook of Medicine, 13th Ed.*, Philadelphia, 1971, W. B. Saunders Co.

Beland, I. L., *Clinical Nursing, 2nd Ed.*, New York, 1970, The Macmillan Co.

Bergersen, B. S., *Pharmacology in Nursing, 12th Ed.*, St. Louis, 1973, The C. V. Mosby Co.

Blake, F., Wright, F., and Waechter, E., *Nursing Care of Children*, Philadelphia, 1970, J. B. Lippincott Co.

Chatton, M. J., Margen, S., and Brainerd, H., *Handbook of Medical Treatment, 12th Ed.*, Los Altos, California, 1970, Lange Medical Publications.

Conn, H. F., et al., *Current Therapy 1974*, Philadelphia, 1974, W. B. Saunders Co.

Goodman, L. S., and Gilman, A., *Pharmacological Basis of Therapeutics, 4th Ed.*, New York, 1970, The Macmillan Co.

Marlow, D., *Textbook of Pediatric Nursing, 4th Ed.*, Philadelphia, 1973, W. B. Saunders Co.

Meltzer, L., Abdellah, F., and Kitchell, J. R., *Concepts and Practices of Intensive Care for Nurse Specialists*, Philadelphia, 1970, The Charles Press.

Metheny, N., and Snively, W., *Nurses' Handbook of Fluid Balance*, Philadelphia, 1967, W. B. Saunders Co.

Meyers, F., Jawitz, E., and Goldfien, A., *Review of Medical Pharmacology*, Los Altos, California, 1968, Lange Medical Publications.

Miller, B. F., and Keane, C. B., *Encyclopedia and Dictionary of Medicine and Nursing*, Philadelphia, 1972, W. B. Saunders Co.

Rodman, N. J., and Smith, D. W., *Pharmacology and Drug Therapy in Nursing*, Philadelphia, 1968, J. B. Lippincott Co.

Shafer, K. N., et al., *Medical-Surgical Nursing*, St. Louis, 1971, The C. V. Mosby Co.

Watson, J. E., *Medical-Surgical Nursing and Related Physiology*, Philadelphia, 1972, W. B. Saunders Co.

Journal Articles

Cummings, J., "The pressures and how the patients respond," *Am. J. Nurs.* 70:1:70 (January, 1970).

Cummings, J., "Two days of every week," *Am. J. Nurs.* 70:1:77 (January, 1970).

Davis, J., "Drugs for urological disorders," *Am. J. Nurs.* 65:8:107 (August, 1965).

Downing, S., "Nursing support in early renal failure," *Am. J. Nurs.* 69:6:1212 (June, 1969).

Foy, A., "Dreams of patients and staff," *Am. J. Nurs.* 70:1:80 (January, 1970).

Fulton, B. J., et al., "Symposium on patient care in kidney and urinary tract diseases," *Nurs. Clin. North Am.* 4:3 (September, 1969).

Hirchman, J. L., and Herfindal, E. T., "Current therapeutic concepts—Urinary tract infections," *J. Am. Pharm. Assoc.* NS 11:11:619 (November, 1971).

Kasselman, M. J., "Nursing care of the patient with prostatic hypertrophy,"*Am. J. Nurs.* 66:5:1026 (May, 1966).

Lonsdale, K., "Human stones," *Sci. Am.* 219:6:104 (December, 1968).

MacKinnon, H., "Urinary drainage: the problem with asepsis," *Am. J. Nurs.* 67:2:336 (February, 1967).

O'Neil, M., "Peritoneal dialysis," *Nurs. Clin. North Am.* 1:2:309 (June, 1966).

Read, M., and Mallison, M., "External arteriovenous shunts," *Am. J. Nurs.* 72:1:81 (January, 1972).

Santora, D., "Preventing hospital-acquired urinary infections," *Am. J. Nurs.* 66:4:790 (April, 1966).

Sapperstein, M., "Dialysis," *Am. J. Nurs.* 72:1:85 (January, 1972).

Schlatter, L., "What do you teach the dialysis patient?" *Am. J. Nurs.* 70:1:82 (January, 1970).

Shea, E., "Peritoneal dialysis," *Nurs. Forum* 4:3:33 (1965).

Shea, E., "Hemodialysis—Feelings, facts and fantasies," *Am. J. Nurs.* 70:1:70 (January, 1970).

CHAPTER 23

DRUGS USED FOR DISORDERS OF THE SKIN

CORRELATION WITH OTHER SCIENCES

I. ANATOMY AND PHYSIOLOGY

1. The integumentary system consists of the skin, and mucous membranes with the blood vessels, sebaceous (oil) and sudoriferous (sweat) glands, the ends of the sensory nerves and the appendages—the hair and nails.

2. The skin serves as a protective covering and as an organ of sensation, heat regulation, excretion and absorption.

3. The skin is made up of several layers of tissue, the outer or stratum corneum being a relatively heavy, rough layer often referred to as the horny layer.

III. MICROBIOLOGY

1. The skin is the natural habitat of many organisms such as bacteria and fungi. Any break in the skin is a potential source of infection, since microorganisms which are harmless on the surface may become deleterious upon entrance into the body.

2. Higher forms of organisms such as *Sarcoptes scabiei* and pediculi occasionally infest the skin as ectoparasites.

IV. PHYSICS

1. The skin is active in the transfer of heat from the body by conduction and radiation. It also aids in the conservation of heat.

2. To a slight degree, materials rubbed onto the skin are absorbed through the skin cells into the deeper tissues.

3. Any break in the skin will cause a loss of fluid, since the horny cells which retain this fluid have been destroyed.

V. PSYCHOLOGY

1. Undesirable conditions which are chronic often lead to emotional depression, since the individual becomes overwhelmed by the possibility of a long-term battle.

2. Disfiguring skin conditions can and do produce emotional disturbances. No person wants to be repulsive to those around him.

3. Chronic illness or prolonged enforced idleness produces adverse emotional reactions.

4. Emotional shock is caused by any unpleasant experience, and the more disturbing the experience the greater the shock.

5. Psychologic trauma may cause a retardation in the normal development and in the normal reactions of the individual.

VI. SOCIOLOGY

1. Social stigma due to certain types of diseases may make the patient delay seeking medical advice. This may result in a much more severe condition than would otherwise have occurred.

2. The thought of disfigurement or of severe scarring of any kind will produce a fear of public reaction to the unattractiveness and also the fear of inability to perform one's regular routines. Fear is a strong emotion.

3. Fear of social ostracism is a potent factor in the life of everyone. Every person desires to be liked by his peers. He will avoid almost anything which might lower him in the eyes of the public.

4. Fear of being unable to compete with the average person produces an unfavorable reaction in the individual, especially if he is the breadwinner of the family.

5. The patient with a chronic illness who will require long-term therapy may find the cost of medications, treatments and physicians' fees a severe burden on the family budget. All possible means of continuing the treatment should be investigated.

INTRODUCTION

Diseases and disorders of the skin present many problems to the physician, the nurse and the patient. If the area involved is on the exposed portions of the body, the problems are greatly increased, but even if usually covered areas are the parts affected, there are still many difficulties, emotional as well as physical. The young girl with a disorder characterized by ugly lesions may have a genuine social problem. If the trouble involves the face it is with her all the time; if on the body it becomes important on such occasions as the senior prom or the beach party. Many times the condition may seem minor to the nurse or the doctor, but it is not minor to the patient (V-2, 4).

Of course, many skin conditions are acute and are quickly cured, but some skin disorders are chronic or recurrent, and it is these which present the greatest problems. Some skin disorders are basically emotional in etiology, and many others are made worse by emotional disturbances. The nurse should be aware of the psychologic problems involved in the various skin conditions and do all in her power to minimize the effect upon the patient (V-1).

Patients with disorders of the integumentary system are not usually acutely ill in the same sense as many other patients (I-1, 2). They are rarely confined to bed, and still more rarely are they hospitalized. This fact sometimes makes the nurse feel that the condition is unimportant, but to the patient it is of major dimensions in that he is uncomfortable, unattractive and sometimes unable to pursue his normal occupation.

The main treatment for most skin disorders is the use of drugs, and the number of drugs used is almost limitless. There are, however, some basic medications that form the treatment for most of these conditions. One interesting fact that is of importance for the nurse to remember in this connection is that the same drug may be used for many purposes—often exactly opposite in action—with the strength of the drug making the difference. For example, salicylic acid 1 to 2 per cent is keratoplastic (tending to increase the thickness of the horny layer of the skin); in a 5 to 20 per cent solution it is keratolytic (tending to decrease the thickness of the horny layer of the skin) (I-3).

Many of the drugs and treatments used for one skin disease are also useful in the treatment of many others, and it is possible to find one drug being ordered for several different skin disorders. This fact may need to be explained to the patient. It also should be a warning for, although the drug in question can be used for several different conditions, it does not necessarily follow that it is useful in all conditions. Only the dermatologist is capable of deciding what disorders will respond to what drug. The diagnosis of skin disorders is extremely difficult since many conditions resemble each other.

GENERAL TREATMENTS

The nurse must be familiar with all the basic treatments used for conditions of the skin, since one type of treatment may be used for a large number of disorders. Details concerning these treatments are, no doubt, already familiar so only a brief review will be needed.

Baths

Baths, local or general, plain or cleansing, to remove scabs, crusts and medications may be required before treatment is begun or new treatment started. Medicated baths, also either local or general, may be used for cleansing and, at the same time, to apply any number of drugs.

The temperature of the water should be 95 to 100° F (35 to 38° C) and the patient usually remains in the tub for one-half hour. In most skin diseases the skin is dried by gentle patting with soft towels and no rubbing.

Wet Dressings

Wet dressings are used chiefly when redness, edema, crusting, pruritus, infection or weeping lesions are present. The open type rather than the closed type (covered with some watertight material) are more often used in dermatology. The dressings are made of some soft material, one layer thick (to allow for evaporation), and should be thoroughly moistened with the appropriate medication before being applied to the skin. Dressings should not be remoistened while on the patient because it is difficult to wet the bandage evenly and also because complete resoaking is necessary to remove the accumulated detritus. Dressings are usually changed every five to ten minutes for one to two hours three times a day to provide the maximal results.

Powdery Suspensions

As the name implies, powdery suspensions are combinations of an insoluble substance with a fluid base. The suspensions, often called lotions, are mainly emollient and antipruritic in action; however, other substances are often added which will broaden their effectiveness. Powdery suspensions are usually applied by daubing with absorbent cotton wet with the solution and they are not covered.

Ointments, Creams, Pastes and Similar Preparations

Ointments are oily, semisolid preparations containing various drugs and are by far the most commonly used preparations for the relief of skin disorders. They are probably one of the oldest forms of medications, since chemicals, solutions from herbs and other substances have been added to goose grease or lard since the beginning of history. The oil used in the ointment may be animal, vegetable or mineral. They are nonhydrophilic – do not attract water. Some of the newer preparations are water soluble, yet of an oily consistency.

A *cream* is similar to an ointment. These preparations are hydrophilic. Greaseless creams and vanishing creams may also be used as a medium for medications.

A *paste* is a preparation containing 40 to 50 per cent of a powdery material in an oily base.

GENERAL MEDICATIONS

Since it is often the type of lesion rather than the disease that is treated, a brief consideration of the purposes for which drugs are used on the skin will aid in the understanding of why certain medicines are used in so many varied skin diseases.

Types of Medications

Anodynes and *anesthetics* are drugs which allay sensations, wholly or in part. These are usually the same drugs used to lessen sensations in any part of the body.

Antipruritics are drugs used locally to relieve itching, probably the most consistent and distressing symptom of skin disorders. Systemically this is treated by the use of antihistamines or corticosteroids.

Antiseptics are drugs used to retard the growth and reproduction of microorganisms. These were considered in Chapter 7 in the discussion of drugs used for infections of the skin and mucous membranes.

Astringents are substances which change the surface tension of body cells.

Emollients are oily substances which are soothing in action. They aid in the reduction of itching and pain and so help to increase healing.

Demulcents are similar preparations which are not oils but colloids.

Keratolytic agents are those that reduce or decrease the thickness of the horny layer of the skin.

Keratoplastic agents are those that increase the thickness of the horny layer of the skin.

Protectives are substances used to cover raw surfaces.

MAJOR SKIN DISEASES

Exfoliative Dermatitis

DEFINITION. Exfoliative dermatitis is a condition in which a great amount of the epidermis is shed (I-3). This condition is usually secondary to other diseases or follows the administration of certain toxic drugs. Exfoliative dermatitis is an acute, serious condition requiring immediate treatment.

MAJOR SYMPTOMS. Beginning with a patchy erythema, this gradually spreads to become universal. Scaling (fine or coarse) is present, and thickening of the skin soon develops. The skin is hot and dry, and the patient complains of chilliness (I-2). Scalp hair thins and the nails become dystrophic and may be shed. Itching may be prominent. The course is always protracted (V-1, 2; VI-1).

DRUG THERAPY. There are no specific remedies. The application of a vegetable grease is usually well tolerated. *Antihistaminic drugs* orally in full dosage are often helpful in controlling pruritus. *Starch* baths every other day may be tried and soap is contraindicated. Cool wet dressings of *aluminum acetate* 1:10 to 1:40 solution or 1 to 4 Domeboro tablets to a liter of water, *potassium permanganate* 0.1 Gm. per liter (1:10,000 solution) or cool water alone may be helpful in the relief of itching in the early, acute, "wet" stage. Baths with colloidal oatmeal (Aveeno) (1 cup to tub) or *potassium permanganate* (1 teaspoon of crystals to tub) may also be used. Some dermatologists use topical corticosteroid sprays, foams or lotions in the acute phase and creams and ointments in the drier stage. Systemic corticosteroids are used for devastating exfoliative dermatitis.

Erythema Multiforme

DEFINITION. This disease syndrome is manifested by the development of erythematous and edematous lesions. This condition may be acute or chronic, mild or severe, and recurrence is not uncommon. There are several types.

MAJOR SYMPTOMS. Itching is not usually present. Eosinophilia or purpura may be found. The even distribution of the lesions, often vesicobullous in type, with later drying and crusting, is the most outstanding symptom. A burning sensation is often present. Mucous membranes may be involved. Systemic symptoms include fever, malaise or arthritis or all.

DRUG THERAPY. The general drug intake of the patient should be checked as this may be the etiologic factor. The nurse may be able to aid the physician here since she may find out for the doctor what the patient is taking. Many people do not consider aspirin, cascara, the antihistamines or similar preparations as "drugs."

If there is a disturbance in the fluid and electrolyte balance as might occur after severe vomiting or diarrhea, it should be corrected as soon as possible.

Topical applications of *calamine,* 0.25 to 1.0 per cent *hydrocortisone lotion* or *fluocinolone acetonide cream* (Synalar) 0.01 to 0.025 per cent are often prescribed. Colloidal baths help some patients. Mild cases may be helped by a long-acting antihistamine orally.

If the disease is widespread and severe, one of the systemic steroids (often *prednisone,* 5 mg., or equivalent) is started with five to 12 tablets daily. Then this is decreased by one tablet every two days over a ten day period. If this severe condition persists, the steroid is given every other day to lessen pituitary depression.

For the burning sensation *brompheniramine maleate*, N.F. (parabromdylamine [C]) (Dimetane) 4 to 12 mg. or *diphenhydramine*, U.S.P. (Benadryl) 50 to 100 mg. every six hours may be given.

One of the broad-spectrum antibiotics such as *tetracycline* or *erythromycin* or equivalent is used if the disease is suspected to be of bacterial origin.

A mouthwash with warm water helps relieve the bothersome mouth lesions.

Psoriasis

DEFINITION. Psoriasis is a chronic, nonscarring skin disorder which most frequently affects the scalp, face, elbows and knees, but all parts of the body may be involved.

MAJOR SYMPTOMS. Psoriasis is characterized by "silver scaling" of the epidermis, with fine bleeding after the peeling and healing without scarring (I-3). The affected areas are very unattractive, even repulsive at times (V-2).

Psoriasis is apt to be most severe during puberty and adolescence and again during the climacteric. The condition is also usually more severe in the winter months. There is some indication that the disorder may have certain allergic or glandular relationships, but the exact cause of the disease is unknown.

DRUG THERAPY. Each individual varies in his response to treatment. What helps one may not help another; those medications which are useful once may not produce any effect another time. Severe attacks can usually be controlled, but relapses are the rule (V-1). Drugs are used both locally and systemically.

LOCAL TREATMENT

THE DRUGS. When there are a moderate number of lesions, a keratolytic drug may be used in gradually ascending concentrations. Some dermatologists use a combination of 3 per cent *salicylic acid* and 5 per cent *liquor carbonis detergens* (tar) in an ointment base, gradually increasing the percentage as tolerance is established. This ointment is applied several times a day. Coal tar preparations are messy, have an objectionable odor and stain the skin and clothing.

Some good results may be obtained if after an overnight application of distilled *tar* in an ointment base, the affected skin is irradiated with ultraviolet rays.

Good results have been obtained in many cases by using the surface depot method of administration of corticosteroid creams. The cream is spread over the surface of the lesion and covered with pliable plastic or polyethylene film (plastic wrap, such as that used in the kitchen, will suffice) taped around the edges. It remains in place for several hours, often overnight. If folliculitis or other heat retention phenomenon occurs, the treatment should be stopped. Drugs which have proved effective include *fluocinolone acetonide* (Synalar) 0.01 per cent, *flurandrenolone* (Cordran) 0.025 per cent and *triamcinolone acetonide* (Kenalog or Aristocort) 0.025 to 0.1 per cent. Many lesions can be cleared within 10 to 12 days' treatment, but periodic retreatment is usually necessary.

Anthralin 0.1 per cent with salicylic acid 0.4 per cent in Lassar's paste may be used topically. Five to 10 per cent paraffin may be added to form a firmer mixture. The paste is applied generously to the lesions, not the uninvolved skin. Stockinette used for the extremities and cotton underwear will minimize the staining of the clothing. The paste is left on for 24 hours. Then the patient is bathed and the lesions are exposed to ultraviolet light. A course of three weeks is recommended. The anthralin concentration may be increased at weekly intervals to a maximum of 0.3 to 0.6 per cent. This preparation will stain the skin, but only temporarily.

SCALP PSORIASIS. The scales on the scalp may be softened with a vegetable oil which is massaged into the scalp and covered with a warm towel for 30 minutes or with a soft head covering which is left on overnight. The hair is then washed with a psoriatic shampoo (there are a number of these on the market). If the medicated shampoo leaves an odor, the hair may be washed again with a mild shampoo.

PSORIASIS OF THE NAILS. Psoriasis of the nails is very resistant to treatment. Any crumbling material or debris should be removed and a topical corticosteroid cream applied into the nail fold and occluded for several hours. This should be done every two or three days for as long as three months. A finger cot makes a good occlusive bandage. This is often done at night and left on overnight.

In all instances, scales should be removed before the topical application is used.

Preparations containing hydrocortisone should not be used on infected areas unless a suitable specific antibiotic or chemotherapeutic agent is given concomitantly. Coal tar extracts are contraindicated in infected or impetiginized lesions. The nurse must be aware that prolonged use of coal tar may cause irritation of the skin.

There are no restrictions on bathing or use of soap for psoriatic patients. In fact, it does help remove scales. Alcohol rubs and the application of astringents should be used with caution as they may produce much irritation in patients with generalized erythroderma and when the lesions are fissured or crusted.

EXTENSIVE PSORIASIS. If at all possible the patient with widespread psoriasis should be hospitalized. The treatment follows much the same regimen as for localized lesions. The patient is given a warm bath to which is added about 30 ml. of a tar preparation or liquor carbonis detergens. The scalp is shampooed daily as stated previously. The lesions are exposed to ultraviolet radiation after the bath. A 1 per cent crude tar and 2 per cent salicylic acid in petrolatum is massaged into all lesions except those on the face or in the axillae and groin. This is done every two hours and at bedtime. The face and intertriginous areas are treated with a corticosteroid cream, also every two hours.

SYSTEMIC TREATMENT

THE DRUGS. Mild sedation may be required, usually phenobarbital 15 mg. three times a day is sufficient. If insomnia is a complication a hypnotic may be used or the last dose of the phenobarbital increased. Tranquilizers are not usually required, but may be of value in some cases.

Treatment by systemic therapy has not proved universally effective. *Vitamin A* orally 50,000 to 100,000 units daily will almost always reduce the amount of scaling. If this helps it should be given for three out of every four weeks indefinitely. Liquid potassium arsenite (*Fowler's solution*), 1 drop three times a day after meals increasing 1 drop each week and ending after four to six weeks, has aided some people. *Antihistamines* are helpful if itching is a problem.

Oral corticosteroids are used only in very severe conditions. Their withdrawal is difficult and often results in a relapse. Inveterate solitary lesions respond to intralesional injection with *triamcinolone* suspension. Improvement is usually noted within a week.

Methotrexate may be useful. It is given 15 to 50 mg. weekly or biweekly. It may control resistant lesions. This antimetabolite is a potent folic acid antagonist and its action in psoriasis is not yet well understood. It should not be given during the child-bearing years, during pregnancy or when there is a history of a peptic ulcer. This drug is used cautiously, if at all, for children or the older patient. When the drug is used frequent blood count, urinalysis and liver function tests should be done.

THE NURSE. The nurse will usually see the patient with psoriasis only during the acute stage, and she will be very busy trying to take care of the immediate situations as they occur. The local medications must be applied regularly and often. The systemic drugs are also given regularly. During the administration of the medicines the nurse should take the opportunity to teach the patient to care for himself. She should explain how the drugs help and how they are used, especially the local ones and those systemic drugs which may be continued after the patient has been dismissed from the hospital for home care. The nurse should shield the patient from other patients and from "inquiring" visitors (V-2).

When the isolated lesions are injected, very strict aseptic technique must be observed. The same area must not be reinjected for several weeks or atrophy may result.

THE PATIENT. The patient with psoriasis is faced with a severe emotional problem. The condition is likely to affect more or less widespread areas of his body for the rest of his life. If the individual is an adolescent, and this is the usual time for the first appearance, the social and psychologic impact is great (V-1, 2). No one wants to be "ugly," and the lesions of psoriasis are anything but pretty. If on the exposed portions of the body, they cannot very well be covered, and uninformed people may shun the afflicted person as if he had a communicable disease (VI-1). The nurse can help the patient by showing him ways to cover the lesions, explaining to visitors and relatives that the disease cannot be transmitted and encouraging the patient to keep up the treatments which usually control even if they do not cure the disorder. If the physician approves, the nurse may tell the patient of some of the cosmetics which will cover the lesions. These preparations should be used only when it is essential to do so.

Herpes Zoster

DEFINITION. Herpes zoster, or shingles, is a virus infection of the sensory ganglia of the spinal cord (III-1). Postherpetic neuralgia often occurs following the acute attack, especially in the older patient. Strictly speaking, herpes zoster is not a skin disease, but it is usually discussed under that heading since its main manifestation is a skin rash.

MAJOR SYMPTOMS. Herpes zoster is manifested by a vesicular rash along the course of the nerve or nerves involved, especially along the nerve fibers which end in the skin. This is a very painful condition. The pain follows the course of the nerve, and the patient will complain of a burning, stinging sensation as well as actual pain. The rash is raised, red, tender to touch and has many small vesicles. In postherpetic neuralgia, there are recurring attacks of burning and pain along the course of the nerve.

DRUG THERAPY

LOCAL APPLICATIONS. During the acute phase, cooling and antiseptic lotions such as 0.25 per cent *phenol*, 0.1 to 2 per cent *menthol in Acid Mantle* (Dome), *Lubriderm lotion* or *calamine* and *neocalamine lotion* every two to three hours may be helpful. Some dermatologists add *iodochlorhydroxyquin* (Vioform) 3 per cent to prevent secondary infections. *Hydrocortisone* 0.5 per cent may also be added for its antipruritic and anti-inflammatory effects.

When applying any of these topical applications, the area should be left uncovered, if possible. If, because of the location of the eruption, it must be covered, a smooth cloth should be used, since any rough material will add to the patient's discomfort. Silk, rayon, nylon or similar cloth is best. The part should be kept warm, but not hot, as extremes of temperature increase the pain.

Those who are afflicted with herpes zoster should understand the nature of the disease and that they will have pain. They should understand the reason for all treatments. Since the rash is the part of the disease that "shows," the patient will be most concerned about it. The nurse may explain to the patient that it is the external evidence of an internal disorder and that, as soon as the internal condition improves, the external disorder will clear. She may explain that the local treatment is helpful mainly because it aids in the control of pain and in drying the vesicles.

SYSTEMIC DRUGS. To relieve pain and discomfort, analgesics are needed. In the milder forms, aspirin, 0.3 to 0.6 Gm. every three hours, may suffice. *Propoxyphene* (Darvon), 30 to 65 mg., or *codeine*, 30 mg. every three to four hours, may be needed to control the severe pain some patients have. Occasionally, *meperidine* (pethidine [C]) or *morphine* may be necessary. Sedation is usually needed for sleep and *chloral hydrate*, 0.5 to 1.0 Gm. or *secobarbital* (Seconal; quinalbarbitone [C]), 0.1 Gm. is often used.

Cyanocobalamin (vitamin B_{12}), in doses of 300 micrograms intramuscularly daily for three to five days, helps prevent postherpetic neuralgia and reduce pain in some patients. This also seems to aid in the re-establishment of nerve function.

The systemic steroids ordinarily are not used in the first seven days of the eruption but may be useful for postherpetic neuralgia. *Corticotropin* gel intramuscularly usually is given in 40 unit doses on three to four consecutive days or every other day for one to two weeks. Should this drug be used, the usual precautions are necessary and the patient must be observed closely for untoward effects. See Rheumatoid Arthritis for more details.

The antibiotics are useful if secondary infection occurs.

Acne Vulgaris

DEFINITION. Acne vulgaris is a slowly progressive infection of the skin, usually of the face, which is most prevalent in the adolescent and young adult. The basic cause is unknown, but may be endocrinologic. It is especially resistant to treatment.

MAJOR SYMPTOMS. The most prominent symptom of acne is the pimple, which may or may not suppurate. The lesions often last for several days and when they heal often leave discoloration and pitting of the skin. The pitting may produce a permanent scar.

DRUG THERAPY. The choice of treatment depends in part on the extent and severity of involvement and the age and sex of the patient. Both systemic and topical treatments are usually employed.

TOPICAL TREATMENT. The topical therapy is designed to keep the skin dry, the pores open and the skin as free of bacteria as possible. Antiseptic soaps and mildly abrasive soaps such as Lava, Dial, Palmolive Gold and the like may be used. Some physicians prefer to use preparations such as Fostex soap or Acme-Dome brasivol as a cleanser. Cosmetics, especially creams, are to be avoided. Hair should be shampooed at least twice a week. There are many topical drugs that may be employed. Those containing sulfur seem to be more effective than others. However, saturated lotio alba (white lotion) is still an effective agent as are preparations containing retinoic acid or benzoyl peroxide. There are also compounds containing antibiotics such as neomycin, bacitracin, polymyxin B. The list of topical drugs is almost limitless. Some contain only one, but by far the majority contain several, active ingredients. Once or twice a week, the doctor may order hot compresses of well diluted sulfurated lime (Vleminckx' solution). When this is used, the eyelids and lips should be protected by a heavy layer of petroleum jelly. The diluted solution (the strength depending upon the individual order) is heated and kept hot, but not hot enough to burn. The compresses are changed every minute for about twenty minutes.

SYSTEMIC TREATMENT. One of the most effective medications is tetracycline which is usually given orally 250 mg. twice daily for as long as required. Most doctors also prescribe a vitamin compound, since many of these young patients do not eat a well rounded diet. Sometimes the diet is restricted, omitting such foods as chocolates, nuts and some fats. However, many doctors feel that the diet has little to do with the condition. Hormones may be prescribed. The most helpful appears to be estrogen or an oral contraceptive agent given to the female patient whose acne is worse at the time of menstruation. The corticosteroids are usually reserved for the severe case that does not respond to more conservative treatment.

Ultraviolet light and/or x-ray may be used, but they are supplemental to other therapy. These should be used only by a competent therapist. The patient should not try to treat himself with ultraviolet lights or sunlamps.

Most acne patients are not hospitalized, but the office nurse, the school nurse and other nurses dealing with outpatients will see a great deal of the condition. The most important point for the nurse is to aid these young people to understand the "why" of their diet and treatment and to show them how to apply or take the prescribed medicines. The nurse should explain the reasons for taking the drugs and how to use them properly.

Acne produces a severe emotional strain on the patient since the lesions are often very disfiguring at a time in life when the individual most wants to be attractive (V-2). It is of little help, and not too scientifically accurate, to tell these young people that the condition will clear automatically in a few years. Many cases will, but that does not aid the afflicted person. Instead of giving false hopes of spontaneous cures, the patient should be encouraged to persist in the treatment and the diet prescribed, as most cases can be materially helped, even though not entirely cured, by careful following of orders. The patient should understand that the disease is apt to be chronic and that he should not hope for an immediate cure.

Ulcers (Stasis and Decubitus)

DEFINITION. An ulcer is a break in the continuity of the tissues, occurring upon the surface of the skin or mucous membranes, resulting from necrosis of the tissue and loss of the covering epithelium (I-2, 3). The most common skin ulcers are those due to the disturbance of circulation, such as the decubitus ulcer (bedsore) from pressure and varicose ulcers from impaired venous drainage. Ulcers may be superficial, with only the upper layers of the skin denuded, or they may be deep, with necrosis of underlying structures.

MAJOR SYMPTOMS. The symptoms of an ulcer are those of a sore (usually oozing), sometimes, especially if secondarily infected, with pus formation. Ulcers are painful and tend to be chronic and difficult to heal. Deep ulcers will present the symptoms associated with any severe wound.

DRUG THERAPY. The treatment of ulcers varies widely according to the etiology, extent and other factors. There are, however, a few general methods used. Most physicians first try to remove the cause of the ulcer, and this process may or may not be medical. After the cause has been removed, actual healing of the ulcer becomes the major problem. Obviously, treatment will depend upon the depth of the ulcer and the structures involved. The most common process is to do a surgical excision first, if possible, or a surgical or biologic debridement if excision is not considered advisable. Only biologic debridement is medical.

Biologic debridement involves the use of one of the digestive enzymes. Various preparations are available to the physician such as *sutilains* (Travase), *fibrinolysin-desoxyribonuclease* (Elase), *streptokinase-streptodornase* (Varidase) and *collagenase* (Santyl). The enzymes are usually applied directly to the ulcer in strength and for the length of time desired, according to the specific conditions encountered. The type of preparations used, the depth of the wound and the amount of the necrotic tissue to be removed are the deciding factors. When debridement has been accomplished, any number of healing preparations can be used. Among such preparations are *scarlet red ointment, cod liver oil ointment,* or *vitamin A and D ointment* (the last two are practically the same). Other medicines which may be used are *compound tincture of benzoin, balsam of Peru, bismuth* and *oil.* The purpose of all these drugs is to cover the raw surface and to promote healing by stimulating cell growth. Any of these drugs may be used without debridement, especially on small or entirely superficial ulcers. The *corticosteroid creams* are useful also.

In many ways the most important duty of the nurse is to aid in the prevention of the ulcer. This is especially true of the decubitus ulcer (bedsore) or of ulcers caused by the pressure of orthopedic appliances. When the ulcer has occurred, the nurse must be very careful to see that the area is kept dry and clean and that the drugs ordered are applied exactly as the physician has directed.

The patient will need assurance that the ulcer can be healed and that, by proper care, other ulcers can be prevented. The changing of the dressings may be very painful, and the nurse should do everything possible to keep this pain to a minimum.

LUPUS ERYTHEMATOSUS

Discoid Lupus Erythematosus

DEFINITION. Lupus erythematosus is usually divided into two conditions, the chronic discoid type, which is primarily a skin disease, and the disseminated or systemic type which may affect any organ or many organs of the body. The types sometimes coexist; the discoid may evolve into the disseminated type, or they may be distinct. The former are the more common.

MAJOR SYMPTOMS. Discoid type. Lupus erythematosus is characterized by persistent localized erythema, scales, telangiectasis, follicular plugs and atrophy usually with scarring. It most commonly affects the exposed portions of the body, but may occur in other areas. Chief symptoms include rash, itching, scarring and loss of hair over scarred areas. It is adversely affected by sunlight, natural or artificial.

DRUG THERAPY

LOCAL TREATMENT. The local treatment consists of prevention of exposure of the lesions to sunlight or any form of radiation. When the patient goes out into sunlight, lesions on the face may be protected by a broad brimmed hat; those on the hands may be shielded by gloves. This may be sufficient, especially if exposure is to be of short duration, less than a half hour. There are commercial preparations that can be applied to cover the lesions, with the physician's permission. Since the lesions are often unsightly, the same preparations may be used for social occasions as well. Medical therapy consists of the application of corticosteroid creams. The cream may be covered with a thin plastic covering taped around the edges. This is especially helpful at night. The physician may inject the lesions with one of the steroid compounds. Cosmetics are usually contraindicated.

SYSTEMIC TREATMENT. Medicines, exclusive of those used as therapy, are to be avoided as much as possible, since some drugs appear to intensify the trouble. Drugs are given systemically only if the local treatment is ineffective. The antimalarial drugs are used most frequently. *Hydroxychloroquine* (Plaquenil) 200 mg., is often given three times a day for one or two weeks, gradually decreasing until the patient is taking 200 mg. once daily or every other day. There is also a triple preparation containing *atabrine* 25 mg., *chloroquine* 65 mg. and *hydroxychloroquine* 50 mg. One tablet is given on the same regimen as the single drug.

Systemic Lupus Erythematosus

MAJOR SYMPTOMS. Since systemic lupus may involve almost any organ or organs, symptoms are highly variable. However, weakness, malaise, weight loss, musculoskeletal pain and fever are common.

DRUG THERAPY. The *salicylates* (aspirin or sodium salicylate) sometimes help. Their use here is the same as in rheumatoid arthritis. (See Chapter 21.) The *antimalarial* drugs are used as with the discoid type mentioned earlier.

Seriously ill patients are treated with the *corticosteroids.* The dose may be well above the average adult dose. As much as 120 mg. daily of *prednisone* may be given. The patient must be carefully watched for toxic symptoms. (See Chapter 27 and Current Drug Handbook.) If mental aberrations occur, it must be remembered that this can be either a result of the disease or a toxic reaction to the drug.

The immunosuppressive drug, *azathioprine,* the antimetabolite, *6-mercaptopurine,* the alkylating agent, *nitrogen mustard* and *cyclophosphamide* may be tried. However, the use of these drugs is experimental for this disease. Results are inconclusive.

OTHER DRUGS OCCASIONALLY USED FOR LUPUS ERYTHEMATOSUS. The heavy metals such as *bismuth subsalicylate* or *gold sodium thiosulfate* have been tried with varying success. Crude *liver extract* seems to help some patients, as does *Vitamin A.* It is not particularly clear why any of these drugs help.

THE NURSE. Although hydroxychloroquine (Plaquenil) is considered to be less toxic than the parent drug—chloroquine (Aralen)—it is still not without possible side effects, especially in long-term use in such diseases as lupus erythematosus. Some of the side effects the nurse should be alert for are gastrointestinal disturbances (these may be minimized by giving the drug with food), visual difficulties (regular ophthalmological examinations are important), pruritus, headache and psychic stimulation. Since the adverse symptoms are dose related, the nurse will need to discuss this with the physician if side effects become distressing.

Side effects of corticosteroid therapy are discussed in Chapter 27. The antimetabolite preparations are discussed in Chapter 30.

Lupus erythematosus is a very discouraging disease and the patients become very depressed. The nurse must try to understand the value of continued therapy. Although cure is not the rule, prolongation of a useful life is usually possible if the treatment regimen is followed.

The family may need counseling as to their role in the much-needed care and support of the patient.

THE PATIENT. The patient with lupus erythematosus should be taught why he should not use a sunlamp or sun-bathe. He need not be made a "sun cripple," but should be warned that excessive exposure to the rays of the sun or a sun lamp will adversely affect his condition. If drugs are to be taken at home, the patient must know the undesirable side effects which may occur. He must know to stop the drug and to contact his doctor if these side effects occur.

The patient and his family should be reminded that these medications, like any other drug, should be kept out of the reach of children.

These patients should avoid excessive fatigue because it tends to activate the disease. Since this is a chronic condition, the nurse should do everything in her power to help the patient to adjust to his condition and to encourage him to continue treatment, even though it may not seem to be effective.

He should understand why he has to have periodic blood counts and examinations by his physician.

This is a very discouraging disease and the patient is prone to be depressed. It is wise for his family and friends to understand just why the patient is anxious and depressed and to help him in as many ways as they can.

VIRAL INFECTIONS OF THE SKIN

Herpes Simplex

DEFINITION. Herpes simplex is a viral infection of the skin and mucous membranes occurring most frequently on or around the lips and nares. It may occur spontaneously or may accompany certain diseases, usually those which are febrile in nature. Some patients are especially prone to the infection, and there appears to be a tendency to a breakdown rather than an upbuilding of immunity so that the person who has had herpes simplex is more apt to have it again than one who has never had the disorder. The infection is commonly referred to as a fever blister or cold sore.

MAJOR SYMPTOMS. Multiple small vesicles which tend to coalesce are the predominant symptoms of the condition. The vesicles often become pustules which later crust and crack. Herpes is a very painful disorder. A burning sensation often accompanies development of blisters. Predisposing factors include fever, gastrointestinal upsets, sunburn, and mechanical irritation.

DRUG THERAPY. There is no specific treatment for herpes simplex, but antibiotic or steroid ointments may be used, especially if the condition is severe.

Many topical preparations, especially those which form a covering or are drying in nature are helpful. Such medications as compound tincture of *benzoin, camphor-ice* and various commercial products for "chapped lips" may be used. These tend to allay the pain and prevent crusting and cracking.

A synthetic antiviral agent which is used for ocular lesions of herpes simplex is *idoxuridine* (IDU). Optimal results seem to be obtained when one drop is instilled in the infected eye every hour. During sleeping hours, it can be reduced to one drop every other hour, or the ointment may be used every two hours, and therapy should be continued for three days after the lesion heals.

BACTERIAL DISEASES OF THE SKIN

Impetigo Contagiosa

DEFINITION. Impetigo contagiosa is a streptococcal or staphylococcal infection of the superficial layers of the skin (III-1).

MAJOR SYMPTOMS. The disease manifests itself in a crusty, exudative series of sores, often on the face, especially around the mouth, but which may occur on any skin surface. The lesions are superficial and usually with an adherent, light brownish-yellow crust surrounded by erythema. The disease is autoinoculable and quickly spreads. It is often epidemic among children. Constitutional symptoms are rare; no immunity is conferred by an attack.

DRUG THERAPY. A form of isolation should be imposed on the patient for there is danger of transmission of the disease as long as any crusts remain. The infected individual should not use anyone else's towels, dishes, clothing or toys (with children).

Systemic antibiotics are used to treat impetigo. *Penicillin* is the drug of choice, but *erythromycin* or one of the *tetracyclines* may be substituted for the penicillin, especially in patients sensitive to penicillin.

Locally, various baths and/or compresses may be used. Some physicians use local medications after all crusts have been removed. Drugs used include *ammoniated mercury, gentian violet, chlorquinaldol* (Sterosan, Dermaspred-Q [C]) or an antibiotic ointment may be used.

Bacterial Pyodermas

DEFINITION. Since most of the pyodermic infections are treated medicinally in the same manner, they can be discussed together. The pyodermas (pus-forming infections) here include folliculitis, an inflammation of the hair follicle which may be either streptococcal or staphylococcal; furunculosis, or boils, usually staphylococcic; carbunculosis, similar to furunculosis but extending over a much larger area; paronychia, an infection around the nail, usually a staphylococcic infection, but sometimes streptococcic.

MAJOR SYMPTOMS. The symptoms of these conditions vary somewhat with the area involved, but all are those of acute inflammation; redness, heat, pain, swelling and complete or partial loss of function.

DRUG THERAPY. Treatment of the pyodermic infections is both local and systemic. *Penicillin, ampicillin, erythromycin* or one of the *tetracyclines* is usually given systemically. The usual doses apply. The topical antibiotics such as *bacitracin, neomycin,* or *gentamycin* are used locally.

The pyogenic skin infections are also treated by x-ray locally, and by either stock or autogenous vaccines. The vaccines are especially valuable for those patients who have repeated attacks of the same type of infection.

If the oral penicillin G is prescribed, it should be taken on an empty stomach.

The nurse has the responsibility to see that isolation practices are enforced when caring for these patients and this should be continued until the crusted or open lesions are resolved.

Fungal Infections of the Skin

DERMATOPHYTOSIS

DEFINITION. Dermatophytosis (athlete's foot) is a fungus infection of the feet and hands usually beginning as an invasion of the toe web and later often spreading to soles, groin, hands and nails.

MAJOR SYMPTOMS. This condition begins as an interdigital maceration and scaling. There may be considerable erythema, vesiculation and soreness followed by fissuring of the skin.

DRUG THERAPY

TOPICAL APPLICATIONS. When the infection is not severe and is confined to the toes, 3 per cent *salicylic acid* in alcohol at bedtime applied to the infected area and a 10 per cent *boric acid* foot powder in the morning often suffice. If there is considerable inflammation, the doctor may order the feet soaked in *potassium permanganate* 1:8000 for 30 minutes in the morning and afternoon. The highly inflamed cases may be treated by painting with 1 per cent *gentian violet* in water. *Whitfield's ointment* is an old remedy still useful in some cases.

After the condition has been cleared, it is advisable for the patient to use a foot powder daily to prevent recurrences. Often prescribed are salts of *propionic* and *caprylic acids* (Anafung or Sopronol) and *undecylenic acid* and *zinc undecylenate* (Desenex). The chronic form of this disease responds very poorly to treatment and cure is extremely difficult.

The nurse must take care to secure the exact strength ordered and prevent staining of articles of bedding and clothing when gentian violet or potassium permanganate is used.

The nurse should show these patients how to prevent a recurrence of the condition. The feet should be thoroughly washed at least once each day, taking special care not to break the skin by excessive rubbing with rough towels or washcloths. The feet should be carefully dried and, as an additional aid to the control of the condition, various antiseptic and drying powders may be applied. These powders are also put into the shoes. Hose should be changed daily, and shoes rotated so that one pair is not worn continuously. These things will aid in controlling perspiration, which seems to increase the tendency for the condition to reappear after apparent recovery. No drug treatment will be effective if there are no general remedial procedures accompanying its use. Only in the acute stage will the patient be under the direct care of the nurse, but she should give the patient directions for applying the drugs prescribed for use at home.

The nurse should explain to the patient that though the condition is infectious and chronic it can be controlled. He should not walk barefooted at all, not even at home, lest some member of his family do the same thing and acquire the fungus from the carpet, rug or other floor covering. The fungus may remain viable in a dry state away from the body for many weeks or months. After the patient takes a bath or shower, the tub should be thoroughly washed with a disinfectant before being used by others.

Since potassium permanganate stains the skin a dirty brown, the patient should be assured that this stain is not permanent. On unaffected areas, the stain may be removed by the use of a weak acid such as lemon juice or vinegar. No attempt should be made to remove the stain on affected parts since the acid may be harmful.

The Patient. The patient with dermatophytosis should be assured that if he follows the rules given to him by the physician, the condition will neither bother him nor be transferred to those about him. The fact that the condition tends to last a long time and to recur should be explained so that the patient is not under any misapprehension. He should be on the lookout for the very first sign of a reappearance so that treatment can be instituted quickly to prevent a severe relapse.

Dermatophytosis tends to recur in warm weather and at any time the feet become warm enough to perspire. The use of rubber boots, especially in the summer, is to be avoided.

Systemic Treatment. In the last few years, there have been developed several antibiotics which can be given orally to help eradicate fungus infections. One such drug when taken internally prevents the fungus from burrowing into the skin's outer keratin layers. As the new skin cells form and move to the surface, the infected cells are shoved outward, taking the infection with them. *Griseofulvin* (Fulvicin, Grifulvin; Grisovia [C]); and the microcrystalline forms, Fulvicin UF, Grifulvin V and Grisactin are in this group. They have proved moderately effective in "athlete's foot" but best results are obtained when the infection is treated concomitantly with topical therapy. The microcrystalline forms are more effective and are used more frequently. The usual dose is 0.5 Gm. daily in two to four divided doses, from four weeks to several months.

Severe side effects from these drugs are infrequent. However, some patients complain of a severe headache but this disappears after a week or two even though the drug is continued. Other side effects which may be noted are epigastric distress, heartburn, nausea, diarrhea, abdominal cramps, breathlessness, neuritic pain, vertigo, fever, insomnia and urticaria.

To raise blood and skin levels of the drug even further, sometimes the drug is given right after the patient has eaten a meal rich in fats, for the drug is soluble in lipids.

RINGWORM (TINEA CIRCINATA AND OTHER FORMS)

DEFINITION. Ringworm is a fungal infection of the skin which may affect any portion of the body but is most commonly found on the scalp, face and trunk.

MAJOR SYMPTOMS. Ringworm is characterized by the formation of a rough scaly area, usually circular in form, which spreads peripherally with clearing in the center. It is itchy, but not so much so as many other skin disorders.

DRUG THERAPY. Most ringworm on the body (Tinea corporis) responds well to the application of 5 per cent *ammoniated mercury, sulfur, iodine, thymol, undecylenic acid, salicylanilide* or *Whitfield's ointment* one-fourth to one-half strength. The area should be painted about one inch around the actual lesion as well as the area of involvement since the fungus grows in a circular form, spreading in a ring. Tinea corporis is not usually treated with griseofulvin unless topical applications fail.

The Nurse. Ringworm of the scalp, tinea capitis, responds rapidly to *griseofulvin* with relief from itching in a few days. (See Dermatophytosis for details of action.) Other objective signs of improvement are subsidence of erythema and scaling and loosening of infected hairs within two weeks of starting therapy. Some dermatologists believe it helpful to clip the hair at weekly intervals, use a protective cap and remove scales and crusts with keratolytic agents and shampoos, but others do not believe topical antifungal therapy is needed.

Tinea unguium (onychomycosis) affects the nails and responds slowly to griseofulvin. The faster a nail is replaced, the more amenable it is to this type of treatment. Fingernails grow much more rapidly than do toenails. The antibiotic is deposited in the matrix of the nail, and by its fungistatic action the keratinized nail is replaced gradually by noninfected tissue.

The dose of griseofulvin for adults is the same as in dermatophytosis (0.5 Gm. daily in two to four divided doses). For children, the dose is calculated on 10 mg. per kilogram (5 mg. per pound) of body weight per day, given as a single dose or in divided doses.

The Patient. In all cases, the drug is continued until the causative fungus has been eliminated by natural exfoliation of skin or by clipping infected portions of hair or nails. The average time required is four to eight weeks in tinea capitis, with the return of normal hair growth, four weeks in tinea corporis, four to five months for tinea unguium of fingernails and six months to a year for tinea unguium of the toenails.

For most fungal infections of the skin, *tolnaftate* (Tinactin) is often used. The drug comes as a solution, ointment or powder. The drug is gently massaged into the affected areas twice daily for two to three weeks. If the condition is not relieved, the physician may order a second course of the same length. It may be continued for as long as six weeks. The medicine appears to be relatively nontoxic. However in some cases it is ineffective. If this happens the drug is discontinued. It is not effective against *Candida albicans (Monilia). Nystatin* (Mycostatin) ointment may be used for the monilial infections.

SKIN INFESTATIONS WITH HIGHER ORGANISMS

There are two common skin infestations: scabies and pediculosis. Both of these are caused by higher organisms, though the *Sarcoptes scabiei* is barely macroscopic. However, under low-power microscopic examination, its animal characteristics are clearly visible. Pediculi (lice) are, of course, easily seen without magnification.

Scabies

DEFINITION. Scabies (seven years' itch) is an infestation of the skin by the *Sarcoptes scabiei*. It has world-wide distribution. It does not, as the name implies, last seven years, but it is very persistent and can be of relatively long duration unless the patient is properly treated and his clothing properly cleaned as well. Reinfection from contaminated clothing is not uncommon.

MAJOR SYMPTOMS. First noted are reddened areas with minute dark spots which are very itchy. Signs of scratching are usually apparent. The disease affects mainly the folds of the body, between the fingers and the toes. It is rarely seen on the face. It is typically symmetrically distributed.

DRUG THERAPY. Several drugs have been found effective in treating scabies but little is accomplished unless all infested members of the family are treated at the same time. Those drugs recommended are *sulfur, benzyl benzoate* (Albacide, Benylate), *crotamiton* (Eurax) and *gamma benzene hexachloride* (Gexane, Kwell, Kwelada [C]) in the form of ointments or liquids. There are several commercial preparations available for the treatment of scabies, but they usually contain one of these chemicals.

The Nurse. Gamma benzene hexachloride is commonly used in the treatment of scabies and pediculosis. In the latter disorder, it is used to kill the nits (eggs) as well as the adult forms. The drug is irritating to the eyes, mucosa and sometimes the skin. If the skin becomes irritated, the drug should be stopped. Any portion on the skin should be thoroughly washed off and another drug substituted. It should not be applied near the eyes or any body opening lined with mucous membranes (nose, mouth). Gamma benzene hexachloride is applied to the entire body, except the face. It comes in a cream or lotion 1 per cent (20 to 30 Gm. is usually required). The medication is left on for 24 hours and then removed by a warm bath. Treatment is usually repeated in 8 days. For pediculosis capitis, the hair and scalp are moistened with water. The drug (15 per cent solution) is worked into the hair and left for five minutes. The hair is then rinsed thoroughly. This may be repeated in 4 days.

Care of clothing, bedding, towels, combs and so forth by washing or dry cleaning—as indicated by the material—is most important.

The Patient. The patient suffering from scabies is very uncomfortable, and the treatments, no matter what drug is used, are apt to be arduous. Every possible means of allaying the patient's distress must be used. He must be encouraged to undergo the needed treatment and assured that the treatment will be effective. Protection of friends, relatives and, if in the hospital, other patients must be maintained and the need for this explained to the patient.

Pediculosis

DEFINITION. Pediculi (lice) may infest the body (pediculosis corporis), the pubic area (pediculosis pubis) or the head (pediculosis capitis). The pubic louse may also infest the axillary region. The organisms are similar but are not identical.

Body Lice and Pubic Lice. In order to kill body and pubic lice, the hairy areas may be shaved preliminary to treatment and the patient given a cleansing bath. All clothing should be washed or cleaned to destroy the organisms. Sometimes the clothing is sprayed with *pyrethrum, rotenone, naphthalene* or *gamma benzene hexachloride*. These procedures may be sufficient to get rid of the lice. However, if this does not accomplish the desired results, *sulfur, creosote* or *iodoform* ointment may be used.

For body or pubic pediculi, *gamma benzene hexachloride* is usually the drug of choice. A warm soap and water bath is given utilizing a soft brush. After thorough drying, the drug is applied directly to the skin in concentrations up to 1 per cent. It is not applied to the face. If the scalp is involved gamma benzene hexachloride (*Kwell shampoo*) is used. Care must be taken to avoid contact of the drug with the eyes or mucous membranes. Twelve hours later a second application is made. At the end of 24 hours a second bath is taken and clean clothes are donned. After another 24 hours the process is repeated. This is usually sufficient to complete the removal of the organisms.

When the body lice affect a large group of people, a "delousing" house may be set up. The people are passed through the house in sequence. In the first room the individual is stripped and his clothing taken into another room and sprayed. The patient is then taken into a second room where a shower bath is given. He goes to a third room where either the freshly sprayed or clean clothing is put on. He is then released. With a regular staff of attendants, a large number of people can be treated in a relatively short time. This procedure is usually used to prevent the spread of louse-borne diseases such as typhus fever. Sometimes, when very large numbers of people are involved, the spraying of the individual and his clothing is done in one procedure, and only those known to be actually infested are given the aforementioned extra treatment.

Head Lice. Pediculosis capitis (head lice) is by far the most common form of lice infestation in this country. Children are most frequently affected.

The treatment of head lice is somewhat different from that of the body lice since it is not practical to shave the head, and the hats and hair utensils would be the only items needing delousing.

DRUG THERAPY. Several drugs are used to kill head lice, such as *larkspur, petroleum* products, *benzyl benzoate, gamma benzene hexachloride* (Gexane, Kwell), *isobornyl thiocyanoacetate-technical* (Bornate) and *xylene ointment* 10 per cent. All of these preparations, and many more, have been found effective. At present gamma benzene hexachloride (Kwell) shampoo is the preparation most often used for pediculosis capitis. One treatment is usually sufficient, but it may be repeated in one week if needed. Specific directions come with each product and these should be carefully followed. If any of the petroleum products are used, they should be mixed with oil lest they burn the scalp.

If a dermatitis is present, soothing ointments such as 10 per cent zinc oxide or neocalamine lotion may be applied.

The Nurse. The usual procedure for the treatment of head lice is first to wash the hair with a mild soap or shampoo, dry, and then apply the drug ordered, unless gamma benzene hexachloride (Kwell) shampoo has been used in washing the hair. The head is then wrapped in a clean cloth and left for the time limit of the preparation being used. Larkspur is usually left on about 12 hours or overnight. After the required time has elapsed, the hair is again washed, and vinegar is put into the rinse water, which should be warm. The warm vinegar solution will dissolve the nits (eggs) and prevent recurrence. Fine combing the hair will remove the dead lice and nits, if the washing has failed to remove them completely. One treatment is usually sufficient, but in some cases the treatment will have to be repeated.

When isobornyl thiocyanoacetate-technical is used, about 30 to 60 ml. (cc.) is applied to the hair and worked into a lather and allowed to remain for ten minutes. The hair is combed with a fine-tooth comb and washed with a bland soap and water. When applied to the body, the preparation is worked well into the body hair and washed off with bland soap and water. Care should be taken not to allow the drug to remain in contact with the skin too long for it may act as a mild primary irritant to the skin.

Xylene ointment may be applied to the hair daily for several days, the hair then combed with a fine-tooth comb and shampooed. This drug dissolves the cement substance holding the nits to the hair shaft.

The Patient. The patient with either scabies or pediculosis may be very embarrassed or even feel disgraced at such a condition (VI-1). The nurse must lessen the distress of the patient as much as possible. A stock expression which really applies here is, "It is no disgrace to get, but it is to keep pediculi (or scabies)." The nurse can assist the patient and his family in controlling the spread of rumor and social stigma associated with these infestations. Sometimes it is wise to isolate the patient to avoid transfer of the organisms, which might occur before the treatment is completed. With these patients, especially children, the skin becomes irritated, and the nurse should do what she can to lessen the patient's discomfort.

BURNS

DEFINITION. The cause, extent and severity of burns vary widely. They may be caused by dry heat, moist heat, the sun's rays, other penetrating rays, chemicals or extreme cold. The burn may be very limited, involving a small portion of the body, or it may be extensive, involving most of the body. Burns are often classified as to severity by indicating the depth of tissue damage. A first degree burn is one that affects only the outer layer of the epidermis (stratum corneum), causing erythema. A second degree burn is one that involves the epidermis but not usually the deeper portion of the stratum germinativum. This results in vesicle formation. A third degree burn is very severe and the entire dermis and corium down to the subcutaneous fat are destroyed by coagulation necrosis (I-1). Burns are also classified as to the percentage of body surface covered by the trauma. See Figure 39.

SYMPTOMS. The symptoms of the burn will depend upon the cause, degree, extent and length of time since the accident. A reddened area with some local swelling accompanied by some pain may be all that is felt in first degree burns. In second degree burns there is redness of the skin, blister formation accompanied by loss of tissue fluid, and considerable pain. In third degree burns there is actual tissue destruction, a severe loss of tissue fluid and severe shock. As the area of the burn increases, so does the pain. If the burn is extensive, the emotional reaction is usually severe enough to add to the shock (V-4).

The Severely Burned Patient

FIRST AID TREATMENT. For severe or extensive burns, medical aid should be sought promptly because the longer treatment is delayed, the more serious the burn becomes. While awaiting the arrival of aid, the nurse, in lieu of further instructions, should treat the patient for shock by covering him, keeping him quiet, warm and in a reclining position. Since one of the primary causes of pain in severe burns is exposure of the exposed nerve endings to air drafts, the burned area should be covered with a clean sheet, pillow case or towel held in place with strips of bandage. This helps, also, to prevent further contamination of the wound.

Ordinarily no fluids should be given by mouth. No greases or ointments should be applied unless the burn is a very minor one. The nurse has another important responsibility here to attempt to allay the patient's apprehension, which is often very severe (V-2). The patient should be transported to the hospital or, if near, to a burn center, at the earliest possible moment, for the sooner adequate fluid replacement can begin, the

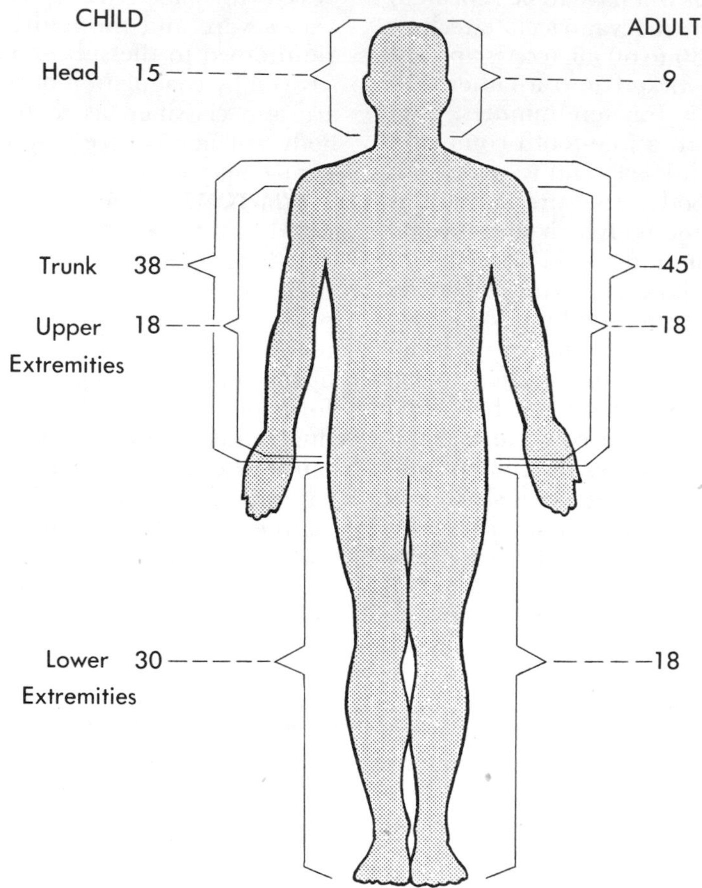

FIGURE 39. To aid in the estimation of the amount of body surface involved in burns.

better are the patient's chances of recovery.

DRUG THERAPY. On arrival at the hospital, there is a definite priority list of activities to be carried out. The order may vary a little according to the condition of the patient, the routine of the hospital and that of the physician. However, all will include a determination of whether a tracheostomy is required to assure an adequate airway. In a general hospital, the emergency room may be by-passed and the patient taken directly to surgery. Where a burn center is available, the emergency room is usually equipped for surgical procedures. The second treatment is usually to start an intravenous infusion. A cutdown may be done and an indwelling catheter installed. Blood is taken for laboratory analysis, and fluid is started. The patient is given tetanus immunization – a toxoid booster if he has been immunized previously. Otherwise, he is given tetanus human immune globulin. The wound is then cleaned, but no dressing is applied, since most physicians prefer the "open method."

Usually, no narcotics are given after the first 24 hours except for surgery. With full-thickness burns, pain perception is often decreased due to destruction of the pain receptor nerve endings. After the first three or four days, most patients can be maintained on short-acting barbiturates.

Fluid Therapy. The sooner fluid therapy can be started, the better chance for recovery for the patient. The deeper the burn, the greater is the fluid loss and the greater is the state of shock. This fluid loss is composed of protein, electrolytes and erythrocytes so the replacement therapy is aimed at these. The physician's first attention is directed to the electrolyte balance.

The fluid replacement therapy is planned by the doctor to cover a period of at least the first 48 hours after the burn. He will calculate the amount of fluid replacement to be given and the rate at which it is to be administered and will watch the results closely. He usually tries to plan to give one-half of the total fluids for the first 24 hours after the burn in the first eight hours (no matter when therapy is started); then one-quarter of the total fluid volume during the second eight hour period and the remaining quarter during the third eight hour period. Adequate fluid therapy reduces the chances of acute renal failure.

The type and amount of fluids given depend upon many factors. There are several accepted formulas for determining replacement. The following is one formula suggested as a guide for the adult.

1.5 ml. of crystalloid/kg. body weight/per cent burned area

0.5 ml. of colloid/kg. body weight/per cent burned area

Enough fluid must be given to insure 25 to 50 ml. per hour of urine output.

A second formula is 4 ml. of crystalloids/kg. body weight/per cent burned area and no colloid
(crystalloid – lactated Ringer's solution)
(colloid – Plasmanate) (Refer to Chapter 10 for details.)

A third formula is 1 ml. of colloid/kg. body weight/per cent burned area (plasma or dextran)
3 ml./kg. body weight/per cent burned area electrolyte (lactated Ringer's solution).

Total fluids for adults – 1500 to 2000 ml.
Total fluids for a child:
6 months – 100 ml./kg. body weight
1 year – 80 ml./kg. body weight
5 years – 60 ml./kg. body weight
8 years – 40 ml./kg. body weight

After the patient's condition is stabilized, the physician will decide, from laboratory reports and observation, if there has been sufficient erythrocytic loss to warrant whole blood transfusion. For the first three or four days, the colloids and electrolytic solutions are usually sufficient.

Tetanus Prophylaxis. Burns are always considered as contaminated wounds and all patients should receive adequate tetanus prophylaxis. If the patient has been known to have been previously immunized against tetanus, 0.5 cc. of toxoid booster is given. To the unimmunized and those not definitely known to have been, 250 to 500 units of the tetanus immune globulin is given intramuscularly.

Topical Therapy. The burned area is left open until treatment is begun. The first treatment is usually debridement, which is done under anesthesia, with surgical technique. This may need to be repeated several times. In the later procedures, anesthesia may not be required, and some physicians use biological debridement if the area burned is not extensive. Biological products used for this purpose are the same as those used for ulcers and discussed previously. Here, fibrinogen 10 units with desoxyribonuclease 6666 units (Elase) or sutilians 82,000 units per gram (Travase) are the ones most commonly used. Both are proteolytic and are applied once daily.

Various preparations are used on the burned area. The doctor selects that which is best, considering mainly the extent and depth of the burn area involved. Some drugs commonly used include silver nitrate 0.5 per cent solution, antibiotic ointments such as gentamicin or often either mafenide acetate (Sulfamylon) or silver sulfadiazine cream (Silvadine). Another preparation in common use is providone iodine (Betadine) ointment.

Other Treatment. As soon as a culture and sensitivity test can be done, the proper anti-infective drug is given intravenously or orally as indicated by the preparation used and the condition of the patient.

Oxygen in a hyperbaric chamber at 2 ATA (atmospheric pressure twice normal) has been shown to increase healing and diminish scarring. However, such treatment is possible only where such a chamber is available.

The use of homographs and heterographs aids in promoting healing. However, human skin for such purposes is in limited supply and is relatively expensive. Porcine heterographs have been proved to be as effective as human heterographs, are much easier to obtain and are less expensive. These heterographs are usually changed every four days and have reduced healing time materially.

Various symptoms are treated as they occur. Sedative-hypnotics may be needed for daytime sedation as well as for sleep. Analgesics are not usually required but are often given before surgery or before applying dressings, to reduce the pain of the procedures.

Corticosteroids are not given, except in specific cases such as a known deficiency, since they tend to promote invasive infection, destroy granulation tissue and mask other signs and symptoms.

The Nurse. Correct calculations and preparation of the intravenous fluids are vitally important. This is a very complex situation and it is absolutely imperative that all fluids be properly and adequately labeled. This label should include the patient's name and kind of fluid in the bottle with notation on it of any additions to it with their amounts. An absolutely accurate record of all fluids taken and the route used must be kept. When the protein hydrolysates are used, extreme care must be taken to insure the cleanliness of the equipment and to see that the fluid is not administered too rapidly.

The nurse must be constantly on the alert for any untoward signs. Vomiting may be an indication of circulatory collapse, acute gastric dilatation, paralytic ileus or a nonspecific result of injury. Indications of inadequate fluid replacement are restlessness, disorientation, circulatory collapse, hypotension and decreased urinary output. Sometimes the blood pressure cuff cannot be applied so the nurse must rely on central venous pressure readings, pulse rate and urinary output to determine circulatory maintenance. The urinary output should be checked on an hourly basis. An hourly outflow of urine through the indwelling catheter of 25 to 50 cc. is usually considered adequate for adults. An outflow of 10 to 25 ml. per hour for children 1 to 10 years of age and 5 to 10 ml. per hour for infants from birth to 1 year is generally considered adequate. Any alterations in this urinary outflow or any other unusual signs should be reported to the physician immediately. Signs of circulatory overload include venous distention, moist rales, dyspnea and an increase in the blood pressure (CVP). The nurse must also be alert for the possible development of pneumonia, for if the burn is so severe as to immobilize the patient, this predisposes him to such a complication.

It is wise for the nurse to remember that the patient is very sensitive to others' attitudes toward him and his potential disfigurement. Any sign of distaste or revulsion on the part of attendants is immediately noticed and reacted to by the patient. The nurse can do much to allay the fears and apprehensions of these patients.

The Patient. The severely burned patient initially is so seriously ill that his physical care is all important. However, when the acute stage is over, emotional shock may be severe. The nurse will need to be patient and understanding with the patient and his family. In most cases an entire life style must be changed, and adjustment is very difficult. If the burned area involves the face and/or the hands, plastic surgery will be required to give as good a cosmetic effect for the face and as much restoration of function for the hands as is possible. The patient will need help in reeducation and rehabilitation. Various public health and social agencies can be contacted to aid the patient when he is discharged from the hospital.

Minor Burns

For those minor burns which do not require medical attention, ointments of various kinds are usually applied. Some ointments contain vitamins A and D to stimulate tissue repair. Many proprietary ointments contain either picric acid or tannic acid. Both of these are potentially dangerous and should not be used without the consent of a physician. Most of the ointments prepared for the treatment of burns contain some form of a local anesthetic which helps to deaden the pain and makes the patient more comfortable.

Radiation Burns

Skin damage from radiation usually does not constitute the same type of burn as occurs from heat or sunburn. It develops slowly and forms a rather definite type of dermatitis. It is not treated as are heat burns but more as other skin disorders.

Chemical Burns

Chemical burns present peculiar problems, especially in emergency treatment. The first procedure in any chemical burn is to wash off as much of the offending chemical as possible. Then, if it is known, the chemical antidote should be used to reduce the burning action of the chemical (II-2). The initial washing with water will remove the material and also dilute it so that it is less caustic. If an acid has been spilled on the skin, the immediate application of a weak alkali will counteract the burning action of the acid by forming an inert salt. Naturally the reverse is true, a weak acid being used for burns caused by alkali. In the home, a weak vinegar or lemon juice solution may be used to counteract a known surface alkali burn, and a solution of sodium bicarbonate (baking soda) may be used if it is known that the chemical is an acid. If the nurse does not know the antidote, or the chemical that has caused the burn, she should continue to wash the area with copious amounts of plain water. This washing will not aid in repairing the damage already done but it does stop further injury. As soon as emergency care has been completed, the burn is treated as any other burn would be. It is unwise to use any drugs before orders are received from the physician, since the chemical and the drug applied might form an undesirable compound. A wet dressing of plain sterile water or normal saline should be used if any dressing is required before the physician arrives.

Many chemicals tend to cause ulceration, and these ulcers may need special treatment. The same drugs are used as would be employed for decubitus ulcers, namely, antiseptics, protectives and drugs which stimulate growth of cells.

PROBLEMS OF THE BURNED PATIENT

The burned patient, no matter what the cause of the burn may be, will need special care from the nurse. These patients are emotionally upset, afraid for their very lives and also for the damage the burn may have done. They are in great need of reassurance (V-1). It is usually helpful if the patient can be led to discuss his disability with the nurse and come to accept the help offered to him through the psychiatrist, clergyman, social worker and others. If the burn involves the face, hands, arms or other exposed parts, loss of attractiveness as well as loss of function is a concern of the patient and may even result in psychotic behavior. The nurse needs to explain, often over and over, that plastic surgery will be able to overcome most, if not all, of the scarring that may result from the burn. If a functional part of the body, such as the hands, has been burned, it is important that the nurse help the patient to realize that many possibilities for rehabilitation exist (VI-2, 4). Naturally, the nurse should not be too optimistic or promise what she knows cannot be realized, but she should be as encouraging as is possible under the circumstances. She can be most helpful in reducing the anxiety of the patient by her attitude as well as by what she may say.

Caring for the severely burned patient taxes the ingenuity of the nurse to the utmost. She must be ever on the alert for changes in the patient's condition, emotional as well as physical. She must know all the medications being used and be able to note the adverse as well as the beneficial results from these drugs. She must be ready to explain what the treatments and the medications are expected to do in order to achieve the cooperation of the patient and his family. Sometimes the nurse will be called upon to amplify the patient's own knowledge and clarify points which he does not understand. The nurse must always try to help the patient (and his family) maintain an optimistic viewpoint, since this will greatly aid recovery. Any treatment produces better results if the patient has confidence in it.

SUMMARY

All skin conditions, from whatever cause, are distressing disorders, and they upset the patient emotionally as well as physically. The nurse must try to understand the patient's problem and to shield him from misunderstanding people. Many skin disorders are chronic and are rarely, if ever, cured, but most of them can be controlled if the patient, his family and those aiding him persist in the often rigorous routine required to control the disease. It is not easy to realize that one may have to continue such a program for years, or even for the rest of one's life, but neither is it easy for the heart patient to live within his limits or for the gastric ulcer patient to keep on his diet (V-1). The nurse can help these people to accept their situation and encourage them to keep using their drugs regularly so that the disease does not interfere with the normal processes of life.

IT IS IMPORTANT TO REMEMBER

1. That many skin disorders are chronic and need the same care as other chronic conditions—persistence in treatment and rearrangement of the person's routine to meet the new situation.

2. That the patient has a very real emotional problem since many skin diseases reduce the attractiveness of the individual markedly, often at a time when the person most wants to be attractive.

3. That if the condition is chronic, there may be financial problems since the patient may have to change his occupation and buy expensive drugs.

4. That the same drug is often used for many conditions, even for conditions exactly opposite in character, the difference being one of strength. The importance of the correct strength cannot be overemphasized.

5. That most preparations used on the skin contain not just one, but several ingredients. The vehicle is usually something which will stay on the skin easily, such as ointment.

TOPICS FOR STUDY AND DISCUSSION

1. A young girl has just been admitted to the medical division with a severe attack of psoriasis, her first. She is in for treatment of the acute condition and to plan a routine for the future.

How can the nurse aid in:

a. Treatment of the acute condition.
b. Planning the future regimen.
c. Helping the young girl to become adjusted to her condition.

What drugs might be used in the treatment and why?

2. What drugs are used systemically to aid in treating skin disorders? What are the purposes of these drugs?

3. Show how the same drug may be used for more than one purpose in the treatment of skin disorders.

4. What are some of the emotional disturbances encountered in the patient with a skin disease? Does this have any effect upon drug therapy? Explain your answer.

5. The order for a wet dressing of aluminum acetate is 1 per cent. You estimate that two quarts will be needed. How should this be prepared from the crystals?

6. Check the daily newspapers for a week for reports of accidents. Note the following: What were the diagnoses, if given? How many were burns? Of these, how many might be considered to be severe burns?

7. If possible, visit a dermatologist's office or visit a dermatological clinic. Report to the class on the types of skin conditions seen. What treatments and medications were given? Did these agree with what you had been taught or with what is in the text? If different, try to reconcile this difference.

8. What per cent is the solution formed when five gr. 5 tablets of aspirin are dissolved in 200 ml. of water?

BIBLIOGRAPHY

Books and Pamphlets

American Medical Association Council on Drugs, *Drug Evaluations*, Chicago, 1971, American Medical Association.
Beeson, P. B., and McDermott, W., *Cecil-Loeb Textbook of Medicine, 13th Ed.*, Philadelphia, 1971, W. B. Saunders Co.
Beland, I. L., *Clinical Nursing, 2nd Ed.*, New York, 1970, The Macmillan Co.
Chatton, M. J., Margen, S., and Brainerd, H., *Handbook of Medical Treatment, 12th Ed.*, Los Altos, California, 1970, Lange Medical Publications.
Conn, H. F., et al., *Current Therapy, 1974*, Philadelphia, 1974, W. B. Saunders Co.
Goodman, L. S., and Gilman, A., *Pharmacological Basis of Therapeutics, 4th Ed.*, New York, 1970, The Macmillan Co.
Shafer, K. N., et al., *Medical-Surgical Nursing*, St. Louis, 1971, The C. V. Mosby Co.
Watson, J. E., *Medical-Surgical Nursing and Related Physiology*, Philadelphia, 1972, W. B. Saunders Co.

Journal Articles

Daniels, F., Jr., et al., "Sunburn," *Sci. Am.* 219:1:39 (July, 1968).
DiPalma, J. R., "Enzymes used as drugs," *R.N.* 35:1:53 (January, 1972).
Fraser, R. D. B., "Keratins," *Sci. Am.* 221:2:87 (August, 1970).
Gaul, A. J., Thompson, R. E., and Hart, G. B., "Hyperbaric oxygen therapy," *Am. J. Nurs.* 72:5:892 (May, 1972).
Hall, N. A., "O.t.c. products for rhus dermatitis," *J. Am. Pharm. Assoc.* NS 12:12:576 (August, 1972).
Hallsell, M., "Moist heat for relief of postoperative pain," *Am. J. Nurs.* 67:4:767 (April, 1967).
Larson, D., and Gaston, R., "Current trends in the case of the burned patient," *Am. J. Nurs.* 67:2:319 (February, 1967).
Margen, M. J., "Life on the human skin," *Sci. Am.* 220:1:108 (January, 1967).
Ritchie, J. M., and Ritchie, B. R., "Local anesthesia: effect of pH on acidity," *Science* 162: 3860:1394 (1968).
Ross, R., "Wound healing," *Sci. Am.* 220:6:40 (June, 1967).
Ryan, R. F., "Topical therapy of burns," *Postgrad. Med.* 52:4:105 (1973).
Satos, F. F., "Trials with cyclophosphamide in systemic lupus erythematosus," *Am. J. Nurs.* 72:6:1077 (June, 1972).
Shaw, B. L., "Current therapy for burns," *R.N.* 34:3:33 (March, 1971).
Torosian, G., and Lembuger, M., "O.t.c. suncream and suntan products," *J. Am. Pharm. Assoc.* NS 12:11:571 (November, 1972).

CHAPTER 24

DRUGS USED FOR DISORDERS OF THE EYES AND EARS

CORRELATION WITH OTHER SCIENCES

I. ANATOMY AND PHYSIOLOGY

1. The organ of hearing is divided into three major divisions, the external ear and auditory canal, the middle ear, and the inner ear.

2. Hearing results from a stimulation of the nerve cells of the inner ear and an interpretation of these impulses in the brain. Sound waves enter the external auditory canal and set the tympanic membrane in motion; these vibrations are transmitted across the ear ossicles to the cochlea and, in turn, to the organ of Corti which communicates impulses to the auditory nerve.

3. Deafness occurs when sound waves from the outside are not transmitted to the brain for interpretation. Abnormal conditions of any structure along the path of the sound waves will, therefore, result in deafness.

4. The eye, a very delicate and complex organ, is composed of the coats of the eyeball, the retina, the lens and vitreous body, the muscles, the cornea, the conjunctiva, the eyelids and the lacrimal apparatus.

5. The exposed portion of the eye as framed by the eyelids is an ellipse. The two ends of this ellipse are called the canthi. The one next to the nose is the inner or medial canthus, and the one on the outer end, the outer or lateral canthus.

6. Due to the anatomic structure of the eye, rays of visible light reflected from outside objects are brought to focus on the retina. This is accomplished by the refractive surfaces of the cornea and lens as well as by the refractive fluids, the aqueous humor and the vitreous humor inside the cavity of the eye.

7. Because the eye contains a confined fluid, pressure to the surface of the eye during treatment will be transmitted undiminished to the retina and blood vessels at the back of the eye.

III. MICROBIOLOGY

1. Besides the common microorganisms like the staphylococci, streptococci and pneumococci, fungi may also cause diseases of the ear.

2. Infections of the eye may be caused by viruses, staphylococci, pneumococci, gonococci and streptococci. Other organisms may also cause diseases of the eye.

V. PSYCHOLOGY

1. Treatment of some diseases of the eye and ear is often long and some diseases tend to recur. This is often discouraging to the patient.

2. In eye diseases, the chances of disfiguration are rather large in some instances and may make the patient extremely sensitive about his condition. This situation requires thoughtful education of the patient by the doctor and nurse and consideration by the patient's family.

VI. SOCIOLOGY

1. The prolonged treatment necessary in some of these diseases, especially glaucoma and trachoma, may prove a serious financial burden to the patient and his family.

2. The public should be informed about the importance of early and proper treatment of acute conditions of these organs as they involve two of our sense organs—the ears and the eyes—which cannot be replaced.

INTRODUCTION

Diseases of the eyes and ears are common throughout life. Early, they occur frequently as extensions of the common cold or other infection. Later in life, hearing and vision are often impaired owing to many causes. Treatment of diseases of these vital organs is imperative. Neglect in childhood can easily handicap the individual for life. Early diagnosis is especially important. With the eyes, slight trauma to the cornea, treated early, usually causes no permanent damage, but if it is left untreated too long, infection, ulceration and scarring with resultant diminution of vision can occur. The same is true of trachoma or incipient glaucoma. Hearing acuity may be permanently reduced if an upper respiratory infection is allowed to progress until sinusitis and/or otitis media sets in.

DISEASES OF THE EAR

Dermatitis of the Auricle and External Canal

DEFINITION. An inflammation of the skin, the dermatitis may be confined solely to the external ear or to the external auditory canal or both. It may be caused by a bacterium or result from a dermatosis. The responsible organisms may be *Proteus vulgaris*, staphylococci, streptococci, with *Pseudomonas aeruginosa* (*pyocyanea*) being especially common.

MAJOR SYMPTOMS. The acute form has a rapid onset with intense pruritus, redness and edema of the skin of the ear canal. Small blisters form early and rupture, releasing quantities of serum; crusting follows. In the chronic form, the itching is so intense that the patient usually scratches and picks at his ears constantly. Erosions are formed and yield a purulent discharge with large crusts filling the ear canal.

DRUG THERAPY. In the acute stage, the ear canal is irrigated with a solution of one per cent *acetic acid.* It is then dried, usually with *isopropyl alcohol* 85 per cent (acetic acid 5 per cent may be added). There are a number of solutions and ointments which may be used, depending upon the type of infection or irritation present. Most preparations are combinations, often containing an anesthetic, an antiseptic and a drying agent. One of the *corticosteroids* may also be included. The physician usually does a culture and sensitivity test and then gives the appropriate antibiotic locally, systemically or both, as circumstances indicate.

Solutions are the preferred form, but they must be given as drops at frequent intervals, since it is difficult to keep the drug in contact with the area. Most doctors do not approve of putting any cotton or other "plug" in the canal, since this blocks drainage. If the area is very dry and crusty, an ointment may be used.

It is not often that these patients are in the hospital, but the nurse will meet them in the doctor's office or in the outpatient department. They should be encouraged to avoid scratching their ears. If the patient is a small child, he may have to be forcibly restrained. The nurse may help the mother by showing her how to make a tongue blade splint for the child's elbows. The nurse should also show the mother how to administer the ear drops. The nurse should remember that soap should not be used in the area of infection. If crusts and secretions need removal, an applicator dipped in mineral or olive oil should be used.

The treatment of this condition is a long and tedious process. The patient should be encouraged by every means available to pursue treatment if at all possible. Though the treatment may not cure, at least the patient can be made more comfortable.

Otomycosis

DEFINITION. Otomycosis is an inflammation of the skin of the ear canal and frequently of the drum. It is caused by a fungus, frequently pityrosporon or one of the aspergilli (niger, flavus). This organism is almost invariably introduced by scratching the ear canal.

MAJOR SYMPTOMS. While the chief symptom is itching, there is usually some slight pain and soreness of the ear. There is a thin, watery and often musty-smelling discharge. When the growth has filled the canal or the drum is involved, there is tinnitus and deafness. If the growth is allowed to go unchecked, the pain is intense, the canal swells shut and some constitutional symptoms appear.

ANTISEPTICS AND CHEMOTHERAPEUTIC AGENTS. Before any treatment is very effective, cleansing of the ear canal must be done to remove as much of the fungus as possible. After this, the doctor may wipe the ear canal with 70 per cent alcohol and dry it. Acetic acid 2 per cent in aluminum acetate solution (Burow's solution) 1:10 may be used. This helps to make the skin reaction acid and markedly interferes with the growth of fungus and *Bacillus pyocyaneus*. In the chronic forms where scaling is marked, the doctor may prefer to insert into the ear canal for 24 hour intervals cotton tampons moistened with *cresatin* plain or with 1 per cent thymol. This is followed by the patient's using 2 per cent *salicylic acid in alcohol* drops in the ear once or twice daily.

Preparations containing corticosteroids are contraindicated in fungal infections.

The antibiotic *nystatin* (Mycostatin) may be helpful, especially if the infection is caused by monilia. This is usually applied in a concentration of 100,000 units per gram several times daily.

There are several accepted methods of administering ear drops and the nurse should know these before administering the drops. The drugs should be neither very hot nor very cold and are usually best at room temperature. Usually the drug is allowed to remain in the canal for some time and the patient is then allowed to sit up. Unless so ordered, no cotton should be placed in the ear canal or auricle.

The patient who has a fungus infection of the ear canal must thereafter avoid wetting the canal (as in bathing or swimming) since recurrence is common (V-1; VI-2). Watery ear drops are to be avoided. Reinfection of the ear canal by scratching the canal with hairpins, matches, etc., should be avoided. If cresatin, plain or with thymol, is used, there is considerable burning, but its use should be continued until a cure is certain.

Furuncles of the Canal

Furuncles (boils) may occur in the external auditory canal either from a middle ear infection or from an external infection in an abrasion in the canal. Staphylococcus is the most common causative organism (III-1). The canal becomes swollen and very painful and may be occluded completely by debris and the edema present. Pain on movement of the jaw is noted and there may be malaise and a slight fever.

The systemic use of one of the antibiotics after culture and sensitivity testing is indicated. To aid in suppuration, the physician may insert into the ear canal a tampon moistened with alcohol and *acetic acid* 2 per cent, 2 per cent *aluminum acetate (Burow's) solution, metacresylacetate* (Cresatin) or 8 per cent *salicylic acid in boroglyceride*. These should be remoistened every four hours. Analgesics such as aspirin are given for the pain.

Triethanolamine polypeptide oleate condensate (Cerumenex) may be instilled into the external auditory canal to aid in liquefaction and removal of debris. It is rarely, if ever, used if there is an opening in the tympanic membrane.

Acute Otitis Media

DEFINITION. Acute otitis media is an acute inflammation of the mucosa of the tympanic membrane almost invariably accompanied by an inflammation of the mucosa of the auditory tube and the mastoid cells. The organisms most commonly responsible are the hemolytic streptococci, pneumococci and staphylococci. (III-1). The organism usually reaches the middle ear by way of the eustachian tube.

MAJOR SYMPTOMS. Depending upon the severity of the infection, the symptoms will vary from very mild and transient to extremely severe. The patient usually has sudden pain in and about the ear which rapidly becomes more severe and often spreads to other parts of the head and is worse on swallowing. Fever soon follows, varying from 101 to 104° F. Headache, malaise, anorexia and other constitutional symptoms are usual. On examination, the physician finds a typical picture of congestion and inflammation. The eardrum may be bulging. If unchecked, mastoiditis is a common result.

DRUG THERAPY. If one of the anti-infective agents is given early enough, the need for a myringotomy may be obviated. At least, early and sufficient doses of one of these drugs will assist greatly in preventing the development of mastoiditis. *Ampicillin*, by intramuscular injection or orally, is the drug of choice. If no marked improvement is noted within 72 hours, another antibiotic, often tetracycline or a sulfonamide, may be used.

Warm drops (5 to 10) of *Auralgan* (antipyrine and benzocaine in glycerin) every two hours help relieve the pain and aid in reducing the inflammation. Some specialists subscribe to the use of mild nasal shrinkage with 0.25 per cent *phenylephrine* (Neo-Synephrine) in normal saline three or four times a day. One of the systemic decongestants such as *pseudoephedrine* or *phenylpropanolamine* may be used.

THE NURSE. The nurse must be alert to signs and symptoms which may indicate that otitis media is developing, e.g., fever, headache, vomiting, inattentiveness (due to decreased hearing) and ear pain. Ear pain may be reflected in infants and younger children by such behavior as rolling the head from side to side or pulling at the ear. If infection has developed, the nurse should thoroughly wash her hands before doing any treatments so that "mixed" infections of the middle ear are avoided. Sterile cotton should be used for cleaning and removal of drainage. In a young child, the earlobe must be pulled downward and back to straighten the canal. For older children, the earlobe should be pulled up and back. Zinc oxide may be applied to external skin and auricle to prevent excoriation of the skin from excessive drainage. Aspirin may provide temporary relief from pain.

DISEASES OF THE EYE

Drug therapy plays a large and important role in the treatment of eye conditions, of which there are many. However, some serious eye conditions, such as cataracts and detached retina, are treated surgically.

Blepharitis

DEFINITION. Blepharitis is a very common, chronic, bilateral inflammation of the lid margins (I-4). It occurs in two forms: ulcerative type caused by staphylococci and nonulcerative (seborrheic) type (III-2). Mixed infections are common. Contributing factors may be refractory errors, a debilitating disease or malnutrition.

MAJOR SYMPTOMS. The chief symptoms are irritation, burning and itching of the lid margins. The eyes are red rimmed, and many scales are seen clinging to the lashes. In the staphylococcic form, small ulcers can be seen about the attachments of the lashes.

DRUG THERAPY. Sometimes this condition responds readily to simple treatment and at other times it may prove resistant to many forms of therapy. Removal of the cause, if possible, is of importance. Improvement of general health and regulation of diet are of equal importance.

The scalp, eyebrows and lid margins must be kept clean, especially in the seborrheic types, by means of soap and water shampoos. Scales must be removed from the lid margins daily with an oily preparation on a damp cotton applicator or therapy will not be effective. In the ulcerative type, local use of a sulfonamide ophthalmic ointment, such as *sodium sulfacetamide* 10 per cent or *sulfisoxazole diolamine* 4 per cent may be used. *Bacitracin* or *neomycin ophthalmic* ointment is also helpful. Sometimes the physician may massage the lids after cleansing with 1 per cent *yellow oxide of mercury* or 3 per cent *ammoniated mercury* ointment. For seborrheic blepharitis, *selenium sulfide* (Selsun) seems to be most effective. This is applied by the physician for ten minutes once a week until the disease is under control. Because selenium sulfide (Selsun) is apt to be toxic to the cornea, it must be removed with a dry applicator after ten minutes.

Hordeolum

Hordeolum (stye) is a circumscribed purulent infection of a sebaceous gland along the lid margin, usually caused by a staphylococcal organism (III-2). There is a strong tendency for styes to recur and this should warrant a complete examination of the patient to determine if there is a focal point for this infection.

This condition starts as a markedly hyperemic area on the edge of the lid increasing in size until it is a typical boil-like lesion. Gradually it localizes and breaks through, discharging yellowish pus.

In order to hasten suppuration, hot moist compresses of either *physiologic saline* or plain water are applied. During the day, a combination of *neomycin, bacitracin* and *polymyxin*, 2 drops every hour, is advised. At night, *sulfacetamide ointment* or an ointment of the same combination used during the day is used. Local applications of 10 to 30 per cent *sodium sulfacetamide* are also effective. When the infection is localized, surgical incision is indicated to establish adequate drainage. Antibacterial therapy should be continued for at least a week to suppress the occurrence of another stye from self-infection.

Acute Catarrhal Conjunctivitis

DEFINITION. Acute catarrhal conjunctivitis is an inflammation of the conjunctiva caused by organisms which are only virulent enough to produce excessive secretion of mucus (not pus); common offenders are the Morax-Axenfeld diplobacillus, the Koch-Weeks bacillus or the pneumococcus. It may also be caused by trauma or other organisms (III-2). It is transmitted from person to person and is more frequent in children.

MAJOR SYMPTOMS. The patient usually complains of burning, smarting and itching of the eyes, photophobia and a feeling of a foreign body in the eye. There is intense redness of the conjunctiva (pink eye). There is a mucoid discharge from the eyes which causes the lid borders to become adherent during the night. Usually both eyes are involved.

DRUG THERAPY. Although the disease is self-limiting (two to eight days), active treatment will shorten the period of infectivity and relieve symptoms. Iced compresses applied frequently during the day add to the comfort of the patient.

The eyes should be washed with normal *saline* four to five times a day. It is recommended that after each irrigation, an antibiotic or a sulfonamide be instilled. See Hordeolum, covered previously, for details. These may be used with or without steroids.

THE NURSE. It is extremely important for the nurse to administer eye drops and ointments properly. Of primary importance is the fact that great gentleness must be used whenever doing anything about the eye. The nurse should try to gain the patient's confidence before attempting any eye procedure—she should explain what is to be done and why. With the patient's cooperation it may be done painlessly with only a momentary smarting of the eyes resulting. Before performing any eye procedure, the nurse should thoroughly wash her hands with soap and water.

When giving eye drops, the nurse should ask the patient to look up while she pulls gently down on the lower lid with the left index finger. With the medicine dropper in the other hand, she should drop the required number of drops at the edge of the lid and allow the medication to enter the conjunctival sac by capillary attraction. The dropper should never come in contact with the eye and the solution should never be allowed to fall directly on the sensitive cornea. Only sterile solutions should be used and, before using, the nurse should be sure that the solution is not cloudy and that there is no precipitate present.

Ointments for ophthalmic use are always plainly labeled *ophthalmic* and are almost invariably marketed in sterile tubes from which the ointment is allowed to escape through a minute opening when the tube is pressed. It is usually best to hold the eye open with the thumb and forefinger of one hand and squeeze the ointment out of the tube in a fine line on the edges of the lids. The lids are then closed and gently massaged.

The patient and his family must be instructed regarding the contagiousness of the disease and shown how to prevent its spread.

Purulent Conjunctivitis

DEFINITION. An inflammation of the conjunctiva, this disease invariably is caused by the gonococcus or the pneumococcus (III-2). The term purulent conjunctivitis includes gonorrheal ophthalmia and ophthalmia neonatorum. The gonococcal forms are highly contagious. Ophthalmia neonatorum will be considered with the care of the newborn in Chapter 28.

MAJOR SYMPTOMS. The symptoms may be mild at first but they progress rapidly to a severe infection with redness and marked edema of the eyes. At first, the discharge may be watery but it soon becomes thick and purulent. Intense ocular pain and constitutional symptoms are present. There may be corneal involvement unless treatment is instituted early.

DRUG THERAPY

Ophthalmia neonatorum is best prevented by instilling *penicillin* ointment (100,000 unit per Gm.) in the conjunctival sac at birth. However, in some states, *silver nitrate* 1 to 2 per cent is legally required. If 2 per cent is used, it must be followed within 30 seconds by neutralization with normal saline. Penicillin ointment has the distinct advantage over silver nitrate in that it is painless and does not injure the eye. However, it tends to produce resistant forms, and some physicians feel that silver nitrate is more consistently effective.

A usual method of treating the infected eye is to irrigate it thoroughly with *saline* solution and instill two drops of 1 per cent silver nitrate which is neutralized with saline in 30 seconds. This is followed by penicillin 100,000 units per Gm. ointment every hour during the day and night. In addition, the patient should receive at least 300,000 units of penicillin intramuscularly each day. If any pus forms, the eye should be carefully irrigated with saline.

For the patient who is sensitive to penicillin, bacitracin or one of the sulfonamide drugs may be substituted.

Extreme care must be used in caring for patients with gonorrheal conjunctivitis. To avoid contamination of the nurse's eyes, protecting goggles may be worn. Scrupulous handwashing and strict isolation techniques must be carried out. The eye irrigations may be done by allowing the prescribed solution to trickle between the lids from a piece of absorbent cotton dripping with the medication.

Herpetic Keratoconjunctivitis

Herpetic keratoconjunctivitis is an infection of the conjunctiva and cornea caused by the herpes simplex virus. It usually follows an upper respiratory infection or fever with "cold sores." The eye is infected and there is pain, excess lacrimation and a burning sensation. If untreated, it may cause corneal ulcers and scarring with loss of vision if the central portion of the cornea is affected. It is treated topically with idoxuridine (Dendrid, Herplex, Stoxil) (Kerecid [C]).

Acute Uveitis

DEFINITION. Inflammation of the uveal tract (choroid, ciliary body, iris) has many causes and may involve any portion singly or any two or all three parts simultaneously. Acute anterior uveitis (iridocyclitis and cyclitis) is the most frequent form and is believed to be due to a sensitivity phenomenon (endogenous) rather than to some specific organism. Posterior uveitis (choroiditis, chorioretinitis, retinochoroiditis) is usually more serious. Although the etiology may be difficult to establish, most cases are thought to be due to a direct invasion by a microbial agent. Acute uveitis is characterized by repeated attacks over a period of years.

MAJOR SYMPTOMS. Subjective symptoms consist of pain, photophobia, lacrimation and interference with vision. The pain, often severe, is referred to the eyeball itself, radiates to the forehead and temple and is worse at night. The pupil is small and reacts sluggishly to light; the cornea is injected. Most often the disease is unilateral and it occurs mainly in young and middle-aged people. Complications are common.

DRUG THERAPY. ANALGESICS. *Aspirin* may not be sufficient in some cases to control the pain and a stronger analgesic, such as *codeine* in the usual doses, may be needed.

Moist, hot compresses for several hours each day help to diminish the pain and the inflammation.

ADRENAL CORTICOSTEROIDS. The adrenal corticosteroids are used because of their anti-inflammatory reactions. The results of their administration may be quite dramatic, with relief of pain, subsiding of hyperemia and mobilization of exudate and edema fluid taking place within a few hours. There are many different preparations on the market and about the only difference in them is the collateral metabolic changes they produce. In both anterior and posterior uveitis it is advisable to administer these drugs by three channels—topically, subconjunctivally and systemically.

For topical application in both conditions, physicians often use a suspension of *prednisolone* 0.25 to 0.5 per cent, *prednisolone ointment* 0.1 to 0.25 per cent, *dexamethasone* solution 0.1 per cent or ointment 0.1 to 0.5 per cent. By the subconjunctival route, *prednisone* 0.25 per cent, 0.5 ml.; *dexamethasone* 0.1 per cent, 0.5 ml.; or *methylprednisolone*, 0.1 per cent, 0.5 ml., are employed. Systemically *prednisone* is given, 5 mg. a day in anterior uveitis, with the dose increased to 30 to 80 mg. a day in posterior uveitis. *Methylprednisolone*, 4 mg., is used in anterior uveitis. *Dexamethasone* is given in 0.25 to 0.75 mg. a day dosage in anterior uveitis; in posterior uveitis the dose is 2 to 4 mg. a day. Sometimes, for an unknown reason, one corticosteroid does not cause the usual effects so another should be tried. The usual precautions should be observed when any corticosteroid is used. (See Chapter 27 or Current Drug Handbook for details.). There may also be certain ocular side effects from these drugs. A superficial punctate staining similar to that caused by other local drugs has been noted. There may also be an enhancement of herpetic, bacterial or fungal conjunctivitis or keratitis.

MYDRIATICS AND CYCLOPLEGICS. The main objective of treatment in uveitis is to prevent the formation of synechiae (adhesion of iris to lens and cornea). This is accomplished by the use of a mydriatic or a cycloplegic drug or both, which not only dilate the pupil but help to diminish congestion of the iris and put the part at rest (Fig. 40). They also help relieve ciliary spasm and pain. *Atropine sulfate solution* 1 to 4 per cent or *homatropine* 2 to 5 per cent may be used from two to six times a day as needed to keep the pupil dilated. The ointment may be preferable to the solution. It is possible for this drug to cause irritation of the eye, especially on long administration, or the patient may be allergic to it. Sometimes *scopolamine hydrobromide* (hyoscine) 0.2 per cent is used two to six times a day in preference to atropine because there is a lower incidence of allergic reactions to it.

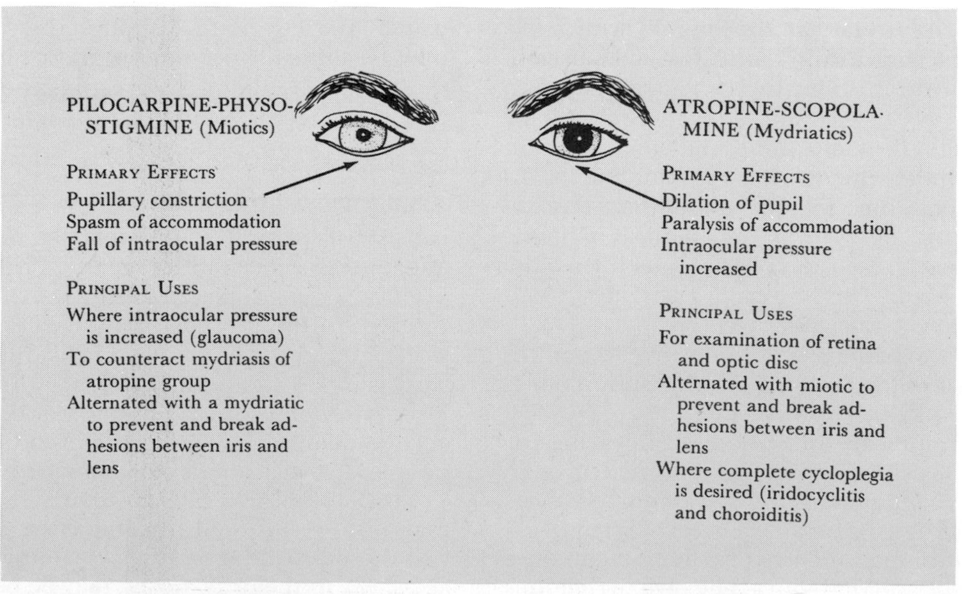

FIGURE 40. Comparison of effects of miotics and mydriatics.

Other solutions which may be used include *eucatropine hydrochloride* 2 to 5 per cent or *cyclopentolate hydrochloride* (Cyclogyl) 0.5 to 2 per cent two to six times a day. The shorter duration of action of the latter two requires that they be administered more frequently. Cycloplegics and mydriatics should not be administered over long periods, and they should not be used if the patient has glaucoma.

Whenever any of these mydriatics are used, the nurse should apply slight pressure to the inner canthus for a few minutes after putting in the drops to prevent the drug from reaching the nasal cavities, from which systemic absorption would occur (I-5). It is extremely important that the eye drops be instilled at the prescribed times to keep the pupil well dilated, thus preventing formation of adhesions.

This condition recurs often and the patient may become discouraged at the repetition of the inflammation (V-2). It is often desirable for the patient to wear dark glasses most of the time to help relieve the photophobia.

Corneal Ulcers

DEFINITION. An infection of the cornea (I-6), these ulcers are of two general types —serpiginous (creeping) and catarrhal. The serpiginous ulcers are infected ulcers and may be caused by pneumococci, streptococci, Morax-Axenfeld diplobacillus, *Klebsiella pneumoniae, Pseudomonas aeruginosa, Staphylococcus aureus* or various fungi. The catarrhal type is more often caused by Morax-Axenfeld diplobacilli or Koch-Weeks bacilli and occurs more frequently in older people who are debilitated from some general disease.

MAJOR SYMPTOMS. A gray area appears on the cornea with dilation of the circumcorneal blood vessels and great pain which seems out of proportion to the size of the lesion in the serpiginous type. If untreated, hypopyon (pus in the anterior chamber) develops. Pain and lacrimation are severe with the lids swollen and the conjunctiva inflamed. In the catarrhal type, the pain and congestion is less marked and hypopyon rarely develops. If untreated, in either case, the ulcer may result in perforation and loss of the eye.

DRUG THERAPY. The treatment for both types is similar except that in the catarrhal type it is less radical. The choice of drug to be used depends upon identifying the causative organism and using the drug both topically and systemically.

Pneumococci and other gram-positive organisms respond to *penicillin*, 1,200,000 units every 4 to 6 hours intramuscularly, or *erythromycin propionate* orally, 2 Gm. as an initial dose followed by 1 Gm. every eight hours. If there is no improvement, *chloramphenicol* may be given either orally or intramuscularly in an initial 3 Gm. dose and then 1 Gm. every eight hours. Topically, the treatment may include 0.5 per cent *chloramphenicol ophthalmic solution*, one drop every half hour, *chloramphenicol ointment* 1 per cent instilled three times a day or *neomycin* ointment (5 mg. per Gm.) three times a day.

Ulcers caused by the pseudomonas organism require heroic measures quickly. *Gentamicin sulfate* (Garamycin) or *carbenicillin* (Geopen) is given by injection in the usual dosage. (See Chapter 7.) Topically, gentamicin ophthalmic solution is administered one or two drops every 1 to 4 hours during the acute stage. Then gentamicin ophthalmic ointment is instilled two or three times daily.

Ulcers caused by the diplobacilli usually respond well to topical *zinc sulfate* 1 per cent and *chloramphenicol*.

Homatropine sulfate, one drop of a 2 per cent solution used three times a day or oftener, causes dilation of the pupil. This has a sedative effect and helps to promote healing by diminishing the iritis and by paralyzing the sphincter iridis and ciliary muscle. Hot compresses applied for ten minutes at a time every three hours help relieve pain and discomfort.

Analgesics and sedatives should be given for the pain and sleeplessness.

As in administering any medication to the eye, extreme care and gentleness are important. It is very important, too, to give the medications on time for if the ulcer proceeds, there may be corneal scarring, perforation and endophthalmitis and loss of the eye.

The patient's eyes are not bandaged but the patient should be in bed and his eyes shielded from the light.

Glaucoma

DEFINITION. Glaucoma, a fairly common disorder of the eye, is characterized by increased intraocular tension. This, if allowed to continue, will cause at the least permanent visual defects and, if unchecked, irreversible blindness. The fundamental cause is an interference with the flow of the aqueous humor (fluid) from its secretion by the ciliary body into the posterior chamber, through the pupillary opening and into the anterior chamber. From there the fluid passes through the openings in the trabeculum and Schlemm's canal and thence to the venous circulation. Any blockage of this circulation will cause an increase in intraocular pressure which can result in glaucoma. There are several forms of the disease. The most common form is simple, chronic, open-angle glaucoma. Next in frequency is angle-closure glaucoma. It may be either acute or subacute. Less common forms are congenital glaucoma and glaucoma due to trauma or infection.

MAJOR SYMPTOMS. In the acute phase angle-closure glaucoma comes on suddenly, with headache, pain in the eye and a rapid failure in vision. Gastrointestinal symptoms may be present. The attack may be severe and persistent, requiring immediate treatment, or less severe (lasting only a short time), but there may be repeated attacks until treatment is started or there is serious visual loss. This latter type is called "subacute." In the chronic or gradual type (open-angle), the symptoms come on more gradually and the patient frequently complains of colored rings around sources of light. The cornea is cloudy and the pupil is stiff and dilated; the eyeball feels hard on manual examination.

DRUG THERAPY. Drugs form the basis of treatment for chronic, open-angle glaucoma and sometimes for the subacute angle-closure type. However, acute angle-closure glaucoma is usually treated surgically to re-establish drainage. Surgery is more frequently used than drugs for the subacute type. Medications are used to prepare the eye for the surgical procedures. A combination of drugs and surgery may be used for congenital cataracts depending upon circumstances. Glaucoma caused by infection or trauma usually clears up as soon as the cause is removed.

MIOTIC DRUGS

Parasympathomimetic (Cholinergic) Agents.

THE DRUGS. The parasympathomimetic drugs may be divided into several subgroups according to source (either the plant alkaloids, pilocarpine and physostigmine, or one of the many synthetic compounds), length of effectiveness, (those whose effective time is relatively short—again pilocarpine and physostigmine—and those that are relatively long acting such as carbachol, demecarium, isoflurophate and echothiophate) or mode of action plus time element. This is the most commonly accepted method of classification. The cholinergic drugs which mimic the natural parasympathomimetics are short-acting pilocarpine (the most commonly used drug in this group) and the long-acting carbachol. The other drugs inhibit the action of cholinesterase—short-acting physostigmine, long-acting demecarium, isoflurophate and echothiophate.

Physical and Chemical Properties. Pilocarpine, now produced synthetically, is a tertiary amine. The synthetic compounds are choline esters. The salts of these preparations are readily soluble in water and body fluids. Physostigmine is an alkaloid derived from the plant *Physostigma venenosum* or Calabar bean.

Action. Parasympathomimetic agents all, to a greater or lesser degree, have the following action: by stimulating the parasympathetic nervous system they cause increased heart rate, contraction of smooth muscle tissue, increased glandular secretion and contraction of the pupils of the eyes. It is this last action which is important in glaucoma. They constrict the ciliary muscle, allowing the canal of Schlemm to drain the aqueous fluid and thus diminish the intraorbital pressure. Those that inhibit cholinesterase prolong the action of acetylcholine. The net result is practically the same as with direct cholinergic agents.

Therapeutic Uses. Cholinergic drugs have three main uses: stimulation of smooth muscle tissue, especially of the gastrointestinal and urinary tracts, increase in perspiration and contraction of the pupils of the eyes. These drugs are also used in certain cardiac disorders and in the treatment of peripheral vascular disease.

Absorption and Excretion. The fate of

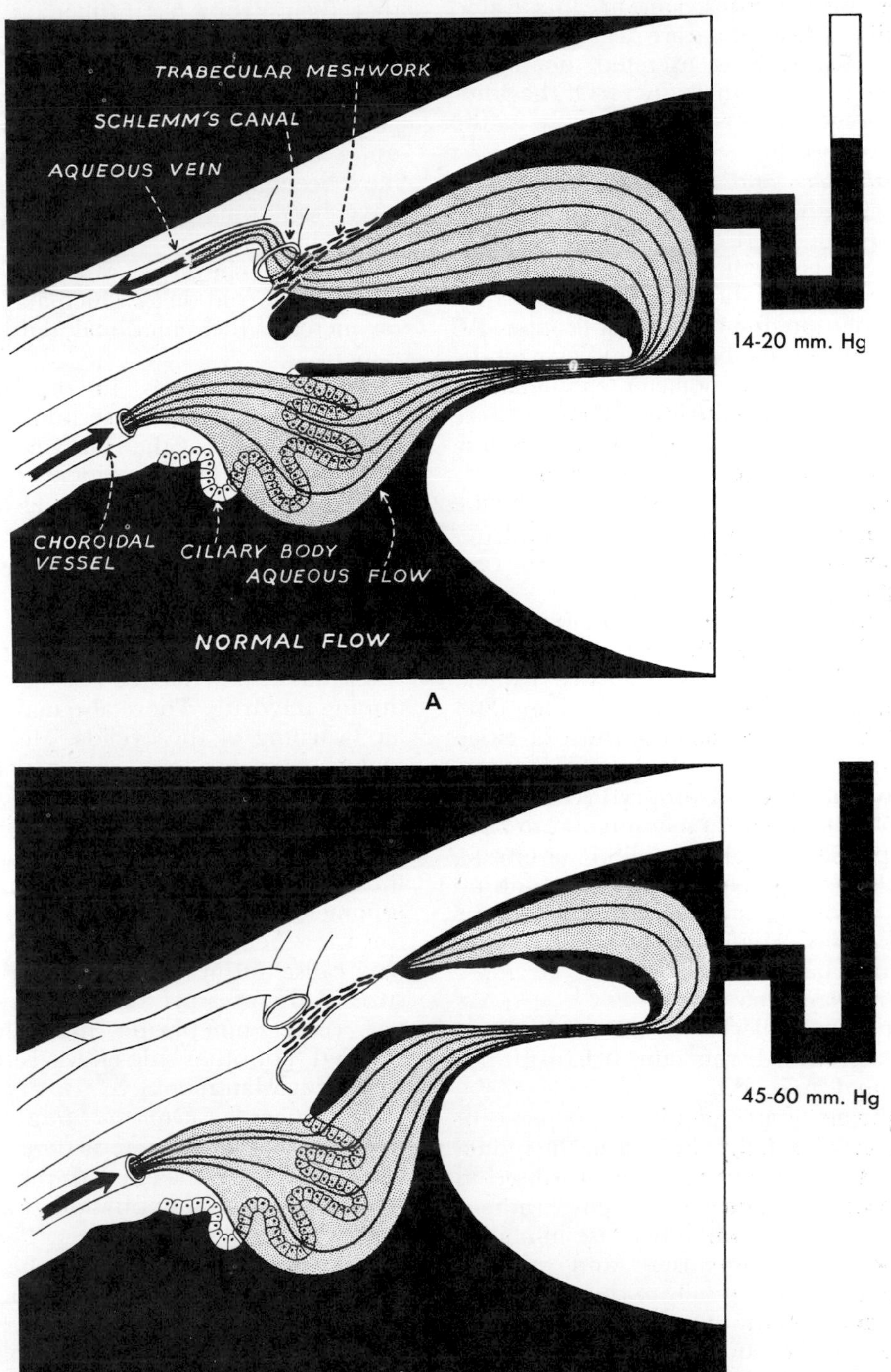

FIGURE 41. *A,* Trabecular obstruction as the mechanism of rise in intraocular pressure in open-angle glaucoma. *B,* Mechanism of the rise in intraocular pressure in angle-closure glaucoma. (From Kolker, A. E., and Hetherington, J., *Becker-Shaffer's Diagnosis and Therapy of the Glaucomas, 3rd Ed.,* St. Louis, 1970, The C. V. Mosby Co.)

these drugs in the body varies with the different preparations. Some are inactivated by cholinesterase. Some are degraded by the liver. Pilocarpine is excreted mainly in combined form by the kidneys. Of the other drugs, some are excreted partially in the feces, but mostly in the urine.

Preparations and Dosages. Only those cholinergic drugs used primarily for glaucoma are included here. There are many others. See Current Drug Handbook. The cholinergic medications used for glaucoma are in solution for topical application. All doses are prescribed by the physician on the basis of frequent tonometer examinations and must be individualized. One to three drops are instilled in each eye as directed. This may be as often as every 3 hours.

Carbachol, U.S.P., B.P. (carbamylcholine chloride, Carcholine) (Carbamiotin, Isopto-Carbachol [C]) 0.75 to 3.0 per cent solution every 8 to 12 hours.

Demecarium bromide (Humorsol) (Tosmilen [C]) 0.125 to 0.25 per cent solution every 12 hours to once or twice a week.

Echothiophate iodide (Phospholine) 0.03 to 0.25 per cent solution, once or twice a day.

Isoflurophate, N.F. (Floropryl) (Dyflos [C]) 0.025 to 0.1 per cent solution q 12 to 72 h.

Pilocarpine hydrochloride, U.S.P. or nitrate, U.S.P., (Almocarpine, Carpine nitrate [C]) 0.5 to 6.0 per cent solution up to four times a day. Higher doses up to 10 per cent may be used preoperatively in angle-closure glaucoma.

Physostigmine salicylate, U.S.P., B.P. (Eserine salicylate) (Esromiotin) 0.1 to 1.0 per cent b.i.d. to q.i.d.

Epinephrine bitartrate 1.0 to 2.0 per cent once or twice daily, also aids in the reduction of intraocular pressure. It is used in open-angle glaucoma usually with a miotic or a carbonic anhydrase inhibitor.

Epinephrine, ephedrine and phenylephrine are used topically in the eyes as decongestants in any eye disorder in which there is need for such medication.

THE NURSE. ***Mode of Administration.*** It is extremely important that the drops be given as ordered, and the nurse must teach the patient the importance of following directions regularly. Maintenance of adequate miosis is of prime importance or further loss of eyesight will occur.

Glaucoma patients are often in the hospital for other diseases. It is *very important* that their drops be instilled at the times directed. It is not only that the skipping or late timing of them may adversely affect the eyes; it can greatly diminish the vision. It is also important for the emotional effect upon the patient. These patients usually have been giving themselves the drops and have been timing them accurately. They know that blindness can occur if the drops are missed. The nurse must do everything possible to avoid delay which may aggravate or increase the emotional tension of the patient.

Side Effects. Early in the administration of the cholinesterase inhibitors, there may be a spasm of the ciliary body and the iris sphincter. This is evidenced by aching of the eyes, brow pain, headache, photophobia and blurring of vision. Echothiophate can cause papillary blockage in angle-closure glaucoma, and it is contraindicated preoperatively (iridectomy). Though these disturbances usually disappear after a few days, they may be reason for discontinuing the drug. There also may be muscular twitching of the eyelids. Most ophthalmologists prefer to have the patient take his eye drops at bedtime if possible, to minimize the photophobia and blurring of vision. After the first dose of either isoflurophate or demecarium bromide, a tonometer reading should be done hourly for a few hours. Paradoxically, these drugs may cause an increase in intraorbital pressure. If the pressure does not lower 1 to 2 per cent, epinephrine hydrochloride is instilled. For other side effects refer to Current Drug Handbook.

Interactions. *Cholinergic drugs* in general exert the following interactions. They decrease the mydriatic effect of the sympathomimetic agents and physiologically antagonize the nitrites and nitrates. Their cholinergic action is enhanced by the antihistamines, but decreased by the corticosteroids.

Direct-acting cholinergics have the following interaction effects. Acetylcholine, when given with procainamide, antagonizes the depolarizing effect of acetylcholine. Pilocarpine prolongs the action of ethyl alcohol.

Cholinesterase inhibitors have the following interactions. Neostigmine reduces the neuromuscular blockage toxicity of the aminoglycoside antibiotics, antagonizes the muscle relaxant effect of curare, increases the intensity and duration of the analgesic effect of morphine, meperidine and methadone and reduces the exacerbation of myasthenia by tetracycline. Physostigmine antagonizes the curare like effect of the aminoglycoside antibiotics. Echothiophate iodide (an organo-phosphate cholinesterase inhibitor) is potentiated by other cholinesterase inhibitors and potentiates the action of succinylcholine.

Patient Teaching. Because the patient will need to use drops the remainder of his life, he must learn to give the drops to himself. This is not easy to do as the blink reflex is a strong one. The nurse will have to teach the patient when to use the drops and how many to use. She must also show him how to instill them.

Most of these eye drops cause a momentary stinging sensation in the eyes when given, but this ceases after a few seconds. This should be explained to the patient.

It is helpful to close the eyelids once lightly after the drops are introduced. Tightly squeezing the eyelids may cause the medication to be expressed and lost from the eye. The patient should also be taught how to maintain sterility of the eyedropper and the solution being used.

THE PATIENT. The patient should be told by his doctor the nature of the disease and that even though it is a chronic disease, it usually can be controlled, provided he continues treatment for the rest of his life. He must also understand that he must have regular periodic examinations by the ophthalmologist (every three to six months) for the rest of his life. Because a person with glaucoma will have to use eye drops frequently and probably for the remainder of his life, he must learn to give the drops to himself. This is not easy to do, but with encouragement he may accomplish this procedure without incident.

Patients often react adversely to imposed restrictions which they consider unnecessary. It is important for the nurse to explain the reasons for these. Some precautions include extra care in daytime driving, probable prohibition of night driving and extra light for all close work such as reading. Other restrictions will depend largely upon the amount of vision lost.

It is important that the patient understand that lost vision cannot be regained, but that further loss can be largely prevented by faithfully following the prescribed regimen.

Other Drugs. *Glycerin* 60 to 120 ml. in orange juice may be given orally presurgery to aid in the reduction of the intraocular pressure.

CARBONIC ANHYDRASE INHIBITORS. The drugs in this class have their effect in glaucoma by depressing the rate of secretion of aqueous humor. The carbonic anhydrase inhibitors are not used as the primary therapy but as a supplement to miotic medications. They may be instrumental in avoiding or postponing surgical intervention. It is recommended that they be given intermittently (but concurrently) rather than continuously.

Acetazolamide, U.S.P. (Diamox), a heterocyclic sulfonamide compound, is a potent carbonic anhydrase inhibitor. It is helpful in some cases of glaucoma in reducing the intraocular pressure when the standard miotics have been unsuccessful. It is also useful in certain patients with cardiac disturbances (see Chapter 18). The usual dose in glaucoma is 250 mg. orally every four to six hours. The most important action of this drug is the inhibition of carbonic anhydrase in the renal tubule, which results in the tubular reabsorption of bicarbonate rather than the chloride ion. *Sodium acetazolamide* (Diamox Sodium) is the sodium salt of the parent drug and has the same actions, potency and dosage as equivalent amounts of acetazolamide. It is given parenterally (either by the intramuscular or intravenous method) and should be reserved for those who cannot take the oral preparation.

Dichlorphenamide (Daranide; Daramide [C]), also a sulfonamide derivative, is considered to be the most potent of these drugs but its action varies somewhat from that of acetazolamide and ethoxzolamide. It appears to increase urinary excretion of electrolytes, with sodium and potassium the principal cations affected. Bicarbonate (an anion) is also excreted, as is chloride. This then means that a metabolic acidosis is less frequent than with the other drugs in this group. The use of this drug is limited mainly to the treatment of glaucoma. In patients who are responsive to the drug, the intraocular pressure begins to fall within one hour after oral administration, reaches a minimal level within two to four hours and is sustained at a reduced level for six to 12 hours. As with all of the drugs in this group, it must be emphasized again that they are only supplements and do not replace the standard miotic drugs. Given orally, the initial dose for adults is 50 to 200 mg. every 6 to 8 hours until the desired response has been obtained. Maintenance dosages range from 25 to 50 mg. one to three times daily with individual adjustments often necessary.

Still another sulfonamide derivative, *ethoxzolamide* (Cardrase) is similar to acetazolamide and shares with it the same kind of urinary excretion of electrolytes as well as the side effects. The effects last about 8 to 12 hours after a single dose. In glaucoma, the oral dosage ranges from 62.5 to 250 mg. two to four times daily, depending on individual response. On a weight basis, this drug appears to be approximately twice as active as acetazolamide.

THE NURSE. The development of side effects is common when these drugs are administered and some are shared by all of them. They are not usually serious and are usually rapidly reversible. Generally, the rate of excretion of these drugs is rapid and certain compensatory mechanisms seem to prevent a serious distortion of the acid-base balance. The intermittent but concomitant administration of one of these drugs with a miotic helps contribute to this acid-base balance. Acetazolamide may frequently produce drowsiness, paresthesias of the face and extremities, fatigue, excitement, gastrointestinal upsets and polydipsia. Side effects from dichlorphenamide and ethoxzolamide include anorexia, nausea, vomiting, confusion, ataxia, tremor, tinnitus, dizziness, depression, lassitude and paresthesias. If methazolamide is the drug used, the nurse should be alert for drowsiness, fatigue, malaise and minor gastrointestinal upsets.

When the carbonic anhydrase inhibitors are used, the patient should be advised of the increase in urinary output and what it means. He would then not become alarmed when diuresis occurs. The patient should also be taught about the side effects (especially for the ambulatory patient) the drug may produce and told to stop the drug and notify the doctor immediately if they occur.

THE PATIENT. These patients are usually instructed by their physicians to abstain from taking large quantities of fluid and some may even be advised against the use of coffee or tea and all alcoholic beverages.

If any of these drugs are to be given for a long time, the doctor will probably request frequent determinations of the patient's blood cell counts and electrolyte balance. The patient should be advised of the reasons for this. The patient may also keep a daily weight record as an index of his response to the drug. Precautions for hypokalemia must be reported and a potassium-rich diet may be ordered, as may potassium supplements.

HYPEROSMOTIC AGENTS. Unlike most other drugs that are given for glaucoma, these drugs are systemic, and not topical, preparations. Their purpose is to increase the osmolality of the blood and thus withdraw fluid from the trabeculum and Schlemm's canal. They are administered either orally or intravenously.

Glycerin (Osmoglyn) 1.5 Gm. per Kg. of body weight of a 50 per cent solution dissolved in 0.9 per cent sodium chloride solution is given orally several times a day if needed. Lemon juice may be added to increase palatability. Glycerin is safer than the intravenous preparations but somewhat less effective. Side effects are rare, but headache, nausea and diarrhea occur occasionally. Its main use is before surgery.

Mannitol (Osmitrol) is given intravenously 0.5 to 2.0 Gm. per Kg. of body weight in a 20 per cent solution infused slowly over a period of 30 to 60 minutes. It is used as is glycerin but is more effective. Side effects are more common than with glycerin and include dehydration, diuresis, headache, nausea, vomiting, chills and dizziness.

Urea for injection (Urevert, Ureaphil) is also given intravenously 0.5 to 2.0 Gm. per Kg. of body weight of a 30 per cent solution administered at a rate of 60 drops per minute. Use and side effects as above.

(See Current Drug Handbook for further information on these drugs.)

Trachoma

DEFINITION. Caused by an intracellular organism called *Chlamydia* belonging to the psittacosis—lymphogranuloma venereum group, trachoma is a chronic, infectious, granular disease of the conjunctiva (III-2). The *Chlamydia* has a special affinity for the eye and has no effect on other body tissues. It produces an increase in the small vessels of the cornea with a resulting overgrowth of scar tissue (I-4). Both eyes are affected and the ultimate effect is usually blindness. Predisposing causes include crowded and unsanitary living conditions, malnutrition and lack of proper personal hygiene.

MAJOR SYMPTOMS. At the onset, the disease resembles acute catarrhal conjunctivitis with a thickening of the conjunctiva and a moderate amount of secretion. After seven to ten days, a number of small follicles appear in the upper tarsal conjunctiva and in the upper retrotarsal folds. The follicles increase in size and number and after three to four weeks changes become evident. A month to six weeks later the follicles of the palpebral conjunctiva are much enlarged and surrounded by inflammatory tissue so that they form papillae. At first they are beefy red but later they change to gray or yellow. Gradually, the papillae are replaced by scar tissue with resulting entropion. There is pain, photophobia and lacrimation and ptosis is not uncommon. Eventually, if the condition is untreated, the lacrimal apparatus is blocked and corneal opacities and diminished vision (even to blindness) are present (V-2). Secondary eye infections are common.

DRUG THERAPY. The aim of therapy is to reduce the inflammatory symptoms and sections, check and remove granules and reduce hypertrophy of the conjunctiva, thus reducing the duration of the disease and lessening the chances for cicatrization of the cornea and development of sequelae.

Topically, *tetracycline ophthalmic suspension* or ointment is usually used. At the same time, *tetracycline* 1 to 2 Gm. daily, orally in divided doses is ordered or a triple *sulfonamide* preparation is given 4 Gm. daily in divided doses. Treatment is usually continued for six to eight weeks.

In addition to teaching the patient how to give his own eye medication, the nurse should try to teach the patient some elements of personal hygiene and how to prevent spread of the disease.

Injuries to the Eye

BURNS

Burns of the eye are caused either by extreme heat or by chemical compounds and it is extremely important that they be given prompt and proper care. The nurse, by being aware of what to do, may save the eyesight of the patient. Though the symptoms will vary somewhat with the type of burn, pain, photophobia and blepharospasm are usually present. Complete removal of the caustic substance should be done at the earliest possible moment. The conjunctival sac should be washed out with great quantities of water immediately, whether the foreign material is acid or alkaline. The water should be directed from the inner canthus toward the outer canthus with the patient's head turned so the fluid will flow away from the nose. This is to avoid the possibility of the chemical's reaching the unaffected eye. It also aids in keeping any of the chemical from entering the nasal cavity. If both eyes are affected, it is best for the patient to be lying on his back without a pillow. The water can then be directed into each inner canthus and flow outward. Burns with acids are not usually as serious as those caused by alkalis. The extent of the injury depends upon the length of time the agent has been allowed to act. A local anesthetic such as *tetracaine* or *proparacaine* may be instilled to help alleviate the pain. If the burn was caused by an alkali, a weak solution of 0.5 per cent *acetic acid* may be instilled by the physician. When the burn is due to an acid, 3 per cent *sodium bicarbonate* will often be used for further washing of the eye. An anti-infective ointment such as a *sulfonamide* or antibiotic may be useful in preventing secondary infections. Local corticosteroid therapy helps to retard the inflammation and decreases the formation of scar tissue. An eye patch is usually used during the acute stage.

WOUNDS: NONPERFORATING AND PERFORATING

While almost any object may injure the eye, the wound may vary from a slight abrasion to a laceration or complete perforation of the eyeball. There is sudden severe pain, photophobia and blepharospasm. In perforating wounds, a visible disruption in the continuity of the sclera or cornea may be observed.

The use of a local anesthetic agent on the doctor's orders may relieve pain in nonperforating wounds. *Tetracaine* (Pontocaine) 0.5 per cent may be used. The eye is usually patched. An antibiotic ointment helps to prevent infection.

Perforating wounds are treated surgically and should be the responsibility of an ophthalmologist. Often a prophylactic dose of one of the antibiotics is given to prevent a secondary infection. If there has been gross contamination, tetanus and gas-gangrene prophylaxis is usually indicated.

OTHER CONDITIONS

There are several eye conditions in which there is a lack of the normal amount of lacrimal secretions (tears). This causes dryness and a tendency for the eyelids to adhere to the anterior surface of the eyeball, causing irritation. In such cases, "artificial tears" are instilled as often as is necessary on a temporary basis. The basic ingredient in such preparations is either methylcellulose or polyvinyl alcohol. These same substances may be included in solutions used for contact lenses. They are viscous (methylcellulose more than polyvinyl alcohol), and they lubricate the eyelids and the surface of the eye.

IT IS IMPORTANT TO REMEMBER

1. That drugs of the atropine-belladonna (parasympatholytic) group should never be given to patients with glaucoma.
2. That the patient with glaucoma must continue to use his eye drops regularly for the rest of his life.
3. That trachoma is infectious.
4. That acute otitis media, unless promptly and intensively treated, frequently causes acute mastoiditis. It can endanger hearing.
5. That fungus infections of the ear canal are often difficult to eradicate.
6. That extreme gentleness is essential when performing any procedure concerned with the eye.

TOPICS FOR STUDY AND DISCUSSION

1. Why is it important that eye drops be given as scheduled in the medical therapy for glaucoma?
2. What drugs are used most effectively in glaucoma? What is their action?
3. Demonstrate to the class the proper method of giving eye drops, eye ointments and eye irrigations.
4. Demonstrate how you would teach a patient to use eye drops and eye ointments.
5. Prepare a 5 per cent solution—100 ml. from glacial acetic acid.

BIBLIOGRAPHY

Books and Pamphlets

American Medical Association Council on Drugs, *Current Medical Terminology, 3rd Ed.*, Chicago, 1966, American Medical Association.

American Medical Association Council on Drugs, *Drug Evaluations*, Chicago, 1971, American Medical Association.

Beland, I. L., *Clinical Nursing, 2nd Ed.*, New York, 1970, The Macmillan Co.

Bergersen, B. S., and Goth, A., *Pharmacology in Nursing, 12th Ed.*, St. Louis, 1973, The C. V. Mosby Co.

Goodman, L. S., and Gilman, A., *Pharmacological Basis of Therapeutics, 4th Ed.*, New York, 1970, The Macmillan Co.
Miller, B. F., and Keane, C. B., *Encyclopedia and Dictionary of Medicine and Nursing*, Philadelphia, 1972, W. B. Saunders Co.
Mueller, C. G., *Light and Vision*, New York, 1966, Life Science Library, Time Inc.
Rodman, N. J., and Smith, D. W., *Pharmacology and Drug Therapy in Nursing*, Philadelphia, 1968, J. B. Lippincott Co.
Shafer, K. N., et al., *Medical-Surgical Nursing*, St. Louis, 1971, The C. V. Mosby Co.
Stevens, F. W., *Sound and Hearing*, New York, 1965, Life Science Library, Time Inc.
Vaughan, D., Cooke, R., and Asbury, T., *General Ophthalmology, 6th Ed.*, Los Altos, California, 1971, Lange Medical Publications.
Watson, J. E., *Medical-Surgical Nursing and Related Physiology*, Philadelphia, 1972, W. B. Saunders Co.

Journal Articles

Botelho, S., "Tears and the lacrimal glands," *Sci. Am.* 211:4:78 (1964).
Cockerill, E., "Reflections on my nursing care," *Am. J. Nurs.* 65:5:63 (May, 1965).
DiPalma, J. R., "Enzymes used as drugs," *R.N.* 35:1:52 (1972).
Gordan, D., "The inflamed eye," *Am. J. Nurs.* 64:11:113 (November, 1964).
Harris, C., and Rock, I., "Vision and touch," *Sci. Am.* 216:5:96 (1968).
Leary, J., Vessella, D., and Yeau, E., "Self-administered medication," *Am. J. Nurs.* 71:6:1193 (June, 1971).
Nilo, E., "Needs of the hearing impaired," *Am. J. Nurs.* 69:1:114 (January, 1969).
Nordstrom, W., "Adjusting to cataract glasses," *Am. J. Nurs.* 66:7:1578 (July, 1966).
Ohno, M., "The eye-patched patient," *Am. J. Nurs.* 71:2:271 (February, 1971).
Rosborough, J., "Ocular emergencies," *Hosp. Med.* 7:11:46 (1971).
Tong, T. G., and Inoffo, R. J., "Glaucoma," *J. Am. Pharm. Assoc.* NS 12:10:520 (1972).
Vaughn, D. G., "Common Ocular Disorders," *Hosp. Med.* 7:10:22 (1971).
Walike, J. W., and Snyder, J. M., "Recognizing and avoiding ototoxicity," *Postgrad. Med.* 52:4:141 (1973).
Wesseling, E., et al., "Symposium on patients with sensory defects," *Nurs. Clin. North Am.* 5:3 (1970).

CHAPTER 25

DRUGS USED FOR AN ALTERED ANTIGEN-ANTIBODY RESPONSE

CORRELATION WITH OTHER SCIENCES

I. ANATOMY AND PHYSIOLOGY

1. The lumen of a tube is the space within the tube.
2. The skin is made up of several layers of cells divided into two main parts, the epidermis or outer skin, and the derma or inner "true" skin. Blood vessels are found only in the derma.
3. The respiratory tract includes the nose, nasopharynx, pharynx, larynx, trachea, bronchi and bronchial tubes and alveoli of the lungs. It is roughly divided into upper and lower divisions. The larynx is usually considered as the lower end of the upper respiratory tract.

III. MICROBIOLOGY

1. An antigen is a substance which, when it enters the body, stimulates the production of an antibody.
2. An allergen is an antigen that triggers an allergic response.

IV. PHYSICS

1. Air is a combination of many gases. The principal ones are nitrogen 79 per cent and oxygen 20 per cent. The remaining 1 per cent is made up of many gases, including helium, carbon dioxide, ozone, neon and krypton.

V. PSYCHOLOGY

1. Disfiguring skin conditions create emotional disturbances. No person wants to feel that he is repulsive to those around him.

VI. SOCIOLOGY

1. Fear of social ostracism is a potent factor in the life of everyone. Every person desires to be liked by his peers. He will usually avoid anything which might lower him in the eyes of the public.

INTRODUCTION

An altered antigen-antibody response means an abnormal reaction of the body's antibodies to an antigen (allergen) (III-1). It is essential to define the terms before discussing the conditions caused by the altered response. Antigens (allergens) are chemical compounds, usually proteins or polysaccharides. They may be intrinsic (within the individual) or extrinsic (from the outside). Most intrinsic antigens produce chronic disorders and often do not appear until adulthood or middle age is reached. Extrinsic antigens tend to cause acute conditions, and the altered response is apt to be noted in infancy through adolescence. Antibodies are blood serum constituents. As a group they are called gamma-globulins. There are several known types, but the divisions are not of significance here.

The altered antigen-antibody response may be divided into two groups. Allergies (allergic reactions) occur in otherwise nonallergic individuals, and usually there is no history of allergies in the family. The conditions under this classification include serum sickness, dermatitis venenata, drug anaphylaxis and tuberculosis sensitization. Atopic disorders, sometimes called "natural or spontaneous allergies," occur in persons whose family history usually includes others with the same or similar disorder. Conditions include hay fever (allergic rhinitis), eczema, urticaria, angioneurotic edema, allergic purpura, allergic migraine, allergic asthma and anaphylactic reaction (shock).

For many years the only condition classified as an allergy was bronchial asthma. Now there are any number of conditions known to be due to an altered antigen-antibody response, and many more that are suspected.

ALLERGIES

Since the medical treatments for many allergic conditions are the same or similar, some of the drugs used in those treatments will be discussed before the disorders themselves are considered.

MAJOR SYMPTOMS. Most allergic conditions have similar basic symptoms, and these are treated by similar drugs whether the allergy is severe or mild. Allergy produces swelling of the sensitive membranes with an increase in secretion. There is a tendency to oozing and, with the edema of the membranes, there is a narrowing of the lumen if tubular organs are involved (I-1). The exact mechanism of the antigen (allergen)-antibody reaction is not entirely understood. However, research would indicate that the antigen-antibody reaction may activate a chymotrypsin-like enzyme which liberates histamine. It is known that excessive amounts of histamine are liberated.

ALLERGENS (AS A TEST)

THE DRUG. Allergens are used both to test for specific allergies and to treat the condition. It is very important to determine, if possible, the cause of the allergy, which is usually done by skin tests.

Physical and Chemical Properties. The physical and chemical properties of allergens vary widely. They are weak solutions of various substances known to cause allergy. Allergens include pollens, molds, dust, feathers, fur, food and chemicals. Most allergens (antigens) are proteins or polysaccharides and, as used medically, water soluble.

Action. The action of the allergen (or antigen) is dependent upon the presence or absence of the specific antibodies in the body. The reaction of the body to the allergen in a susceptible individual is very complex and therefore incompletely understood. If the patient is not allergic to the substance for which he is being tested, there is no observable reaction. If the individual is allergic to the substance, a wheal is produced locally.

Therapeutic Uses. Allergens are used to test an individual's susceptibility to various substances known to produce an allergic reaction.

Absorption and Excretion. In testing, the amount of allergen used is so small that it is usually inactivated at the point of contact and is not absorbed. Absorbed antigens are usually inactivated by the body enzymes. The length of time required for inactivation is in relation to the presence or absence of antibodies and the number of such antibodies.

Preparations and Dosages. Allergens (antigens), although they vary in substance, are usually standardized in units on their protein nitrogen content. One unit is 0.01 microgram of protein nitrogen. The dosage is usually 0.01 to 0.1 ml. of a dilute solution, 1 to 100 units/ml., and is given intradermally (intracutaneously).

The Nurse. Ordinarily the physician performs the tests, although the nurse may, under his direction, carry them out. Two common methods are employed, the scratch test and the intracutaneous test. The former is considered safer, but the latter more accurate. In the former test, a small scratch is made in the epidermis (shallow enough not to draw blood) and a minute amount of the allergen is gently rubbed into it (I-2). The test is read in 20 minutes and usually again in 48 hours. Local irritation denotes a positive reaction. If the reaction is immediate, a wheal is formed; if delayed, an area of induration and redness occurs.

The intradermal test is carried out by introducing 0.01 to 0.2 ml. of the allergenic solution into the outer layers of the skin. Care must be taken not to put the drug into the derma (I-2). The intradermal test is watched as is the scratch test and the reactions are the same. It is customary to use a short 1/4 to 1/2 inch needle of about 25 gauge with a syringe calibrated in 1/100 ml. for this procedure.

Usually a number of tests are made at a time, a chart being kept to show the allergens that have been used. As many as 100 to 150 allergens may be used in a series of tests. The physician may use the inner surface of the forearm or of the thigh for the tests. In this way, if an acute reaction occurs, a tourniquet can be applied to the extremity to delay absorption and allow time for treatment. Other doctors feel that this is not a real problem and use the back for the tests, thereby gaining a larger surface area. Immediate and delayed wheal reactions to each allergen are measured (in millimeters) and recorded on the chart.

Side Effects, Toxicity and Treatment. If the reaction to the tests is positive, a local wheal will occur which ordinarily requires no treatment. However, the possibility always exists that some of the allergen will be absorbed, causing a reaction in the allergic patient that may be mild, moderate or severe. The usual treatment is administration of epinephrine hydrochloride (Adrenalin) 0.3 to 1.0 ml. of a 1:1000 solution subcutaneously; it should be available whenever allergens are being given, whether for tests or for treatment.

The Patient. The allergic patient is usually well aware of his condition and is often very apprehensive. He should be told what the tests are designed to do, how they are done and what reactions may be expected. The tests are relatively expensive, but if they point the way to relief, they are worth all the trouble as well as the money expended. The allergic patient is apt to be an individual who might be described as emotional or high-strung, but this is not always the case. He is fearful, always expecting an attack, and trying to do everything to avoid becoming ill, yet knowing that sooner or later the trouble will return. He needs constant reassurance and encouragement to pursue as nearly normal a life as possible. He must be helped to persist in the tests once they are started since only by completing them can any value be obtained.

ALLERGENS (AS A TREATMENT)

The Drug. When the doctor has determined the offending allergens, two courses are open to him: when possible, the allergens can be removed from the environment of the patient; in cases in which this is not feasible, the physician may endeavor to desensitize (immunize) the patient by giving repeated small, but progressively increasing, doses of the allergen over a period of time, usually weeks, not uncommonly months or even years. The allergen is an antigen which stimulates the body to produce antibodies (III-1). The exact dose is determined individually and is usually increased as the course of treatments continues. If these two courses are successful the patient will be free of this particular allergy.

The Nurse. The nurse may assist with the collection of data demonstrating the cause-effect relationship after contact with an allergen and the appearance of allergic symptoms. Diaries or records of activities, clothing worn, cosmetics used and food eaten are frequently helpful. After allergy testing and record-keeping, the nurse can aid the patient and his family in making whatever adjustments in living and eating habits are indicated.

If the allergen is a food, it will need to be eliminated from the diet. The nurse may be able to suggest substitutes. At the same time, she can check to see that an adequate, nutritious diet is being followed.

Other possible changes in environment usually include removal of carpets (especially if wool), the use of bare wood or linoleum floors with washable throw rugs, elimination (insofar as is possible) of tobacco smoke, use of nonallergic clothing (synthetics or cotton fabrics), use of plastic covers over pillows and mattresses, damp dusting and avoidance of pets and indoor flowers. These changes can cause considerable disruption of the family members as well as the patient, and may create emotional stress. The nurse can do much to avoid this by explaining the reasons for the alterations and suggesting alternatives where possible.

The Patient. It sounds as if the treatment of allergies would be simple—either remove the offending allergen or desensitize the patient—but in practice it is extremely difficult to immunize against or remove from the environment all the allergens to which the patient is sensitive. Even when this can be accomplished, it is not uncommon that in a manner of months or possibly years the patient becomes sensitive to other substances. So although the sensitivity tests and the desensitizing injections are a great help in the control of allergy, they do not afford any panacea.

Patients must not be made to feel that cure is easy or complete but should be encouraged to continue with the treatment in the hope that it will help even if it does not completely cure the condition. The patient should also be advised to carry a card or wear a bracelet indicating his specific allergies. Allergens which create severe reactions can be recorded with Medic Alert or similar organizations.

VASOCONSTRICTORS AND DECONGESTANTS

The Drugs. The drugs considered as vasoconstrictors and decongestants are of the sympathomimetic (adrenergic) group (see Current Drug Handbook). Epinephrine hydrochloride (Adrenalin) has already been discussed in detail. Refer to Chapter 15 for details. However, it must be understood that epinephrine is commonly used for allergy, especially if the allergic reaction is severe and the patient's condition critical. Ephedrine (source vegetable *Ephedra vulgaris* and *E. equisetina* [Ma Huang] and synthetic) and certain of the synthetic adrenergic drugs will be discussed here.

Physical and Chemical Properties. The physical and chemical properties vary with each preparation, but they are all amines, and readily soluble in water and share with epinephrine a basic formula including a benzene ring and an aliphatic portion. Ephedrine is an alkaloid and its salts are used medicinally.

Action. They constrict the small blood vessels, causing local decongestion and systemic rise in blood pressure. They all, to a greater or less degree, produce mydriasis, lessened tone of smooth muscle tissue (bronchial, intestinal and urinary), and constriction of the blood vessels other than those of the heart. However, they tend to increase the output of the heart. Some of them, most markedly ephedrine, stimulate the central nervous system. The most important action in allergy is the constriction of the small blood vessels and the relaxation of the bronchioles, which causes the lumen to dilate (Fig. 42).

Therapeutic Uses. Topically, these drugs are used for decongestion and mydriasis; systemically, they elevate blood pressure and relieve the symptoms of allergy.

Absorption and Excretion. The exact fate of these drugs in the body is not completely understood. Some of them are doubtless deaminized by the liver and excreted by the kidneys; others are excreted unchanged. When administered systemically, they are widely distributed in the body fluids. Some of them pass the blood-brain barrier, especially ephedrine.

Preparations and Dosages

Cyclopentamine hydrochloride, N.F. (Clopane), 0.5 to 1.0 per cent solution, topically.

Ephedrine sulfate, U.S.P., Ephedrine hydrochloride, N.F., B.P., 25 to 50 mg. q 3 to 4 h orally; 3 per cent solution topically.

Isoproterenol hydrochloride, U.S.P., Isoproterenol sulfate, B.P. (Isuprel, Norisodrine, Iso-Intranefrin, Isovon [C]), 10 to 15 mg. orally. Also available for topical and parenteral use.

Phenylephrine hydrochloride, U.S.P., B.P. (Neosynephrine, Isophrin [C]), 10 mg. q 3 to 4 h orally; 0.5 to 1.0 per cent solution topically.

The Nurse

Mode of Administration. As already indicated, these drugs are given by diverse routes. The difference lies chiefly in the preparation selected and the urgency of the case. Applied topically, as a respiratory decongestant, the drug may be in the form of a

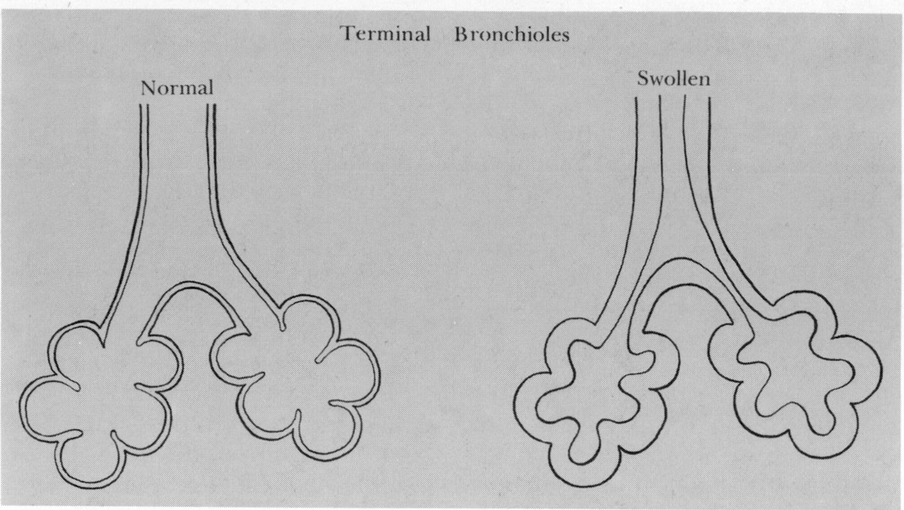

FIGURE 42. Swelling of the mucous membranes of the respiratory system, no matter what the cause, may be reduced by several medicinal means. The most commonly used are the decongestants, vasoconstrictors and diuretics. The first two act by constricting the capillaries and thus reducing the amount of fluid in the area. Diuretics act by decreasing the total volume of the circulating fluids.

spray, nose drops, an aerosol or combined with oxygen as the carrier. Parenterally, the drug may be given in an aqueous or oil solution. The intramuscular oil preparation is given in higher doses and should not be repeated for approximately 8 hours. Subcutaneous dosage is usually 0.2 to 0.5 mg. of a 1:1000 aqueous solution. Patients subject to acute allergic asthmatic attacks may be instructed in emergency self-administration of the drug by subcutaneous injection. The tissue directly beneath the needle site will appear blanched owing to vasoconstriction. Local massage will restore the normal skin color.

Epinephrine is destroyed by the digestive juices, so other routes such as inhalation of 1:1000 solution and topical sprays 1:1000 to 1:10,000 in strength must be used.

Side Effects, Toxicity and Treatment. If the dosage is within therapeutic limits, undesirable side effects are rare. However, headache, dizziness, palpitation, anxiety and elevated blood pressure may occur. Reducing the dosage will usually eliminate the symptoms, but if they persist, the drug may have to be discontinued, and another preparation substituted. Treat toxic symptoms as they occur.

Interactions. As a group, the adrenergic (sympathomimetic) drugs interact with a large number of other drugs. Only the more important ones can be included here. Adrenergic drugs given with the monoamine oxidase inhibitors or the oral contraceptives may cause a hypertensive crisis. They potentiate the nitrates and the nitrites, and they decrease the hypotensive effect of drugs such as methyldopa and reserpine. With the antihistamines, the pressor effect is increased. Specific drug interactions include the following. Isoproterenol is antagonized by propranolol. Ephedrine with nialamide may cause a subarachnoid hemorrhage or a postpartum hemorrhage with ergonovine. Phenylephrine eye drops may cause a reversal of mydriasis when used in the eyes of patients taking guanethidine.

Patient Teaching. It has been found that in many instances an increase in dosage does not produce an equal increase in effect. For example: Epinephrine (Adrenalin) 1:1000 solution in a dose of 0.6 ml. will not give twice the results of 0.3 ml. Many times no benefit can be observed from the higher dose. This may need to be explained to the patient and his family, since in an attack they may think that an extra amount will bring quicker relief.

Epinephrine (Adrenalin) produces a tolerance sooner or later in practically all patients. They become "Adrenalin-fast"; that is, the drug no longer gives relief—in any amount. This is very distressing to the patient. Withholding the drug for a varying amount of time will usually overcome this rebound congestion, and the patient can again receive benefit from it. This should be explained to the patient, and he should be advised to use the drug only when needed or as ordered by the doctor so as to prevent loss of efficiency as long as possible.

THE PATIENT. The vasoconstrictors are probably the most effective drugs for use in allergic emergencies, but they do not cure, and this must be understood by the patient. The patient and his family should also be aware of the signs of excessive use of such drugs, such as severe headache. They should know that extra dosage not only will not benefit the patient, but may even be undesirable.

ANTIHISTAMINES

THE DRUGS. When it was discovered that histamine was liberated during an allergic attack, workers began looking for blocking agents, and a safe antihistamine was eventually synthesized. Since that time a large number of preparations have appeared, and although they are effective and safe, only a few have gained popularity.

Physical and Chemical Properties. All of the antihistamines have similar chemical formulas. The core of their structure is usually a substituted ethylamine. There are three groups: ethylenediamine derivatives, an alkylamine and—producing greater depression of the central nervous system than either of these—an aminoethyl ether. They are white crystalline substances, the salts of which are readily soluble in water and in body fluids.

Action. The antihistamines antagonize the action of histamine, apparently by occupying the "receptor sites" on the effector cells, and in this way denying them to histamine.

The antihistamines are not so effective against the secretory action of histamine as against its other actions, although some of them do decrease nasal secretions.

Therapeutic Uses. Of proven value in many conditions, not all of which are allergic in nature, the antihistamines are useful in combating seasonal hay fever, urticaria, angioneurotic edema, serum sickness and pruritus, but are ineffectual against asthma and severe anaphylactic reactions. It is well to remember that they do not cure allergy but only relieve its symptoms. Certain of the preparations are effective against motion sickness and parkinsonism. Some of them induce cerebral depression that is useful in sedation and hypnosis. Their effectiveness against the "common cold" is questionable.

Absorption and Excretion. The antihistamines are readily absorbed from the intestinal tract or from parenteral sites. Effects vary with preparations, usually appearing in 15 to 60 minutes after oral administration and lasting from six to eight hours. The drugs are widely distributed in the body, the highest concentration being in the lungs. Progressively lower concentrations occur in the spleen, kidneys, brain, muscles and skin. Most of the drug is changed by the liver; some is altered by the lungs. Excretion is chiefly by the kidneys, although a small amount of the degradation products may be excreted in the bile.

Preparations and Dosages. Listed here are a few representative preparations. For a more complete list see Current Drug Handbook.

Brompheniramine maleate, N.F. (Dimetane, Parabromdylamine [C]) 4 to 12 mg. q.i.d. orally; 5 to 20 mg. parenterally.

Chlorpheniramine maleate, U.S.P., B.P. (Chlor-Trimeton, Chlorphenamine, Chlor-Tripolon [C]) 4 to 12 mg. q.i.d. orally, 10 mg. parenterally.

Diphenhydramine hydrochloride, U.S.P. (Benadryl) 25 to 50 mg. orally, parenterally, topically.

Pyrilamine maleate, N.F. Mepyramine maleate, B. P. (Neo-Antergan-Dexahest [C]), 25 mg. up to q.i.d. orally.

Tripelennamine citrate, U.S.P. (Pyribenzamine) 25 to 75 mg. t.i.d. orally.

Tripelennamine hydrochloride, U.S.P., (Pyribenzamine) 50 to 100 mg. t.i.d. orally.

Dosages of all antihistamine drugs are individually adjusted to suit the patient.

THE NURSE

Mode of Administration. Most of these drugs are given orally three or four times a day. The hours of administration should be spaced so as to cover as much of the twenty-four hours as possible. The first dose should be given as soon as the patient is awake and the last just before he retires.

Many of these drugs are prepared in solutions for parenteral use and also in solution or ointments for topical application. The antihistamines are often ingredients in drug combinations for the treatment of allergies, colds and other similar conditions.

The effect of these drugs is either all or nothing; they do not work halfway to relieve the symptoms. The nurse must check carefully, and record and report to the physician the results obtained.

Side Effects, Toxicity and Treatment. In general the antihistamine drugs are nontoxic, but side effects do occur often. They include dizziness, drowsiness, dryness of mouth and throat, disturbed coordination and occasionally nausea, vomiting and insomnia. Reducing the dosage or changing the preparation is usually all the treatment that is required. Some preparations cause considerable sedation.

Interactions. As a group, antihistamines react with the central nervous system depressants (alcohol, narcotics, hypnotics, analgesics, anesthetics, rauwolfia derivatives, tranquilizers, bromides and scopolamine) as follows. They have an additive sedative effect, enhance anesthetics and may impair visual discrimination, but they do not potentiate analgesia. Some of the group antagonize the steroids by enzyme induction, and their effects are enhanced by the monoamine oxidase inhibitors through hepatic microsomal enzyme inhibition.

SPECIFIC INTERACTIONS. *Antazoline* enhances the cardiovascular effect of norepinephrine by inhibiting tissue uptake, thus causing a concentration of unbound drug. With the addition of the monoamine oxidase inhibitors there can be further potentiation of this interaction by their inhibiting the enzyme which degrades norepinephrine.

Chlorcyclizine decreases the effectiveness of the barbiturates, oral anticoagulants, diphenylhydantoin, griseofulvin and phenylbutazone by enzyme induction. It decreases the activity of testosterone, estradiol, progesterone and desoxycorticosterone by increasing the metabolism of the hormone.

Chlorpheniramine See Antozoline.

Diphenhydramine (See Antazoline and Chlorcyclizine.) In addition, it will react with itself, causing decreased activity (tolerance) as enzyme action speeds up metabolism. Other reactions include an additive effect with phenobarbital to enhance sedation. It decreases other antihistamine and barbiturate activity by enzyme induction and decreases the steroid effects of hydrocortisone.

Contraindications. Most preparations have no contraindications. However, chlorpheniramine is contraindicated in severe cardiac conditions.

Patient Teaching

The nurse should explain to the patient what the drugs will usually do, as well as what they cannot be expected to do. Many people use these drugs without the physician's advice or knowledge and may do themselves more harm than good. Like many other drugs, the antihistamines may mask important symptoms, allowing a condition to become worse without the patient's realizing it. However, antihistamines do help real allergies and are used in the treatment of most allergic conditions.

THE PATIENT. The patient should be encouraged to take these drugs if and when they are ordered by the doctor, but excessive self-medication should be discouraged. There are many reasons for this, not the least of which is that an excessive amount of a drug may produce tolerance so that the drug will not be effective when it is really needed. The nurse should explain to the patient taking the antihistamine drugs that they may produce side effects such as sedation, inability to concentrate, dizziness and disturbed coordination of movement and vision. If any of these symptoms occur, the next dose should be withheld until the physician can be consulted. If hesitancy in urination is noted, this symptom can be reduced by having the patient develop a practice of micturating at the time of drug administration. It is also inadvisable for an individual taking these medications to engage in any hazardous occupation, or driving an automobile, especially until the drugs have been taken long enough to test the patient's reaction to them.

HORMONES. One of the *adrenocortical steroids* (cortisone or hydrocortisone or the newer synthetic or semisynthetic cortical steroids) may be given in any severe allergy. Usually the therapy is started intramuscularly with cortisone. Later, when the acute stage is past, the drug is given orally (cortisone, hydrocortisone or similar product). The dosage is very gradually decreased. Dosage is regulated to suit the individual patient. The cortisone may be started with a dose of 25 mg. o.d. to q.i.d. The reduction will be over a period of weeks, until the patient may be receiving as little as 5 mg. two or three times a week.

The Nurse. The nurse must explain to the patient the reason for the gradual withdrawal. She should watch for and report any signs of excessive dosage, such as euphoria, edema, headache and rise in blood pressure.

The Patient. It is important that the patient not be allowed to become dependent upon these drugs and that he understand that they are for emergency use. He will often obtain so much relief that he will want to continue using them, and the nurse may need to emphasize that, although they may sometimes be used for long periods, this is not the usual procedure. These drugs are discussed in more detail in Chapter 27 and in Current Drug Handbook.

SPECIFIC ALLERGIES

Upper Respiratory Allergies

DEFINITION. Allergic rhinitis (hay fever), allergic sinusitis and other allergies of the upper respiratory tract are perhaps the most common of all allergic disorders (I-3). Certainly they occur very frequently and are most annoying. Some are seasonal, and the sufferer can tell almost to a day when the affliction will begin. Often these are the easiest to treat, for it is relatively simple to find what pollens are liberated in a particular season and to give the individual, well in advance of the date, immunizing treatments, which will usually prevent the recurrence of the symptoms. However, most nasal and sinus allergies are difficult to diagnose.

SYMPTOMS. The symptoms of this condition are similar to those of the common cold, so much so that many physicians give an antihistamine in treating a cold. Sometimes the allergy is part of the cold but not the entire cause of the symptoms. The outstanding symptoms are lacrimation, excessive nasal secretions, sneezing, headache and a general feeling of discomfort. If the sinuses are affected, there will be pain in that area.

DRUG THERAPY. In addition to the antihistamines, the nasal allergies are treated by local applications of the vasoconstrictors—decongestants—which tend to shrink the mucosa, reduce the swelling and secretions and make the patient much more comfortable. Systemically *ephedrine sulfate,* 25 mg., *phenylpropanolamine hydrochloride* (Propadrine) 25 to 50 mg. or a similar drug may be used. When there is infection as well as allergy, *penicillin* or other antibiotic drugs may be given. In very severe and persistent nasal or sinus allergy *cortisone* may be used. This drug is also employed in severe allergic reactions involving the conjunctivae of the eyes. The dosage varies widely according to the condition of the patient—5 to 25 mg. may be used. It may be given as often as every four hours or as seldom as once daily.

Decongestants may be used as drops in the nose or they may be given through nebulizers or "sniffers." These last two methods are also used for various combinations of drugs such as *camphor, pine tar, eucalyptol* and *menthol.* These are pleasant and will often aid in opening the air passages so that breathing is easier. They do not give permanent relief but can be repeated frequently.

Lower Respiratory Allergies

ASTHMA

DEFINITION. Asthma is probably the most severe of the general allergic conditions. It occurs alone or is complicated by other conditions. In uncomplicated asthma, the patient has an "attack" whenever he comes into contact with an allergen to which he is sensitive. Asthma causes a narrowing of the lumen of the bronchial tubes, which produces difficulty in breathing, especially in expiration (I-3). There is an asthmatic condition which is persistent and which does not respond to the treatment that has previously been effective. This is called status asthmaticus.

MAJOR SYMPTOMS. The main symptoms of asthma are dyspnea, cyanosis and "wheezing" respirations. The patients become very apprehensive during an attack. The symptoms of status asthmaticus are the same as for any asthmatic attack except that they are more severe and more difficult to treat.

DRUG THERAPY

The Drugs. The present theory that asthma is a decrease of beta-adrenergic receptor blockage gives credence to the use of those drugs that stimulate the beta-receptors—*epinephrine, isoproterenol* and *ephedrine.* Epinephrine or isoproterenol is usually used during an acute attack. Epinephrine is given in doses of 0.2 to 1.0 ml. of a 1:1000 solution parenterally. Isoproterenol is usually given by inhalation 1:200 or 1:100 solution, one to five inhalations at intervals of 5 to 30 minutes. No more of the drug should be used than is required to secure relief. Ephedrine may then be used, or it may be the main drug in less acute circumstances. The dose is 25 mg. up to four times a day orally. A mild sedative such as *phenobarbital* 15 to 60 mg. two to four times a day orally, may aid in overcoming the stress which makes the asthmatic attack worse. No opiates should be given since they tend to constrict the bronchial tubes which are already overconstricted. There is one exception to this; *codeine phosphate,* 15 to 60 mg., may be used since it decreases the frequency of the cough.

In severe asthmatic attacks one of the prime requisites is adequate rest. If these drugs do not secure this, some more powerful analgesics and hypnotics may be required. *Meperidine hydrochloride* (Demerol; pethidine [C]), 50 to 100 mg., or similar drug will probably be ordered. The medium-acting barbiturates such as *amobarbital* (Amytal), *secobarbital* (Seconal) and *pentobarbital* (Nembutal) may be given for sleep. Some physicians use *chloral hydrate* instead of the barbiturates. In addition, the antiemetic-type antihistamine tranquilizers are helpful, such drugs as promazine hydrochloride (Sparine), proclorperazine (Compazine) and promethazine hydrochloride (Phenergan).

Oxygen, by mask or nasal catheter, is used if there is cyanosis. It may be given by any means, but the mask is usually most effective for these patients. The oxygen may be given with helium in place of air. Helium is much lighter than nitrogen—the main constituent of air—and this makes breathing easier since the patient does not need to put forth so much effort (IV-1). Some hospitals have special rooms for such cases. These rooms are hermetically sealed, the air is filtered to remove all extraneous material, and the amount of oxygen, air, helium or other gases that enters the room is accurately controlled. The patients are very comfortable in these rooms, but naturally their use is limited to those suffering an acute attack. Sometimes the patient becomes much worse the minute he is removed from the controlled atmosphere.

When the sputum is very tenacious, it is necessary to give the patient something which will aid in liquefying it to make expectoration easier. Several drugs may be given for this purpose. *Potassium iodide,* 0.3 Gm., and *ammonium chloride,* 0.3 Gm., have long been favorites and are still used. The iodides may be given alone or in combination with other drugs in an expectorant cough syrup. *Acetylcysteine* (Mucomyst) is used to aid in the removal of mucus. This preparation may be given by intermittent positive pressure or other apparatus. Refer to Chapter 17. Most physicians feel that the positive pressure gives the best results.

AMINOPHYLLINE

The Drug. Aminophylline is a synthetic drug which is related to the xanthine alkaloids, caffeine, theophylline and theobromine. Aminophylline and some preparations of theophylline used primarily for asthma will be discussed here. See also caffeine, Chapter 9, the xanthine diuretics, Chapter 18, and Current Drug Handbook for further information.

Physical and Chemical Properties. Aminophylline is a combination of roughly 81 per cent anhydrous theophylline and 14 per cent ethylenediamine. A white or light yellow powder with an ammoniacal odor and a bitter taste, it is readily soluble in water.

Action. Aminophylline relaxes smooth muscle tissue, relaxes the bronchial tubes, and increases urinary output and excretion of sodium. It tends to stimulate skeletal and cardiac muscles, increases cardiac output and causes some peripheral vasodilation. It also stimulates the central nervous system, although not as deeply as caffeine.

Therapeutic Uses. Aminophylline is widely used in the treatment of bronchial asthma, some other allergies and pulmonary edema. It increases the flow of urine in edema, lowers blood pressure, relaxes the coronary vessels and dilates the bronchial tubes not only in asthma, but also in emphysema and bronchitis.

Absorption and Excretion. Aminophylline is erratically absorbed from the gastrointestinal tract. Well distributed in the body, some of the drug is degraded in the body and excreted through the kidneys.

Preparations and Dosages

Aminophylline, U.S.P. (several trade names) 100 to 200 mg. t.i.d. or q.i.d. orally; 200 to 500 mg. I.M. or I.V. (I.V. given very slowly) p.r.n.; 250 to 500 mg. rectally, p.r.n.

Oxtriphylline (choline theophyllinate [C]; Choledyl) 100 to 400 mg. orally, t.i.d. or q.i.d.

Theophylline (Elixophyllin) 200 to 300 mg. orally, t.i.d. or q.i.d. (a solution).

THE NURSE

Mode of Administration. Aminophylline can be given by many different routes, although the oral, rectal and intravenous are the ones most commonly used. The drug is relatively irritating to the tissues, so if it is to be given intramuscularly, it should be given deep into the muscle. Intramuscular and intravenous preparations cannot be interchanged. When the drug is given intravenously, the medication should be given very slowly—0.25 Gm. every 15 minutes to prevent a severe drop in blood pressure, subjective awareness of heartbeat, headache, dizziness or nausea. Oral preparations are bitter and irritating, so administration is often planned with or after meals to reduce the evidence of gastric distress. If oral doses are administered more frequently than every 8 hours, cumulative effects may be noted.

When rectal suppositories are to be administered the nurse should encourage the patient to empty the bowel of feces prior to administration, so that uniform drug absorption may be expected. After insertion of the suppository, the patient may be advised to remain recumbent for 15 to 20 minutes, or until the desire to expel the medication has passed.

Side Effects, Toxicity and Treatment. Side effects, ordinarily, are not severe when the drug is administered in therapeutic dosage. However, gastric as well as urinary irritation may occur. Following intramuscular injection, local irritation may develop. Headache and a feeling of fullness may follow any route of administration.

Patient Teaching. As with any drug, the patient should be instructed as to time and mode of administration. If the rectal suppository form of the drug is prescribed, the patient should understand that the rectum should be empty before the suppository is inserted, and should be shown how the suppository is to be inserted. The suppository is usually inserted at bedtime to insure against respiratory distress during sleep.

The patient will also need to be instructed to expect increased urinary output since aminophylline has a diuretic effect. If the patient is hospitalized, an intake or output record may be maintained. Nocturnal micturition may be an annoynace when the medication is given at bedtime and should not be misinterpreted as another physiological problem.

THE PATIENT. By relaxing the tension of the bronchial tubes, the medication permits easier respiration, and gives the patient the chance of obtaining much needed rest.

Any attack of asthma will be associated with fear and anxiety on the part of the patient. The patient often feels as though he is unable to get enough air—a feeling of suffocation. Reaction to these fears often increases the symptoms and prolongs the attack. The patient may be so fearful that he will insist on someone's staying with him for reassurance that help is nearby. These fears are "real" and the patient will need to feel staff support and help during these times. Confidence that his call for help will be quickly responded to will often be a large step in developing a secure feeling. Family members can be encouraged to give emotional support to the patient and perhaps to stay with him for periods in the late evening and night, when feeling alone is such a problem.

OTHER DRUGS USED FOR THE TREATMENT OF ASTHMA

Asthma, during an attack, may be treated with *cortisone* or *hydrocortisone* or other adrenocortical steroid. At first the drug is given intramuscularly and, later, orally. As the patient recovers, the dosage of the cortisone is very gradually reduced. These drugs must not be stopped abruptly or the patient may have a severe relapse. Cortisone will usually bring about rather prompt improvement, but there is one important reason why many physicians hesitate to start it: it is much easier to start than to stop. The patient feels much better; the dyspnea lessens; the appetite improves; and the patient wonders why this drug has not been used before. However, edema due to sodium retention, headaches due to rise in blood pressure and other such disturbances may occur. Then, when the physician tries to reduce or discontinue the drug, the patient reverts to his asthmatic condition—a very discouraged, unhappy individual. Some patients, once they have had cortisone must continue with it indefinitely. In these cases, the dosage is very gradually reduced until a maintenance dose is established, and this is then used as long as required. There are several newer preparations similar to, but more potent than, cortisone that are very helpful in the treatment of asthma. They can be given in much lower dosage.

The Nurse. The nurse's duties in the case of the asthmatic are varied and exceedingly important. During the acute attack she will not only need to prepare the drugs and administer them as she would for any patient, but she must also reassure the patient and his relatives. The nurse must watch the asthmatic patient constantly for the least sign that the drugs either are not giving relief or are making the condition worse. In either event the physician should be notified immediately.

If corticotropin or cortisone is employed, the nurse should explain to the patient and his relatives the possibility of the patient's feeling better than his actual condition warrants. This will help to prevent the patient's overexertion. A relapse is a very discouraging setback.

As with all drugs the nurse must be aware of and watch for adverse symptoms. If the patient is to be cared for at home, the patient or some responsible member of his family should be told what untoward symptoms there may be and to notify the doctor should they occur.

If the patient has status asthmaticus, he is extremely apprehensive. Suddenly the drugs he has been taking, often for years, do not afford relief. He is afraid, and rightly so, that nothing can be done to help him. The nurse must first of all reassure the patient by telling him that other drugs are available and that the physician will keep on trying until one is found that will give relief.

Many combined drugs are available for the treatment of the asthmatic patient. These are very good in that they allow several drugs to be administered at one time and the patient has to take only one dose. Most of these medications contain one of the xanthine drugs, ephedrine and phenobarbital. Another combination contains aminophylline, aluminum hydroxide and ethyl aminobenzoate.

Asthma may be complicated by infection or other diseases. In such cases treatment of the complicating disease is the same as if it were not associated with asthma. Some physicians routinely give an anti-infective drug in severe asthma, especially if there is an associated bronchiectasis, atelectasis or similar condition. Refer to Chapter 17. This is to prevent the development of severe infections and aid the patient in his fight to regain health. The patient can be advised to avoid those individuals with apparent upper respiratory infections and to avoid crowds during the "cold season."

The various drugs mentioned have been covered in detail in other areas and in the Current Drug Handbook. The student should check any that are not clear to her.

Cutaneous Allergies

Allergies of the skin are relatively common and often very difficult to treat. The manifestations of skin allergy are varied, but three types predominate—eczema, urticaria and angioedema and the contact dermatitides.

Urticaria and angioedema are acute manifestations of allergy. They are similar in cause but somewhat different in reaction. Urticaria (hives) is familiar to almost everyone. The itching wheal is characteristic and may be caused by any number of things. If the condition is mild, elimination of the causative agent and antihistamine therapy may be sufficient to correct the trouble. With the antihistamine, many physicians give calcium, which reduces the permeability of the capillaries, and this in turn reduces the swelling. However, if the urticaria is severe, one of the vasoconstrictor drugs—*epinephrine* or *ephedrine*—may be needed. *Aminophylline* intravenously is also helpful in severe conditions. The usual doses prevail.

In angioedema (angioneurotic edema) there is acute swelling of the skin and mucous membranes. It often occurs around the lips, nares, buccal membranes and pharynx. If the swelling extends into the larynx or trachea, breathing may be impaired, and this may call for heroic action to maintain life. It is possible that some cases of "choking to death" have resulted from closure of the lumen of the respiratory tract due to angioedema. These cases are treated similarly to severe urticaria, with *epinephrine* subcutaneously or *ephedrine* orally. Either of these may be used topically as a spray. *Aminophylline* may be given intravenously. The patient with angioedema is very apprehensive since he suddenly finds himself in a rather critical condition and, if it is the first attack, he does not understand the reason for the condition or what to do about it. If a nurse is available she should do what she can with whatever antiallergic drugs she may have, but her first duty is to get the patient to a physician or a physician to the patient. As in other emergencies, the nurse may be able to have some relative or friend call the doctor while she stays with the patient. Often the patient who has an attack of angioedema is subject to other allergic conditions and may, therefore, have medications with orders available, but he may not realize the allergic nature of his condition. The nurse will be able to explain the situation to the patient and aid him in the use of the medications at hand.

Eczema

DEFINITION. Eczema (atopic dermatitis, allergic eczema) is a chronic skin condition exhibiting a variety of lesions and generally considered to be caused by either external or internal allergens. It may affect any age group. The face, folds of the skin (cubital and popliteal) and the nuchal region are the most common sites, or the eczema may be disseminated in character.

MAJOR SYMPTOMS. Most of the skin lesions are dry, scaly and lichenified, although vesiculation may occur. Pruritus and burning are usually present. Scratching may produce an infection in the lesions (III-1).

DRUG THERAPY

SOAP SUBSTITUTES. Most patients with eczema are sensitive to soaps because of their high pH and cleansing action which irritates and damages the skin. Neutral soaps and soap substitutes which may prove useful are Lowila, Dermolate, pHisoderm (pH 5.5) and Soy-Dome. If the eczema is disseminated, soap is prohibited.

TOPICAL APPLICATIONS. Steroid creams and ointments are the local treatment of choice. *Triamcinolone* (Aristocort or Kenalog) is effective as a cream or ointment 0.025 to 0.1 per cent in strength. Others that might be used are *fluocinolone acetonide* (Synalar) or *flurandrenolone* (Cordran). The systemic use of steroids is not recommended unless the condition is critical, for they do not cure but merely suppress the condition.

Open, cold, wet dressings during the day are cooling and soothing when used in the acute stages to help stop the oozing so often present. *Burow's solution* (aluminum acetate) 1:20 is often used, and if the lesions are infected, *potassium permanganate* 1:10,000 may be helpful. At night, Lassar's paste (compound paste of zinc oxide) applied on a closely woven cloth of cotton is substituted for the wet dressings.

In the chronic stage, the skin is usually dry and the use of an ointment such as *iodochlorhydroxyquin* 3 per cent and *hydrocortisone* 1 per cent (Vioform-Hydrocortisone) may be of use.

If there is secondary infection, many dermatologists use one of the broad-spectrum antibiotic creams along with a steroid cream.

Colloid baths may be employed if the skin is highly inflamed and rather large areas are involved. *Colloidal oatmeal* and *starch* (Aveeno), *colloidal oatmeal oleated* (Aveeno Oilated) or *Soyaloid Colloid Bath* (from soy beans) may be used with some success. *Cornstarch* (cooked) baths are also used.

THE NURSE. One of the major tasks of the nurse when eczema is first diagnosed is to reassure the patient (or parents if it is a child) that this disease is not contagious and usually is self-limited (V-1) (VI-1). The skin will probably heal without scarring if there is no secondary infection.

In babies and children, it is important to prevent them from scratching. The nurse may instruct the parents how to apply occlusive dressings made of old, soft sheeting secured with bandage. In some cases, it may be necessary to apply arm and leg restraints to prevent scratching and removal of the occlusive dressings.

Should *colloidal oatmeal* (Aveeno) baths be used, the usual proportion is 1 cup to a bathtub of water. This oatmeal preparation will be apt to make the bathtub slippery, and necessary precautions should be taken and the patient (or parents) instructed about this when giving the baths at home.

In administering wet dressings to elderly or debilitated patients, undue chilling should be prevented by covering only a small area. The wet dressings should be left open, not wrapped in plastic.

Eczema is aggravated by emotional strain and the nurse should do everything possible to make the patient comfortable, both physically and mentally, avoiding anything which causes emotional tension and helping the patient to relax (V-1, VI-1).

The nurse should be alert for possible development of a local sensitivity reaction when antibiotics are used.

THE PATIENT. The patient will have to live with this condition for some time and he often becomes discouraged and feels a social outcast because of the unsightly lesions. The family should understand and accept the patient and give him support at all times. Patients in the acute phases should avoid direct exposure to sunlight as this aggravates the condition.

SYSTEMIC THERAPY. In treating eczema in the disseminated form, oral antihistamines are quite good and effective to combat the pruritus. Even infants tolerate this form of therapy. Of the many antihistamines on the market, *diphenhydramine* (Benadryl) and *chlorpheniramine* (Chlor-Trimeton; Chlor-Tripolone [C]) are the most popular. The usual dose for *diphenhydramine* (Benadryl) is about 25 mg. three times a day; for *chlorpheniramine* (Chlor-Trimeton) it is 4 mg. three times a day.

Another drug is *Trimeprazine tartrate* (Temaril; Panectyl [C]), which is related to the phenothiazine group of drugs and does produce some depression of the central and sympathetic nervous systems. Its action is not completely understood but it does interrupt the itch-scratch-itch cycle, which encourages healing of lesions. The dosage is individually adjusted but the usual dose for adults is 2.5 mg. four times a day or 5.0 mg. (as a sustained release capsule) every 12 hours. For children up to the age of two years, 1.25 mg. is given at bedtime or, if needed, 1.25 mg. three times a day.

Cyproheptadine hydrochloride (Periactin) is said to work well against serotonin and histamine. It is given to adults in doses of three or four tablets daily (each tablet contains 4 mg. of the drug). Children from 2 to 14 years may receive one and a half to four tablets daily.

When either of these drugs is used, a mild and transient drowsiness is frequently encountered but this usually disappears after several days of administration.

Because trimeprazine is a phenothiazine derivative, the patient should be observed for signs of possible agranulocytosis.

SEDATIVES AND TRANQUILIZERS. Some sedative or tranquilizing drugs may be used to calm the patient who is disturbed not only by the sight of the lesions, but by the continued itching present. Almost any of the tranquilizers may be used; *meprobamate* (Equanil, Miltown and others; Tranquilate and others [C]) and *chlordiazepoxide hydrochloride* (Librium) are the most frequently used (see Chapter 30 for more details). The tranquilizers relax the patient and take the "edge" off the itching. Some doctors use small doses of phenobarbital instead of tranquilizers. *Hydroxyzine hydrochloride,* N.F. (Atarax, Vistaril), has also been somewhat successful. The usual oral dose for adults is 25 to 100 mg. three to four times daily. Adverse reactions are low in incidence; the drowsiness that may appear shortly after administration is transient.

Contact Dermatitis

DEFINITION. Possibly one of the most frequent forms of dermatitis is that which is caused by contact with substances to which the individual is sensitive. These may range through the animal, mineral or vegetable kingdom (plants such as poison ivy, poison oak, even oleander and geranium). Certain fabrics, dyes used in clothing, cosmetics and almost anything can be the cause of a reaction.

MAJOR SYMPTOMS. The symptoms are those of an acute dermatitis with redness, itching, burning and progression through the vesicular or "weeping" stage in the affected areas.

DRUG THERAPY. Obviously, the first treatment is to remove the cause. As soon as this has been accomplished (if possible), any number of treatments may be used to aid the recovery of the patient. Soap is contraindicated for these patients.

Open wet compresses, baths or soaks provide for evaporation from the skin surface and promote drying and decongestion of the affected tissue. Wet compresses of 1:40 liquid ammonium acetate *(Burow's solution)* during the acute stage for two to three hours twice a day may be alternated with *calamine* or *neocalamine lotion.* As the reaction subsides, the compresses may be continued but the time is shortened to 15 to 30 minutes every three to four hours.

If the dermatitis is generalized, baths may produce relief from the itching and general state of being uncomfortable. *Colloidal oatmeal baths* (Aveeno), *hydrolyzed starch* (Linit or Argo), *soy bean* (Soy-Dome) or plain water may be used.

For small areas (foot or hand) a soak using an aqueous solution of hydrolyzed starch or colloidal oatmeal may be effective.

A steroid cream along with calamine lotion may be applied locally. Other lotions which contain solids suspended or dissolved in alcohol or water, or a mixture of the two, allow secretions and exudates to pass fairly well. Calamine or neocalamine lotion is widely used, If there is a caked accumulation of lotions or pastes, the use of a water-miscible lotion with hydrocortisone or other steroid is effective in helping remove them.

Antihistaminic drugs orally may help alleviate the pruritus. Antibiotics topically or systemically are indicated for infections.

Several layers of soft white muslin (old sheeting) may be used for the compresses. The cloths are soaked in the prescribed solution, wrung out lightly and placed on the involved areas for one hour on and one hour off during the acute stages. The solution should be warm or cool. Any loose surface debris, crusts or scales should be removed with sterile forceps or scissors between applications. As the exudation decreases, the time of application of the compresses is shortened to 30 minutes every two hours. Once drying has occurred, wet compresses of plain water, for five to ten minutes once or twice a day, may be ordered to soften crusts.

The temperature of baths should be from warm to cool and the time spent in them from 20 minutes to one hour, depending upon the degree of comfort of the patient. They may be taken from one to four times a day during the acute stages.

Considerable reassurance must be given the patient and the family that this is not a contagious disease, and with time and treatment he will be well.

Plant dermatitis may be prevented or at least minimized by following a prescribed routine. When a known contact has been made, the part should be washed with a bar of laundry soap. After this, the entire body, with special attention to the exposed areas, should be sponged with rubbing alcohol.

There is some question as to the efficacy and advisability of prophylaxis against such plant dermatitides as poison ivy or poison oak. It is generally agreed that this is beneficial largely in those who are extremely sensitive to these plants. The protection is not complete but may lessen the severity of the dermatitis, shorten the course and reduce the dissemination.

Drug Dermatitis

Drugs produce diverse sensitivity reactions varying from profound anaphylactic shock and asthmatic type reaction to a mild skin redness. Treatment is pointed to (1) stopping and, if possible, removing the drug, and (2) relieving the symptoms. Here only skin reactions are being considered. If the results are mild, removal of the offending drug may be sufficient. Other symptoms are treated as they occur.

Various Allergic Conditions

MIGRAINE HEADACHES

Although the migraine or "sick" headache is considered by many physicians to be basically allergic in nature, it does not respond favorably to the usual antiallergic medications. One of the most effective treatments consists of the use of *ergotamine tartrate* (Gynergen), 0.25 to 0.5 mg. given by hypodermic injection. *Caffeine citrate* or *sodium benzoate,* 0.2 to 0.3 Gm., given at the same time increases the effectiveness of the ergotamine. *Dihydroergotamine,* a derivative of ergotamine, is also used. It is less toxic and has fewer side effects than the parent drug, and can be given intramuscularly or intravenously in dosages of 1 mg. The reason for the relief afforded by the drug is not well understood, but a majority of patients receive relief from 15 minutes to two hours after the drug has been given. The drug is almost dramatic in action. *Methylsergide maleate* (Sansert) is occasionally used as a preventative for vascular headache, 2 mg. orally t.i.d.—usually—with meals, although it is contraindicated in certain cardiac conditions, severe hypertension, pregnancy, peripheral vascular disease and atherosclerosis.

Ergotamine and related drugs interact with the sympathomimetics to increase the blood pressure. They should be used with caution if the patient is hypertensive.

Diuretics may be helpful in reducing cerebral edema and thus lessening the pressure and the pain. The diuresis also tends to lessen the nausea and vomiting which are a part of the syndrome. *Aminophylline,* the mercurial diuretics or the synthetic oral diuretics such as *hydrochlorothiazide* (Esidrix) or *acetazolamide* (Diamox) may be given. The antiemetic-antihistamine tranquilizers may give relief, either alone or more often in combination with other medications.

GASTROINTESTINAL ALLERGIES

Many physicians feel that various gastrointestinal disorders may be of allergic origin. However, it is often difficult to differentiate between those of allergic nature and other gastrointestinal conditions. If in doubt, a small dose of epinephrine hydrochloride may be given. If symptoms subside, the cause is allergy. It is then essential to determine the allergen and either remove it from the patient's environment or desensitize the patient. During an attack the symptoms are treated as they occur. Usually the vasoconstrictors will help.

SERUM REACTIONS

Serum reactions are reactions of the same antigen-antibody types as the allergies. The distinction lies in the fact that the reaction is induced by the introduction of a foreign material (serum, drug) into the body. The symptoms and treatment are not unlike other allergic reactions. However, serum reactions do vary and this should be understood. There are two main forms of serum reactions, anaphylactic shock and serum sickness.

ANAPHYLACTIC REACTION OR ANAPHYLACTIC SHOCK

DEFINITION. Anaphylactic reaction usually occurs within a short time after the administration of the serum or drug. (The antibiotics, particularly penicillin, are prime offenders.) It may occur within minutes. With a serum, this condition can usually be avoided by the preadministration of a skin sensitivity test. The reaction depends upon the presence of antibodies developed from a previous exposure in the recipient's blood. However, in many cases, no known previous exposure has occurred. In these instances, it is probably induced hypersensitivity and may be fatal within a few minutes.

MAJOR SYMPTOMS. The patient often first complains of apprehension or a feeling of impending death. There is cyanosis, paresthesia, a wheezing cough, incontinence, fall in blood pressure, fever, dilation of the pupils, loss of consciousness, laryngeal edema, bronchospasms, vascular collapse and, unless treated, death.

DRUG THERAPY. *Epinephrine* here is life saving. An initial dose of 1 ml. of a 1:1000 solution should be given intramuscularly with the first symptoms if it is available. It is repeated in 5 or 10 minutes if required. If there is no response, 0.1 to 0.4 ml. of a 1:1000 solution diluted in 10 ml. of saline solution is given slowly intravenously. The patient should be put in shock position, kept warm and an airway kept open by tracheostomy if required. Other drugs that may be used include *diphenhydramine hydrochloride* (Benadryl), *hydrocortisone* or *methylprednisolone* given intravenously. Oxygen under positive pressure is used, especially if cyanosis is marked. *Aminophylline* by slow intravenous route may help. If hypotension is severe, one of the antihypotensive drugs is given. The usual emergency doses of these various medicines prevail.

Anaphylactic shock is a condition in which an ounce of prevention is worth several pounds of cure. Always skin test before giving a serum. Ask the patient if he has ever had the serum or drug to be given, and what the result was. Remember, a patient may have taken penicillin, for example, several times without difficulty, but in the meantime he may have built up antibodies to it. Ask the patient if he has any allergies, and if he has had conditions such as hay fever, asthma and the like. Some individuals seem prone to allergic reactions. When giving a drug known to cause allergic reactions, detain the patient or stay with him until the possibility of anaphylactic shock is over. There are histories of patients' dying of anaphylactic shock on their way home from doctors' offices.

SERUM SICKNESS

DEFINITION. Serum sickness is a delayed reaction to the introduction of an antigen. It usually occurs one to two weeks following the injection or ingestion of the serum or drug.

MAJOR SYMPTOMS. Serum sickness usually manifests itself by a patchy or generalized rash, malaise, lymphadenopathy, nausea and vomiting, muscular aches and pains and abdominal pain. It rarely lasts more than two or three days.

DRUG THERAPY. The oral antihistamines are usually sufficient, but if they are not effective, *ephedrine* and/or *epinephrine* are used. The usual doses apply.

There is a condition which is between this and the anaphylactic reaction. It occurs nine to twelve hours after the antigen has entered the body. Not as severe as anaphylactic shock, it is more severe than serum sickness. It usually starts with urticaria. It is initially treated with epinephrine or ephedrine and then an antihistamine until the condition clears.

DRUGS USED TO PREVENT REJECTION OF AN ORGAN TRANSPLANT

DEFINITION. An organ transplant involves the process of grafting an entire organ from a donor into a recipient. As with skin grafts, blood transfusions or bone marrow infusion, the sensitive immune mechanism of the recipient recognizes the foreign antigens (nonidentical tissue) of the donor and, depending on the degree of difference from the recipient's antigens, produces antibodies that attempt to destroy or reject the transplant. Prior to organ transplants, tests are done to determine and match the antigenic makeup of donor and recipient as nearly as possible. The greatest problem is to prevent rejection of the new organ. Still under investigation at this time is the theory that the rejection of the new organ is a complex phenomenon which may involve both circulatory antibody and cell-borne immunity of the delayed hypersensitivity type.

MAJOR SYMPTOMS. In the rejection syndrome no one symptom is predominant, but the general condition of the patient deteriorates. However, certain symptoms especially related to the specific organ are apt to occur.

With kidney transplant patients, the symptoms of renal failure will be manifest. Physical changes include anorexia, oliguria or anuria, hypertension, tenderness over the site of the transplant and blood changes due to the retention of substances normally excreted by the kidneys. The patient is apathetic and lethargic.

With the liver transplant patient, the signs of hepatic failure occur, such as jaundice, lightening of the color of the feces and increases of bilirubin, transaminase and alkaline phosphatase in the blood. There is tenderness over the affected organ.

In the heart transplant patient, there will be symptoms associated with some type of heart disease, usually cardiac failure.

DRUG THERAPY. The usual preoperative and postoperative drugs (analgesics and anti-infectives) are used, and the nurse is referred to Chapter 15, "Drugs Used in Surgical Intervention" for them. Here the discussion will be limited to those drugs known at this time to be of use in preventing rejection of the new organ.

Drug therapy is directed at the suppression of the immunological system of the body. The nurse must remember that the immunological system in the normal individual helps to prevent infections, and when it is suppressed, there is always the grave danger of the occurrence of an overwhelming infection. The immunosuppressive drugs are absolutely essential for all organ transplants. If it is possible, the treatment may be started three to five days prior to the transplant. The length of time the drug will be needed may be days, weeks, months but more likely years, depending upon the progress of the patient.

AZATHIOPRINE (IMURAN)

THE DRUG

Azathioprine is a synthetic, but potent, helpful adjunct for the prevention of rejection in organ transplants. Much more needs to be learned about it.

Physical and Chemical Properties. This drug is an antimetabolite and is an imidazolyl analogue of 6-mercaptopurine (6-MP). Chemically it is 6-[(1-methyl-4-nitroimidazol-5-yl) thio] purine.

Action. The precise mode of action of azathioprine is unknown, but it apparently works by blocking the conversion of inosinic acid to adenylic acid, preventing the synthesis of nucleic acids. It also serves as a general enzyme inhibitor by binding sulfhydryl groups.

Absorption and Excretion. Azathioprine is readily absorbed from the gastrointestinal tract. In the body, the drug is split into 6-mercaptopurine which is then subjected to catabolic degradation forming a variety of oxidized and methylated derivatives among which 6-thiouric acid predominates. About eight hours after ingestion, there is little or no unchanged azathioprine or mercaptopurine in the urine. Although elimination of the drug is mainly by metabolic destruction, small amounts of the unchanged drug and mercaptopurine are eliminated by the kidney. Especially in kidney transplants, the biological effectiveness and toxicity may be doubled in the anuric patient. Some of the azathioprine is bound to the serum proteins but this does not appear, at this time, to have significant therapeutic importance.

Preparations and Dosages. Azathioprine (Imuran) is given in doses of 1 to 5 mg. per kg. body weight once a day. The dose is adjusted for each individual patient so as to suppress the immune response without undue depression of the bone marrow as judged by the daily white blood count. Alterations in dosage are indicated if there are signs of rejection.

THE NURSE

Mode of Administration. This drug is given orally once daily and is supplied in 50 mg. scored tablets.

Side Effects. Many side effects have been reported but the percentage of these is not high. These include nausea, vomiting, diarrhea, anorexia, oral lesions, skin rash, drug fever, alopecia, pancreatitis, and arthralgia. Jaundice has occurred in a few patients. For most of these, reduction of dosage level is sufficient to overcome the difficulty.

Toxicity and Treatment. An extremely toxic drug, Azathioprine (Imuran) should never be used unless the patient is under very close medical supervision. The most serious toxic effects are bone marrow depression with leukopenia, anemia, thrombocytopenia and bleeding. This, of course, lowers the patient's resistance to infection and he must be guarded carefully against *any* type of infection. A reduction in dosage may halt the depression, but it may be necessary to discontinue the drug.

Contraindications and Precautions. Hypersensitivity to the drug is the only important contraindication to the drug. However, the safety of its use during pregnancy has not been established, a factor which should be weighed against the possibility of its teratogenic activity. It is important that the benefits and risks involved be weighed very carefully before use in women of childbearing potential.

The dosage should be reduced in the following conditions: (1) lowered renal function; (2) the concomitant use of allopurinal; (3) persistent negative nitrogen balance; and (4) an infection.

Patient Teaching. Azathioprine (Imuran) is believed to be necessary for the rest of the patient's life so it will be necessary that he be knowledgeable about the drug. He should be taught the importance of the regular administration of the drug. If any questions arise, most particularly about medication, the family is to telephone the physician immediately. Missed doses of azathioprine (Imuran) have been known to trigger rejection. The recipient is instructed to report any unusual signs or symptoms to his doctor and he must understand the importance and reason behind the regular blood counts for himself. Commonly, the patient and his family become so concerned about the essential blood work, that they may be very anxious and often demanding at this time. It is essential that the patient and his family understand *why* he must be under the close supervision of his physician at all times, even long after he leaves the hospital.

The nurse's main responsibility while the patient is still in the hospital is to provide emotional support in addition to the regular nursing care. She must be a good listener, allowing the patient and the family to express their fears and doubts without becoming too emotionally involved. It is not easy. She should be as encouraging as the patient's condition warrants, but she must not be overly optimistic. Perhaps most important of all is that the patient and his family thoroughly understand the importance of preventing *any* kind of infection.

The Patient. The person who is to have or who has had an organ transplant is first of all an extremely ill person. He is physically ill and emotionally disturbed; there are so many factors involved. Not only are these physical, they are moral and spiritual as well. The nurse must try to help the patient and his relatives bridge this trying time. They all know that without the new organ, the patient cannot live much longer. They also know that organ transplant surgery has had only limited success to this date. The drugs will give each case a better hope of recovery.

Other Drugs Useful for These Cases

Antilymphocytic Globulin (serum) (ALG) or (ALS) is a biological preparation. This drug is investigational as of 1973. Lymphocytes from the blood or thymus tissue are injected over a period of time into the blood stream of a horse. When sufficient antibodies to the foreign lymphocytes are produced, the serum is collected and refined. Its mode of action seems to be to clear the lymphocytes from the blood stream and cause the lymph nodes to shrink. This then prevents the immediate immune response from occurring. This immunosuppressive drug is used with other medications and allows for a lower dosage of the corticosteroids.

It is recommended that ALG (ALS) be given intramuscularly 4 to 5 ml. three to five days preoperatively, if this is possible. It should then be given daily for two weeks postoperatively, then twice weekly for one month and, finally, once a week for another month.

Precautions include a skin sensitivity test *before* the first dose is given since this is an animal serum. If the test is positive, this must be reported. For these patients the serum may be prepared in rabbits.

Side effects include severe pain, fever, edema and swelling at the site of the injection. A sterile abscess may form at the site of the injections. Some muscle cramping has been reported. It has been reported that up to 20 per cent of the transplant patients develop anaphylactic reactions such as shortness of breath, flushing or cyanosis, decreased blood pressure accompanied by a weak and rapid pulse and rapid respirations, anterior and posterior chest pain and nausea and vomiting. Dosage may need to be lowered should any of these appear.

Actinomycin C is a cytostatic drug which affects lymphoid tissue. At the present, its use is extremely limited as it is not manufactured in the United States. It is invariably used in conjunction with local irradiation over the area during the initial crises. The dose is 200 mcg. per vial given daily, intravenously for three days. The most common side effect is irritation of mucous membranes. Toxic reactions rarely occur with controlled dosage.

Corticosteroids also play an important role in organ transplants. More commonly, prednisone by mouth or prednisolone by intramuscular injection may be used interchangeably in doses up to 200 mg. per day. These doses should be evenly divided to be given throughout the day and as is usual in corticosteroids, must be withdrawn gradually. The actions of the drug which are important in preventing organ rejection are reduction of vascular endothelial reactions, moderation of plasma cell and lymphocyte infiltration; and, in addition, reduction of arteriolar constriction during the active rejection process. For more details of the actions, precautions and other information see Chapter 27.

IT IS IMPORTANT TO REMEMBER

1. That in all allergies the basic symptoms are congestion with dilation of capillaries, increased interstitial fluid and, when glands are involved, increased secretion.

2. That in all allergies there are some psychosomatic factors. This varies widely in different allergic conditions, in different patients and in the same patient at different times.

3. That for the immediate treatment of most allergies vasoconstrictors are used. Later treatments vary, including antihistamines, hormones, sedatives, diuretics, analgesics and other drugs as indicated by the symptoms.

4. That all patients with allergies will need reassurance and encouragement to persist in their treatments since the condition does not appear to be curable. It can, however, be allayed, if not arrested.

5. That in all cases of organ transplants there is an emotional problem, not only with the patient and his family, but also with the donor's family.

6. That organ transplant cases are usually terminal and that this surgery really is a "last resort."

TOPICS FOR STUDY AND DISCUSSION

1. Atropine sulfate is sometimes an ingredient of multiple antiallergic drugs. What would be its value—especially in asthma?

2. Look up several charts of patients suffering with allergies. List all the drugs used. Compare with those given in this chapter. Why was each ordered? Did the patient secure the desired effect from the drugs? Explain.

3. Epinephrine hydrochloride has many uses. List the more important ones and explain how all are due to certain basic effects the drug has in the body.

4. Differentiate between corticotropin and cortisone and tell in what conditions each is most apt to be used and why.

5. Try to visualize a patient with angioneurotic edema of the lips and cheeks. How might the patient be aided by the nurse emotionally? Do the same for asthma.

6. You find the following orders on the chart of a newly admitted patient with status asthmaticus. Which should be done first, second and so on? Explain your reasons for your selection. What is the purpose of each order?

Orders:
a. Bed rest
b. Phenobarbital gr. $1/2$ b.i.d.
c. Seconal suppository gr. 3 h.s.
d. Soft diet, low salt, no stimulating drink, but patient may have decaffeinated coffee or weak tea if desired.
e. Prednisone 5 mg. t.i.d.
f. Oxygen per mask.
g. Aminophylline gr. $3^3/_4$ in 1000 ml. 5 per cent glucose I.V., o.d.
h. Adrenalin m. 5 p.r.n.

7. Refer to Topic 6. The nurse finds that the phenobarbital is in scored tablets marked 60 mg. each. How should she proceed?

8. Refer to Topic 6. The aminophylline is in ampules marked 0.25 Gm. per 10 ml. How much should be used for each dose?

9. Since only a few student nurses will have the opportunity to actually care for a patient with an organ transplant, a class or seminar on the subject might be beneficial.

BIBLIOGRAPHY

Books and Pamphlets

American Medical Association Council on Drugs, *Drug Evaluations*, Chicago, 1971, American Medical Association.

Beeson, P. B., and McDermott, W., *Cecil-Loeb Textbook of Medicine, 13th Ed.*, Philadelphia, 1971, W. B. Saunders Co.

Beland, I., *Clinical Nursing, 2nd Ed.*, New York, 1970, The Macmillan Co.
Conn, H. F., et al., *Current Therapy, 1974*, Philadelphia, 1974, W. B. Saunders Co.
Falconer, M. W., Patterson, H. R., and Gustafson, E. A., *Current Drug Handbook, 1974–1976*, Philadelphia, 1974, W. B. Saunders Co.
Goodman, L. S., and Gilman, A., *Pharmacological Basis of Therapeutics, 4th Ed.*, New York, 1970, The Macmillan Co.
Hartshorn, E. A., *Handbook of Drug Interactions*, Cincinnati, 1970, University of Cincinnati Press.
Meltzer, L., Abdellah, F., and Kitchell, J. R., *Concepts and Practices of Intensive Care for Nursing Specialists*, Philadelphia, 1970, The Charles Press.

Journal Articles

Albright, J. F., Omer, T., and Deitchman, J., "Antigen competition: Antigens compete for a cell occurring with limited frequency," *Science* 167:3915:196 (1970).
Child, J., Collins, D., and Collins, J., "Blood transfusions," *Am. J. Nurs.* 72:9:1602 (September, 1972).
Clapin, A. J., and Smithies, O., "Antibody producing cells in division," *Science* 157:3796:1561 (1967).
Craven, R. F., "Anaphylactic shock," *Am. J. Nurs.* 72:4:718 (April, 1972).
DiPalma, J. R., "Drugs used in organ transplants," *R.N.* 32:53 (1969).
____________ "Oxygen as drug therapy." *R.N.* 34:8:49 (August, 1971).
Doolittle, R. F., "Antibody active sites and immunoglobulin molecules," *Science* 153:3131:13 (1966).
Echlin, P., "Pollen," *Sci. Am.* 218:68:4 (1968).
Edelman, M. J., "The structure and functions of antibodies," *Sci. Am.* 223:2:34 (September, 1969).
Feinberg, S., "Allergens and air conditioning," *Am. J. Nurs.* 66:6:1333 (June, 1966).
Feinberg, S., "Immunology," *Nurs. Times* 64:1244 (1968).
Hildreth, J., "Some common allergen emergencies," *Med. Clin. North Am.* 50:3:1313 (1966).
Kahn, D. B., and Reisfeld, A. R., "Transplantation antigens," *Science* 164:3879:514 (1969).
Lister, J., "Nursing intervention in anaphylactic shock," *Am. J. Nurs.* 72:4:720 (April, 1972).
Miller, M. W., "The comprehensive approach to the allergen patient," *Nurs. Clin. North Am.* 49:5:1415.
Nye, A. W., et al., "Sixteen patients: postgraduate nursing experience with heart transplantation," *Am. J. Nurs.* 69:12:2630 (December, 1969).
Peterson, M. H., "Understanding defense mechanisms: a programmed instruction unit," *Am. J. Nurs.* 72:9:1651 (September, 1972).
Rodman, M. J., "Drugs for allergic disorders," *R.N.* 34:6:63 (June, 1971).
Rodman, M. J., "Drugs for allergic disorders," *R.N.* 34:7:53 (July, 1971).
Rodman, M. J., "Drugs for allergic reactions," *R.N.* 29:6:66 (June, 1966).

CHAPTER 26

DRUGS USED FOR DISORDERS OF THE REPRODUCTIVE SYSTEM

CORRELATION WITH OTHER SCIENCES

I. ANATOMY AND PHYSIOLOGY

1. The functions of the reproductive system of both male and female are controlled by the pituitary gland with other glands involved.
2. The female reproductive organs are divisible into two groups. In the external group are usually included the vagina, the vulva and the clitoris. The internal organs include the uterus, tubes and ovaries.
3. In the female the menstrual cycle is influenced by all the endocrine glands and is actually a preparation of the uterus for pregnancy. When this does not occur, the menstrual flow results.
4. The male reproductive system includes the testes, the epididymis with the accessory glands (seminal vesicles and prostate gland) and the supporting structures (the scrotum, penis, and spermatic cords).
5. At the time of menopause (approximately 45 to 55 years of age) there is a gradual cessation of the function of the reproductive glands of the female. This covers a period of several years.
6. The male also experiences a period corresponding to the cessation of menstruation in the female. The male sex organs become less active and general regressive changes begin. The male climacteric occurs later than that of the female.
7. The male does not have abrupt spectacular changes to correspond with the onset of the menstrual function in the female. However, the male does undergo gradual developmental changes.
8. The period of senescence is the period when the physical powers wane. The regressive changes may be mental as well as physical. The entire body undergoes these changes and the process may be relatively rapid, or it may be very slow.

II. CHEMISTRY

1. The normal pH of the vaginal secretion is acid (4.5 to 5.0) which acts as a natural defense against certain infections.
2. When tissue changes, even to the slightest degree, there will also be chemical changes.
3. Neutralization is the formation of a salt from an acid and a base. If both the acid and the base are either weak or strong, the salt will be neutral. If there is a strong acid with a weak base, the result will be an acidic salt, the reverse will result in a basic salt.

III. MICROBIOLOGY

1. Viruses are very small organisms which are capable of producing disease. They are too small to be seen under the light microscope but are visible under the electron microscope. Viruses vary in length from 12 to 400 millimicrons. A millimicron is one thousandth of a micron and a micron is one thousandth of a millimeter. Viruses depend upon the living cell for part of their metabolic processes; hence, they live only in the living cell of the host organism (intracellular).
2. Bacteria are organisms which are visible under the light microscope by staining. They are classified in various ways such as shape (bacilli, cocci, spirilla), staining reaction (gram-positive, gram-negative, acid-fast), spore formation, oxygen requirement and so forth.

3. Spirochetes are slender, flexible coiled organisms that resemble both protozoa and the spiral bacteria.
4. Fungi are plants of a lower order. They do not produce chlorophyll.
5. Protozoa are minute one-celled animals.
6. The normal flora of the vagina may include many types of organisms. Some of the ones more commonly found are streptococci, staphylococci, Döderlein's bacillus and diphtheroids.
7. Infections of the reproductive organs may be caused by almost any organism or fungus.

V. PSYCHOLOGY

1. Many physicians believe that a great many cases of dysmenorrhea are of psychogenic origin.
2. One of the causes of sterility in both the male and female is probably mental or emotional stress.
3. Many of the problems of the female menopause are believed to be psychogenic.

VI. SOCIOLOGY

1. Society has produced barriers and taboos in relation to sex. Any person who crosses the accepted limits is open to social ostracism.

INTRODUCTION

When discussing the diseases of the reproductive system, we must consider those of both the male and female. The largest proportion of drugs used in these conditions are endocrine preparations and, before discussing the diseases and their drug therapy, it would be wise to clarify the action of some of these drugs.

Recalling the menstrual cycle, it will be remembered that the growth of the ovarian follicle is induced by the follicle-stimulating hormone of the anterior pituitary gland. This follicle produces an estrogenic hormone which causes certain changes in the accessory organs. These substances have been isolated and synthesized and are referred to in medicine as estrogens.

At ovulation there is a release of the luteinizing hormone of the pituitary. The corpus luteum then secretes a hormone called progesterone. This term has been adopted to describe this particular hormone as used in medicine. In turn, this hormone induces secretory changes in the endometrium. In summary, then, estrogens are the hormones of the first part of the cycle and progesterone is the hormone of the latter part of the cycle.

Female sex hormones were formerly standardized in terms of international units, but more recently these dosages have been expressed in terms of weight. However, some preparations are still marketed on the basis of units.

DISEASES OF THE FEMALE REPRODUCTIVE SYSTEM

Amenorrhea

DEFINITION. There are many causes of amenorrhea (the absence of menstruation), but we are concerned here only with those of endocrine origin (I-1, 3, 5). In many instances, the thyroid gland is responsible; other cases are due to a lack of ovarian function; and still others are related to the pituitary gland. Primary amenorrhea is the failure of menstruation to occur well beyond the age of puberty. Secondary amenorrhea is a cessation of the menstrual function after it has previously been present. Both are due to an endocrine dysfunction.

MAJOR SYMPTOMS. Aside from the absence of menstruation, the symptoms will

OVARIES

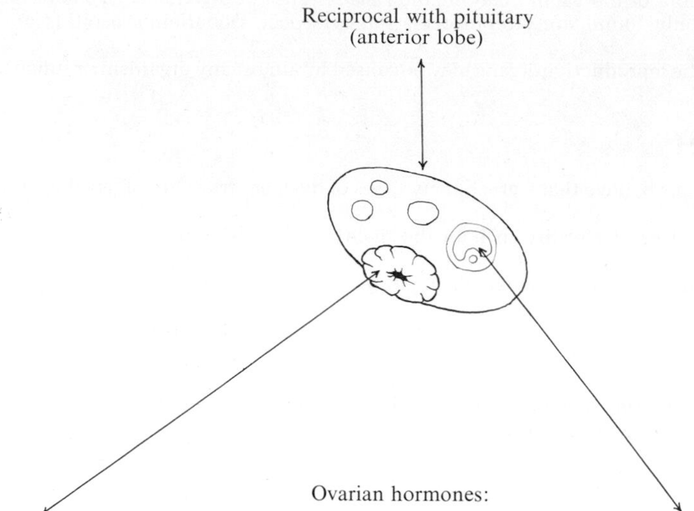

Ovarian hormones:

Progesterone or luteal: Maintain pregnancy

Estrogen: Maintain secondary sex characteristics
Stimulate production of ova

Drug therapy: Used for above conditions and also to treat many conditions

Progesterone or luteal:
Ethisterone, U.S.P.
Progesterol, U.S.P.

Estrogen:
Estradiol benzoate, U.S.P.
Estrone, U.S.P.
Diethylstilbestrol, U.S.P. (synthetic)

There are many nonofficial natural and synthetic preparations of these hormones.

Refer to Current Drug Handbook and to Pituitary Gland diagram and discussion.

FIGURE 43. Endocrine system in drug therapy.

vary somewhat with the origin of the endocrinopathy.

DRUG THERAPY. Constitutional factors play a role and measures taken here are essential and helpful. When anemia is present, hematinic treatment with *iron* and even *liver* preparations is indicated. Dietary errors must be corrected and any associated or related constitutional disease alleviated. If obesity exists, the patient should reduce since this is one known cause of amenorrhea. Before treatment can be instituted with drugs, tests must be done to see if it can be determined which one of the endocrine glands is at fault. Drug therapy will then revolve around the endocrine gland which is responsible, but it is a well recognized fact that the results of treatment are often disappointing.

THYROID THERAPY. In those cases of amenorrhea directly attributable to hypothyroidism, the administration of *thyroid extract* is indicated and yields the best results of all the groups. The administration of this drug is then a replacement therapy. Thyroid extract in small doses, 30 to 60 mg. daily, is usual.

FEMALE HORMONE THERAPY. In primary amenorrhea in which ovarian dysgenesis is proved, estrogens are given, not necessarily to induce menstruation, but to provide the patient with the secondary sex characteristics. It is treated in the same way as delayed menarche for other reasons. *Diethylstilbestrol* is administered orally in 3 to 5 mg. doses daily for 20 days. Withdrawal bleeding usually occurs within five to ten days. This may be repeated for two or three cycles followed by a rest to see if this stimulation will trigger the onset of a menstrual cycle, but this does not always prove to be the case. *Stilbestrol* is contraindicated during pregnancy. For those who cannot take stilbestrol, *conjugated estrogenic substance* (Premarin), one of the water-soluble estrogens, may be used. The dose is 2.5 to 7.5 mg. daily, orally. *Ethynyl estradiol* (Estinyl, Lynoral; Nadestyl, Nylestin [C]), is a semisynthetic estrogen of high potency and may be given in oral doses of 0.05 mg. daily. There are many preparations available, some for oral administration and others for the parenteral route. (See Current Drug Handbook for further details.)

Progesterones will sometimes prove helpful in the secondary type of amenorrhea. These drugs are given orally or intramuscularly or, in larger doses, sublingually. Some gynecologists give progesterone simultaneously with the estrogen for the last five days of the course described in the preceding paragraph. *Progestogens* are synthesized compounds which reproduce most (but not all) of the effects of progesterone. They have a greater potency when given orally and an increased duration of action when given parenterally. The rationale behind the use of progestogens is based on the production of the progestational changes in the endometrium which are characteristic of the secretory phase of the menstrual cycle. Many gynecologists do not like to use the intramuscular preparations of progestogens because of their long action—from one to four weeks.

Dydrogesterone (Duphaston) is one of the more commonly used progestogens and is useful in the diagnosis of primary amenorrhea. Withdrawal bleeding indicates a relatively normal genitoendocrine system. Intermittent therapy frequently causes spontaneous menses but if it does not occur, priming with estrogens may be tried. If menses still does not occur, endometrial failure is probably present. In secondary amenorrhea, withdrawal bleeding will occur in the absence of pregnancy. This drug is relatively nontoxic and seems to have no androgenic or estrogenic activity. It is usually given orally 5 to 10 mg. daily from the fifth to the twenty-fifth day of the menstrual cycle and may be repeated.

Another progestogen which may be useful is *medroxyprogesterone acetate* (Provera). Cyclic oral therapy of from 2.5 to 10 mg. daily for five to ten days beginning on the assumed sixteenth to twenty-first day of the menstrual period is usual. *Norethindrone* (Norlutin), *norethindrone acetate* (Norlutate) is a potent, orally effective progestogen which has some estrogenic and androgenic activity. The onset of action is as rapid as parenterally administered progesterone. The dosage for norethindrone acetate (Norlutate) should be one half that of norethindrone (Norlutin). Cyclic therapy is used with 5 to 20 mg. of Norlutin or 2.5 to 10 mg. of norethindrone acetate (Norlutate) daily starting on the fifth day of the menstrual cycle and continuing through the twenty-third day. Withdrawal bleeding should occur within five days.

Hydroxyprogesterone caproate (Delalutin) may also be used intramuscularly in doses of 125 to 250 mg. This usually induces withdrawal bleeding from estrogen-primed endometrium within seven to ten days. (See Current Drug Handbook for other drugs which may be used.)

The oral contraceptive agents are also used in the treatment of primary amenorrhea. Usually given in regular routines for three to six months, they will often start the normal menstrual cycle. These drugs are discussed in detail under Family Planning in Chapter 28.

Side effects that may occur on administration of estrogens and progesterone include nausea, vomiting, headache and dizziness. If dydrogesterone (Duphaston) is used, the patient may complain of mild gastrointestinal difficulties such as nausea, diarrhea or constipation but these do not usually necessitate withdrawal of the drug. If spotting or break-through bleeding occurs before the calculated onset of menstruation, it usually means the dosage level is too low. Medroxyprogesterone (Provera) may occasionally cause somnolence. Norethindrone (Norlutin) has been known to cause a

ESTROGENS
Hormone of first part of menstrual cycle–during growth of ovarian follicle
PRIMARY EFFECTS
On sex organs:
Stimulates proliferative changes in uterus but this is also influenced by progesterone
Given early in menstrual cycle, delays ovulation and prolongs cycle
On skeletal muscles:
Large amounts inhibit growth of cartilage and longitudinal osseus growth
Augments proliferation of medullary bone, presumably by stimulating osteoblasts
On electrolytes and water retention:
On prolonged administration may cause a positive electrolyte and water balance and edema
PRINCIPAL USES
Menopause
Atrophic (senile) vaginitis
Postmenopausal osteoporosis
Dysmenorrhea
Amenorrhea
Functional uterine bleeding
Ovarian agenesis
PROGESTERONE
Hormone of latter part of menstrual cycle–from the corpus luteum. Is secreted all through pregnancy and is necessary for its continuation
PRIMARY EFFECTS
Complete proliferative changes in uterus started by estrogens (action almost solely on uterus)
PRINCIPAL USES
In threatened and habitual abortion
Functional uterine bleeding
Amenorrhea

FIGURE 44. Estrogens and progesterones as therapeutic agents.

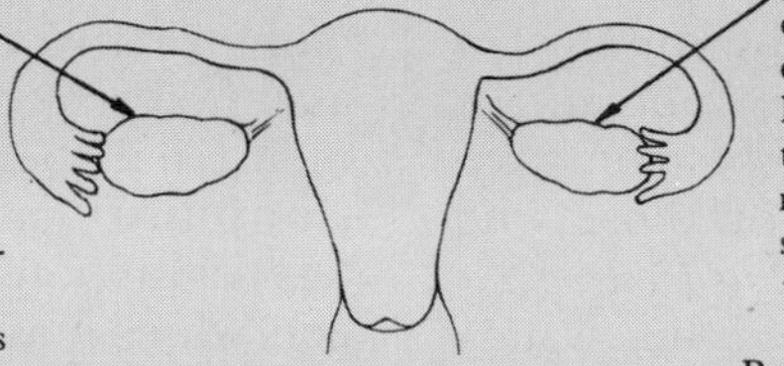

transient lethargy and nausea, hirsutism, voice change and acne. Hydroxyprogesterone (Delalutin) is used with caution in patients with asthma, migraine or epilepsy.

These drugs are relatively expensive and their frequent failure to produce a satisfactory result may make their use unwarranted. Quite often, nature itself takes care of the condition.

Dysmenorrhea

DEFINITION. The most common of all symptoms of gynecologic disorders is menstrual pain or dysmenorrhea. In some cases there is a demonstrable pelvic disease present (secondary dysmenorrhea) but in others, no known cause can be found (essential primary dysmenorrhea). Essential dysmenorrhea is in some cases believed to be of psychogenic orgin.

MAJOR SYMPTOMS. In the primary type, the pain may not appear until the beginning of menstruation and may persist for one to two days. Occasionally, it may precede the onset by a few days and sometimes the pain may persist throughout the period. The pain is described as colicky or severe aching in character, and it may be so severe as to cause the patient to go to bed. It may be accompanied by nausea and vomiting in addition to extreme nervousness.

DRUG THERAPY

ANALGESICS AND ANTISPASMODICS. A simple analgesic such as aspirin or *acetaminophen* (Tylenol) in doses of 0.6 Gm. orally repeated in one to three hours may be effective for those patients whose pain is not too severe. *Phenobarbital* 15 to 30 mg. given alone or with one of the above may also give relief from pain and tension.

Adiphenine hydrochloride (Trasentine) in doses of 50 to 75 mg. orally may be used with or without phenobarbital. This is an antispasmodic with papaverine-like action on smooth muscle tissue. It is usually given three times a day.

These drugs are effective in the milder conditions but are usually only partially effective for those patients with severe pain.

Many of the pain remedies on the market for dysmenorrhea are simple salicylic acid compounds and the extra cost of buying these proprietary preparations is not justified.

DIURETICS. A more vigorous routine based on the physiology of ovulation and menstruation calls for the reduction of body fluid content preceding the period. For seven days prior to the expected onset of menstruation, the patient is requested to restrict the salt content of her diet. A diuretic is given, often one of the thiazide preparations. When menstruation starts, the patient is given *isoxsuprine hydrochloride* (Vasodilan) 10 mg. with a phenobarbital-belladonna combination drug four times a day. This routine is effective in a large percentage of cases.

THE NURSE. It is important to give the patient counseling in the treatment of dysmenorrhea. She should understand the physiology of menstruation. The nurse, being a woman herself, is often better equipped to give the young patient support than is the physician. Being overly sympathetic is not the answer. These patients need a great deal of patience. They must be taught what is required of them, what the drugs will do and how they can aid in overcoming the problem. Their general health is important; maintenance of normal weight, a well-rounded diet, exercise (but not to the point of fatigue), ample rest and sleep are all essential. Menstruation must be understood as a normal physiological process and not a "disease" (V-1).

Since the nurse herself may have suffered from dysmenorrhea, she may be more understanding than the physician (most often a man). However, excessive sympathy is not the answer, but the nurse may assist the patient greatly by teaching her some sound health practices which may help in overcoming the difficulty (V-1).

THE PATIENT. Those who suffer from very severe dysmenorrhea may in desperation cling to any hope for relief. The often temporary relief provided by endocrine therapy may give the patient some psychic relief by providing freedom from pain for a time at these periods.

ENDOCRINE THERAPY. In some instances, endocrine therapy is indicated but it is not always effective. It has been found that an anovulatory cycle is devoid of pain. Since the pain is less or absent when there is no ovulation, one of the oral contraceptive drugs may be tried. See Chapter 28 and Current Drug Handbook for details. Any one of these preparations may be helpful.

The drug is given for two or three consecutive menstrual cycles and then stopped. This is often sufficient to afford a "permanent cure." However, if the pain returns, the doctor may give the contraceptive for six months, but rarely for any longer period. Some physicians use an estrogen alone, but this is usually not as effective as the combination given as oral contraceptives, such as *norethynodrel with mestranol* (Enovid), *norethindrone with mestranol* (Ortho-Novum) or other similar products.

Dysfunctional Uterine Bleeding

DEFINITION. Dysfunctional uterine bleeding may be metrorrhagic, menorrhagic or a combination of the two and may be due to one of several causes. This condition is regarded as the endometrial reflection of disturbances in normal cyclic ovarian activity. In a majority of cases, there is ovulatory failure with a resulting absence of progesterone, the product of the corpus luteum, and an excess of estrogens. There is little consensus as to the cause. Some cases occur in the so-called menopausal years (roughly the fifth decade of life); there are some few in young women at the age of puberty or early adolescence; the larger number fall into the "in-between" years.

MAJOR SYMPTOMS. Depending upon the type of bleeding, menorrhagic, metrorrhagic, or a combination of both, the symptoms will vary. In metrorrhagia, there may be only bleeding between periods, varying in amounts. In menorrhagia, the cycle may be well preserved but the flow may be prolonged and continue for many weeks or even months.

DRUG THERAPY. Two factors influence the treatment of these patients: first, the age of the patient; and, second, the importance or unimportance of preserving the reproductive function. In the young girl near adolescence, nature may remedy the situation of its own accord. In the menopausal group, it may be the outward sign of uterine malignancy. In any event, no endocrine therapy should be tried until malignancy has definitely been ruled out as the cause. Irradiation or hysterectomy is usually best for the menopausal group of patients.

ENDOCRINE THERAPY. Much of the hormone therapy today is empirical and it must be remembered that all hormone therapy is a substitution process and does not of itself cure. Frequently this substitution therapy proves disappointing but does seem to be satisfactory if there is evidence of anovulatory bleeding and a progestin lack. The aim of treatment is to establish a regular cycle.

If the bleeding is severe, it may be controlled rapidly by giving a conjugated estrogen such as *Premarin* by the intravenous route. It is usual to give 20 mg. intravenously and repeat every four to six hours until bleeding has subsided. At the same time, an oral estrogen is started. (See Current Drug Handbook for individual estrogens available.) The actual mechanism of the very effective action of the conjugated estrogens is little understood, but they are thought to raise the blood level of estrin, which is believed to have fallen below the critical point beyond which bleeding occurs. When the bleeding is controlled, a progestational agent is added to the regimen. The aim now is to influence the endometrium so that it will shed completely after the hormone is discontinued (so-called medical curettage). There are numerous drugs available and all are about equally effective. *Norethindrone* (Norlutin) in 15 mg. doses daily from the fifth through the twenty-fourth day of the menstrual cycle may be used. This drug has potent progestogen activity with some estrogenic and androgenic activity as well. *Norethindrone acetate* (Norlutate), 2.5 to 10 mg., is given orally in the same schedule as norethindrone.

Also useful is *medroxyprogesterone acetate* (Provera), 2.5 to 10 mg. given orally for five to ten days beginning on the assumed sixteenth to twenty-first day of menstrual period. *Hydroxyprogesterone caproate* (Delalutin) has a slow onset of action and so is less useful in controlling bleeding but is useful in establishing normal cycles. It is often given in 250 mg. doses I.M. every four weeks. Still another is *dydrogesterone* (Duphaston), given orally in 5 to 10 mg. doses daily in the usual fifth to twenty-fifth day of the cycle. After the drug is discontinued, withdrawal bleeding is expected within three to five days.

The oral contraceptive agents are valuable here because they have the ability to bring about changes in the endometrium, producing a more physiologic balance in hormonal activity after the excessive vaginal bleeding has been controlled. They have the advantage, too, of combining both a progesterone and an estrogen in one drug. *Norethindrone with mestranol* (Ortho-Novum) is given in oral doses of 2 to 10 mg. daily from the fifth through the twenty-fourth day of the cycle. Another drug in use is *norethynodrel with mestranol* (Enovid). It is given in 5 to 10 mg. doses daily from the fifth through the twenty-fourth day of the cycle. These two latter drugs are discussed in more detail under Family Planning, Chapter 28.

In the last few years several long-acting injectable estrogens and progestins have been introduced. They have the advantage that the physician can control the dosage more accurately, but they do require more visits to the doctor's office.

Some physicians use *estradiol valerate* (Delestrogen) 20 mg. I.M. as an initial dose to control bleeding. A single injection lasts two to three weeks. After two weeks the combination of hydroxyprogesterone caproate 250 mg. and *estradiol valerate* 5 mg. is given I.M. Withdrawal bleeding occurs within two weeks.

Androgens may even be tried but their results are unpredictable and disappointing usually. If used, they are often given as *methyltestosterone* linguets, 10 mg. daily for 14 days.

No matter what method is used, it is important that after the initial withdrawal bleeding the cycle length and amount of flow can be controlled in most instances with a progestin alone.

Sometimes the uterine bleeding may be caused by a state of hypothyroidism. Thyroid extract as indicated is likely to be curative in most cases.

THE NURSE. Side effects from most of these drugs are negligible. Medroxyprogesterone acetate (Provera) occasionally produces somnolence. Norethindrone (Norlutin) and norethindrone acetate (Norlutate), because of the androgenic activity, may cause a deepening of the voice, hirsutism and acne occasionally. Other side effects sometimes observed include weight gain, mild nausea, lethargy and breakthrough bleeding. The side effects of norethindrone with mestranol (Ortho-Novum) and norethynodrel with mestranol (Enovid) are discussed under Family Planning, Chapter 28.

The main role of the nurse in dysfunctional uterine bleeding is to encourage the patient to follow the schedule outlined. A careful explanation of the aim of the therapy may be needed and the patient should be assured that therapy will not continue indefinitely. The nurse should also carefully record the amount and character of the menstrual flow daily.

THE PATIENT. The estrogen-progesterone therapy may be very effective for some patients, but to many, the side effects are often worse than the disease itself. For such patients the expense and discomfort outweigh the benefits. However, most physicians feel that the therapy should be tried.

MISCELLANEOUS THERAPY. In some few cases, the abnormal uterine bleeding may cause an iron deficiency anemia. This in turn may contribute to repeated menorrhagia. If this is the case, improvement is usually noted in two to four weeks after *iron* in doses of 1.0 to 1.5 Gm. daily is started. This may be supplemented with *vitamin* B_{12}. This is discussed in detail under Pernicious Anemia, Chapter 19.

Endometriosis

DEFINITION. Endometriosis means the presence of functioning endometrial tissue outside its normal environment, but usually confined to the pelvis. These patches of displaced tissue are susceptible to the hormone influences and will bleed during the menstrual cycle.

MAJOR SYMPTOMS. This disease is more common in those women who have never been pregnant and although it is largely a disease of the reproductive years, it may be seen occasionally in adolescence or after the menopause. The patient suffers from dysmenorrhea, and there may be abnormal bleeding, backache, rectal pain and dyspareunia.

DRUG THERAPY. The management of endometriosis depends on several factors: the severity of the symptoms, marital status, age and desire to have children. Drug therapy is only palliative and surgery is usually the ultimate result. A mild analgesic such as *codeine* may be needed to control pain.

It has been found that during the periods of anovulation the disease subsides, so the aim in drug therapy is to produce an amenorrhea for an interval of three to six months. The results are somewhat unpredictable and recurrences are often noted when the hormones are discontinued.

Drugs used as oral contraceptives are employed since they not only produce amenorrhea and inhibit ovulation but also produce a decidual response in the endometriosis, thereby effecting a state of pseudopregnancy. Some physicians start the patient on *norethynodrel with mestranol* (Enovid), 2.5 or 5.0 mg. daily for seven to ten days, then 10 mg. daily for two weeks, followed by 15 mg. daily for two weeks. Then 20 mg. daily is given for the duration of therapy unless breakthrough bleeding occurs, in which case the dosage should be increased by 10 mg. *Norethindrone* (Norlutin) or *norethindrone acetate* (Norlutate) may be substituted in similar doses as for Envoid. Other physicians use *medroxyprogesterone acetate* (Provera), 50 mg. intramuscularly weekly or 100 mg. every two weeks. If breakthrough bleeding occurs, an estrogen may be added. The regimen varies with the physician and with the patient's response to the drug. It may be continued for three to six months.

THE NURSE. The nurse should explain to the patient that she will be infertile during the period of therapy, unless the androgens are used, but that pregnancy may occur after withdrawal of the drugs.

THE PATIENT. To some of the patients with endometriosis who wish to have children, the diagnosis may be a severe emotional blow. Some reassurance can be given, however, if the patient follows closely the schedule set for her. She should check with her doctor frequently so he may follow the progress of the condition.

Vaginitis

An inflammation of the vaginal canal, vaginitis may be caused by the gonococcus, staphylococci, streptococci, the colon bacillus or a diphtheroid (III-6, 7). Other causes may be foreign bodies (neglected pessaries) or too hot or chemically irritating douches. The appearance of a milky or mucopurulent vaginal discharge usually sends the patient to the physician. This discharge causes itching and burning, especially on urination.

Mild antiseptic douches of *acetic acid* 1 per cent (vinegar may be used in the home, 60 ml. per liter of water) are often ordered for local relief. If the condition is severe, a culture and sensitivity test are done and the appropriate anti-infective drug is used. It may be given systemically, locally or both.

In nonspecific forms, in addition to mild antiseptic douches, relief may be obtained by first drying the vagina and then applying *nitrofurazone* (Furacin) vaginal cream.

Mycotic Vaginitis

DEFINITION. Also called monilial vaginitis, this is an infection due to a fungus of the yeast group—the monilia or *Candida albicans.*

MAJOR SYMPTOMS. The vaginal discharge varies from a thin, watery type to a thick, purulent material and is characterized by intense pruritus, local irritation and marked reddening of the entire vaginal or vulvo-vaginal mucous membranes. It is often difficult to clear.

DRUG THERAPY

ANTIBIOTICS. *Nystatin* (Mycostatin) is one antibiotic which is helpful in monilial vaginitis. It is relatively nontoxic and the few side effects that occur are transitory when the usual doses are used. It is most commonly used as vaginal tablets inserted one or two each day (100,000 units each). In very resistant cases, this may be augmented by oral administration of nystatin, 500,000 units three times a day. This is done to help reduce the possibility of reinfection from the intestines where this organism is normally found. Large oral doses have occasionally produced diarrhea and gastrointestinal distress.

Mild douches preceding the insertion of the tablet are usually recommended. If there is severe irritation, a bland ointment may be used on the external genitalia.

THE NURSE. The nurse should explain to the patient what is being done and why. If she is to take the douches, insert the tablet and use the ointments at home, the nurse should instruct the patient in all the details.

The douche might be of saline solution or tap water. Medicated douches should not be used. It is a good time to give the patient information about douches and cleanliness of the genital area. Some physicians believe that douches should not be used too often, especially if various medicinal substances are used.

The Patient. The patient may be taught (if needed) to modify and correct her douche habits. She should be encouraged to continue therapy, since it is often long (three to six months). She must understand that stopping, even temporarily, may make it very difficult to effect a cure, since stopping allows the organisms to grow unchecked during the interim. Persistence in therapy must be rigidly adhered to until the physician gives permission for discontinuance. Patients may be told that it is advantageous to wear panties and that these should not be pulled over slippers or shoes. A daily change is best. Careful hygiene after voiding or defecating is important. Tissue should always be used from anterior to posterior and discarded. After defecation a mild soap and water wash may be used. If an ointment is being used for the external genitalia, it may need to be reapplied.

Trichomonas Vaginitis

DEFINITION. Probably one of the most common causes of an inflammation of the vagina is the trichomonas organism, a parasitic protozoan (III-5).

MAJOR SYMPTOMS. The outstanding symptoms of this type of vaginitis are leukorrhea with associated vaginal soreness, burning and often itching. The discharge is usually very thick and white or yellowish white. It is often resistant to treatment.

DRUG THERAPY

Metromidazole (Flagyl) (Trichazol, Trikamon [C]) is the drug of choice for trichomonas vaginitis. It is given orally 250 mg. three times a day for 10 days. At the same time a mild douche is usual, often once a day. Trichotine (sodium lauryl sulfate, sodium perborate and sodium borate) is often ordered for the douche. The directions on the commercial package should be followed. If the condition persists, metronidazole vaginal inserts may be added to the therapy regimen. However, the oral dosage is reduced to once or twice a day. If the patient cannot take metronidazole, a powder or suppository of *furazolidone* and *nifuroxime* (Tricofuron) may be substituted. The male partner should be treated with one tablet of metronidazole 250 mg. twice daily for ten days. Patients taking this drug should be warned not to take any alcoholic drink at the same time, since it can act similarly to *disulfiram* (Antabuse).

Metronidazole (Flagyl) is contraindicated during the first three months of pregnancy and in those with evidence of or a history of blood dyscrasias or disease of the central nervous system. Side effects of a change in taste, furring of the tongue, slight nausea and darkening of the urine have been reported.

The Nurse. The nurse will need to teach the patient how to maintain the therapeutic regimen. She can also help the patient to overcome her embarrassment, feelings of guilt, "uncleanliness" or shame. Occasionally, some women confuse a trichomonas infection with venereal disease. It is transmitted from one sexual partner to another, but the organism is not related to the causative agent of either gonorrhea or syphilis.

The Patient. The patient may find the daily regimen of suppositories (once or twice a day), oral medication and douching difficult. She should not douche more often than the physician has directed and the water temperature should not exceed 100° F., since the already inflamed mucosa might be further traumatized by hotter water.

Some physicians feel that tight girdles and pantyhose which cause perspiration may lead to a climate favorable for growth of the organism. Wearing apparel should be thoroughly cleansed after daily wear to remove all traces of vaginal discharges and organisms.

Acute Pelvic Inflammatory Disease

DEFINITION. An infection of bacterial origin which affects the upper genital organs (uterus, tubes, ovaries and pelvic peritoneum) is referred to as pelvic inflammatory disease. It may be either acute or chronic and the more common causative organisms are the gonococcus, various pyogenic organisms (streptococci, staphylococci) and that of tuberculosis (III-2, 6).

MAJOR SYMPTOMS. In many cases, the acute symptoms appear during or immediately following a menstrual period. There is severe pain in the pelvic and lower abdominal region, muscular rigidity and tenderness in the abdomen, distention, nausea and vomiting, fever, leukocytosis, a rapid pulse, prostration and particularly an elevated sedimentation rate.

DRUG THERAPY

ANTI-INFECTIVES. *Penicillin, ampicillin* or one of the *tetracyclines* is usually given. The regular dosage prevails. *Streptomycin* may be used occasionally. The use of these drugs tends to curb the acute infection. Other supportive measures such as fluids are often needed.

The Menopause or Female Climacteric

DEFINITION. The cessation of menstruation as the normal course of events is referred to as the menopause but this is only a part of the change that takes place at this time of life. For that reason, the term climacteric is probably more descriptive and inclusive. This may occur roughly between the ages of 45 and 55 years (I-5).

MAJOR SYMPTOMS. There is usually a gradual diminution in the menstrual flow, with the skipping of a month or two and then its resumption. This may continue for several years before there is a final cessation of the flow. Ovulation usually ceases at this time. Various vasomotor symptoms of varying intensity occur. These include hot flashes and profuse diaphoresis (frequently following the flashes). The cause of these is the cessation of ovarian function, which causes a relative increase in the gonadotropic activity of the anterior lobe of the pituitary. The ovary has a definite life span and, when this is reached, no form of pituitary stimulation will reactivate it.

DRUG THERAPY. A large part of the treatment of patients going through the menopause is psychologic. About 70 per cent of women respond to explanation, reassurance, a revision of living habits, exercise, re-evaluation of their point of view on life supplemented with mild sedation or tranquilizing drugs. Many physicians believe that drug therapy should be resorted to only when and if vasomotor symptoms are extremely troublesome (V-3).

ENDOCRINE THERAPY

Estrogens

THE DRUGS. It was established about 1900 that there was a hormone secreted by the ovaries which controlled the functioning of the female reproductive system. By 1929, the substance, estrogen, had been isolated. Later it was determined that the ovaries secreted two hormones, estrogen and progesterone.

Physical and Chemical Properties. The natural estrogens, estradiol, estrone and estriol, are steroid compounds. However, the synthetic preparations such as diethylstilbestrol, hexestrol and dienestrol are non-steroid compounds. All these preparations are readily soluble in body fluids.

Action. The action of the estrogens is varied and wide, but their main function is the development and maintenance of the female sex characteristics.

Therapeutic Uses. As would be expected, the estrogens are used primarily in the treatment of gonadal disorders in the female. They are used to lessen the adverse symptoms of the menopause. Estrogens are also used to produce a mild "feminization" state in the treatment of certain male disorders such as cancer of the prostate. This is palliative, not curative. Estrogens have been tried as a prophylaxis in myocardial infarctions in men since women have this condition less often. Results have been varied and not always satisfactory.

Absorption and Excretion. Most estrogens are readily absorbed through the gastrointestinal tract as well as through the skin and other mucous membranes. A few lose potency when given orally. Apparently they are either changed by the digestive juices or degraded by the liver before they reach the blood stream. Oral drugs are absorbed into the blood capillaries and enter the liver via the portal vein. Some are excreted in the bile and then again pass to the liver. The exact fate of these products is not known. Some are degraded rapidly; for others, such as ethinyl estradiol and some of the synthetic compounds, the process of degradation goes on very slowly. Of course, these have a slower and more prolonged action. The estrogens are mainly metabolized by the liver and excreted in the urine as various metabolites.

Preparations and Dosages. See Current Drug Handbook for details concerning these drugs and other preparations. A few representative ones are:

Diethylstilbestrol, U.S.P., Stilboestrol, B.P. (Many trade names) 0.1 to 25 mg. Orally.
Ethinyl estradiol, U.S.P., B.P. (Many trade names) 0.01 to 0.5 mg. Orally.
Estrogenic substances, conjugated (Premarin) 0.3 to 2.5 mg. Orally.
Chlorotrianisene, N.F. (Tace) 12 to 72 mg. Orally.
Estradiol valerate, U.S.P. (Delestrogen) 10 to 40 mg. I.M.

A combination of an estrogen and an androgen may be ordered. The ratio of the androgen to estrogen is between 1:15 and 1:20. This minimizes the chance of bleeding. Some physicians feel that the use of the androgen, usually testosterone, as well as having protein sparing effects, is good as an anabolic stimulant. These all tend to make the patient feel better.

THE NURSE. ***Mode of Administration.*** Most estrogens are given orally, once a day for three weeks and then omitted for a one week "rest period." The estrogens may also be administered parenterally (usually I.M.). These are longer acting, so the injections may be given only once or twice a week. The "tablet implant" is a still longer-acting form. The tablet is placed under the skin either by using an injector or a small (2 mm.) incision, usually on the infrascapular region or the postaxillary line. This method may provide substantial therapy for as long as 3 months. Too much estrogen in the postmenopausal patient may reactivate menstruation, sometimes called withdrawal or breakthrough bleeding.

Side Effects. Side effects from estrogen therapy are usually mild. However, too much can cause vaginal bleeding. Diethylstilbestrol may cause various gastrointestinal disturbances such as anorexia, nausea, vomiting, epigastric distress and occasionally diarrhea. Dizziness has also been reported. If any of these occur, the drug is discontinued and another preparation used in its place.

Patient Teaching. Probably the most important thing for the nurse to do is to aid the patient to adjust to her condition. The nurse should explain what is happening and what the medication will do. The patient should understand the need for and the importance of the rest period. Some doctors suggest that the patient omit the drug the first five to eight days of each month. This gives the patient an easy way of remembering when to take the drug and when not to take it.

THE PATIENT. This is a most distressing time in a woman's life. She feels as if she were losing her femininity, which of course she is not. She also thinks that she will be less attractive. This also is not true. Many women are more beautiful and have more energy after menopause than they had for the years just previous to its onset. Naturally, it is an indication of the passing of years, but this has been going on since birth.

It may be advisable for the patient to keep a weekly weight chart. This will help the physician to detect early any signs of edema. Monthly examination of the breasts and yearly or semiannual vaginal examinations and Papanicolaou smear are important to indicate any possible incipient disease.

SEDATIVES. The conservative use of *phenobarbital* in 15 to 30 mg. doses two or three times a day or the use of one of the tranquilizers (see Chapter 27) often helps calm the patient. It seems to make everyday activities more bearable.

Kraurosis Vulvae

DEFINITION. Kraurosis (shrinkage) vulvae is a condition marked by atrophy of the vulva (I-2). It most frequently follows the menopause and would seem to be connected with the cessation of ovarian function (I-5), but it may be seen occasionally in younger women in whom the menstrual function is intact.

MAJOR SYMPTOMS. The skin of the vulva shrinks markedly and becomes thin and reddened. The skin is dry, brittle, light gray or whitish in appearance, and a severe pruritus accompanies the condition.

DRUG THERAPY. THE ESTROGENS. Because it is believed that kraurosis is the result of the lack of ovarian function, *estrogens* may be used as replacement therapy but are not always effective. There are many preparations on the market. They may be given orally, intramuscularly or intravaginally, with the latter usually preferred. If this method is used, it is usually recommended that *dienestrol cream* or similar product be used daily for ten days. Antiseptic ointments or suppositories are used if there is bacterial invasion. The amounts used orally and parenterally will vary with the preparation used. Among the many preparations which may be used are: *estradiol valerate, piperazine estrone sulfate, hexestrol* (hexital [C]), *benzestrol, diethylstilbestrol dipropionate* (orestrol [C]), *methallenestril* (Vallestril) and *conjugated estrogenic substances* (Premarin).

The Nurse. It is often the responsibility of the nurse to instruct the patient in the insertion of the vaginal suppository. All suppositories are made of material which melts rather easily at body temperature and so the suppositories should be kept in a cool place. Most are encased in a protective covering of foil or glass and it should be demonstrated to the patient that the removal of this covering is important before insertion in a body cavity.

The Patient. The patient should understand that this treatment may help but may not necessarily cure. These drugs may cause various side effects (See "Menopause" in this chapter and Current Drug Handbook.) The side effects seldom require withdrawal of treatment; adjustment of dosage or change of preparation is usually sufficient. Cyclic therapy may be initiated as in menopausal disorders—three weeks of therapy followed by one week without the medication (as discussed under Menopause, this chapter). Withdrawal bleeding may be observed during the week when the medication is not given. The patient should understand that any of these side effects might occur and that she should report them to the physician.

Antipruritic Drugs. There is no drug which will consistently relieve itching. *Calamine lotion* may help, and others that may provide relief are *cold cream, sodium bicarbonate* solutions, or *sulfur* or *crude tar* ointments. Various other topical preparations are available as solutions, ointments and creams. Those containing a corticosteroid either alone or in combination have some value.

Cool, wet dressings with *acetic acid* 1 per cent or saline 0.9 per cent or tepid sitz baths have proved helpful to some patients. Tucks (soft flannel pads with a solution of witch hazel 50 per cent, glycerin 10 per cent and distilled water) exert a soothing, antipruritic effect but this relief is relatively brief.

Scrupulous cleanliness of the area will help, but excessive rubbing should be avoided lest it damage the fragile tissues. Only a mild soap (not a deodorant one) should be used unless the physician orders a medicated soap.

Pruritus Vulvae

DEFINITION. Pruritus vulvae is the term for intense itching of the external genitals in the female. There are many causes for the condition, which is baffling and intractable.

MAJOR SYMPTOMS. Intense itching is present and there may be associated skin lesions which might account for the symptoms. In some instances, serious emotional reactions may result from its continuance.

DRUG THERAPY. To a great extent, the treatment will be directed at the cause. General health and cleanliness measures are important and local applications of cold or hot compresses may help.

Local hygiene is very important. The vulva and the perianal areas should be washed after each stool, being sure that all feces is removed from hair and skin.

Local Treatment. Ointments, creams and lotions may be applied. *Dimethindene maleate* (Forhistal) 1 per cent with either *gammacorten* 0.05 per cent or *hydrocortisone* 1 per cent has proved effective in some instances. Preparations containing local anesthetics, gentian violet and Castellani paint are usually avoided as they tend to increase the difficulty. Sitz baths and/or wet dressings may help. Superficial x-ray therapy, six to eight treatments, may be given. If these do not help, additional treatments are valueless.

Local injection of the corticosteroids, particularly triamcinolone acetate or diacetate, may give temporary or even lasting relief. The injection must be done very carefully. If too superficial, sloughing may occur and if a blood vessel is entered, a nitritoid reaction can result.

SYSTEMIC TREATMENT

Antipruritic Drugs. There are several orally effective antipruritic drugs, the antihistamines and two phenothiazine derivatives, *trimeprazine tartrate* (Temaril, Alimemazine, Panectyl [C]) and *methdilazine* (Tacaryl; Dilosyn [C]). The antihistamines are often tried first in their usual doses. (See Chapter 27 and the Current Drug Handbook.) Trimeprazine (Temaril) and methdilazine (Tacaryl) are potent antipruritics. The dose of the former is 2.5 to 5.0 mg. three to four times daily. Methdilazine is given also three to four times a day in doses of 4 to 8 mg. All of these drugs are given orally for this condition. Trimeprazine is said to have antagonistic activity against histamine and serotonin. After the initial starting dose, the amount is changed according to the response of the patient.

As with any of the phenothiazine derivatives, the nurse must be alert for possible occurrence of agranulocytosis, liver toxicity, neuromuscular (extrapyramidal) symptoms or other serious side effects. Side effects, however, are rarely seen with the recommended dosage. Overdosage involves the gastrointestinal and central nervous systems. Drowsiness, dizziness, dryness of mucous membranes and gastrointestinal upsets may occur. Refer to Chapter 30 and the Current Drug Handbook for further information on the phenothiazine drugs.

Mild and temporary drowsiness may be encountered when the drug is first started, but the patient should be reassured that this usually disappears after a few days of medication. Those who receive this drug must understand that they should be under frequent medical observation.

Sedatives and Tranquilizers. The continued and unrelenting itching usually makes the patient very nervous and irritable. The use of tranquilizers or sedatives or both is usually advisable to help the patient through her ordeal. Some physicians believe that small doses of *phenobarbital* (phenobarbitone [C])—usually in elixir form—three times a day are best. Almost any of the tranquilizers may be used; they are discussed in detail in Chapter 30. If these are used, frequent blood counts should be taken and the patient questioned about side reactions.

Miscellaneous Therapy. The use of an estrogen such as *conjugated equine estrogen* (Premarin) 0.625 to 1.25 mg. daily may be helpful. If the condition is due to a fungal infection *griseofulvin,* U.S.P. (Fulvin, Grisactin) may be given. Some physicians use *vitamin A,* 50,000 to 100,000 units daily, when there are scaling lesions of the vulva, with good results. The injection of 95 per cent alcohol immediately beneath the skin is helpful but, like the local injection of corticosteroids, may produce a sloughing of the skin. Sometimes the repository form of 6-methylprednisolone or triamcinolone may be used. Oral corticosteroids are not usually effective. In severe idiopathic pruritus, procaine hydrochloride may be given intravenously. If these methods fail to give results, the patient should be referred to a psychiatrist. Many patients fear that the condition is evidence of cancer and others develop obsessions that it follows infection from public toilets or other such sources. These patients should be encouraged to establish a regimen conducive to general health, including a bland diet, sufficient recreation and the avoidance of alcohol and excessive smoking.

Atrophic or Postmenopausal Vaginitis

Following the menopause, there is an atrophy of the vaginal mucosa making it thin and pasty and more prone to infections. Almost any organism can be the cause (III-7).

The more common symptoms are a discharge, itching, burning and soreness in the vaginal region. The discharge is usually rather thin and may be blood tinged.

Estrogenic drugs produce some stimulation of the normally present defense mechanisms of the vaginal mucosa, and for this reason *estrogens* may be of value in senile vaginitis. The relief that follows the use of one of these drugs is often temporary (lasting from about six months to one and a half years in some cases) and there frequently is an exacerbation later. There are many preparations available and it is felt by some physicians that the drug should be used intravaginally. Others believe that it is best to combine vaginal application with either oral or parenteral administration. The amount used will vary with the drug used and the clinical response and health of the vagina.

DISEASES OF THE MALE REPRODUCTIVE SYSTEM

Disorders of the male reproductive system are somewhat less numerous than are those of the female, and of these only a few are amenable to drug therapy.

Hypogonadism

DEFINITION. Hypogonadism is that condition in which the testes fail to function properly, due either to some inherent defect in the testes themselves (primary) or to lack of adequate stimulation, largely by the anterior lobe of the pituitary (secondary hypogonadism). The absence of this pituitary function results in an atrophy of the testes and genitalia (I-1, 4).

MAJOR SYMPTOMS. The symptoms will vary somewhat, depending upon whether the condition develops before or after puberty, the chief difference being in the effect on the body contour. The voice is usually high pitched, and secondary sex characteristics fail to develop or are greatly diminished. In those in whom the condition occurs before puberty, there is a rather characteristic body contour, with the extremities long in proportion to the trunk and narrow chest and shoulders. The ability to perform the sex act is absent or greatly diminished.

DRUG THERAPY

ENDOCRINE THERAPY. Two types of therapy are now used in the treatment of hypofunction of the testes. One is substitution therapy with androgens and the other is stimulation therapy with gonadotropic drugs. Androgens are those substances, such as the testes hormone, which produce or stimulate male sex characteristics. Androgens are discussed in Chapter 27. Chorionic gonadotropin is the preparation often used for hypogonadism.

Testosterone

THE DRUG. It had been known for hundreds of years that the testes produced a masculinizing substance, however, it was not until between 1927 and 1935 that the hormone was isolated. Andosterone had been isolated previously, but it had also been shown to be an adrenal cortex secretion.

Physical and Chemical Properties. Testosterone and its many derivatives are all steroid compounds. Various substitutions are made, but there is not much difference in the basic structure. These preparations are freely soluble in body fluids.

Action. The action of testosterone is primarily the development and maintenance of the male gonads and the male secondary sex characteristics. These medications also have an anabolic effect.

Therapeutic Uses. Testosterone is used for any number of conditions both in the male and in the female. Its prime uses are in the treatment of hypogonadism, cryptorchidism and the male climacteric which can cause distressing symptoms.

In the treatment of various disorders of the female, testosterone is used both with estrogen and alone, such as in the treatment of breast cancer. (See Chapter 27.)

Testosterone is sometimes used, in either sex, for its anabolic effect. Research goes on to try to find an anabolic drug without masculinizing properties which can be used more freely for the female patient.

Absorption and Excretion. Most of the testosterone preparations are given parenterally and are readily absorbed by this route. They are degraded by the liver and excreted by the kidneys. Some of the drugs are given sublingually with rapid absorption. Oral compounds are readily absorbed, but some of the drug is degraded by the liver before it enters the blood stream.

Preparations and Dosages. See Current Drug Handbook.

Testosterone propionate, U.S.P., B.P., in oil 10 to 75 mg. I.M.
Testosterone cypionate, U.S.P., 50 to 100 mg. I.M. A long-lasting form.
Testosterone enanthate, U.S.P., 200 mg. I.M. A long-acting form.
Methyltestosterone, N.F., B.P., 5 to 20 mg. Orally.

All doses of these drugs are individually adjusted as to times and amounts.

THE NURSE

Mode of Administration. Various preparations of testosterone are given by different routes: buccal, sublingual, subcutaneous (pellet implants), oral and intramuscular. The last two are by far the most common methods. There are no specific problems in giving these drugs.

Side Effects. The main side effect of testosterone therapy is edema with sodium and water retention. Some compounds have been known to cause a reversible jaundice. This usually clears when the drug is withdrawn. Very occasionally, chills and fever may occur. Another side effect which may be seen is a rise in blood calcium.

THE PATIENT. These patients need a great deal of psychological as well as medicinal care. However, because of the sex ratio in the professions, the physician, not the nurse, usually gives this support. The nurse should be ready to augment any information given by the physician.

Demonstrable improvement in testosterone therapy is very slow in appearing; effects may not be observed for two or three months.

Cryptorchidism

DEFINITION. Failure of the testes to descend by puberty from the abdominal cavity to the scrotum is called cryptorchidism. The descent is dependent on the normal anatomy of the parts involved and hormonal stimulation (I-4).

MAJOR SYMPTOMS. There is an absence of one or both testes from the scrotum. It is not usually noticed until about puberty. When the condition is bilateral and allowed to remain untreated, it almost invariably results in atrophy of the testes, arresting the development of the secondary male sex characteristics.

DRUG THERAPY. Most authorities agree that the best procedure is to try hormone therapy followed by the necessary surgical procedures. It is the consensus that the therapy must be instituted before puberty is advanced to prevent irreparable testicular damage. Hormone therapy is successful only when there is no mechanical obstruction to the descent.

Chorionic gonadotropin is usually used first. It is given two to three times a week 1000 to 2000 I.U. subcutaneously. If this is not effective, some form of *testosterone* is given intramuscularly daily for three days or three times a week for three weeks. Sometimes when the testes are finally in the nor-

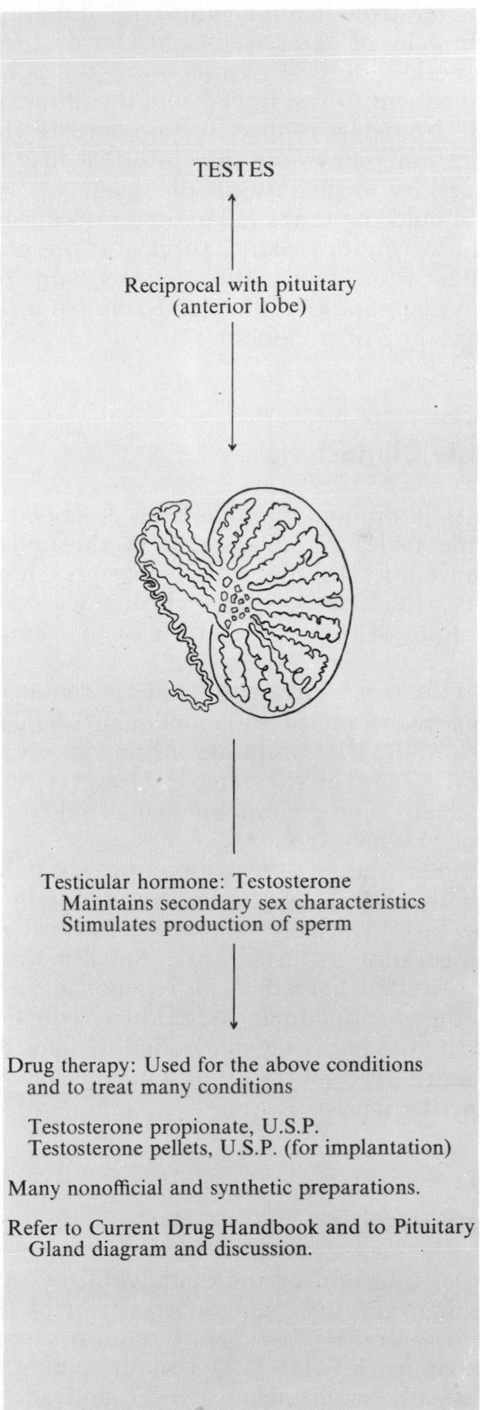

FIGURE 45. Endocrine system in drug therapy.

mal position and fail to develop, a course of testosterone will stimulate them to activity. (See Hypogonadism, this chapter.)

Some patients under this type of therapy complain of temporal headache or fever or both. The best treatment for this is for the patient to rest in bed, and the physician will probably reduce the dosage. If this does not relieve the discomfort, it may be necessary to discontinue the drug.

Should the testes fail to descend with this type of therapy alone, surgery is the only other resort and the patient (and his parents) should understand this from the beginning of treatment.

Male Climacteric

A condition which has been described in some males resembles that of the female climacteric. In the male climacteric, however, there is no definite chronological age or time of onset as there is in the female (I-6, 7, 8).

This condition in the male is characterized by vasomotor and emotional instability. Generally, the symptoms are not so severe as they are in the female. However, it is probably more common than would generally be believed.

When the signs of vasomotor instability manifest themselves and prove troublesome, they are invariably relieved by the oral administration of *testosterone*. Smaller doses are needed here than in hypogonadism in younger individuals. A gradual reduction in the dosage is recommended to allow for a more gradual transition into the state of gonadal inactivity.

Epididymitis

An infection of the epididymis, by pyogenic organisms, the gonococcus or by the *Mycobacterium tuberculosis,* is known as epididymitis (I-4, III-1, 2). Usually coming on suddenly with malaise, fever and severe localized pain, the scrotum is hot, swollen and very sensitive, especially over the epididymis. Occasionally an abscess may form. A broad-spectrum antibiotic such as *tetracycline*, 250 mg. four times a day for five days or longer, is usually effective in those of pyogenic cause. *Penicillin* or *ampicillin* is the drug of choice if the cause is the gonococcus and if tuberculosis is at fault, it is treated as any other such infection (see Tuberculosis, Chapter 16). If early treatment is not effective, a culture and sensitivity test should be done and the proper anti-infective drug then used. Bed rest, forced fluids and elevation of the scrotum are extremely important. The patient should be warned that the epididymis will not return to normal size in less than six weeks after the infection has subsided.

PROSTAGLANDINS. Prostaglandins, which are normal body secretions, are being investigated for use as medicines in a number of different diseases, especially disorders of the male and female genital organs. At present, their main use is in the induction of labor and to produce abortion, which is discussed in Chapter 28.

VENEREAL DISEASES

The social stigma attached to the venereal diseases needs no emphasis (VI-1). It is so great that many patients forego treatment because they do not want to acknowledge even to themselves that one of these diseases might be the cause of their feeling ill. They fear the worst and so postpone consulting a physician. This goes on until the condition becomes so severe they can no longer delay treatment and then, of course, it is difficult—often impossible—to effect a cure. Even if the disease can be cured (that is, if the organisms causing the disease can be destroyed), irreparable tissue damage may have taken place.

THE NURSE. Sometimes the nurse may be able to advise a particular patient concerning the need for early treatment of these conditions, but more often she can spread general information concerning the early symptoms, effectiveness of early treatment and the seriousness of delay in securing treatment. She can also help in dispelling the social stigma and ostracism associated with the venereal disease. The nurse must realize that so far as the medical professions are concerned it is just another communicable disease requiring control. How the disease has been acquired is none of the nurse's concern, but from whom it was acquired may be, since it is important to remove the source of the infection by treating all infected individuals.

The nurse must be willing to evaluate her own attitudes toward sex and sexual behavior. This must be accomplished before she can work objectively with patients, families and other health professionals. The nurse may also be involved in various sex education programs.

THE PATIENT. The patient may delay seeking treatment for a venereal disease because he does not recognize the symptoms or wish to reveal his sexual practices. Many problems may underlie the patient's behavior. The nurse must always attempt to instill confidence and trust and to assure the patient that she will respect the confidential nature of the situation. She must try not to add to the guilt and fear already existing.

With the generally permissive attitude toward sex and sexual practices and the ready availability of contraceptives and abortions, venereal disease has reached epidemic proportions. There has been an increase in the efforts of federal, state and local authorities to control this. The nurse can aid by personal contact with patients (teaching, recognizing possible causes and contacts) and by aiding in community programs.

There are many venereal diseases, but by far the most important ones are syphilis and gonorrhea since they are the most prevalent and the most serious.

Syphilis

DEFINITION. Syphilis is caused by a spirochete, *Treponema pallidum.* At various stages it may produce almost any symptom—so much so that it has been called the "great imitator." It is a disease which usually is transmitted by sexual contact and which may affect any organ of the body.

MAJOR SYMPTOMS. Syphilis has three main stages: first or primary, when the organisms are localized and a sore, called a chancre, appears at the site of the infection; second or secondary, when the infection becomes systemic and symptoms such as fever, malaise, rash and sore throat are noted; and third or tertiary, when the onset of symptoms produced by damage to a specific organ or organs such as the heart or brain occur. A latent period of from a few months to several years occurs between the second and third stages.

The chancre is relatively painless and may go unnoticed in the female if it is intravaginal. The disease is communicable during the primary and secondary stages.

DRUG THERAPY. It is now generally believed that if adequate treatment is given in the first and second stages, the patient can be assured that his chances of clinical recovery are excellent.

Penicillin is the drug of choice unless there are definite contraindications. There are several different schedules of administration and all are about equally satisfactory. One frequently used schedule requires a total dosage of 6,000,000 units of *procaine penicillin.* When possible, it should be given in ten daily doses of 600,000 units. The physician may find it more convenient to give the injections twice a week. Using the aforementioned preparation, 2,400,000 units are given in the first injection, followed by three more injections of 1,200,000 units at three to four day intervals. Still others prefer to use *benzathine penicillin* (Bicillin, Neolin; Benzethacil [C]) because a single injection produces an effective blood level for one to four weeks or longer, depending on the size of the dose. A total dosage of 4,800,000 units is given in two injections of 2,400,000 units a week apart.

For those who cannot tolerate penicillin, the broad-spectrum antibiotics are imperfect substitutes but will have to be used. The tetracyclines are probably best, though others may be tried. A minimal effective dose has not been definitely established. It is usually recommended that the total dosage be 40 to 60 Gm. given at the rate of 0.25 to 0.5 Gm. four times daily, according to tolerance.

During pregnancy, penicillin 1,200,000 units is given weekly for four weeks if the syphilis is diagnosed during the first or second trimesters, and 300,000 units of procaine penicillin three times a day for eight days if the diagnosis is not made until the third trimester.

Whenever massive doses of penicillin are given, the patient must be watched closely for the "Herxheimer reaction," caused by the rapid disintegration of untold numbers of spirochetes. It is characterized by chills, fever, malaise, edema and localized swellings. The patient should be put to bed and the symptoms treated as they occur. It is also important to reassure the patient that there is nothing seriously wrong. He will be very apprehensive. The nurse can do much to allay the patient's fears and to make him more comfortable.

OTHER DRUGS. Now that the efficacy of penicillin in curing syphilis in the first and second stages has been proved, the heavy metals are seldom used. These included arsenicals, bismuth and mercury. *Potassium iodide* is still used in the tertiary stages to aid in the reduction and elimination of gumma, but the results are not striking.

Gonorrhea

DEFINITION. Gonorrhea is an acute or chronic communicable disease, usually involving the mucous membranes and, later, various internal organs. The disease is caused by the *Neisseria gonorrhoeae*, a gram-negative intracellular diplococcus, which is a pyogenic organism (III-2).

MAJOR SYMPTOMS. The organisms cause much irritation of mucous membranes and produce copious mucopurulent drainage. The drainage is very distressing and highly infectious. Systemic symptoms of gonorrhea include arthritis, arthralgia, fever and other symptoms of an acute infection.

The nurse should be aware of the fact that a patient may have gonorrhea and yet be asymptomatic. In some cases, this appears to be a long incubation period. In others, it is more like the "carrier" condition. This is true of both the male and the female. These asymptomatic cases constitute a reservoir of the infecting agent, and their detection and treatment are extremely important. The nurse can work with other health personnel in the identification of these patients and their contacts and aid in bringing them into a clinic or physician's office for treatment.

DRUG THERAPY. Uncomplicated gonorrhea can be cured by an intramuscular injection of *benzathine penicillin G* (Bicillin; Benzethacil [C]), if the organism is not resistant to penicillin. The dose is 1,200,000 to 2,400,000 units and it may show measurable concentrations in the blood for three to four weeks. For gonorrheal urethritis, a single intramuscular dose of 600,000 units of procaine penicillin will cure most patients. For insured results, this is usually followed by a similar dose for two to three days in men and for four to seven days in women. (See Chapter 7 for details of these drugs.)

If the use of penicillin is contraindicated, one of the broad-spectrum antibiotics, usually one of the tetracyclines, in doses of about 0.5 Gm. orally every six hours gives satisfactory results in uncomplicated cases.

Another antibiotic drug used in the treatment of gonorrhea is *spectinomycin dihydrolchloride pentahydrate* (Trobicin). It is given deep intramuscularly in doses of 2 to 4 Gm. in a special diluent supplied with the drug. Usually one dose is sufficient. The drug is not effective against syphilis and if syphilis is suspected, proper tests should be made and appropriate treatment instituted.

Gonorrheal Vulvovaginitis in Children

A gonorrheal infection in the young female, vulvovaginitis is commonly spread by way of infected persons. The vaginal mucosa of the young child is immature and as yet has not developed all the normal flora which seem to protect the adult female from many infections.

The persistence of a vaginal discharge of varying consistency is often the chief symptom. Attendant to this is some irritation which may lead to masturbation.

The treatment of choice is *penicillin* in doses of 100,000 units intramuscularly for three successive days, which clears the condition easily. The *sulfonamides* may be used if the patient cannot take penicillin, or the organism is resistant to it. These drugs have been discussed in detail elsewhere. See Chapter 7.

Chancroid

Chancroid, caused by *Hemophilus ducreyi*, is characterized by a lesion resembling the chancre of syphilis. The lesions may be treated by the local application of an antibiotic cream such as *chloromycetin* or *erythromycin*. Orally, the *sulfonamides* are the drugs of choice in doses of 2.0 Gm. a day for five days and then 1.0 Gm. daily for five days. The tetracyclines and streptomycin may also be used effectively but these two drugs tend to mask the symptoms of syphilis, which is often present. Penicillin is of no value.

Granuloma Inguinale

Granuloma inguinale, caused by a microorganism called *Donovania granulomatis* (a bipolar, gram-negative bacillus) is both a local and a systemic disease. It is treated successfully with the tetracyclines, chloramphenicol or erythromycin. The *tetracyclines* are usually given orally, 2 Gm. daily in divided doses for at least two weeks. *Chloramphenicol* is recommended to be given 10 to 40 Gm. in a ten day interval and *erythromycin* should be given twice a day in doses of 100 mg. for two weeks. *Streptomycin*, 2.0 Gm. daily in divided doses for two weeks, is equally effective, but organism resistance develops rapidly.

Lymphogranuloma Venereum

Lymphogranuloma venereum is a *Chlamydia* disease characterized by local, regional and sometimes generalized adenitis. It is best treated with the sulfonamides. Some clinicians believe *sulfisoxazole* (Gantrisin; sulphafurazole [C]), 4.0 Gm. daily in divided doses for two to three weeks, is best. *Tetracycline* in doses of 500 mg. orally, four times a day is also effective. During treatment with tetracycline, dairy products, antacid and iron supplements should be eliminated, since they reduce its absorption. The broad-spectrum antibiotics are useful also but are more expensive and more apt to produce side effects. Most physicians agree that complete eradication of the organism from the body is probably accomplished only rarely.

IT IS IMPORTANT TO REMEMBER

1. That medications are usually ineffective if the patient does not have confidence in their usefulness.
2. That the influence of the pituitary gland upon the menstrual cycle is always to be considered in understanding the functioning of the female reproductive system.
3. That with adequate mental hygiene, many cases of dysmenorrhea can be prevented and corrected.
4. That adequate mental hygiene is of great value to men and women approaching the climacteric.
5. That the indiscriminate use of endocrines must be discouraged.
6. That in the treatment of any communicable disease the nurse is confronted with two or more problems—the care of the patient, the prevention of further spread of the disease and possibly the determination of how the patient became infected in order to eliminate the focus.
7. That the prime purpose of the nurse, as well as other health workers, is to keep people well rather than to get people well.
8. That health teaching is one of the most important duties of every nurse, and nowhere does she have a better opportunity for health teaching than in the field of venereal disease control.
9. That in venereal diseases drugs form the main therapy.

TOPICS FOR STUDY AND DISCUSSION

1. Describe the part played by the endocrine secretions in the menstrual cycle and why estrogens and progesterones are helpful in drug therapy.

2. What is the role of the endocrine secretions in the proper functioning of the male reproductive system? What endocrine drugs might be helpful?
3. Describe some of the factors that are responsible for the present "venereal disease epidemic."
4. What procedures are used by your local and state health departments in the control of venereal disease?
5. Plan a talk to give to a group of junior high school students on the subject of venereal disease, its prevention, treatment and control.

BIBLIOGRAPHY

Books and Pamphlets

American Medical Association Council on Drugs, *Drug Evaluations*, Chicago, 1971, American Medical Association.
Beeson, P. B., and McDermott, W., *Cecil-Loeb Textbook of Medicine, 13th Ed.*, Philadelphia, 1971, W. B. Saunders Co.
Beland, I., *Clinical Nursing, 2nd Ed.*, New York, 1970, The Macmillan Co.
Bergersen, B. S., *Pharmacology in Nursing, 12th Ed.*, St. Louis, 1973, The C. V. Mosby Co.
Chatton, M. J., Margen, S., and Brainerd, H., "*Handbook of Medical Treatment, 12th Ed.*, Los Altos, California, 1970, The Lange Medical Publications.
Conn, H. F., *Current Therapy, 1974*, Philadelphia, 1974, W. B. Saunders Co.
Goodman, L. S., and Gilman, A., *Pharmacological Basis of Therapeutics, 4th Ed.*, New York, 1970, The Macmillan Co.
Miller, B. F., and Keane, C. B., *Encyclopedia and Dictionary of Medicine and Nursing*, Philadelphia, 1972, W. B. Saunders Co.
Rodman, N. T., and Smith, D. W., *Pharmacology and Drug Therapy in Nursing*, Philadelphia, 1968, J. B. Lippincott Co.
Shafer, K. M., et al., *Medical-Surgical Nursing*, St. Louis, 1971, The C. V. Mosby Co.
Watson, J. E., *Medical-Surgical Nursing and Related Physiology*, Philadelphia, 1972, W. B. Saunders Co.

Journal Articles

Ahern, C., "I think I have V.D.," *Nurs. Clin. North Am.* 8:1:77 (January, 1973).
Alford, O. M., et al., "Symposium on the woman patient," *Nurs. Clin. North Am.* 3:2:193 (February, 1968).
American Health Association, "V.D. control measures," *J. Am. Pharm. Assoc.* NS 11:8:424 (August, 1971).
American Health Association, "V.D. around the world," *J. Am. Pharm. Assoc.* NS 11:8:428 (August, 1971).
Bacon, W. R., Lofholm, P. N., and Mayer, F. S., "V.D. in California," *J. Am. Pharm. Assoc.* NS 11:8:429 (August, 1971).
Bacon, W. R., Lofholm, P. N., and Mayer, F. S., "Education and awareness," *J. Am. Pharm. Assoc.* NS 11:8:434 (August, 1971).
Brenner, L. R., "Pharmacy's response to the challenge of venereal disease," *J. Am. Pharm. Assoc.* NS 13:4:185 (April, 1973).
Brenner, L. R., "V.D. prevention—Pharmacy's challenge and opportunity," *J. Am. Pharm. Assoc.* NS 11:8:438 (August, 1971).
Brown, M. A., "Adolescents and V.D." *Nurs. Outlook* 21:2:99.
Brown, W. J., "Acquired syphilis—Drugs and blood tests," *Am. J. Nurs.* 71:4:713 (April, 1971).
Brown, W. J., "V.D.—Everyone's concern." *J. Am. Pharm. Assoc.* NS 11:8:422 (August, 1971).
Casinelli, M., "The Rhode Island program—Beyond expectations," *J. Am. Pharm. Assoc.* NS 11:8:436 (August, 1971).
deLeon, R., "Current drug concepts—Syphilis and gonorrhea," *J. Am. Pharm. Assoc.* NS 13:4:190 (April, 1973).
Editorial, "V.D.—Education, prevention, treatment." *J. Am. Pharm. Assoc.* NS 13:4:177 (April, 1973).
Eichner, E., "Progestins," *Am. J. Nurs.* 65:9:78 (September, 1965).
Hamilton, T. H., "Control of estrogen of genetic transcription and translocation," *Science* 161:3842:649 (1968).

Lammert, A., "The menopause: a physiologic process," *Am. J. Nurs.* 62:56 (February, 1962).
Lammert, A., "The female sex hormones," *R.N.* 31:41 (1968).
Lenz, P., "Women, the unwitting carriers of gonorrhea," *Am. J. Nurs.* 71:4:717 (April, 1971).
Mathews, R., "T.L.C. with penicillin," *Am. J. Nurs.* 71:4:721 (April, 1971).
Pharriss, B., "The possible vascular regulation of luteal function," *Perspect. Biol. Med.* 13:3:434 (1970).
Schwartz, W. F., "Communities strike back," *Am. J. Nurs.* 71:4:724 (April, 1971).
Vandermeer, D. C., "Meet the V.D. epidemiologist," *Am. J. Nurs.* 71:4:722 (April, 1971).

CHAPTER 27

DRUGS USED FOR DISORDERS OF THE ENDOCRINE SYSTEM

CORRELATION WITH OTHER SCIENCES

I. ANATOMY AND PHYSIOLOGY

1. The glands of the endocrine system secrete substances directly into the blood stream rather than secreting them through ducts.
2. The secretions of the endocrine (ductless) glands are called hormones and are responsible for orderly body functioning.
3. The pituitary gland's secretion is essential for the production of the adrenal cortex and other glandular hormones.
4. Estrogens and androgens affect extracellular fluid as well as the retention of protoplasm and bone.
5. Adrenocortical insufficiencies are characterized by deficiencies in renal function which lead rapidly to distortions in the volume and composition of body fluids.

II. CHEMISTRY

1. The endocrine glands secrete hormones, chemically active substances which react on body organs and tissues in specific ways, thus regulating their activities.

IV. PHYSICS

1. The more concentrated a fluid, the higher will be its specific gravity or its weight in relation to distilled water.

V. PSYCHOLOGY

1. Chronic illness or prolonged idleness produces adverse emotional reactions.
2. Fear of being unable to compete with the average person can cause an unfavorable reaction in an individual, especially if he is the breadwinner of the family.

VI. SOCIOLOGY

1. The patient with a chronic disease requiring long-term therapy may find the cost of medications, treatments and physicians' fees a severe burden on the family budget. All possible sources should be investigated so that treatment can continue.

INTRODUCTION

Endocrinology, the science of the endocrine or ductless glands, is, in the general history of medicine, a relatively new study (II-1). It is only in recent years that the importance of these glands and their effect upon health, and even life, have been understood. Most scientists will agree that there is still much to learn about these organs. A few basic facts, however, are accepted. The most important point to remember is the interdependence of all the endocrine glands. Since no one gland acts entirely independently of the others, disturbance of one of these essential organs sets up a relative disturbance in the others. This may be very pronounced or so slight as to cause very few symptoms. The severity will depend upon the type of disorder and the glands involved. This spreading of symptoms may be difficult to explain to the patient, and usually the physician will be the person to make such an explanation, but the nurse must be prepared to answer questions relative to the situation if she is asked. If the nurse is unable to answer the patient's questions, she should refer the patient to his doctor. The function of the endocrine glands is extremely complex, and the nurse will often find her knowledge inadequate.

Hormones, the secretions of the endocrine glands, are used medicinally in two main ways: first, in replacement therapy when the patient's own glands are not elaborating a sufficient quantity of the hormone and, second, in the treatment of various diseases and disorders for which experience has demonstrated the remedial value of hormones (I-2, II-1).

Hormones, as drugs, are derived from a variety of sources. Some are secured from animals, while others have been synthesized. The synthetic hormones do not always act exactly as the normal hormones of the body, but usually their action is similar. The figures and the accompanying discussions show the uses of the hormones of the normally functioning human body.

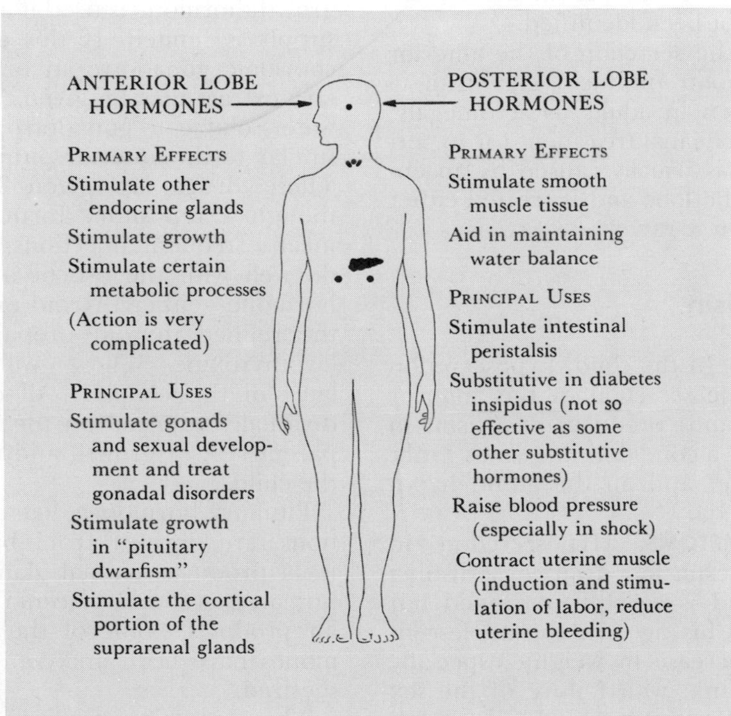

FIGURE 46. Pituitary (hypophysis) hormones as therapeutic agents.

PITUITARY GLAND (HYPOPHYSIS)

The pituitary gland consists of two main portions—the anterior lobe and the posterior lobe joined by the pars intermedia. The secretion of the intermediary portion is under research. Its exact nature is still to be determined. The two main lobes of the gland secrete different hormones with decidedly different functions (Fig. 46).

Anterior Pituitary

The anterior lobe has been called the "master gland" since its varied hormones have a regulatory effect upon the other endocrine glands. For this reason, in any condition involving malfunction of this gland, there is a relative malfunction of other glands as well. The secretion of the anterior pituitary gland is not one single hormone but a combination of many hormones. Some of these hormones have been isolated, and some have been synthesized. Others are known to exist because of the action of the secretion, but the actual substances have not been identified.

Increase in the secretion of the anterior lobe in childhood produces gigantism, a condition known in adults as acromegaly. There is no medicinal treatment for hyperpituitarism. It is usually caused by an enlargement of the lobe and is treated either by surgery or by x-ray.

Hypopituitarism

DEFINITION. In the child, hyposecretion (decrease in the secretion of the anterior lobe of the gland) produces dwarfism; in the adolescent, a condition known as Fröhlich's syndrome; and, in the adult, hypopituitary cachexia.

MAJOR SYMPTOMS. Hyposecretion in the child will result in a dwarf of a distinct type. The child is well proportioned but very small for his age. In the adolescent there is an increase in weight, especially around the trunk, with failure of the sex glands to develop properly. In the adult there may be impotency, sterility, amenorrhea, hypoglycemia and other signs of cortical failure such as lowered metabolism. Reference to Figures 46 and 47 will aid in clarification of these points.

DRUG THERAPY

ANTERIOR PITUITARY HORMONES. In the treatment of hypopituitarism, except in certain specific conditions to be discussed later, most physicians do not give the entire anterior pituitary hormone. In place of this, they give the hormones of the main target glands—the adrenal cortex, the gonads and the thyroid. Since treatment of the various age groups varies somewhat, they will be discussed separately.

Infant and Preadolescent Hypopituitarism. The nurse is often the first person to notice that a child is not developing as well as he should and to suggest to the parents that a physician should be consulted to determine the cause of the delayed growth. The earlier the child is treated for hypopituitarism, the better the results. When a child is under the constant care of a pediatrician or family doctor, the nurse will, of course, not be needed in this capacity, but many children are not so fortunate.

Any single hormone or combination of three hormones may be used to stimulate growth and development. The human growth hormone is used if available, but the supply is limited. If this cannot be used, chorionic gonadotropin or anterior pituitary extract may be given. The former is a water-soluble gonadotropic substance similar to the anterior pituitary hormones. These drugs are given I.M. and even though a repository form is available, it means frequent injections. Some children do well with the use of only the thyroid hormone—either thyroid extract or one of the refined thyroid preparations such as levothyroxine. These will be discussed later in this chapter. All dosages are individually adjusted on the basis of the apparent lack of growth and the response of the child.

Pituitary hormones, like all such medications, are derived from biologic sources, meat products, animal glands, animal and human excretions, placenta and other similar products. Some of the endocrine hormones have been analyzed and later synthesized.

The parents must be impressed with the fact that whatever medication is ordered must be given continuously, and that the child must have frequent medical checkups to insure continuous, adequate growth and development.

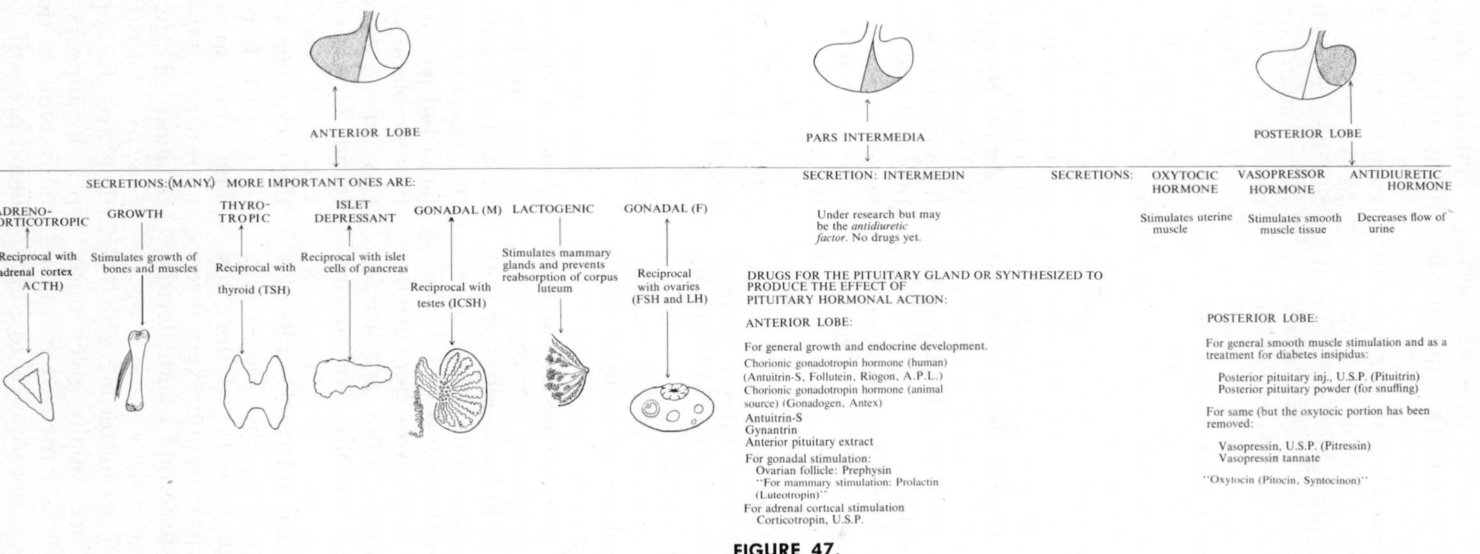
ENDOCRINE SYSTEM IN RELATION TO DRUG THERAPY
(HYPOPHYSIS OR PITUITARY GLAND)
ANTERIOR LOBE
PARS INTERMEDIA
POSTERIOR LOBE
SECRETIONS: (MANY) MORE IMPORTANT ONES ARE:
ADRENO-CORTICOTROPIC
Reciprocal with adrenal cortex ACTH)
GROWTH
Stimulates growth of bones and muscles
THYRO-TROPIC
Reciprocal with thyroid (TSH)
ISLET DEPRESSANT
Reciprocal with islet cells of pancreas
GONADAL (M)
Reciprocal with testes (ICSH)
LACTOGENIC
Stimulates mammary glands and prevents reabsorption of corpus luteum
GONADAL (F)
Reciprocal with ovaries (FSH and LH)
SECRETION: INTERMEDIN
Under research but may be the *antidiuretic factor*. No drugs yet.
SECRETIONS:
OXYTOCIC HORMONE
Stimulates uterine muscle
VASOPRESSOR HORMONE
Stimulates smooth muscle tissue
ANTIDIURETIC HORMONE
Decreases flow of urine
DRUGS FOR THE PITUITARY GLAND OR SYNTHESIZED TO PRODUCE THE EFFECT OF PITUITARY HORMONAL ACTION:
ANTERIOR LOBE:
For general growth and endocrine development.
Chorionic gonadotropin hormone (human)
(Antuitrin-S, Follutein, Riogon, A.P.L.)
Chorionic gonadotropin hormone (animal source) (Gonadogen, Antex)
Antuitrin-S
Gynantrin
Anterior pituitary extract
For gonadal stimulation:
Ovarian follicle: Prephysin
"For mammary stimulation: Prolactin (Luteotropin)"
For adrenal cortical stimulation
Corticotropin, U.S.P.
POSTERIOR LOBE:
For general smooth muscle stimulation and as a treatment for diabetes insipidus:
Posterior pituitary inj., U.S.P. (Pituitrin)
Posterior pituitary powder (for snuffing)
For same (but the oxytocic portion has been removed:
Vasopressin, U.S.P. (Pitressin)
Vasopressin tannate
"Oxytocin (Pitocin, Syntocinon)"

FIGURE 47.

Adolescent Hypopituitarism. Hypopituitarism presents a psychologic as well as a physiologic problem for the patient, especially the adolescent. Fröhlich's syndrome is apt to be a significant social stigma for a youth, and he may even be ostracized by his peers. He may turn to eating to satisfy his emotional needs, thus aggravating the already present problem of obesity. Often, by working with him, the nurse can get the patient to reduce to such a weight that he is no longer an object of criticism by his group.

Diet is important for the patient with a low pituitary output since obesity is usually a complication, especially in the adolescent or adult. The nurse can do much to aid the patient in understanding that his problem is one which, though chronic, is by no means hopeless. She can encourage the patient to persist in the diet and the drugs as prescribed by the physician.

Most physicians give the hormones of the target glands rather than the whole anterior pituitary extract to the adolescent and the adult. With the adolescent, from a short prepubertal period through postadolescence and into adulthood, three hormones are generally employed. Thyroid hormone is continued, and adrenal corticosteroids and gonadal hormones are added. For the adrenal cortex hormone, any one of many preparations can be given. Cortisone is not used as much for this purpose as it once was, and the synthetic or semisynthetic preparations appear to be as effective and have fewer side effects. Prednisolone 2.5 to 10.0 mg. or dexamethasone 0.5 to 2.0 mg. may be given. The doses given here are the total initial daily doses. They are usually divided t.i.d. and given orally. The adrenal cortical hormones are discussed later in this chapter. (See also Current Drug Handbook.)

For the male patient, the long-acting form of testosterone is often used, since this therapy requires injections only every three to four weeks. Testosterone (methyltestosterone) may be given daily. The dose is 10 to 20 mg., or fluoxymesterone 2 to 10 mg. orally. These are usually given once daily. For the female, any form of estrogen may be used, and it is not unusual to add a small amount of testosterone to the drug. As with the above, the drug is given orally once daily. The size of the dose will depend upon the preparation used and the response of the individual patient.

For the male patient, the gonadal hormone is given continuously; for the female, it is usually given about twenty days out of each month or three weeks out of every four weeks with a rest period of from seven to ten days. For a more complete discussion of the gonadal hormones, refer to Chapter 26 and the Current Drug Handbook.

This condition is chronic, and the patient will need help from every available source. There may be need for rehabilitation, as well as psychologic and spiritual care. The nurse can be of great assistance in directing the patient to the proper persons or agencies for help and in encouraging him to continue medical care.

Adult Hypopituitarism. The treatment for this disorder is the same as for adolescent hypopituitarism. However, if infertility is a problem and if children are desired, human gonadotropin may be given to either sex. The "fertility" drug *clomiphene citrate* (Clomid) may also be given to the female. This is discussed under Family Planning in Chapter 28, "Drugs Used During Pregnancy, Delivery and Lactation."

Posterior Pituitary

The posterior portion of the pituitary gland is embryonically distinct from the anterior portion. It has direct connections with the hypothalamus. The secretions of the posterior pituitary are elaborated in the latter but pass to the gland and are secreted into the blood stream from there. There are two hormones of the posterior pituitary gland. One, *oxytocin* (Pitocin, Syntocinon, Uteracon), has direct stimulating action on the uterine musculature, causing the uterus to contract. This is discussed in Chapter 28. The other, posterior pituitary hormone, is known as *vasopressin* (Pitressin). The combination of the two hormones, *posterior pituitary extract* (Pituitrin), is less often used than are the separate preparations. Vasopressin appears to have two distinct functions. One, as the name implies, is to raise blood pressure by stimulating the muscle in the walls of the arteries. The second action is antidiuretic. The main pharmaceutical use of vasopressin is for this action.

Diabetes Insipidus

DEFINITION. A relatively rare disease, diabetes insipidus is the result of a deficiency of the antidiuretic hormone (vasopressin).

SYMPTOMS. The most prominent symptoms of diabetes insipidus are excessive thirst and diuresis. These patients drink gallons of water every day and void large amounts of urine with a very low specific gravity since the salts are so greatly diluted (IV-1). Sleep is often interrupted to a serious degree as the patient must have water and must void at frequent intervals.

DRUG THERAPY

THE DRUGS. Vasopressin is the pressor and antidiuretic hormone of the posterior pituitary gland.

Physical and Chemical Properties. This hormone is a polypeptide.

Action. Pitressin tannate has the ability to increase the reabsorption of water from the distal convoluted tubules and the thin portion of Henle's loop in the kidneys.

Therapeutic Uses. The most valuable use of pitressin tannate is in diabetes insipidus. It may also be used postoperatively in abdominal distention. The aqueous preparation is usually used in diagnostic procedures.

Preparations and Dosages.

Desiccated posterior pituitary powder, N.F., B.P., 5 to 40 mg. intranasally (snuffed). Comes plain and in capsules with a special inhalator. This last is much the easier and pleasanter to use.

Lypressin (8-Lysine vasopressin) is an intranasal spray which is used as needed.

Posterior pituitary injection (Vasopressin) Inspidin [C], N.F. (20 units per ml.) 0.3 to 1.0 ml. subcutaneously, p.r.n. Used mainly as a test to determine the reason for the excessive diuresis.

Posterior pituitary injection in oil (Vasopressin tannate) (five units per ml.) 0.25 to 0.5 ml. intramuscularly every one to three days depending upon the response of the patient.

THE NURSE

Mode of Administration. The aqueous preparation of vasopressin may be given subcutaneously. Vasopressin tannate (5 units per ml.) is given intramuscularly and the posterior pituitary powder (10 to 20 units) as a snuff inhalation.

Side Effects. Nasal irritation frequently occurs and prevents continued use of the powder. This occurs less frequently with the nasal spray, lypressin. If the aqueous preparation is used in therapy subcutaneous injections are required at four to twelve hour intervals. Some unpleasant musculotropic effect may appear in the gastrointestinal tract. Occasionally patients will exhibit allergic reactions. Large doses may cause intestinal and uterine cramps.

Toxic Effects. It is well to remember that this drug can cause spasm of the coronary arteries; it is administered with caution to those with coronary circulation problems.

Patient Teaching. The patient must be instructed in the proper self-injection methods. The nurse must also teach the patient that the hormone sediments to the bottom of the vial and so it must be briskly (but not vigorously) agitated and warmed (usually by holding in the hand except in very cold weather, when the vial should be warmed by placing it in warm water) before it can be injected.

The drug comes in 1 ml. ampules and the usual dose is from 0.25 to 0.5 ml. at one time, the remainder can be placed in a disposable syringe with a 22-gauge needle (with cover and well labeled) until needed. It keeps well at room temperature.

Patients with diabetes insipidus are usually advised to limit their intake of salt and some proteins to decrease the strain on the kidneys. Daily weight records may be helpful in indicating incipient water intoxication. Rapid weight gain usually precedes other symptoms such as headache, listlessness and drowsiness.

If vasopressin is used to clear the bowels of gas prior to x-ray examination, the drug is usually given two to two and a half hours in advance. The placement of a rectal tube for twenty minutes every hour will facilitate the passage of gas.

THE PATIENT. It may be inconvenient for the patient to take an injection at the time when the last dose wears off. Short-term relief can conveniently be obtained with vasopressin snuff (posterior pituitrin powder). A pinch of the powder is placed in the nostril. Unfortunately, this powder is somewhat unpleasant to smell and may cause nasal irritation with frequent use. Two other intranasal forms are available. One is a capsule containing vasopressin powder which comes with a special inhalator. The other is the synthetic nasal spray, lypressin. These are much easier and pleasanter to use than vasopressin snuff.

Paradoxically, many mild cases can obtain reasonable control of the polyuria by the use of a diuretic agent, especially thiazide derivatives. Specifically, *chlorothiazide* (Diuril), 0.5 to 1.0 Gm. a day, or *hydrochlorothiazide* (Hydrodiuril, Esidrex, Oretic), 50 to 100 mg. daily, will reduce the urinary output to approximately 3500 ml. a day. *Ethacrynic acid* may also be used 25 to 50 mg. four times a day. The patient must be watched closely for any signs of electrolyte imbalance, especially potassium deficiency. Foods rich in potassium should be included in the diet.

Since some patients do not tolerate the use of vasopressin for any appreciable length of time, the intervals of rest must be frequent and often longer than desirable. Some patients, however, do tolerate it fairly well, and for these the intervals of rest need not be so frequent or so extended and their lives may be made much more comfortable by the use of the drug.

The patient with diabetes insipidus is faced with a real economic problem since the drug is relatively expensive and must be used intermittently for the remainder of his life. He may also need to readjust his routine of living, even to the extent of securing a new job. The nurse can aid the patient by reassuring him that such readjustments can be and have been made by many other patients. She can often tell the relatives ways of aiding the patient and direct them to agencies which will help in rehabilitation.

THYROID

The thyroid gland secretes a hormone whose active principle is thyroxin, a complex substance that contains iodine. Two hormones, triiodothyronine and thyroxin, are believed to be the only significant secretion products of the thyroid gland. It is believed that thyroxin may be elaborated by other tissues, but the main source is the thyroid gland. The secretion of the thyroid gland is essential for the proper functioning of the general body metabolism (Fig. 48). Any

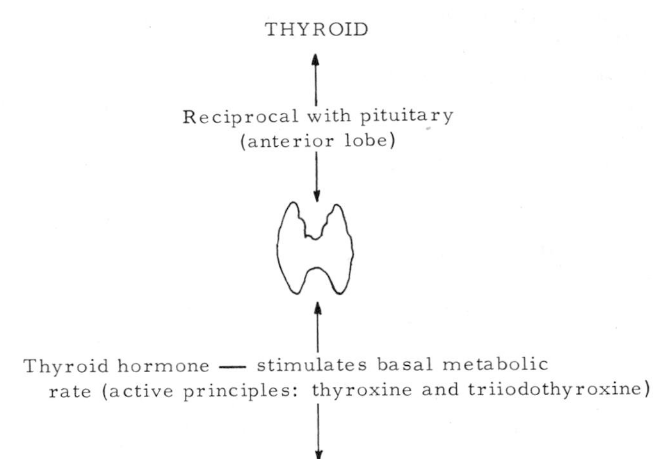

Drug therapy: Used to stimulate basal metabolic activity and to treat many conditions

For stimulation or substitution:
- Thyroid extract, U.S.P.
- Refined thyroid, U.S.P
- Thyroxine, U.S.P.
- Sodium liothyronine, U.S.P. (Cytomel)
- Sodium levothyroxine, U.S.P. (Synthroid)

To depress activity of gland:

- Strong iodine sol., U.S.P.
- Sodium iodide, U.S.P.
- Potassium iodide, U.S.P.
- Sodium radioiodide sol., U.S.P.
  - tracer — 1-100 microcuries
  - therapy — 1-100 millicuries
- Thiouracil
- Propylthiouracil
- Methylthiouracil (Methiacil
- Iothiouracil sodium (Itrumil)
- Methimazole, U.S.P. (Tapazole)
- Carbimazole

FIGURE 48. Endocrine system in relation to drug therapy.

enlargement of the thyroid gland is known as a goiter. This condition may be accompanied by either hyposecretion or hypersecretion, or there may be no appreciable change in the output of the thyroid hormone. It is only when there is a change in the normal amount of the hormone that drug therapy becomes important.

Hypersecretion

DEFINITION. An increase of the secretion of the thyroid gland, hyperthyroidism, if marked, produces a condition known as thyrotoxicosis (Graves' disease or exophthalmic goiter).

MAJOR SYMPTOMS. The symptoms of thyrotoxicosis include loss of weight, tremors, palpitation, tachycardia, nervousness and irritability. If it is very severe, exophthalmos and diarrhea may occur. If the increase in the secretion is mild, the symptoms will be relatively less pronounced.

DRUG THERAPY. The control of thyrotoxicosis by continuous administration of antithyroid drugs is not so effective as removal of the gland because it is difficult to maintain precise control and also because of the high rate of recurrence after the drug is discontinued. However, irradiation or some form of drug therapy is usually used before surgery. Also there are patients who cannot tolerate surgery or irradiation and for these medical treatment is necessary.

ANTITHYROID DRUGS

THE DRUGS. The four drugs in this group are usually called the antithyroid drugs. They are *propylthiouracil, Iothiouracil sodium, methimazole* and *methylthiouracil.*

Physical and Chemical Properties. These drugs are classed as thiocarbamides. The compounds have a bitter taste and are only slightly soluble in water. They are absorbed readily through the gastrointestinal mucosa.

Action. Basically, all four of these drugs inhibit thyroxin synthesis but not the iodine-concentrating ability of the thyroid gland. They are believed to reduce free iodine or to compete with the iodide-oxidizing enzymes. They appear to block the reactions which require free iodine. Preformed thyroxin continues to be secreted. Subsequently, the thyroxin secretion diminishes as the stored organic iodine becomes exhausted. Iothiouracil contains iodine, so it does not produce the extreme vascularity and friability that occur when the other thiouracil compounds are given alone.

Therapeutic Uses. The only use of these drugs is to reduce the hypersecretion of the thyroid gland.

Absorption and Excretion. These drugs are absorbed rapidly from the gastrointestinal tract. They are also excreted and metabolized fairly rapidly.

Preparations and Dosages

Propylthiouracil, U.S.P., B.P. (Propyl-Thyracil [C]), 50 to 800 mg. daily, orally, in divided doses.

Iothiouracil sodium (Itrumil), 50 to 300 mg. daily in three or four divided doses, orally.

Methylthiouracil, N.F., B.P. (Antibason, Methiacil), 50 to 200 mg. daily, orally in four divided doses for two months. Then the basal metabolism should be checked and dosages adjusted to suit the rate. Oral.

Methimazole, U.S.P. (Tapazole) (Thiamazole [C]), 10 to 30 mg. daily, orally.

THE NURSE

Mode of Administration. These drugs are always given by mouth.

Side Effects. Reported side effects for all include skin rashes, urticaria, swelling of the cervical lymph nodes, gastrointestinal disturbances, arthralgia, visual disturbances, headache, drowsiness and vertigo. Methylthiouracil seems to produce a higher incidence and greater severity of side effects than does propylthiouracil or methimazole. These drugs may mask the results of certain laboratory examinations such as the protein bound iodine test.

Toxic Effects. Agranulocytosis is the most serious toxic effect, but leukopenia and thrombocytopenia may also occur. These occur with great frequency with the administration of methylthiouracil. Hepatic damage has also been reported.

Contraindications. None of these drugs should be given during pregnancy or lactation unless absolutely necessary for the health or survival of the mother. These drugs pass the placental barrier.

Patient Teaching. The patient must understand that improvement may not occur for several weeks. Dosage adjustments may be required, especially if signs of hypothyroidism appear. These include weight gain – the patient should keep an accurate record of weight, recorded every other day or at least once a week—sensitivity to cold, constipation, sluggishness, dryness of skin and hair, nonpitting edema, hoarseness and muscle weakness. Periodic medical checkups are essential. Because of the possibility of blood dyscrasias, the checkup will usually include a complete blood count. The patient must learn to report any sore throat or fever to the physician.

Other Nursing Problems. These drugs, especially propylthiouracil, may be altered by prolonged exposure to light and should be stored in light-resistant containers.

THE PATIENT. It is important that the patient continue his medication until the doctor decides that it can be discontinued. The patient should know that allergic reactions may occur and should be reported immediately. The drug may produce marked improvement. If surgery has been planned, the patient may feel it is unnecessary. The nurse may explain that the surgery will provide permanent relief. For mild hyperthyroidism (especially in the older patient) surgery is not performed if the drug is effective.

The family must also understand that the irritability of the patient with hyperthyroidism is a part of the disorder and that they should be tolerant of this and other symptoms, such as nervousness and restlessness. Some few patients may be unable to tolerate one of these drugs, but another drug in this same group may prove effective. There seems to be no cross-sensitization among them.

THE IODIDES

THE DRUGS. In large doses, iodides can decrease the functional activity of the thyroid gland in thyrotoxicosis. This is the oldest form of therapy but is now seldom used alone; its best use is with one of the antithyroid drugs.

Physical and Chemical Properties. These drugs are either elemental iodine or the salts of iodine.

Action. The way these drugs act in reducing the hypersecretion of the thyroid gland is not completely understood. It seems that they exert their influence by preventing the liberation of thyroxin into the bloodstream and by decreasing the vascularity of the thyroid gland. They are seldom used alone but enhance the action of the previously mentioned antithyroid drugs.

Therapeutic Uses. These drugs are used in hyperthyroidism and a variety of other conditions.

Preparations and Dosages. Iodine may be utilized by the body either as the elemental iodine in solution or as one of the salts of iodine. For antithyroid therapy it is usually given as one of the following:

Strong iodine solution, U.S.P. (Lugol's Sol., Lugol Caps), aqueous iodine solution, B.P., 0.3 ml. three times a day, orally.

Potassium iodide solution, saturated, N.F., 0.5 to 1.0 ml. daily, orally.

THE NURSE

Mode of Administration. These drugs are always given by mouth but may present a problem to the nurse. Strong iodine (Lugol's) solution is a dark brown solution, resembling tincture of iodine and will stain the skin. Both saturated solution of potassium iodide (S.S.K.I.), and strong iodine (Lugol's) solution, because of their potency, are prescribed in doses small enough to be lost in the medicine cup; this, and the drug's unpleasant taste, make its inclusion in some form of food essential. Patients differ in their reactions to drugs, but some bland drink should be used as a vehicle for giving the drug. There are many things that will suffice—fruit or tomato juice, milk or half and half (half milk and half cream).

The latter has proved best in many cases. The drug should be put into a small amount of the drink being used. Immediately after taking the drug, the patient should be given the same or some other food.

Side Effects. If taken for a long period of time, iodine in any form can produce adverse and unpleasant symptoms. Some symptoms are similar to those of a cold or allergic rhinitis, skin eruptions and gastrointestinal disturbances.

Contraindications. The iodine preparations should not be given to patients with tuberculosis lesions because it is believed that iodine causes a breakdown in the healing of these lesions. They are also contraindicated in those with laryngeal edema, swelling of the salivary glands or increased salivation for they will aggravate the condition.

THE PATIENT. The patient will need to learn how to best take his medicine and should be encouraged to keep taking it as long as it is prescribed, despite its taste.

RADIOACTIVE IODINE (I^{131})

THE DRUG. Radioactive iodine, also

called radioiodine, is perhaps the most important and most useful of the radioisotopes. It is the preferred form of therapy in some cases of hyperthyroidism.

Physical and Chemical Properties. I^{131} has a half-life of eight days and is chemically indistinguishable from the natural non-radioactive iodide.

Action. Radioactive iodine emits both gamma and beta rays and is handled in the body in the same manner as ordinary iodine. The destructive effect on thyroid tissue is due to the beta rays. Its effectiveness is due to its preferential localization in the thyroid. The degree of damage of a given dose depends upon the size of the dose, the uptake by the gland, the rate of turnover of the isotope, and the radiation sensitivity of the cells.

Therapeutic Uses. Radioactive iodine (I^{131}) may be used as a diagnostic measure to determine the presence of thyrotoxicosis and as treatment for both thyrotoxicosis and malignancy of the thyroid gland. The gamma rays are taken up by the gland and can be detected there by means of a scintillation detector held at the surface of the body near the neck. Radioactive iodine may also be used to tag other iodine containing substances to determine their absorption, distribution and excretion.

Absorption and Excretion. Because of its composition (presence of iodine) it is absorbed in the thyroid gland in the same manner as ordinary iodides. It is excreted via the urine.

Preparations and Dosages. Radioactive iodine is available as *sodium radioiodide* U.S.P., B.P. (Radio-iodide, Iodotope, Radio Caps, Tracervial) and is usually taken orally. It is in a clear liquid form that resembles water. Doses are, of course, individualized. For testing iodine uptake about 1 to 100 μc. (microcuries) are taken orally; for therapeutic uses the dose may range from 4000 to 10,000 μc. A repeat dose is not usually given until after an interval of several months to ensure that the initial dose was not sufficient to control the disease. There is an intravenous preparation available, but it is seldom used.

THE NURSE

Mode of Administration. It is suggested that the nurse review in Chapter 30, the necessary precautions when radioactive materials are used. The drug is usually given in a glass or the dose may be put in a gelatin capsule to facilitate its administration and to be sure none of the dose is lost.

Side Effects. Immediate effects from radioactive iodine (I^{131}) are usually mild with some slight pain and tenderness over the gland. Dysphagia for a few days is usually experienced after a therapeutic dose.

Toxic Effects. The most potent effect is a state of hypothyroidism because of too much destruction of the gland. Usually this lasts a few months and then the gland gradually returns to euthyroidism.

Contraindications. Pregnancy is an absolute contraindication for administering this drug for any reason. The drug crosses the placental barrier and the fetus is exposed to a higher concentration than the mother. The fetal thyroid begins to pick up iodide at about 12 to 16 weeks of gestation and the developing gland would be destroyed or damaged.

The administration of radioactive iodine is avoided if at all possible in patients below the age of 25, because the still-growing tissues may be damaged irreparably.

Patient Teaching. Special precautions need not be taken when a diagnostic dose is given, but, if a therapeutic dose is given, the patient should be instructed in the necessary precautions. (See Chapter 29.)

Other Nursing Problems. Special precautions must be taken when therapeutic doses are given, and the regulations will vary from hospital to hospital. Particular precautions are taken with the urine of the patient and in some cases, the linen. If the drug is spilled or the patient vomits the drug, the directions of the radiology department should be followed.

If the drug is placed in a gelatin capsule it may dissolve into the capsule and it may look empty. Do not discard it—the material is still there.

THE PATIENT. The patient who is to receive radioactive iodine should have a detailed explanation of what is to be done and why certain things are done. Without this explanation, the already excitable patient may become completely uncooperative. The family should also understand what is being done for the patient and why.

OTHER IMPORTANT DATA. Usually, drugs are used to prepare the patient for surgery or treatment with radioactive iodine. Most of the antithyroid drugs are not considered curative.

At almost any stage in the treatment of

hyperthyroidism, a patient may develop a thyrotoxic crisis. This calls for immediate and stringent treatment. Bed rest, sedation and a reduction of the elevated temperature are the first steps. The physician will probably order a full dose of methimazole (Tapazole) orally or parenterally if the patient is vomiting. This is followed in a few hours by full doses of iodine. Shock and dehydration are combated by transfusions of blood or balanced electrolyte solutions or both. Adrenal failure may play a role in thyroid crisis and so a corticosteroid preparation may be given.

Hypothyroidism

DEFINITION. Hypothyroidism is caused by absence of the thyroid gland or a reduction of the gland's secretion from disease, trauma, surgery or other cause. In the infant a lack of the thyroid hormone produces cretinism or infantile myxedema; in the adult, hypothyroidism results in myxedema.

MAJOR SYMPTOMS. Hypothyroidism in the infant, if untreated, will produce a dwarf with relatively short legs and arms, a stocky trunk and a rather large head. There is mental as well as physical retardation. Adult hypothyroidism, or myxedema, is a condition in which there is a decrease in metabolic rate, with weight gain, dry skin, coarse and dry hair, thickening of the subcutaneous tissues, mental sluggishness and a general slowing of all body processes.

DRUG THERAPY. Hypothyroidism responds favorably to the administration of thyroid extract or thyroxin. In the infant or the young child, delay in giving the drug may produce irreparable damage since it is not possible to increase stature after the rapid growth period has passed. Treatment is always beneficial; but to secure normal growth and development the hormone must be given early. It should be started as soon as symptoms indicate its need.

For the adult with myxedema, the administration of thyroid extract in adequate amounts will usually produce startling results. The return to normal is rapid and usually complete (Fig. 49).

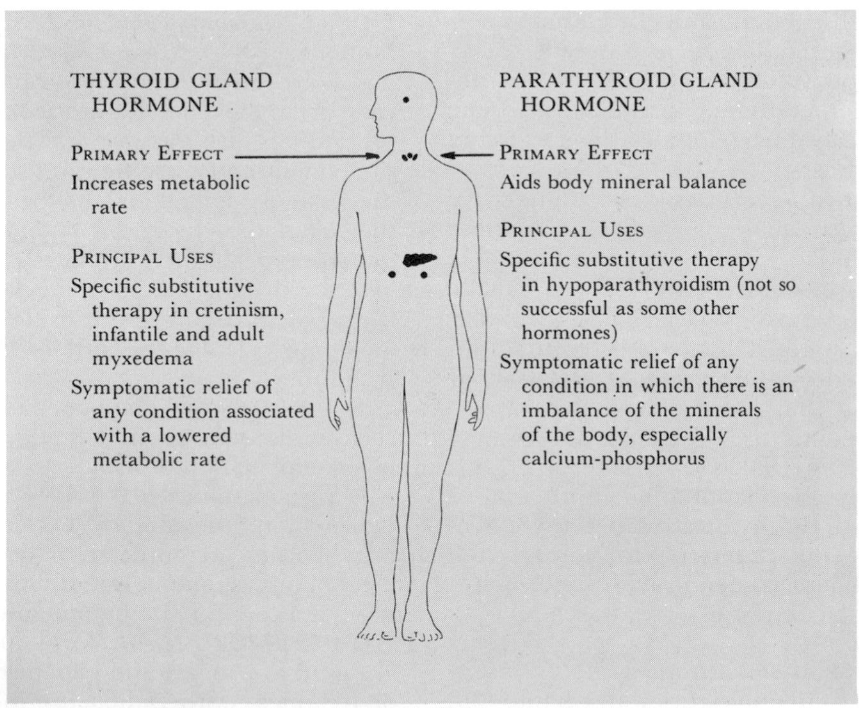

THYROID GLAND HORMONE
PRIMARY EFFECT
Increases metabolic rate
PRINCIPAL USES
Specific substitutive therapy in cretinism, infantile and adult myxedema
Symptomatic relief of any condition associated with a lowered metabolic rate
PARATHYROID GLAND HORMONE
PRIMARY EFFECT
Aids body mineral balance
PRINCIPAL USES
Specific substitutive therapy in hypoparathyroidism (not so successful as some other hormones)
Symptomatic relief of any condition in which there is an imbalance of the minerals of the body, especially calcium-phosphorus

FIGURE 49. Thyroid and parathyroid hormones as therapeutic agents.

THYROID PREPARATIONS

THE DRUGS. There are several thyroid preparations available to the physician giving him a choice for each patient and condition. They are derived either from domestic animal glands, properly prepared, or by synthesis.

Physical and Chemical Properties. Thyroid hormones, soluble in water and body fluids, are iodine-containing amino acids—thyroxine and triiodothyronine. They are incorporated in a red-staining material, thyroglobulin, a protein with a molecular weight of about 670,000.

Action. Basically all the preparations are for replacement therapy. When sodium levothyroxine is used, there is a lag of one or two days before results are noted. The effects are not as predictable as those of the other preparations.

Therapeutic Uses. The widest use of these preparations is in states of hypothyroidism but they are helpful in some other conditions. Diabetes insipidus has already been mentioned. Other uses are in certain gynecological conditions, in sterility in both male and female and in some cases of extreme obesity.

Absorption and Excretion. These drugs are readily absorbed from the gastrointestinal tract and are used by the thyroid gland to supplant the lack. They are cumulative in the body and are excreted via the feces.

Preparations and Dosages. For other preparations see Current Drug Handbook.

Dextrothyroxine (Cholaxin sodium) (d-thyroxine sodium [C]), 1 to 8 mg.

Sodium levothyroxine, U.S.P. (T_4, Letter, Synthroid) (Eltroxin [C]), 0.05 to 3 mg. orally, 0.05 mg. injection.

Sodium liothyronine, U.S.P. (Cytomel) (Tertoxin [C]), 5 to 50 μg.

Thyroglobulin (Proloid, Thyrar, Thyroprotein) 60 mg.

Thyroid, U.S.P., B.P., (Novothyroid, Thyronol [C]), 15 to 300 mg.

All doses are the total daily dose which may be given once or divided as suits the patient's condition.

All of these preparations are for oral administration except as indicated. The amount of medication that will be needed depends upon how much hormone the patient produces and also upon the individual needs of the patient as well as other factors. Some patients appear to require more of the hormone than others. If there has been complete destruction or removal of the gland, the patient will require a great deal more than if there is some glandular substance remaining and still functioning. The choice of the drug depends upon the particular requirements of the patient or the preference of the physician.

It is customary to begin administering any of the thyroid preparations with a minimal dose. This is increased gradually at intervals of seven to ten days until optimal response occurs. Then a maintenance dose is established.

THE NURSE

Mode of Administration. See above.

Side Effects. Most of the side effects are related to the early symptoms of hyperthyroidism. These include tachycardia, excitability and hyperhidrosis. After the dosage has been adjusted to the patient's requirements, checks should be made as the physician deems necessary. Dextrothyroxine sodium potentiates the oral anticoagulants, probably by enzyme induction.

Toxic Effects. Toxic effects are due to the cumulative effects of the drug and are similar to that of acute hyperthyroidism. Included in these are: hypertension, chest pain, dyspnea, nervousness, tremor, insomnia, and increased basal metabolic rate with weight loss. In most cases, if the dosage is reduced, the symptoms disappear.

Patient Teaching. The nurse should explain the major symptoms of both hypothyroidism and hyperthyroidism to the patient and his family, emphasizing that, should either occur, the patient should consult his physician at once. She should explain why it is essential that the patient have yearly physical examinations as a means of maintaining health. The drugs used as a substitute for the patient's own glandular products probably never completely take the place of the normal secretions; hence, the general physical condition of such patients is somewhat more precarious than that of the individual whose glands function adequately.

THE PATIENT. Many patients learn to judge their needs accurately, but the physician will need to re-examine even such patients at regular intervals.

Usually the patient taking thyroid will need this drug for the rest of his life, and this may pose a problem especially if the patient's means are limited (VI-1). Thyroid extract is much less expensive than the other preparations and is believed by some doctors to be as good or better than the others. Thyroid extract purchased in quantities of 100 or even 1000 tablets is much less expensive in the long run than is the same drug in smaller amounts. This should be explained to the patient. Another thing should be considered: different lots of thyroid extract may vary slightly in potency so that the patient may see more results from one prescription than from another. The nurse should explain to the patient that unless there is great variation, no change in dosage is indicated but if the variation seems excessive, the doctor should be notified. All of these drugs accumulate in the body and this fact should also be understood by the patient. Some physicians advise withholding the drug every so many days, such as once every seven to ten days.

PARATHYROID GLANDS

Controlled by blood chemistry

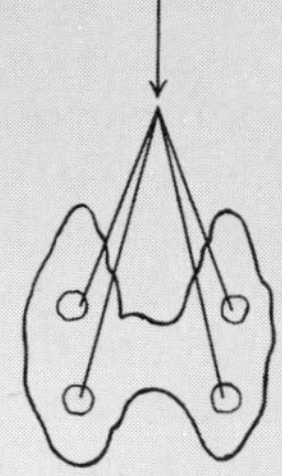

Parathyroid hormones (Control calcium metabolism)

Drug therapy: Used to treat deficiency and calcium-phosphorus imbalance

Parathyroid extract (Parathormone)
Parathyroid inj., U.S.P.

Usually used in conjunction with calcium and vitamin D.

Refer to Current Drug Handbook

FIGURE 50. Endocrine system in relation to drug therapy.

PARATHYROID

The hormone secreted by the parathyroid gland is essential for proper metabolism of calcium. It is associated with vitamin D and aids in the maintenance of the calcium-phosphorus balance.

Hyperparathyroidism, an increase in the hormone, causes a condition known as von Recklinghausen's disease. This disorder is usually treated by surgery or x-ray. In preparing the patient for surgery or irradiation, diuresis with saline cathartics is used to aid in the excretion of the excess calcium, but only if other conditions of the patient permit such treatment. Milk, milk products and any calcium-containing food are eliminated from the diet. Temporary reduction in the hypercalcemia may be obtained by hemodialysis. This lasts about three days.

In those cases that cannot be treated by surgery or irradiation, phosphate salts may be effective. One regimen is to give 24 ml. of a 1 molar dibasic sodium phosphate solution four times a day, orally, to provide 3 Gm. of phosphorus. Potassium phosphate may be substituted for the sodium salt when sodium should be restricted. See Chapters 10 and 18 for further details.

Hypoparathyroidism

Hypoparathyroidism may result from a variety of causes—injury to the parathyroid gland during any kind of extensive neck surgery or congenital absence of the glands. Treatment is directed at preventing tetany and the other sequelae of hypocalcemia.

In acute tetany, it is common to give calcium gluconate, 20 ml. of a 10 per cent solution slowly, intravenously, and repeat when necessary. Other clinicians prefer to give 30 to 60 ml. of calcium gluconate in a liter of physiologic saline solution, intravenously, over a prolonged period (12 to 24 hrs.). Calcium gluconate (Neo-calglucon) is also begun by mouth in doses of 2.0 Gm., or calcium lactate, 1.2 Gm., every four hours is given. Vitamin D, 100,000 units, is also given. (See Chapter 10 for more details.)

The treatment of chronic patients is much the same as for the oral treatment of acute tetany. Blood tests to determine calcium and phosphorus levels should be done at regular intervals during therapy.

PANCREAS—ISLETS OF LANGERHANS

Diabetes Mellitus

DEFINITION. Diabetes mellitus is a disorder of carbohydrate metabolism characterized by hyperglycemia and glycosuria resulting from a disturbance in the insulin-producing mechanism of the body. The exact role of the islets of Langerhans of the pancreas is not entirely clear, and it is now believed that other endocrine glands may play a part. There is a genetic predisposition to diabetes caused by a Mendelian recessive trait.

MAJOR SYMPTOMS. This disease has many symptoms, with polyuria being the most common and characteristic. Polydipsia, polyphagia, weight loss or loss of strength and hyperglycemia are also present.

DRUG THERAPY

INSULIN. THE DRUG. Isolated in 1922 by Banting and Best in Toronto, Canada, insulin has saved an untold number of lives since that time. Many diabetic patients are alive and relatively well because of it. However, insulin has not replaced the dietary treatment of diabetes; it has only supplemented such treatment; nor is it a cure for diabetes. Diet is a major aspect of treatment, but, with the use of insulin, the patient is able to eat many more foods than he could otherwise.

Physical and Chemical Properties. Insulin, molecular weight 6000, is made up of two chains of amino acids joined together by disulfide linkages. Insulin is freely soluble in body fluids. Because of its chemical nature, insulin is destroyed by the digestive juices and hence cannot be given orally.

Action. The main action of insulin is believed to be its power to increase the transport of glucose into the cells, especially those of the muscles and fatty tissue.

Therapeutic Uses. The principal use of insulin is in the treatment of diabetes mellitus. It is also used to produce a comatose state in certain psychoses. Occasionally, insulin is given to stimulate the appetite in debilitated or cachectic patients.

Absorption and Excretion. Insulin is rapidly absorbed from parenteral sites and is widely distributed throughout the body. Insulin is degraded by the liver and the kidneys. Little is excreted unchanged.

Preparations and Dosages. Insulin potency is expressed in terms of International Units (I.U.). It is usually marketed in 10 ml. vials labeled with potency per ml. as 40, 80 or 100 units. These strengths mean that each ml. contains the stated amount of insulin. Thus, in a 40 unit, 10 ml. vial, there will be 400 units. If U-100 vials are ordered, the patient will have to secure a U-100 syringe. The use of any other insulin syringe could cause a variation in the dose. This could result in the patient's receiving too much or too little insulin, with detrimental consequences. Insulin dosages are individualized. Some preparations act quickly, some have an intermediate period of activity and some are relatively long acting. Insulin sometimes causes hypersensitivity. In such cases another form of the drug can be used. The type and amount of the insulin to be used is usually determined by serial blood sugar estimation levels. After the dosage has been established, repeated urinalysis aids in evaluating each day's requirements within limits set by the physician. (Refer to Fig. 51 and the Current Drug Handbook for further details.)

QUICK-ACTING

Insulin injection, U.S.P., B.P. (regular, unmodified).

Insulin zinc suspension, prompt, U.S.P. (Semi-Lente).

INTERMEDIATE-ACTING

Globin insulin with zinc, B.P.

Insulin isophane suspension, U.S.P., B.P. (NPH Iletin).

Insulin zinc suspension, U.S.P. (Lente Iletin).

LONG-ACTING

Insulin zinc suspension, extended, U.S.P. (Ultra-Lente Iletin).

Insulin protamine zinc suspension, U.S.P., B.P.

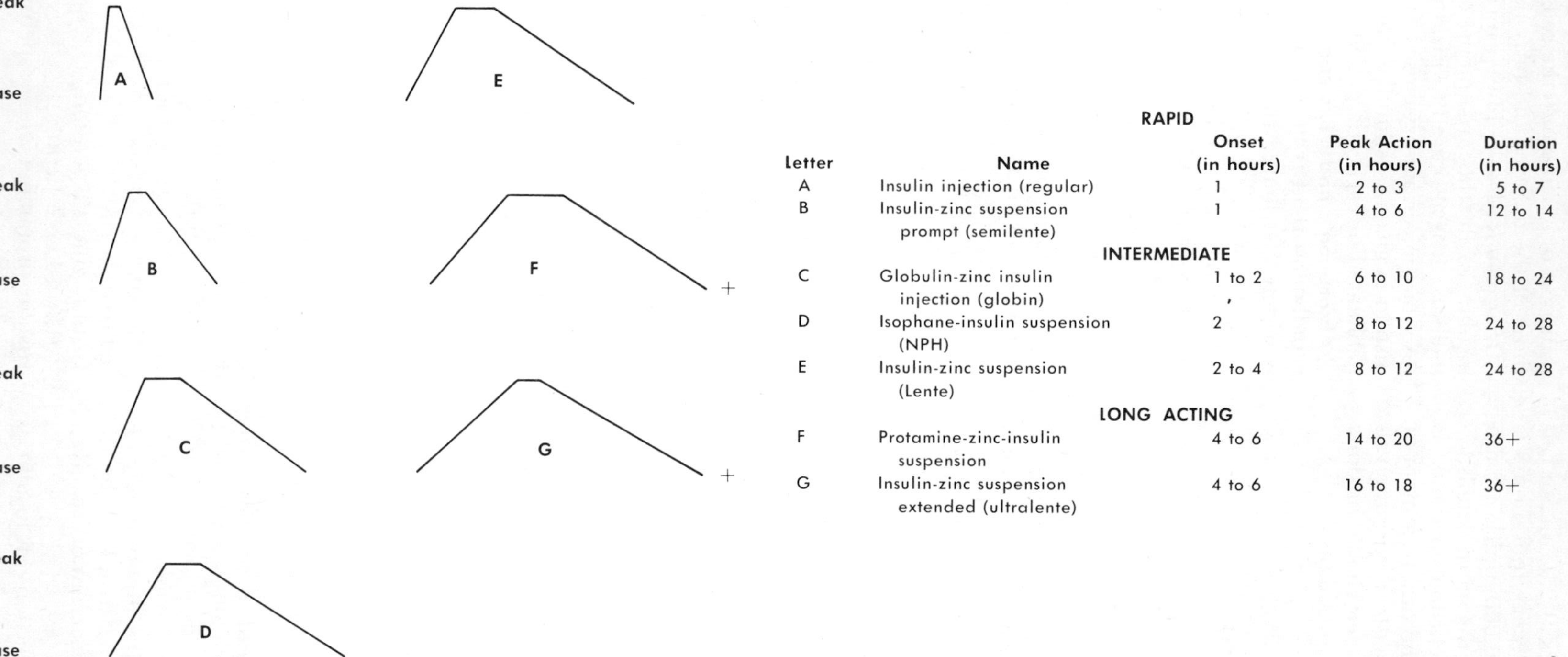

Letter	Name	Onset (in hours)	Peak Action (in hours)	Duration (in hours)
	RAPID			
A	Insulin injection (regular)	1	2 to 3	5 to 7
B	Insulin-zinc suspension prompt (semilente)	1	4 to 6	12 to 14
	INTERMEDIATE			
C	Globulin-zinc insulin injection (globin)	1 to 2	6 to 10	18 to 24
D	Isophane-insulin suspension (NPH)	2	8 to 12	24 to 28
E	Insulin-zinc suspension (Lente)	2 to 4	8 to 12	24 to 28
	LONG ACTING			
F	Protamine-zinc-insulin suspension	4 to 6	14 to 20	36+
G	Insulin-zinc suspension extended (ultralente)	4 to 6	16 to 18	36+

FIGURE 51. Times of insulin action as based on blood reports. (Adapted from *Drug Evaluations*, Chicago, 1971, American Medical Association and Goodman, L. S., and Gilman, A., *Pharmacological Basis of Therapeutics, 4th Ed.*, New York, 1970, The Macmillan Co.)

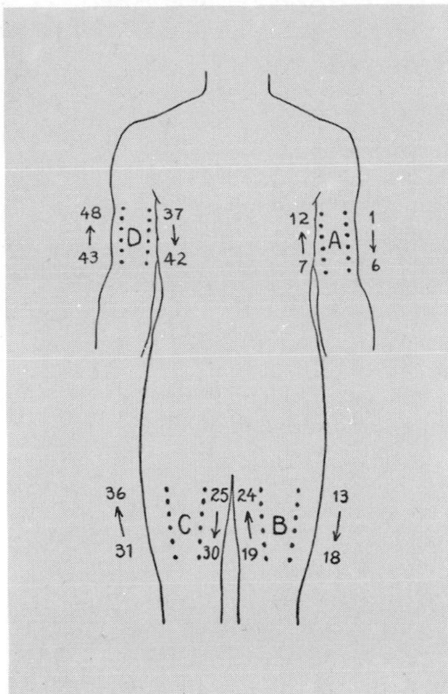

FIGURE 52. A diagram to illustrate one possible rotation of injection sites for insulin. This would allow more than six weeks before the same area would be used a second time. Areas on the abdominal wall may also be used.

THE NURSE

Mode of Administration. All forms of insulin can be given subcutaneously. Insulin injection (regular, unmodified) can also be given intravenously. This insulin cannot be mixed with other insulins, except the lente variety, without changing times and duration of effect.

All insulin, other than regular, must be thoroughly mixed before using. This should be done by gently rotating the vial—vigorous shaking must be avoided. Some patients have quick- and long-acting insulin given at the same time. The physician should be asked if he prefers to have these given separately. If not, the short-acting insulin should be drawn up first to avoid contaminating the regular insulin with the long-acting form. Then the long-acting form is drawn into the syringe, and the syringe is gently rotated to mix the two. Both the long- and the short-acting forms should be in the same unit form; that is, both either U-40, U-80 or whatever has been ordered, so there is less chance of error.

The time of the administration of insulin in relation to that of the meals is very important. It is usual to give the short-acting forms about 20 to 30 minutes before eating. The meal should be served promptly at the time indicated so as to avoid the possibility of an insulin reaction. The longer-acting forms of insulin also will have a definite time schedule, depending upon the type of the preparation. However, whatever the time ordered, it is important that it be given exactly as ordered and that the meals be taken at the proper interval after the drug has been given.

The urine is usually tested for sugar and acetone before each dose of insulin is administered. Some physicians order insulin dosage to be estimated on a fractionated urine sliding scale which indicates the presence of glycosuria. Usually, glycosuria indicates an insufficient insulin dose, dietary imbalance and other factors which may result in uncontrolled hyperglycemia.

Side Effects and Toxicity. Insulin, when used as directed, is relatively nontoxic. However, some patients are allergic to insulin, especially the regular, unmodified form. For these patients another form of the drug (sulfated bovine insulin or porcine insulin) must be used. The toxicity of insulin occurs mainly when the dosage has not been established, when the patient becomes ill from some other cause or when the patient receives another drug which interacts with the insulin, and the dosage is not readjusted. Hypoglycemia (insulin shock) occurs if too much insulin has been given; hyperglycemia (diabetic coma) may be the result of too little insulin or incorrect timing of insulin in relation to serving time of the meal. Table 15 gives the symptoms of these conditions. Any nurse caring for a diabetic patient should be familiar with the early signs of either too much or too little insulin. Emergency orders should be obtained ahead of time so that in case of need no time will be lost in obtaining relief. In cases of excessive insulin, some form of carbohydrates should be given such as fruit juice, sugar or candy. With hyperglycemia, insulin is given, the amount, kind and method of administration determined by orders from the physician.

The early signs of various reactions to insulin therapy should be familiar to every nurse caring for a diabetic patient. Diabetic acidosis can be suspected if the patient develops symptoms such as thirst, polyuria, glucosuria, and/or weakness. The most common causes are acute infections or gastrointestinal disorders.

Resistance to insulin can be caused by

TABLE 15. *MAJOR SYMPTOMS OF DIABETIC COMA AND HYPOGLYCEMIC SHOCK*

DIABETIC COMA (HYPERGLYCEMIA)	HYPOGLYCEMIC SHOCK
Early	
Clouding of the sensorium	Nervousness
Lethargy	Tremors
Irritability	Clammy perspiration
Anorexia	Hunger
Nausea and vomiting	Faintness
Flushed face	Ashen color
Hyperpnea	
Later	
Increased desire to sleep	Psychic disturbances
Abdominal pain	Emotional and mental disorder
Deep, rapid breathing	Complete disorientation
Acetone breath	
Fully Developed	
Deep respirations (may be either Cheyne-Stokes or Kussmaul)	Unconsciousness
	Convulsions
Deepening coma	Coma
Death is not uncommon	*Death* is rare

many disorders, some of which are severe adrenal-cortical hyperfunction, acromegaly, thyrotoxicosis, intestinal disorders (nausea, diarrhea) or an antigen-antibody reaction. This last comes on slowly, usually after several weeks or months of therapy, and is due to the fact that insulin is a foreign protein against which the body produces antibodies. This reaction is more common with bovine insulin than with porcine insulin.

Hypoglycemia may occur in any diabetic patient receiving insulin or one of the oral hypoglycemic drugs. If a patient is ill and not eating, the insulin should be omitted. If it has been given and the patient cannot take his food, glucose in some form must be given. Other causes of hypoglycemia include excessive amounts of exercise, an overdose of insulin, gastrointestinal disturbances or an improvement in the patient's ability to utilize glucose. Early symptoms of hypoglycemia include sweating, tremor, apprehension, hunger, weakness, tachycardia, and palpitation.

Interactions. Known interactions include the following. With the monoamine oxidase inhibitors, insulin is enhanced. With propranolol (Inderal) or biguanidine (Phenformin), the hypoglycemic action is increased.

Alcohol can cause a marked hypoglycemia in some patients with diabetes. The overall effect of alcohol can vary with total consumption, adequate diet and other factors.

Patient Teaching. The first and most important thing for the patient to realize is that insulin is not a substitute for a properly regulated diet. The patient may be allowed a wider variety of foods, but it does not allow unlimited intake of carbohydrates.

The nurse will need to teach the patient, or a member of his family the entire process of giving the injections. It is usual for the patient to give his own injections, even if the patient is a child. This makes him independent. The nurse must teach him not only how to give the hypodermic injections, but also the care of the hypodermic, or the use of a disposable one, the measurement of the insulin and where to give the injections. (See Fig. 52.) There are special insulin syringes which make the calculation and measuring of the drug easy.

The patient and his family need to know the signs and symptoms of both insulin shock and diabetic coma. It is wise for the patient to carry with him, at all times, a card or tab stating that he is a diabetic and what to do in case of an emergency. This card should include his home address and phone number and the name and phone number of his physician. The patient and his family must realize the seriousness of both hypoglycemia and hyperglycemia and understand that the doctor should be contacted at once should the early signs occur.

THE PATIENT. The patient who has just been informed that he has diabetes will present many problems. It is usually not easy for him to accept the fact that he will be on a restricted diet and will have to take injections for the remainder of his life. The nurse can do much to ease the emotional shock by explaining how many people have lived normal happy lives in spite of diabetes. She can also show the patient how the diet can be regulated so that it is not too restrictive. Economics may also play a part in the patient's difficulty. The nurse can often tell the patient of agencies that will help him to secure employment again or, if necessary, learn a new trade or vocation.

The patient who is receiving insulin regularly has many problems, one of which is the repeated hypodermic injections. If these are all given in the same area, the skin and subcutaneous tissues become less elastic because of fibrous tissue development, and this makes giving the injections difficult and may delay absorption of the drug. The person who is administering the injections should make a chart and follow it regularly. There are many variations, but Figure 52 shows one possibility. If this routine is followed, 48 injections will be given before the first area must be reused. Even for the patient taking regular insulin three times a day, this will allow 16 days before a part is used the second time, and this will permit healing of the skin and the subcutaneous tissue before it is necessary to inject into that part again. Following such a procedure will prevent the formation of excessive amounts of scar tissue and will promote the comfort of the patient. In addition to the areas given (Fig. 52), the anterior surface of the abdomen is often used, especially if the patient is giving his own injections, which is common.

The nurse must be ready to teach the patient or some member of his family how to give insulin, how to care for syringes and other pertinent information essential for the proper care of the diabetic patient. Simple well-illustrated books are available that will aid the patient materially, but the nurse should be ready to clarify any details which the patient may need explained. Most important points include the types of insulin, which one is used in preference to another, why the various strengths of insulin are marketed and how to calculate dosage. If the physician has not already done so, the nurse should be able to explain the nature of diabetes mellitus, the symptoms of insulin shock and diabetic coma and the emergency procedures to be used until the physician can be reached. The prevention and recognition of possible complications and a regimen of general health measures will also need to be discussed with the patient and his family.

SYNTHETIC HYPOGLYCEMIC AGENTS

THE DRUGS. Since the discovery of insulin there has been hope that someday a drug would be developed that could be taken orally. The drugs discussed here have partially solved that problem. They are not "oral insulin." However, for many patients they eliminate the need for insulin and for others they allow a lower insulin dosage. Research into these agents has revealed a great deal of information about the mechanism by which insulin acts and about the disease. The ideal drug has yet to be discovered.

Physical and Chemical Properties. There are two chemically different types of synthetic hypoglycemic agents: the first type is the sulfonylureas, similar to the sulfonamide drugs, the second is a biguanide. The sulfonylurea drugs are arylsulfonylurea with substitutions on the benzene and urea groups. The biguanide is derived from two molecules of guanidine with the elimination of one molecule of ammonia. These drugs are all marked in tablet forms which are soluble in water and in body fluids.

Action. The sulfonylurea drugs (acetohexamide, chlorpropamide, tolazamide and tolbutamide) all act in approximately the same manner. They either stimulate the beta cells of the pancreas to produce more endogenous insulin or trigger the release of it. Obviously, these drugs will succeed only in those patients who have viable pancreatic beta cells which are capable of responding to stimulation. This eliminates their use in most juvenile, difficult or unstable diabetic patients.

The action of biguanide (Phenformin) is not well understood. It is not insulinogenic. It seems to allow more effective use of insulin in a number of ways including decreased gluconeogenesis. In those patients who are insulin dependent (having little or no endogenous insulin) this preparation, if used alone, will be ineffective.

Therapeutic Uses. These drugs are used exclusively for the hyperglycemic patient.

Indications for Use. Recent onset of diabetes mellitus. (Rarely used for patients who have had diabetes for more than ten years.)

Onset of diabetes after the age of forty.

An insulin requirement of less than 40 units per day.

Absorption and Excretion. The sulfonylurea preparations are all readily absorbed from the gastrointestinal tract. They are widely distributed throughout the body. Some, such as tolbutamide, are rather rapidly degraded by the body (half-life of about five hours) and are excreted in the degraded form by the kidneys. Others, such as chlorpropamide, are not metabolized to any appreciable degree and are excreted slowly, mainly unchanged. It has a half-life of about 36 hours.

The biguanide (Phenformin) is readily absorbed from the gastrointestinal tract. The exact fate of the drug in the body is not entirely understood, but its duration of action is about six to fourteen hours.

Preparations and Dosages. All the synthetic hypoglycemic drugs are administered orally. Dosage is individually adjusted, usually started low, with increases as indicated by the patient's response. The drug may be given once in the morning before breakfast or divided into two or three doses. Since the sulfonylurea compounds stimulate the release of insulin and the biguanides appear to decrease gluconeogenesis and with other mechanisms render small amounts of insulin more effective, the combination of these drugs has proved to be effective in many patients who have shown decreasing response to maximum doses of one alone. See accompanying table.

The Nurse

Mode of Administration. All the synthetic hypoglycemic agents are given orally. As with insulin, these drugs are administered in relation to meals. It is important that the patient keep to the prescribed diet and that he eat all the food allowed.

Side Effects. Side effects with the sulfonylurea drugs are usually not serious and can be overcome by either a dosage change or use of another preparation. Side effects may include: skin rashes and eruptions; gastrointestinal disturbances, such as flatulence, nausea, vomiting; dizziness or a general feeling of malaise.

Phenformin side effects, also usually not serious, are associated with the gastrointestinal tract, such as a metallic taste, anorexia, nausea, vomiting, flatulence or diarrhea. These occur less with the delayed-release form than with the prompt-acting preparation.

Toxicity. The longer acting sulfonylurea drugs are more apt to cause toxic symptoms than those of shorter duration. Jaundice due to liver dysfunction is most common. If this occurs, the drug should be stopped and another one substituted. Some blood dyscrasias have been reported, but the number is small. Phenformin does not appear to produce any serious toxic symptoms. In all cases, toxic symptoms rarely occur with the use of recommended dosages. A study of patients taking tolbutamide has linked the drug with a possible increase in cardiovascular deaths.

Interactions. The interactions of the sulfonylureas with other drugs are as follows. Coumarin potentiates the hypoglycemic effect of tolbutamide probably by inhibiting its conversion to carboxytolbutamide in the liver. The action of the sulfonylureas is enhanced by phenylbutazone, sulfonamide compounds, the salicylates and the thiazide diuretics. The sulfonylureas potentiate the action of the barbiturates and alcohol. With the latter, an antabuse like reaction can occur.

Hypoglycemic Reactions. Hypoglycemic reactions due to oral hypoglycemic agents are less severe and occur less frequently than with insulin, since the reduction of blood sugar is less precipitous.

Such reactions happen most frequently

Name	Usual Daily Dosage (mg.)	Usual Effective Time (hrs.)
Sulfonylurea Compounds		
Acetohexamide, N.F. (Dymelor) (Dimeler, Ordimel [C])	250 to 1000	12 to 24
Chlorpropamide, U.S.P., B.P. (Diabinese) (Chloronase, Stabinol, Mallinase [C])	100 to 500	24 to 60
Tolazamide, U.S.P. (Tolinase) (Diabenase [C])	250 to 1000	6 to 16
Tolbutamide, U.S.P., B.P. (Orinase) (Delipol, Tolbutol [C])	500 to 3000	5 to 10
Biguanide Compounds		
Phenformin, U.S.P. (D.B.I., Dibotin) (Insoral [C])	25 to 200	4 to 6
Phenformin (delayed release form)	50 to 200	8 to 12

with the long-acting sulfonylurea medications than with others of this group. Many physicians find it best to reduce the dosage slightly after reaching the optimal effect. This aids in preventing hypoglycemic reactions.

Advantages of the Oral Hypoglycemic Agents. These preparations, if the response is adequate, allow for use of the patient's own insulin. This is usually as good, if not better, than injected insulin. If the drugs are completely effective it is possible to maintain the blood sugar within normal limits for a long time. The medicines avoid the necessity of hypodermic injections.

Disadvantages of the Oral Hypoglycemic Agents. Once the patient has received the oral drug, it is difficult to switch to the injection of insulin. There is probably greater risk of self-medication and the changing of dosage without the order from the physician. With long-term use there is more danger of toxicity than with insulin since the latter is a normal body hormone.

Patient Teaching. This is the same as with insulin except there is no need to discuss hypodermics or injection techniques. If the physician has not already done so, the nurse should explain to the patient that these oral medications are not insulin and cannot be expected to help if the patient has no endogenous insulin. She should explain that it may be necessary to substitute insulin if the oral medication is not effective. See Insulin for further teaching.

THE PATIENT. For the patient, the most important thing about these drugs is that they relieve him of injections. Many patients will seek medical advice if they have symptoms of diabetes (most are generally known) if they feel they can be treated without insulin. (See Insulin for further discussion.) Patients who use the oral hypoglycemic agents must understand that these are not a cure and that they will probably have to take them for the rest of their lives. This in no way releases them from responsibility regarding diet, weight control, personal hygiene or testing of urine. They must still be followed by the physician or nurse practitioner. Perhaps more so than when insulin is used, these patients are apt to become careless about their diets or about taking the drug.

If a patient is being switched from insulin to an oral hypoglycemic agent, it is best for him to be hospitalized where he can be watched carefully. The urine is tested three times daily for sugar and acetone and a fasting blood sugar determined before and four hours after the first dose. If the patient is not hospitalized, he should be seen daily by his physician for the first week and alerted to watch for signs of reactions.

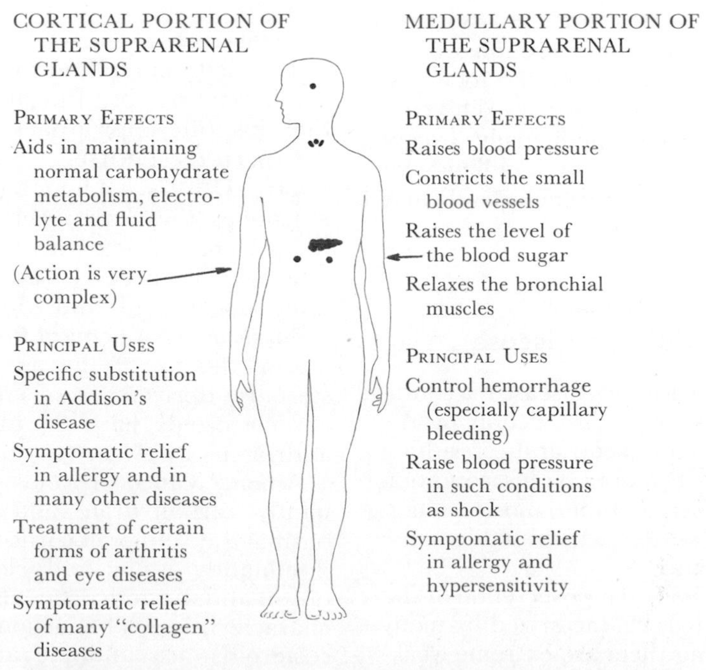

CORTICAL PORTION OF THE SUPRARENAL GLANDS
PRIMARY EFFECTS
Aids in maintaining normal carbohydrate metabolism, electrolyte and fluid balance
(Action is very complex)
PRINCIPAL USES
Specific substitution in Addison's disease
Symptomatic relief in allergy and in many other diseases
Treatment of certain forms of arthritis and eye diseases
Symptomatic relief of many "collagen" diseases
MEDULLARY PORTION OF THE SUPRARENAL GLANDS
PRIMARY EFFECTS
Raises blood pressure
Constricts the small blood vessels
Raises the level of the blood sugar
Relaxes the bronchial muscles
PRINCIPAL USES
Control hemorrhage (especially capillary bleeding)
Raise blood pressure in such conditions as shock
Symptomatic relief in allergy and hypersensitivity

FIGURE 53. Suprarenal (adrenal) gland hormones as therapeutic agents.

The patient should be checked once a month after the proper dosage is established.

As noted under *Interactions*, alcohol can react with the sulfonylurea to cause severe adverse symptoms. While a small amount of alcohol may not be contraindicated, the patient should be advised of this possibility. He might be wise in allowing several hours to elapse between the taking of the drug and the ingestion of even a small amount of alcohol.

SUPRARENAL GLANDS (ADRENAL GLANDS)

The suprarenal glands, located one above each kidney, like the pituitary gland are divided into two parts, the medulla and the cortex, each with specific and somewhat unrelated functions (Fig. 53). The secretion of the medullary portion, epinephrine (Adrenalin), was isolated and used medicinally many years before those of the cortex. (This is discussed in detail in Chapter 25.) The hormones of the suprarenal glands are used for many diseases and disorders not associated with the gland itself. These uses are discussed with the diseases for which they are used.

Hypersecretion of the Suprarenal Glands

Cushing's syndrome, which is associated with an increase in the secretion of the gland, appears to be secondary to a disturbance of the anterior pituitary. This condition is not treated medicinally except symptomatically. Surgery or irradiation of the pituitary or the suprarenal glands may be performed.

Chronic Adrenal Cortical Insufficiency (Addison's Disease)

DEFINITION. Addison's disease is a condition in which there is destruction of the gland (partial or complete) and a resulting decrease in the secretions. This condition may be the result of tuberculosis, malignancy or any disorder which reduces the activity of the gland.

MAJOR SYMPTOMS. Hyposecretion of the suprarenal glands is characterized by many symptoms. Among them are extreme weakness, a very low blood pressure, excessive pigmentation of the skin, anorexia, nausea and vomiting, weight loss and, sometimes, lumbar pain.

This insufficiency is definitely diagnosed by giving pituitary corticotropin (ACTH) and then checking the urine for 17-ketosteroids and 17-hydroxycorticoids and the eosinophil count. Pituitary corticotropin (corticotrophan C), 25 to 50 U.S.P. units, is infused intravenously in 500 ml. of 5 per cent dextrose or saline over an eight-hour period on each of three successive days. The urinary 17-ketosteroids and 17-hydroxycorticoids are determined on a 24-hour collection of urine on the control day and on each successive day during the administration of the drug. The eosinophil count is determined at the beginning and end of each infusion. Normal subjects exhibit an increase of 8 to 16 mg. per day in the excretion of 17-hydroxycorticoids and 4 to 8 mg. per day of 17-ketosteroids. Those with Addison's disease show virtually no response. In normal subjects, there is an eosinopenia of 80 to 90 per cent; those with Addison's disease show little or no change. An alternative method of administration is to give corticotropin gel intramuscularly, 40 units, twice a day for two days.

DRUG THERAPY. The main form of therapy in this dysfunction is to provide adequate replacement for the vitally important adrenal cortical secretion. The physician will first attempt to find some possible cause —tuberculosis or fungal infection—and then institute appropriate therapy.

CORTICOSTEROIDS

THE DRUGS. Though there are many hormones that have been extracted from the adrenal cortex, these are usually put into one of three classes: glucocorticoids, mineralocorticoids and androgens.

Physical and Chemical Properties. All of the secretions of the adrenal cortex are steroids derived from cholesterol. The corticosteroids have 21 carbons, and the androgens 19. All are soluble in body fluids.

Action. Glucocorticoids affect predominantly carbohydrate and protein metabolism; the mineralocorticoids affect predominantly water and electrolyte metabolism; and the androgens affect the male sex characteristics. The actions of the corticosteroids are multiple and not easy to understand. In Addison's disease, their administration is directed to replacement therapy, for without that, the patient soon dies.

Glucocorticoids promote the conversion of some proteins to carbohydrate and its deposition as glycogen in the liver; they promote a loss of protein from many organs producing a negative nitrogen balance in the body. Fat metabolism is interfered with by the inhibition of lipogenesis in the liver resulting in an atypical deposit of fatty tissue in the abdomen, shoulder areas and face ("moon face"). The electrolyte balance is affected because there is retention of sodium and excretion of potassium; the excretion of creatinine and uric acid via the urine is increased. Even the lymphatic system is affected, causing a leukopenia and reduction of enlarged lymph nodes. Still further, the circulating eosinophils and antibody production are decreased. These drugs also alter the normal inflammatory response.

The mineralocorticoids also cause increased retention of sodium and water and increased potassium excretion. The water retention causes an increased blood volume which in turn increases the cardiac output and the blood pressure. They share with the glucocorticoids the effects of promoting a negative nitrogen balance and increasing the absorption of fat and glucose from the gastrointestinal tract. Patients with Addison's disease cannot be kept in electrolyte balance with glucocorticoids alone.

The androgens from the cortex of the adrenal gland (adrenosterone and dehydroepiandrosterone) may or may not be used. If the male patient has normal testicular function, they are not needed; in the female with very low ketosteroid excretion they might help. There is a wide variability in response to them.

Therapeutic Uses. Besides being a lifesaving measure in Addison's disease, these drugs (the corticosteriods) have a wide variety of uses. Some of the most notable are: rheumatoid arthritis and bronchial asthma. They are often tried in many other conditions primarily for their anti-inflammatory or antiallergic effect.

Absorption and Excretion. Several of the glucocorticoids can be given by mouth, producing a plasma level as high as that produced by parenteral administration. This implies practically complete absorption from the upper gastrointestinal tract and absorption primarily into the lymph stream instead of the bloodstream. In doing so, it by-passes the liver which is important in the transformation of steroids. Apparently, evidence shows, the drug is excreted via the urinary system.

Preparations and Dosages. All dosages are very strictly individualized. The number of adrenal cortex hormone preparations is extensive. Only a few representative ones will be mentioned here. See Current Drug Handbook for more details.

For Addison's disease, the glucocorticosteroids are used. Doses given are for maintenance in Addison's disease in the adult.

Cortisone acetate, U.S.P., B.P., Novocort [C]) 25 to 100 mg. daily, orally or I.M.

Hydrocortisone acetate, U.S.P., B.P., (Bio-Cort, Cortanal [C] 20 to 40 mg. daily, orally or I.M.

Prednisolone, U.S.P., B.P. (metacortandrolone, Inflamase, Cormalone, [C]) 5 to 15 mg. daily, orally or I.M.

Prednisone, U.S.P., B.P., (metacortandiacin, Colisone, Prednisol [C]) 5 to 15 mg. daily.

The mineralocorticosteroids are also used for Addison's disease. The more important ones are:

Desoxycorticosterone acetate, N.F. (Cortate, DOCA Percorten) 2.0 to 5.0 mg. daily, orally or parenterally.

Fludrocortisone acetate (Florinef) 0.05 to 0.2 mg. daily, orally or parenterally.

Aldosterone (Electrocortin, Aldocertin), investigational as of 1973.

THE NURSE

Mode of Administration. The way the drugs are given varies slightly with the preparation, but most are given orally. Desoxycorticosterone acetate is given intramuscularly or buccally (placed under the tongue or against the cheek and allowed to dissolve) because it is destroyed in the gastrointestinal tract. The nurse should consult the accompanying literature for proper means of administration in the aqueous or lipid (sesame oil) forms.

A 19-gauge needle may be used to withdraw the lipid form. The drug should be given slowly and deeply intramuscularly (the gluteal muscles or the lateral aspect of the thighs). The site should be noted and recorded and rotated. When the buccal route is preferred, the tablet should be placed as previously described. Eating, drinking, chewing or smoking should be avoided until the tablet has dissolved completely. It may be helpful to use a mouthwash or brush the teeth after the administration of this drug.

Side and Toxic Effects. It is often difficult to distinguish between side effects and toxic effects when these drugs are given; the distinction is one of degree. Fluid retention (edema) and facial rounding ("moon face") are common; there are usually increased fat deposits with an increase in appetite and weight gain. An increase in body hair with a thinning of scalp hair is often noted; acne or skin pigmentation may appear. Ecchymosis with stria is not uncommon. The blood pressure is elevated and the patient may complain of tachycardia. There is a decreased resistance to infections and delayed wound and fracture healing; osteoporosis with fractures may occur. Laboratory tests show negative nitrogen balance, increased blood glucose and increased coagulation. Mental symptoms such as euphoria or depression may occur. If the patient has a history of peptic ulcer, the condition will be aggravated.

Interactions. Possible interactions of the adrenal cortical steroids with other drugs include the following. With the barbiturates, the metabolic rate is increased. Barbiturate action is enhanced, but that of the mineralocorticoids is inhibited. With the antihistamines, metabolic rate is also increased. With an anticholinergic there may be, on long-term use, an increase in ocular pressure. The steroids are inhibited by some antituberculosis drugs, the cholinergic compounds and the antiviral eye preparations.

The action of desoxycorticosterone is inhibited by phenobarbital, chlorcyclizine and phenylbutazone by enzyme inhibition. With the latter, the metabolic rate is increased.

Contraindications. Because of the sodium-retaining property of the corticosteroids, these drugs are given with caution when there is heart disease, hypertension or renal insufficiency. These drugs are used with extreme caution if diabetes mellitus is present for it is well known that the glucocorticoids raise the blood sugar. Other complicating conditions in which they should be used with caution include osteoporosis, convulsive disorders, treated peptic ulcers, and tuberculosis.

Absolute contraindications include psychoses, severe psychoneuroses, active peptic ulcers, herpes simplex of the eyes and some infections that cannot be controlled by chemotherapy. They should rarely, if ever, be used in pregnancy or during lactation.

Patient Teaching. Patient teaching of the Addisonian patient must be complete and detailed, for continual medication means life to him. He will undoubtedly have to take this hormone for the rest of his life and if the doctor does not explain this to the patient, the nurse should do so. Some patients, because they feel so much better, think they can do without the medicine, but the nurse must impress upon them that only the physician can decide when the drug can be stopped. The family should know as much about the disease and its treatment as the patient. For those with little or no adrenal function, it is wise to carry a kit containing 100 mg. of hydrocortisone for intravenous use, and/or 10 to 20 ml. of cortisone acetate for intramuscular use. The patient should always carry a card bearing his name and address, next of kin, doctor's name and address and phone number, and stating that he has Addison's disease. This should help establish prompt and correct treatment at the earliest possible moment should a crisis occur or if emergency surgery becomes necessary.

The doctor usually instructs the Addisonian patient to supplement his daily maintenance dose with an additionally prescribed dose when there is greatly increased activity or unusual stress – physical, emotional or psychological, which would be manifested by nausea, vomiting, arthralgia and lowered blood pressure.

The patient must know what the side effects and toxic symptoms are and must be instructed to call his doctor immediately if any of them appear.

The patient should take his oral medications with or immediately after eating to decrease gastric irritation.

Other Nursing Problems. An accurate, daily record should be kept of the patient's intake and output, his weight and blood pressure. The patient should be observed closely for any edema or symptoms of potassium depletion (muscle weakness, nausea and vomiting, depression, cardiac

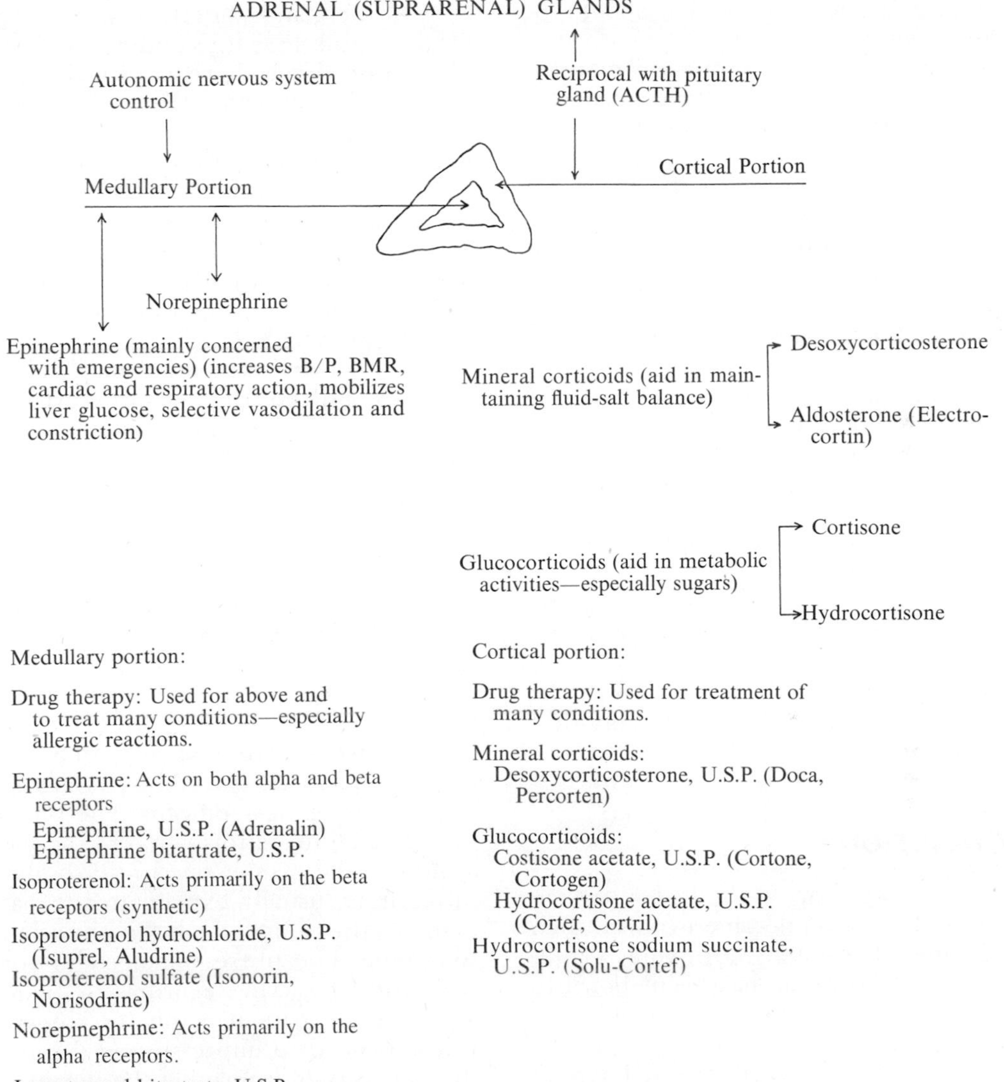

Medullary portion:

Drug therapy: Used for above and to treat many conditions—especially allergic reactions.

Epinephrine: Acts on both alpha and beta receptors
Epinephrine, U.S.P. (Adrenalin)
Epinephrine bitartrate, U.S.P.

Isoproterenol: Acts primarily on the beta receptors (synthetic)

Isoproterenol hydrochloride, U.S.P. (Isuprel, Aludrine)
Isoproterenol sulfate (Isonorin, Norisodrine)

Norepinephrine: Acts primarily on the alpha receptors.

Levarterenol bitartrate, U.S.P. (Levophed) (synthetic)

Cortical portion:

Drug therapy: Used for treatment of many conditions.

Mineral corticoids:
Desoxycorticosterone, U.S.P. (Doca, Percorten)

Glucocorticoids:
Costisone acetate, U.S.P. (Cortone, Cortogen)
Hydrocortisone acetate, U.S.P. (Cortef, Cortril)
Hydrocortisone sodium succinate, U.S.P. (Solu-Cortef)

Many similar preparations.

Refer to Current Drug Handbook and to diagram and discussion of Pituitary Gland.

FIGURE 54. Endocrine system in relation to drug therapy.

arrhythmias). The diet may be low in sodium, and potassium supplements may be ordered; even a high protein diet may be indicated. The nurse should check the urine routinely for sugar and acetone, since a "steroid diabetes" may result from the increased blood glucose level. Complete blood count and serum electrolytes should be done periodically.

Any patient receiving one or more of these steroids should be protected from sources of infection for the usual signs of inflammation are masked by their action. Some patients who receive these steroids are subject to emotional or psychological changes. It is important that the nurse observe and record these changes.

THE PATIENT. These patients should be able to lead a normal active life if given adequate replacement therapy and instructed in the nature of the disease. Of course, they should have regular check-ups by their physician.

The patient and his family will need to take special precautions to avoid conditions that add stress, such as emotional upsets. Coping with chronic illness is difficult. The nurse can be very valuable in helping the patient and his family solve the many problems it brings about. Continued contact with community health agencies can be arranged to aid them during the period of transition to new life styles.

CONCLUSION

There are other organs in the body which are thought to be endocrine in form, such as the pineal body and the thymus gland. However, no hormone has been shown to be elaborated by these organs, and no drugs are derived from them.

Glandular diseases have attracted a great deal of attention in recent years. It is very popular to have "gland" trouble, and many people blame all their ills upon these important organs. However, not nearly all the conditions thought by laymen to be of glandular origin are really caused by the endocrine glands. Most obesity, for instance, is caused by overeating, not by any disturbance of the glands, but the obese individual likes to think that the condition is due to a gland disorder rather than to his inability to curb his appetite (II-1). The patient who really does have a glandular disorder may be a psychologic as well as a physical problem. The hormones are as essential for the proper emotional balance of the person as for normal physical condition. The nurse must be aware of these emotional disorders and try to aid the patient in his adjustment to his condition.

Glandular disorders are usually relatively chronic, and the patient must learn to live with his condition and to maintain as nearly a normal life as possible. The patient should understand the interdependence of the various glands (that any disorder upsets the fine balance which nature normally maintains) and that this imbalance must be counteracted either by the use of the needed hormone or by whatever other method the physician may indicate. The patient must understand that he cannot expect this balance to be obtained overnight and that he will have to help the physician by noting and reporting all symptoms, even though they may seem insignificant. The physician may give all this information to the patient and he is the proper one to do so, but the nurse must usually explain to the patient many of the things which the physician has told him. The nurse will need to consult with the physician regarding a plan for teaching the patient about his illness. She will also need to impress upon the patient the necessity of informing the doctor of all the symptoms he notices.

IT IS IMPORTANT TO REMEMBER

1. That the secretions of the endocrine glands are essential to the proper functioning of the body.
2. That there is no quick cure for the patient with a disorder of the endocrine glands.
3. That all the endocrine glands are interdependent, and that malfunction of one will produce, to a greater or lesser degree, malfunction in others.

4. That the substitutive drugs, though of great value, probably never completely replace the patient's own glandular secretion, which is uniquely suited to his own metabolic physiology.

5. That the indiscrimate use of the secretions of the endocrines must be discouraged.

TOPICS FOR STUDY AND DISCUSSION

1. What are some of the social problems that may be encountered by the patient with a gland disorder? Select one disturbance and discuss the resulting problem in detail.
2. What might be the economic impact on the family budget of a patient with diabetes mellitus requiring insulin?
3. Prepare to give in class the instructions which might be given to a patient with diabetes mellitus, myxedema, Addison's disease or other endocrine condition when the patient is discharged.
4. Make a list of all the known hormones, and then those that have been used as drugs. List the conditions for which these drugs can be used. Are the disorders in the list all of endocrine origin? Explain, briefly, the exceptions.
5. From Sources of Drugs in the Appendix and from references in the library find out the sources of the endocrine drugs. Take any group which the teacher assigns or which interests you. Why are some of the hormones so much more expensive than others?
6. Why do the dosages of the same hormone vary so widely in different patients? (For instance, one patient may receive 1½ grains of thyroid extract daily whereas another one is getting 6 grains.)
7. The order for insulin is U. 12 three times a day before meals. How is this dose prepared from a U. 20 vial using a regular 2 ml. hypodermic?
8. The vial states that each ml. contains cortisone acetate 25 mg. How could the nurse give gr. ⅙ from this vial?

BIBLIOGRAPHY

Books and Pamphlets

American Medical Association Council on Drugs, *Drug Evaluations*, Chicago, 1971, American Medical Association.

Beeson, P. B., and McDermott, W., *Cecil-Loeb Textbook of Medicine 13th Ed.*, Philadelphia, 1971, W. B. Saunders Co.

Conn, H. F., et al., *Current Therapy, 1974*, Philadelphia, 1974, W. B. Saunders Co.

Feldman, E. G., *Evaluations of Drug Interaction*, Washington, D.C., 1971, American Pharmaceutical Association.

Goodman, L. S., and Gilman, A., *Pharmacological Basis of Therapeutics, 4th Ed.*, New York, 1970, The Macmillan Co.

Hartshorn, E. A., *Handbook of Drug Interactions*, Cincinnati, 1970, University of Cincinnati Press.

Rotenberg, G. N., *Compendium of Pharmaceutical Specialties*, Toronto, 1972, Canadian Pharmaceutical Association.

Watson, J. E., *Medical-Surgical Nursing and Related Physiology*, Philadelphia, 1972, W. B. Saunders Co.

Journal Articles

Arky, R. A., et al., "Irreversible hypoglycemia. A complication of alcohol and insulin," *J.A.M.A.* 206:639 (October, 1968).

Bernstingl, M., "Subtotal thyroidectomy," *Nurs. Times* 63:1333 (1967).

Burke, E. L., "Insulin injection, the site and the technique," *Am. J. Nurs.* 72:12:2194 (December, 1972).

Coates, F. C., and Fabrykant, M., "An insulin injection technique for preventing skin reactions," *Am. J. Nurs.* 65:2:127 (February, 1965).

Croft, D. N., "Radioisotopes in clinical medicine. 1. The physics, thyroid function and treatment," *Nurs. Times* 64:1416 (October 18, 1969).
DiPalma, J. R., "Drugs for diabetes mellitus," *R.N.* 30:71 (October, 1967).
DiPalma, J. R., "Diabetes mellitus, current concepts," *Am. J. Nurs.* 66:3:510 (March, 1966).
Ellis, M., "Assessment of thyroid function," *Can. Nurse* 61:881 (November, 1965).
Hawkins, P., "Hypophysectomy with yttrium 90," *Am. J. Nurs.* 65:10:122 (October, 1965).
Herfindal, E. T., and Hirschman, J. L., "Current therapeutic concepts—Hypothyroidism," *J. Am. Pharm. Assoc.* NS 11:9:493 (1971).
Hornbock, M., "Diabetes mellitus, the nurse's role," *Nurs. Clin. North Am.* 5:1:3 (1970).
Hummel, K. P., et al., "Diabetes, a new mutation in the mouse," *Science* 153:1127 (September, 1966).
Jones, F. E., "Chronic adrenal insufficiency—Addison's disease," *J. Am. Pharm. Assoc.* 13:2:99 (February, 1973).
Kirshner, N., et al., "Release of catecholamines and specific protein from adrenal glands," *Science* 154:529 (October 28, 1966).
McFarlane, J., and Nikerson, D., "Two-drop and one-drop test for glycosuria," *Am. J. Nurs.* 72:5:939 (May, 1972).
Moore, M. L., "Diabetes in children," *Am. J. Nurs.* 67:1:104 (January, 1967).
Munck, A., "Glucocorticoids inhibition of glucose uptake by peripheral tissues—Old and new evidence, molecular mechanisms and physiological significance," *Perspect. Biol. Med.* 14:2:265 (1971).
Nikerson, D., "Teaching the hospitalized diabetic," *Am. J. Nurs.* 72:5:935 (May, 1972).
Selye, H., "Adaptive steroids: retrospect and prospect," *Perspect. Biol. Med.* 13:3:343 (1970).
Selye, H., "The thyroid and antithyroid drugs," *R.N.* 31:55 (February, 1968).
Selye, H., "Oral drugs for diabetes," *R.N.* 26:35 (December, 1963).
Shea, K. M., et al., "Teaching a patient to live with adrenal insufficiency," *Am. J. Nurs.* 65:12:20 (December, 1965).
Stuart, S., "Day-to-day living with diabetes," *Am. J. Nurs.* 71:8:1548 (August, 1971).
Trainer, L., Killiam, P., and Nahas, G. G., "Ouabain hypoglycemic: insulin medication," *Science* 162:3853:560 (1969).

CHAPTER 28

DRUGS USED DURING PREGNANCY, DELIVERY AND LACTATION

CORRELATION WITH OTHER SCIENCES

III. MICROBIOLOGY

1. Many microorganisms are found on the skin and mucous membranes that are entirely harmless there but which become pathogenic when introduced into the deeper tissues.

V. PSYCHOLOGY

1. Mental and emotional satisfaction and a happy outlook depend not only upon psychogenic factors but also on physical factors as well.
2. To aid others to obtain personal satisfaction is one of the most satisfying of all achievements.

INTRODUCTION

This part of pharmacology has been almost completely ignored in published textbooks, and touched upon only lightly in books dealing with obstetrics. It has been assumed that since pregnancy and delivery are natural processes, drugs do not play a major part in the care of these patients. This assumption is, of course, true, but the authors of this book believe that this fact does not warrant omission of this area. The maternity patient usually receives some medications from the very beginning of her pregnancy, through labor, delivery and the puerperium. Modern medicine has made this normal process ever so much safer for both the mother and the infant. Much of this is a result of better techniques, but some certainly is the result of newer drugs, newer forms of old drugs and better understanding of the actions of these drugs.

Since this chapter is designed to be studied in conjunction with theoretical and clinical study of obstetrics, the headings usually used in obstetric books have been given to the divisions of the chapter. It should be remembered that there will be some overlapping since many drugs used in one situation are also used in others.

PREGNANCY—UNCOMPLICATED

Throughout the entire nine months of pregnancy, the mother is maintaining the metabolism for herself and for the developing infant. The resultant strain on the mother's system may be so slight that she may not notice any change, or it may be severe enough to cause many discomforts and disturbances. During the normal progress of pregnancy most of the treatment is directed toward proper general hygiene and diet. In addition to the diet, most physicians advise *multiple vitamin* preparations to insure that the mother receives enough of these essential chemicals. Many of these preparations also include minerals such as *iron, phosphorus, calcium* and the *trace elements* as well as the *vitamins.*

Early in the first trimester, the patient often complains of morning sickness. This is one of the first and the most consistent of the discomforts of pregnancy. Various treatments have been suggested for this, mainly dietary. To prevent injury to the fetus, most obstetricians prefer not to give any medications during the first trimester. Drugs ordinarily are not required for morning sickness. Vitamin preparations, especially B, C and pyridoxine, may be administered if dietary amounts are insufficient. Antacids may also be prescribed. However, if the nausea and vomiting do not respond to these measures, a combination drug (Bendectin) may be used. It is a combination of *dicyclomine* (Bentyl), *doxylamine succinate* (Decapryn) and *pyridoxine,* 10 mg. each. The patient takes two tablets at bedtime. The tablets are coated so as to release the medicine in the morning. If nausea persists during the day, one or two tablets may be taken as required.

Another rather common disorder of pregnancy which causes the patient a great deal of pain and often interferes with rest is muscle cramps. Any muscle of the body may be affected but those of the legs and feet cause the most frequent complaints. Most physicians agree that an insufficient amount of calcium in the blood is the main cause of the muscle cramps, but the method of overcoming that deficiency varies with different doctors. Some patients do well on a preparation containing *calcium, phosphorus* and *vitamin D,* but in other instances this does not overcome the cramps. For these individuals the physician uses *calcium lactate* or *calcium gluconate* with *aluminum hydroxide gel* given before meals. The theory behind this procedure is that there is a shortage of calcium with an excess of phosphorus. The aluminum hydroxide gel will decrease the absorption of phosphorus. The doctor usually reduces or eliminates milk in the diet since it is a source of phosphorus as well as calcium.

The obstetric patient may suffer from any disease or disorder, but usually the treatment is the same as for the nonpregnant patient. Thus for anemia, often iron deficiency anemia, various iron preparations are used such as *ferrous sulfate, ferrous gluconate* and *ferrous glycinate.* These are given orally. If the oral administration does not prove satisfactory, *iron-dextran complex* may be administered intramuscularly. Infections are treated as with the nonpregnant woman.

Disturbances of the gastrointestinal tract other than nausea and vomiting are relatively common, especially in the latter months of pregnancy. Gastric distress and constipation occur very frequently. The main treatment of these is dietary. Laxative foods will aid in overcoming constipation, and the use of frequent small feedings in place of three large meals may be sufficient to control gastric distress. Gas-forming foods should be eliminated. If these measures are not effective, medications will be used.

Aluminum hydroxide or *magnesium hydroxide* or a similar drug may be used for gastric disturbances. Sodium bicarbonate is not usually used since it is readily absorbed from the intestinal tract. It can cause some sodium retention with water and a resultant edema, or it may tend to cause a systemic alkalosis. See Chapter 10 for details. For constipation any one of a number of laxative medications may be given, such as *milk of magnesia, agar* or *agar* and *mineral oil* combined, *dioctyl sodium sulfosuccinate* (Colace, Doxinate). If edema exists, the saline cathartics are usually ordered. *Bisacodyl* (Dulcolax), which stimulates the colon mucosa, can be given either orally in enteric-coated tablets, 5 mg., or rectally by suppositories, 10 mg. *Glycerin* suppositories may also be used.

COMPLICATIONS OF PREGNANCY

Varicosities

For varicosities the same drugs are used as for leg cramps, since both are circulatory disturbances. In addition, *vitamin C* appears to aid in reducing the size of the varicose veins and in preventing ulceration and bleeding. If the condition is severe, the physician may feel it necessary to inject the veins with one of the sclerosing solutions such as *sodium morrhuate.* The use of support or elastic hosiery is usually recommended.

Hemorrhoids or rectal varicosities are a rather common accompaniment of pregnancy, especially in the later months when there is increasing pressure of the developing fetus on the hemorrhoidal veins. Very few physicians care to correct these surgically until after the termination of the pregnancy. Occasionally, the hemorrhoids are injected with a sclerosing solution, but more often conservative, palliative treatment is used. The most effective treatment is the use of suppositories containing an *analgesic* and an *astringent*. These aid in shrinking the hemorrhoids, thus reducing the inflammation and relieving pain. Any one of a number of preparations may be used.

Hyperemesis Gravidarum

Vomiting during pregnancy is common and may occur in any degree from an occasional morning nausea and vomiting to vomiting so persistent that it endangers life. The treatment of morning sickness has been discussed. If vomiting continues, especially after the first trimester, various medications are employed. The first drugs tried are those mentioned earlier under Pregnancy—Uncomplicated. If the condition is moderately severe, and the tablets do not give relief, other antiemetic drugs are used when, in the doctor's opinion, the possible adverse effects are less important than stopping the nausea and vomiting in the pregnant patient. Examples include drugs such as *dimenhydrinate* (Dramamine) and *phenobarbital*. If these do not suffice, *chlorpromazine* (Thorazine), *promazine* (Sparine) or *prochlorperazine* (Compazine) may be required. *Vitamin B-complex* plus extra amounts, 50 to 100 mg., of *vitamin* B_6 (pyridoxine) may be given. These drugs may be given intravenously if there is a probability that the oral drugs may be vomited. *Vitamins C* and *K* are also used. When the condition is very severe, all drugs and fluids are given intravenously until the tendency to vomit is reduced. The fluids must contain not only water but *nutrients (glucose* and *amino acids)* and the *electrolytes*. Often the intravenous route is the only one used for several days. Total parenteral nutrition may be employed for a few days to allow the gastrointestinal tract to rest and recuperate. Sedatives are given, often in large amounts. *Sodium amobarbital* (Amytal), 0.2 Gm. intravenously is often employed, but any of the usual sedatives may be used.

Bleeding—or Threatened Abortion

Vaginal bleeding is one of the serious complications of pregnancy, though occasionally a patient does have some menstrual bleeding during all or part of her pregnancy without any apparent detrimental effects. In most cases the bleeding signifies an impending loss of the fetus. Everything possible should be done to prevent this. Bed rest is usually ordered, and any one of a number of drugs may be given. The drug therapy is usually a combination of the gonadal hormones and vitamins. Sedatives are given as indicated. The hormones include *progesterone, estrogen* or *lututrin* (Lutrexin) or combinations of the three. Lututrin also tends to relax the uterus. The long acting progesterones such as hydroxyprogesterone caproate (Delalutin) and methoxyprogesterone acetate (Provera) may be used. These drugs are given intramuscularly and because absorption rate is slow, their action is prolonged. *Vitamins E, C* and *K*, all or any one, may be used since vitamin E is believed by some physicians to aid in the maintenance of pregnancy and vitamins C and K in the control of bleeding. The value of vitamin E in humans has not been definitely established. A synthetic drug has been used to delay premature labor; this is *isoxsuprine* (Vasodilan). Reports indicate that it is effective in some cases in preventing loss of the fetus before viability. Ethyl alcohol given intravenously is being used to stop or delay premature labor on a clinical trial basis, and it has shown some good results.

If there is any reason to suspect infection, the antibiotics (principally penicillin or one of the broad-spectrum oral antibiotics) are used. Sometimes the physician may order these drugs as a means of preventing possible infection.

Hypertension—Pre-eclampsia—Eclampsia

Hypertension, pre-eclampsia and eclampsia may be discussed together since medications used are the same or similar in each

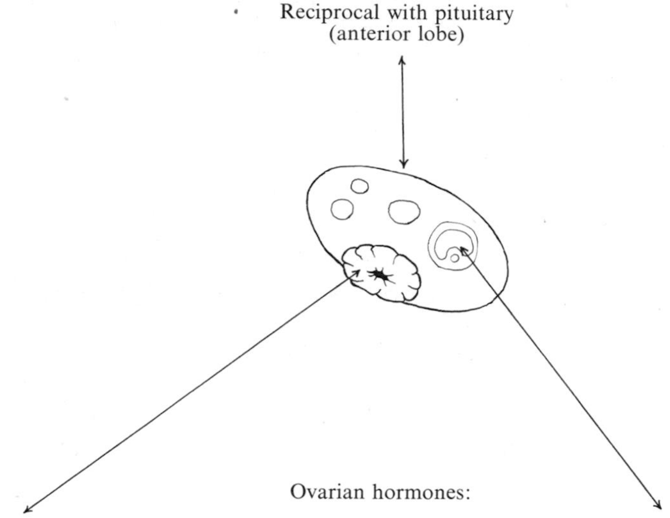

Ovarian hormones:

Progesterone or luteal: Maintain pregnancy

Estrogen: Maintain secondary sex characteristics
Stimulate production of ova

Drug therapy: Used for above conditions and also to treat many conditions

Progesterone or luteal:
- Ethisterone, U.S.P.
- Progesterol, U.S.P.

Estrogen:
- Estradiol benzoate, U.S.P.
- Estrone, U.S.P.
- Diethylstilbestrol, U.S.P. (synthetic)

There are many nonofficial natural and synthetic preparations of these hormones.

Refer to Current Drug Handbook and to Pituitary Gland diagram and discussion.

FIGURE 55. Endocrine system in drug therapy.

condition. Many physicians feel that these conditions are, in reality, phases of the same disorder, varying only in degree. Certainly one condition commonly leads to another.

Hypertension or high blood pressure is discussed in detail in Chapter 18. The patient suffering from hypertension may be entirely unaware of her condition but she will have symptoms which point to the fact that the pressure is above normal. The most prominent symptom is a persistent throbbing headache. The patient may also complain of palpitation, vertigo and, if a pre-eclamptic state has been reached, pain in the epigastrium. Often the patient will take various headache remedies for some time before she realizes that they are giving no real relief. She may even fail to tell the physician of the headache, not thinking it worth mentioning, and the first intimation he has is an elevation of the blood pressure. Until the blood pressure can be lowered, the physician will probably order some of the analgesics along with the hypotensive medications.

The list of drugs which may be used to lower blood pressure is long. They all have advantages and, to a greater or lesser extent, disadvantages. The drugs used include the veratrum veride derivatives such as cryptenemine (Unitensin), the Rauwolfia serpentina derivatives—often reserpine (Serpasil)—or the synthetic drug hydralazine hydrochloride (Apresoline). Any one of the drugs may be used. These have been discussed in detail in Chapter 18. (See also Current Drug Handbook.)

Pre-eclampsia is a condition characterized by the symptoms of hypertension, blurred vision, albuminuria and a rapid increase in weight as a result of edema. The condition is dangerous. It requires immediate and energetic treatment to avoid the onset of true eclampsia. The medical treatment includes, in addition to the antihypertensive drugs, medications which will reduce the edema. Many different routines exist, but one or all of the following may be given: *magnesium sulfate* in water each morning before breakfast; *calcium chloride* or *magnesium sulfate* intravenously (especially if cerebral edema is suspected); or *glucose* 20 to 50 per cent, 100 to 250 ml., may also be given intravenously for the same purpose. *Vitamins*, especially *C* and *B* and sometimes *D* with *calcium gluconate*, are given. If anemia is a complicating circumstance, which is not unusual, some form of iron will be given. See Anemia, Chapter 19.

The oral diuretics such as *acetazolamide* (Diamox), *chlorothiazide* (Diuril), *hydrochlorothiazide* (HydroDiuril, Esidrix), *ethoxzolamide* (Cardrase) or *ammonium chloride* often prove to be all that is required to reduce the blood pressure and overcome the edema. Other potent diuretics may include *furosemide* (Lasix) and *ethacrynic acid* (Edecrin). (See Current Drug Handbook.)

When sedation is desired the opiates are usually avoided in pre-eclampsia and the barbiturates favored. *Chlorpromazine* (Thorazine), *Promazine* (Sparine), *prochlorperazine* (Compazine) and *promethazine* (Phenergan), combined with small doses of the barbiturates, are used by some obstetricians because of their sedative action and their tendency to enhance the effectiveness of the accompanying drug. The first three drugs also lower blood pressure, dilate blood vessels and tend to increase renal output with consequent reduction of the edema.

If the condition progresses to eclampsia with convulsions, in addition to the drugs already mentioned, some sedative or hypnotic or both are given to control the convulsions. This is often thiopental sodium. Any drug used is given either parenterally or rectally, since it may be dangerous to administer anything by mouth because of the possibility of choking. A combination of drugs may be ordered to produce sedation, such as *amobarbital sodium*, 0.25 Gm. intravenously or subcutaneously, *chloral hydrate*, 3.0 Gm. rectally given in a starch solution, *magnesium sulfate*, 1 or 2 Gm. of a 25 or 50 per cent solution intramuscularly. Additional 1 Gm. doses may be given at 30 minute intervals until relief is obtained. Magnesium sulfate, given parenterally, is a strong cerebral nervous system depressant. It can be given intravenously, but great care must be exercised. Injection rate should not exceed 3 ml. per minute of a 5 per cent solution. Magnesium sulfate, given parenterally, potentiates other central nervous system depressants, so doses of such drugs given concurrently may need to be reduced to prevent respiratory depression or paralysis. When this drug is given either I.M. or I.V., a calcium salt should be available for

IMMUNIZATION DURING PREGNANCY†

	TETANUS-DIPHTHERIA	POLIOMYELITIS	MUMPS	MEASLES	RUBELLA	INFLUENZA	TYPHOID
RISK FROM DISEASE TO PREGNANT FEMALE	Severe morbidity. Tetanus mortality 60%, diphtheria mortality 10% unaltered by pregnancy.	No increased incidence in pregnancy, but possible increased risk of more severe disease.	Low morbidity and mortality, not altered by pregnancy.	Significant morbidity, low mortality, not altered by pregnancy.	Low morbidity and mortality, not altered by pregnancy.	Possible increase in morbidity and mortalty during epidemic of new antigenic strain.	Signficant morbidity and mortality, not altered by pregnancy.
RISK FROM DISEASE TO FETUS OR NEONATE	Neonatal tetanus mortality 60%.	Anoxic fetal damage reported. 50% mortality in neonatal disease.	Questionable association with fibroelastosis in neonate.	Signifcant increase in abortion rate. No malformations reported.	High rate of abortion and congenital rubella syndrome in first trimester.	Possible increased abortion rate. No malformations confirmed.	Unknown.
VACCINE	Combined tetanus diphtheria toxoids preferred: request adult DT from pharmacist.	Live, attenuated virus (Sabin) vaccine.	Live, attenuated virus vaccine.	Live, attenuated virus vaccine.	Live, attenuated virus vaccine.	Inactivated type A and type B virus vaccines.	Killed bacterial vaccine.
RISK FROM VACCINE TO FETUS	None confirmed.	None confirmed.	None confirmed.	None confirmed.	None confirmed.	None confirmed.	None confirmed.
INDICATIONS FOR VACCINATION DURING PREGNANCY	Lack of primary series, or no booster within past 10 years.	Not recommended routinely for adults in USA. In epidemics, mandatory to immunize all adults.	Contraindicated.	Contraindicated.	Contraindicated.	Recommended only for patients with serious underlying diseases.***	Not recommended routinely except for close, continued exposure or travel to endemic areas.
DOSE/SCHEDULE	**Primary:** 3 doses at 1-2 month intervals. **Booster:** 0.5 cc per 10 years.	Monovalent or trivalent OPV. Primary series of 3 doses at 1-2 month intervals, or booster dose.	———	———	———	**Primary:** 2 doses 6-8 weeks apart in early fall. **Booster:** Single dose.****	Primary immunization 2 injections 4 weeks apart. Booster injection every 3 years as indicated.
COMMENTS	Updating of immune status should be part of antepartum care.	Vaccine indicated for susceptible women traveling in endemic areas.	———	2.0 cc Immune Serum Globulin to exposed, susceptible female.	Teratogenicity of vaccine virus suspected but not confirmed.*	Vaccination of pregnant women before new virus strain left to discretion of physician.	———

†From American College of Obstetricians and Gynecologists, *Technical Bulletin No. 20:* March, 1973.

*To determine the teratogenicity of rubella virus and rubella vaccine virus, the Center for Disease Control maintains a registry of *Congenital Rubella Syndrome* and of *Rubella Vaccination During Pregnancy.* This surveillance allows continuing evaluation of the rubella vaccination program. Therefore, all cases concerning either one of these problems should be reported to the CDC.

**Though congenital vaccinia and abortion following smallpox vaccination are not unknown, they are certainly rare events. The safest procedure for primary smallpox vaccination during pregnancy is to administer a simultaneous, separate injection of vaccinia immune globulin (VIG). But when VIG is not available and vaccination is mandatory, during epidemics or travel in endemic areas, vaccine should not be withheld. The risk of maternal and fetal death from smallpox under such conditions far outweighs the risks from vaccination itself. Complications following smallpox *revaccination* are very rare, and VIG is not indicated.

***All influenza vaccines presently available are highly purified and minimally reactogenic. As prevention of influenza is desirable in the pregnant woman, immunization should be considered (Infectious Disease Section, California State Department of Health).

****The primary series of bivalent influenza vaccine has traditionally been 2 doses. Preliminary data indicate that with the more potent influenza vaccines available in recent years, the second dose provides little additional benefit. It is therefore reasonable to give a single dose of vaccine for either primary or annual booster vaccination. MMWR, 22(24): 207, 1973.

	SMALLPOX	YELLOW FEVER	CHOLERA	PLAGUE	RABIES	HEPATITIS-A (Infectious)	VARICELLA ZOSTER
RISK FROM DISEASE TO PREGNANT FEMALE	Mortality increased to 90% during pregnancy (variola major).	Signficant morbidity and mortality, not altered by pregnancy.	Signficant morbidity and mortality, not altered by pregnancy.	Signficant morbidity and mortality, not altered by pregnancy.	Near 100% fatality not altered by pregnancy.	Significant morbidity, low mortality, not altered by pregnancy.	Low morbidity and mortality, not altered by pregnancy.
RISK FROM DISEASE TO FETUS OR NEONATE	Possible increased abortion rate. Congenital smallpox reported.	Unknown.	Unknown.	Unknown.	Determined by maternal disease.	Transmission to fetus and possibility of neonatal hepatitis.	Possible increased risk of severe disease in neonate, especially if premature.
VACCINE	Live vaccinia virus vaccine.	Live, attenuated virus vaccine.	Killed bacterial vaccine.	Killed bacterial vaccine.	Killed virus vaccine (Duck embryo). Rabies immune globulin.	Pooled immune serum globulin.	Zoster immune globulin or convalescent zoster plasma.
RISK FROM VACCINE TO FETUS	Rare cases of congenital vaccinia.	Unknown.	Unknown.	None reported.	Unknown.	None reported.	None reported.
INDICATIONS FOR VACCINATION DURING PREGNANCY	Not recommended routinely in U.S.A. except for at risk populations (hospital and public health workers). Avoid in pregnancy except in cases of probable exposure.	Contraindicated except for unavoidable exposure.	Only to meet international travel requirements.	Very selective vaccination of exposed persons.	Pregnancy does not alter indications for prophylaxis. Each case must be considered individually.	Household or institutional exposure. Travel in developing countries.	Experimental drug. No PHS recommendation for use in pregnancy.
DOSE/SCHEDULE	Give VIG (0.3cc/kg) with primary vaccination, when available. Revaccination without VIG.	Single injection per 10 years.	2 injections 4-8 weeks apart.	Consult public health authorities for indications and dosage.	Consult public health authorities for indications and dosage.	2.0 cc IM for adults for exposure or short-term foreign travel.	———
COMMENTS	**	Postponing travel preferable to vaccination.	Vaccine of low efficacy.	———	———	Not recommended for protection against hepatitis-B (serum).	CDC is maintaining surveillance of varicella during pregnancy.

Inquiries for additional information or assistance can be directed to:

Center for Disease Control
Immunization Branch
State and Community Services Division
Atlanta, Georgia 30333
Telephone: 404/633-3311 Extension 3736

intravenous use in case of magnesium intoxication. See Chapter 10 for details. *Morphine sulfate* may or may not be included, depending upon circumstances. In place of chloral hydrate, some obstetricians prefer paraldehyde given in oil rectally. Hypertonic *glucose* solution intravenously may be given to control cerebral edema. *Oxygen* is usually given continuously during and after a convulsion. Eclampsia is such a serious condition, often proving fatal to either the mother or the infant or both, that every effort should be made to detect the early symptoms and to institute preventive treatment.

Other Complications of Pregnancy

The patient should be specially guarded against infections by every possible means. During an epidemic of certain communicable diseases, many physicians feel that the maternity patient should have *immune serum globulin* if she has not had that disease. This is especially true of rubella, which, it is believed, causes congenital anomalies, especially if it occurs in the first trimester. If a young woman has not had rubella in childhood, some doctors advise that she be vaccinated against it before she becomes pregnant, since the vaccine is not used during pregnancy.

Since the number of available vaccines has greatly increased in recent years, guidelines for their use in specific groups are now necessary. In the case of pregnant women, the goal of such guidelines is to protect the woman and the fetus from serious disease and/or unnecessary vaccination. (See accompanying table, Immunization During Pregnancy.)

Another complication of pregnancy is the so called Rh discrepancy, occurring when the mother is Rh negative and the father and the unborn child are Rh positive. With the first pregnancy, if the mother has not had a blood transfusion with Rh positive blood the infant is usually normal. However, the mother builds up antibodies against the infant's Rh positive blood and in subsequent pregnancy the infant, if it is Rh positive, may develop erythroblastosis fetalis, a serious and often fatal disease of the newborn. To prevent it, the mother is given intramuscularly one dose of Rh_0 (D) immune globulin (human) (Rhogam) within 72 hours after the delivery of the normal Rh positive infant; the inoculation arrests formation of antibodies in her blood. It is repeated after every pregnancy if the infant is Rh positive. The commercial circular should be read carefully and the directions followed exactly in giving this preparation. The drug is valueless if the mother has already developed antibodies against blood containing the Rh positive factor.

Pregnancy ought to be a happy time for the mother, and every effort should be made to make it as pleasant as possible. Often there is no need for medications, but when drugs can help the mother to be more comfortable or can prevent complications, they should be used (V-1).

Since the disastrous results of the use of the tranquilizing drug Thalidomide in Europe, much research and thought have been given to the use of various drugs during pregnancy. Many obstetricians hesitate to order even the "simplest" medications. Just how many drugs adversely affect the fetus is difficult to estimate. However, some are known. Conn, H. F., *Current Therapy, 1972,* Philadelphia, 1972, W. B. Saunders Co., lists the following drugs. (Martin, *Hazards of Medication,* Philadelphia, 1971, J. B. Lippincott Co., has a more complete list.)

TOXIC AGENT (DRUG)	EFFECT ON FETUS
Quinine	Deafness
Streptomycin	Deafness
Chloroquine	Deafness
Tetracycline	Abnormal teeth
Iodides	Congenital goiter Secondary tracheal compression

TOXIC AGENT (DRUG)	EFFECT ON NEWBORN
Sulfonamide derivatives Sulfonamide and acetazolamide Tolbutamide Aspirin	Displace or interfere with bilirubin-albumin binding

OTHERS: Contraceptives in breast milk may cause sterility in the female infant.
Oxygen to the newborn may cause retrolental fibroplasia and blindness, especially if given too long or in too concentrated a dose.

LABOR—FIRST STAGE

The first stage of labor extends from the onset until complete dilation of the cervix. The length of this stage varies from a few minutes to several days, but with many patients it is about 12 to 18 hours. In the early stage the patient should be encouraged to rest as much as possible to conserve her strength. To insure this rest, most physicians order narcotic or hypnotic drugs. The following are some of the analgesic drugs that may be used:

Meperidine (Demerol; pethidine [C]) 50 to 100 mg. intramuscularly.

Alphaprodine (Nisentil) 40 mg. subcutaneously.

Opium derivatives such as Pantopon, Dilaudid, or, for some cases, morphine sulfate subcutaneously. The usual dosage prevails.

The following are the most commonly used hypnotics:

Pentobarbital sodium (Nembutal) 50 to 100 mg. orally.

Seconal 0.1 to 0.2 Gm. orally.

Chloral hydrate is also used by some obstetricians for certain patients.

All these drugs have advantages and disadvantages. The barbiturates tend to cause restlessness but are relatively safe for both mother and child (if the dosage is not excessive and the drug is given early in labor); chloral hydrate is relatively safe and gives good sedation; the bromides are safe but give less sedation than some of the other drugs; opium derivatives may cause uterine inertia if given too soon, and may cause respiratory depression in the infant if given too late; meperidine and alphaprodine give good analgesia and are relatively safe.

There are other drugs that can be used to aid in relieving the distress of the mother which do not seem to cause depression in the infant. Among these are the synthetic analgesics *pentazocine* (Talwin) and *piminodine* (Alvodine) and the phenothiazine-type tranquilizer *propiomazine* (Largon). The action of this latter drug is about the same as other similar preparations. It also enhances the action of accompanying analgesic or hypnotic drugs.

When any of the sedative or hypnotic drugs is administered, the nurse must watch the patient very carefully since she will not realize the strength of the contractions, and labor may progress rapidly. The drug will relieve the patient's worry and tension, thus relaxing the muscles of the pelvic floor so that the infant can pass through more easily.

Scopolamine hydrobromide (hyoscine), 0.4 to 0.6 mg., may be given alone or with other drugs for the same purposes as when used preoperatively (to dry secretions and to tranquilize). Scopolamine acts best when it is given with other medication. It may be given with any of the aforementioned drugs and also with *methadone.* The combination of methadone, 10 mg., and scopolamine, 0.4 mg., gives good analgesia and amnesia, usually without ill effects to either mother or infant.

For many years "twilight sleep" was very popular, and some obstetricians still use it, wholly or in part, to produce an amnesia during the first stage of labor, especially when this stage is apt to be prolonged as with a primipara. In its entirety this routine (also called Gwathmey's oil-ether anesthesia) requires three drugs given together as follows: *Quinetherol (Ether* 2 ounces, *alcohol* 2 ounces, *olive oil* 1½ ounces and *quinine sulfate* 1.2 Gm.) rectally; *morphine sulfate,* 15 mg. subcutaneously; and *magnesium sulfate,* 2 ml. of a 50 per cent solution intramuscularly. The morphine and the magnesium sulfate are repeated if needed. This combination is rarely, if ever, used now, but drugs given for essentially the same purpose are used. One such combination has been discussed under Eclampsia. As with any use of analgesic medications, any of the antiemetic tranquilizers may be used to enhance the analgesic and reduce the tendency to nausea. These also reduce the patient's anxiety. Many doctors give small doses of *levallorphan* (Lorfan), usually about 0.3 mg., *nalorphine hydrochloride* (Nalline), 5.0 mg. or *naloxone hydrochloride* (Narcan) 0.4 mg. These are most often employed when the doctor is giving one of the strong analgesics and especially with the opiates. This is to lessen the possibility of respiratory depression in either the infant or the mother. The patient under this type of analgesia needs very careful nursing since she will not be able to tell the nurse how she feels. The obstetrician will usually limit the number of examinations since the patient is to be disturbed as little as possible.

This will make essential a close watch on the contractions (type, duration, frequency) and fetal heart tones.

During the latter stage of pregnancy or at the onset of labor many physicians give *vitamin K*, either orally or parenterally. This is to aid in preventing excessive blood loss during and after delivery, and also to prevent bleeding in the infant. Of course, vitamin K is especially important if there is any indication that the patient has a tendency to bleed.

To institute labor, when this is desirable, *castor oil* with or without *quinine* may be used. One to two ounces of the oil is given any way that will help the patient to take it without discomfort. One method is to put together an equal amount of the oil and orange juice, then add a small amount (1/4 teaspoonful) of sodium bicarbonate to the mixture just before the patient takes it. This is stirred and the resulting "fizz" is not at all unpleasant to drink. Of course, if the patient is on a low sodium or salt free diet, sodium bicarbonate should not be used. A little ice held in the mouth before taking the drug will also aid in disguising the taste. There is a form of castor oil which is almost odorless and tasteless and this should be used when possible. The quinine sulfate is given in capsules usually 0.3 to 0.6 Gm. each.

POSTERIOR PITUITARY HORMONES. (See Chapter 27 and Current Drug Handbook.) There are two hormones secreted by the posterior portion of the pituitary gland, *vasopressin* (Pitressin) and *oxytocin* (Pitocin). The former is primarily an antidiuretic and hypertensive agent, the latter an ecbolic, stimulating uterine muscle. Oxytocin (Pitocin, Syntocinon, Uteracon) is given intranasally or intrabuccally to induce labor. It may be added to an intravenous solution. The dose is usually determined by the uterine contractions and the route by which it is given. Oxytocin is often given intravenously in labor induction at term, giving 1 ml. (10 units) per liter of either physiological sodium chloride solution or 5 per cent glucose solution. The intravenous must be given very slowly. The rate can be adjusted to assure that the amount used is only what is required. It may also be given intramuscularly in doses of 0.3 to 1.0 ml. at the time the anterior shoulder is delivered. Given at this time, it will help check blood loss.

A synthetic preparation, *sparteine sulfate* (Tocosamine), is also used to induce or stimulate labor. Its action is similar to that of oxytocin. Initial dose is 150 mg. in 1 ml. It is given intramuscularly and repeated every three or four hours as required. This drug, like oxytocin, should not be used when there are obstetrical complications. See Current Drug Handbook for contraindications and toxicity. If sparteine is ineffective and oxytocin is to be employed, several hours should elapse between the drugs because their action is synergistic.

THE NURSE. The posterior pituitary hormone is a very potent oxytocic agent, and the nurse must be constantly on the alert when it is being administered. Labor may progress very rapidly and the contractions may become severe. The obstetrician should be notified frequently as to the progress of labor.

When an intravenous infusion containing oxytocin is being given, a nurse must be in constant attendance. The condition of the baby (rate and rhythm of the heart) must be constantly monitored. At any sign of fetal distress or a sustained uterine contraction, the infusion should be stopped and the doctor notified. He should be readily available when this treatment is performed.

The nurse must watch for increased bleeding or signs of water intoxication during oxytocin therapy. This drug may exert an antidiuretic effect, especially in patients receiving intravenous fluids. It may also reduce the amount of the circulating fibrinogen. A careful record of uterine bleeding is important.

THE PATIENT. The patient receiving these drugs should be told what to expect from the drug. The patient will be happy to know that at last her period of waiting is nearly over, even if the contractions do become much more severe.

PROSTAGLANDINS. Prostaglandins are modified unsaturated fatty acids which are synthesized in the body in a variety of tissues. The parent compound is named prostanoic acid and is derived from the essential fatty acid, arachidonic acid.

There are any number of compounds that have been identified as prostaglandins. They have been given letter designations. Some of them are PGA, PGA_2, PGE, PGE_2, PGF and PGF_3. The prostaglandins are rapidly inactivated in the lungs. These compounds are believed to be formed and to act locally and are deactivated quickly to prevent a build-up in the body.

The exact action or actions of the prostaglandins are, as yet, only partially understood. However, their therapeutic potential appears to be great, since they seem to affect a variety of organs. The highest concentration is found in semen, and they are therefore considered to be important in reproduction. Prostaglandins are extremely potent and are active even when present in minute amounts. Research and investigation are being done to ascertain just what their actual clinical application may be.

There are two compounds marketed in Great Britain, Prostin E_2 and Prostin $F_2\ \alpha$. Recently, Prostin F α has been released for use in the United States. They are used to induce labor and for abortion. Other possible uses are as antihypertensive agents, for allergic reactions, for infertility of the male and in the treatment of arthritis. At present these preparations are given intravenously. For abortion, however, the drugs have been inserted into the vaginal vault with some success.

DELIVERY—SECOND AND THIRD STAGE OF LABOR

Whether the actual delivery takes place in a hospital or in a home does not materially alter the procedure, though the nurse in the home will need to anticipate which medicines will probably be used and see that they are at hand. The physician may bring all needed drugs with him, but the nurse must ascertain if he is preparing to do this and, if not, she must secure prescriptions and obtain the drugs.

If the first stage of labor is prolonged, or if the patient does not seem to be able to take enough fluids and nourishment during the first stage or the first part of the second stage, it may be necessary to supply the patient with additional fluids. For this purpose any of the common intravenous preparations is used, such as the *electrolyte* solutions, *glucose, amino acids* or *vitamin B* or combinations of them.

During the latter part of the first stage or in the beginning of the second stage, preparations for delivery are made. Among the major preparations is the painting or spraying of the vulva and perineal area with an antiseptic solution (III-1). Physicians and institutions vary as to the exact chemical used, but any of the usual skin and mucous membrane antiseptics will be satisfactory.

With the end of the first stage, the complete dilation of the cervix is accomplished, the contractions become more severe, and the patient begins to feel "as if she were getting somewhere." She now needs less of the analgesic, and more of the anesthetic drugs. Any of the standard general anesthetics—*chloroform, ether, ethylene, cyclopropane, nitrous oxide* or other inhalatory drug—may be administered. No matter what anesthetic is employed, care must be exercised to be sure that the patient receives no more than is absolutely necessary since the anesthetic may delay the process of delivery if it is too strong and may also have adverse effects upon the infant. Respiratory paralysis of the infant may result if the anesthesia of the mother is too deep or too prolonged. Many physicians use only a local or nerve block anesthetic, believing that these are less dangerous for the mother and the baby. Of course, there are some patients who do not want or need any anesthetic at all. This is especially true of patients being delivered by the natural childbirth procedure.

A local or regional anesthetic may be used for a spinal, caudal, pericervical or pudendal nerve block or perineal anesthesia. Any of the common local anesthetics may be used. The nurse should have ephedrine, epinephrine or phenylephrine (Neo-Synephrine) ready for use if the patient has an allergic reaction to the drug used. In some cases the nurse will be asked to give the anesthetic, but usually an anesthetist will administer it. The physician will always give the local anesthetic. The nurse must, of course, prepare the anesthetic agent for him. Before an episiotomy is to be done, the physician will use a local anesthetic in the area of the incision, unless a caudal, spinal or nerve block anesthetic has already been employed or the patient is under a general anesthesia. *Lidocaine hydrochloride* (Xylocaine) 0.5 per cent, *mepivacaine hydrochloride* (Carbocaine) 1.0 per cent and *procaine hydrochloride* (Novocain) 0.5 to 1.0 per cent or similar medication with or without *epinephrine* (Adrenalin) will be used. The exact drug will depend upon (1) the condition of the patient, (2) the individual doctor's preference, (3) the routine of the institution.

If during any stage there is delay in the process of labor as a result of uterine inertia, *oxytocin* may be ordered either intranasally or intravenously.

In obstetric emergencies, symptoms are treated as they occur. These are similar to those encountered in the operating room.

Following the birth of the infant, most doctors give some form of ergot. Others repeat the oxytocin to reduce postpartum bleeding.

ERGOT

THE DRUG. Ergot, the dried sclerotinum (mycelium) of a fungus, *Claviceps purpurea*, growing on grain, usually rye, has been known since early recorded times. Ergot poisoning due to the ingestion of contaminated grain or flour has been a problem for centuries. It occurs most often when the growing season has been warm and moist. Even though it is now known what the use of moldy grain can do, epidemics of ergot poisoning have occurred as late as 1953 (France). However, epidemics are now rare. Ergot poisoning, especially the acute form, occasionally happens when it is used to induce abortion.

Physical and Chemical Properties. Ergot is an extremely complex substance, and at least twelve alkaloids as well as other substances have been isolated from it. Both levorotatory and dextrorotatory forms are known, but only the former is pharmaceutically important. These are derivatives of lysergic acid. There are three important ergot alkaloids: ergotamine, ergonovine and ergotoxine (the last being a mixture of three alkaloids, ergocristine, ergocrytine and ergocornine). Ergotamine and ergotoxine upon hydrolysis yield amino acids and lysergic acid, ergonovine yields lysergic acid and amines. The diethylamide derivative of lysergic acid (LSD) is not used medicinally and was discussed previously in the chapter on drug abuse. Originally, the ergot preparations were used in crude form; now produced synthetically or semisynthetically, they are in purer form. The salts of the alkaloids are soluble in water, but not all are readily absorbed from the gastrointestinal tract, ergonovine being better absorbed than ergotamine or ergotoxine.

Action. The alkaloids of ergot have many actions, but the important ones are stimulation of smooth muscle tissue, especially the uterus and the muscles of the blood vessels, and decreasing the cerebral blood supply. The result of these actions is stimulation of the uterus (oxytoxic), rise in blood pressure with a decrease in peripheral blood supply, and cerebral hypotension. Ergotamine especially reduces the cerebral blood supply. Ergonovine acts primarily on the uterus. These are the drugs used most frequently in therapy.

Therapeutic Uses. Ergotamine is used to relieve migraine and other vascular headaches. Ergonovine is used to stimulate the uterus, usually for the control of postpartum hemorrhage.

Absorption and Excretion. Because both ergotamine and ergotoxine are poorly absorbed from the gastrointestinal tract, they are usually administered parenterally. Ergonovine is absorbed from the gastrointestinal tract and may be given orally or parenterally. The fate of the ergot alkaloids in the body is incompletely known. They are believed to be detoxified by the liver and excreted by the kidneys.

Preparations and Dosages. Only the oxytoxic agents are given here. See Chapter 9 and Current Drug Handbook for more information.

Ergonovine maleate, U.S.P. (Ergotrate), Ergometrine maleate, B.P., 0.2 mg. orally or parenterally.

Methylergonovine maleate, U.S.P. (Methergine), Methylergometrine maleate, B.P. 0.2 mg. orally or parenterally.

THE NURSE

Mode of Administration. Ergonovine or the synthetic, methylergonovine, may be given orally, intramuscularly or intravenously. Subcutaneous injection should be avoided because the drug irritates tissue. In the discussion of oxytocin, it was stated that it might be given at the time of the delivery of the anterior shoulder of the infant. Ergonovine maleate (Ergotrate) 0.2 mg. may be given intramuscularly in the place of oxytocin. However, many obstetricians prefer the oxytocin, since there "seems to be less danger of a retained placenta." Ergonovine is usually given after the delivery of the placenta. The drug is given either intramuscularly 0.2 mg. or orally 0.2 to 0.4 mg. The oral administration is continued two to four times a day for 48 to 72 hours post partum to prevent excessive blood loss. It is discontinued when uterine atony is controlled. Prolonged use is not advised.

Since the trade name of ergonovine is Ergotrate, there has been confusion of this drug with ergotamine tartrate, used for vascular headaches. The nurse should check carefully the drug ordered. Ergonovine preparations for parenteral use should be checked for expiration date since they deteriorate with age.

Side Effects, Toxicity and Treatment. Side effects and toxicity are rare in therapeutic dosage. However, with continued use of the ergot preparation, chronic toxicity may occur and with an overdose, acute poisoning is possible. It has been found that patients with liver or renal disorders are more likely than others to develop toxic symptoms.

In acute toxicity, there is likely to be tingling of the extremities, nausea, vomiting, diarrhea, uterine bleeding and—if the patient is pregnant—abortion. Subsequently edema, abnormal sensations, pallor and a fall in temperature may develop. These symptoms may be followed by convulsions and coma. Treatment is largely symptomatic. If there is reason to believe that the drug is still in the gastrointestinal tract, lavage and purgation are indicated.

With chronic ergot poisoning, there is dry gangrene of the extremities preceded by tingling and coldness. Sometimes, cataracts develop. Other symptoms include vertigo, headache, muscle tremors and various abnormal skin sensations. Treatment is to stop the medication completely and treat symptoms as they occur.

Contraindications. Ergot preparations should not be given to patients with infections, peripheral vascular disease, hepatic or renal dysfunction, severe hypertension or during pregnancy.

THE PATIENT. Ergonovine and methylergonovine are used to control postpartum hemorrhage and to speed involution. The nurse can take this time to explain to the patient the process of involution, its importance and why the medication is continued. The patient will need to understand that the medication should be used only as long as it is required. However, many women know the effect of ergot during pregnancy and they may ask the nurse about its use to produce abortion in an unwanted pregnancy. The nurse should emphasize the grave danger this use entails. Any number of deaths from acute poisoning have been reported from the use of ergot in just such cases.

PUERPERIUM

For the first few days postpartum, most physicians routinely order certain drugs to make the patient's recovery more rapid and complete. Drugs usually employed are the following:

To control bleeding and facilitate involution: methylergonovine, 0.2 mg. orally every four to six hours for six doses, or ergonovine, 0.2 mg. in same routine.

To aid in securing adequate rest: *Pentobarbital sodium, secobarbital, amobarbital* or *phenobarbital,* 0.1 Gm., for sleep, or *phenobarbital,* 30 mg., for restlessness may be given.

To ease discomfort, especially from sutures or after-pains: Any of the antipyretic-analgesics may be used with or without *codeine*; or one of the stronger analgesics such as *meperidine* (Demerol) or *morphine* may be given. The usual dosage prevails.

To prevent infection: *Penicillin* or one of the other antibiotics or chemotherapeutic drugs may be used.

To prevent constipation: Any one of a number of drugs may be used. (See the medications discussed under Pregnancy—Uncomplicated.)

If the infant is not to be nursed, one of the gonadal hormones is used to prevent lactation, such as testosterone or estrogen or a combination of them.

Puerperal fever, once a great menace to the life of the mother, is now relatively uncommon. It is, of course, caused by the introduction of pathogenic microorganisms into the birth canal and the uterus at the time of labor and delivery. Various organisms may be responsible for this condition, but different strains of streptococci and staphylococci predominate. The major symptoms are high fever, malaise, arthralgia and profuse foul-smelling lochia. The condition is treated with *penicillin, ampicillin,* the *tetracyclines* or the *sulfonamides* or combinations of the four. The exact drug will depend upon the known or suspected organism.

When the mother recovers from the immediate strain of delivery, she often needs some help to rebuild her strength. The usual antianemic medications are used together with a general vitamin preparation. If the mother is nursing the infant, these may be given as long as lactation continues.

THE NEWBORN INFANT

The newborn infant requires separate care from the instant of birth, and some of this care is medicinal. Usually the infant's first introduction to drugs is the application of the antigonorrheal (Credé's) treatment to the eyes. All states require that some form of preventive, antiseptic drug be used. If the state law specifies the actual preparation to be used, no variation can be made, but if the law simply requires that an antiseptic drug be used, the physician or institution may choose any one of several drugs. Two drugs that may be used are silver nitrate 0.5 to 1.0 per cent followed in 15 to 20 minutes with a saline wash or a combination ointment containing neomycin, bacitracin and polymyxin.

If the newborn infant is not breathing effectively, oxygen is administered. For absolute asphyxia neonatorum, in addition to the oxygen, *epinephrine* may be ordered. Oxygen should be given continuously even if there is no apparent breathing, until death has been established or the child has begun to breathe and is maintaining good color without the extra oxygen supply. Oxygen is used only as long as is absolutely essential, since retrolental fibroplasia with loss of vision can occur if too much oxygen is used for too long a time.

Newborn infants are often given *vitamin K* to aid in preventing undue loss of blood, especially if any surgical procedure such as circumcision is contemplated.

The newborn infant may become ill as may any child, and in such cases treatment is the same as it would be for the older infant. Infections which at one time were relatively common are now rare, thanks to better techniques.

In most cases, diseases of the newborn are the same as or similar to those of the older child and medical therapy is the same with reference to the size and maturity of the infant. Newborn babies' immune systems are not as well developed as those of the older child or the adult. This means that the invasion of microorganisms which might cause little or no damage in the adult can be devastating for the newborn at term and even more disastrous for the premature infant. A brief discussion of some of the problems follows.

The possibility of an RH factor discrepancy has already been considered. It is now possible to monitor the blood condition of the fetus through testing of the amniotic fluid in addition to the more frequently used checking of antibody development by the mother and to prepare for difficulty should it arise. If there is imminent peril, intrauterine transfusion may be done. If gestation is at or near term, labor may be induced and preparations made for a complete transfer transfusion as soon as the infant is delivered.

Congenital syphilis is usually encountered in cases where there has been no prenatal care or the care came too late to treat the mother sufficiently. Congenital syphilis is usually treated with *penicillin* in doses appropriate to the size of the infant. Doses for infants are usually calculated on the basis of the surface area. See Chapter 13.

Prevention of ophthalmia neonatorum (gonorrheal ophthalmia in the newborn) has been mentioned. Babies born without adequate medical attention may not have the benefit of this preventive measure and may develop this condition. Incidentally, these infants are often born of mothers who might well have gonorrhea, either active or silent. Ophthalmia neonatorum requires vigorous treatment, usually with penicillin parenterally and a combination ointment (neomycin, bacitracin and polymyxin) topically. These infants are usually seen in the isolation wards of the pediatric department rather than in the hospital's newborn nursery.

Infantile infections from such organisms as *E. coli,* staphylococcus, streptococcus or viruses may take various forms—gastrointestinal (usually with severe diarrhea), skin (with persistent multiple small abscesses), pulmonary (pneumonitis) or blood (septicemia). Such infections have been caused by "carriers" among the hospital personnel. These organisms may be entirely harmless for the adult but can cause very severe illness and sometimes death for the newborn baby. Drugs used will depend upon many factors. Usually, penicillin or ampicillin is used to start treatment. A culture is taken before or at the start of therapy to avoid inhibition of the organism during culture. As soon as a report of the culture and the sensitivity test is in, the appropriate anti-infective drug is used. Supportive therapy must be started immediately. If there is severe diarrhea, potassium loss is apt to result in hypokalemia and can be serious. Electrolyte monitoring is essential, with intravenous fluids used as indicated by the reports. Strict separation of infants in a nursery will aid in preventing spread of the infection to other infants. In many cases, the organisms seem to gain in virulence as they pass from one infant to another. Thus the later cases, if they occur, may be more severe than the earlier ones.

The hospital-acquired infection is extremely difficult to justify or to explain to parents and to the public. Every effort should be made to see that nursing personnel (especially those in the newborn nursery) are well, and that they are not "carriers" of any potential disease organisms, that newborn infants are kept separate and that those handling the infants wash their hands thoroughly after handling each infant. Briefly, this is isolation technique.

Probably no field of nursing is a greater challenge to the nurse than is the area of maternal and child care. So much can now be done to prevent the loss of mother or baby, and so much of this is done by the nurse that this is one of the most pleasant and most satisfying of all types of nursing. It is a great privilege to be able to help in this great work of saving lives at their very beginning (V-1, 2).

PLANNING A FAMILY

Although the term "Family Planning" has come to be associated with the limiting of the number of children, it can also be applied to the attempt by the couple to have children. Too few or no children can be as disturbing as having too many children. Hence infertility may be a very distressing problem. Both conditions will be discussed as they relate to medicinal treatment.

Infertility—Female

DEFINITION. The inability to initiate the reproductive process is referred to as infertility, and the difficulty may lie with either the female or the male partner. When existing conditions are known to make conception clearly impossible, the term absolute sterility is used. Relative sterility implies that there are various factors which make conception difficult but not impossible (V-2).

MAJOR SYMPTOMS. The definition of infertility gives the symptoms of this condition. Few, if any, symptoms can be said to be characteristic.

DRUG THERAPY. Although constitutional factors—mental stress and nutritional deficiencies—cannot be overlooked, drug therapy may possibly be of assistance in infertility if a hormonal deficiency can be demonstrated. There are no drugs which are extremely valuable, but several may play an important role when used judiciously. The proper treatment depends upon adequate diagnosis.

Thyroid extract is probably one of the most useful of these drugs. This is often used when there is no real evidence of hypothyroidism in small doses of about 50 mg. daily by mouth. Apparently, the thyroid, in some way, improves the character of the germ plasm.

If the failure of ovulation is due to an adrenal dysfunction, there are usually signs of masculinization. These patients may respond to *prednisolone,* 30 mg. daily gradually reduced to a maintenance dose of from 5 to 10 mg. daily in divided doses. This may re-establish the menstrual cycle, ovulation and fertility. Those who do not respond to this may respond to estrogens. *Diethylstilbestrol,* 1.0 mg. daily for one week, is given, 2.0 mg. daily for the second week and then 3.0 mg. daily for the third week. Ovulation may occur after such therapy.

Another hormone approach is to give *chorionic gonadotropin,* 5000 units daily for six days, in the immediate postovulative period.

There have been some attempts to use one of the "birth control pills" with the hope of inducing a rebound ovulation reaction. This is based on the report that fertile women who have been placed on birth con-

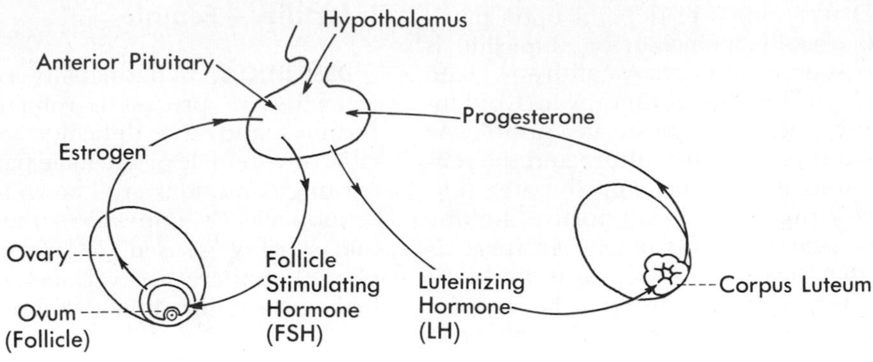

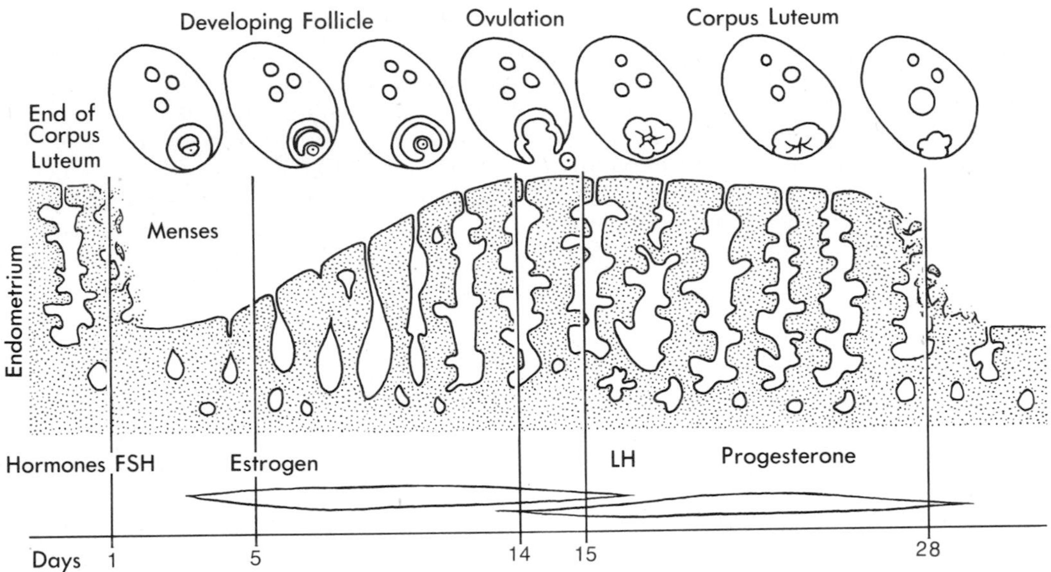

FIGURE 56. Hormonal control of menstrual cycle.

trol pills regain their fertility as soon as the pill is stopped. This method has not produced encouraging results.

Clomiphene citrate (Clomid), a nonsteroid analogue of chlortrianisene, is a drug that has been used to promote fertility. It appears to increase the output of the pituitary gonadotropins, which in turn stimulate maturation and endocrine activity of the ovarian follicle. This is followed by the subsequent development of the corpus luteum.

The drug should be given only to selected patients. Liver function evaluation should be done and the drug withheld if evidence of liver damage or malfunction is found. It is contraindicated in the presence of an ovarian cyst because further enlargement of the ovary may occur. Basal body temperature should be recorded all through the treatment cycles to determine whether ovulation occurs because it is contraindicated in pregnancy.

The patient and her husband should be warned that the incidence of multiple pregnancies (including triplets, quadruplets and quintuplets) is ten times greater if conception takes place during a cycle in which clomiphene is used.

The dose is usually 50 mg. orally daily for five days. It may be started at any time in a patient who has had no recent uterine bleeding. If spontaneous uterine bleeding occurs prior to therapy, the five day regimen should be started on or about the fifth day of the cycle. If ovulation appears not to have occurred after the first course, a second course of 100 mg. daily for five days may be given. This may be started as early as 30 days after the previous course. At no time should the dosage or duration go over 100 mg. for five days.

The patient should be warned about the possible side effects—some of them serious. Blurring and other visual symptoms occasionally occur during therapy, so the patient should be warned about driving a car or operating machinery. Other less serious effects include hot flashes, abdominal or pelvic discomfort, nausea and vomiting, breast discomfort, increased nervous tension, headache, dizziness and a heavier menstrual flow. More serious side effects are allergic dermatitis, weight gain and reversible loss of hair.

Infertility—Male

As previously stated, infertility is the inability to initiate the reproductive process. It has been determined that in 40 to 50 per cent of all cases, the male is the infertile partner.

Generally, it is believed that fertility is uncommon in the male when the sperm count is below 20 million, when any considerable percentage are nonmotile or when a stained smear shows a high percentage of morphologically abnormal forms. If the sperm count is low, a full urologic and medical investigation is warranted.

No method of treatment in use today is very satisfactory. *Thyroid extract* may be helpful but there seems to be some indication that *sodium liothyronine* (Cytomel; tertoxin [C]), is more effective in producing an increase in sperm count and motility. This drug is closely related chemically to thyroxin, but is more rapid in action and about three to four times as potent. The drug is started at 5 mcg. (micrograms) daily and the semen is examined every four weeks. The dose is increased by 5 to 10 mcg. per day at four week intervals according to sperm count and motility. Maintenance dosage is usually 25 mcg. daily but if there is no improvement after six months, the drug is discontinued.

Then a "rebound" type of therapy is attempted. *Testosterone propionate* in large doses, 100 mg. twice weekly, is given to depress spermatogenesis. When the sperm count is very low, the drug is stopped. Occasionally a rebound sperm production occurs.

FAMILY PLANNING

Called by a variety of names—Planned Parenthood, Family Planning, Responsible Parenthood—family planning has been with us for some time. The rhythm method, based on the "safe period" of the menstrual cycle, has been and still is used by many. Success with this method has been qualified. Mechanical devices are also used. A variety of intrauterine devices (IUDs) are available and are usually successful, but occasionally the device is lost through the cervical os. Another mechanical device, the diaphragm, is used with a special jelly or foam. It is moderately successful, but inconvenient. The condom is also used rather widely and is usually successful.

The development of the hormonal control of ovulation has allowed women to avoid the mechanical devices, and for many women this method is more successful than the rhythm method. Since this is the only method in which drugs form the main basis of control, they will be discussed in some detail.

Whatever the belief of the nurse, it is her responsibility to know a great deal about all methods of family planning. It is not her place to recommend any one way of doing this; it is up to the woman and her sexual partner to decide on the method they want. The nurse's role in the use of oral contraceptives lies in her knowledge of how the medication works, how it is administered and the side effects.

Steroidal oral contraceptives may be given to any adult female who desires them *provided* there is no past history of 1. thrombophlebitis or thromboembolic disorders; 2. hepatocellular disease; 3. known or suspected carcinoma of the breast; 4. known or suspected estrogen-dependent neoplasia; and 5. undiagnosed abnormal genital bleeding. It is given with caution to those with a history of epilepsy, migraine, asthma and cardiac or renal dysfunction because of its fluid retention properties. It should *never* be prescribed without a thorough physical examination including breast examination, a vaginal examination and a Papanicolaou smear, the last repeated yearly.

At this point, the nurse should review the hormonal control of menstruation in the human female. The basic action of the oral contraceptives is to maintain a high blood level of both estrogen and progestin, causing a reciprocal inhibition of the follicle stimulating hormone (FSH) so that the ova cannot mature. Specifically, estrogen in sufficient amounts blocks the FSH and progestin prevents a sharp rise in the luteinizing hormone (LH). These two preparations imitate nature's method of establishing so-called "safe periods." When the drug is withdrawn, uterine bleeding occurs as in menstruation but the flow is often less than usual or scanty. The use of a progestin changes the cervical secretion to a thick and tenacious mucus which is hostile to sperm. After an interval of five to seven days, the tablets are resumed for another cycle.

There are two main types of hormone preparations. One is a combination type with both an estrogen and a progestin together; the other is a sequential type. In the latter, an estrogen is given for 14 to 16 tablets (days) and for the last five to six days a combination of estrogen and progestin tablets is taken. It should be noted here that an estrogen is included in every preparation whether combined or sequential to achieve greater menstrual regularity and more complete shedding of the endometrium. There are more pregnancies resulting from use of the sequential type than in the combined type (Table 16).

It is very important that the tablets be taken regularly. The possibility of ovulation increases with each successive day that tablets are missed. If a woman missed one tablet, the missed tablet should be taken as soon as it is remembered and the next tablet at the regular time. It is usually best to take the tablets regularly at the same time of the day to avoid "forgetting." For many women, taking the tablet when they brush their teeth before retiring at night is a good time. If pregnancy results, especially with the combined type, it is almost always due to human error—a forgotten tablet or two. Manufacturers now prepare their preparations in specially marked boxes to assist the woman in remembering.

The most common side effects associated with oral contraceptives are nausea, edema, weight gain, spotting, breakthrough bleeding, discoloration of the skin, especially the face, and breast tenderness. These are usually mild and transient and occur most often during the first few cycles. Nausea can be controlled by having the patient take her tablet with meals, with a glass of milk at bedtime or with an antacid. If it continues, she can be changed to another preparation. The weight gain in some women is due partly to sodium retention, whereas in other women it is a real weight gain due to the protein building effect of the drugs. Facial discoloration is due to the estrogens and women who have experienced it should avoid direct sunlight.

Other side effects encountered include gastrointestinal symptoms such as abdominal cramps and bloating, amenorrhea during and after treatment, chloasma or melasma, migraine, allergic rash, rise in blood pressure in susceptible individuals and mental depression.

There is a long list of other side effects such as headaches, dizziness, fatigue, nervousness and so on but none of these has been shown to be directly related to oral contraceptives.

There is some indication that these drugs increase the incidence of thrombophlebitis and possibly carcinoma. This has not been definitely proved to be the case. Further research probably will confirm or refute this. However, it is known that approximately eight million women in the United States are now using this form of contraception.

Most physicians will prescribe the tablets at the first postpartum examination whether or not the patient has had a spontaneous menses. Others order it to be started on the first Sunday after delivery or immediately following delivery. It does depress lactation, however. If withdrawal flow fails to appear in two consecutive cycles, a test for pregnancy should be done.

Some physicians believe that a woman should not remain on the oral contraceptives indefinitely and will recommend a

TABLE 16. *STEROID ORAL CONTRACEPTIVES**

COMBINED METHOD			
Trade Name	**Estrogen**	**Progestin**	**Schedule of Administration**
Enovid 5 mg.	mestranol 0.075 mg.	norethynodrel 5 mg.	One 5 mg. tablet daily for 20 days beginning on day 5 of cycle, counting first day of menstruation as day 1. Withdrawal flow usually in 1 to 3 days. Next cycle as before.
Enovid-E	mestranol 0.1 mg.	norethynodrel 2.5 mg.	One tablet daily for 20 days beginning day 5 of cycle. Withdrawal flow usually in 1 to 3 days. Next cycle as before.
Loestrin	ethinyl estradiol 0.02 mg.	norethindrone acetate 1.0 mg.	One white table daily for 21 days beginning on day 5 of cycle. Days 22 through 28, one brown tablet daily, ferrous fumerate 75 mg. Withdrawal flow in 2 to 3 days after stopping white tablets.
Norinyl	mestranol 0.5 mg.	norethindrone 1 mg.	One tablet daily for 21 days starting on day 5 of cycle. Withdrawal flow in 2 to 3 days.
Norinyl 2	mestranol 0.1 mg.	norethindrone acetate 1.0 mg.	One tablet daily for 20 days of each cycle, beginning on day 5 of cycle and continuing through 24th day. Withdrawal flow in 2 to 3 days, but may be as late as 4 to 5 days.
Norlestrin 21 1 mg.	ethinyl estradiol 0.05 mg.	norethindrone acetate 1 mg.	Norlestrin-21 1 mg. Three weeks on and one week off. Start day 5 of cycle and daily for 21 days. Next course 7 days after last tablet taken. Withdrawal flow in 2 to 3 days but may be as late as 4 to 5 days.
Norlestrin 28 1 mg.			Norlestrin-28 1 mg. provides continuous regimen with 21 yellow tablets of Norlestrin 1 mg. and 7 white inert tablets. No need to count between cycles. Start on day 5 of cycle one yellow tablet and follow with 7 white tablets. Taken without interruption menstruation usually begins 2 to 3 days (or as late as 4 to 5 days) after white tablets started. If taken continuously, no mix-up in dates.

*These charts are not meant to be all-inclusive since new products are constantly being introduced.

Table 16 continued on following page.

TABLE 16. *STEROID ORAL CONTRACEPTIVES (Continued)*

COMBINED METHOD			
Trade Name	**Estrogen**	**Progestin**	**Schedule of Administration**
Ortho-Novum 1/80-21	mestranol 0.08 mg.	norethindrone 1 mg.	One tablet daily from 5th through 25th day of cycle. Omit for 7 days and then new schedule started. Three weeks on and one week off.
Ortho-Novum 1 mg.	mestranol 0.05 mg.	norethindrone 1 mg.	One tablet daily from 5th day of cycle through 24th day. Subsequent cycles, first tablet taken 7th day following completion of previous 20 day course (6 days without medication).
Ortho-Novum 2 mg.	mestranol 0.10 mg.	norethindrone 2 mg.	One tablet daily from 5th day of cycle through 24th day. Subsequent cycles, first tablet taken on 7th day (6 days without medication). Also used for hypermenorrhea – dosage the same. After three months, discontinue for evaluation.
Ortho-Novum 10 mg.	mestranol 0.06 mg.	norethindrone 10 mg.	One tablet daily from 5th through 24th day of each cycle. Subsequent cycles, first tablet on 7th day following completion of previous 20 day course (6 days without medication). Also used in hypermenorrhea (dosage the same) and in endometriosis – dosage different. Discontinue after 3 months for evaluation.
Ovulen	mestranol 0.1 mg.	ethynodiol diacetate 1 mg.	20 tablet dosage schedule: 1 tablet daily for 20 consecutive days beginning on day 5 of cycle. Withdrawal flow in 2 to 3 days. Next cycle as before.
Ovulen-21			Ovulen-21 – three weeks on and one week off. One tablet daily for 21 consecutive days beginning on day 5 of cycle. Withdrawal flow in 2 to 3 days. Off for 7 days. User begins new cycle on same day of week she began first course.

COMBINED METHOD (*Continued*)			
Ovulen-28			There are 21 tablets (white) containing the drug and 7 pink placebo tablets. One tablet (white) on first Sunday after onset of menstruation. If onset on that Sunday, start same day. Take a tablet a day for 28 days. Subsequent cycles begin always on Sunday. Should use additional protection until after first week in initial cycle. Withdrawal flow usually occurs during week taking the pink placebo tablet – often 2 to 3 days after last white tablet taken.
SEQUENTIAL METHOD			
Norquen	mestranol 0.08 mg. 14 tablets – white	mestranol 0.08 mg. and norethindrone 2.0 mg. 6 tablets – blue	One white tablet daily for 14 days starting with day 5 of cycle and continuing through 18th day; then one blue tablet daily for 6 days starting on 19th day and continuing through 24th day. Withdrawal flow usually begins within 4 days.
Oracon	ethinyl estradiol 0.1 mg. 16 tablets – white	ethinyl estradiol 0.1 mg. and dimethisterone 25 mg. 5 tablets – pink	One white tablet beginning on 5th day of cycle and take one daily in sequence. Additional contraceptive methods are recommended for first 7 tablet days of first cycle. Withdrawal flow should take place by 7th day – if not resume therapy on that day (6 days without medication).
Ortho-Novum SQ	mestranol 0.08 mg. 14 tablets – white	mestranol 0.08 mg. and norethindrone 2 mg. 6 tablets – blue	One white tablet for 14 days starting on 5th day of cycle and continuing through the 18th day; then one blue tablet for 6 days through 24th day. Subsequent cycles – first white tablet on 7th day following completion of previous 20 day course (6 days without medication).
SINGLE METHOD			
Micronor	none	norethindrone 0.35 mg.	Taken one tablet daily on a continuous basis.

substitute (such as foams and jellies) for a few months. But, an undesired pregnancy conceived during the "rest period" can cause much unhappiness. Other doctors have had patients on the tablets for six to eight years without observable ill effects. Fertility does not seem to be affected, for many women after stopping the medication can conceive within three to six months.

There are a large number of vaginal creams and foams on the market and all should be used with a diaphragm for best results. These medications contain a variety of drugs claimed to be spermacidal in action but there is a high rate of patient failure with their use largely because the instructions are not followed.

Unwanted pregnancies may, of course, be terminated by abortion. However, this is usually a surgical procedure, not involving medications other than those generally used for other operative therapy. Drugs are used in two techniques. The use of prostaglandins (experimental in this country) has already been mentioned. The other is the "saline technique." Hypertonic saline is introduced into the amniotic sac. As soon as labor starts, the patient is given oxytocin, often in much larger doses than are used to induce labor at term. The drug is repeated as needed until the abortion is complete. Fetuses delivered by this method are often born alive. The fetal death may occur within minutes or be delayed for as long as four days, according to various circumstances. This is mainly determined by the length of gestation at the time of the abortion.

In caring for the patient having an abortion, the nurse will need to examine her own feelings in the matter if she is to care for the patient objectively. The nurse must realize that this is just another patient who needs good nursing care and support during what is, at best, a trying and stressful time for her. This may be an excellent period in which to teach the patient means of obtaining and maintaining good health habits, both physical and emotional.

IT IS IMPORTANT TO REMEMBER

1. That though pregnancy and delivery are normal physiologic processes, both can be made more comfortable and safer for the mother and the baby by the judicious use of drugs.
2. That the nurse will usually administer the drugs used during labor and delivery, but less often during pregnancy and the later puerperium.
3. That though the nurse may not actually give the drugs used during pregnancy and the puerperium, she will be called upon to explain to the patient the purpose of the medications and the methods of administration.
4. That some of the reduction in maternal and infant mortality is a direct result of the use of drugs.
5. That the care of the mother and her infant is one of the most rewarding fields of endeavor.

TOPICS FOR STUDY AND DISCUSSION

1. Check the charts of the obstetric division and see what drugs are being used; also check the out-patient department. Compare these drugs with those mentioned in the text. Add to your card file any that differ from the ones in the book. What changes do you note?
2. Plan for a home delivery—what medicines would you need? How would you obtain them?
3. Plan a talk to a group of prospective mothers, paying special attention to the maintenance of the health of the mother during pregnancy and to the care of the baby for the first few months of life. This might be a project for a group.
4. What are the main hormones in posterior pituitary extract? What is the use for each in the body? When might the use of the entire extract be contraindicated?

BIBLIOGRAPHY

Books and Pamphlets

American Medical Association Council on Drugs, *Drug Evaluations*, Chicago, 1971, American Medical Association.

Bergersen, B., *Pharmacology in Nursing, 12th Ed.*, St. Louis, 1973, The C. V. Mosby Co.

Conn, H. F., *Current Therapy, 1972*, Philadelphia, 1972, W. B. Saunders Co.

Goodman, L. S., and Gilman, A., *Pharmacological Basis of Therapeutics, 4th Ed.*, New York, 1970, The Macmillan Co.

Miller, B. F., and Keane, C. B., *Encyclopedia and Dictionary of Medicine and Nursing*, Philadelphia, 1972, W. B. Saunders Co.

Rodman, N. T., and Smith, D. W., *Pharmacology and Drug Therapy in Nursing*, Philadelphia, 1968, J. B. Lippincott Co.

Smith, C. S., *Maternal Child Nursing*, Philadelphia, 1963, W. B. Saunders Co.

Journal Articles

Aure, B., "Intrauterine transfusions, the nurse's role with expectant parents," *Nurs. Clin. North Am.* 7:4:817 (December, 1972).

Bancroft, A. V., "Pregnancy and the counterculture," *Nurs. Clin. North Am.* 8:1:67 (January, 1973).

Cochran, L., et al., "Symposium on the care of the newborn," *Nurs. Clin. North Am.* 6:1:1 (January, 1971).

Connell, E., "The pill and the problems," *Am. J. Nurs.* 71:2:326 (February, 1971).

DiPalma, J. R., "Prostaglandins, the potential wonder drug," *R.N.* 35:1:51 (November, 1972).

Gonzales, B., "Voluntary sterilization," *Am. J. Nurs.* 70:12:2581 (December, 1970).

Gordon, E. S., "Prostaglandins: physiologic action and clinical potential," *Postgrad. Med.* 52:4:75 (1973).

Greiss, F., "Obstetric anesthesia," *Am. J. Nurs.* 71:1:67 (January, 1971).

Greiss, F., "Birth control, current technology, future prospects," *Science* 179:4079:1222 (1973).

Guttmacher, A. F., "Family planning: the needs and the methods," *Am. J. Nurs.* 69:6:1229 (June, 1969).

Kopp, L. M., "Ordeal or ideal—The second stage of labor," *Am. J. Nurs.* 71:6:1140 (June, 1971).

Krotoski, W. A., and Wynn, R. N., "Intrauterine devices—Contraceptives or abortifacients," *Science* 157:3795:1465 (1967).

Lammert, A., "Oral contraceptives," *R.N.* 29:51 (1966).

Lammert, A., "The female sex hormones," *R.N.* 31:41 (1968).

Lammert, A., "The menopause—a physiologic process," *Am. J. Nurs.* 62:56 (February, 1962).

Laros, R. K., Work, B. R., and Witting, W. C., "Prostaglandins," *Am. J. Nurs.* 73:6:1001 (June, 1973).

O'Leary, J. A., and Spellacy, W. N., "Serum copper alteration after ingestion of an oral contraceptive," *Science* 162:3854:682 (1968).

Ostering, T. O., Marozovich, W., and Roseman, T. J., "Prostaglandins, scientific edition," *J. Am. Pharm. Assoc.* 12:61:1861 (1972).

Rains, A. P., et al., "Symposium on maternity nursing," *Nurs. Clin. North Am.* 3:2:275 (March, 1968).

Rubin, R., Erickson, F., et al., "Symposium on nursing care of the mother and child," *Nurs. Clin. North Am.* 4:1:1 (January, 1969).

Salk, L., "The role of the heartbeat in the relations between mother and infant," *Sci. Am.* 228:5:24 (April, 1973).

Sasmor, J. L., Castor, C. R., and Hassid, P., "The childbirth team during labor," *Am. J. Nurs.* 73:3:444 (March, 1973).

Smith, B. A., Priore, R. M., and Stern, M. K., "The transition phase of labor," *Am. J. Nurs.* 73:3:448 (March, 1973).

Upjohn Co., "Prostaglandins go commercial," *Sci. News* 102:18:102 (October, 1972).

CHAPTER 29

DRUGS USED FOR MALIGNANT CONDITIONS

CORRELATION WITH OTHER SCIENCES

I. ANATOMY AND PHYSIOLOGY

1. Hormones are the secretions of the endocrine or ductless glands which have regulatory action in the maintenance of body functions.
2. Mitosis is the process of cell replication in which the cellular elements undergo intricate changes.

IV. PHYSICS

1. An isotope is an element which has the same atomic number as another element but a different atomic weight.
2. A radioactive isotope is an isotope which is undergoing spontaneous decomposition and giving off energy in the form of radiation.
3. Radioactive substances can give off three types of radiation: alpha, beta and gamma.
4. The half-life of a radioactive substance is the length of time it takes to give off one-half of its total radioactivity.

V. PSYCHOLOGY

1. Fear is an emotional reaction which is both physical and psychologic in nature.
2. Worry is a process of mental anxiety brought about by adverse situations, or the fear of such situations, when the individual is unable to do anything concrete to remedy the situation.
3. An individual's beliefs are a powerful factor in his life.

INTRODUCTION

Cancer has been and still is one of the major causes of death. Even though early treatment has saved many patients, it is a dreaded disease, and the fear it engenders is often one of the major problems to be faced by the physician and nurse. This fear has been responsible for many premature deaths. Some individuals, faced with the symptoms of cancer, have denied the existence of their illness to themselves and their relatives and have postponed going to the physician until it was too late. Others have delayed through ignorance, since the early symptoms of the condition are often insignificant and misleading. Some physicians also have disregarded these early signs and sometimes have found it difficult to differentiate the real from the imagined symptoms. If the patient had been a "neurotic complainer," the doctor may have felt that this was just another complaint without foundation. However, most physicians do, and nurses should, understand that symptoms of any kind must be heeded, for it is far better to treat an imagined ailment than it is to let cancer progress. The physician and nurse also know that psychosomatic pain hurts just as much as physical pain and that it, too, must be treated. The physician today investigates any sign which might indicate the beginning of any cancer.

The public now understands that most cancer treated early can be cured, since this has been stressed through the press, radio and television. When left untreated until the late stages, it cannot be cured. Since this has become common knowledge many more lives are being saved each year by early, accurate diagnosis and early treatment. Medicine, of course, does not play a large part in cancer therapy. Surgery and radiation still form the basis for the treatment of the actual condition. Drugs are used in the major portion of the palliative and supportive measures.

An unexplained phenomenon that occurs in rare cases is the spontaneous remission. In these patients, the malignant process is interrupted and a normal state of health is regained. It is not unusual for such a patient to attribute his recovery to supernatural intervention and it is likewise not unusual for unscrupulous "quacks" to capitalize on this rare event by holding out false hopes to other patients.

Patients with cancer, whether they are aware of their condition or not, are usually very uncomfortable, for pain is often continuous and severe. The tumor mass often interferes with the normal functioning not only of the organ directly involved but also with those in the surrounding area. When the cancer is slow growing and the patient is ill for a long time, he needs to build up his weakened body. This is one way in which drugs can help. There are those who may argue that it is wrong to try to keep these patients living, but for the nurse and the doctor, conservation of human life is the first consideration. Who knows when a cure for cancer will be discovered? It may come before this book is published. The patient should be brought to the best possible state of health and kept there for as long as is possible.

Cancer appears in many forms. The more common forms are carcinoma (which means cancer to most people), sarcoma and the blood disorders such as leukemia. Briefly, these can be distinguished by the anatomic structures involved. Carcinoma affects epithelial tissue, sarcoma connective tissue and the blood disorders either bone marrow or the lymphatic system—the blood-forming organs. The malignant disorders of the blood and the blood-forming organs were discussed in Chapter 19.

Carcinoma is the most common form of cancer and affects the skin, mucous membranes and the glands. It usually starts insidiously, often without any really significant symptoms and is relatively slow growing, though this varies greatly. Relatively uncommon in the early years, the incidence of carcinoma rises slowly until about the third decade when it becomes more prevalent. From 40 years on it rises rapidly until between 60 and 70 years when it gradually declines. Some of the more common forms of carcinoma are those of the breasts and uterus in the female, the prostate gland in the male, the stomach, sigmoidal area of the large bowel, the skin, lips and lungs. Carcinoma tends to metastasize early and easily by way of the blood and lymph streams. It causes few or no symptoms in the very early stages but is apt to cause severe pain, bleeding and interference with functioning as it progresses. An open ulcerative sore is apt to occur if the tumor is on the surface of the body.

Sarcoma is a highly malignant, rapidly growing tumor of connective tissue. It is more common in youth and early adult life than it is in the later years. Sarcoma causes severe pain and, because its progress is rapid, quickly reduces the patient's vitality. The patient is more acutely ill with sarcoma than with carcinoma. There is much less time for consideration of the best possible treatment, and the physician is faced with making a quick diagnosis and then acting on it since otherwise the disease will progress to a fatal termination in a short time.

Carcinoma and sarcoma are treated by surgery, radiation or both. Chemotherapy plays a less important role here than in leukemia, although it is now being used with increasing frequency. More medicinal therapy is palliative and supportive. The main reason that early diagnosis is so important is that surgery can be effective only if it is done before the tumor has metastasized. If this can be accomplished and the entire tumor and the surrounding areas removed, the condition can be cured. When there is doubt about the complete removal, the operative area is subjected to radiation either by x-ray or radium. Of course, if metastasis has taken place, the growth will continue in a new place even though the primary tumor has been removed.

RADIATION THERAPY

When surgery cannot be done either because of the type or location of the tumor, or when there is indication that metastasis has made surgery inadvisable, radiation becomes the treatment of choice. X-ray, radium, radon, radioactive isotopes or linear accelerator may be used (IV-1, 2). The choice will depend upon the type of tumor and its location.

Radioactive Chemicals

The Drugs. More of today's cancer patients can expect relief of pain and a moderate lengthening of life because of drug therapy. Promising new drugs are appearing frequently, along with more effective and new methods of administering both the old and new drugs. The advent of controlled nuclear fission has made possible an ever increasing group of drugs of value in certain selected conditions. A large proportion of their use is in the treatment of malignancies and in diagnostic tests.

Radioactive isotopes are chemical elements or compounds whose atoms have unstable nuclei which attempt to reach a more stable state by releasing excess energy in the form of nuclear radiations. They are created in an atomic reactor by bombarding selected elements with neutrons (IV-1, 2). Immediately, these isotopes begin to disintegrate, emitting ionizing radiation for a predictable length of time. The term nuclide refers to all species of isotopes.

This predictable length of life is expressed in terms of time called half-life. This is a physical constant which expresses the time required for an isotope to expend half of its radioactive atoms. For example, I^{131} (radioiodine) has a half-life of eight days; thus 100 mc. (millicuries) of I^{131} will decay to 50 mc. in eight days and to 25 mc. in 16 days (IV-4). The unit of measurement of radioactive isotopes is the millicurie (mc.), one thousandth of a curie, and the microcurie (μc.), or one millionth of a curie. The curie is named after Madame Curie, the discoverer of radium. This decay rate serves as a guide to determine safe working times and distances when working with patients who have received a radioactive isotope.

There are three kinds of radiation (IV-3). Alpha particles (helium nuclei) are weak and penetrate only a fraction of a millimeter of tissue. Beta particles are electrons and penetrate tissues only to the extent of a few millimeters of tissue. Gamma rays are electromagnetic radiations similar to x-rays and both these rays are highly penetrating. The accompanying schematic diagram shows the approximate depth of penetration of the types of radiation.

Tables 14 (Chapter 19) and 17 show the various drugs used in the treatment of various malignant conditions.

In addition to these, several other radioisotopes are useful as diagnostic measures. *Radioiodinated serum albumin,* U.S.P. (Albumotope I^{131}, RISA) is used as an adjunct to other diagnostic procedures in the detection and localization of brain tumors and as a tracer substance for tests of circulatory action, circulation time and cardiac output. *Radioactive chromium* (Cr^{51}), U.S.P. (Chro-

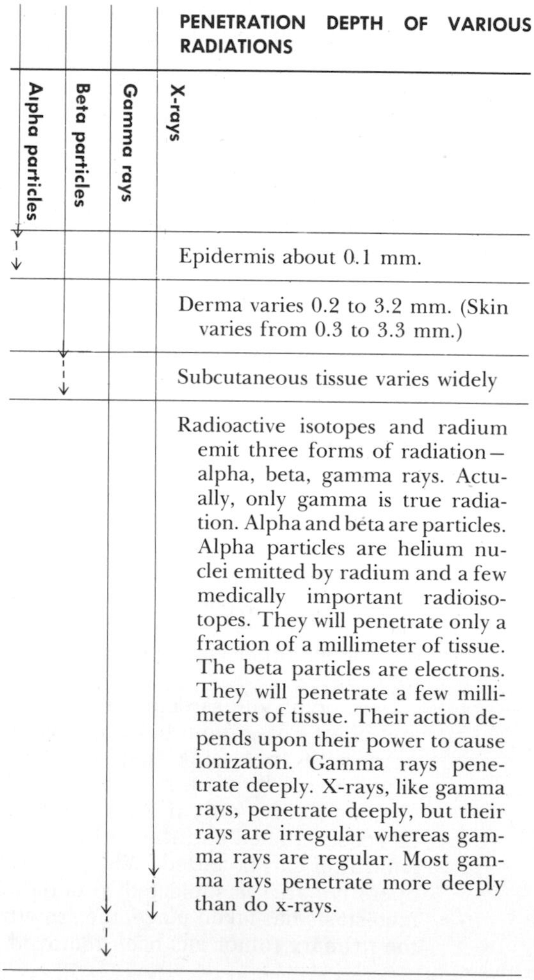

Alpha particles	Beta particles	Gamma rays	X-rays	PENETRATION DEPTH OF VARIOUS RADIATIONS
				Epidermis about 0.1 mm.
				Derma varies 0.2 to 3.2 mm. (Skin varies from 0.3 to 3.3 mm.)
				Subcutaneous tissue varies widely
				Radioactive isotopes and radium emit three forms of radiation—alpha, beta, gamma rays. Actually, only gamma is true radiation. Alpha and beta are particles. Alpha particles are helium nuclei emitted by radium and a few medically important radioisotopes. They will penetrate only a fraction of a millimeter of tissue. The beta particles are electrons. They will penetrate a few millimeters of tissue. Their action depends upon their power to cause ionization. Gamma rays penetrate deeply. X-rays, like gamma rays, penetrate deeply, but their rays are irregular whereas gamma rays are regular. Most gamma rays penetrate more deeply than do x-rays.

mitope Sodium-Cr 51, Rachromate-51), is used in tests for red blood cell survival, red blood cell volume and fecal blood loss determination. *Radioactive cobalt* (C^{60}) with vitamin B_{12} is employed in testing for pernicious anemia. This isotope is used in teletherapy machines to provide a precise localized area for irradiation of tumor tissue. Both the nurse and the patient should be aware that the markings on the skin should not be washed away for they act as a guide to the radiologist in administering the cobalt therapy. *Radioactive iron* (Fe^{59}) is used in the iron turnover test, and *radioiodinated rose bengal* solution is used as a liver function test. *Radioactive mercury* (Hg^{203}) is useful in locating brain tumors. There are many more being developed all the time and they are too numerous to list here.

Newer techniques of administration also hold out more hope. To be effective, the anticancer drug should reach into the complex molecular structure of cancer cells and kill them or retard their growth mechanism. The newer methods of administration attempt to concentrate the chemical in the cancer itself, preventing normal tissues in the rest of the body from being affected. The technique of isolation perfusion is just such an attempt and is proving more and more successful.

The Nurse. The nurse has many responsibilities when radioactive isotopes are used. Some of the more important ones are summarized in the following paragraphs.

1. Precautions necessary will vary, depending on whether a tracer dose or therapeutic dose has been given.

2. The nurse must know the nature of the radioisotope with which she is working. She should know the particular procedure used in this hospital. The potential danger in the use of these drugs lies in the fact that they emit radiation which cannot be seen or otherwise detected without special equipment. If oral or implanted therapeutic doses of radioisotopes are to be given, it is a good rule to minimize the time spent close to the patient by each individual—about 20 minutes per day at 6 feet.

3. Just as surgical asepsis is concerned with preventing bacteria from getting into a wound, radiologic safety is concerned with the protection of people from harmful radiation. There are three methods of protection which can be used alone or in combination; they are distance, shielding and time. The effect of distance is usually expressed in geometric terms as the inverse square law: the amount of radiation is inversely proportional to the square of the distance from the radiation source. Shielding requires the use of a lead barrier between the patient and the person caring for him. This is seen in the x-ray department. The technician goes behind a cubicle of lead and heavy glass to activate the machine. To avoid radiation of areas not involved by the tumor, lead shelding may also be used. Time has two connotations: (1) the rapidity of decay (radiation decreases in direct proportion to the length of time the isotope is radioactive) and (2) the time of exposure. The nurse who stays with a patient for a half hour will have half the time exposure (half the radiation) she will have if she remains with the patient for an hour.

4. The nurse must help to prepare the patient physically and psychologically for the treatment.

5. Solutions of radioactive drugs are most often clear, watery solutions. This increases the possibilities of error since the solution may be mistaken for plain water. The nurse must be extremely careful that these solutions are not spilled. Even a few drops may be important. If an accident occurs, the laboratory which supplied the drug and the physician should be notified immediately so that proper steps may be taken to handle the situation safely.

6. It is well for the nurse to remember that there are numerous potential sources of radiation hazard in the nursing care of these patients. Aside from the drug itself, the others include equipment used for administration and handling of the drug, the patient himself, urine, feces, vomitus, perspiration, secretions from the mouth and lungs, the bedpan and urinal, the linen, food trays, needles, syringes and dressings. When and to what extent each of these items may be a real danger will vary with the drug used, the modes of administration and other factors.

7. Specific precautions such as the following may be required with some radioisotopes.

a. The patient is usually in a single room with a sign on the door identifying him as a radiation hazard and stating NO VISITORS.

b. The nurse and all who come in direct contact with the patient for any length of

TABLE 17. RADIOACTIVE ISOTOPES

ISOTOPE	METHOD OF ADMINISTRATION	USUAL DOSE	USES	ACTION AND FATE	PRECAUTIONS AND COMMENTS
Radioactive Iodine, U.S.P. (I^{131}) Other names: Iodotope Oriodide Radiocaps Theriodide Tracervial Half-life: 8 days Emits: Beta and gamma rays	Orally I.V.	Diagnostic: up to 30 μc. Treatment: 15 to 30 mc.	Diagnostic of: Thyroid function Iodine uptake Location of cancerous thyroid metastasis Cardiac output Palliative in Ca of thyroid Treatment of hyperthyroidism	Thyroid becomes less active With less thyroid secretion, most of body cells slow down biochemically Body cells do not take as much oxygen from blood, thus heart is able to slow down	Contraindicated in pregnancy Side effects: None for diagnostic tests Others: Mild febrile reaction Local radiation effects—swelling and soreness in neck Thyroid crisis Depression of hematopoiesis See special precautions listed in this chapter
Radioactive Phosphorus, U.S.P. (P^{32}) Other names: Phosphotope Sodium Radio-Phosphate Half-life: 14.3 days Emits: Beta rays	I.V. Orally Local application	2.5 to 5 mc.	Locating tumors (particularly in eye and brain if skull is open) Blood dyscrasias, such as polycythemia vera, chronic myelogenous leukemia, chronic lymphatic leukemia Applied locally to skin cancers, keloids, keratoses	Slows down blood cell production for longer time than x-rays May produce remissions and leave patient symptom-free for months Has preferential uptake in neoplastic tissues	Seldom causes radiation sickness None of material should be allowed to come in contact with skin of patient, doctor or nurse as it will cause radiologic burn; have adequate monitoring devices convenient Radiation precautions unnecessary as only beta rays emitted
Radioactive Gold (Au^{198}) Other names: Radio-Gold Colloid Aurcoloid	Intracavity injection (all fluid removed from cavity first)	35 to 150 mc.	Into pleural or abdominal cavity in cancer patient as palliative treatment in ascites and pleural effusion	Reduces excessive fluid formation by direct radiation and thus contributes to comfort of patient	Drug diluted with isotonic sodium chloride Do not need strict isolation of patient Film badge and rubber gloves worn

Table 17 continued on facing page.

TABLE 17. RADIOACTIVE ISOTOPES (Continued)

ISOTOPE	METHOD OF ADMINISTRATION	USUAL DOSE	USES	ACTION AND FATE	PRECAUTIONS AND COMMENTS
Aureotope Half-life: 2.7 days Emits: Beta rays				N.B.: If patient dies, prominent notation on tag on body for protection of mortician	when changing dressings Dressings burned or saved until deemed safe Red stain appearing at site of injection means material escaping – notify doctor immediately Patient turned every 15 min. for 2 hrs. to help spread evenly within cavity Not used unless cavity is strictly closed May have mild radiation sickness after 3 or 4 days Should not be repeated at intervals of less than 4 weeks and then only as reaccumulation of fluid may require
Radioactive Iridium (IR^{192}) Emits: Gamma rays	Intracavity delivered at 1 cm. distance for 5 to 16 days	300 to 1000 r. daily	Cancer of skin, lip, tongue, tonsil, palate, cervix uteri, endometrium	May be both curative and palliative	New preparation of nylon ribbons holding stainless steel cylinders (seeds) of the drug – better mechanical way to give small areas of radiation
Radium and *Radon* Emits: Gamma rays	Surface and local application Seeds, tube, needles, plaque or wire, gas enclosed within metal: gold, silver, platinum or brass	–	Cancer of skin, lip, tongue, tonsil, palate, cervix uteri, endometrium	May be both curative and palliative	Radiation sickness or dermatitis may occur Radon seeds may be permanently implanted

time must wear isolation gowns and rubber gloves and film badges under gowns to determine amount of exposure received.

c. The nurse explains to the patient that she will take care of his needs but will work quickly and remain only long enough to carry out essential nursing activities.

d. The nurse should learn from the patient what he understands about the treatment and she should advise the doctor if she thinks further information is needed.

e. If most of the radioactive element is eliminated in the urine, the care of it is very important. It is usually placed in a lead-encased container and it is important that all urine be saved. It is the quantitative determination of the amount of radioactive substance secreted that determines when the patient is to be removed from isolation (at least 96 hours).

f. The amount of contamination of equipment in the room is determined by monitoring with a Geiger counter.

g. Linen is usually put in metal containers and stored until deemed safe.

h. Dishes are washed in the room and kept there. Some institutions permit sending them to the main kitchen if when monitored the reading is less than 6 milliroentgens per hour. Disposable plates and utensils may be used and discarded as are other disposable materials with possible radiation contamination.

i. If the nurse should contaminate her skin, it should be washed thoroughly with a soft brush, soap and water and monitored. If monitoring still shows contamination, a mixture of 25 per cent detergent, 25 per cent corn meal and 50 per cent water may also be used. If that is not sufficient, a potassium permanganate in 0.2N sulfuric acid solution may be used—and the stain removed with sodium bisulfite. This technique will also remove layers of skin. If monitoring still shows contamination, the skin should be washed until monitoring indicates that additional cleansing will not be effective.

j. When the patient is removed from isolation, all equipment is monitored and carefully scrubbed by attendants instructed in safe methods and then remonitored. The room is aired for at least 24 hours.

k. Should death occur, the body is carefully tagged, and the mortician is notified to follow special precautions.

The Patient. The nurse should explain the routine to the patient. He is to remain in bed for the period of isolation so that the danger of contamination of others is minimized and so that his reaction to the radioactive substance can be better studied and controlled. He should know that no visitors will be permitted for at least 48 to 72 hours when radioactive iodine is used. An intercom system and telephone communications may be helpful in reducing some anxieties. The patient should be made as comfortable as possible and have sufficient reading material, a radio and a television to keep him occupied. The patient should know how the substance is eliminated and for how long. Otherwise, he may fear he will be dangerous to others indefinitely and may become panicky about the social isolation or harming his loved ones when he returns home. Refer to Chapter 19, Table 14, for Chemotherapy of Malignancies.

RADIATION SICKNESS

DEFINITION. Whenever radiation is used extensively, radiation sickness is apt to occur. This condition, according to present theory, is brought about by the liberation of the products of protein decomposition due to the death of a large number of cells at one time.

MAJOR SYMPTOMS. The symptoms vary considerably, but anorexia, nausea and vomiting, and mental depression are common. The patient feels very uncomfortable.

DRUG THERAPY

Sedative and Antiemetic Drugs. Antiemetic-tranquilizing drugs are widely used and also serve an additional purpose of providing some sedation. Most of the drugs used are phenothiazine derivatives and as such share to a varying extent the dangers of damage to the hematopoietic system.

Almost any of the phenothiazines used as tranquilizers can be used as antiemetics. See Chapter 30, Table 18, for the drugs and dosages. One phenothiazine that is used almost exclusively as an antiemetic is *thiethylperazine maleate* (Torecan), which may be given orally, intramuscularly or rectally in doses of 10 to 30 mg. per day. The single optimal antiemetic dose for adults is 10 mg.

Some of the other drugs used primarily for motion sickness are useful here. *Dimenhydrinate* (Dramamine), in 50 to 100 mg. doses, is usually effective. It may be given orally, rectally or intramuscularly. *Meclizine hydrochloride* (Bonine; Gravol [C]), may be given orally in doses of 25 to 50 mg. *Trimethobenzamide hydrochloride* (Tigan) is useful also, for it does not have the autonomic, extrapyramidal or sedative effects of the phenothiazine group. It is given orally, rectally or by intramuscular injection in doses of 100 to 300 mg. four times a day.

The nurse can do much to aid in overcoming the patient's fear of the radiation treatments by assuring him that, although he may have some discomfort from the treatments, the difficulties rarely last more than a few hours and the doctor will order medicines to stop most of the symptoms. The nurse should consult Chapter 30 for the adverse reactions of the phenothiazines. There are few side effects when *Dimenhydrinate* (Dramamine) is used, but prolonged administration may result in toxic effects on the hematopoietic system. Side effects from *thiethylperazine maleate* (Torecan) are infrequent but may include drowsiness, dizziness, dryness of mouth and nose, tachycardia and anorexia. *Meclizine hydrochloride* (Bonine) is an antihistamine and may cause such side effects as drowsiness, blurred vision, dryness of the mouth and fatigue.

To the patient, the tranquilizers render a real service. Many people know that surgery, x-ray and radium are standard treatments for cancer and, when these are used to treat them, they suspect cancer to be the reason even though they may not have been told so by their doctor. These patients are fearful and disturbed and, even if the tranquilizer does not actually counteract the untoward symptoms, it will relieve the patient by reducing his fears and worries (V-1, 2).

When drowsiness is a presenting adverse sign, the patient should not operate machinery, including automobiles, or participate in any activity in which constant alertness is needed.

Supportive and Other Drugs Used for Radiation Sickness. During the long course of radiation, such as might be used in deep x-ray therapy, the patient may need supportive drugs to aid in maintaining adequate nutrition. The drugs used are the same ones that are used for anemia, plus vitamins and often amino acids. Refer to Chapter 19 for other drugs used in anemia. Since there is considerable breakdown of cells with radiation, there is an increase in protein waste in the body. To avoid its retention in the blood stream for a long time, the doctor may order a diuretic. This should be explained, very briefly, to the patient if he becomes alarmed by the increase in urinary output.

PALLIATIVE AND SUPPORTIVE MEASURES

The cancer patient always presents an emotional as well as physical problem. Of course, the same thing can be said of most patients, but it is especially true of patients suffering from inoperable or terminal cancer. The nurse usually realizes that the patient cannot be cured, and the patient often suspects this to be true. Whether the patient is told of his condition or not depends upon the philosophy of medical and nursing care practiced in that community.

Analgesics

The Drugs. Cancer does not always produce severe pain in the early stages and, even when the condition is far advanced, the suffering may result from any number of causes which may take precedence over the pain. Dyspnea, cough, nausea and vomiting, exhaustion or the fear of invalidism, disfigurement or impending death may be reasons for extreme discomfort in the patient (V-1, 2, 3). Each particular patient presents a problem to the doctor and the nurse, and this must be approached individually with proper evaluation. The personality of the patient is as important to consider as is his general physical status. Under most circumstances, pain serves as a protective mechanism for the individual.

The antipyretic drugs—*aspirin* or *acetaminophen*—are very effective and useful analgesics for the less severe forms of pain. These are always tried first and continued as long as reasonably effective. Combinations of these drugs may possess some advantages in terms of pain relief. Some of the *barbiturates* are often useful in relieving some of the milder types of discomfort.

If the pain becomes more severe as the disease advances, codeine or propoxyphene

(Darvon) may be added to the aspirin for relief. Subjective phenomena such as pain are often readily influenced by various positive forms of suggestion and this may well be confused with the drug effect (V-3). Patients complaining of pain and known to have valid cause for pain may sometimes be relieved by inert placebos.

Narcotics are reliable and effective drugs to control the more severe forms of pain. A large proportion of them have addicting properties. The list of usable drugs for these more severe forms of pain is most impressive, ranging from opiates and their derivatives to synthetic preparations and various compounds. Some of them may be given orally and/or parenterally. Probably the more commonly used are *pentazocine* (Talwin), codeine, morphine and *meperidine hydrochloride* (Demerol; pethidine [C]). The reader is referred to the Current Drug Handbook and Chapter 9 for others and for further information about routes of administration, dosage and side effects.

Tolerance to many of these drugs is common and requires ever-increasing dosages. A drug once used to tolerance can later be used again if the patient has had other drugs in the interim. Some patients lose the tolerance for a drug rather rapidly; others do not.

In a patient with advanced, incurable cancer, the problem of abuse and probable addiction becomes a philosophic or academic question. The important thing to discover and remember is whether or not the patient is compulsively demanding a narcotic for its pleasurable effects and as an escape from reality. It is possible for a patient with pain to become psychically dependent on a drug merely because it relieves his pain.

Chlorpromazine (Thorazine; Chlor-Promanyl [C]), *promazine* (Sparine; Promwill [C]) or *prochlorperazine* (Compazine; Stemetil [C]) may be given with the various analgesics. For most patients, they enhance the action of the analgesic to such a degree that it can be given in lower dosages and at longer intervals. This is a distinct advantage, for it increases the period of usefulness of each drug.

THE NURSE. The frequency with which the drugs will be given will depend upon many factors, some of which have already been discussed. Most physicians leave timing of doses to the discretion of the nurse. In other words, the order for the medication is written with "p.r.n." (whenever necessary) after it. Sometimes this is written q. 3 or 4 h., p.r.n. (every 3 or 4 hours, as necessary). In the first instance, the nurse must decide when the drug is needed. This may be a very difficult thing to do since it is not always easy to determine when subjective complaints are majorly identified as pain. Many patients become restless and uncomfortable, even lonesome, and translate this feeling as pain. If the nurse can satisfy the emotional or physical need, the pain may lessen or disappear and the medication not be required. It is the nurse's duty to do all in her power to make the patient comfortable without medication, but she should not make a patient in real pain wait for relief. When the order is for every three or four hours, if necessary, the nurse must wait at least three hours after the last dose before giving the analgesic. Of course, if the nurse is unable to get the patient relaxed or comfortable, she will need to consult the physician to determine alternative measures.

It is often the duty of the nurse to explain the home care of the patient to the member of the family who will be giving the nursing care. She should explain what the medications are used for, when and how to give them.

THE PATIENT. When terminal care is to be given in the home, the family will need considerable support in dealing with the steady deterioration of the patient. Families should be thoroughly aware of what symptoms or events to expect. The patient is often aware of the process that is occurring. Often, much support and thoughtfulness will be required to help him (and his family) cope with this grieving process.

Hypnotics

Hypnotics, or sleep-producing drugs, are usually ordered for the patient with a malignancy since these patients usually do not sleep well and some means of securing rest is essential. The barbiturates are the drugs most often used for this purpose. Since these drugs also produce some tolerance, the kind and amount will need to be varied from time to time. It is not unusual to give very small doses of one of the milder barbiturates two or three times a day and thus aid the patient to rest during the day as well as to get to sleep at night. The drug may be given orally, rectally or parenterally, as the condition of the patient and the type of drug used may indicate.

Supportive Drugs

The patient with a malignant disorder, especially the one who has had surgery or radiation, will need medicines to aid in building up the body gradually. Everything possible must be done to repair the damage caused by the tumor. Drugs may form only a small part of this repair process, but it may be a very important part. The drugs used will vary somewhat with the type of condition encountered.

If, as is not unusual following radiation, there is some urinary disturbance, one of the urinary antiseptics and sedatives is given, such as potassium citrate, methenamine or similar drug. If there is a tendency to oliguria, one of the zolamide, thiazide, xanthine or mercurial diuretics may be used. Refer to Chapter 18 for details.

To combat general debility, which is common, some of the amino acid preparations may be ordered. Also the multiple vitamin preparations are given. These are especially good as they improve the appetite as well as supply needed chemicals. If the patient is an older person, some of the so-called "tonics" may help. These also improve the appetite, and they have an excellent psychologic effect upon the patient. He feels that these are really beneficial and consequently they do improve his condition (V-3).

It is often necessary in the course of cancer to combat intercurrent infection. For instance, with any form of gastrointestinal cancer it may be desirable to "sterilize" the contents of the tract to avoid gastroenteritis. This is also done pre- and postoperatively. Some of the anti-infective drugs are effective for this purpose. It may be desirable to use anti-infective drugs in lung cancer to avoid extra strain on the patient from other diseases. The usual drugs are used, the antibiotics either orally or parenterally, or the sulfonamides. For lung cancer the drugs may be given by aerosol or by inhalation.

The patient with cancer may, of course, develop any other disease during the course of the cancer, but these would be treated in the same manner as they would be if the patient did not have cancer. The only difference is that the patient will not be in good condition and will, therefore, need extra care.

Nursing the patient with cancer requires all the skill and ingenuity the nurse is able to employ. It is a test of her ability to understand the problems of the patient and to rightly interpret his feelings. It is not enough just to be technically competent. She must have an understanding of the emotional and the spiritual needs of the patient and be able to meet these needs, at least in part.

IT IS IMPORTANT TO REMEMBER

1. That, at present, there are no drugs to cure malignancy. It can only be cured by eradication through surgery or radiation (x-ray, radium or radioactive chemicals).
2. That most patients with cancer are ill for a long time and that drugs used to alleviate pain must be used with discretion since tolerance will usually be built up in time.
3. That though the medicines used to make the patient more comfortable must not be given in excess of requirements, the nurse must never deny the patient a needed drug. It takes expert judgment to know when to give and when not to give the drug.
4. That the patient suffering from cancer needs spiritual aid, and the nurse should see that this need is met.
5. That remissions in malignancy do occur. They are an infrequent and unexplained phenomenon.

TOPICS FOR STUDY AND DISCUSSION

1. Look in various recent medical publications and reports for the most recent developments in the treatment of all forms of cancer. Are these drug treatments? If so, compare with the drugs listed in this chapter. Several students might work on this, each taking one of the more common forms of cancer.

2. Check the charts in the medical and surgical departments for patients with malignancies and report to the class on the drugs used. List the drugs, dosage and so forth. Tell why each drug was given in the particular condition, and what the results were. Several students might report on this also, each taking one case or a group of similar cases.

3. Explain how an element is made radioactive. (Refer to a physics text—be brief and do not try to explain in too much detail.) What does half-life mean? Is there any radioactivity left at the end of twice the half-life of the radioactive isotope? Explain your answer.

4. Why does the radioactive element not affect all body cells equally? How does this influence the treatment of cancer?

5. In what types of cancer do drugs form an important treatment? Why?

6. The dose of nitrogen mustard is 0.1 mg. per kilogram of body weight. If the patient weighs 120 pounds, how much drug should the nurse prepare for each dose?

7. Methyl testosterone has been ordered for a patient with inoperable carcinoma of the breasts. The dose ordered is gr. 1½ daily in divided doses—four times a day. The nurse finds that the drug is in scored tablets marked 25 mg. each. How should she proceed?

BIBLIOGRAPHY

Books and Pamphlets

American Medical Association Council on Drugs, *Drug Evaluations*, Chicago, 1971, American Medical Association.

Beeson, P. B., and McDermott, W., *Cecil-Loeb Textbook of Medicine, 13th Ed.* Philadelphia, 1971, W. B. Saunders Co.

Beland, I., *Clinical Nursing: Pathophysiological and Psychosocial Approaches*, New York, 1970, The Macmillan Co.

Bevan, J. A., *Essentials of Pharmacology*, New York, 1969, Harper & Row.

Conn, H. F., *Current Therapy, 1974*, Philadelphia, 1974, W. B. Saunders Co.

Goodman, L. S., and Gilman, A., *Pharmacological Basis of Therapeutics, 4th Ed.*, New York, 1970, The Macmillan Co.

Meyers, F. E., and Goldfien, J. A., *Review of Medical Pharmacology*, Los Altos, California, 1968, Lange Medical Publications.

Rodman, N. J., and Smith, D. W., *Pharmacology and Drug Therapy in Nursing*, Philadelphia, 1968, J. B. Lippincott Co.

Watson, J. E., *Medical-Surgical Nursing and Related Physiology*, Philadelphia, 1972, W. B. Saunders Co.

Periodicals

Backer, E. D. (Ed.), "Symposium on radiation uses and hazards," *Nurs. Clin. North Am.* 2:1:3 (1967).

Barckley, V., "The crises in cancer," *Am. J. Nurs.* 67:2:278 (February, 1967).

Dulbecco, R., "The induction of cancer by viruses," *Sci. Am.* 216:4:28 (1967).

Editorial, "How to protect patient and physician during x-ray examinations, 1. Effects of radiation," *Am. Fam. Physician-G.P.* 1:113:28 (1970).

Editorial, "How to protect patient and physician, during x-ray examinations, 2. Responsiible use of diagnostic x-rays," *Am. Fam. Physician-G.P.* 1:105:22 (1970).

Edwards, P., "Regional cancer clinic therapy," *Can. Nurse* 63:4:41 (1967).

Grimes, O. F., "Neuromuscular syndrome in patients with lung cancer," *Am. J. Nurs.* 71:4:752 (April, 1971).

Henderson, I. W. D., "Current status of cancer chemotherapy," *Can. Nurse* 63:4:37 (1967).

Livingston, B. M., "The patient's right to know the facts," *Can. Nurse* 58:1:25 (1962).

Moore, G., "Cancer: 100 different diseases," *Am. J. Nurs.* 66:4:749 (April, 1966).

O'Dell, A. J., "Radical neck dissection," *Nurs. Clin. North Am.* 8:1:159 (1973).
Rogers, A., "Pain and the cancer patient," *Nurs. Clin. North Am.* 2:4:682 (1967).
Rosillo, R. H., et al., "Psychologic aspects of maxillo-facial cancer," *Nurs. Clin. North Am.* 8:1:153 (1973).
Rummerfield, P., and Rummerfield, M., "What you should know about radiation hazards," *Am. J. Nurs.* 70:4:780 (April, 1970).
Schafer, W. P., "Centrioles in human cancer: intracellular order and intracellular disorder," *Science* 164:3885:1300 (1969).
Taylor, M. C., Phillips, G. C., and Young, R. C., "Pion cancer therapy: positron activity as an indicator of depth doses," *Science* 169:3943:377 (1970).
Welty, M. J., et al., "Treatment and nursing care of maxillo-facial cancer," *Nurs. Clin. North Am.* 8:1:137 (1973).

CHAPTER 30

DRUGS USED FOR PSYCHOGENIC DISORDERS

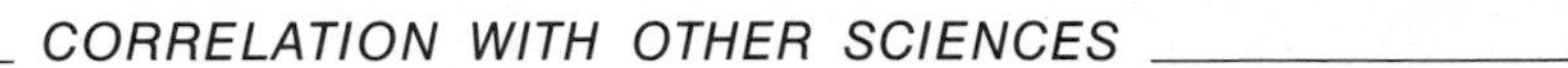

CORRELATION WITH OTHER SCIENCES

Since this chapter is devoted to the discussion of patients with psychogenic disorders and the drugs used in the treatment of such conditions, a brief review of the subject of psychology would be valuable to the student.

I. ANATOMY AND PHYSIOLOGY

1. Mental processes depend upon a physically active nervous system, including the brain, spinal cord, cranial and spinal nerves and the end organs.

V. PSYCHOLOGY

1. Psychogenic disorders may be the exaggeration of normal or customary (socially accepted) behavior. They may be either organic (based upon actual pathology) or functional (without any apparent physical basis). The latter appear to be the more common.
2. The individual's characteristic behavior is the result of the effect of his environment on his inherited traits.
3. Habit is a form of acquired response which is relatively invariable and is readily elicited. It is often the result of a conditioned reflex.
4. The subconscious mind is a storehouse of repressed and suppressed ideas. Often these ideas are of an undesirable character, and their existence produces various complexes. When these ideas are brought into consciousness their force is lessened.

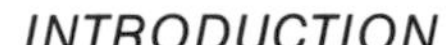

INTRODUCTION

Patients suffering with definite psychoses and neuroses form a large segment of the total patient population, and many more people not under active treatment have tendencies toward neurotic or psychotic behavior. However, even though these disorders are very widespread, drug therapy is limited. There are many reasons for this. Psychogenic disorders appear to be functional rather than organic (V-1). Many functional disorders do not respond to medicinal therapy though the number that do is increasing each year. Organic psychoses are treated as any other physical condition would be treated. Patients with organic disorders form only a small part of the total number of patients with emotional disturbance.

Contrary to popular belief, the nurse should be absolutely frank and truthful with the psychoneurotic patient. It may not be advisable to tell the whole truth, but what is said should be true. To illustrate, it might be unwise to tell what drug is being given, but the purpose of the drug, and the advantages of taking it should be explained. The nurse should endeavor to secure the patient's cooperation. Writing "refused" on the chart is an admission of failure. It may be a lot easier than persuading the patient to take the drug but it is not good nursing, especially in a psychiatric ward. Needless to say, there will be times when the nurse cannot get the patient to cooperate but these should be the exception and not the rule.

The same rules for giving drugs p.r.n. (whenever necessary) to the patient with a physical disorder apply to the patient who has an emotional disturbance. Drugs for pain, real or imagined, or for sleep may be given only after all other methods of control have failed, since the chronic nature of mental illness makes drug addiction or habituation more of a threat than it is in acute diseases. The nurse must always remember that the patient with any form of mental illness is apt to be ill for a relatively long time; rarely is relief effected in a matter of weeks—more often it is months, and even years, before the patient is "cured." Furthermore, the word "cure" is being used less and less. It is better to say "improved" or "condition arrested."

Needless to say, this places an even greater responsibility on the nurse in the use of drugs. If the patient has had to have analgesic or sedative drugs or, in fact, any medication that might lead to habituation, most physicians advise gradual reduction in the dose rather than the substitution of another drug or the use of a placebo. If another drug is used the result may be the substitution of one habit for another (V-3). Even more dangerous may be the use of the placebo, since the time usually comes when the patient finds out that he has been deceived. This makes the patient distrust the nurse and may lead to a distrust of all nurses, an attitude which may ultimately extend even to the physicians and other health professionals.

The administration of medications in the units for the mentally ill presents many problems not found in the general hospital divisions. First, the nurse must always remember that many of her patients have suicidal tendencies. Besides those patients who are known to have this desire, there are many who have thought of suicide but have never made this feeling known. Then there are some mentally ill patients with excessive desire for attention who feel that the other patients are getting more of the nurses' time than they. In that case, snatching the other patients' medicines for themselves appears to them to bring the attention they desire. Some patients may think that the drug ordered for someone else should be given to them, that they need it more than the one for whom it has been ordered. These are a few illustrations which partially explain a few simple rules for the administration of drugs usually followed in the units for the mentally ill.

1. Keep *all* medications under lock and key in an area of the nurses' station that cannot be seen from the ward. The drugs are doubly locked. First, the door to the nurses' station is locked. Second, the cupboard in which the drugs are kept is locked. The patients should not see the nurse pouring the medicines and, therefore, cannot learn where the drugs are kept or their arrangement on the shelves.

2. Use only unbreakable equipment. Trays are usually plastic; medicine cups, spoons, straws and so forth are paper or plastic. This will avoid the dangers inherent in the use of glass or metal containers.

3. Take one drug into the ward at a time. Use a small tray and watch carefully that another patient does not snatch the medicine.

4. Give the medicine to the patient with a small amount of food or water, unless contraindicated, as with cough syrup. Do not disguise medicines with food, for if the patient finds out he may fear his food is being poisoned and then refuse all food. *Never* leave the drug with the patient. The nurse should always stay with the patient until it is obvious the medication has been swallowed. Patients have been known to swallow just the water, keeping the capsule or tablet in the mouth. Repeating this lets the patient accumulate enough of the drug to commit suicide if he has this tendency. The nurse may prick holes in capsules or suggest liquid preparations if drug hoarding is suspected.

5. If the patient vomits or expectorates the drug, do not repeat until the physician has been advised of the situation.

6. The nurse must make the usual record of all drugs given, plus the following:

a. Was it easy to give, was persuasion needed or was the drug refused?

b. Did the patient make any remarks about the drug? What did he say? Be brief, but be specific.

c. Does the patient request medications? Does he request any specific medication?

d. Does he want to know what drug he is getting?
e. Is the patient suspicious of medications?
f. Was the drug effective? Were there any unexpected or unusual reactions?

These questions should be answered when the nurse charts the medications given to the patients.

ORGANIC PSYCHOSES

The organic psychoses are mental disorders which result from physical causes, such as specific diseases, trauma or drugs (I-1). Mental disturbances resulting from or accompanying disease will be discussed with the specific disease, since in these cases the mental condition is really only one manifestation of the over-all picture.

Mental disorders resulting from trauma are relatively rare and are not usually treated by means of any definite drug therapy. This leaves to be considered here only those mental illnesses which result from drugs. Some mention has already been made of the treatment of drug addicts in Chapter 6. A brief review of that section will make this one more meaningful.

Alcoholism

Of all the patients admitted to psychiatric institutions for "drug psychoses," by far the greatest number are alcoholics and as such this constitutes a major health problem. Some are in acute alcoholic mania, some in delirium tremens, some in a chronic drunken state and others are suffering from alcoholic deterioration of the brain (Korsakoff's syndrome). For the last, drug therapy is of little, if any, value.

For the acute or the chronic alcoholic patient in whom mental deterioration has not yet occurred, much can be done. Ultimate cure usually does not depend upon medicines, but upon psychologic and sociologic rehabilitation. Drugs are used to get the patient well enough physically so that other therapy may be instituted.

ACUTE ALCOHOLISM

The patient in alcoholic coma presents an immediate medical emergency for the margin of safety between an anesthetic and a lethal dose is so narrow as to be almost nonexistent. The first thing is to maintain an adequate airway, lavage the stomach and administer an enema. *Caffeine* and *sodium benzoate,* 0.5 to 1.0 Gm. intramuscularly, is often ordered. An intravenous infusion of a saline solution containing 5 per cent dextrose may be given in 1000 to 2000 ml. doses over the course of 12 to 24 hours. Vitamin B-complex and ascorbic acid are usually added to the solution. It may be necessary to repeat this for two or three days. This provides several needs of the patient in one administration: energy-giving glucose, replenishment of body salts and water and the regulatory action of vitamin B.

If the coma persists, *doxapram* (Dopram) or *ethamivan* (Emivan) may be given. The usual doses prevail. (See Chapter 9 and Current Drug Handbook.) When the coma lightens and restlessness appears, *chlorpromazine* (Thorazine; Chlor-Promanyl [C]), 50 mg. or *chlordiazepoxide* (Librium), 50 to 100 mg. intramuscularly, is useful. Extreme restlessness or insomnia is usually well controlled by *chloral hydrate,* 1 to 2 Gm., *flurazepam* (Dalmane) 15 to 30 mg. or, in some cases, *paraldehyde,* 5 to 15 ml. in ice water by mouth.

CHRONIC ALCOHOLISM

Chronic alcoholism is a disease. The chronic alcoholic habitually relies on alcohol and is unable to abstain from taking excessive amounts of the drug. He may be a steady drinker or a spree drinker. Several drugs have been suggested for the treatment of alcoholism, but most physicians feel that drugs alone are not completely effective. Other therapies should be included for best results.

ATARACTICS. In order to help control the tension, motor restlessness and agitation of the patient, one of the ataractic drugs is often given. The term ataractic means "without disturbance"—calmness without depression of mental faculties or clouding of consciousness. There is a wide range of choice here but some of the more commonly used include *reserpine* (Serpasil; Alserin [C]), 0.5 to 2.0 mg.; *chlorpromazine hydrochloride* (Thorazine; Chlor-Promanyl [C]), 25 to 200 mg. daily in divided doses; *meprobamate* (Miltown, Equanil and others; Tranquilate and others [C]), 400 to 1600 mg. daily; *promazine hydrochloride* (Sparine), 25 to 200 mg. daily.

SEDATIVES. Though the ataractic drugs do have some sedative action, this may not be sufficient for the patient. The dangers with the sedative drugs are that the patient may learn to substitute an addiction to sedatives for the alcohol addiction. Useful drugs are *barbiturates* and some of the nonbarbiturates such as *chloral hydrate,* Ph.I., 0.5 Gm.; *ethchlorvynol* (Placidyl; Serenil [C]), 0.5 Gm.; *glutethimide* (Doriden), 0.5 Gm.; *flurazepam* (Dalmane), 15 to 30 mg.; *paraldehyde* 5 to 15 ml.

ABSTINENCE-PRODUCING DRUGS. Quite by accident several years ago it was discovered that after the administration of *disulfiram* (Antabuse) the ingestion of alcohol produced uncomfortable and alarming symptoms. This drug is now used as a basis for part of the treatment to help produce an aversion to alcohol. When the drug is taken daily, no significant effects are usually noticed unless the patient consumes an alcoholic beverage. The drug acts by interference with the excretion of acetaldehyde which is an intermediate product in the oxidation of alcohol.

The drug is slowly absorbed from the gastrointestinal tract, and it takes about three weeks of daily administration before it can be expected to produce satisfactory results. Then should the patient use alcohol in any form, he will within a short time experience flushing, palpitation, dyspnea, hyperventilation, nausea, vomiting, an increase in pulse rate and a fall in blood pressure. Following this, drowsiness occurs; the patient is usually completely recovered after sleep. This experience is very disturbing to the patient and in a large number of cases this may be a strong deterrent to taking the first drink. The sensations are so severe the patient would rather do without alcohol. Symptoms will follow the ingestion of alcohol taken as long as one week after a single large dose of the drug.

Though the drug has a low toxicity, it is used with extreme caution because very severe reactions indicating impending collapse may occur. The antihistaminic drugs are a specific antidote to these serious symptoms. This drug should not be used in patients who have recently been treated with paraldehyde nor should paraldehyde be given to patients receiving disulfiram.

The Nurse. Formerly, it was believed that a "drying out" period was necessary before starting Antabuse therapy, but this has been proved generally not to be needed. For about three weeks daily doses of disulfiram, 500 mg., are given. A test dose of alcohol is then given to the patient to allow the physician and the patient to determine what will happen and to act as a guide to proper dosage levels. The usual maintenance dose of disulfiram ranges from 125 to 500 mg. daily. It is important that the administration of the drug be uninterrupted and continued until the patient has been assisted by psychotherapy to be able to exercise permanent self-control. This may take from several months to several years. During the first couple of weeks after initiating the therapy, the patient may experience a metallic or garlic-like aftertaste. This usually disappears spontaneously but occasionally requires a reduction in dose level. Another drug with action similar to disulfiram is calcium carbamide (Temposil). Excreted more rapidly, its effectiveness is short-lived.

The use of this drug should always be initiated in the hospital where the patient will have close medical and nursing supervision. The nurse should understand the symptoms which will occur after the test dose of alcohol and should have oxygen ready for administration in case of the occurrence of a severe reaction. Antihistaminic drugs should also be readily available. The nurse may assist the patient greatly with her understanding attitude and encouragement of continued therapy.

This drug cannot be used without the consent and full knowledge of the patient and must be accompanied by psychotherapeutic measures. The patient must know the symptoms to be expected (even before the test dose) if drinking is resumed. The family must know these symptoms as well and be warned against the secret administration of the drug (without the patient's knowledge). Family members and close associates may need to be cautioned against encouraging or pressuring the patient to drink.

The Patient. Patients receiving disulfiram should avoid contact with alcohol in ANY form—even in the disguised forms such as cough syrups or other medications containing it. They should not use alcoholic lotions on the skin as they may cause a skin rash.

There is invariably a nutritional depletion in the chronic alcoholic. The patient has been too busy with drinking to eat properly, if at all. The vitamins in the B complex are especially helpful for they are not stored in the body except in small amounts. Usually the physician orders *polyvitamins, polyprotein* and *carbohydrate* supplements generously.

All drug treatment for the alcoholic patient is accompanied by other therapy—psychological, sociological and occupational. The patient is encouraged to seek help from any source which may be beneficial. This includes his spiritual advisors, if he is of a religious nature or if he will accept such advice. Alcoholics Anonymous is often a most useful medium for help if he can be convinced to join. Since it is important to use all possible sources of help, the patient's family should be included in the planning of treatment. Of course, such advice is given by the physician attending the case, but the nurse may be called upon to aid in clarifying certain details.

While receiving disulfiram, the patient should carry an identification card or wear an identification bracelet in case of an emergency situation.

For further information on drug dependency refer to Chapter 6.

FUNCTIONAL PSYCHOSES

In the treatment of functional psychoses, as in organic psychoses, drug therapy is rarely the major treatment. However, drugs can be used as adjuncts to other therapy, to build the patient physically, to combat some specific symptoms or as a means of determining the patient's basic psychologic problems.

VITAMIN THERAPY. Of the drugs used to aid the patient physically, the most common are the *vitamins.* These drugs are used here for the same purposes and in the same way as for the physically ill person. They give the patient needed chemicals, and they also aid psychologically since the patient feels that "something is being done for me," and this may be of more value than the action of the chemicals in the body. Any general vitamin product may be used. It will usually contain *vitamin B*, and often *iron*, especially when there is iron deficiency anemia. (Refer to Chapter 19 for details.)

CATHARTICS AND LAXATIVES. Certain physical symptoms, that may or may not be due to the mental disturbance of the patient, often require medicinal treatment before other therapy can be instituted. For example, cathartics may be needed before the patient can be given a diet which will eliminate the necessity for them. *Mineral oil, cascara, saline* purgatives or one of the fecal softeners may be used. (See Chapter 18.) Oil retention enemas, and later tap water cleansing enemas, will help if there is a tendency to impaction. Sometimes with the catatonic schizophrenic patient there is a persistent tendency to bowel retention since these patients just do not think about such things. The severely depressed patient may also be too engrossed with his own sad thoughts to make the effort to have a bowel movement. These types of patients do not bother to go to the toilet. Even if they are taken they may not have the strength or attentiveness to have a movement. Cathartics may be needed to tide them over the worst period but, as is the case with all constipation, dietary treatment should be instituted as soon as possible.

APPETITE STIMULANTS. For the patient who does not want to eat, small doses of *insulin* (decided upon an individual basis) may be given before meals and often produce very satisfactory results. These patients often eat much better, gain weight and after a short time have the eating habit re-established to a point where the insulin is no longer needed.

TRANQUILIZING DRUGS. Since the introduction, in 1952, of the phenothiazine type drugs and other new compounds, the management of psychoses and psychoneuroses has altered significantly. These drugs are called ataractic or tranquilizing drugs and provide generally a calming and quieting action without clouding of consciousness or mental faculties. The use of these drugs has made many more patients amenable for psychotherapy and has helped many to resume more normal activities. As calmative agents, tranquilizers are chemically different, pharmacologically selective and have a broad range of use greater than previously used drugs. Their effects last longer than those of sedatives. Classification of this large group of drugs is difficult, since the same drug may be used for several different conditions, the distinction being one of dosage. Several classifications have been used, such as major and minor tranquilizers, antipsychotic and anxiety drugs, but there is no consensus of opinion as to where specific drugs should be placed. In Table 18, the divisions are based on the derivations of the drugs. Consult the Current Drug Handbook for others not listed in Table 18.

THE PHENOTHIAZINES

THE DRUGS. The largest group of the major tranquilizers (antipsychotic drugs) is the phenothiazine derivatives. These have been separated into subgroups. See Table 18.

Physical and Chemical Properties. All the phenothiazine drugs are structurally similar and vary only by minor substitutions in the basic molecules.

Action. Just how the phenothiazines act is not completely understood as yet, but it is believed that they depress the subcortical area of the brain. Apparently, they selectively inhibit the chemoreceptor "trigger" zone, the thalamus and the reticular formation, interrupting the passage of impulses coming through this area to the cortex. This has a calming, quieting effect. Many of them also possess antiemetic and antipruritic qualities.

Therapeutic Uses. All these preparations are effective tranquilizers for a wide number of disturbed psychiatric and psychoneurotic patients. In addition, they have proven to be valuable in some psychophysiologic conditions. Because of their tranquilizing and antiemetic effects, these drugs potentiate the action of general anesthesia.

Absorption and Excretion. All these preparations are well absorbed from the intestinal tract and are widely distributed throughout the body tissues. They are metabolized in the liver by hydrolysis and glucuronidization.

Preparations and Dosages. All of the phenothiazine drugs have their dosage adjusted individually. See Table 18 for further details.

THE NURSE

Mode of Administration. All the phenothiazine drugs can be given by mouth and some can be given by the parenteral route (see Table 18 for details). When a phenothiazine preparation is given intramuscularly, it should be injected deep into the muscle; if it is given superficially, a sterile abscess may result. The site should be massaged gently after giving to relieve irritation and pain. Intravenous preparations must be given with caution. Infiltration is to be avoided since sloughing may occur. Phenothiazine drugs should not be mixed with any other drug(s) in an intravenous solution. Phenothiazine solutions should be protected from light.

Side Effects. Most of the phenothiazines share the same side effects—some more than others. Drowsiness, relatively common, usually disappears after one or two weeks of therapy. Nasal stuffiness and orthostatic hypotension occur frequently after parenteral administration. Other side effects include dry mouth, unpleasant taste in the mouth, tachycardia, palpitation, constipation, headaches, pyrexia and pains in the legs and abdomen. The variations are noted in Table 18. The patient who receives these drugs should be advised not to drive a car or operate dangerous machinery during the initial stages of therapy, until the action of the drugs has been evaluated.

Toxic Effects. There can be serious effects from taking drugs in this group. Liver damage is not uncommon as evidenced by jaundice. Periodic liver studies should be done. Agranulocytosis or other blood dyscrasias have also occurred. When one of these drugs is taken, tardive dyskinesia or even parkinsonian symptoms may occur. (See Parkinsonism, Chapter 32.) Tardive dyskinesia may even require the administration of antiparkinsonian drugs. Sometimes, the tardive dyskinesia is reversible, but it may persist after the drug has been withdrawn. Tonic convulsions have been noted especially in children.

Contraindications. Sensitivity to any one of the phenothiazines is a contraindication for use of any of the others.

Interactions. The phenothiazine tranquilizers are enhanced by the thiazide diuretics through additive hypotensive

TABLE 18. *TRANQUILIZERS*

DRUG	TRADE NAMES	METHOD OF ADMINISTRATION	USUAL DAILY PSYCHIATRIC DOSE	PRECAUTIONS AND SIDE EFFECTS	COMMENTS
Phenothiazine Derivatives					
DIMETHYLAMINE SUBGROUP					
Chlorpromazine hydrochloride, U.S.P., B.P.,	Thorazine (Clor-Promanyl, Largactil, Megaphen [C])	Oral: Tablets, Spansules, Syrup, Concentrate; I.M.; I.V.; Rectally	30 to 1200 mg.	Postural hypotension strongly possible after parenteral use. Blood pressure taken before and after giving drug. Patient should lie down for at least 30 minutes after parenteral administration.	Suppository form not useful for repeated use. Syrups and suppositories used mainly for children. Maximum effect in one hour, duration about six hours. Potentiates barbiturates and narcotics.
Promazine hydrochloride, N.F.	Sparine (Promwill [C])	Oral: Tablets, Syrup; I.M.; I.V.	50 to 1000 mg.	Postural hypotension occurs more often than with chlorpromazine. Patient should remain in bed for ½ to 1 hour after parenteral administration.	Not usually used for long-term therapy; best use when temporary tranquilizing effect desired. Arteriolar spasms and gangrene have occurred following I.V. administration.
Triflupromazine hydrochloride, N.F.	Vesprin, Vespral (fluopromazine [C])	Oral: Tablets, Concentrate; I.M.	20 to 200 mg.	Higher incidence of Parkinsonian symptoms than in other drugs of this group.	
PIPERAZINE SUBGROUP					
Butaperazine maleate	Repoise	Oral	5 to 100 mg.	Not used in the presence of circulatory collapse or in patients with history of jaundice, blood dyscrasias or bone marrow depression. Used with caution in those about to have a general anesthetic, in glaucoma, cardiovascular disease, hypotension or epilepsy.	Antiemetic, as well as tranquilizing, action.
Carphenazine maleate, N.F.	Proketazine	Oral: Tablets, Concentrate	40 to 400 mg.	Contraindicated in excessive psychomotor agitation and comatose states and in severe anxiety.	Has short duration of action. Potentiates action of many drugs. Used with care in conjunction with central nervous system depressants.

Fluphenazine dihydrochloride, N.F.	Permitil Prolixin (Moditon, Permitel [C])	Oral Tablets Elixir I.M.	0.5 to 20 mg.	Parkinsonian symptoms observed with prolonged use or high dosage.	
Fluphenazine enanthate, N.F.	Prolixin enanthate injection	I.M.	12.5 to 100 mg. q 1 to 3 weeks		
Fluphenazine decamoate	Prolixin decamoate	I.M.	12.5 to 100 mg. q 2 weeks		
Perphenazine, N.F., B.P.	Trilafon	Oral Tablets Repeat action tablets Syrup Concentrate Suppositories I.M.	6 to 64 mg.	Contraindicated in psychic depression and depression of the central nervous system from drugs and in the presence of bone marrow depression.	Suppositories and injectable preparations are seldom used.
Prochlorperazine maleate, U.S.P., B.P.	Compazine dimaleate (Stemetil [C])	Oral Tablets Sustained release capsules Syrup Concentrate I.M. I.V.	15 to 150 mg.	Subcutaneous administration is not advisable because it produces local irritation. Extrapyramidal symptoms, motor restlessness and dystonias are relatively common with prolonged use.	
Trifluoperazine dihydrochloride, N.F., B.P.	Stelazine	Oral Tablets Concentrate I.M.	2 to 30 mg. in graduated increments	Should not be given in greatly depressed states, in blood dyscrasias, bone marrow depression or preexisting liver disease. Extrapyramidal symptoms occur frequently in higher doses.	Should be given deeply I.M.

Table 18 continued on following page.

TABLE 18. *TRANQUILIZERS (Continued)*

DRUG	TRADE NAMES	METHOD OF ADMINISTRATION	USUAL DAILY PSYCHIATRIC DOSE	PRECAUTIONS AND SIDE EFFECTS	COMMENTS
Thioxanthene Derivatives					
Clorprothixene, N. F.	Taractan	Oral Tablets Concentrate I.M.	30 to 200 mg.	Used with caution in conjunction with anesthetics, hypnotics, analgesics and other central nervous system depressants. It intensifies the actions of these drugs. Also used with caution in patients with a history of convulsive disorders and agitated states accompanying depression. Transitory hypotension may occur but recovery is usually spontaneous. Most frequent side effect is drowsiness.	Closely related chemically to the phenothiazines.
Thiothixene	Navane	Oral Capsules Concentrate I.M.	6 to 30 mg.	Contraindicated in circulatory collapse, comatose states, central nervous system depression and blood dyscrasias. Used with extreme caution in those with history of convulsive disorders. Drowsiness less frequent than with most of these drugs.	A new drug with side effects similar to phenothiazines.
Butyrophenone Derivatives					
Haloperidol, N.F.	Haldol (Serenase in Europe)	Oral Tablets Concentrate I.M.	2 to 25 mg.	In high dosage, extrapyramidal symptoms are frequent. Contraindicated in coma, those severely depressed by alcohol or other central nervous system agents and with Parkinson's disease. Given with caution in those patients with heart disease and those receiving anticoagulant drugs. Sometimes even small dosages will set off severe extrapyramidal symptoms such as spasms and seizures. An antiparkinsonian drug may be given to control the spasms.	Good for patients who cannot take the phenothiazines. Best in the manic phase of manic-depressive psychoses and in paranoia. Does not potentiate anticonvulsant drugs.

Rauwolfia Derivatives					
Rescinnamine hydrochloride, N.F.	Moderil	Oral	3 to 12 mg.	Used with caution in those patients with a history of peptic ulcer. Patients are less prone to mental depression, somnolence, tachycardia and weakness than with some other ataractic drugs.	Medication should be given before meals in order to obviate possible discomfort from increased gastric secretion.
Reserpine, U.S.P.	Raurine Rau-Sed Serpasil Many others (Alserin, Serpone [C])	Oral I.M.	5 to 15 mg. Individually adjusted	Overdose may produce confusional state. Contraindicated in patients with history of peptic ulcer as it increases volume and acidity of gastric secretion. Some patients show signs of hydration which may cause confusion.	Optimal level of dosage proportional to severity of emotional disturbance. Acts more slowly than chlorpromazine. If no improvement after 2 months, discontinue. If chronic psychotic patient improves with use, it can be given indefinitely.
Benzodiazepine Derivatives					
Chlordiazepoxide hydrochloride, N.F.	Librium	Oral I.M. I.V.	20 to 100 mg.	Common side effects are drowsiness and limitation of spontaneity with impaired concentration. Those receiving this drug should not operate a car or machinery. Concomitant use with other psychotropic agents not recommended.	Muscle relaxant and anticonvulsant. Stimulates appetite. Not given to those prone to drug addiction. Especially potentiated by monoamine oxidase inhibitors, phenothiazines and alcohol.
Chlorazepate dipotassium	Tranxene	Oral	15 to 60 mg.	See Chlordiazepoxide. Contraindicated in patients with acute narrow angle glaucoma.	Prolongs effect of central nervous system depressants and increases inhibitory effect of chlorpromazine.
Diazepam, N.F.	Valium	Oral I.M. I.V.	6 to 30 mg.	Dosage should be limited to the smallest effective dose for the elderly or debilitated patient to prevent development of ataxia or oversedation. Contraindicated in infants, patients with history of convulsive disorders and with those having glaucoma.	Helpful in alcohol withdrawal; may be helpful in alleviation of muscle spasm associated with cerebral palsy and athetosis. Potentiates action of phenothiazines, barbiturates, monoamine oxidase inhibitors and alcohol.

Table 18 continued on following page.

TABLE 18. *TRANQUILIZERS (Continued)*

DRUG	TRADE NAMES	METHOD OF ADMINISTRATION	USUAL DAILY PSYCHIATRIC DOSE	PRECAUTIONS AND SIDE EFFECTS	COMMENTS
Oxazepam, N.F.	Serax	Oral	30 to 120 mg.	Not given to those known to be sensitive to oxazepam. Used with caution in patients in whom a drop in blood pressure might be serious. Patient should not drive a car or operate machinery until effect of drug is known not to cause drowsiness or dizziness. Transient mild drowsiness is apt to occur in the first few days of therapy.	Not indicated in psychoses. Tolerance to alcohol may be lowered. Careful supervision of those patients known to take excessive amounts of drugs.
Miscellaneous					
Acetophenazine maleate, N.F.	Tindal	Oral Tablets Repetabs Syrup Concentrate I.M.	40 to 80 mg.	Excessive drowsiness may be seen at first but this usually clears in a few weeks. Used with caution in patients with a history of convulsive episodes. Not used with epinephrine because acetophenazine reverses its action.	Often used in outpatients with anxiety and tensions. When insomnia is a factor, last tablet should be taken 1 hour before retiring.
Ethchlorvynol, N.F.	Placidyl	Oral	200 to 500 mg.	Contraindicated in those with known hypersensitivity to the drug and in those patients with porphyria. Given with caution in those patients with suicidal tendencies. Used with caution as daytime sedation. Reversible toxic amblyopia has been reported with long-term use.	There is a possibility of physical dependence. Drug may exaggerate effects if combined with alcohol, barbiturates or other central nervous system depressants.
Hydroxyzine hydrochloride, N.F.	Atarax Vistaril	Oral I.M.	100 to 200 mg.	No serious side effects. Transitory drowsiness, dryness of mouth, headache, itching and increased peristalsis have been reported.	Potentiated by meperidine and the barbiturates; dosage must be adjusted when these drugs are used concomitantly.

Mepazine hydrochloride	Pacatal (Pecazine [C])	Oral I.M. I.V.	75 to 400 mg.	Most common side effects are atropine-like, although leukopenia and agranulocytosis have been reported with long continued use.	Intermediate between more potent tranquilizers, such as chlorpromazine, and milder agents, such as meprobamate. Less drowsiness, sedation and depression than with chlorpromazine.
Phenaglycodol	Ultran (Alcalo [C])	Oral	600 to 1200 mg.	Given with caution to depressed patients.	Appears not to impair speed of fine movements, alertness, attention, eye coordination, reaction time, etc.
Meprobamate, U.S.P., B.P.	Equanil, Miltown, Wyseals, Meprospan, Metrotabs (Tranquilate [C])	Oral	1200 to 1600 mg.	Dependence and habituation have been reported, especially in such patients as former drug addicts, alcoholics and other severe psychoneurotics. Drug should be withdrawn gradually. Tolerance to alcohol is lowered with slowing of reaction time and impairment of judgment and coordination.	Also useful as a skeletal muscle relaxant, for use in the management of anxiety and tension either alone or with other symptoms, petit mal epilepsy, and prior to electroconvulsive therapy.
Tybamate, N.F.	Solacen	Oral	250 to 1000 mg.	Not given to those patients known to be sensitive to the drug. Used with caution with phenothiazines or other central nervous system depressants and with patients having history of convulsive seizures. Abrupt withdrawal to be avoided.	Useful also in agitation in the elderly patient and some cases of adverse emotional reactions in the aged. Used in some depressive states such as those associated with anxiety.

action. They potentiate reserpine, central nervous system depressants, anticholinergic drugs and antihistamine compounds, all by additive sedation, hypotension or atropine like effect. The phenothiazine drugs antagonize the monoamine oxidase inhibitors.

Patient Teaching. Patients receiving phenothiazine therapy are often also receiving interpersonal or group therapy. The nurse must be ready to help the patient cope with his behavioral problems. She must also observe closely for signs of adverse reactions to the medical regimen so that dosage adjustments may be made. Tolerance to these drugs occurs with some patients who may require larger doses. When the drug is to be discontinued, it should be withdrawn slowly, since abrupt stoppage can cause untoward symptoms such as dizziness and/or gastrointestinal disturbances.

THE PATIENT. If the patient can cooperate, he should be advised to tell his physician of any unusual occurrences. Everyone receiving these drugs should be guarded against exposure to sunlight for any appreciable length of time for this may aggravate the side effects.

The nurse will need to instruct the patient in the possible interactions of the drug with other medicines, especially when the patient is going home. She should remind him that many remedies sold without a prescription might contain drugs which he should avoid. (See Interactions above.) A conference with the patient, his family, the hospital nurse and the public health nurse can secure continuity of care, which gives the patient a sense of security.

Other Tranquilizers

The Rauwolfia derivatives were first introduced as hypotensive agents but were soon found to produce a state of mental quietude and relaxation as well. The mechanism and site of tranquilizing action is not known. (See Chapter 17.) Table 18 shows the drugs most often used, their trade names, methods of administration and dosages within certain accepted ranges. Their use in psychiatry has diminished because of their delay in action, their tendency to induce or intensify depression and the possibility of gastrointestinal hemorrhage.

SEDATIVE-HYPNOTICS. Insomnia is a common symptom in many mental illnesses. In all manic and in certain of the agitated depressions, it becomes a real problem. Various sedative treatments such as packs, baths and back rubs form the main means of overcoming sleeplessness. However, some patients require drugs to secure rest, and most of the sedative and hypnotic drugs previously discussed are used. The same dosages, precautions and methods of administration apply to the mentally disturbed patient as to the physically ill. The danger of habituation is, if possible, even greater with the patient who is emotionally upset than with the physically sick person, so the nurse must do all in her power to secure rest without the use of drugs (V-2).

Some drugs tend to increase the confusion of these patients, and the nurse should be aware of this. Since the patient suffering from psychosis is apt to be ill for a relatively long time and since, by the very nature of the condition, he is in a state of mental confusion, some sedative drugs are much better than others. *Chloral hydrate* and *paraldehyde* are the drugs of choice in many instances as they are less habit forming and do not tend to increase the confusion of the patient. *Bromides* are used sparingly because of their cumulative toxicity. The effectiveness of the *barbiturates* is limited since they tend to produce "drug delirium." Sedatives are usually given in, or with, a cup of hot milk. After a short time the drug can be reduced and later eliminated, the hot milk being all that is needed to produce sleep (V-2).

ANTIDEPRESSANT DRUGS. The antidepressant drugs also might be classified as indirect stimulants because their action on the central nervous system is not believed to be due to direct excitation of neural cells. They have been shown to increase concentrations of serotonin and norepinephrine in the brain. There are a few drugs which have often been found helpful. (See Table 19 – Antidepressant Drugs.)

Untoward effects are common when the antidepressant drugs are given. The monoamine oxidase inhibitors (see Table 19) may induce restlessness, insomnia, postural hypotension and headache. Jaundice with hepatic toxicity has been noted with the hydrazine derivatives – *isocarboxazid* (Marplan) and *phenelzine dihydrogen sulfate* (Nardil). Transient jaundice has been noted

TABLE 19. ANTIDEPRESSANT DRUGS

DRUGS	TRADE NAMES	METHOD OF ADMINISTRATION	USUAL DAILY PSYCHIATRIC DOSE	PRECAUTIONS AND SIDE EFFECTS	COMMENTS
MONOAMINE OXIDASE INHIBITORS—PSYCHIC ENERGIZERS					
Isocarboxazid, N.F.	Marplan	Oral	10 to 30 mg.	May cause hepatitis, blood dyscrasias and skin disorders. Patient should be warned to avoid cheese, beer, wine and chicken livers for these foods contain tyramine and may precipitate a hypertensive crisis. Hypotension, dizziness, vertigo and fainting are common. Contraindicated in known sensitivity to the drug, severe liver or renal impairment, congestive heart failure and pheochromocytoma.	
Phenelzine dihydrogen sulfate	Nardil	Oral	40 to 60 mg.	Not given to elderly or debilitated patients, those with cardiovascular defects or diseases, hypertension, significant history of headache, pheochromocytoma, liver disease or abnormal liver function tests. Hypomania has often been reported.	Precautions—See *Isocarboxazid.* More effective than Niamid. Said to cause fewer hypotensive symptoms than other monoamine oxidase inhibitors.
Tranylcypromine sulfate, N.F.	Parnate	Oral	10 to 30 mg.	May cause postural hypotension or overstimulation. Contraindications: confirmed or suspected cardiovascular defects or disease. Avoid use with the sympathomimetics or other stimulants. Very serious side effects are not uncommon.	Usual precautions as with other monoamine oxidase inhibitors. Has fast and sustained action. Consult commercial brochure for information.

Table 19 continued on following page.

TABLE 19. *ANTIDEPRESSANT DRUGS* (Continued)

DRUG	TRADE NAMES	METHOD OF ADMINISTRATION	USUAL DAILY PSYCHIATRIC DOSE	PRECAUTIONS AND SIDE EFFECTS	COMMENTS
NON-MONOAMINE OXIDASE INHIBITORS **Tricyclic Type (Psychostimulants, Psychoanaleptics)**					
Amitriptyline, U.S.P.	Elavil	Oral I.M.	75 to 200 mg.	Contraindicated in glaucoma or urinary retention. May cause drowsiness, nausea, hypotension, excitement, fine tremors, jitteriness, weakness, headache, heartburn, anorexia, increased perspiration and incoordination. Patients should not drive a car or operate machinery during therapy.	Related to imipramine with less untoward reactions. Has hypnotic action and is helpful in sleep disturbance during depression. Should not be given to patients who have been receiving monoamine oxidase inhibitors for at least two weeks after stopping the other drug.
Desipramine hydrochloride, N.F.	Pertofrane, Norpramin	Oral	150 mg.	Contraindicated in glaucoma, urethral or ureteral spasms, recent myocardial infarction, active epilepsy, patients with manic depressive psychoses; may induce hypomanic state after depressive phase is over.	Not given with or within two weeks of any monoamine oxidase inhibitor. Used with caution in those receiving sympathomimetic drugs or thyroid hormone since potentiation of these may occur.
Imipramine hydrochloride, U.S.P.	Tofranil	Oral I.M.	75 to 300 mg.	Common side effects: dryness of mouth, difficulty with accommodation, perspiration around head and neck. Used with caution in patients with cardiovascular disturbances. Insomnia is often seen when first given.	Change in mood and behavior seldom noticed in first week; maximum benefits usually occur in two to three weeks. May remain on drug for 3 to 6 months. After improvement, drug is gradually withdrawn.
Nortriptyline hydrochloride, N.F.	Aventyl	Oral Pulvules Liquid	25 to 100 mg.	Used with caution in patients with convulsive or hypotensive states, glaucoma or urinary retention.	Usually started with a small dose and increased gradually. Given after meals and at bedtime. Minimum dose given for about a week; if neither adverse reaction or benefit, dose is increased. Usually continued for several months after improvement.

Protriptyline	Vivactil	Oral	15 to 40 mg.	See amitriptyline.	Should not be used in the acute recovery stage after myocardial infarction.
Miscellaneous Types					
Deanol acetamidobenzoate	Deaner	Oral	100 to 300 mg.	Relative contraindications: grand mal or mixed epilepsy.	Best use is in the alleviation of abnormally shortened attention span in school age children and those with learning problems.
Lithium carbonate		Oral	300 mg.	Contraindicated in renal disorders, heart disease, epilepsy and the elderly. Drug withdrawn if diarrhea and vomiting occur or if tremulousness is very severe and associated with drowsiness, ataxia or dizziness.	Serum lithium concentration must be maintained below levels of 2 mEq per liter. Helpful in those who do not respond to phenothiazines or electroconvulsive therapy.
Methylphenidate hydrochloride, U.S.P.	Ritalin hydrochloride	Oral	20 to 60 mg. b.i.d. or t.i.d. preferably 30 to 45 minutes a.c.	Contraindicated in marked anxiety, tension, agitation, glaucoma, epilepsy. Used with caution with patient with hypertension and concomitantly with pressor agents or the monoamine oxidase inhibitors.	Effective also in overdosage and in hastening recovery from anesthesia. Last dose should be taken before 6 P.M. to prevent interference with sleep. This drug has many uses (see Chapter 9).
Pipradrol hydrochloride	Meratran	Oral	5 to 10 mg.	Contraindicated in hyperactive, agitated or severely anxious patients and in chorea or obsessive convulsive states.	Overdose may cause nausea, tension, exacerbation of pre-existing anxiety or agitation.

with the use of *imipramine hydrochloride,* N.F. (Tofranil). The tricyclic type drugs (see Table 19) are not usually given with or immediately after any of the monoamine oxidase inhibitors, for this combination may produce severe atropine-like reactions. However, under very close supervision and in special cases they may be given concurrently. The tricyclic depressants and reserpine probably should not be used in combination owing to their potential for precipitating a manic reaction.

Most of these drugs require several days to several weeks of administration before noticeable effects are seen. The dosage should not be increased until there has been sufficient time to evaluate the patient's response.

These drugs are potentially hepatotoxic, possibly because of hypersensitivity. During therapy, frequent liver function tests and blood counts should be taken.

Interactions. When patients are started on tricyclic antidepressant therapy, they should be warned about the enhanced central nervous system depression with alcohol, especially for the first three or four days. These drugs can increase the impairment of motor function when given with drugs such as *chlordiazepoxide* (Librium) or *diazepam* (Valium). Such combinations can be used, but only under close supervision. The patient should be warned of this possibility.

Other interactions include the following. The tricyclic medications can be potentiated by thyroid preparations, especially in the hypothyroid patient. They antagonize the effect of propranolol on the heart, probably because of the anticholinergic effect of the drug.

The monoamine oxidase inhibitors interact with many other drugs in many ways. See Chapter 9 for details.

The tricyclic antidepressants potentiate the monoamine oxidase inhibitors and the phenothiazine tranquilizers. They antagonize reserpine and guanethidine.

THE NURSE. The nurse will need to be able to instruct the patient about which foods and drugs to avoid while taking the monoamine oxidase inhibitors. The patient may be taking nonprescription drugs, not realizing that it is inadvisable to take them with the tranquilizers. Remedies such as those for hay fever, colds and weight reduction should be avoided. Patients often fail to realize that the nonprescription remedies may contain potent medications. The list of foods that should not be taken is long, but it is most important to avoid strong cheeses, wine, beer, tea, coffee, cola drinks and beans (various legumes).

Changes in the patient's mood, which might be reflected by an increased concern for his environment and easier verbalization, should be recorded and reported to the physician.

THE PATIENT. As the patient improves, it is well to remember that though he may appear better, the improvement may be more apparent than real. He still needs therapy. If he has suicidal tendencies, he may now be able to mobilize his energies enough to accomplish this end. Close supervision is required. The nurse must aid and support him in continued psychiatric therapy. It often takes many months to bring the patient to a point of being able to cope with his problems without the help of others.

SHOCK THERAPY. Some years ago it was noted that the grand mal seizure of epilepsy had a beneficial effect upon patients with certain mental disorders. It had also been observed that the epileptic patient was not often afflicted with severe psychoses. These two observations made psychiatrists look for some way of producing the grand mal seizure in an effort to aid in the treatment of the severe psychoses. Various drugs were tried that would produce a convulsion similar to that of epilepsy but only *pentylenetetrazol* (Metrazol; Leptazol [C]) became popular. Pentylenetetrazol is rarely used now. It has been largely replaced by *flurothyl* (Indoklon). Flurothyl is given by inhalation. The precautions, routines and general use of flurothyl are the same as for the electric convulsive therapy.

Insulin has also been used in a form of shock therapy. With this there is no true convulsion, but an unconsciousness is established. This, too, has been largely abandoned.

Electric convulsive therapy (E.C.T.) can bring about symptomatic improvement in some severe depressions. Frequently a muscle relaxant such as *succinylcholine* (Anectine; suxamethonium chloride, Scoline [C]), 30 to 50 mg. is given intravenously shortly before the treatment to diminish the risk of breaking bones during the convulsion. A sedative may be given about one-half hour before the treatment to help allay fears. When the succinylcholine (Anectine) is given, a small dose of *sodium thiamylal* (Surital) may be added in place of the sedative. Usually, electroconvulsive therapy is administered by passing an alternating current of 70 to 130 volts between temporal electrodes for 0.1 to 0.5 second. A severe convulsion immediately appears and is over shortly, after which the patient sleeps for a while. He may remain slightly confused for several hours after the treatment. This form of therapy is seldom given oftener than three times a week.

Both shock and electric convulsive therapy are contraindicated for patients receiving reserpine. They are used with caution, if at all, if the patient has an upper respiratory infection, increased cranial or intraocular pressure or severe cardiovascular, hepatic or renal disease. Flurothyl has not been proven safe for use during pregnancy.

The nurse should be with the patient for some time before the treatment to help reassure him and should remain with him until his confusion is gone. Maintenance of an airway during the actual shock and resulting convulsion is imperative.

IT IS IMPORTANT TO REMEMBER

1. That the use of drugs in the treatment of psychogenic conditions is expanding, and new scientific knowledge may change the picture greatly in the near future.

2. That the use of drugs for the treatment of the patient who is emotionally disturbed may seem unreasonable, but it may well be that the emotional disorder is due, at least in part, to a physical condition which will respond to medical therapy.

3. That many cases previously thought to be entirely hopeless have responded, to a greater or lesser degree, to drugs, and as our understanding of these conditions expands it is hoped that more of these disorders will be corrected.

4. That though drug therapy does not play the major role in the treatment of the psychoneurotic patient, when used, its role is important, and that to administer a drug properly in these conditions the nurse must understand the drug and its properties as well as the disorders and their symptoms.

5. That as with all drug therapy, but possibly more in this area than in some others, the specific reaction of the individual patient to the drug is extremely important, and that this reaction may be emotional as well as or in addition to being physical.

TOPICS FOR STUDY AND DISCUSSION

1. Why is the physician reluctant to give sedative drugs to the excited psychotic patient? What substitutes may be used?

2. Discuss the use of the placebo in both the general and the mental hospital. Give reasons for and against its use.

3. Why is drug therapy not the major form of treatment for the patient suffering with a psychosis? Discuss, as well as you can, all phases of the problem.

4. One of the bulk laxatives has been ordered for a depressed patient. The patient does not want to take the medicine. What means might you use to secure cooperation? Why do you think that the drug was ordered?

5. How is disulfiram (Antabuse) used? Why is it effective? What psychotherapy might be used to aid in this therapy? Suppose you are assigned to give directions to the relatives of a patient going home to continue disulfiram. Describe in detail how you might carry out the assignment.

BIBLIOGRAPHY

Books and Pamphlets

American Medical Association Council on Drugs, *Drug Evaluations*, Chicago, 1971, American Medical Association.

Beeson, P. B., and McDermott, W., *Cecil-Loeb Textbook of Medicine, 13th Ed.*, Philadelphia, 1971, W. B. Saunders Co.

Bergersen, B., *Pharmacology in Nursing, 12th Ed.*, St. Louis, 1973, The C. V. Mosby Co.

Conn, H. F., *Current Therapy, 1974*, Philadelphia, 1974, W. B. Saunders Co.

Goodman, L. S., and Gilman, A., *Pharmacological Basis of Therapeutics, 4th Ed.*, New York, 1970, The Macmillan Co.

Watson, J. E., *Medical-Surgical Nursing and Related Physiology*, Philadelphia, 1972, W. B. Saunders Co.

Journal Articles

Ayd, F. J., Jr., "The chemical assault on mental illness: the major tranquilizers," *Am. J. Nurs.* 65:4:70 (April, 1963).

Ayd, F. J., Sr., "The chemical assault on mental illness: the minor tranquilizers," *Am. J. Nurs.* 65:5:89 (May, 1965).

Ayd, F. J., Jr., "The chemical assault on mental illness: the antidepressant," *Am. J. Nurs.* 65:6:78 (June, 1965).

Canning, M. C., "Care of alcoholic patients," *Am. J. Nurs.* 65:11:113 (November, 1965).

Carter, A. B., "Rural emergency psychiatric services," *Am. J. Nurs.* 73:5:868 (May, 1973).

Fischer, L. R., et al. "Symposium on the nurse in community mental health," *Nurs. Clin. North Am.* 5:4:1 (1970).

Goshen, C., "The placebo effect—For whom," *Am. J. Nurs.* 66:2:293 (February, 1966).

Kline, N. S., and Davis, J. M., "Psychotropic drugs," *Am. J. Nurs.* 73:1:54 (January, 1973).

Leidig, R. M., "Narcolepsy: Jody's story," *Am. J. Nurs.* 73:3:491 (March, 1973).

Lennard, H. L., et al., "Hazards implicit in prescribing psychoactive drugs," *Science*, 169:438, (July, 1970).

Paul, M., Cramer, H., and Bunney, W., Jr., "Urinary adenosine 3′-5′-monophosphate in the switch process from depression to mania, *Science* 171:300 (January 22, 1971).

Reid, W. D., et al., "Tricyclic antidepressants: evidence for an interneural site of action," *Science* 164:3878:437 (1969).

Tupin, J., "The use of lithium for manic-depressive psychoses," *Hosp. Community Psychiatry* 21:3:17 (1970).

CHAPTER 31

DRUGS USED FOR COMMUNICABLE DISEASES

CORRELATION WITH OTHER SCIENCES

III. MICROBIOLOGY

1. Insects that transfer disease organisms are known as vectors.
2. The pathogenic virus is a very small organism which is capable of producing disease. Viruses grow only in living cells, and are too small to be seen with the light microscope. They are visualized with the electron microscope.
3. Viruses vary in length from 12 to 400 millimicrons. The millimicron is one thousandth of a micrometer, and a micrometer is one thousandth of a millimeter or one twenty-five thousandth of an inch.
4. Coxiella are organisms lying in complexity between the viruses and the rickettsiae. They are small, intracellular organisms, as are the viruses.
5. Rickettsiae are small organisms, some of which can be seen with the aid of the ordinary microscope, but are better seen under the electron microscope. They live only in living tissue. The pathogenic rickettsiae are transmitted by various vectors.
6. Bacteria are classified in several ways: shape—bacilli, cocci, spirilli; staining reaction—gram-negative, gram-positive, and acid-fast; spore formation—form spores, do not form spores; oxygen requirements—aerobic, anaerobic, facultative, obligate.
7. Microorganisms occurring in chains are given the prefix "strepto"—thus streptococci (cocci in chains), streptobacilli (bacilli in chains).
8. Staphylococci are microorganisms of the coccal group that appear as bunches of grapes.
9. The prefix "diplo" refers to grouping of two—thus diplococci (cocci in pairs).
10. The Gram stain is a general stain used to separate bacteria into two great groups: those that are "gram-positive" retain the dark stain, appearing bluish-black under the microscope; those that take the counterstain, appearing pink or reddish under the microscope, are "gram-negative."
11. The term hemophilus means "blood loving."
12. Many microorganisms move by means of flagella—hair-like appendages—which wave rapidly, propelling the organism through its fluid environment.
13. Actinomycetes are organisms between bacteria and the molds. They have some of the characteristics of each group. They have been called the "higher, mold-like bacteria."
14. Fungi are plants of a lower order. They include yeasts and molds. Fungi do not produce chlorophyll.
15. Spirochetes are slender, flexible, coiled organisms that resemble both protozoa and the true spiral bacteria.
16. Fusiform bacilli are spindle-shaped organisms with pointed ends.
17. The tendency for two or more microorganisms to associate together for the benefit of both is symbiotic or mutualistic action.
18. Protozoa are minute one-celled animals.
19. Most protozoa reproduce asexually, but some species at particular stages in their morphologic development produce gametes (which correspond to the sex cells of higher organisms) and these unite to form a zygote or new organism.
20. Pyogenic organisms are organisms which cause the production of pus in the host.
21. Microorganisms which may cause an infection in the intestinal tract include the colon-typhoid group (probably the largest group), staphylococci, streptococci and pneumococci.
22. The skin is the natural habitat of many organisms such as bacteria and fungi. Any break in the skin is a potential source of infection since microorganisms which are harmless on the surface may become deleterious upon entrance into the body.
23. Higher forms of organisms such as *Sarcoptes scabiei* and *pediculi* occasionally infest the skin as ectoparasites.

V. PSYCHOLOGY

1. "What man does not understand, man fears."
2. Treatment of some diseases in this group is often a prolonged procedure. This may be very discouraging to the patient.
3. The realization that one has a serious illness that is communicable and likely to be prolonged is a serious emotional shock.

VI. SOCIOLOGY

1. Fear of social ostracism is a potent factor in the life of everyone. Every person desires to be liked by his peers. He will usually avoid anything which might lower him in the eyes of the public.
2. Social stigma attached to certain diseases may make the patient delay seeking medical advice. This may result in a much more serious condition which may then be harder to treat.
3. The cost of prolonged treatment may become a financial burden to the patient with a disease lasting for a long time. He and his family should be assisted by every means possible to continue treatment.

INTRODUCTION

Diseases which can be transmitted from one person to another have always formed an important segment of the disorders of mankind, especially since the development of urban population centers. The close contact of many individuals facilitated transfer of these diseases and, as concentration became greater, this tendency increased to continue unabated until about the time of the French and American Revolutions. All too well known are the plagues of the Middle Ages; nothing seemed to stop a communicable disease once it got started. Many factors, in addition to the massing of people, combined to make these scourges possible —including almost complete absence of sanitary facilities and lack of knowledge about the cause, prevention, mode of transfer and cure of disease.

The first real break in this wall of ignorance was the famous observation and experimentation by Dr. Edward Jenner in the use of cowpox lymph to prevent smallpox. From that time until the present an ever-increasing number of diseases have been nearly eliminated by various control measures. Some diseases, like smallpox, are prevented by proper inoculation, and the list of these is growing each year. Other diseases have been prevented largely by the elimination of their method of transfer from one person to another. This is especially true of the diseases transmitted by vectors and those due to unsanitary conditions (III-1). Adequate sanitation has greatly reduced the incidence of water-borne diseases, as well as reducing the prevalence of flies that carry many organisms. In addition to the use of drugs as specific preventives, the general anti-infective medications have tended to decrease the amount and the severity of many of the communicable diseases so that today it is often possible to "cure" the diseases before an accurate diagnosis has been made.

All these and many other factors have combined to lessen the number of communicable diseases, so that both mortality and morbidity rates have been markedly reduced from what they were even 20 or 30 years ago. However, the picture is not entirely bright. A relatively new problem is presented by rapid transportation. Since people now go thousands of miles in a few hours and can easily travel from one continent to another during the incubation period of almost any communicable disease, a traveler might conceivably carry an infection into an area whose residents have little or no natural immunity, and the disease could become epidemic. Obviously, this means that the medical profession must become aware of the symptoms and treatments of the diseases common in all areas of the world. Our own knowledge of diseases prevalent in other parts of the world has been greatly increased through the movement of the armed forces. But even though this rapid and multiple transfer of people would appear to be a potent source of epidemics, it has not seemed materially to change the picture; communicable diseases are less prevalent now than ever before. Some of this reduction is due to border controls at the points of entrance and exit. Certain specific restrictions are set up, varying with the countries and the incidence of endemic communicable diseases.

Individuals differ in their physical resistance to disease and also in their psychologic approach to disease. Many people still feel that certain communicable diseases are a disgrace. The specter of the "pest" house and the "lazaretto" is still vivid in the minds of many, and just to mention the word leprosy brings a shudder of horror to the majority of people. The Biblical cry "unclean, unclean" still seems to be heard even in our "enlightened" age. Many diseases were mistakenly diagnosed as leprosy, especially before microbiology became a science (V-1). In fact, many lay people still mistake one type of disease for another; the leper and the person with an entirely noncommunicable skin disease are still shunned equally by society (V-1).

Any disease which can be transmitted from one individual to another is the potential source of serious trouble and should be treated as quickly and completely as possible not only for the sake of the patient involved but for the protection of society at large. For another reason, too, it is very important to reduce the danger of epidemic diseases. Many of these diseases are contracted in childhood and, therfore, endanger citizens of the future. One of the greatest savings of human lives has been in the younger age groups, and it is the hope of all concerned that more and more can be done to prevent the epidemic diseases of childhood.

Drugs useful in the treatment of a number of diseases have already been discussed. In this chapter these drugs will be mentioned only briefly in the areas to which they apply, and the so-called "specific" drugs will be emphasized. The "specifics" are drugs used to treat or cure a single disease or only a relatively limited number of diseases. Since there are so many diseases and conditions to be considered, and also such a great number of drugs, this chapter has been divided into sections according to the type of organism causing the disease. This method was selected since it is not uncommon to find that one drug is effective against a type of organism, rather than one specific disease. No system of classification has any real advantage over another. The arrangement used should be varied to suit the sequence of the study of communicable diseases, which this is intended to accompany.

To give the student a brief overall picture of these diseases and the drugs used to treat them, tables have been included with each group of organisms responsible for most infectious diseases. Certainly they do not contain all diseases that are transmissible, but in these outlines will be found the major ones encountered in the United States and Canada, with some of the more important ones prevalent in other countries. Certain diseases will be considered in more detail.

Some of the infectious (communicable) diseases have already been covered in other chapters with the various systems affected. These are mentioned here only in the tables.

VIRAL DISEASES

The list of diseases caused by the viruses is one of the longest of the communicable diseases (III-2, 3). They do not all have the same characteristics, and a few subgroups are helpful in understanding them. The diseases discussed in detail here are mainly those affecting children and young adults.

For most viral disease there is no specific treatment. Interferon, a protein produced by tissue cells in response to stimulation by some viruses and chemicals, prevents the reproduction of certain other viruses and thus, infection. Interferon is species-specific (that produced in animals is ineffective in humans). Thus, for prevention of infection in humans, a human source is required. For this reason it is not generally available. Passive artificial immunity is used when available. If an individual has been exposed to one of these diseases or when it has actually occurred, immune serum globulin may be used to prevent its development

TABLE 20. *VIRAL DISEASES*

VIRAL DISEASES	DRUG THERAPY
Dermatropic	
Chickenpox (varicella)	Symptomatic; antibiotics for complications
Smallpox (variola) (Also cowpox and vaccinia)	Thiosemicarbazones early; antibiotics for secondary infections; symptomatic
Herpes zoster (shingles)	Symptomatic
Herpes simplex (cold sores)	Symptomatic
Rubella (German measles)	Symptomatic; antibiotics for complications
Rubeola (red measles)	Same
Other viral exanthema such as exanthem subitum, erythema infectiosum and Duke's disease	No specific treatment
Pneumotropic	
Common cold	Symptomatic
Influenza (la grippe)	Symptomatic
Viral pneumonia (atypical) (Organism is similar to one causing lymphogranuloma venereum)	Symptomatic
Psittacosis	Tetracyclines
Viscerotropic	
Infectious hepatitis	Symptomatic and supportive
Infectious mononucleosis	Same as above
Infectious parotitis (mumps)	Same as above; complications treated if and as they occur
Phlebotomus fever (pappataci or sandfly fever) (Transmitted by sandfly)	Symptomatic and supportive
Lymphogranuloma venereum (See viral pneumonia above)	Tetracyclines or sulfonamides may help
Oculotropic	
Epidemic keratoconjunctivitis	Symptomatic
Inclusion blennorrhea	Sulfonamides, tetracyclines, chloramphenicol
Herpetic keratitis	Idoxuridine, topical
Trachoma	Sulfonamides, tetracyclines, chloramphenicol
Neurotropic	
Poliomyelitis	Symptomatic
Coxsackie disease	Same as above
Encephalitis lethargica	Same as above
Encephalitis equine Eastern	Same as above
Encephalitis equine Western	Same as above
Encephalitis Japanese	Same as above
Encephalitis St. Louis	Same as above
Encephalitis, postinfection	Same as above
(Equine Eastern, Equine Western, Japanese, and St. Louis encephalitis are transmitted by vectors—mosquitoes or mites)	Same as above
Rabies	No treatment—sedation as required
Lymphocytic choriomeningitis	Symptomatic

or to reduce its severity. Other treatment is largely symptomatic and supportive (Table 20). There is an increasing amount of research into drugs that might be helpful in curing various viral diseases and in stimulating interferon production. Some of the broad-spectrum antibiotics are helpful, and several other chemicals are being tested.

Microbiologists are in the process of assigning names to the various viruses, but since these have not received universal acceptance, they have not been included.

Some of the more common viral diseases are discussed on the following pages.

Rubella

DEFINITION. Rubella (German measles) is a relatively mild viral disease occurring mainly in childhood.

MAJOR SYMPTOMS. Rubella is characterized by a mild prodrome of fever and generalized aching followed by a punctate rash. During the prodrome and throughout the course of the disease, cervical adenopathy, especially of the postauricular glands, occurs. This glandular swelling is almost as diagnostic as the rash.

DRUG THERAPY. No specific drug therapy is required for rubella unless complications occur.

THE NURSE. Symptoms are treated as they appear, and the child does not often complain of discomfort. Occasionally, mild analgesics and antipyretics may be needed.

If rubella occurs in a woman during pregnancy, or if a prospective mother who has never had the disease is exposed to it, she is given immune serum globulin. It has been found that rubella occurring during pregnancy, especially during the first trimester, may have serious effects upon the fetus. Various congenital anomalies have been attributed to this source. The immune serum globulin should be given in sufficient quantities to prevent or curb the disease. Before the full dose is given, the patient should be checked for serum sensitivity by an intradermal skin test. About 0.1 ml. is put into the layers of the skin of the forearm and watched for 20 minutes. If there is no reaction the drug is given. The usual dose is 2.2 ml. per kg. of body weight intramuscularly for prevention. If, however, there is a reaction, redness and wheal formation, the physician should be advised of the situation and his orders secured.

A vaccine for rubella, believed to confer a long term immunity, is available and many pediatricians give it routinely to small children. Others wait until just prior to puberty. Then if the child has not had rubella, the vaccine is given. Efforts to reduce the incidence of rubella have been disappointing to the public health officials. It appears that immunization of all children will be essential if the disease is to be eliminated.

THE PATIENT. Concern has been expressed by many over the uncertainty surrounding the question of rubella and its effect upon the developing fetus. There are still many unanswered questions such as, if a child is immunized upon or before entering school, will this immunity carry over into the childbearing years? Does vaccination during pregnancy have the same effect upon the fetus as having the disease? It is possible to allay these fears by testing the would-be mother to determine her level of immunity (hemagglutination-inhibition test for rubella antibodies). In this way, safe vaccination or the use of immune serum globulin may be recommended.

Rubeola

DEFINITION. Rubeola, unlike rubella, can be and often is a very serious viral disease for the child or the adult unlucky enough to contract it.

MAJOR SYMPTOMS. Rubeola, or red measles, is characterized by a prodrome in which coryza and a persistent hacking cough are the predominant symptoms. Toward the end of the prodromal stage, Koplik's spots appear. These are bluish-white spots in a reddened area and are found on the inside of the cheeks and over other portions of the buccal mucosa. On the third to the fifth day after the first symptoms, the rash begins. It is a macular rash occurring first on the neck and chest and spreading rapidly over the entire body. There is fever, photophobia and general discomfort, with a continuation of the prodromal symptoms.

Complications of rubeola are common. The most important ones are bronchopneumonia and otitis media.

DRUG THERAPY. As with rubella, there is

no specific treatment for this disease. Vaccines are available for rubeola. The Edmonston "Schwarz" strain attenuated measles vaccine may be administered without concurrent use of immune serum globulin. However, the immune serum globulin should be given with the Edmonston B strain vaccine to reduce the reaction. The immune serum globulin should be given at a different site and with separate equipment. Immune serum globulin is used to prevent the disease and to reduce the severity of an attack if the patient has not received the vaccine. It may be given upon exposure to prevent the occurrence of the disease or to reduce its severity so the child will have only a mild attack. Immune serum globulin for the treatment of the disease is of limited value, but some doctors believe that these preparations do shorten the duration of the disease and reduce the possibility of serious complications.

For treatment of a regular attack of rubeola, most physicians will order either the sulfonamides or the antibiotics to aid in the prevention of complications. These drugs do not have any effect upon the virus but they will often prevent or cure such severe complications as pneumonia or ear infection. Since the child is usually very uncomfortable with fever, headache and similar complaints, the analgesics-antipyretics are often used. Cough mixtures with or without codeine are used to control the distressing cough. Calamine lotion may be used if the rash begins to itch.

Epidemic Parotitis

DEFINITION. Epidemic parotitis (mumps) is one of the common viral diseases of childhood affecting the parotid glands.

MAJOR SYMPTOMS. Parotitis causes swelling of the parotid and other salivary glands. One or all six of the glands may be involved. The swelling produces difficulty in swallowing and chewing. Even to open the mouth may be very painful. If mumps is uncomplicated, the inflammation and swelling begin to subside after a few days, and recovery is uneventful. However, if complications do occur, the patient may be very ill for a protracted period of time. The most common complication is an involvement of the gonads. This is especially true with the male, during or after puberty. However, any of the glands of the body, especially the exocrine saccular glands, may be affected.

DRUG THERAPY. There are vaccines available for the prevention of mumps. One is incorporated in the M-M-R—mumps, measles and rubella combined vaccine. (Refer to Chapter 7.) Whether given alone or in a combination, the vaccine is usually given before puberty. The commercial brochure should be consulted before administering any of these preparations. If, during or after puberty, an individual who has not had either the disease or the vaccine is exposed to mumps, *mumps immune globulin* (Hyparotin) may be used as a temporary agent to lessen the severity of the disease and to aid in the prevention of complications which are not uncommon in the adult, especially the male. Symptomatic treatment with the analgesic-antipyretic drugs is used as may be indicated for the relief of fever and pain. Complications are treated as they occur.

Varicella

DEFINITION. Varicella (chickenpox) is a relatively benign viral disease, usually of childhood.

MAJOR SYMPTOMS. Varicella is characterized by a papular eruption occurring in crops. The lesions are very itchy but, unless scratched, rarely cause any real difficulty.

DRUG THERAPY. There is no specific preventive or treatment for varicella. Immune serum globulin is occasionally used to prevent an exposed child from becoming ill, especially if the child is not in good health, such as a child with acute rheumatic fever. In such a case it might be very serious for the child to have any extra physical burden, even as simple and usually uncomplicated a disease as chickenpox. During the course of the disease various antipruritic drugs are used either as ointments, lotions, washes or pastes. The systemic antipruritic drug, trimeprazine tartrate (Temaril) (alimemazine, Panectyl [C]) may be used to relieve the itching. Since the main complication of varicella is the infection of the vesicles (usually from scratching) some physicians routinely order antibiotics to prevent this. Any soothing ointment will help: *calamine* lotion, with or without *phenol*, is beneficial, as is *sodium bicarbonate* as a wash or paste.

Some doctors, especially those engaged in public health activities, order *penicillin* or antibiotics, but other doctors feel that these are of little value in the treatment of this condition.

Variola

DEFINITION. Variola (smallpox) needs only a brief discussion in spite of the fact that it is a relatively severe viral disease, since it is much better prevented than treated. Smallpox vaccination is an effective, relatively long-term preventive and, when used consistently throughout the population, reduces the number of cases almost to zero. In countries where routine vaccinations have been done on the entire population for a number of years, the disease has disappeared, except for an occasional imported case that enters the country during the incubation period. The United States Health Service no longer recommends routine vaccination for smallpox. If an imported case occurs, the contacts are vaccinated. It is recommended that persons travelling in countries where the disease is still endemic be vaccinated before entering such countries, and that physicians, nurses and other health personnel be preventively immunized and revaccinated every three years as a precaution against their possible exposure to the imported case.

MAJOR SYMPTOMS. Smallpox has a prodromal period of about five days with symptoms similar to those of influenza: fever, headache, backache and malaise. On about the fifth day the eruption appears. It is a papular eruption and comes out all at one time. The lesions go through all the classical stages of skin lesions: macule, papule, vesicle, pustule, scab or crusting and healing with or without cicatrization. During the pustular stage secondary infection of the skin is not uncommon. At this time there is a return of the fever which has usually subsided after the prodromal period.

DRUG THERAPY. Early treatment, before the eruption takes place, includes the use of the investigational thiosemicarbazones such as *amithiozone* (Tibione, Panrone). The earlier in treatment these are given, the more effective they are. Symptoms are treated as they occur. If the disease is mild, antipruritic and colloidal baths may be given during the scabbing stage. Analgesic-antipyretics are helpful in controlling pain and fever.

Severe cases are treated much as a serious thermal burn would be. Baths and ointments are to be avoided. *Silver nitrate* may be applied to the lesions, before secondary bacterial invasion has taken place. *Penicillin* is the drug of choice in infected cases. The broad-spectrum antibiotics should be avoided and chloramphenicol should not be used.

Poliomyelitis

DEFINITION. Poliomyelitis is a disease in which the virus attacks the motor cells of the spinal cord. It occurs in all degrees from a mild upper respiratory condition to a death-dealing bulbar infection.

MAJOR SYMPTOMS. Poliomyelitis is characterized by muscle spasms and pain, with muscle weakness or paralysis resulting. Nausea and vomiting are common during the early stages of the disease. Tenderness over the affected muscles may be very disturbing.

DRUG THERAPY. The efficacy of the Salk and Sabin vaccines has been established. Their use helps to control this crippling disease which is much better prevented than cured. However, as the incidence of epidemics decreases, there appears to be a decrease in preventive immunizations. This could result in an increase in the disease. As with many other diseases, adults traveling in countries where poliomyelitis is endemic should have a booster immunization before entering those countries.

Poliomyelitis is treated with *immune serum globulin;* however, there is a difference of opinion as to its effectiveness. It is also sometimes used for short-term immunity. It does reduce the incidence of paralysis. In bulbar poliomyelitis (affecting the upper spinal cord and the medulla oblongata) *penicillin* may be given to prevent complications, especially penumonia, which often occurs. The salicylates may help in overcoming some of the pain. Narcotic analgesics and most sedative-hypnotics should be avoided because of their adverse effect upon respirations; nor do the muscle relaxants seem to be of any real value. For most symptoms and complications, treat-

TABLE 21. RICKETTSIAL DISEASES

DISEASE	CAUSATIVE AGENT	VECTOR
Typhus, epidemic	*Rickettsia prowazeki*	Louse *(Pediculus humanus)*
Typhus, benign (Brill-Zinsser's disease, recurrent typhus)	*Rickettsia prowazeki*	Louse *(Pediculus humanus)*
Typhus, endemic (murine typhus)	*Rickettsia typhi*	Flea *(Xenopsylla cheopis)*
Typhus, tick-borne (boutonneuse fever)	*Rickettsia conorii*	Tick *(Rhipichalus,* various strains)
Typhus, scrub (tsutsugamushi)	*Rickettsia tsutsugamushi (R. orientalis, R. nipponica)*	Mite *(Trombicula akamushi* and *T. deliensis)*
Rocky Mountain spotted fever	*Rickettsia rickettsii*	Tick *(Dermacentor andersoni, Dermacentor variabilis)*
Rickettsialpox	*Rickettsia akari*	Mite *(Allodermanyssus sanguineus)*
Q fever	*Coxiella burnetti (Rickettsia burneti)*	Tick *(Ixodes holocyclus* and others, also through dust and milk)

ments are used rather than drugs, such things as diet (fruit juices and so on) for constipation, respirator for respiratory involvement, extra fluids for urinary retention and so on. Sometimes a drug such as urecholine may be used. Catheterization is to be avoided, if possible.

Supportive treatment forms the basis for most of the care given to the patient suffering from poliomyelitis, with drugs being used to augment the treatment and to overcome adverse symptoms as they occur.

Infectious Mononucleosis

DEFINITION. Infectious mononucleosis is probably caused by a virus known as the Epstein-Barr virus (EBv), or an agent similar to it. It is a fairly common condition which may be either acute or chronic.

MAJOR SYMPTOMS. Infectious mononucleosis is characterized by both acute and chronic states. In the former there is sore throat, fever and malaise; in the chronic condition there may be no symptoms. In both cases the characteristic blood picture which gives the disease its name will be found.

DRUG THERAPY. There is no specific treatment for mononucleosis. Short courses of steroids may be used for moderate to severe cases. Usually *prednisolone* is given, 80 mg. the first day, 60 mg. daily for the next two days and then 40 mg. each day for another two days, after which the drug is discontinued.

Unless streptococcal sore throat develops, antibiotics are contraindicated. If the complication arises, however, *penicillin* is usually the most effective agent.

RICKETTSIAL DISEASES

Diseases caused by the Rickettsia and the Coxiella can be considered together as they all have similar characteristics (III-4, 5). These diseases have many things in common: they all have animal reservoirs, most are transmitted by vectors and they usually produce fever and a rash (III-1). The same drugs are used in treating all of them. The drug of choice is one of the *tetracyclines. Chloramphenicol* is also effective. With some, especially epidemic typhus and Rocky Mountain spotted fever, *para-aminobenzoic acid* is beneficial. There is an immune serum available for Rocky Mountain spotted fever, but it is used only in very serious cases. Active immunization can be secured for epidemic typhus and for Rocky Mountain spotted fever.

Rocky Mountain Spotted Fever

DEFINITION. Rocky Mountain spotted fever, transmitted by the wood tick, is the most important rickettsial disease in this country (Table 21). This is a serious disease that is not confined, as the name would imply, to the Rocky Mountain area but also occurs in other parts of the country, including areas of the eastern part of the United States.

MAJOR SYMPTOMS. Rocky Mountain spotted fever is characterized by fever, malaise, rash and a tendency to bleed easily.

DRUG THERAPY. There is a vaccine available, and it should be used by anyone apt to be in the area in which infected wood ticks exist. When the disease occurs it is treated with the oral antibiotics, preferably the *tetracyclines* and *chloramphenicol*. Symptoms are treated as they occur. Various supportive measures may be required, especially in severe cases.

BACTERIAL DISEASES

This area, like that of the viral disorders, includes a large number of diseases (Table 22). The organisms vary widely in size, form, infectiveness and response to chemotherapy. As with all the communicable diseases, some of the bacterial diseases have been discussed in previous chapters. Since each group of organisms responds to a different group of drugs, there has been an attempt to put similar ones together even though the diseases produced sometimes vary greatly. Antibiotic resistance is a phenomenon of increasing significance in antibacterial therapy. New drugs are continuously sought to cope with the situation.

Diseases Caused by Cocci

Most of the diseases caused by the cocci (either gram-positive or gram-negative) can be successfully treated either with the sulfonamide drugs or the antibiotics (III-6). The severity of these diseases and their complications has been greatly reduced with the advent of these drugs. The dramatic effect of chemotherapy has been most apparent in its action on these and certain of the gram-positive, rod-shaped organisms.

Scarlet Fever, Erysipelas and Streptococcal Sore Throat

DEFINITION. Scarlet fever, erysipelas and streptococcal sore throat are all caused by the hemolytic streptococci and have many things in common (III-7). They are acute, serious diseases which have been more prevalent in the past than they now are.

MAJOR SYMPTOMS. These conditions all have an abrupt onset, with high fever, malaise, general aches and pains and skin manifestations. In scarlet fever and streptococcal sore throat there is an acute sore throat with a diffuse "scarlet" rash which may or may not appear in streptococcal sore throat. In erysipelas the area of the skin involvement is elevated, red and hot to touch and there is a clear line of demarcation with the adjoining uninvolved skin.

DRUG THERAPY. There is a satisfactory vaccine for erysipelas alone. It is used mainly for those patients who have had more than one attack of the disease.

These diseases respond favorably to *penicillin*. There is an antiserum (antitoxin) available for both erysipelas and scarlet fever, but since sulfonamide drugs and antibiotics became common the antisera are rarely needed. However, in very toxic conditions some physicians feel that it is best to give the antiserum in addition to other therapy. Other drugs used include *lincomycin, erythromycin* and rarely, *triacetyloleandomycin.*

Locally erysipelas is treated with ultraviolet and x-ray therapy. Wet dressings of *magnesium sulfate* or aqueous *ichthyol* are helpful in reducing the inflammation.

Scarlet fever may be diagnosed by the use of the Schultz-Charlton test. A minute amount of the antitoxin is introduced into an area of skin which has a definite rash. If there is a blanching in the area after the injection the test is positive and the patient does have scarlet fever.

Diseases Caused by Gram-Negative Rods

BRUCELLOSIS

DEFINITION. Brucellosis is a disease, transmissible to man, most commonly found in goats but also occurring in cows and pigs. In each case the causative agent is a different species of the bacterium. *Brucella melitensis*—goats, *Brucella abortus*—cows, *Brucella suis*—pigs (III-6, 10). The agent is fre-

TABLE 22. BACTERIAL DISEASES

DISEASE	CAUSATIVE AGENT	DRUG THERAPY
Pneumonia (pneumococcal meningitis)	*Diplococcus pneumoniae (D. lanceolatus)*	Penicillin, tetracyclines
Infections	*Staphylococcus* (various strains)	Penicillin (staphylococcic resistant forms), vancomycin
Infections, scarlet fever, erysipelas, puerperal fever, septicemia	*Streptococcus pyogenes* (various strains)	Penicillin, erythromycin, triacetyloleandomycin, lincomycin
Bacterial endocarditis, septicemia	*Streptococcus viridans* (and other organisms)	Penicillin, or antibiotic indicated by sensitivity test
Brucellosis (undulant fever, Malta fever, Bang's disease)	*Brucella melitensis, abortus, suis*	Tetracyclines, streptomycin
Typhoid fever and paratyphoid fever A & B	*Salmonella typhosa* and other species	Chloramphenicol, ampicillin
Bacillary dysentery (Shigellosis)	*Shigella,* various species	Ampicillin, chloramphenicol, sulfadiazine
Cholera	*Vibrio cholera*	Supportive, tetracyclines, streptomycin, chloramphenicol, erythromycin
Gonorrhea	*Neisseria gonorrhoeae*	Penicillin, tetracyclines, spectinomycin, ampicillin
Cerebrospinal meningitis	*Neisseria meningitidis* (intracellularis)	Penicillin, sulfonamides
Influenzal meningitis	*Hemophilus influenzae*	Ampicillin, chloramphenicol
Pertussis (whooping cough)	*Bordetella pertussis*	Ampicillin, tetracyclines, chloramphenicol
Diphtheria	*Corynebacterium diphtheriae*	Antitoxin, antibiotics for complications
Tetanus	*Clostridium tetani*	Tetanus immune globulin (human); antibiotics for complications; sedation; some use muscle relaxants
Gas gangrene	*Clostridium welchii,* etc.	Same as above
Botulism	*Clostridium botulinum*	Same as above, but sedatives are rarely used; mainly symptomatic and supportive treatment
Anthrax	*Bacillus anthracis*	Penicillin, tetracyclines, erythromycin, hyperimmune serum
Tularemia	*Pasteurella tularensis*	Streptomycin, tetracyclines
Plague	*Yersinia pestis*	Tetracyclines, chloramphenicol, streptomycin
Granuloma inguinale	*Donovania granulomatis*	Tetracyclines
Syphilis	*Treponema pallidum*	Penicillin, tetracyclines, erythromycin; previously preparations of arsenic, bismuth, and mercury were employed
Yaws	*Treponema pertenuae*	Penicillin, tetracyclines, and as above
Rat-bite fever	*Spirillum minus* or *Streptobacillus moniliformis*	Penicillin. Same as above
Relapsing fever	*Borrelia recurrentis (B. obermeieri)*	Same as for syphilis
Vincent's angina	*Borrelia vincentii* and a fusiform bacillus	Penicillin, or other antibiotics
Weil's disease (leptospirosis)	*Leptospira icterohaemorrhagiae*	Penicillin
Tuberculosis	*Mycobacterium tuberculosis*	Streptomycin, viomycin, cycloserine, isoniazid, aminosalicylic acid (calcium, potassium and sodium salts), pyrazinamide, ethambutal, ethionamide, kanamycin
Leprosy	*Mycobacterium leprae*	Sulfones – dapsone, glucosulfone sodium, sulfoxone sodium, sulfetrone, etc., streptomycin may be used; amithiozone is also given

quently transmitted to man in raw milk from infected goats or cows.

MAJOR SYMPTOMS. Brucellosis in man produces a wide variety of symptoms, the most prominent being a series of attacks of fever with afebrile periods between. The disease is often called undulant fever from this tendency for the fever to occur in "undulations." The disease is chronic and many complications and sequelae occur.

DRUG THERAPY. Drugs of all types are used to treat the symptoms and the complications. For the destruction of the organisms and their toxins, various preparations have been employed. The drug of choice is *tetracycline*. Other effective drugs are *chloramphenicol, streptomycin* and the *sulfonamides. Convalescent serum* and *Brucellin* (a preparation containing the antibodies) have been useful in some cases. In acute conditions *corticotropin* or *cortisone* may be used. The dosage of Brucellin is individually established according to the condition of the patient. The other drugs are used in their usual dosages. During the acute attack, intravenous fluids may be required. Vitamins and antianemic drugs are of value between attacks and during convalescence.

TULAREMIA

DEFINITION. Tularemia, so called because it was first identified in Tulare County, California, is a plague-like disease of rodents that is sometimes transmitted to man. Tularemia has also been called "rabbit fever." It is caused by the *Pasteurella tularensis*, a gram-negative rod (III-6, 10). There are several types of the organisms, some of which produce a fatal disease, whereas others produce relatively mild conditions.

MAJOR SYMPTOMS. The symptoms of tularemia vary greatly from one patient to another, the more serious types simulating typhoid fever and pneumonia, the less severe showing glandular involvement without major systemic symptoms.

DRUG THERAPY. An antiserum is available which is especially indicated in the more severe forms of the disease. Transfusions are used when the condition is acute. *Streptomycin* and the *tetracyclines* are helpful, but penicillin is of little use except in complicated cases. Streptomycin is the drug of choice. In severely ill patients who do not respond to streptomycin or tetracycline, *chloramphenicol* is usually given. There is no preparation available for long-term immunity.

PERTUSSIS

DEFINITION. Pertussis (whooping cough) is a severe disease of childhood. It is caused by a gram-negative rod called *Bordetella pertussis* (III-11).

MAJOR SYMPTOMS. Pertussis is characterized by paroxysmal spells of coughing. There is congestion of the mucosa of the respiratory tract and usually bronchopneumonia. With the severe coughing spells vomiting often occurs, making nutrition a problem.

DRUG THERAPY. An effective vaccine is available for pertussis and, with its increasing routine use, less and less of the disease is seen. The vaccine is usually administered along with that for diphtheria and often also for tetanus at two to six months of age, with booster doses at three and six years of age. It is much better to prevent than to attempt to cure this disease, but if it does occur, many drugs can be used. There is a *hyperimmune serum* (Hypertussis) which is often given, especially in the early stages of the disease. *Ampicillin,* the *tetracyclines* or *chloramphenicol* is used for treatment. The last-named is usually given only in severe cases which do not respond to the other drugs.

Symptoms are treated as they occur. Sedatives and hypnotics are often required to insure rest, with *phenobarbital,* 30 to 100 mg., the most commonly used drug of this type. *Potassium iodide* and *ammonium chloride,* 0.3 to 0.6 Gm. for either drug, are used to liquefy the mucus and make its removal easier. *Benzoin* steam inhalations may be helpful, and in severe cases *oxygen* will be needed. Supportive measures must be used, including the various vitamins and other drugs as indicated by the symptoms.

Diseases Caused by Spore-Forming Rods

Botulism, gas gangrene and tetanus are caused by toxins produced by different species of the genus *Clostridium* (III-6).

These are gram-positive, anaerobic, spore-bearing rods that produce potent exotoxins under appropriate conditions.

Botulism was discussed in Chapter 17 with the gastrointestinal disorders.

GAS GANGRENE

DEFINITION. Gas gangrene is a condition caused by any one or more of a number of organisms of the genus *Clostridium*.

MAJOR SYMPTOMS. As the name implies, gas gangrene is characterized by the formation of "gas" in the tissues surrounding an infected wound, and later producing gangrene of the tissues. Gas gangrene also produces a severe systemic toxemia.

DRUG THERAPY. Until the perfection of an effective antiserum, the disease was usually fatal. The disease now is treated with the serum. The use of the antiserum has reduced the mortality rate dramatically, but the disease is still considered serious. Blood transfusions are used to help maintain the patient until the medications can effect a cure. These patients require expert nursing care throughout the entire course of the disease. The patient and his relatives are rightfully very apprehensive and should be encouraged only insofar as the condition of the patient warrants encouragement.

TETANUS

DEFINITION. Tetanus (lockjaw) is probably the most common of this group of diseases. It has long been one of the most dreaded complications of any wound, especially one infected with dirt. It is a severe toxemia, affecting mainly the nervous control of the muscles.

MAJOR SYMPTOMS. Tetanus produces symptoms of muscle involvement, usually beginning with difficulty in swallowing. Later other muscles become involved until convulsions occur. The patient is very sensitive, and the least sensory stimulation will result in a convulsion.

DRUG THERAPY. Tetanus toxoid provides effective immunity and is usually included with pediatric immunizations. Boosters are recommended when the child enters school and at five-year intervals or upon potential exposure. In the event that the patient has not had the toxoid and is injured in such a manner as to make the physician feel that tetanus might occur, temporary passive immunity can be secured by the use of human *tetanus immune globulin* (TIG) or *tetanus antitoxin* of bovine or equine origin. If the patient has had the toxoid, a boster injection may be given.

THE NURSE. In giving this or any antitoxic serum, an intradermal skin test for serum sensitivity should be done. A very small amount, 0.1 ml., is introduced into the skin of the forearm and watched for about 20 minutes. If there is no reaction the antitoxin is given, but if a wheal occurs, the nurse should notify the doctor and secure his orders before giving the serum. Usually it is administered in small doses at intervals of 20 to 30 minutes until the entire amount ordered is given. *Epinephrine* (Adrenalin) 1:1000 solution should be available for use if indicated, since the patient may have a reaction which will be similar to an asthmatic attack. About 0.3 to 1.0 ml. of epinephrine is ordered if needed for a reaction. The nurse must be very careful in giving the antitoxic serum, if the equine preparation is used, to see that the drug is for prophylactic and not for therapeutic use. The latter, used in the treatment of the disease, is a different strength. Usually, 1500 to 10,000 units are given intramuscularly or subcutaneously for prophylaxis. The therapeutic dosage may range from 10,000 to 100,000 units.

Should the disease occur, it requires (as do all the clostridial infections) almost heroic work to save the patient's life. Certainly these diseases are ones in which "an ounce of prevention is worth several pounds of cure."

Tetanus is often classified as mild, moderate or severe. Obviously, treatment will not be the same for all three types. However, the same drugs may be used in different doses. If the patient is seen early enough, most physicians give either the tetanus immune globulin (TIG) or tetanus antitoxin in relatively large doses. The antitoxin does not remove any toxin already attached to the nerves, but it will react with and detoxify any still in the blood stream. If available, the human immune serum is preferred. Up to 100,000 units may be given, if it is necessary to use the tetanus antitoxin. As with any such administration, a serum sensitivity test is done before the antitoxin is given. If the patient shows sensitivity, specific orders must be obtained from the physician.

Sedation is essential. The drugs used and the dosage will depend upon circumstances. Some drugs which may be used include the *barbiturates, chlorpromazine, diazepam, chloral hydrate* or *paraldehyde.* The method of administration will depend upon the drug and the severity of the condition. If the patient cannot swallow, and an oral drug is to be ordered, it is given through a nasogastric tube. The muscle relaxants, *mephenesin* and *meprobamate,* are used in mild or moderately severe tetanus. They are not employed for the very severe form. The dosage necessary to obtain any help in the latter case would be almost or actually toxic. Even in such heavy dosage they might not secure needed muscle relaxation. In such cases, *curare,* or a similar drug is employed. If such a drug is used, it may be necessary to maintain respiration by artificial means. In the more severe cases, aspiration pneumonia is a not uncommon complication. A suitable anti-infective drug is used to control the infection. One of the urinary antiseptics is often employed to aid the kidneys in the excretion of body wastes.

Electrolyte and fluid balance must be maintained, as must nutrition. In severe cases, total parenteral nutrition may be required. In all cases a close watch must be kept on the electrolytes, and usually intravenous fluids are used to correct any deficiency.

The Patient. Tetanus is a very frightening condition, both for the patient and his relatives, and the nurse should do all in her power to lessen the strain for them. Reassurance will help greatly, and with modern medicinal therapy, it can honestly be given in the vast majority of cases. Of course, if the nurse has any doubt of the outcome, she should refer all questions to the physician.

To aid in the effectiveness of the drugs, the nurse should see that the environment of the patient is the best possible. This means that there must be nothing to cause stimulation; noise should be reduced to a minimum, the light should be subdued but not eliminated and everyone entering the patient's room should be careful to do so without exciting the patient. Even jarring the bed may cause a convulsion.

Since tetanus is such a serious disease the patient should have all possible aid, including not only medicinal but psychologic and spiritual as well. The nurse should endeavor to see that the patient secures mental and emotional as well as physical rest.

A calm, soothing voice and an unhurried manner are very helpful in supporting relaxation. Clear explanations must always be given prior to nursing intervention. Severe loss of muscular control produces a tremendous sense of helplessness and hence, anxiety.

The patient's family may also need support. There may be feelings of guilt due to the accidental injury which brought on the disease.

Other Bacterial Diseases

DIPHTHERIA

DEFINITION. Diphtheria is a severe disease caused by *Corynebacterium diphtheriae* which has in the past caused untold numbers of deaths, especially in infants and small children.

MAJOR SYMPTOMS. Diphtheria is characterized by local inflammation and membrane formation and by a systemic toxemia. It occurs most often on the oropharynx, but may affect any mucous membrane.

DRUG THERAPY. Diphtheria is much less prevalent now than it once was thanks to a very effective toxoid which produces a fairly long active immunity. The toxoid along with tetanus toxoid and pertussis vaccine, is usually given to the infant at about two to six months of age and then is repeated at about three, and again at about five or six years of age, just before the child enters school. Later in life the Schick test (an intradermal skin test for susceptibility) can be used to ascertain susceptibility, and further toxoid given if the need is indicated. A sort-term passive immunity may be secured by the use of the antitoxin. The same procedure should be used as was discussed under Tetanus to be sure the patient is not allergic to the serum.

Diphtheria now is relatively rare since most of the susceptible individuals have been immunized, but there is still an occasional case. When this does occur it calls for prompt and energetic treatment. The patient often rapidly becomes acutely ill and must have the advantage of every available help to overcome the infection. *Penicillin*, often in large doses is usually given with the *antitoxic serum*, 20,000 units or more as indicated by the patient's condition. The penicillin will destroy the organism and at the same time the antitoxic serum will neutralize the toxin. If the patient is allergic to penicillin, *erythromycin* is usually used. The *tetracyclines* are also effective. The drugs are never a complete substitute for the serum since the toxemia is the most serious part of the disease.

Diphtheria tends to cause cardiac disorders, and it may also cause paralysis. These and other symptoms are treated as they appear: sedatives for restlessness, intravenous fluids for support and *epinephrine* (Adrenalin) if the patient reacts unfavorably to the antitoxin. If the patient's breathing is difficult, steam inhalations with or without *compound tincture of benzoin* may be used.

LEPROSY

DEFINITION. Leprosy is caused by *Mycobacterium leprae*—an acid-fast bacterium similar to *Mycobacterium tuberculosis* which causes tuberculosis (III-6). Leprosy is one of the oldest known diseases. It has been mentioned in the very earliest writings. It is a chronic disease which, if untreated, cripples the patient, who usually dies either from the disease itself or from some intercurrent infection.

MAJOR SYMPTOMS. Leprosy is a mildly communicable disease which is characterized by skin and nerve involvement with anesthesia, terminal vasoconstriction, nodular enlargements of subcutaneous areas and often gangrene of the terminal phalanges.

DRUG THERAPY. Although authorities vary as to dosage amounts and schedules, all agree that the sulfone preparation, *dapsone,* U.S.P. (Avlosulfon) (diaphenylsulfone [C]), is the drug of choice for the treatment of leprosy. It is given orally starting with a low dose and increasing gradually to a maintenance level established individually. The beginning dose may be as low as 10 mg. weekly, increasing to a maximum of 400 mg. twice weekly. The drug has few side effects except in high dosage and these are usually avoided by the gradual increase in the size of the dose. If the drug does upset the gastrointestinal tract as sometimes occurs, *solapsone* (Sulphetrone) may be given either deep subcutaneously or intramuscularly. This drug is not now available in the United States. *Glucosulfone sodium,* U.S.P. (Promin) given intravenously or sulfoxone sodium (Diasone) given intramuscularly may be substituted for dapsone. In acute exacerbations and/or when the eyes are involved with iritis or keratitis, some physicians use a steroid preparation for a short period. The steroid is rarely given for long periods, whereas the sulfone drugs may be administered over a period of years. It is thought best to continue the sulfone medication even after apparent cure to prevent a relapse which is very discouraging to the patient.

Diphenylthiourea (DPT) has been used as has streptomycin, but most doctors consider these drugs too toxic for long-term use and they appear to have no advantage over the less toxic sulfone drugs. Experience has shown that in most cases they are less effective.

THE NURSE. Since leprosy is a long-term, chronic disease, the nurse will need to keep the patient interested in continuing treatment. Often the symptoms of the disease will all but disappear, with a relapse later if treatment is withdrawn. It is important for the nurse to see that the drugs are continued even in the face of an apparent recovery.

The nurse's main responsibility in relationship to leprosy, is probably the dispensing of accurate information concerning the disease and dispelling the superstitions which surround it.

THE PATIENT. The stigma of leprosy has persisted for centuries and, in spite of modern knowledge, is still strong (IV-1). Leprosy is not easily communicable; only in terminal cases is it disfiguring; and it is now responding well to modern treatment. In spite of all this, patients with this disease, or with an arrested condition, are often treated with less consideration than is given to criminals. The nurse can do much to dispel the superstitions which surround the disease and help the patient who has or who has had leprosy to overcome the adverse attitude of the public toward him.

There are not many cases of leprosy in the United States, but because of the social stigma attached to it, it is important. The public should be informed that this disease is not a horrible plague, that it is curable and that patients with the disease are not dangerous to others. Physicians who have studied the disease feel that direct transfer from one person to another is rare except when the predisposing factors are the same for both people. There are many, many more diseases that are infinitely easier to pass from one individual to another.

Leprosy is a chronic, long-term disease that has been and still is surrounded by superstition and misunderstanding. With modern therapy, the disease is not disfiguring, rarely debilitating enough to require hospitalization or even bed rest at home. Most cases are now treated in the physician's office or in an outpatient clinic. The United States does maintain two leprosy sanitariums, one on the island of Molokai in Hawaii, and the other at Carville in Louisiana. Because of the attitude of so many people toward the "leper," some patients prefer to stay in the sanitaria.

FUNGAL INFECTIONS

The mycotic diseases are of two main types, dermal and systemic (III-14). There are certain similarities to all systemic fungal infections; they are all relatively rare, slow in developing and very difficult to eradicate because of the tendency to form spores. Many patients with fungal diseases succumb to intercurrent infection rather than to the primary mycotic condition. Refer to Table 23 and Chapter 23 for drug therapy.

PROTOZOAL INFECTIONS

Of the major protozoal infections, only amebic dysentery and malaria are endemic in the United States. Most of the protozoal infections are tropical and subtropical in locale. There is not much similarity among the various protozoal infections except that of the causative agents and also the fact that no effective agent for active immunization has been found for them (III-18, 19).

Malaria

DEFINITION. Malaria has been said to be the most widespread and the most prevalent disease in the world. It is a great killer, but more than that it is a very debilitating condition which saps the strength of its victim long before it kills. It is caused by a protozoan known as the plasmodium which is transmitted by the mosquito (III-1).

MAJOR SYMPTOMS. Malaria is characterized by paroxysms of chills and fever, occurring at regular or irregular intervals according to the type of organism infecting the patient. The malarial parasite destroys the red blood cells, which not only produces anemia but also lessens the effectiveness of all the organs by reducing their available oxygen supply.

TABLE 23. *MYCOTIC DISEASES*

DISEASE	CAUSATIVE ORGANISM	DRUG THERAPY
Actinomycosis	*Actinomyces bovis* (intermediary between bacteria and fungi)	Penicillin, sulfadiazine, tetracyclines, chloramphenicol
Moniliasis	*Candida albicans*	Nystatin (Mycostatin), tetracycline, amphotericin-B
Coccidioidomycosis	*Coccidioides immitis*	Amphotericin-B, Ethyl Vanillate, and hydroxystilbamidine
Blastomycosis	*Blastomyces dermatitidis*	Amphotericin-B, hydroxystilbamidine, stilbamidine, iodides
	Blastomyces brasiliensis	Same as above and sulfonamides
Histoplasmosis	*Histoplasma capsulatum*	Ethyl Vanillate, amphotericin-B
Cryptococcosis	*Cryptococcus neoformans (Torula histolytica)*	Amphotericin-B
Chromoblastomycosis	*Phialophora verrucosa* *Hormodendrum compactum*	Same as other mycotic infections; no really specific drug
Aspergillosis	*Aspergillus fumigatus*	Same as above

***TABLE 24.** PROTOZOAL INFECTIONS*

DISEASE	CAUSATIVE AGENT	DRUG THERAPY
Amebiasis (amebic dysentery)	*Entamoeba histolytica*	Many drugs are used: salts of arsenic glycobiarsol (Milibis; bismuth glycolyl arsanilate [C]), etc., emetine hydrochloride, metronidazole (Flagyl; Trikamon [C]), diiodohydroxyquin (Diodoquin; diiodohydroxyquinoline, Direxide [C]), carbasone (Ameban), iodochlorhydroxyquin (Vioform; iodochlorhydroxyquinoline, Domeform, Quinambicide [C])
Malaria	*Plasmodium vivax, ovale, malariae* and *falciparum*	Chloroquin phosphate (Aralen; Quinochlor [C]), Amodiaquin hydrochloride (Camoquin; Flasoquin [C]), hydroxychloroquine sulfate (Plaquenil), quinine sulfate or hydrochloride, quinacrine hydrochloride (Atabrine; mepacrine hydrochloride [C]), pyrimethamine (Daraprim) and others
Toxoplasmosis	*Toxoplasma gondii*	Sulfonamides, pyrimethamine (Daraprim)
Leishmaniasis (kala-azar)	*Leishmania donovani*	Stilbamidine and hydroxystilbamidine; organic antimonials
Trypanosomiasis (African sleeping sickness)	*Trypanosoma gambiense, rhodesiense*	Melarsoprol, Suramin, pentamidine. These drugs may be obtained from: Parasitic Disease Drug Service, National Communicable Disease Center, Atlanta, Georgia.

DRUG THERAPY. Malaria has been treated with *quinine sulfate* for many, many years with the usual dosage being 0.6 Gm. It is given orally as often as is indicated. Quinine sulfate effectively destroys the malarial parasite, but it causes several undesirable side effects such as ringing in the ears, reduction of auditory acuity, headache, dizziness and sometimes nausea and vomiting. There are any number of synthetic drugs similar to quinine; these are usually used in preference to quinine since they are more effective and less toxic.

The treatment of malaria depends partly upon the type of plasmodium involved, since some drugs are more effective against one kind than against another. For *P. vivax, malariae* and *ovale*, the agents of choice are *chloroquine diphosphate* (Aralen) given 600 mg. initially, 300 mg. six hours later and then 300 mg. daily for two days; *Amodiaquine dihydrochloride* (Camoquin), dosage 600 mg. initially, then 400 mg. daily for two days; or *hydroxychloroquine sulfate* (Plaquenil) in the same dosage as chloroquine (Table 24). To eliminate tissue forms of the plasmodia, *primoquin diphosphate* 26.4 mg. is given daily for 14 days. The drug can cause hemolytic anemia in some patients, although commonly of a transient and mild nature.

In malaria caused by *P. falciparum*, the same drugs are used unless the organism is known to be resistant to them, in which case the patient is usually treated with *quinine sulfate* 0.6 Gm. given every eight hours for 10 days and *pyrimethamine* (Daraprim) 50 mg. daily for three days, administered parenterally. In severe cases *quinine dihydrochloride* may be given intravenously 0.6 Gm. one to three times a day. Not more than 2.0 Gm. should be given in any 24 hour period.

Other drugs that may be given for malaria include *quinacrine hydrochloride* (Atabrine, Mepacrine hydrochloride [C]). Most of the malarial drugs are relatively nontoxic, although quinacrine causes a reversible jaundice, clearing as soon as the drug is withdrawn. *Pamoquine* (Plasmochin) is sometimes used with one of the other drugs. It is rarely used alone since it is effective only against the gametes (III-19). *Vitamins,* especially the B-complex, *iron* and other antianemic drugs are given to improve the blood picture.

Interactions. The acidifying agents antagonize quinine and chloroquine, whereas the alkalinizing agents potentiate them. Pamoquine is enhanced by quinacrine by displacement at the binding site.

Since there is no effective vaccine for malaria, *quinine* or *quinacrine* is often given in small daily doses to people who have to live in or go into known malarial districts. These drugs destroy the organism upon its entrance into the body before it has a chance to make the person ill. If the dosage is accurately estimated, the individual suffers no ill effects from the drug yet does not become ill if bitten by an infected mosquito.

TABLE 25. HELMINTHIC INFESTATIONS*

DISEASE	CAUSATIVE ORGANISMS	DRUG THERAPY
Nematodes (roundworms)		
Ancylostomiasis (hookworms)	*Ancylostoma duodenale* *Necator americanus*	Bephenium hydroxynaphthoate, pyrantel pamoate, chenopodium, thymol, tetrachloroethylene (most commonly used)
Ascariasis (giant intestinal roundworms)	*Ascaris lumbricoides*	Piperazine (Antepar), hexylresorcinal, bephenium hydroxynaphthoate, pyrvinium pamoate (Povan; viprynium, Pamovin [C]), pyrvinium chloride (Vanquin)
Enterobiasis (pinworms)	*Enterobius vermicularis* *Oxyuris vermicularis*	Piperazine, pyrvinium pamoate (Povan), pyrantel pamoate, thiabenzole (Mintezol), diphenan, quassia as enema
Strongyloidiasis (threadworms)	*Strongyloides stercoralis*	Thiabenzole (Mintezol)
Trichinosis	*Trichinella spiralis*	No specific treatment. (See below.[1])
Trichuriasis (whipworms)	*Trichuris trichiura*	Thiabendazole or hexylresorcinol (0.1 per cent solution) 500 ml. as rectal enema
Platyhelminths (flatworms)		
Cestodes (tapeworms)		
American or dwarf	*Hymenolepis nana*	All are treated with niclosamide (drug obtained from Communicable Disease Center—see Table 24)
Beef	*Taenia saginata*	
Pork	*Taenia solium*	
Fish	*Diphyllobothrium latum*	
Hydatid disease (echinococcosis)	*Echinococcus granulosus*	No effective therapy for this last one; surgery may be used to excise the affected areas
Trematodes (flukes)		
Schistosomiasis	*Shistosoma haematobium* (blood flukes—bilharziasis) *Schistosoma mansoni* (intestinal flukes) *Schistosoma japonicum* (Oriental flukes)	Antimony (tartar emetic), stibophen (Fuadin), Anthiomaline, lucanthone hydrochloride All are treated alike

*Refer to Chapter 17 for discussion of these diseases.

[1]For severe symptoms—steroids. Alternate drug—thiabendazole. It appears to allay symptoms and reduce eosinophilia, but its effect on larvae that have migrated to muscle is questionable.

TABLE 26. REVISED SCHEDULE FOR ACTIVE IMMUNIZATION AND TUBERCULIN TESTING OF NORMAL INFANTS AND CHILDREN IN THE UNITED STATES

2 mo.	DTP[1]	TOPV[2]
4 mo.	DTP	TOPV
6 mo.	DTP	TOPV
1 yr.	Measles[3]	Tuberculin Test[4]
1–12 yr.	Rubella[3]	Mumps[3]
1½ yr.	DTP	TOPV
4–6 yr.	DTP	TOPV
14–16 yr.	Td[5]	and thereafter every 10 years

[1]DTP—diphtheria and tetanus toxoids combined with pertussis vaccine.

[2]TOPV—trivalent oral polio virus vaccine. The above recommendation is suitable for breast-fed as well as bottle-fed infants.

[3]May be given at 1 year as Measles-Rubella or Measles-Mumps-Rubella combined vaccines.

[4]Frequency of repeated tuberculin tests depends on risk of exposure of the child and on the prevalence of tuberculosis in the population group.

[5]Td—combined tetanus and diphtheria toxoids (adult type) for those over six years of age in contrast to diphtheria and tetanus (DT) containing a larger amount of diphtheria antigen.

Tetanus toxoid at time of injury: For clean, minor wounds, no booster dose is needed by a fully immunized child unless more than 10 years have elapsed since the last dose.

For contaminated wounds, a booster dose should be given if more than 5 years have elapsed since the last dose.

Routine smallpox vaccination is no longer recommended.

Approved by the Committee on Infectious Diseases, October 17, 1971 American Academy of Pediatrics

IT IS IMPORTANT TO REMEMBER

1. That in the treatment of any communicable disease the nurse is confronted with two or more problems—the care of the patient, the prevention of the further spread of the disease and possibly the determination of how the patient became infected in order to eliminate the focus.
2. That it is important for the nurse to know all the diseases for which preventives are available, both for active and for passive immunization, and the circumstances under which these should be used. In this way she will be in a position to advise those who may be exposed to a specific disease or who wish information about control of various diseases.
3. That the prime purpose of the nurse, as well as all health workers, is to keep people well rather than to get people well.
4. That health teaching is one of the most important duties of every nurse, and nowhere does she have a better opportunity for health teaching than in the field of the communicable diseases.
5. That in most communicable diseases drugs form the main therapy and are, therefore, very important.

TOPICS FOR STUDY AND DISCUSSION

1. Make a list of diseases for which active immunizing agents are available. Give name of agent, dosage, routine for administration and any other important data. Refer to Chapter 7.
2. Make a list of diseases for which passive immunizing agents are available. Give name of agent, dosage, routine for administration and any other important data. Refer to Chapter 7.
3. Secure from the local school department or the country, state or provincial health department a list of immunizations required for entrance into the public schools. Why do you think these immunizations are required? Why not others listed in this chapter or in Chapter 7?
4. Outline a talk that might be given before a mothers' group on the immunization of children or on an immunization program for infants and small children.

5. Describe factors that are responsible for the marked decrease in communicable diseases over the past 100 years.

6. If possible, secure from several state or provincial health departments in various parts of the country lists of the communicable diseases reported in that area for the previous year. Compare the lists and try to explain similarities and differences among them.

7. Quinacrine hydrochloride has been ordered for a patient with malaria. The dose is to be gr. 1½ b.i.d. The nurse finds that the drug is in scored tablets marked 0.1 gm. each. How should she proceed?

8. Describe in detail how to give a potassium permanganate foot bath in the home. Presume you are giving directions to someone else who is to do the treatment.

9. The physician orders a foot bath of 1:8000 potassium permanganate solution. The drug is found to be in tablets of 0.12 Gm. each. How should the solution be prepared?

BIBLIOGRAPHY

Books and Pamphlets

American Medical Association Council on Drugs, *Drug Evaluations*, Chicago, 1971, American Medical Association.

American Pharmaceutical Association, *Evaluation of Drug Interactions*, Washington, 1972, American Pharmaceutical Association.

Beeson, P. B., and McDermitt, W., *Cecil-Loeb Textbook of Medicine, 13th Ed.*, Philadelphia, 1971, W. B. Saunders Co.

Beland, I., *Clinical Nursing: Pathophysiological and Psychosocial Approaches, 2nd Ed.*, New York, 1970, The Macmillan Co.

Conn, H. F., et al., *Current Therapy, 1974*, Philadelphia, 1974, W. B. Saunders Co.

Falconer, M. W., Patterson, H. R., and Gustafson, E. A., *Current Drug Handbook, 1974-76*, Philadelphia, 1974, W. B. Saunders Co.

Goodman, L. S., and Gilman, A., *Pharmacological Basis of Therapeutics, 4th Ed.*, New York, 1970, The Macmillan Co.

Hartshorn, E. A., *Handbook of Drug Interactions*, Cincinnati, 1971, University of Cincinnati Press.

Shafer, K. M., et al., *Medical-Surgical Nursing*, St. Louis, 1971, The C. V. Mosby Co.

Watson, J. E., *Medical-Surgical Nursing and Related Physiology*, Philadelphia, 1972, W. B. Saunders Co.

Journal Articles

Ager, E., "Current concepts in immunization," *Am. J. Nurs.* 66:9:2004 (September, 1966).

Brachman, P. S., et al., "Symposium on infection and the nurse," *Nurs. Clin. North Am.* 5:1 (March, 1970).

Bruton, M. R., "When tetanus struck," *Am. J. Nurs.* 65:107 (1965).

Calafiore, D. C., "Eradication of measles in the United States," *Amer. J. Nurs.* 67:1871, (1967).

Coriel, L. L., "Smallpox vaccination. When and whom to vaccinate," *Pediatrics* 37:493 (1966).

"Current immunization data: active immunization for common infectious diseases," *Nurs. Clin. North Am.* 1:2:346 (March, 1966).

Frances, B. J., "Current concepts in immunization," *Am. J. Nurs.*, 73:4:645 (April, 1973).

Gamer, M., "Is smallpox vaccination still necessary?" *R.N.* 31:46 (April, 1968).

Gregg, M. B., "Communicable disease trends in the United States," *Amer. J. Nurs.* 68:88 (1968).

Gunn, A. D. G., "Tetanus," *Nurs. Times* 63:752 (June, 1967).

Hallstrom, B. J., "Contact comfort: its application to immunization injections," *Nurs. Research* 17:130 (March-April, 1968).

Hutchinson, D. A., "Measles vaccine," *Can. Nurse* 64:26 (January, 1968).

Rodman, M. J., "Drugs for treating tetanus," *R.N.* 34:12:43 (December, 1971).

Smith, S., "Biological drugs and vaccines," *Nurs. Times* 63:311 (March, 1967).

van Heyningen, W. E., "Tetanus," *Sci. Am.* 218:69 (April, 1969).

Wexler, L., "Gamma benzine hexachloride in treatment of pediculosis and scabies," *Am. J. Nurs.* 69:565 (1969).

Williams, R. F., "Clinical infection. 1," *Nurs. Times* 63:1572 (November, 1967).

CHAPTER 32

DRUGS USED FOR MISCELLANEOUS DISORDERS OF THE NEUROLOGICAL SYSTEM

CORRELATION WITH OTHER SCIENCES

I. ANATOMY AND PHYSIOLOGY

1. The nervous system is made up of the brain, spinal cord, ganglia and peripheral nerves.
2. Anatomically it has two divisions, the central nervous system and the peripheral nervous system.
3. Physiologically it also has two parts, the cerebrospinal nervous system and the autonomic nervous system.
4. Its function is to integrate the functions of the body through communication among various parts and to make the person aware of his surroundings.
5. Nerves may be either sensory (having afferent fibers), motor (having efferent fibers) or mixed (having both afferent and efferent fibers).

III. MICROBIOLOGY

1. Nerve tissue apparently is more susceptible to infections from the viruses and bacteria than from the other classes of organisms.

IV. PHYSICS

1. The nerve impulse is a combination of physical-electrical-chemical changes.
2. The brain emits weak but measurable electrical impulses. The normal or usual pattern of these rhythmic vibrations has been established.

V. PSYCHOLOGY

1. Chronic illness or long enforced idleness produces adverse emotional reactions.
2. Every normal individual wants to feel that he has a great deal of will power, and he must bolster his ego whenever he feels that he is losing this power.

VI. SOCIOLOGY

1. Fear of being unable to compete with the average person produces an unfavorable reaction in the individual, especially if he is the bread winner of the family.
2. Ridicule and ostracism are powerful social weapons which are often used against any member of a social group who deviates physically, emotionally or in any other way from the accepted pattern of the group.
3. The long-range therapy needed by some of these patients may prove expensive. Every possible attempt should be made to ensure continued therapy.

INTRODUCTION

The study of disorders of the nervous system, including the brain, spinal cord and peripheral nerves, has become increasingly important during recent years (I-1, 2, 3, 4). Because of better methods of diagnosis, conditions that had not been clearly understood previously are now known to be neurologic in nature. Available to the neurologist are many new diagnostic procedures which will often pinpoint the disturbance, thus allowing much more effective treatment.

Although its use usually does not constitute the largest portion of the treatment of these conditions, the role of medicine is an important one. Medicines are used alone in some diseases and in conjunction with other therapy in other disorders. Diseases of the nervous system, exclusive of the communicable diseases and the neoplasms, are not so numerous as are conditions caused by trauma or those which are secondary to other disease.

Neurology and neurosurgery are important specialties in the general field of medicine, and the nurse must be qualified to aid the physician in the care of the neurologic patient. The nurse caring for these patients must be especially alert to observe all symptoms, for the smallest detail may be exceedingly important. Changes in expected results from medicines may be very important to the physician and should be noted and reported promptly. Medicines ordered for these patients are given to aid in diagnosis, for treatment and as supportive measures.

TRAUMATIC INJURY TO THE CENTRAL NERVOUS SYSTEM

Most traumatic injuries are treated surgically; however, drugs may be used to ameliorate the condition. There has been a great increase in such injuries in recent years caused by machines, including the automobile. Many of these cause serious damage to the brain, the spinal cord and the nerves as well as to the skeletal system. Head injuries are an all too frequent result of automobile accidents.

Brain Injury

Since the brain injury often causes intracranial hemorrhage, the treatment outlined under Cerebrovascular Accident would apply. Most physicians do not order opiates, especially morphine sulfate, as it is believed that these drugs increase the difficulty by depressing the respirations and also tend to mask other symptoms which might aid in diagnosis. Every effort is made to give the patient rest, but since marked depression must be avoided, the depressant drugs are used sparingly. Occasionally small doses of the barbiturates are ordered, but the nurse must watch carefully and report immediately any adverse symptoms. The respiratory and the cardiac stimulants are also used with care, especially if there has been hemorrhage, since they may increase the bleeding.

Hypertonic solutions, such as *mannitol* 10 to 20 per cent, are commonly used. This is given intravenously 100 to 500 ml. over a period of one to several hours. It reduces intracranial pressure. However, the pressure may again rise after the therapy. Some physicians use the corticosteroid, dexamethasone, to aid in the reduction of cerebral edema.

Spinal Cord Injury

Most spinal cord injuries are also treated surgically, medicines forming only a supportive, but essential, role in therapy.

Each symptom is treated as it occurs. Thus, *neostigmine methylsulfate* (Prostigmin) may be required for retention and flatulence, stimulants for cardiac or respiratory depression, narcotics for pain and hypnotics for sleep. Often *penicillin* or another antibiotic is given to prevent infection—especially pneumonitis which is apt to occur as a result of reduction of movement in such cases.

The nurse must remember that, with the spinal cord injury, the patient does not have normal sensation, and the usual skin sensations cannot be depended upon to tell how the medications are acting. It is necessary to observe closely to determine the results of the drugs and treatments given.

TRAUMATIC INJURY TO PERIPHERAL NERVES

Trauma of the peripheral nerves is not uncommon, but therapy is surgical and not medical. However, some surgeons give the broad-spectrum antibiotics to cure or to prevent infection and vitamin B-complex to aid in the reparative process. Vitamin B seems to increase the healing of nerves, but even with the best of surgery and medical care the repair of a nerve is always a very slow process, and the patient should be warned that such is the case (V-1). He must not expect too rapid a recovery. If the nerve has been badly damaged it will be several months before function will be restored, and there may never be complete recovery (VI-1).

INFLAMMATORY DISORDERS OF PERIPHERAL NERVES, CRANIAL AND SPINAL

There are a large number of peripheral nerves which branch from the main root nerves, the 12 pairs of cranial and the 31 pairs of spinal nerve roots. The spinal nerves are all mixed nerves, carrying both afferent and efferent fibers. Cranial nerves may contain both types of fibers, or they may be entirely sensory containing only afferent fibers, or all motor containing only efferent fibers. Disturbance of the mixed nerves may cause either sensory or motor disturbances or both (I-5, IV-1).

Neuritis and neuralgia are the principal disorders of the nerves, and the nurse must be aware of the distinct difference between these two conditions. The words are often misused. Neuralgia, nerve pain, may be the chief symptom of neuritis or inflammation of the nerve, or it may occur without there being any real infection of the nerve or any inflammatory process in the nerve. The treatment of neuritis is directed toward the cure of the inflammatory process, and the treatment of neuralgia is the relief of pain. The pain may be relieved by giving an analgesic, thereby dulling the brain so that it does not "feel" the sensation of pain, or it may be relieved by the blocking of the impulse anywhere along the course of the nerve or by removal of the cause of the pain, if that is possible.

Simple Neuritis

Simple neuritis, when one or a small group of nerves is affected, is usually treated by mild analgesics and the broad-spectrum antibiotics. Since neuritis is often the result of some other infection, the medicinal treatment will be directed toward the cause.

Polyneuritis

DEFINITION. Polyneuritis is usually caused by one of two things: metallic poisons or vitamin deficiency, frequently of the B-complex. It is an inflammatory process in several of the peripheral nerves.

SYMPTOMS. Polyneuritis is a very painful condition since many nerves are involved. Function may be impaired as it is painful to contract the muscles. In some cases edema may be a complicating factor. Sensory manifestations include a pain that may be described as deep and aching, sharp, pricking or burning or a mixture of these.

DRUG THERAPY. This, naturally, varies according to the cause of the condition and also the urgency of the case. The offending agents should be removed if possible. Therapy then is directed to care of the limbs, relief of pain and restitution.

VITAMIN THERAPY. It is likely that when the condition arises from a nutritional deficiency, more than one vitamin is concerned. *Vitamin B-complex* is the group most strongly involved, with *thiamine* usually the most important one. The recommended daily allowance for this vitamin has been determined, but in treating deficiency states, this amount must be greatly increased. No exact dosage can be given since it is regulated to suit the individual patient.

Thiamine chloride may be given either orally or parenterally. This is a water soluble vitamin and is not stored in the body so there should be no side or toxic effects.

Bedrest is usually advisable at least during the acute stage. The diet of these patients should be rich in vitamin B, and the nurse, after consulting with the physician, can aid the patient to make the right selection of foods to meet his needs. Most physicians order a diet high in all the vitamins since the patient is often undernourished. Like many malnourished people, the patient may not wish to eat the proper foods, and every effort must be made to secure his cooperation.

Analgesics. If the pain is mild, aspirin, 0.65 Gm. as often as every two hours, may be sufficient. When the pain is very severe, stronger analgesics such as *codeine*, 32 mg., *pentazocine* (Talwin) 30 to 60 mg. or *meperidine* (Demerol; pethidine, Pethidone [C]), 75 to 100 mg. every four hours, may be ordered. The narcotics should be used cautiously because the long duration of the condition may predispose the patient to addiction. Sedatives are given as needed for sleep.

Dimercaprol

The Drug. Dimercaprol (BAL) is the result of extensive research to find a drug which would be an antidote for war gases, hence, its other name—British-Anti-Lewisite.

Physical and Chemical Properties. Dimercaprol, a chemical compound, is a dithiol analogue of glycerol. It is a clear, colorless, viscous liquid with a pungent, disagreeable odor, often described as garlic-like or skunk-like. It will form a 7 per cent aqueous solution and is also soluble in plant oils, alcohol and other organic solvents.

Action. Because it is a dithiol, it competes with physiologically essential cellular sulfhydryl groups for arsenic, mercury or gold, thus preventing the combination of the heavy metal with the tissue sulfhydryls.

Therapeutic Uses. Its primary use is in treatment of arsenic poisoning but it may be effective in mercury or gold poisoning.

Absorption and Excretion. Clinical evidence indicates that when given intramuscularly, the highest systemic concentrations are attained within one-half to two hours, and absorption and detoxification are essentially complete within four hours. It is believed that some of the dimercaprol is excreted in the urine in the form of the glucuronide.

Preparation and Dosages. Dimercaprol, U.S.P., B.P., (British Anti-Lewisite, BAL), is marketed in 4.5 ml. ampules which consist of a solution of 10 per cent dimercaprol in peanut oil. To be maximally effective, it must be given in courses.

The Nurse

Mode of Administration. This compound is administered almost exclusively by deep I.M. injection. Topical application is limited to the treatment of local lesions of the skin and eyes produced by arsenical vesicants.

Side Effects. There may be local pain and tenderness at site of injection following administration but severe local reactions do not occur.

Toxic Effects. The toxic effects, although sometimes alarming, do not usually endanger life. The nurse must be alert for an increased pulse and respiratory rate, tremors or even convulsions, nausea and vomiting, headache, a burning sensation of the mucous membranes, conjunctivitis, a sense of constriction in the chest. The blood pressure (both systolic and diastolic) rises within a few minutes after injection and falls to normal levels within two hours. Most symptoms subside in one-half to two hours.

Contraindications. There is no absolute contraindication to the use of dimercaprol (BAL).

Patient Teaching. Many physicians order vitamin B for these patients, especially during convalescence, since it aids in the repair of nerves, and also in the general rebuilding of the patient's health. The nurse should use great care to avoid spilling or even getting the fumes of dimercaprol on her hands or other articles since it will be obnoxious to the patient and to other people as well.

The Patient. The multiple neuritis which accompanies metallic poisoning is a much more severe condition than that caused by vitamin deficiency. The neuritis is, of course, only one symptom of the poisoning, which is a medical emergency. However, the neuritis may be the most distressing symptom to the patient, and he will want relief as soon as it can be secured. The removal of the poisonous chemical will afford some relief, but it must be remembered that the nerves will need time to recover from the damage done by the poison. The patient must understand that recovery may be very slow.

Neuralgia

TIC DOULOUREUX (TRIFACIAL OR TRIGEMINAL NEURALGIA)

DEFINITION. Tic douloureux is a condition in which there is pain along the course of the trigeminal nerve (fifth cranial nerve). It may involve any of the three main branches of the nerve, or all may be affected. However, the more common forms involve either the mandibular or the maxillary branch. It is not often that the ophthalmic branch is primarily affected, and still less common for all three to be affected at one time.

MAJOR SYMPTOMS. The major symptom of trifacial neuralgia is repeated attacks of severe pain and burning along the course of the nerve. As the name implies there may be a "tic" accompanying the pain. Twitching of the eyelid on the affected side is not an uncommon "tic." The pain of trifacial neuralgia is one of the most severe possible.

DRUG THERAPY. No completely successful medicinal therapy has been established for tic douloureux. Some medications help one patient but not another. The following have proven valuable in at least a small percentage of cases:

Vitamin B_{12} may be given parenterally in doses of 1000 μg. daily for two weeks. If there is no improvement, it is then discontinued. Some physicians also order a general vitamin B compound. Though this may not effect any material change in the condition, it often makes the patient feel better.

Diphenylhydantoin (Dilantin) 100 mg. three or four times a day may help. If successful the drug should be continued for several weeks following the last episode of pain.

Mephenesin may be used. It is started with a relatively low dosage, such as 1 Gm. every four to six hours. This is gradually increased as indicated by the patient's reaction. As much as 4 Gm. every four hours may be given. This drug is best given before meals or followed by milk or fruit juice. This aids in avoiding gastric distress.

Carbamazepine (Tegretol) has been used with considerable success for the treatment of tic douloureux. It is given orally 200 to 1200 mg. daily, usually divided doses every 12 hours. When the patient has become pain free, the dosage is gradually reduced over several weeks. This drug is contraindicated in patients receiving the monoamine oxidase inhibitors and during pregnancy and lactation. Patients with liver, renal or significant cardiovascular diseases should not receive the drug. Since the drug has known hemopoietic damage potential, blood tests should be done at frequent intervals during therapy.

Analgesics. Because of the chronic nature of this disease, analgesics are used sparingly, if at all. *Aspirin* may help some patients. During a very severe attack, *pentazocine* (Talwin) may be given. Since this is a nonnarcotic analgesic, it is less apt to cause dependency. The narcotics are usually avoided.

Some physicians inject absolute *ethyl alcohol* into the nerve. This will give relief from the excruciating pain, but it is not a permanent cure. The effect of the alcohol lasts from three to four months and, occasionally, as long as three years. The treatment can be repeated.

THE NURSE. The main problem for the nurse in the care of these patients is to assist them to accept the fact that there may be recurrence of pain and how to avoid this. The patient should stay out of drafts, use care in shaving and washing of the face (use warm water and a mild soap, if any), avoid extremes of either heat or cold about the face, not use harsh material for pillow cases and the like, be careful chewing (especially hard substances) and even avoid talking too long or too loudly. The patient can help to identify stimuli which trigger the pain and learn how to avoid these. The nurse can aid the patient in planning his routines so as to maintain good health.

THE PATIENT. The patient with tic douloureux is faced with a very difficult problem. He is in severe pain a great deal of the time, but there is no lasting help for him, except surgery. Most neurologists recommend surgery, either severing the nerve or removing the gasserian ganglion to which the nerve is attached. If conservative measures are used, the drugs must be administered with caution, especially the analgesics, as the condition is chronic and habituation or even addiction may develop. The fear of the return of the excruciating pain is always present. The family must understand that some of the patient's actions are affected by this.

Sciatica

DEFINITION. Sciatica, pain or inflammation of the sciatic nerve, is a rather common and distressing condition. It is usually caused by trauma or infection. As with most neuralgias, removal of the cause will afford relief. If the condition is the result of trauma, the treatment is surgical; if caused by infection, medical. There are cases of sciatica which do not appear to be caused by either.

MAJOR SYMPTOMS. The major symptoms of sciatica are neuralgia and, to a greater degree than produced by other neuritis, loss of function. The patient with sciatica may not be able to walk or to change position easily. Bending is especially painful.

DRUG THERAPY. The drugs used for sciatica are the same ones that have already been discussed in relation to other forms of neuritis and neuralgia. In addition, the salicylates may give relief.

THE DRUG. *Sodium salicylate* or *aspirin* may be given. The dosage for either of these drugs is 0.3 to 0.6 Gm. every three or four hours.

CONVULSIVE DISORDERS

Epilepsy

DEFINITION. Epilepsy is the most common of the convulsive disorders and is one of the most distressing. The seizures range from a momentary lapse of consciousness to severe convulsive attacks, which most people think of as characteristic of epilepsy. The cause and cure of epilepsy are not known, but, when not complicated by other conditions, it can be fairly well controlled so that the epileptic can lead a relatively normal life. Drugs play a major role here.

MAJOR SYMPTOMS. There are three major kinds of epileptic seizures: petit mal, in which there is momentary loss of consciousness with little or no motor involvement; grand mal, in which there is loss of consciousness complicated with convulsions; and the so-called "epileptic equivalent" or psychomotor attack, in which the individual has some impairment of consciousness and may also exhibit temperamental changes. Thus, the symptoms vary with the type of epilepsy (IV-2). Less frequently seen are seizures which are called myoclonic and akinetic. Some authorities classify them as subdivisions of petit mal.

DRUG THERAPY. The drugs used in the treatment of these conditions are the anticonvulsants, the sedatives and the palliative drugs.

ANTICONVULSANT MEDICATIONS

THE DRUGS. The aim of all anticonvulsant therapy is to establish and maintain a reservoir of drug sufficient to control the seizures with a minimum of side reactions. There are a number of drugs available for the control of seizure disorders but none of these is effective in all types of conditions and each has some degree of undesirable side effects. These drugs have no fixed dosage and are started at what is assumed to be a minimal dose and gradually increased until reasonable control of the seizures is attained or the patient shows signs of overdosage. Not infrequently patients can be maintained better if a combination of two drugs is used, even when only one type of seizure is present. If it becomes necessary to substitute another drug for one of these, the previously used drug is discontinued gradually as the new drug is added. This produces an overlapping of effects and serves to prevent onset of seizures before the new drug can reach effective blood levels. These drugs are thought to raise the threshold of responsiveness of normal neurons which tend to be triggered into activity by excessive discharges of impulses.

There are several types of drugs used as anticonvulsants. Mainly these are the *barbiturates, phenobarbital* (Luminal), *mephobarbital* (Mebaral) and *metharbital* (Gemonil); the diuretics, usually *acetazolamide* (Diamox) and the synthetic anticonvulsant drugs. The latter will be discussed here. A brief consideration of the first two divisions will be given later covering their use in epilepsy. The barbiturates were discussed in detail in Chapter 9, the diuretics in Chapter 18. See also Current Drug Handbook. In some cases of epilepsy the tranquilizers are used. These drugs are discussed in Chapter 30.

Physical and Chemical Properties. There are several anticonvulsant drugs and the chemical properties differ with each group. *Diphenylhydantoin* (Dilantin), *mephenytoin* (Mesantoin) and *ethotoin* (Peganone) are hydantoin derivatives. *Ethosuximide* (Zarontin), *methsuximide* (Celontin) and *phensuximide* (Milontin) are succinimide derivatives. *Trimethadione* (Tridione) and *paramethadione* (Paradione) are ethoxyzoladine compounds. *Phenacemide* (Phenurone) is a cogener of diphenylhydantoin and *primidone* (Mysoline) is a cogener of phenobarbital. All these preparations are soluble in body fluids.

Action. The action of the medication varies with the different compounds and with some the exact method is not known. Most exert their influence directly on the central nervous system raising the threshold of stimulation and thus preventing the seizures.

Therapeutic Uses. The primary use of all these drugs is in the treatment of the various forms of epilepsy. Some are also used in the treatment of certain types of psychoses.

Absorption and Excretion. The fate of these drugs in the body also varies with the different forms. All are readily absorbed from the gastrointestinal tract or parenteral sites and distribution with most preparations is widespread. These drugs are usually degraded by the liver and the metabolites are excreted by the kidneys. See Current Drug Handbook for more information.

Preparations and Dosages. All dosages are individually adjusted.

Diphenylhydantoin, U.S.P., Phenyltoin, B.P. (Dilantin) (Eptoin [C]) 30 to 400 mg. a day, orally.

Diphenylhydantoin sodium 30 to 750 mg. orally, intramuscularly or intravenously.

Mephenytoin (Mesantoin) (Phenantoin [C]) 200 to 600 mg. orally.

Ethotoin (Peganone) (Nirvanol [C]) 2 to 3 Gm. orally.

Ethosuximide, U.S.P., B.P. (Zarontin) (Suxinutin [C]) 0.5 to 3.0 Gm. orally.

Methsuximide, N.F. (Celontin) (Petinutin [C]) 150 to 900 mg. orally.

Phensuximide, N.F. (Milontin) 1 to 3 Gm. orally.

Paramethadione, U.S.P., B.P. (Paradione) 300 to 900 mg. orally.

Trimethadione, U.S.P., Troxidone, B.P. (Tridione) (Trimedone [C]) 0.9 to 2.4 Gm. orally.

Primidone, U.S.P., B.P. (Mysoline) (Mylepsine [C]) 50 to 1000 mg. orally.

Phenacemide (Phenurone) (Epiclase [C]) 2 to 3 Gm. orally.

All dosages are the total daily dose; some are given once each day. However, if not well tolerated, the dose can be divided as needed.

THE NURSE

Mode of Administration. All anticonvulsant drugs may be given orally. They may be given with one glass of water or after meals to minimize gastric distress. Diphenylhydantoin Sodium (Dilantin) can also be given intravenously. It is not given subcutaneously since it is irritating to the tissues. Care should be exercised not to allow infiltration in giving the drug intravenously because of this. The intravenous infusion should be given slowly.

Side Effects. As might be expected the side effects vary with the type of drug used. Usually they are similar in the various groups. *Diphenylhydantoin* (Dilantin), given orally, is a relatively nontoxic drug and adjustment of dosage usually will overcome any undesirable symptoms. These include gingivitis, skin rash, change in color of urine from pink to red to red-brown, gastrointestinal disturbances and central nervous system disorders such as ataxia, giddiness, tremors, visual disturbances and nervousness. If diphenylhydantoin is given too fast intravenously, it can cause cardiovascular collapse, central nervous system depression, cardiac arrhythmias (including ventricular fibrillation) or cardiac arrest. The intravenous infusion rate should not exceed 50 mg. per minute. *Mephenytoin* (Mesantoin) has the same side effects as above. It also is apt to cause drowsiness and is rarely used with phenobarbital. *Ethotoin* (Peganone) exerts side effects similar to the above, but they are usually mild. *Ethosuximide* (Zarontin) may cause gastrointestinal disorders, headache, dizziness or drowsiness and occasionally a transitory skin rash. *Methsuximide* (Celontin) has side effects similar to the above, but is most apt to cause anorexia. It also sometimes causes a "dream-like" state. Phensuximide also exerts the same symptoms, but has less anorexia than methsuximide. Methsuximide may cause the urine to change color from pink to red-brown. *Paramethadione* (Paradione) has side effects similar to those of the parent drug trimethadione (given next). It is considered to be less toxic and side effects are milder. With *trimethadione* (Tridione) the most common side effects are sedation and visual disturbances. The latter effect can usually be overcome with reduced dosage and the wearing of dark glasses. *Primidone* (Mysoline) has only mild side effects such as drowsiness, ataxia, dizziness and nausea. These usually disappear with continued use. The side effects of *phenacemide* (Phenurone) are psychic changes, gastrointestinal disturbances, skin rash, drowsiness and various somatic and central nervous system disorders.

Toxicity. *Diphenylhydantoin* (Dilantin) very occasionally may cause hepatitis with jaundice or blood dyscrasias. If either of these occurs, the drug should be stopped and another drug substituted. *Mephenytoin* (Mesantoin) is more apt to cause toxicity than the parent drug. It may cause a persistent skin rash or blood dyscrasias. *Ethotoin* (Peganone) is less toxic than diphenylhydantoin but symptoms are similar if they occur. With the suximide drugs: *ethosuximide* (Zarontin) has caused blood dyscrasias, *methsuximide* (Celontin) reversible leucopenia, and *phensuximide* (Milontin) reversible renal damage. These usually clear with the discontinuance of the drug, though the blood disorders may persist. *Trimethadione* (Tridione) can cause serious but relatively rare toxic symptoms which include skin rashes, blood dyscrasias, nephrosis, hepatitis; occasionally, it may precipitate a grand mal seizure. *Paramethadione* (Paradione) is less toxic than the parent drug, but the same toxicity has been reported in rare instances. *Primidone* (Mysoline) is relatively nontoxic, but megaloblastic anemia has been reported. *Phenacemide* (Phenurone) may cause blood dyscrasias, hepatitis, nephritis or psychotic disturbance. However, it is used when other drugs fail in the treatment of some psychomotor disorders.

All the anticonvulsants must be continued for long periods of time; hence it is important to watch for early symptoms of toxicity and accumulation. Toxic symptoms of these drugs can be studied easily by consulting Table 27. It will be noted that there is a great similarity of these effects.

Most of these drugs cause some gastric irritation and therefore should be given with meals or immediately after eating. *Diphenylhydantoin* (Dilantin) is known to cause gingival hyperplasia but this can be minimized and controlled by improved oral hygiene.

The eye disturbances most frequently encountered are diplopia and blurring of vision but these usually disappear after adjustment of the dosage.

It is well to point out here that when phenacemide (Phenurone) is given, the nurse should be very alert for any personality change, no matter how slight. Withdrawal or loss of interest on the part of the patient may presage more serious emotional disturbances such as suicidal tendencies and toxic psychosis. The patient should be encouraged to continue under medical supervision.

Interactions. Diphenylhydantoin interacts with many other drugs. The following drugs may raise the blood level of diphenylhydantoin to toxic amounts: isoniazid (especially in individuals who are "slow" in the inactivation of the isoniazid), methylphenidate, benzodiazepine tranquilizers, bishydroxycoumarin and coumarin, phenylbutazone and oxyphenylbutazone. Diphenylhydantoin can potentiate the activity of the following by displacement from the serum binding sites or enzyme inhibition: propranolol, quinidine, tubocurarine, methotrexate and griseofulvin. Diphenylhydantoin is inhibited by phenobarbital through enzyme induction, and it also antagonizes hydrocortisone by enzyme induction. Caution should be used when initiating therapy with most drugs concurrently with diphenylhydantoin since it does interact with so many drugs, the exact number of which has not been established. The other hydantoin preparations have not shown the interactions of dyphenylhydantoin, but they should be suspect on a structural basis.

The Patient. The person with epi-

TABLE 27. SIDE EFFECTS OF ANTICONVULSANT DRUGS*

	G.I. disturb.	Skin eruptions	Drowsiness, lethargy	Dizziness	Ataxia	Headache	Eye disturb.	Blood dyscrasias	Emotional disturb.	Kidney damage	Liver damage	Gingival hyperplasia	
Diphenylhydantoin (Dilantin, Diphenate [C])	✓	X	X	✓	✓		✓	X	✓ T		X	✓	
Ethotoin (Peganone)	✓	✓	✓	✓	✓	✓	✓	X	✓ T			✓	least toxic of group
Phenantoin (Mesantoin, Mesontoin [C])	✓	✓ H	✓	✓	✓			✓					
Trimethadione (Tridione, Trimedone [C])	X	X		X			X	X		X	X		
Paramethadione (Paradione)	✓	✓		✓			✓	X		X	X		less toxic than parent drug
Phensuximide (Milontin)	✓	X	✓	✓					✓				less toxic than others in this group
Methsuximide (Celontin, mesuximide [C])	✓	X	✓	✓	✓	✓	✓		X				
Ethosuximide (Zarontin)	✓	✓	✓	X			X	X	X		X		
Phenacemide (Phenurone)	✓	✓	✓					✓ S	✓ S	✓ S	✓ S		high incidence of untoward effects
Primidone (Mysoline)	X	X	X	X	X				X			X	
Phenobarbital (Luminal) (phenobarbitone [C])		X	✓		X				X				
Mephobarbital (Mebaral)		X	✓		X				X				
Metharbital (Gemonil)		X	✓		X				X				
Acetazolamide (Diamox)	X	✓						X T		X			

*Code: ✓ = common S = serious
X = infrequent or rare T = transient
H = high

lepsy has a fear of recurrent seizures, and embarrassment at having attacks in public. In addition, the restrictive measures imposed on him by misconceptions of the public produce feelings of inferiority and self-consciousness. These can be largely overcome by reassurance and encouragement by the doctor, the nurse and the family. Complete control or, at the least, a significant reduction in the number of seizures can be obtained in about 75 per cent of all patients (V-1). The patient should understand that he must continue under medical supervision for the rest of his life.

Patients should be warned to report any unusual symptoms including fatigue, pallor, easy bruising, bleeding from mucous membranes and sore throat. Because of the great danger of blood dyscrasias developing when most of these drugs are given, the patient should have routine blood counts and urinalyses fairly frequently. Increasing numbers of attacks have been reported to be initiated by increased physical or emotional stress and the ingestion of alcoholic beverages.

These patients need a patient and understanding nurse. She must be prepared to do all in her power to aid them to adjust to their situation. She should also be prepared to dispel any misconceptions and prejudices the public may have concerning epilepsy. Most of these patients do not present a risk in employment and they are not psychotic or retarded, as so many people think.

Members of the family will need to be instructed about caring for the patient during and after a convulsion. They will have to understand the importance of not restraining the patient during a seizure, but rather of protecting him from injury. A padded tongue blade and a nonmetal airway may be kept available in the home environment, but great care must be exercised so that the teeth and tongue are not traumatized by the use of such objects. Many physicians consider it best not to try to put anything between the teeth during the convulsion. The family members must be taught to observe and record the character, location and duration of the muscular movements and the general reactions of the patient before, during and after the seizure. This data should be reported to the physician so he can adjust therapy to suit the particular situation.

A public health nurse would be very helpful in following through with the family teaching. She would also be able to provide the emotional support needed by the entire family.

The patient should be advised to carry a card identifying him as an epileptic or to wear a similar identification bracelet to aid in case of an emergency.

OTHER DRUGS USED IN THE TREATMENT OF CONVULSIVE DISORDERS

Barbiturate Group. The barbiturate group includes: *phenobarbital* (Luminal), *mephobarbital* (Mebaral) and *metharbital* (Gemonil). By far the most commonly used is phenobarbital. The others are used mainly for those patients who do not respond favorably to phenobarbital. See Chapter 9 and Current Drug Handbook for specific information on these drugs.

Dosages are individually adjusted and usually given three or four times a day. Often the last dose is larger than the others. This aids in preventing insomnia and attacks during the night. All these drugs are given orally, but phenobarbital may be given parenterally. This is used in status epilepticus.

Phenobarbital, U.S.P., B.P. (Luminal) 30 to 500 mg.

Mephobarbital, N.F. (Mebaral) 120 to 800 mg.

Metharbital, N.F. (Gemonil) 100 to 300 mg.

The most common side effect from these drugs is drowsiness. Adjustment of dosage is usually all that is required.

Diuretics. The most common diuretic used in the treatment of epilepsy is *acetazolamide* (Diamox) though others can be and are used. It is given 250 to 500 mg. once daily, orally. See Chapter 18 and Current Drug Handbook for details.

Tranquilizers. The tranquilizers are used mainly in those forms of epilepsy in which there is not a definite seizure such as myoclonic and akinetic types. The physician may use any of a number of these drugs, but those of the benzodiazepines such as *diazepam* (Valium) are most commonly used. These drugs are discussed in Chapter 30. See also Current Drug Handbook.

Meprobamate (Equanil) may be used, especially in petit mal in children. It is given 0.4 to 2.0 Gm. daily, orally. See Current Drug Handbook for further information.

Drugs Usually Preferred for the Different Types of Epilepsy. Naturally, physicians differ in their choice of drugs, and many circumstances go into the selection, but the following are often used in the conditions listed:

Grand Mal

ADULT

Primary—diphenylhydantoin (Dilantin) with phenobarbital (Luminal)
Secondary—primidone (Mysoline) and/or mephobarbital (Mebaral)
Others—mephenytoin (Mesantoin)
phenacemide (Phenurone)

CHILD

Primary—phenobarbital (Luminal). This may be sufficient without other drugs.
diphenylhydantoin (Dilantin)
Secondary—primidone (Mysoline)
mephenytoin (Mesantoin)

Petit Mal

ADULT

(This condition is rare in adults.)
Primary—ethosuximide (Zarontin)
trimethadione (Tridione)
phenobarbital (Luminal) This may be all that is required.
Others—acetazolamide (Diamox) used with one or more of the above.

CHILD

Primary—ethosuximide (Zarontin)
trimethadione (Tridione)
Secondary—paramethadione (Paradione)
phensuximide (Melontin)
methsuximide (Celontin)
Others—meprobamate (Equanil).

Psychomotor Equivalent

ADULT AND CHILD

Primary—sodium diphenylhydantoin (Sodium Dilantin)
Secondary—primidone (Mysoline)

Myoclonic and Akinetic Seizures

(These are rare in adults.)

ADULT AND CHILD

Primary—sodium diphenylhydantoin (Sodium Dilantin)
Secondary—ethosuximide (Zarontin)
acetazolamide (Diamox) with other drugs
diazepam (Valium) or other tranquilizer.

Other drugs which may be used to substitute for those above when the patient cannot use the recommended medicine:
Metharbital (Gemonil)
Ethotoin (Peganone)

Status Epilepticus

Status epilepticus is a medical emergency. This occurs when seizures follow so rapidly that the patient does not recover consciousness between episodes. The patient should be hospitalized if at all possible. The first thing to be done is to be sure there is an open airway and that pulmonary ventilation is adequate.

Then an infusion is started and *phenobarbital* is given in the infusion 5 mg. per kg. repeated at 20 to 30 minute intervals as required. The quick acting barbiturates are not recommended as they do not have as much anticonvulsant action as does phenobarbital.

Diphenylhydantoin (Dilantin) 5 mg. per kg. is given in one dose intravenously. It is less effective alone than when given with phenobarbital. When the seizures cease, the patient is started on a suitable regimen as indicated by circumstances.

OTHER NEUROLOGICAL DISORDERS

Paralysis Agitans (Shaking Palsy, Parkinson's Disease)

DEFINITION. Paralysis agitans is a slowly progressive disease of the central nervous system. Because there is preservation of the pyramidal tract and lower motor neurons, it is designated as an extrapyramidal disease. There are three generally recognized types: arteriosclerotic, idiopathic and postencephalitic. The term "parkinsonism" covers the clinical syndrome consisting of the hyperkinetic and hypokinetic features.

MAJOR SYMPTOMS. Both hypokinetic and hyperkinetic features develop gradually. There is a slowing down of movements, loss of arm swing in walking, diminished eye blinking and a mask-like face with decreased response to emotional stimuli. A cog-wheel rigidity of the trunk and extremities causes a propulsive gait. Sialorrhea is common and may be severe. Hyperkinetic features are evidenced by a characteristic tremor of the hands, commonly called "pill-rolling" movement, and indeterminate moving of the head. These disappear in sleep.

DRUG THERAPY. There is no form of therapy that will alter the course of the disease but medicines are helpful in diminishing the symptoms. Drug therapy is only a part of a total program of physical therapy, exercise, psychological support and recreation. Young patients with idiopathic Parkinson's disease are generally more responsive than elderly patients.

Most of the drugs reduce muscular rigidity, resulting in improved posture, balance and coordination. Tremor is less frequently benefited by drug therapy and in some whose severe spasticity is relieved, it may be made even more perceptible. However, some of the drugs are more specific in their central antispasmodic action and cause fewer peripheral (atropine-like) adverse reactions than the belladonna derivatives. The relief of muscle spasm is not long-lasting or complete but any improvement is beneficial, both physically and psychologically. The use of these drugs does tend to delay somewhat the progress of this chronic, slowly crippling disease. None of these drugs are useful in all cases but about one-half to two-thirds of the patients do respond to therapy. Often these drugs are used in combination or with accessory agents. For example, a drug with strong antispasmodic action is given with one that tends to control tremor, or a drug that has a tendency to cause drowsiness is used with one that is a slight central nervous system stimulant.

Individualization of the drug type and dosage is essential for optimal effect. Controlling factors are the patient's age, the underlying cause and the rate of progress of the disease. New drugs are initially started with small doses and increased gradually to optimal effect. The ultimate dose may be five to ten times the starting dose as refractoriness develops. If large doses are needed and the reactions are proportionate, another drug should be tried. As in epilepsy, sudden substitutions are undesirable when supplementing or supplanting existing medication. The frequency, duration and intensity of undesirable effects are related to the size of the dose.

Drugs useful in paralysis agitans may be put into three general classes: atropine-like agents, congeners of the antihistamines and a miscellaneous group.

SYNTHETIC ANTICHOLINERGIC AGENTS (ATROPINE-LIKE DRUGS)

THE DRUGS. There are several synthetic drugs with atropine-like properties. These include: biperiden, caramiphen, cycrimine, procyclidine and trihexyphenidyl. The latter two are the most commonly used. See Current Drug Handbook also.

Physical and Chemical Properties. The chemical structure varies with the different drugs. Trihexyphenidyl resembles atropine. It was synthesized during research for an antispasmodic drug. Cycrimine, biperiden and procyclidine are congeneric compounds related to trihexyphenidyl.

Action. These drugs all have anticholinergic action similar to that of atropine (see Chapter 15). They decrease salivation and tend to make the patient with parkinsonism better able to control his muscles. At the same time they may not decrease the tremors. Their exact mode of action is not known.

Therapeutic Uses. All these drugs are used primarily in the treatment of Parkinson's disease. However, they may be used for any condition requiring anticholinergic action. The anticholinergic drugs are often used with the phenothiazine drugs to decrease the extrapyramidal side effects.

Absorption and Excretion. All these drugs are absorbed from the gastrointestinal tract. Their exact fate in the body is not known.

Preparations and Dosages. The dosages of these drugs are all individually adjusted. It is customary to start with a low dosage and increase as indicated by the response of the patient. It is often necessary to change medications. As the effectiveness of one wears out, another is substituted. The total daily dose may be given at one time or, more often, divided into three or four equal amounts.

Biperiden, N.F. (Akineton), 1 to 2 mg. orally or parenterally, three or four times a day.

Cycrimine hydrochloride, N.F. (Pagitane) 1.25 to 2.5 mg. orally. (Up to 15 mg. daily may be required.)

Procyclidine hydrochloride (Kemadrin) 5 to 10 mg. three or four times a day, orally.

Trihexyphenidyl hydrochloride, U.S.P.,

Benzhexol, B.P. (Artane, Pipanol) 2 to 5 mg. three or four times a day, orally.

THE NURSE

Mode of Administration. Most of these drugs are given orally. Unless there is a tendency to nausea, they are best given before meals, which will cause less dryness of the mouth. The use of hard candy, gum or fluids will aid in overcoming dryness, if the drug cannot be given before meals.

Side Effects. As with all the anticholinergic drugs, there may be dryness of the mouth and throat, giddiness, nervousness or excitement, dizziness, epigastric distress and drowsiness. Excessive weakness or mental confusion is rare unless the patient has had very large doses. Urinary retention and constipation may become persistent problems. Most of the common side effects will disappear with continued medication or a slight reduction in dosage. Most of these drugs are capable of producing epigastric distress, which usually appears early in the treatment. For this reason, they are usually given in divided doses during or before meals or with liquids (milk).

Toxicity. Severe toxic reactions are rare in therapeutic dosages.

Contraindications. These drugs are all contraindicated in glaucoma.

Interactions. Trihexyphenidyl interacts with imipramine or diphenhydramine to increase dryness of the mouth and possible loss of teeth.

Patient Teaching. As with any chronic condition for which there is no cure, the nurse will need to aid the patient to understand and accept his condition and to know the value of the drugs that are to be used. He must know how and when to take them and side effects that may be expected. The patient should understand that if one drug does not help another may be given. The patient must understand that he will need frequent medical check-ups.

THE PATIENT. Younger patients who drive or participate in other activities which require alertness should be on the drugs which produce no sedation.

This is a discouraging disease for it is slowly crippling, and the patient and his family should receive every encouragement to continue treatment (VI-3). Surgery is now being done in selected cases with some fairly good results. As muscular rigidity, spasm and tremor are relieved, the patient exhibits an increased ability to care for himself and a lessening of the characteristic difficulties of ambulation—propulsive gait and a short, stiff, shuffling step.

OTHER DRUGS USED FOR PARKINSON'S DISEASE

The second group of effective drugs are the congeners of antihistamines (diphenhydramine). *Orphenadrine hydrochloride* (Disipal) relieves mainly the rigidity rather than the tremor. It does have a slight euphoriant effect which is often helpful for fatigued, depressed patients. The initial oral dose is 50 mg. three times a day and subsequent doses are adjusted to meet the response of the patient and his tolerance of untoward effects. *Chlorphenoxamine* (Phenoxene; Histol [C]) has actions similar to those of orphenadrine and is given in an initial oral dose of 50 mg. three times daily. Doses up to 100 mg. four times a day may be given if tolerated and required.

The miscellaneous group of drugs include benztropine mesylate, ethopropazine and caramiphen. *Benztropine mesylate,* U.S.P., B.P. (Cogentin) has chemical features of both the atropine-like and antihistaminic drugs. Its action is prolonged but there is no central stimulation. The usual dosage range is from 0.5 to 2.0 mg. orally. If rapid results are needed or there is difficulty swallowing, a very prompt response is obtained by the intramuscular route. It is then started with a single daily dose of 0.5 to 1.0 mg. with 0.5 mg. increments every few days until optimal results are attained.

Ethopropazine hydrochloride, B.P. (Parsidol), a phenothiazine derivative, is a parasympatholytic agent with ganglionic blocking action comparable to that of nicotine, but it produces sufficient depression of the central nervous system to block convulsant activity. It has been found to be helpful in controlling rigidity and has a favorable influence on spasms, tremor, sialorrhea and oculogyric crisis and festination. The medication is usually started at 10 mg. four times a day, increasing by 10 mg. per dose every two to three days to the level of 50 mg. four times a day by the second week.

Caramiphen hydrochloride (Toryn [C]), a synthetic atropine-like agent with weaker mydriatic and antisecretory effects, has potent antispasmolytic effect on smooth muscles. Generally, it seems better suited for postencephalitic parkinsonism than the other two types. It has little effect on tremor but may reduce the rigidity. Although the dosage, like that of the other drugs used, is highly individualized, the doctor may start with 12.5 mg. five times on the first day with increments of 50 mg. in total daily dosage until the disagreeable side effects outweigh the benefits. The maintenance dose may range from 90 to 600 mg. in divided doses at two to three hour intervals.

The antihistamine-type drugs with central sedative action may be preferable for aged patients who cannot tolerate cerebral-stimulating agents well. Some tranquilizers tend to worsen the condition.

Levodopa (Dopar, Larodopa) is a drug based on the knowledge that the level of dopamine (a normal body secretion) in the area of the basal ganglia is lower in patients with parkinsonism than in the normal individual. Dopamine, when administered orally, does not cross the blood-brain barrier, but levodopa, which is the metabolic precursor of dopamine, does cross the barrier. It is presumed that levodopa is converted into dopamine in the basal ganglia. This drug has been most effective in idiopathic parkinsonism, but it has helped in the majority of cases of all types.

There are many adverse reactions, with anorexia, nausea and vomiting being the most common ones. It has been found that patients do best if the usual antiparkinsonism drugs are continued and levodopa is started with a low dose given from four to seven times a day. The dose is gradually increased and the number of times a day decreased until optimum results are obtained or adverse reactions begin. The other drug or drugs that were being given are decreased as the levodopa is increased. Levodopa is usually started with about 300 mg. total daily dose, divided four to seven times. It is given orally. The dosage is increased 50 to 100 mg. a day, every three to four days. Most patients can be maintained on 4 to 6 Gm. per day. Larger doses are not recommended. Before administering this drug, the nurse will do well to read the commercial insert and also to refer to the Current Drug Handbook.

Some patients can be sustained on levodopa alone, but for most, the addition of one of the antiparkinsonism drugs gives the best results. Often, the second drug is one of the atropine-type medications.

Amantadine hydrochloride (Symmetrel) is another drug being used for the treatment of parkinsonism. It is more rapidly effective than is levodopa, but its effectiveness is not as complete and it has not proved to be of as much value for long-term therapy. It is started with 100 mg. given orally after breakfast for five to seven days. Then, an additional 100 mg. is given after lunch. Adverse symptoms include ataxia, tremors, excitability, slurred speech, depression, insomnia and dizziness. Gastrointestinal disturbances may occur, but they are less frequent than with levodopa.

Myasthenia Gravis

DEFINITION. Myasthenia gravis is a chronic disease in which there is progressive muscular weakness. The most commonly involved muscles are the extraocular and other muscles innervated by the cranial nerves. The disease is characterized by exacerbations and spontaneous remissions. It affects most often young females and older males. The cause is often obscure.

MAJOR SYMPTOMS. The symptoms usually develop gradually and there is a definite relationship between exercise and rest. The commonest early sign is ptosis due to involvement of the extrinsic ocular muscles. As the disease progresses, other muscle groups are involved. The patient presents a sleepy appearance, the face is expressionless and apathetic, the voice becomes less and less distinct and swallowing becomes increasingly difficult. Involvement of the muscles of respiration may result in death. The condition varies from day to day and month to month.

DRUG THERAPY. There is no cure but drugs do help lessen the disturbing symptoms. The object here is to restore the patient's strength to the optimal level and to maintain it there with a minimum of deleterious side effects. Management relies mainly on the anticholinesterase compounds.

THE DRUGS. **ANTICHOLINESTERASE AGENTS** Physostigmine (Eserine), a plant alkaloid, was the first of these drugs to be used medicinally. It has a long history of use for many conditions, but espe-

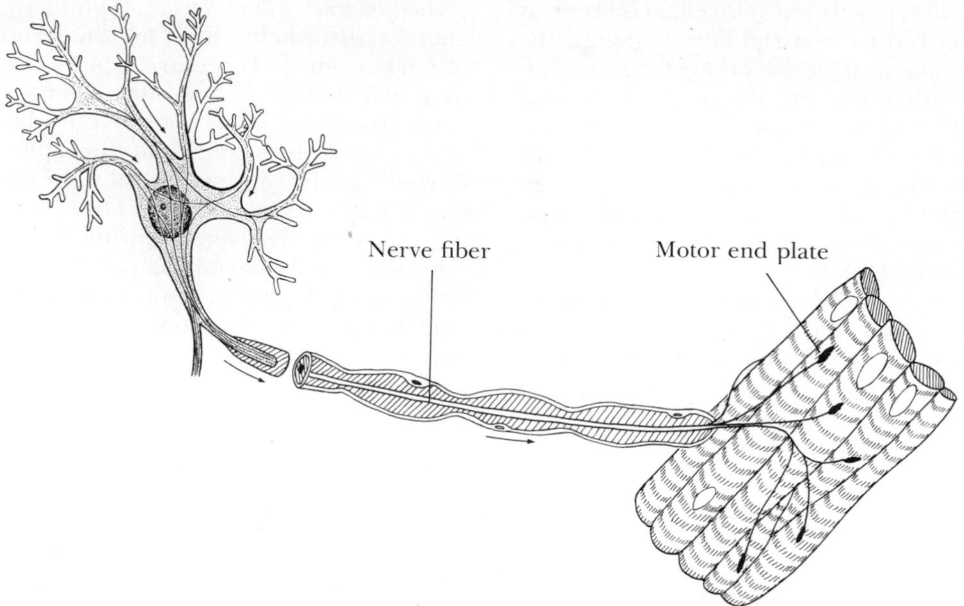

FIGURE 57. The end of the nerve fiber branches so that each muscle cell (fiber) has an end plate.

cially in glaucoma. For myasthenia gravis, the newer synthetic preparations are used. There are any number of these drugs, but the more important ones here are: neostigmine (Prostigmin), pyridostigmine (Mestinon), ambenonium (Mytelase) and edrophonium (Tensilon). See Current Drug Handbook.

Physical and Chemical Properties. All the above compounds except physostigmine contain a quaternary nitrogen. They are relatively soluble, except physostigmine, which is only slightly soluble. Solutions of physostigmine turn pink with time; the more pink the solution, the greater the activity loss. The synthetic compounds with a carbamyl group (neostigmine, pyridostigmine, ambenonium) have greater potency and duration of action than those with just a hydroxyl group (edrophonium).

Action. As the name (anticholinesterase) implies, these drugs inhibit the enzyme cholinesterase, resulting in the accumulation of acetylcholine at the myoneural junction (see Figure 57). In turn this makes the muscle contraction stronger and more prolonged.

Therapeutic Uses. These drugs have many uses. They are used to contract the pupils of the eyes in glaucoma, to diagnose and treat myasthenia gravis and to treat atony of the gastrointestinal and urinary tracts.

Preparations and Dosages. As in so many of these chronic diseases, the type and dosage of the medication is individually adjusted to suit the response of the patient. Each patient reacts differently. A dose suitable for one person may be too much or not enough for another.

Ambenonium chloride, N.F. (Mytelase, Mysuran) 5 to 25 mg. three or four times a day. (Since this is a chloride salt, it can be given to patients who do not respond favorably to the bromide salts).

Neostigmine bromide, U.S.P. (Prostigmin) 15 mg., orally.

Neostigmine methylsulfate, U.S.P. (Prostigmine methylsulfate) 0.25 to 1.0 mg., parenterally.

Pyridostigmine bromide, U.S.P. (Mestinon) (Kalymin [C]) 0.6 to 1.5 Gm. daily, in divided doses, orally. This is considered by many physicians to be preferable to neostigmine because it has a smoother course of action with fewer side effects.

Edrophonium chloride, U.S.P. (Tensilon) 10 mg. intravenously. This is used for diagnosis and in myasthenia crisis—a serious, sometimes fatal episode of the disease.

THE NURSE

Mode of Administration. Treatment is usually started with pyridostigmine 60 mg. or neostigmine 15 mg. If dysphagia is a problem, the drug is given 30 minutes before mealtime. The duration of both of these is four to six hours. The interval will vary from patient to patient and from time to time in the same patient. Dosage is then adjusted to suit the individual patient's response.

Since clinical weakness often increases as the day progresses, dosage may need to be greater in the later part of the day. There is a delayed release form of pyridostigmine available, but it has not always proved to be too reliable. Sometimes, too much of the drug is released at one time and toxic symptoms have resulted.

If the patient is unable to swallow, the tablets may be crushed and dissolved and given by nasogastric tube, or neostigmine methylsulfate may be given intramuscularly.

Side Effects and Toxicity. The side effects of these drugs are due to the excessive accumulation of acetylcholine at the myoneural junction as well as at other synapses. These effects are termed cholinergic reactions, and are of two types: muscarinic or nicotinic. In the muscarinic type of reaction the autonomic nervous system is affected and can cause increased salivation and lacrimation, cold, moist skin, anorexia, nausea, vomiting, diarrhea, abdominal cramps and pupillary miosis. The nicotinic reactions affect both the skeletal muscles, causing fasciculation and weakness, and the central nervous system, causing irritability, anxiety, insomnia, syncope and seizures.

The toxic symptoms may be mild or severe, in which case it is called cholinergic crisis. In some cases it may be necessary to give small doses of atropine to counteract the toxic symptoms, but this is done with care since it masks some of the signs of toxicity.

In either cholinergic or myasthenia crisis, the patient should be hospitalized so that he can be under constant supervision and with emergency equipment available for cardiac or respiratory difficulties.

Interactions. Ambenonium is enhanced by the action of mecamylamine and the two together may cause extreme muscle weakness and an inability to swallow. Edrophonium antagonizes the neuroblocking effect of streptomycin and neomycin. Neostigmine inhibits the neuromuscular blocking toxicity of the aminoglycoside antibiotics and reverses the blocking action of tubocurarine. It enhances the analgesic action of morphine, meperidine and methadone. Physostigmine has much the same activity.

Patient Teaching. The usual things have to be taught, of course, but the nurse has a real responsibility here to explain thoroughly to the patient and his family the side effects that may occur. The patient must know that he should immediately stop the medication and notify his physician.

This is a chronic, long term illness for which, as with so many others, there is no known cure. These patients need help and understanding of their condition. They should realize what the drugs do and that, if one drug does not help, others are available. These patients, as with all such cases, must be encouraged to do all they can and not to become emotionally dependent. Mental health therapy may be very helpful in assisting the patient in adjusting to his situation.

Certain drugs should be avoided in patients with myasthenia gravis because of their deleterious effects. These include curare, quinine, quinidine, ether, chloroform, neomycin, morphine, steroids and sedatives.

Another drug which may help the patient with myasthenia gravis is ephedrine, 25 mg. three or four times a day, which seems to enhance the effect of the other drugs. The adrenal corticosteroids, which may be of some value, do not do much for most patients. With these drugs there are difficulties in using them in a chronic condition. The disadvantages usually outweigh the advantages; however, they may help the patient over a severe episode.

THE PATIENT. It is extremely important that the patient understand the nature of his disease and the objectives of the treatment. Optimal therapy depends upon the knowledge and ability of the patient and his family to alter his medication dosage as needed within limits set by his physician. The remissions and exacerbations should be explained to the patient and he should know of the variability of the disease and that this is a complicating factor. The amount of the drug may vary from day to day and from month to month; the response of the patient to drugs may vary. Factors contributing to variations may include changes in physical activity, menstruation, infection and physical or emotional trauma. The doctor should instruct the patient that any increase in muscle weakness 30 to 60 minutes after taking the drug is a danger signal and he should call his physician immediately.

IT IS IMPORTANT TO REMEMBER

1. That expert nursing care is required for any patient with a disorder of the nervous system because such a patient does not have the normal sensory or motor control and does not react in the usual manner to various stimuli.
2. That these patients are often ill for a long time, since repair of nerve tissue, if possible at all, is a long and tedious process.
3. That in many cases it is necessary for the patient to learn to use other organs for those whose control has been lost.
4. That these patients are often subject to the same disorders and diseases they might have were they not ill with a neurologic condition, but the symptoms may be masked by the neurologic disorder. However, the treatment will be the same as that for a patient who does not have any additional disease.
5. That it is essential first to restore the patient's body to as nearly normal function as possible, and then to secure the correct regimen to keep it in that condition.

TOPICS FOR STUDY AND DISCUSSION

1. Using any news source, note the accidents for one week. How many involved the nervous system? What treatment might be used in the emergency room, during the acute phase and during convalescence? What part might medications have in the treatment?
2. Why does it take longer for nerve tissue to heal than, for example, bones?
3. Plan a discussion (or lecture) which you might give to a parent-teacher association meeting on the care of the child with a long-term neurological disorder such as myasthenia gravis.
4. Why does society (for the most part) tend to ostracize the patient with epilepsy? How might you dispel this attitude if you were in a group and the subject came up?

BIBLIOGRAPHY

Books and Pamphlets

American Medical Association Council on Drugs, *Drug Evaluations*, Chicago, 1971, American Medical Association.

Beeson, P. B., and McDermott, W., *Cecil-Loeb Textbook of Medicine, 13th Ed.*, Philadelphia, 1971, W. B. Saunders Co.

Beland, I., *Clinical Nursing: Pathophysiological and Psychosocial Approaches, 2nd Ed.*, New York, 1970, The Macmillan Co.

Bergersen, B., *Pharmacology in Nursing, 12th Ed.*, St. Louis, 1973, The C. V. Mosby Co.

Chatton, M. J., Margen, S., and Brainerd, H., *Handbook of Medical Treatment, 12th Ed.*, Los Altos, California, 1970, Lange Medical Publications.

Conn, H. F., et al., *Current Therapy, 1974*, Philadelphia, 1974, W. B. Saunders Co.

Feldman, E. G., *Evaluation of Drug Interaction*, Washington, 1973, American Pharmaceutical Association.

Goodman, L. S., and Gilman, A., *Pharmacological Basis of Therapeutics, 4th Ed.*, New York, 1970, The Macmillan Co.

Hartshorn, E. A., *Handbook of Drug Interactions*, Cincinnati, 1970, University of Cincinnati Press.

Miller, B. F., and Keane, C. B., *Encyclopedia and Dictionary of Medicine and Nursing*, Philadelphia, 1972, W. B. Saunders Co.

Rodman, M. J., and Smith, D. W., *Pharmacology and Drug Therapy in Nursing*, Philadelphia, 1968, J. B. Lippincott Co.

Rotenberg, G. N., *Compendium of Pharmaceutical Specialties*, Toronto, 1972, Canadian Pharmaceutical Association.

Shafer, K. M., et al., *Medical-Surgical Nursing*, St. Louis, 1971, The C. V. Mosby Co.

Watson, J. E., *Medical-Surgical Nursing and Related Physiology*, Philadelphia, 1972, W. B. Saunders Co.

Journal Articles

Berlin, R., "Purines: active transport by isolated choroid plexus." *Science* 163:3872:1194 (1969).

Carozza, V. A., "Understanding the patient with epilepsy," *Nurs. Clin. North Am.* 5:1:13 (1970).

Conte, R. R., "Current therapeutic concepts—Epilepsy," *J. Am. Pharm. Assoc.* NS 12:5:230 (1972).

DiPalma, J. R., "L-dopa, new hope for c.n.s. disease," *R.N.* 32:3:63 (1969).

Fongman, A., and O'Malley, W., "L-dopa and the patient with parkinson's disease," *Am. J. Nurs.* 69:7:1455 (July, 1969).

Griffin, C., "Social factors in epilepsy," *Can. Nurse* 61:3:185 (1965).

Hilkemeyer, R., et al., "Nursing care of patients with brain tumors," *Am. J. Nurs.* 64:3:81 (March, 1964).

Hoyle, G., "How is muscle turned on and off?" *Sci. Am.* 222:4:84 (1970).

Huxley, E. H., "The mechanism of muscular contraction," *Science* 164:3886:1356 (1969).

Jontz, D. L., "Prescription for living with m.s.," *Am. J. Nurs.* 73:5:819 (May, 1973).

King, I., et al., "Symposium on neurologic and neurosurgical nursing," *Nurs. Clin. North Am.* 4:2:1 (1969).

Mendell, J. R., Engel, W. L., and Derrer, E. C., "Duchenne muscular dystrophy: functional ischemia reproduces its characteristic lesions," *Science* 172:3988:1143 (1971).

Robb, P., "Epilepsy and its medical treatment," *Can. Nurse* 61:3:171 (1965).

Parson, L. C., "Respiratory changes in head injury," *Am. J. Nurs.* 71:11:2187 (November, 1971).

Rodman, M. J., "Drugs for treating epilepsy," *R.N.* 35:9:63 (1972).

Shimomura, S. K., "Current therapeutic concepts—Parkinsonism," *J. Am. Pharm. Assoc.* NS 12:1:29 (1972).

Trigrano, L. L., "Independence is possible in quadriplegia." *Am. J. Nurs.* 70:12:2610 (December, 1970).

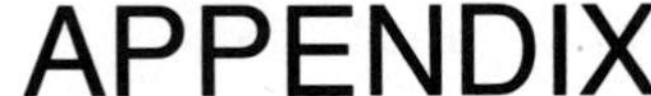

APPENDIX

COMMON ABBREVIATIONS USED IN RELATION TO PHARMACOLOGY

ABBREVIATION	ENGLISH MEANING	LATIN DERIVATION
aa	equal parts	ana
a.c.	before meals	ante cibum
ad	up to	ad
ad lib.	if desired	ad libitum
a.m.	before noon	ante meridiem
aq.	water	aqua
aq. dest.	distilled water	aqua destillata
b.i.d.	twice a day	bis in die
b.i.n.	twice a night	bis in nocte
b.t.	bedtime	
c or c.	with	cum
chart.	powder	chartula
comp.	compound	componere
d.	day	die
D.	give	detur
dil.	dilute	dilue
Div.	divide	divide
dos.	doses	
dr.	dram	
elix.	elixir	
ext.	extract	extractum
fl.	fluid	fluidus
ft.	make	fiat
Gm.	gram	
gr.	grain	granum
gt. (gtt.)	drop(s)	gutta(e)
h.	hour	hora
h.s.	hour of sleep	hora somni
M.	mix	misce
m.	minim	minimum
m. et n.	morning and night	mane et nocte
mist.	mixture	mistura
Noct. or n.	night	nocte
non repetat.	not to be repeated	non repetatur
O.	pint	octarius
o.d.	every day	omne die
o.h.	every hour	omne hora

ABBREVIATION	ENGLISH MEANING	LATIN DERIVATION
Ol.	oil	oleum
o.n.	every night	omne nocte
os	mouth	os
oz.	ounce	uncia
p.c.	after meals	post cibum
p.m.	after noon	post meridiem
pil.	pill	pilula
p.r.n.	when required	pro re nata
q.d.	every day	quaque die
q.h.	every hour	quaque hora
q. 2 h.	every 2 hours (any number may be used)	
q.i.d.	four times a day	quarter in die
q.s.	as much as required	quantum sufficit
q.s.ad	add as much as required	quantum sufficit ad
℞	take	recipe
s or s.	without	sine
S.	mark	signetur
Sig.	write on label	signa
s.o.s.	one dose if necessary	si opus sit
ss.	half	semis
Stat.	immediately	statim
tab.	tablets	tabellae
Tal.	such	talis
t.i.d.	three times a day	ter in die
t.i.n.	three times a night	ter in nocte
tr.	tincture	tinctura
Trit.	triturate	tritura
troch.	lozenges	trochiscus
ung.	ointment	unguentum
ʒ	dram	
℥	ounce	

SOURCES OF DRUGS

Organic

VEGETABLE

PLANTS. All portions of the plants are used.

Root – underground achlorophyllous part; example, rhubarb, belladonna – tuberous; example, aconite, glycyrrhiza.

Bulb – modified stem; example, squill.

Corm – thickened underground stem; example, colchicum.

Wood – hardened portion of tree trunk and limbs; example, quassia, sandalwood.

Rhizome – underground stem with leaves, buds, roots; example, ginger, aspidium.

Bark – outer layer of stem; example, cinchona, cascara.

Leaves – foliage; example, digitalis, belladonna.

Flowers – blossoms; example, chamomile, arnica.

Bud – unopened flowers; example, cloves; juice of these; example, opium.

Fruit – fertilized and ripened ovary; example, colocynth, anise, some vitamins.

Seed – essential part of fruit; example, nux vomica, strophanthin, theobromine.

MICROBIOLOGIC

Fungi – nonchlorophyll-producing vegetation; example, antibiotics such as penicillin.

Bacteria – a low form of nonchlorophyll-producing vegetation; example, antibiotics.

ANIMAL. Note: All portions of the animal are used; the main ones used are as follows.

Glands – endocrine or exocrine; example, hormones, some vitamins, enzymes.

Fluids – blood, lymph, tissue fluid; example, vaccines, sera.

Inorganic

METALS, METALLOIDS, NONMETALS. May be used singly or in compounds.

Inorganic acids, alkalis and salts are all important sources. Radioactive isotopes are an ever-expanding source.

Either Organic or Inorganic

SYNTHETIC

Synthetic preparations may be either organic, inorganic or a combination of these. They are the result of the work of the chemist and form an ever-increasing number of drugs. They may be entirely new products such as the sulfonamides were, or they may be derivatives of other drugs such as thyroxin from thyroid extract, Dilaudid from opium and so forth.

COMPOSITION OF DRUGS

The *active principle* of a drug is the important part to which the drug owes its action.

Alkaloids—organic compounds which react with an acid to form a salt as inorganic acids do (wide source of medicines); example, morphine, atropine, pilocarpine. Note: These usually end in *ine.*

Glycosides—organic compounds in which a sugar is present; example, digitalin, strophanthin. Note: These usually end in *in.*

Saponins—substances, usually glycosides, that act like soaps in water; example, senega.

Fixed Oils—oils from plants that do not evaporate easily (when hydrolyzed these yield fatty acids and glycerin); example, olive oil.

Volatile Oils—oily compounds that give to many plants their characteristic odors, such as lemons, peppermint and juniper (these evaporate easily); example, juniper oil.

Tannins—complex phenolic substances occurring in many plants; example, tannic acid.

Resins—solid or semisolid compounds usually obtained from the sap of certain trees; example, benzoin.

Oleoresins—volatile oils combined with resins; example, copaiba.

Organic Acids—acids occurring naturally in many plants, such as oranges, lemons and grapes; example, citric acid.

Balsams—liquid or semiliquid substances containing resins and other materials; example, balsam of Peru.

Gums—colloidal carbohydrates which swell in water to form a mucilaginous material; example, tragacanth, acacia.

Cellulose—an insoluble form of plant carbohydrates; example, cotton, methylcellulose.

PREPARATIONS OF DRUGS

The number of various forms of drugs is very large. Many previously in common use are rarely used now, and no doubt many now being used will be supplanted by more effective ones in the future. The list here includes the more important ones of both the past and the present.

Liquid Preparations

AQUEOUS SOLUTIONS

These are solutions in which the solvent is distilled water.

FOR INTERNAL USE

Aqua or Waters—watery solutions of a volatile substance (these lose their strength unless tightly closed); example, cinnamon water.

Liquor or Solutions—watery preparations of a nonvolatile substance; example, saline solution.

Mucilage—watery solution of a gummy substance; example, mucilage of acacia.

Syrups—sweetened watery solutions containing medications or flavoring; example, raspberry syrup.

Infusions—aqueous solutions of the active ingredients of plant drugs (they are made by pouring hot or cold water over the powdered drugs and letting steep); example, infusion digitalis, tea.

Decoctions—prepared in a similar way, but the mixture is boiled; example, coffee.

FOR EXTERNAL USE

Lotions—watery solutions or suspensions for local application—a wash; example, calamine lotion.

Solutions—the same as liquors, already defined, except they are intended for external administration.

ALCOHOLIC SOLUTIONS

These are solutions in which the solvent is alcohol.

FOR INTERNAL USE

Elixirs—sweetened alcoholic solutions; example, phenobarbital elixir.

Fluid Extracts—liquid preparations of vegetable drugs that contain alcohol (they are prepared so that 1 ml. of the solution will contain 1 Gm. of the drug); example, fluid extract of cascara.

Spirits—alcoholic solutions of a volatile substance; example, aromatic spirits of ammonia.

Tinctures—alcoholic solutions of drugs that are usually 10 per cent in strength (thus, 1 ml. of the solution will contain 0.1 Gm. of the drug); example, tincture of opium.

FOR EXTERNAL USE

Tinctures—alcoholic solutions of drugs of varying strengths; example, tincture of iodine.

OTHER SOLUTIONS

FOR EXTERNAL USE

Glycerites—drugs dissolved in glycerin; example, tannic acid glycerite.

Collodions—solutions of soluble guncotton (pyroxylin) in ether and alcohol or acetone; example, collodion. Flexible collodion also contains camphor and castor oil.

Sprays or Nebulae—various solutions of antiseptic, astringent or aromatic drugs in an oily or watery base, which are applied to the nose or throat by means of an atomizer or nebulizer; example, compound ephedrine spray.

MIXTURES

FOR EITHER INTERNAL OR EXTERNAL USE

Emulsions—composed of fine droplets of fat or oil suspended in a liquid in which the fat or oil is insoluble; example, liquid petroleum emulsion.

Magmas—thick, milky suspensions of an insoluble (or very slightly soluble) inorganic substance; example, milk of magnesia.

Mixtures—solid material suspended in a watery solution by means of some viscid substance; example, calamine lotions.

FOR EXTERNAL USE

Liniments—solutions or suspensions of irritant substances in oily, soapy or alcoholic vehicle; example, chloroform liniment.

SPECIAL SOLUTIONS

FOR PARENTERAL USE

Injections and Solutions – fluid preparations of drugs especially prepared for injection into the body tissues or cavities (these must be sterile and can contain a preservative); example, caffeine and sodium benzoate injection.

Solid and Semisolid Preparations

FOR INTERNAL USE

Extracts – solid or semisolid preparations made by extracting the active portions of a vegetable or animal drug with suitable solvents and evaporating all or nearly all of the solvent; example, extract of cascara.

Powders. *SIMPLE POWDERS* – finely ground medicinal substances; example, Sippy powders – a mixture of sodium bicarbonate, magnesium oxide or magnesium carbonate and bismuth subcarbonate.

EFFERVESCENT POWDERS – powdered drugs mixed with an acid and an alkaline substance such as citric acid and sodium bicarbonate which will effervesce when dissolved in water; example, compound effervescent powders (Seidlitz powder).

Pills – pellets of drugs molded into spherical or elliptical shape (they contain the drug and an adhesive material such as acacia or flour paste; they are usually coated to disguise the taste); example, pills of aloin, belladonna and strychnine.

GRANULE – very small pill.

BOLUS – very large pill.

Tablets – powdered drugs compressed into round or discoid forms usually uncoated or lightly coated (they contain the drug and usually an excipient such as milk sugar [lactose]); example, tablets of aspirin.

TABLET TRITURATES – small tablets usually intended for oral administration.

HYPODERMIC TABLETS – small readily soluble tablets for parenteral use. Sometimes also called tablet triturates.

Troches or Lozenges – circular or oblong discs containing active substances usually with sugar and mucilage added (they are to be dissolved in the mouth); example, Calcidin troches.

Capsules – small gelatin containers for drugs, usually those having an unpleasant taste; example, Seconal Sodium.

HARD CAPSULES – cylindrical containers, usually for powdered drugs.

FLEXIBLE CAPSULES – containers for liquid drugs, often of an oily nature.

FOR EXTERNAL USE

Discs – small gelatinous discs containing a drug for use on the conjunctiva of the eye.

Dusting Powders – varied inert finely ground substances having adhesive and coating properties, and acting as mechanical protective; example, zinc stearate.

Ointments – semisolid preparations containing an active ingredient and a base, usually an oil such as lard, petrolatum or lanolin (they are rubbed into the skin or applied to the skin); example, sulfur ointment.

Pastes or Poultices – mixtures containing an active ingredient and a base, usually dextrin or flour.

Plasters – thin layers of a drug mixed with resin, wax or lard (the preparation is spread on a cloth or other base; the plaster is solid at ordinary room temperature but becomes soft and adhesive when applied to the skin); example, belladonna plaster.

Suppositories – drugs with a base such as cocoa butter, lanolin, glycerin or gelatin that are solid at room temperature but which melt at body temperature. They are intended for insertion into the vagina, rectum or urethra and are shaped to suit the cavity in which they will be used.

CONICAL SUPPOSITORIES – with at least one end rounded or pointed are for insertion into the rectum.

GLOBULAR SUPPOSITORIES – are for insertion into the vagina.

LONG, NARROW, PENCIL-LIKE SUPPOSITORIES – pointed at one end are for insertion into the urethra.

Other Preparations

Ampules – small hermetically sealed glass containers.

Vials – small glass containers with rubber stoppers.

Ampules and vials contain powdered or fluid drugs intended primarily for parenteral administration. Ampules usually contain one average dose of the drug. Vials contain several doses. Powdered drugs in either ampule or vial are dissolved in either distilled water or isotonic saline solution for use. The amount of the solvent will depend upon the mode of administration, the number of doses to be made from the drug and the solubility of the drug.

Many preparations now in use are designed to extend the time the drug is effective or prevent its release in the stomach or both. Some of these are as follows:

Enteric-coated—preparations which are coated so that they will dissolve in the intestines and not in the stomach.

Delayed-release—may be of many forms—tablets, capsules, fluids—but they are so prepared that the drug will be released a small amount at a time over a relatively longer period of time than would usually be possible.

Tablet within a Tablet—preparations, the outer portion of which dissolves in the stomach for quick action, the inner pill dissolving in the intestines for later effect.

Tablet Implants—drug with very slow solubility which will release the drug over a very long period of time, often weeks or even months. These are designed for insertion under the skin.

TABLES OF WEIGHTS AND MEASURES

APOTHECARIES' SYSTEM OF WEIGHTS

	METRIC EQUIVALENTS	(APPROXIMATE EQUIVALENTS)
1 grain (gr.)	0.0648 gram	(60–65 milligrams)
20 grains = 1 scruple (scr. ℈)	1.296 grams	(1.3 grams)
3 scruples = 1 dram (dr., ʒ) (60 gr.)	3.888 grams	(4.0 grams)
8 drams = 1 ounce (oz., ℥) (480 gr.)	31.103 grams	(30–32 grams)
12 ounces = 1 pound (lb.). (5760 gr.)	373.242 grams (0.3732 kilogram)	(370–375 grams) (0.3–0.35 kilogram)

*Note that in the avoirdupois table there are 16 ounces to 1 pound. In the Troy table there are 12 ounces to a pound as in the apothecaries'.

IMPERIAL SYSTEM OF WEIGHTS (CANADIAN)

	METRIC EQUIVALENTS	(APPROXIMATE EQUIVALENTS)
1 grain (gr.)	0.0648 gramme	(65 mg.)
20 grains = 1 scruple	1.2959 grammes	(1.3 grammes)
3 scruples = 1 drachm (dr., ʒ) (60 gr.)	3.8879 grammes	(4.0 grammes)
8 drachms = 1 troy or apothecaries' ounce (oz., ℥) (480 gr.)	31.1035 grammes	(30–31 grammes)
1 avoirdupois ounce (437.5 gr.)	28.3495 grammes	(28–29 grammes)
16 avoirdupois ounces = 1 pound (lb.) (7000 grains)	453.5924 grammes (0.4536 kilogram)	

METRIC SYSTEM OF WEIGHTS

			APOTHECARIES' EQUIVALENTS
1 microgram (mcg.)	= 0.001 milligram	= 0.000001 Gm.	
10 milligrams (mg.)	= 1 centigram (cg.)	= 0.01 gram	0.15432 gr. (gr. 1/60)
10 centigrams	= 1 decigram (dg.)	= 0.1 gram	1.5432 gr.
10 decigrams	= 1 gram (Gm.)	= 1.0 gram	15.432 gr.
10 grams	= 1 decagram (dkg.)	= 10.0 gram	154.32 gr.
10 decagrams	= 1 hectogram (hg.)	= 100.0 gram	1543.2 gr.
10 hectograms	= 1 kilogram (kg.)	= 1000.0 gram	15432.0 gr. (2.2 lb.)

SHORTENED TABLE (COMMONLY USED MEASUREMENTS)

1000 micrograms	= 1 milligram
1000 milligrams	= 1 gram
1000 grams	= 1 kilogram

VOLUME (USED IN THE UNITED STATES)

		METRIC EQUIVALENTS	(APPROXIMATE EQUIVALENTS)
1 minim (m)		0.06161 ml.	(0.06 ml.)
60 minims	= 1 fluid dram (fl. dr.)	3.697 ml.	(4.0 ml.)
8 fluid drams (480 minims)	= 1 fluid ounce (fl. oz.)	29.5729 ml.	(30.0 ml.)
16 fluid ounces	= 1 pint (pt. or 0.)	473.167 ml.	(500 ml. or 1/2 liter)
2 pints (32 fluid ounces)	= 1 quart (qt.)	946.333 ml.	(1000 ml. or 1 liter)
4 quarts	= 1 gallon (gal. or C.)	3785.301 ml.	(4000 ml. or 4 liters)

IMPERIAL LIQUID MEASURE (CANADIAN)

		METRIC EQUIVALENTS	(APPROXIMATE EQUIVALENTS)
1 minim (m.)		0.0592 ml.	(0.06 ml.)
60 minims	= 1 fluid drachm (fl. dr.)	3.5515 ml.	(4.0 ml.)
8 fluid drachms	= 1 fluid ounce (fl. oz.)	28.4123 ml.	(30.0 ml.)
20 fluid ounces	= 1 pint (pt.)	568.2454 ml.	(600 ml. or 0.6 liter)
40 fluid ounces	= 1 quart (qt.)	1136.4908 ml.	(1100–1200 ml. or 1 liter and 100 or 200 ml.)
8 pints (160 fl. oz.)	= 1 gallon (gal.)	4545.9631 ml.	(4500–5000 ml. or 4.5 or 5.0 liter)

METRIC TABLE SHORTENED

1000 milliliters (ml.) = 1 liter (l.)
1000 liters = 1 kiloliter (kl.)

One cubic centimeter (cc.) is often used in place of 1 ml. A milliliter of water occupies 1 cubic centimeter of space.

APPROXIMATE EQUIVALENTS*

LIQUID

1000 milliliters or 1 liter	= 1 quart
500 milliliters or 0.5 liter	= 1 pint
250 milliliters or 0.25 liter	= 1/2 pint or 8 fluid ounces
30 milliliters	= 1 fluid ounce
15 milliliters	= 4 fluid drams or 1/2 fluid ounce
4 milliliters	= 1 fluid dram
1 milliliter	= 15 minims
0.6 milliliter	= 10 minims
0.2 milliliter	= 3 minims
0.06 milliliter	= 1 minim
0.03 milliliter	= 1/2 minim

WEIGHT

1 kilogram	= 2.2 pounds (avoirdupois)
30 grams	= 1 ounce
4 grams	= 1 dram
1 gram	= 1/4 dram or 15 grains
0.75 gram	= 12 grains
0.6 gram	= 10 grains
0.5 gram	= 7 1/2 grains
0.4 gram	= 6 grains
0.3 gram	= 5 grains
0.25 gram	= 4 grains
0.2 gram	= 3 grains
0.15 gram	= 2 1/2 grains
0.12 gram	= 2 grains
0.1 gram	= 1 1/2 grains
75 milligrams	= 1 1/4 grains
60 milligrams	= 1 grain
50 milligrams	= 3/4 grain
40 milligrams	= 2/3 grain
30 milligrams	= 1/2 grain
25 milligrams	= 3/8 grain
20 milligrams	= 1/3 grain
15 milligrams	= 1/4 grain
10 milligrams	= 1/6 grain
8 milligrams	= 1/8 grain
6 milligrams	= 1/10 grain
5 milligrams	= 1/12 grain
4 milligrams	= 1/15 grain
3 milligrams	= 1/20 grain
2 milligrams	= 1/30 grain
1.5 milligram	= 1/40 grain
1.0 milligram	= 1/60 grain
0.8 milligram	= 1/80 grain
0.6 milligram	= 1/100 grain
0.5 milligram	= 1/120 grain
0.4 milligram	= 1/150 grain
0.3 milligram	= 1/200 grain
0.25 milligram	= 1/250 grain
0.2 milligram	= 1/300 grain
0.15 milligram	= 1/400 grain
0.12 milligram	= 1/500 grain
0.1 milligram	= 1/600 grain
0.05 milligram	= 1/1200 grain

*From the United States Pharmacopeia, XVI.
Canadian students will need to consult individual tables.

ANSWERS TO PROBLEMS IN CHAPTER 5

Pages 54 and 55

B. 1. 2%
2. 12½%
3. 3% or 1:33⅓
4. 0.3%
5. 0.6%
6. 1:500,000
7. 3⅓%
8. 6.3%
9. 0.1% or 1:1000
10. 1:20,000

C. 1. 3 tablets (½ gm.)
2. 1 gm. crystals
3. 5 ml. (cc) in 995 ml. (cc) water
4. 1 tablet (actual figure 9.6 rounded off to 10)
5. 2.5 gm. crystals
6. 1.5 ml. (cc)
7. 2.5 ml. in 997.5 ml. of water (1 l. could be used since the amount is very small).
8. 15 gm. in 1500 ml. water
9. 10 gm. in 60,000 ml. (15 gallons) water (average bathtubful)
10. ½ tablet

Page 55

D. 1. 60 ml.
2. 100 ml.
3. 250 ml.
4. 2 ml.
5. 24 minims

Pages 55 and 56

E. 1. 600 ml.
2. 50,000 ml. or 50 l.
3. 3,200 ml. or 3.2 l.
4. 120 ml.
5. 120 ml.

F. 1. 15,000 ml. or 15 l.
2. 490 ml.
3. 66.6 ml.
4. 1,600 ml.
5. 100 ml.

Page 57

A. 1. Use ½ tablet
2. Use 3 tablets
3. Use 2 tablets
4. Use 2 capsules
5. Use 1 tablet

Page 58

B. 1. 3 ml. or 50 minims
2. 100 ml.
3. 10 ml.
4. 1 minim
5. 30 ml. or 500 minims

Page 58

C. 1. ¾ tablet required. Dissolve 1 tablet in 24 minims and give 18 minims or dissolve in 4 ml. and give 3 ml.
2. 2 tablets required. ⅚ of 2 tablets 1/200 each. Dissolve 2 tablets in 24 minims and give 20 minims or dissolve in 6 ml. and give 5 ml.
3. 3 tablets required. 8/9 of 3 tablets, 1/32 gr. each. Dissolve in 18 minims and give 16 minims or dissolve in 9 ml. and give 8 ml.
4. 3 full tablets required. Dissolve in any amount suitable.
5. ⅔ tablet needed. Dissolve in 18 minims and give 12 minims or dissolve in 3 ml. and give 2 ml.

D. 1. ⅓ tablet required. Dissolve in 24 minims and give 6 minims or dissolve in 3 ml. and give 1 ml.
2. Again ⅓ tablet. See above
3. ⅘ tablet will be needed. Dissolve in 20 minims and give 16 minims or dissolve in 5 ml. and give 4 ml.
4. ½ tablet needed. Dissolve in 24 minims and give 12 minims or dissolve in 2 ml. and give 1 ml.
5. 1 tablet required. Dissolve in any amount suitable.

Page 59

E.
1. 0.5 ml.
2. 1.5 ml.
3. 3.0 ml.
4. 6 minims
5. 2/3 ml. or 0.6 ml.

F.
1. 6 minims
2. 1.2 ml.
3. 0.75 ml.
4. 1.5 ml.
5. 4.0 ml.

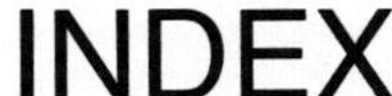

INDEX

INDEX

Numbers in **boldface** refer to the primary discussion of the drug. Numbers followed by *t* indicate tables.

CURRENT DRUG HANDBOOK

PREFACE

This revision, as have past ones, presents specific information on approximately 1500 selected drugs in order to provide a handy source for quick reference. It supplies information supplemental to that in Part II of the textbook, *The Drug, The Nurse, The Patient.* As a general rule, active principles or individual drugs are considered rather than the myriad of mixtures available, and attempts have been made to include only drugs in general use regardless of their recognition by official publications.

Material has been organized with categories of usage similar to that of the *United States Pharmacopeia;* thus, drugs with the same use will be found grouped together in the handbook.

The format has been planned in tabular form for ease in grasping all the pertinent facts at one glance. The material is to be read across the page.

The first column gives the names of the drug–generic, major trade names, and Canadian names when these differ from those used in the United States. The Canadian names are placed in parentheses with the letter "C" at the end. This column also gives the source of the drug, if this is not listed in the heading, the active principles (if any are therapeutically important), and the designation U.S.P. or N.F. if these apply. If should be remembered that there are some drugs with an almost unlimited number of names. Obviously, it has not been possible to include every one. In all cases the official names have been given preference. We have identified main or generic names by underscoring them.

In the second column are given the dosage, method, and times of administration, if the drug is usually given at definite times. The dosages are listed in the metric system. If the apothecaries' dose is desired the reader may consult the list of approximate equivalents in the back of the book.

The third column gives the major uses of the drug and sometimes the minor ones.

The fourth column states the action and fate (absorption, distribution, excretion) of the drug in the body insofar as this is known.

The fifth column covers the toxicity, side effects, contraindications, interactions and when applicable, the treatment of these. The sixth and last column is titled "Remarks" and includes any important information that is not applicable under the other headings. This form has been used with only slight variations throughout, even though in some instances it has not been entirely satisfactory. The variations are self-explanatory. Since the tabular form has been used and brevity stressed, sentences are often incomplete. To conserve space and for clarity, interactions have sometimes been included in column 6 rather than, or in addition to, column 5. When they apply to an entire group, they have been placed across the page with general heading information.

The authors have drawn on a large number of sources for the information used, relying heavily upon such official publications as the *United States Pharmacopeia,* the *National Formulary,* and other sources such as *Drug Evaluations,* the *Modern Drug Encyclopedia,* the *American Drug Index,* and, for the newest drugs, information provided by the pharmaceutical company preparing the medication.

Laws and regulations controlling the dispensing and administration of potentially addicting drugs and narcotics are undergoing intensive scrutiny as legislatures attempt to deal with drug abuse problems. On May 1, 1971, the federal "Comprehensive Drug Abuse Prevention and Control Act of 1970" went into effect in the United States. This act was known as the "Controlled Substance Act." As of October 1, 1973 the name of the control agency is "Drug Enforcement Agency" (DEA).

This act repeals the "Narcotic Acts" as well as the "Drug Abuse Control Amendments to the Federal Food, Drug and Cosmetic Act." The drugs that come under the jurisdiction of the act are divided into five schedules (I, II, III, IV, V). The greater the possibility of abuse and dependence the lower the classification number. Schedule I includes those drugs that have no accepted medical use in the United States and include heroin, marijuana, etc. The remaining schedules have the former Class A, B, X narcotics, the amphetamines and amphetamine-like compounds, the barbiturates and hypnotic drugs.

The people working with these drugs should know in what schedule the various compounds are listed so that they can be handled as required by this act.

State laws are more stringent than federal laws in some cases. The student should become familiar with the local regulations in her area. Canadian students should refer to the books and pamphlets issued by the Department of National Health and Welfare such as *The Food and Drug Act and Regulations, Narcotic Control Act,* and *Controlled Drugs.* As with state laws, provincial laws may be more stringent than the dominion laws, in which case the student will need to know the local regulations. These laws are amended as circumstances indicate.

MARY W. FALCONER
H. ROBERT PATTERSON
EDWARD A. GUSTAFSON

CONTENTS

ANTISEPTICS AND DISINFECTANTS

Drugs included in this group are those which are used to destroy or to inhibit the development of microorganisms in the environment of the patient, or on the body surfaces. Some insecticides also are listed. Systemic anti-infectives are discussed later. These substances are all poisonous to a greater or lesser degree.

Name, Source, Synonyms, Preparations	Dosage and Administration	Uses	Action and Fate	Side Effects and Contraindications	Remarks
HALOGENS. Only two of the halogen elements–chlorine and iodine–are commonly used as antiseptics and disinfectants.					
CHLORINE. *Gaseous element.*		For utensils, skin, mucous membranes, and sometimes food and water. Most common means of making water potable.	In insects, acts as contact and stomach poison. (In man, mainly central nervous system effects.)	Toxic in strong solutions, but poisoning rare in usual strengths. Irritating to skin; protect with oil or petrolatum.	
Chlorinated lime (chloride of lime, bleaching powder).	5-20% solution. Environmental.	For excreta.	Can be caused by presence of chlorine and nascent oxygen liberated.		
Halazone.	4-8 mg. to 1 liter. Environmental.	To render water potable.	Probably due to formation of nascent oxygen by chemical reaction.		After it is mixed with water it should stand 1/2 hour before being drunk.
Sodium hypochlorite diluted solution, N.F. (hychlorite, modified Dakin's solution).(Hygeol [C])	0.5% solution. Topical.	For wounds.	In solution hypochlorites release nascent oxygen and then chlorine.		Hygeol is twice the strength of Dakin's solution.
Sodium hypochlorite solution, N.F.	5% solution. Environmental.			Too strong to use on the skin undiluted.	
Succinchlorimide.	12 mg. to 1 liter. Environmental.	As above.	Same as Halazone.		
OXYCHLOROSENE. *Synthetic.* Derived from hypochlorous acid.					
Oxychlorosene (Clorpactin XCB).	0.5% solution. Topical, with contact time of at least 5 minutes.	Used to kill cancer cells in the operative field.	Thought to be caused by oxychlorination of the free cells.	None unless ingested.	
Oxychlorosene sodium (Clorpactin WCS-90).	0.1-0.4% solution. Topical.	Used as an antiseptic.			

Name, Source, Synonyms, Preparations	Dosage and Administration	Uses	Action and Fate	Side Effects and Contraindications	Remarks
IODINE. *Kelp.*		Antiseptic for skin and wounds.	These compounds are effective because of the presence of elemental iodine but its precise bactericidal action is not presently known.	Topical preparations are toxic if taken internally. Irritating in strong solutions or when skin is wet.	
Iodine solution, N.F.	2% solution. Topical.				
Iodoform, N.F.	Powder. Topical.	Used for infected wounds and on gauze packings.			
Povidone-iodine N.F. (Betadine, Isodine) (Bridine, Provodine, PVP-I. [C])	1% ointment, solution or gel. Topical.	Have longer antiseptic action than most iodine solutions; do not sting. Solutions used for scrubbing, mouth washes and douches. Ointment used for burns.			Various iodopher preparations are available under such trade names as Ioclide and Wescodyne for skin disinfection of minor wounds. These are complexes of iodine and nonionic wetting agents.
Strong tincture of iodine.	7% alcoholic solution. Topical.	For skin; do not use in deep wounds.			
Thymol iodide.	Powder. Topical.	For skin and wounds; contains iodine and thymol from thyme.			
Tincture of iodine, U.S.P.	2% alcoholic solution. Topical.	For skin.			
Undecoylium chloride-iodine (Virac).	0.2-3.2% solution. Topical.	Similar to povidone-iodine.			
HEAVY METALS					
MERCURY. *Mineral.*		For skin, mucous membranes, and utensils.	Mercuric ion will precipitate plasma protein, but its antibacterial action probably results from its ability to inhibit sulfhydryl enzymes.	Local irritation from mercury products is not uncommon; severe dermatitis may occur. Stop drug and treat symptoms.	
Acetomeroctol (Merbak).	0.1% tincture. Topical.	For skin disorders.			
Ammoniated mercury ointment, U.S.P. (white precipitate).	5% ointment. Topical.	For skin disorders.			
	3% ointment. Topical.	For ophthalmic use.			
Merbromin. (Flurochrome K) (Mercurochrome). (Mercurescein [C])	1-5% aqueous solution. Topical.	Used for skin or mucous membranes.			
	1-2% acetone-alcohol solution. Topical.	Used for skin only.			
Mercury bichloride (Mercuric chloride, corrosive sublimate).	1:1000-1:20,000 aqueous solution. Environmental.	Occasionally used as skin wash. Do not use on metals.			
Mercury cyanide.	1:4000 solution. Environmental.	As above; does not corrode metals.			
Mercury oxycyanide.	1:500 solution. Environmental.	As above; does not corrode metals.			

Phenylmercuric nitrate, N.F. (Merphenyl nitrate, Phe-Mer-Nite).	1:1500 ointment or solution. Topical.	For skin.			
	1:3000 ophthalmic ointment.	For eyes.			
Nitromersol, N.F. (Metaphen).	1:1000 aqueous solution. Environmental.				
	1:500-1:2500 aqueous solution. Topical.	For skin and mucous membranes.			
	1:200-1:5000 tincture. Topical.	For skin.			
Mercurial ointment, mild.	1% ointment. Topical.	Mainly for parasites.			
Thimerosal, N.F. (Merthiolate) (Thiomersal [C]).	1:1000 aqueous solution. Environmental.	Also used for mucous membranes.			
	1:1000 alcoholic tincture. Topical.	For skin.			
Yellow oxide of mercury ointment, N.F.	1% ointment. Topical.	For eye infections.			
SILVER. *Mineral.*		For skin and mucous membranes, especially in infections due to the gonococcus.	Silver ion is a protein precipitant, but the concentrations which exhibit bacteriostatic action indicate that silver ions have an effect on some enzyme systems.	Strong solutions are caustic. Normal saline is antidote. If used repeatedly, watch for symptoms of argyria (silver poisoning): pain in throat and abdomen, vomiting, purging, and graying of lips. Stop drug and treat symptoms.	
Toughened silver nitrate, U.S.P. (lunar, caustic, molded silver nitrate).	Pencils or applicators. Topical.	As styptic and caustic.			
Silver nitrate solution.	0.5-2% solution. Topical. 1:2000-1:10,000 solution.	For skin and mucous membranes. Used in a 0.5% solution for treatment of burns.			
Silver picrate.	1-2% solution. Topical.	As above.		Watch also for picric acid poisoning (kidney or liver).	
COLLOIDAL SILVER. *Mineral and protein.*		As above.	As above.	As above.	
Silver protein mild, N.F. (Argyrol, Solargentum).	5-25% solution. Topical.	For skin and mucous membranes.			Mild silver protein contains more silver than strong silver protein, but is less astringent because of difference in ionization of solution. Trade names
Silver protein, strong, (Protargol).	0.25-1% solution. Topical. 1:1000-1:2000 solution. Topical.	For skin and mucous membranes.			

ANTISEPTICS AND DISINFECTANTS (Continued)

Name, Source, Synonyms, Preparations	Dosage and Administration	Uses	Action and Fate	Side Effects and Contraindications	Remarks
COLLOIDAL SILVER (Continued)					
Silver iodide (Neo Silvol).	5% solution. Topical.	For skin and mucous membranes.			listed and others are similar to, but not always identical with, N.F. formula.
OXIDIZING AGENTS. Synthetic. Act by liberating nascent oxygen.			The nascent oxygen liberated from these compounds is capable of oxidizing susceptible components in cellular protoplasm, thereby affording bactericidal effect.		
Hydrogen peroxide, U.S.P.	2.5-3.5% solution. Topical.	Antiseptic for skin and mucous membranes. Especially valuable for anaerobic organisms.		Toxic reactions are rare.	Deteriorates on standing.
Potassium permanganate.	1:5000 solution. Topical.	For gastric lavage in certain cases of poisoning (alkaloid).		Toxic if taken internally, causing gastrointestinal disturbances. Evacuants, demulcent drinks, treat symptoms.	Dyes linens.
	1:1000-1:2000 solution. Topical.	For the skin; dyes skin brown.			
	1:500-10,000 solution. Topical.	For mucous membranes.			
Sodium perborate.	2% saturated solution. 10-20% powder in dentifrices. Topical.	Antiseptic for mouth.		Toxic reactions are rare, but it can cause chronic glossitis from prolonged use.	Constituent of many dentifrices; should be used only on advice of doctor or dentist.
Zinc peroxide, medicinal, U.S.P.	5-25% ointment. 40% aqueous suspension, and as a dusting powder. Topical.	Antiseptic for skin.		Toxic reactions are rare.	Insoluble in water, but gradually decomposed by water to release oxygen.
PHENOL GROUP (carbolic acid). *Coal tar and crude petroleum.*		Disinfectant in strong solutions. Antiseptic in weak solutions.	Effect of phenols thought to result from their ability to denature protein. Some substituted phenols tend to be more effective depending on the position and the substituent.	Caustic if too strong. Wash with alcohol.	
Cresol, N.F. (methylphenol).	1-5% solution. Environmental.	Largely replaced by saponified form.			
Saponated solution of cresol, N.F. (Creolin, Cresol compound, Cresylone, Hydrasol, Phenolor).	2-5% solution. Environmental. 0.25-5% solution. Topical.	For utensils, and for skin and mucous membranes. Disinfectant in strong solutions.			Cresol, vegetable oil, and soap. Cresol content 50%. Phenol coefficient 3.

Liquefied phenol, U.S.P.	85% solution. Topical. 0.5-1% solution. Topical.	As caustic. As antiseptic and antipruritic.			
Phenol, U.S.P.	2-5% solution. Environmental.	Soak for 1/2 hour or more.			
PREPARATIONS MADE SYNTHETICALLY FROM PHENOL					
Arylphenolic compounds (Amphyl, O-Syl, Staphene).	Varied. Topical, environmental. 0.5% strength is usual.	Used for utensils, environmentally, and in weak solutions for skin disinfection.		Some skin irritation in strong solutions.	
Metacresylacetate	Varied. Topical. 0.5% strength is usual.	An antiseptic and analgesic used for ear, nose, and throat.		Relatively nontoxic.	
Betanaphthol.	5-10% ointment. Topical.	Antiseptic for the skin, especially in fungal infections.		Relatively nontoxic.	
Hexachlorophene, U.S.P. (G-11) (Gamophen, pHisoHex, SurgiCen, Surofene) (Hexachlorophane, Dermohex, HexSurg, Ibaderm, Promani, Tersaseptic [C]).	0.5-3% soaps. Topical.	Mainly for skin antisepsis, and also for surgical scrubs.	Active only against gram + organisms, not gram –.	Warning–total body bathing of adults or children can result in absorption of toxic concentrations of hexachlorophene.	
Pyrogallol.	5-10% ointment. Topical.	For skin disorders.		Toxic reactions rare in therapeutic strengths.	
Triacetylpyrogallol (Lenigallol).	6% powder or ointment. Topical.	Keratolytic, keratoplastic, and antifungal.			
RESORCINOL GROUP					
Resorcinol, U.S.P. (Resorcin).	1-10% solution. Topical.	As above.			
Resorcinol monoacetate, N.F. (Euresol).	5-20% ointment and lotion. Topical.	As above.			

Name, Source, Synonyms, Preparations	Dosage and Administration	Uses	Action and Fate	Side Effects and Contraindications	Remarks
QUATERNARY AMMONIUM COMPOUNDS					
(Detergents). *Synthetic.* Soap-like substances.		Used for skin and mucous membranes and for utensils. Especially useful for pre- and postoperative skin disinfection and obstetrical procedures.	The exact mode of action of these agents is not presently known, but they do reduce surface tension.	Toxic reactions rare.	Inactivated by soap. Rinse thoroughly before using after green soap has been used.
Benzalkonium chloride, U.S.P. (Benasept, Germicin, Hyamine-3500, Phencen Roccal, Zephiran Chloride).	1:5000-1:500 aqueous. Environmental. 1:40,000-1:500 aqueous. Topical.	Utensils and skin must be completely rinsed after application.	Effective against gram + and gram – organisms, but some strains of gram – require a longer exposure time. These compounds are not tuberculocidal.		
Benzethonium chloride, N.F. (Hyamine-1622, Phemerol Chloride, Phemithyn).	1:5000-1:1000 aqueous. Environmental or topical. Used full or one-fourth strength as needed.	As above.			
Cetyl pyridinium chloride, N.F. (Ceepryn chloride) (Cepacol, Oracain [C]).	As above.	For skin; not reliable against spores.			
Hexetidine (Sterisol [C]).	0.1% gel. Topical.	Local antiseptic for bacteria, fungi, protozoa. Main use is in the treatment of vaginitis.		Toxic reactions rare in topical application.	
Methylbenzethonium chloride, N.F. (Diaparene Chloride).	1:25,000 solution. Environmental. 0.1% ointment, lotion, or cream. Topical.	Especially for infants' diapers. For skin antisepsis.			
Triclobisonium chloride (Triburon [C]).	0.1% vaginal cream. Topical.	For control of localized bacterial skin and wound infections.	Claimed effective against a wide range of pathogens. Resistant strains have not been observed.	Toxicity rare but low degrees of irritation and sensitization have occurred.	
TAR GROUP					
COAL AND OTHER TARS		For skin antisepsis.	This group has only slight antiseptic action; exact mode of action is not	Toxic reactions rare.	
Coal tar ointment, U.S.P.	1% coal tar in zinc oxide paste. Topical.				

Coal tar solution, U.S.P. (Liquor carbonis detergens, Wright's solution).	20% diluted as required. Topical.		known, but tars are used empirically.		
Ichthammol ointment, N.F. (Ichthymall, Ichthyol).	10% ammonium ichthyosulfonate in petrolatum and wool fat. Topical.	Antiseptic, astringent, and antipruritic.		Toxic reactions rare.	
Juniper tar ointment, N.F. (Cade oil).	15% cade oil in an oily base. Topical.	For skin.		Toxic reactions rare.	
Pine tar ointment, N.F.	5% pine tar in yellow wax and petrolatum. Topical.	For skin.		Toxic reactions rare.	
VARIOUS DYES					
Crude petroleum or *synthetic.*		For mucous membranes and skin antisepsis.	Bacteriostatic and bactericidal.	Harmful to body cells in strong solution but not in therapeutic strengths.	
Acriflavine.	1:8000-1:1000 solution. Topical.	For mucous membranes.			Watch for staining, as with any dye.
Methylrosaniline chloride (gentian, methyl, or crystal violet).	1% solution. Topical. 3-60 mg. Oral enteric-coated tablets are used, often for the relief of pinworms (see page 42).	For pyogenic and fungal skin infections and as an anthelmintic.	Effective against gram-positive organisms but not against gram-negative organisms or acid-fast bacteria. Bactericidal effect thought to result from chemical combination of the dye with vital constituents in bacterial protoplasm.		
Scarlet red ointment.	4-8% ointment. Topical.	For skin—burns, ulcers, and similar conditions.	Bacteriostatic; thought to aid healing and stimulate cell growth.	As above.	As above.
MISCELLANEOUS All of these preparations are synthetic unless otherwise stated.					
Alcohol, U.S.P. (Ethanol).	70% solution. Topical.	For the skin, and utensils.	Action is limited and usually slow.	Toxic reactions rare in topical application.	Wood alcohol (methyl alcohol) is not used except on utensils. Ethyl alcohol is from grain.
Alcohol, rubbing, N.F. (Alcolo, Lavacol, Nor-Co-Hol, Spiritex).	70% solution. Topical.	Used for skin disinfection and as a rubefacient.	As above.	As above. Toxic when taken internally.	Isopropyl alcohol is synthetic.

Name, Source, Synonyms, Preparations	Dosage and Administration	Uses	Action and Fate	Side Effects and Contraindications	Remarks
MISCELLANEOUS (Continued)					
Acrisorcin (Akrinol).	2 mg./Gm. ointment. Topical.	Used to treat mycotic infections caused by tinea versicolor.	Said to have the action of both 9-amino-acridine and hexylresorcinol.	Do not use around eyes. If irritation or sensitization develops, discontinue treatment.	
Aluminum acetate solution, U.S.P. (Buro-Sol, Burow's solution) (Acid mantle [C]). Chemical.	2.5-10% solution. Topical.	Used for treatment of various skin conditions.	An astringent and antiseptic.	None unless ingested.	Used alone and in various combinations either in solutions or ointments.
Benzyl benzoate lotion. (Scabanca, Scabiol [C].	25-30% solution. ointment. Topical.	For skin, especially for scabies and pediculi.	Exact mode of action is not known.	Toxic reactions rare in topical application.	
Boric acid (boracic acid), N.F. Mineral.	2.5% solution and ointment. Topical.	For skin and mucous membranes.	Very weak germicide but can be used because it is non-irritating. It can be used on the cornea without ill effects.	Toxic reactions rare in topical application. Toxic internally; use evacuants.	Do not use on denuded areas.
Chlorquinaldol (Sterosan. [C]).	3% ointment or cream. Topical.	For topical treatment of superficial pyogenic and mycotic infections.	Mode of action is not well understood.	Toxicity low, but skin sensitivity has occurred.	Also available in combinations with hydrocortisone 1%.
Coparaffinate (Iso-Par).	17% ointment. Topical.	Used for mycotic infections of skin and genital or anal mucous membranes.	Same as above.	Toxicity low when used as directed.	Objectionable odor. Do not bandage part.
Crotamiton (Eurax).	10% cream or lotion. Topical.	Used to treat scabies.	Scabicide.	Toxicity low, but hypersensitivity has occurred.	
Diamthazole dihydrochloride.	5% ointment, alcoholic solution, or powder. Topical.	For skin, especially for fungal infections.	For fungal infections. Also keratolytic.	Toxic reactions rare in topical application.	
Formaldehyde solution (Formalin, Formol) 37% solution of gas in water.	1-2%, mucous membranes. 2-10%, surgical instruments and gloves.	Disinfectant for excreta and utensils. (Also used in preparation of toxoids from toxins.)	In high concentration is capable of precipitating protein, and can also preserve tissue. Bactericidal effect thought to be through chemical reaction with protein present.	Irritant to mucous membranes and sometimes to skin. Avoid inhalation. Stop use of solutions; rinse area with water.	Effective disinfectant, but has a disagreeable odor.
Gamma benzene hexachloride, U.S.P. (Gexane, Kwell).	1% cream, soap, or lotion. Topical.	Used to treat scabies and pediculosis.	Exact mechanism of action is not known. Not readily absorbed through intact skin.	Toxicity relatively high, but usually safe in low concentration.	Do not use in concentration greater than 1%. Avoid contact with mucous membranes.

Haloprogin (Halotex)	1.0% cream or solution. Topical. Apply b.i.d. for 2-3 weeks. Interdigital lesions may require 4 weeks.	Treatment of many fungal infections.	Exact mechanism not known.	Local irritation, burning sensation, vesicle formation, and increased maceration, pruritus and exacerbation of preexisting lesions.	If no noticable improvement after 4 weeks of therapy, a rediagnosis is indicated. See insert for exact fungi covered.
Furazolidone, N.F. (Tricofuron) (Furoxone [C]).	0.1-0.25% vaginal suppositories. Topical.	Used mainly for vaginal trichomoniasis.	Action thought to result from inhibition of formation of acetyl coenzyme A from pyruvic acid.	Toxic reactions usually none, but sensitivity reactions may occur in up to 5% of patients. Stop drug and treat symptoms.	
Nitrofurazone, N.F. (Furacin).	0.02-0.2% solution. 0.2-10% ointment. Topical.	For adjunct therapy of patients with second and third degree burns when bacterial resistance to other drugs is a problem. In skin grafting when bacterial contamination may cause graft rejection and/or donor site infection.	Tends to promote healing as well as destroy microorganisms. Nitrofuran derivative effective against certain fungi.		
Nifuroxime (Microfur).	0.1% vaginal suppository. Topical.	See Remarks.		Has been shown to promote development of mammary tumors when fed to female rats in high doses.	Available in combination with furazolidone in Tricofurin vaginal preparations.
Salicylanilide, N.F. (Salinidol).	4.5-5% ointment. Topical.	Antifungal preparation.	Action due to phenolic OH group. Also has some keratolytic effect.	Toxic reactions rare in topical application.	
Sodium borate, U.S.P. (Borax).		For skin and mucous membranes.		Toxic reactions rare in topical application. Toxic internally; use evacuants.	Not so commonly used as boric acid.
Sodium caprylate.	10-20% solution. Topical.	Used to treat mycotic infections of skin.	Exact mechanism is not known.	Toxicity low, but too frequent application may cause skin irritation.	
Sulfur precipitated, U.S.P.	10% ointment. Topical.	For skin, especially in fungal infections.	Must be converted to some other form to be active. Fungicidal properties thought to be owing to conversion of water to pentothionic acid.	Toxic reactions rare in topical application. Occasionally causes local irritation. Stop drug.	
Tolnaftate (Tinactin).	1% solution, powder, ointment or cream. Topical. Apply b.i.d. for from 2-6 weeks.	Treatment of mycotic infections.	Exact mode of action not yet determined.	Keep out of eyes.	Not effective against candidal infections.

Name, Source, Synonyms, Preparations	Dosage and Administration	Uses	Action and Fate	Side Effects and Contraindications	Remarks
MISCELLANEOUS (Continued)					
Triacetin, N.F. (Enzactin, Fungacetin) (glyceryl triacetate [C])	25% aerosol ointment, powder, or solution. Topical.	Used to treat mycotic infections of the skin.	Action due to slow liberation of acetic acid.	Toxicity low when used as directed.	
Copper undecylenate (Decupryl). Undecylenic acid, N.F. (Undecap).	Ointment. Topical. 1-10% ointment. Topical.	For the skin, especially for fungal infections.	Mechanism of action of these compounds is not known.	Toxic reactions rare in topical application.	
Zinc undecylenate, N.F. (Desenex, Undesol).	5% ointment, alcoholic solution, powder. Topical.				

ANTI-INFECTIVES

THE SULFONAMIDES

HISTORY

The first sulfonamide was azosulfonamide (Prontosil). It was a red dye discovered by a German chemist, Gerhard Domagk, about 1932, and could be given only orally. Neoprontosil was produced in 1935 and could be given either orally or parenterally. It was found that these drugs act by the liberation of sulfanilamide in the body. Sulfanilamide was first made in 1937. Since then many variations of the sulfonamides have been synthesized. Some of these preparations are given singly, but now many are given in combinations of two, three, or four. This is thought to be better than any one alone since the dosage of each can be reduced and, with the reduction, the toxicity of each is lessened so that the combined drug is more effective and less toxic than any of its components when given in adequate dosage singly.

THE NURSE'S RESPONSIBILITY IN THE ADMINISTRATION OF THE SULFONAMIDES

The nurse has very important responsibilities in caring for the patient receiving any of these drugs. Some of these are:

1. Maintenance of the blood level of the drug. This means that the drugs must be given in the exact amount ordered at the times directed. Nothing must delay the administration of the drug. If the patient is asleep, he must be awakened. If the drug is vomited, it must be repeated. If the blood level is allowed to fall below the desired level, the organisms have a chance to build up resistance to the drug, which then loses its effectiveness.
2. The fluid balance of the patient must be maintained. Urinary blockage due to the filling of the kidney tubules with the acetylated crystals is serious but uncommon. Accurate intake and output records should be kept. The fluid intake should be high—3000 ml. is considered adequate. If a preference is allowed, the fluids should be alkaline or alkaline-producing, since crystals are less apt to form in alkaline urine. If the urinary output is less than 1500 ml., the physician should be notified.
3. Direct sunlight should be avoided by the patient taking any of the sulfonamide preparations since this increases the tendency for skin rashes to develop.
4. Para-aminobenzoic acid administration is contraindicated during sulfonamide therapy.

SULFONAMIDES. Synthetic. Aminobenzene-sulfonamide rings with various radicals or compounds added.		General anti-infective. Especially valuable against gram-positive organisms (streptococci, staphylococci, pneumococci), *Neisseria* (meningococci, gonococci), *Clostridium tetani, Cl. welchii,* Friedländer's bacillus and others. Used in the treatment of many diseases.	METABOLISM The sulfonamides vary greatly in their rate of absorption. Most of these drugs are given orally, and some rapidly reach a high blood level, while others are so poorly absorbed as to render them useless for therapeutic purposes outside the gastrointestinal tract. The sulfonamides are changed (acetylated–conjugated) in the body, some much more than others. The degree of acetylation is important for in this form they are less effective and more difficult to eliminate. The acetylated sulfonamides tend to form crystals in the urinary tract, and this produces some of the toxic symptoms. The easily absorbed sulfonamides are usually distributed through most or all of the body fluids. Of those absorbed, primary excretion is by the kidneys. The exact way in which the sulfonamide drugs act is not known, but their action is thought to be due to the ability to compete with PABA (para-amino-benzoic acid) for incorporation into PGA (folic acid or pteroyl glutamic acid).	Toxic symptoms include nausea, vomiting; oliguria, anuria, hematuria; cyanosis, anemia, leukopenia, granulocytopenia; dizziness, mental depression, drug fever, jaundice, skin rashes. Treatment symptomatic. If symptoms are serious, drug is stopped; if less serious, dosage is adjusted or type of sulfonamide is changed. Sulfonamides (especially the long-acting type) should not be given during pregnancy or the nursing period because the sulfonamides pass the placental barrier and are secreted with the milk and may cause kernicterus, hyperbilirubinemia and acute liver atrophy. The safe use of the sulfonamides during pregnancy has not been established. The teratogenetic potential of most sulfonamides has not been thoroughly investigated in either man or animals. Sulfonamides should not be given to infants less than 2 months of age, except in the treatment of toxoplasmosis as adjunct therapy with pyrimethamine.	Sulfonamides will not eradicate group A streptococci and have not been demonstrated to prevent sequelae from such infections as rheumatic fever or glomerulonephritis.
PYRIMIDINE DERIVATIVES					
Sulfadiazine, U.S.P. (Diazoline, Solu-Diazine Sulfadets [C]).	0.5-2 Gm. Five to six times daily. Oral.	General anti-infective, relatively nontoxic.			
Sulfadiazine sodium inj., U.S.P., Ph.I.	2.5-5 Gm. q. 6-8 h. I.V.				
Sulfamerazine, N.F. (Sumedine).	0.5-2 Gm. q. 4-8 h. 2-4 Gm. total daily dose. Oral.	General anti-infective, relatively nontoxic.			
Sulfamethazine, U.S.P. (sulfadimidine, sulfadine [C]).	0.5-2 Gm. Maintenance dose 1 Gm. q. 6 h. Oral.	As above.			
Sulfadimethoxine, N.F. (Madribon).	0.25-1 Gm. daily. Oral.	A long-acting sulfonamide that is relatively nontoxic.			Patients on long-term sulfonamides, such as sulfadimethoxine (Madribon) and sulfamethoxypyridazine (Medicel) should be watched for drug rashes; erythema multiforme exudativum (Stevens-Johnson syndrome) has been reported, with serious or fatal results.
Sulfisomidine (Sulfadimetine) (Elkosin [C]).	0.5-4 Gm. Oral.	General anti-infective, relatively nontoxic.			
THIAZOLE DERIVATIVES					
Sulfathiazole (Sulfa-30, Sulfamul, Thiazol [C]).	0.5-1 Gm. q. 4 h. Oral. 5% ointment. t.i.d. Topical. 5% jelly. Topical.	General anti-infective, relatively toxic, but very effective.			
Para-nitrosulfathiazole (Nisulfazole).	10% suspension. Rectal.	As above.			
Phthalylsulfathiazole (Sulfathalidine [C]).	0.5-1 Gm. Four to six times daily. Oral.	As above. Not recommended for bacillary dysentery.			
Succinylsulfathiazole (Sulfasuxidine [C]).	1-3 Gm. Six times daily. Oral.	Poorly absorbed. Used in gastrointestinal surgery or gastrointestinal diseases.			

Name, Source, Synonyms, Preparations	Dosage and Administration	Uses	Action and Fate	Side Effects and Contraindications	Remarks
SULFONAMIDES (Continued)					
Sulfaethidole (Sulfaethylthiadiazole, Sul-Spansion [C]).	130 mg./cc. 10 cc. q. 12 h. Oral. 650 mg. tablet. 2 q. 12 h. Oral.	Similar to sulfamethizole, but more prolonged action.			
Sulfamethizole, N.F. (Thiosulfil) sulfamethylthiadiazole. Ultrasul [C]).	0.25-2 Gm. Oral Adults, 0.5 Gm. q.i.d. oral.	Urinary antiseptic.			
SULFACETAMIDE DERIVATIVES					
Sulfacetamide, N.F. (Blep-10-30, Optiole S; Isopto-Cetamide, [C]).	0.5-2 Gm. Three to four times daily. Oral.	Urinary antiseptic; relatively nontoxic.			
Sulfacetamide sodium, U.S.P. (Sulamyd sodium) (Almocetamide, Solulone [C]).	10% ointment. Ophthalmic. Four to five times daily. Topical. 10-30% solution. Ophthalmic. 1-2 drops three to four times daily. Topical.				
Phthalylsulfacetamide, N.F. (Thalamyd)	0.5-1 Gm. t.i.d. Oral.	Poorly absorbed. Used in gastrointestinal surgery or gastrointestinal diseases.			
OTHERS					
Salicylazosulfapyridine (Azulfidne) (Salozosulazine, sulphasalazine, Salazopyrin [C]).	Therapy. 4-8 Gm. daily in divided doses. Oral Maintenance 2 Gm. daily in divided doses. Oral.	Ulcerative colitis (chronic).		Has caused agranulocytosis. In beginning therapy weekly white blood cell counts should be done. Watch for sudden sore throat or infections. Doctor must weigh risks against benefits in pregnancy and lactation.	Fluid intake should be maintained at 1500 ml. daily or more.
Sulfachlorpyridazine (Sonilyn) (sulfachloropyridazine, Cosulfa, [C]).	1.0 Gm. t.i.d. Oral.	Urinary tract infections.			Continued therapy, at present, should not exceed 180 days.
Sulfaguanidine.	0.05 Gm./kg. of weight. q. 4 h. Oral.	Poorly absorbed.			Has largely been replaced by sulfonamides that are more effective and less toxic.

Sulfameter (Sulla). (Sulfamethoxydiazine [C]).	1.5 Gm. first day then 0.5 Gm. Oral.	Urinary tract infections (acute and chronic).		As with others of this group including Stevens-Johnson syndrome. Contraindicated in renal or hepatic impairment. Not recommended for generalized infections (including meningitis), pregnant women or nursing mothers. Do not use for children under 12 years or less than 100 pounds.	
Sulfamethoxazole, N.F. (Gantanol).	1-2 Gm. 4 tablets stat, then 2 tablets two to three times a day. Oral.	Used for urinary, respiratory, and soft tissue infections. Not recommended for newborn infants.			
Sulfamethoxypyridazine, U.S.P. (Midicel) (Kynex S.M.D. [C]).	1 Gm. stat, then 0.5 Gm. daily. Oral.	Long-lasting blood level due to slow excretion. Also available as the acetyl salt.			See remarks on page 11 under Sulfadimethoxine.
Sulfanilamide (Streptocile, Pronlylin [C]).	0.1 Gm./kg. of weight daily in divided doses every 4 hours. Oral.	General anti-infective, relatively toxic; sodium bicarbonate given to combat acidosis.			Rarely used now.
Sulfaphenazole (Orisul, Sulfabid) (sulphaphenazole [C]).	1-3 Gm. Oral.	Used for urinary, respiratory, and soft tissue infections. Not recommended for newborn infants.			
Sulfapyridine, U.S.P. (Dagenan [C]).	0.5-1 Gm. t.i.d. Oral.	Suppressant for dermatitis herpetiformis.		Toxic reactions frequent; include hematuria, methemoglobin formation, and nausea.	
Sulfisoxazole, U.S.P. Gantrisin) (sulfafurazole, Novosoxazole, Sulfizol [C]).	0.5-2 Gm. Usually 1 Gm. q. 4 h. Syrup, 5 ml. contains 0.5 Gm. Oral.	General anti-infective. Relatively nontoxic. Dissolves in acid urine.			Caution should be observed when sulfisoxazole is given concurrently with methotrexate, since it decreases plasma protein binding of methotrexate and could result in methotrexate toxicity.

Name, Source, Synonyms, Preparations	Dosage and Administration	Uses	Action and Fate	Side Effects and Contraindications	Remarks
SULFONAMIDES (Continued)					
Sulfisoxazole acetyl, (Gantrisin acetyl, Lipogantrisin).	0.5 Gm./9 kg. of body weight in divided doses q. 4 h. 5 ml. equals 0.5 Gm. Lipo solution given b.i.d. Oral.				
Sulfisoxazole diethanolamine (Gantrisin-diethanolamine).	5-10 ml. contains 2-4 Gm. q. 8-12 h. I.V. or I.M. 4% solution. 2-3 gtt. three or more times a day. Ophthalmic.				Must be given slowly.

ANTIBIOTICS

Penicillin was actually discovered by Sir Alexander Fleming at St. Mary's Hospital, London, in 1929. It did not come into general use until the period of World War II, about 1944-45. However, moldy bread has been used as a home remedy for infections for many years. Since the discovery of penicillin many other antibiotics have been discovered, and the search goes on. Antibiotics are all derived originally from molds or bacteria, which usually are soil organisms.

Penicillin is available in an endless number of preparations. Only representative ones are given here. Penicillin is prepared in salts of potassium and sodium. It is also made in a number of types (G, O, V), but type G is the one most commonly used.

Penicillin and streptomycin are known as narrow spectrum antibiotics; some of the others are called broad spectrum antibiotics. The former are effective against a few organisms; the latter are effective against many organisms. Some antibiotics, though very effective in killing organisms in vitro, have only limited use in medicine because of their toxicity.

Some antibiotics can be administered by one route only, which limits their effectiveness. Others may be given by a number of routes. Antibiotics may be grouped according to their usual mode of administration. Thus, penicillin and streptomycin are most often administered parenterally; tetracyclines, chloramphenicol and erythromycin are given orally; and some others are administered topically. Another method of categorizing them is according to the organisms against which they are effective.

Name, Source, Synonyms, Preparations	Dosage and Administration	Uses	Action and Fate	Side Effects and Contraindications	Remarks
PENICILLIN. *Mold. Penicillium chrysogenum.* Also *Synthetic.* **PENICILLIN G.**		Effective against most gram-positive organisms (streptococci, staphylococci, pneumococci); clostridia; some gram-negative organisms (gonococci, meningococci); some spirochetes	Bacteriostatic and bactericidal. It acts by blocking the synthesis of the bacterial wall. Penicillin G 1/3 oral dose is absorbed from the intestinal tract, reaches peak	Actual toxic symptoms are rare, but allergic reactions do occur. These include direct reaction at the point of intramuscular injection, dermatitis of various types, delayed or immediate	Oral penicillin should be given 1 hour before or 2 hours after meals. Injections: After reconstitution, the solution may be stored under refrigeration for 1 week and is

GROUP 1.					
Potassium penicillin G., U.S.P. crystalline buffered (Pentids, Pfizerpen) (benzyl-penicillin potassium, Abbocillin, Crystapen, Falapen, Hylenta, Ka-Pen, Megacillin [C]).	50,000-400,000-20,000,000 U. q. 2-3 h. day and night. Available in varied forms for oral, parenteral, and inhalational use.	*(Treponema pallidum, Treponema pertenue)*; some fungi.	level in 30-60 minutes. After injection reaches maximum level in 15-30 minutes. Widely distributed in body. 60-90% of I.M. dose excreted by the kidneys.	anaphylactic reactions. Local reaction may be due to the vehicle and not to the actual drug. Treatment as for any allergic reaction. Repetition of the drug may be unwise, if the reaction is severe.	stable 24 hours at room temperature. Potassium Penicillin G, U.S.P. inj. contains 1.7 mEq. K and .33 mEq. Na per 1,000,000 units; Sodium penicillin G inj., U.S.P., contains 2 mEq. Na per 1,000,000 U.
Sodium penicillin G. (Crystapen, Unikcrystalline [C]).	100,000-5,000,000 U. Oral, I.M., or I.V.			Hemolytic anemia, leukopenia, thrombocytopenia, neuropathy and nephropathy are rarely observed side effects and are usually associated with high I.V. dosage. In high doses (10,000,000 units) potassium penicillin should be given very slowly I.V. because of adverse effects of electrolytic imbalance due to potassium content.	
GROUP 1. Penicillins G and O, modified chemically and physically to increase duration of action by delay of absorption.					
Procaine penicillin G., U.S.P. Crysticillin, Duracillin, Wycillin) (Ayercillin, Francacilline, Ibacillin [C]).	300,000-2,400,000 U. Given every 12-24-48 hours. Available in crystalline form and in oil; also with potassium penicillin for immediate and delayed action. I.M.				
Procaine penicillin G with aluminum monostearate, U.S.P.	300,000-1,200,000 U.I.M.				
Benzathine penicillin G, U.S.P. (Bicillin) (benzethacil, Ben-P, Duapen, Megacillin [C]).	600,000-2,400,000 U.I.M. Given every 7-14 days; action prolonged due to slow absorption.				
PENICILLIN V					
Phenoxymethyl penicillin (Penicillin V, Pen-Vee, V-Cillin) (Compocillin, Nadopen-V, Therapen V [C]).	200,000-500,000 U. q.i.d. Oral.		Better absorption than penicillin G after oral dose. More acid resistant. Gives measurable blood level up to 4-6 hours after oral dose.		
Potassium phenoxymethyl penicillin, U.S.P. (Compocillin-VK, Pen-Vee K, V-Cillin-K, Veetids).	200,000-800,000 U. q.i.d. Oral.				
Hydrabamine phenoxymethyl penicillin (Compocillin-V).	300,000 U. (180 mg). q.i.d. Oral.				

Name, Source, Synonyms, Preparations	Dosage and Administration	Uses	Action and Fate	Side Effects and Contraindications	Remarks
GROUP 2.					
SEMISYNTHETIC GROUP					
Potassium phenethicillin, N.F. (Syncillin)	250 mg. q.i.d. Oral.		Absorption from gastro-intestinal tract incomplete. Gives peak blood level in about 1 hour. Widely distributed in body. Excreted mainly by kidneys.	Safe use during pregnancy has not been established.	
SYNTHETIC PENICILLIN USED FOR RESISTANT STAPHYLOCOCCAL INFECTIONS					
Methicillin sodium (Staphcillin) (meticillin, Celbenin, Synticillin [C]).	1 Gm. q. 4-6 hr. I.M. or I.V.	Used for resistant staphylococcal infections.	Widely distributed, but not to spinal fluid unless meningeal inflammation is present and then larger amounts are found here. Rapidly excreted by kidneys. Half-life for person with normal renal function, 6 hours.	See above.	Destroyed by stomach acid; must be given by injection. Methicillin should not be physically mixed with other agents. Methicillin, once diluted, should be administered within 8 hours but may be stored in concentrate 1 day at room temperature and 48 hours under refrigeration.
Nafcillin sodium (Unipen).	500 mg. –2 Gm. q. 4 h. I.V. 500 mg. q. 6 h. I.M. 250-500 mg. q. 4-6 h. Oral.	As above.	Peak blood level in 1 hour. 60-70% plasma bound. 90% of I.V. dose excreted in bile.		
Sodium cloxacillin monohydrate (Tegopen) (Orbenan [C]).	250-500 mg. q. 4-6 h. Oral.	As above.			
Dicloxacillin sodium monohydrate (Dynapen, Pathocil, Veracillin).	250-500 mg. q. 6 h. Oral.	See Oxacillin.			Best absorption on empty stomach at least 1 hour before meals.
Sodium oxacillin, U.S.P. (Prostaphlin, Resistopen).	250-1000 mg. q. 4-6 h. Oral, I.M.	As above.	60% of oral dose absorbed. Peak blood level in 1 hour after oral dose. Excreted mainly by kidneys.	Pain at point of injection may occur. Neutropenia and an elevated SGOT have been reported.	Should be taken on empty stomach.

SYNTHETIC PENICILLIN WITH BROAD SPECTRUM ACTIVITY

Ampicillin (Omnipen, Penbritin, Polycillin, Polycillin-N, Principen) (Amgill, Ampen, Ampicin [C]).	250-500 mg. q.i.d. Oral. 250-1000 mg. q. 6 h. I.M. or I.V.	A broad spectrum antibiotic used in a number of infections.	Appear in all body fluids except cerebrospinal. Excreted unchanged by the kidneys. High concentration found in bile.	Pain at point of injection may occur. Allergic reactions (see penicillin) and neutropenia have been reported.	Ampicillin is of no value in penicillinase producing organisms.
Carbenicillin disodium (Geopen, Pyopen).	4-40 Gm. daily I.M. or I.V.	Indicated in infections due to susceptible *Pseudomonas aeruginosa, Proteus species* (particularly indole positive strains) and some strains of *E. coli.* Used in the treatment of severe systemic infections and septicemia, infections of the urinary and respiratory tracts and of the soft tissues.	Not absorbed orally. Following I.M. injections, peak blood levels are reached in two hours. As with other penicillins, probenecid will prolong the serum levels and also increase them somewhat. The drug is rapidly excreted in the urine.	Hypersensitivity (anaphylactic reactions have been seen). Such conditions as skin rashes, urticaria, pruritus, drug fever and nausea may occur. As with other penicillins, anemia, thrombocytopenia, leukopenia, neutropenia and/or eosinophilia can occur. SGOT and SGPT levels may become elevated. With high serum levels, convulsions or neuromuscular irritability may be seen. Vein irritation and phlebitis have been reported. Contraindicated in patients who have known penicillin allergy.	This is a synthetic penicillin with gram negative spectrum. It is a benzylpenicillin derivative. Emergence of resistant organisms may lead to superinfections. When used with gentamycin I.V. the two must not be mixed together in the same infusion fluid.
Carbenicillin indayl sodium (Geocillin).	382-764 mg. q.i.d. Oral.	Upper and lower urinary tract infections caused by susceptible strains of *E. coli, Proteus mirabilis,* and *Pseudomonas.*	This salt is acid stable and well absorbed following oral administration. After absorption it is hydrolyzed to carbenicillin which is primarily excreted in the urine.	See above. Safety during pregnancy has not been established.	
Hetacillin and Hetacillin K (Veraspen and Veraspen K) (phenazacillin [C]).	225-450 mg. q. 6 h. in persons weighing over 90 pounds. Oral. Under 90 lbs. 10-20 mg./lb./day in 4 divided doses. Oral.	See ampicillin.	The drug itself has no antibacterial activity, but it is converted by the body into ampicillin and as such is active against ampicillin-sensitive organisms during the stage of multiplication by inhibition of mucoproteins for cell wall synthesis. Well absorbed orally, but absorption is retarded by food so is best given on an empty stomach.	See ampicillin. It is said to cause fewer gastrointestinal problems because it is converted by the body into the active substance. Periodic assessment of hepatic, hemopoietic and renal systems should be carried out when used on a long-term basis, especially in prematures, neonates and infants.	The possibility of superinfections with mycotic or bacterial pathogens should be kept in mind.

Name, Source, Synonyms, Preparations	Dosage and Administration	Uses	Action and Fate	Side Effects and Contraindications	Remarks
SEMISYNTHETIC GROUP (Continued)					
CEPHALOSPORIN ANTIBIOTICS (Derived from *Cephalosporium sp.*)					
Cephalothin (Keflin).	0.5-1 Gm. q. 4-6 h. I.M. 2-6 Gm. Daily. I.V. Can be given intraperitoneally in concentrations of 0.1 to 4% in saline.	A broad spectrum antibiotic used in a number of infections.	Appear in all body fluids except cerebrospinal. Excreted rapidly in the urine.	Pain at point of injection may occur. Allergic reactions including anaphylaxis have been reported. Also, neutropenia and hemolytic anemia have been seen. Some patients (especially those with azotemia) have developed direct positive Coombs' test. Transient rise in SGOT and BUN and, in some patients, thrombophlebitis have occurred, especially those receiving over 6 Gm. daily I.V.	Solutions may be stored 48 hours under refrigeration. If solution precipitates, they will redissolve on warming.
Cephaloridine (Loridine) (Caporan [C]).	0.5 to 1.0 Gm. I.M. at equally spaced intervals. Range 1.0 to 4.0 Gm. daily. Children 30-50 mg./kg. in divided doses. 100 mg./kg. in severe infections. Do not exceed maximum adult dose.	Used in severe infections of bone, joints, blood stream, genitourinary tract and respiratory system and skin, if the organism is susceptible.	Peak blood levels of 7-15 mcg./ml. reached in ½-1 hour after I.M. injection of 250-500 mg. Measurable amounts persist for longer than 12 hours. These doses produce high urine concentrations (up to 1000 mcg./ml.).	Contraindicated in azotemia and hypersensitivity to cephalothin. Side effects: urticaria, skin rashes, itching, drug fever, rise in eosinophil count, leukopenia, elevation of transaminase and alkaline phosphatase, severe acute renal failure in some cases, especially with high dosage. Nausea and vomiting may occur. Safety during pregnancy, and for premature infants and infants under 1 month has not been established.	Because of renal toxicity dosage should not exceed 4 Gm. daily. After mixture, store in refrigerator for not more than 96 hours. Extemporaneous mixture with other antibiotics not recommended.
Cephaloglycin dihydrate (Kafocin).	250-500 mg. q.i.d. Oral.	Indicated only for urinary tract infections, both acute and chronic, due to	Is said to be acid stable and is absorbed orally. Food does not interfere with total	Gastrointestinal: nausea, vomiting, diarrhea. With allergy: rash, urticaria, etc.	Use with extreme caution in patients known to be sensitive to penicillin.

		susceptible strains of *E. coli, Klebsiella, Aerobacter, Proteus,* staphylococci and streptococci.	absorption, but it can delay the time that peak urinary levels are reached. It is excreted almost entirely as the active metabolite desacetyl-cephaloglycin in the urine. Serum levels are not sufficient to be effective in any infections other than those of the urinary tract.	Others reported: malaise, fever, chills, headache, dizziness and vertigo. Eosinophilia has been reported. Contraindicated in known sensitivity to the cephalosporin drugs. Safe use during pregnancy or in children has not been established.	There is clinical evidence of cross-sensitivity between the penicillins and the cephalosporins. There are instances of patients who have had reactions to both drugs (including fatal anaphylactic reactions after parenteral use).
Cephalexin monohydrate (Keflex).	1-4 Gm. daily in divided doses (usually 250-500 mg. q.i.d.)	Indicated for respiratory infections due to *D. pneumoniae* and hemolytic streptococci; in skin and soft tissue infections caused by staphylococci; and in urinary infections caused by *E. coli, Pr. mirabilis* and *Klebsiella sp.*	It is acid stable and can be given without regard for meals. It is bactericidal because of its effect on cell wall synthesis. Well absorbed orally with peak serum level reached in an hour, and 90% is excreted unchanged in the urine in 8 hours.	Safe use during pregnancy or in infants under one year has not been established. Side effects: see cephaloglycin. Can cause positive Coombs' test and slight elevation of SGPT and SGOT.	Use with extreme caution in patients known to be allergic to penicillin. Allergic reaction to one cephalosporin C derivative contraindicates the use of all such derivatives.

AMINOGLYCOSIDE ANTIBIOTICS

These drugs are organic bases with amino sugar groups. Hence, their group name, aminoglycoside antibiotics. They have similar activities, spectrums and side effects. They are not absorbed to any extent after oral administration. They are obtained from species of *Streptomyces* or are synthetic. They all potentiate gallamine triethiodide and other muscle relaxant drugs used in anesthesia.

Dihydrostreptomycin sulfate.	0.5-1 Gm. daily. I.M.	Most effective against gram-negative organisms and acid-fast bacteria.	Bacteriostatic and bactericidal. Streptomycin is thought to act by inhibiting energy production of microorganisms by interfering with one of the steps in the Krebs cycle.	Vertigo, dizziness, temporary loss of hearing, mental depression; sometimes severe reactions such as fever, skin eruptions, and arthralgia. Treatment: symptomatic. Drug is usually reduced in amount or stopped.	Dihydrostreptomycin is a semi-synthetic preparation. It appears to be more toxic than streptomycin and is therefore used less. Streptomycin sulfate is the most popular form of streptomycin.
Streptoduocin injection, U.S.P.	0.5-1 Gm. daily. I.M.			Crosses placenta and has been associated with hearing loss, multiple skeletal anomalies and eighth cranial nerve damage in the fetus.	

Name, Source, Synonyms, Preparations	Dosage and Administration	Uses	Action and Fate	Side Effects and Contraindications	Remarks
AMINOGLYCOSIDE ANTIBIOTICS (Continued)					
Streptomycin sulfate, U.S.P. (Strycin) (Strepolin [C]).	0.5-1-2 Gm. Daily, but not usually continued on daily basis more than 3 to 4 weeks. Though available for subcutaneous and topical administration, by far the most common mode is I.M.		Widely distributed but mostly in extracellular fluids. After I.M. dose 50-60% excreted unchanged in urine within the first 24 hours, mostly in the first 12 hours.		
Kanamycin sulfate (Kantrex).	15 mg./kg. in divided doses daily. I.M. Should never exceed 1.5 Gm. in one day. 1 Gm. q. 4-6 h. Oral. 15-30 mg./kg. Daily in divided doses. Oral. Also prepared for intravenous or intracavitary use.	For tuberculosis and other infections. Active against a number of organisms. For preoperative disinfection of the intestines. For *Shigella* and *Salmonella* infections. For specific and usually severe infections.	Bactericidal. Action as for streptomycin. Poorly absorbed from GI tract. 50-80% of parenteral dose excreted by kidneys in 24 hours, most in the first 6 hours.	May cause nausea, vomiting, diarrhea. Adjust or stop dosage. Major toxic effect of parenteral kanamycin is its action on the auditory portion of the 8th cranial. Safe use during pregnancy has not been established.	Concurrent use of kanamycin and ethacrynic acid (especially if given I.V.) should be avoided because of possible resulting deafness. In patients with impaired renal function, the dose interval should be adjusted by the use of the following formula: serum creatinine (mg./100 ml.) x 9 = dose interval. As the creatinine clearance changes, dosage interval should be adjusted.
Neomycin sulfate, U.S.P. (Mycifradin, Neobiotic. [C]).	4.5-9 Gm. Divided doses 24-72 hours prior to surgery. Oral. 4-12 Gm. daily in divided doses. Oral. 10-15 mg./kg. in divided doses every 6 hours; not more than 1 Gm./day. I.M. Treatment by I.M. should not be continued longer than 10 days.	Effective against a number of organisms. For preoperative intestinal disinfection. For hepatic coma. For treatment of severe infections that do not respond to less toxic drugs.	Bacteriostatic and bactericidal. For mechanism see Streptomycin. Oral dose poorly absorbed; 97% of such dose excreted in feces. After I.M. injection 30-50% excreted by kidneys.	Mild laxative action with oral use. With parenteral use there may be renal disorders, eighth cranial nerve involvement, or both. Adjust dosage or stop drug and treat symptoms.	With I.M. use, frequent urinalyses and audiometry advised.

Neomycin sulfate ointment and solution, U.S.P. (Myciquent) (Neomycreme [C]).	1% solution or ointment once or twice daily. Topical.	For infections of skin and exposed mucous membrane.			
Paromomycin sulfate, U.S.P. (Humatin).	35-50 mg./kg. Daily in divided doses for 5-7 days. Oral.	Used in treating enteric bacterial and amebic infections, and in preoperative suppression of intestinal flora.	Bacteriostatic.	Diarrhea, abdominal cramps, pruritus ani. Treatment symptomatic.	Poor absorption from G.I. tract precludes systemic use; overgrowth of some organisms may occur.

TETRACYCLINES, including chlortetracyclines, oxytetracycline and others, are all derived directly from a strain of streptomyces, indirectly from chlortetracycline or are produced synthetically. They are mainly bacteriostatic. These drugs are effective against both gram-positive and gram-negative bacteria and many other types of microorganisms. They have a broad spectrum of activity. Tetracycline, oxytetracycline and methacycline may form a stable complex in any bone forming tissue. No serious harmful effects have been reported thus far in humans. However, use of these drugs during tooth development—last trimester of pregnancy, neonatal period and early childhood—may cause discoloration of the teeth (yellow-grey-brown). The effect occurs most often during long-term use of the drug, but it has also been observed with the usual short-term therapy. It has also been associated with inhibited bone growth, micromelia and syndactyly in the fetus. Photosensitivity has occurred with all the tetracyclines and patients taking these drugs should be aware of this.

Chlortetracycline hydrochloride capsules, N.F. (Aureomycin).	50-250 mg. q. 6 h. Oral.				
Chlortetracycline hydrochloride injection, N.F.	50-250 mg. q. 6 h., and only when unable to take medication orally. I.V.				
Demethylchlortetracycline (Declomycin) (demectocycline [C]).	30-150 mg. q. 6 h. Oral.				
Doxycycline hydrate and monohydrate (Vibra).	25-100 mg. Oral. Usually 100 mg. q. 12 h. 1st day then 100 mg, q. d. or 50-100 mg. q. 12 h. Children less than 100 lb. 2 mg./lb. 1st day then 1 mg./lb.		Better absorption than some tetracyclines after oral dose. Absorption is not influenced by food or milk. Excreted slowly. Do not give with antacids.	If renal impairment exists usual dose may accumulate excessively and hepatic toxicity be induced.	Doxycycline hydrate comes in capsules; the monohydrate is a powder for oral suspension 25 mg./ml.
Doxycycline hydrate (Vibramycin Hydrate).	100-200 mg./day I.V. children under 100 lbs. 2 mg./lb/1st day, then 1-2 mg./lb./day.				Avoid rapid administration. Consult brochure before giving this drug. Solutions should be protected from light and used within 12 hours at room temperature or 72 hours if kept under refrigeration.

Name, Source, Synonyms, Preparations	Dosage and Administration	Uses	Action and Fate	Side Effects and Contraindications	Remarks
TETRACYCLINE ANTIBIOTICS (Continued)					
Methacycline hydrochloride, N.F. (Rondomycin).	150 mg. q. 6 h. or 300 mg. q. 12 h. Children: 3-6 mg. per lb. in divided doses b.i.d. to q.i.d.			Side effects: Same as others plus proctitis, vaginitis, dermatitis. If allergic reactions occur, stop drug at once. In renal impairment, dosage should be reduced.	In infants, intracranial pressure has occurred. It clears with discontinuance of drug without known sequelae.
Minocycline hydrochloride. (Minocin).	200 mg. 1st day, then 100 mg. q. 12 h. Oral. or I.V. 300 mg. single dose.	For gonorrhea.			Dairy products have not been shown to noticeably influence this particular tetracycline.
Oxytetracycline hydrochloride, N.F., (Terramycin) (Novoxytetra [C]).	50-250 mg. q. 6 h. Oral. 100-250 mg. q. 6 h. I.M. 250-500 mg. Daily or q. 12 h. I.V.				Also available in preparations for topical use.
Rolitetracycline, N.F. (Syntetrin) (Reverin, Syntetrex [C]).	150-350 mg. q. 6 h. I.M. 350-700 mg. daily, I.V.				
Tetracycline hydrochloride, U.S.P. (Achromycin, Panmycin, Polycycline) (Cefracycline, Muracine, Neo-Tetrine, Tetrosol, Tetradyn, [C]).	50-500 mg. q. 6 h. Oral. Also I.M., I.V., or as ophthalmic ointment.	These drugs are used in the treatment of many diseases caused by microorganisms.	The exact mechanism has not been established, but it is believed tetracyclines act by interfering with protein synthesis.	Slight gastrointestinal disorders, including diarrhea. Treatment: symptomatic. If severe reaction occurs, drug is usually changed for another similar antibiotic.	Any product containing aluminum, magnesium or calcium ions (antacids, milk and milk products) should not be taken the hour before or after an oral dose, since it can decrease absorption by as much as 25-50%.
Tetracycline phosphate complex, N.F. (Panmycin Phosphate, Sumycin, Tetrex).	150-500 mg. q. 6 h. Oral. Also I.M.		Well absorbed and distributed to most body tissues and fluids after oral dose. Tetracyclines are excreted in the urine and bile. Less chlortetracycline is excreted by the kidneys than the others.	They can cause an increase in BUN and depress plasma prothrombin activity. Tetracyclines cross the placental barrier, are found in fetal tissue and can have toxic effects on the developing fetus. They are also found in the milk of lactating mothers.	In renal dysfunction (especially during pregnancy) I.V. tetracycline therapy in daily doses exceeding 2 gm. has been associated with deaths from renal failure.

CHLORAMPHENICOL GROUP					
CHLORAMPHENICOL. *Bacterial. Streptomyces venezuelae.* Also *synthetic.*		Effective against many organisms, but especially the gram-negative organisms (colon-typhoid group). Useful in certain urinary infections and in many other conditions, but should be reserved for serious infections caused by susceptible organisms when less potentially hazardous therapeutic agents are ineffective or contraindicated.	Bacteriostatic and bactericidal. Believed to act by interfering with protein synthesis including enzyme formation. Rapidly absorbed. Widely distributed, but distribution not uniform; highest in liver, lowest in brain and spinal fluid. Excreted by kidneys mainly as the glucuronide, only 5-10% in the biologically active form.	May cause nausea and vomiting. Serious, even fatal, blood dyscrasias may occur. Reduce or stop drug and treat as indicated. See manufacturer's bulletin for specific toxicology and contraindications.	Frequent blood tests should be done during therapy. Can cause Gray syndrome or fetal death, since drug does cross placental barrier.
Chloramphenicol capsules, U.S.P. (Chloromycetin) (Chloroptic, Enicol, Mycinol, Novochlor, Sopamycetin [C]).	50-250-500 mg. q. 6 h. Oral. 50-100 mg./kg. daily is usually adequate.				
Chloramphenicol palmitate, U.S.P. (Chloromycetin palmitate).	50-250 mg. Oral.				
Chloramphenicol sodium succinate, U.S.P. (Chloromycetin succinate).	1 Gm. q. 8 h. I.V.				
POLYPEPTIDES					
BACITRACIN. *Bacterial. Bacillus subtilis.*		Effective against gram-positive organisms, the *Neisseria,* some spirochetes and *Entamoeba histolytica.* Used alone or in combination with other antibiotics.	Bacteriostatic and bactericidal. It has been reported to inhibit the incorporation of amino acids into bacterial protein with the accumulation or uridine nucleotide.	May cause renal disturbance. Adjust dosage, or discontinue and use another antibiotic.	
Bacitracin ointment, U.S.P. (Baciquent)	500 U./Gm. p.r.n. Topical.				
Bacitracin solution, U.S.P. (Topitracin). (Many of these antibiotics are used as powders and sprinkled directly on the wound or in solution as wet dressings.)	10,000-20,000 U. t.i.d. I.M.				
COLISTIMETHATE SODIUM. *Bacterial. Aerobacillus colistinus.*		For the treatment of genitourinary or systemic infections caused by gram-negative organisms, particularly those caused by *Pseudomonas aeruginosa.* Not effective against *Proteus.*	The exact mechanism is not known but is believed to be similar to that of polymyxin B. Not absorbed from gastrointestinal tract. Most excreted by kidneys following injection. Has serum half-life of 2-3 hours following I.M. or I.V. administration.	Toxicity similar to that of polymyxin B. Nephrotoxic, local irritation, nausea, paresthesia, leukopenia, fever, dermatitis, azotemia, pruritus, and vertigo have been reported. *Used with caution in patients with impaired renal function.* This drug is transferred across the placental barrier. Safe use	See interactions with anesthetic muscle relaxants and aminoglycoside antibiotics under Streptomycin. See brochure for dosage calculation.
Colistimethate sodium (Colistin, Colymycin). Colistin Sulfate, N.F.	100-150 mg. I.M. or I.V. daily. Dose on weight basis: 2 to 4 divided doses 2.5-5.0 mg./kg./day.				

Name, Source, Synonyms, Preparations	Dosage and Administration	Uses	Action and Fate	Side Effects and Contraindications	Remarks
POLYPEPTIDES (Continued)					
COLISTIMETHATE SODIUM (Continued)				during pregnancy has not been established. Respiratory arrest has occurred following I.M. injection. Increased BUN has been seen, but returns to normal when drug is stopped.	
GENTAMICIN. *Bacterial. Micromonospora purpurea.*		Used to treat various bacterial skin diseases.	Antibacterial. After injection effective blood levels are seen for 6-8 hours. Most is excreted via glomerular filtration.	If sensitivity reactions occur drug should be stopped. Gentamicin used parenterally is potentially ototoxic (both vestibular and auditory) and nephrotoxic. Monitoring of renal and 8th cranial nerve function during therapy is recommended. Other side effects include elevated SGOT and SGPT, increased bilirubin, anemia, granulocytopenia and thrombocytopenia. Fever, rash, urticaria, laryngeal edema, nausea and vomiting, lethargy, decreased appetite, headache, weight loss.	Not effective against fungi or viruses. Concurrent use of other neuro- and/or nephrotoxic drugs should be avoided. Dose must be adjusted in patients with impaired renal function. Safe use in pregnancy has not been established. See carbenicillin for interactions.
Gentamicin (Garamycin)	0.1% ointment or cream t.i.d. or q.i.d. Topical. Ophthalmic ointment 3 mg./Gm. or solution 3 mg./ml. b. or t.i.d.	Primary: impetigo contagiosa, folliculitis, ecthyma, furunculosis, sycosis barbae, pyoderma gangrenosum. Used for infections of the external eye caused by susceptible organisms. Secondary: infections in acne, pustular psoriasis, excoriations, wounds, burns.			
Gentamicin sulfate, U.S.P.	0.8-3.0 mg./kg. daily in 3 divided doses I.M. Up to 5 mg./kg. in life threatening infections.	Used parenterally in *Pseudomoas aeruginosa, Proteus sp., E. coli, Klebsiella, Enterobacter, Serratia sp.* and *Staphylococcus sp.* for infections of the central nervous system, urinary tract, upper respiratory tract, gastrointestinal tract, skin and soft tissues, including burns.			
POLYMYXIN B. *Bacterial. Bacillus polymyxa.* Polymyxin B sulfate, N.F. (Aerosporin).	1.5-2.5 mg./kg. in divided doses. b.i.d. but not over 200 mg. in any one day. Oral, I.M., or I.V.	Effective mainly against gram-negative organisms. Not given orally for systemic infections.	Bacteriostatic and bactericidal. Acts by rupture of cell membranes through cationic surface effect.	Toxicity usually low in recommended dosage, but neurotoxic and nephrotoxic symptoms may occur. If symptoms are severe, drug	Available in preparations for topical use.

			Not absorbed orally. Slowly excreted by kidneys after I.M. or I.V.	should be stopped and symptoms treated as indicated.	
TYROTHRICIN. *Bacterial. Bacillus brevis.* Tyrothricin, N.F. (Hydrotricine [C]).	0.5-25 mg./cc. Cream, ointment, and spray for topical use.	Effective against gram-positive bacteria and some other organisms.	Bacteriostatic and bactericidal. Acts as cationic detergent which damages all membranes.	Very toxic systemically. Used mainly topically.	Used alone or with other antibiotics.
MACROLIDES					
ERYTHROMYCIN. *Bacterial. Streptomyces erythreus.* Erythromycin (Erythrocin, E-Mycin, Ilotycin) (Chem-Thromycin, Emcin, Ilosone [C]).	100-500 mg. q. 6 h. Oral. 100 mg. q. 8-12 h. I.M. 250-1000 mg. q. 6-8 h. I.V. 5 mg./Gm. ophthalmic ointment.	Effective against a number of gram-negative, gram-positive, and other organisms. Especially useful against penicillin-resistant staphylococci.	Inhibits protein synthesis without affecting nucleic acid synthesis. Bacteriostatic. Widely distributed. Excreted in bile and urine.	Usually slight. Treatment: symptomatic. The estolate ester (Ilosone) has been associated with an allergic type of cholestatic hepatitis (in adults). The effects appear reversible on discontinuing the drug.	Available as several salts and in preparations for parenteral and topical use; also as chewables, especially for children. Safety during pregnancy has not been established.
OLEANDOMYCIN. *Bacterial. Streptomyces antibioticus.* Oleandomycin phosphate, N.F. (Matromycin). Triacetyloleandomycin (Cyclamycin, Tao).	0.25-0.5 Gm. q.i.d. Oral. 0.25-0.5 Gm. q.i.d. Oral.	Uses are similar to those of penicillin, but it has a somewhat wider spectrum.	Bacteriostatic. Exact mechanism is not known. Absorption incomplete. Widely distributed but not to brain and cerebrospinal fluid. Excreted in urine and bile.	Rare, but sensitivity may occur. Stop drug and treat symptoms.	
ANTIFUNGAL POLYENES					
CANDICIDIN. *Bacterial. Streptomyces sp.* Candicidin, N.F. (Candeptin).	3 mg. tablet or ointment b.i.d. intravaginally for 14 days.	Treatment of vaginitis due to Candida.	Fungicidal.	Sensitivity may occur, but this is rare.	Store in a cool place. The tablet form is advised during pregnancy.
NYSTATIN. *Bacterial. Streptomyces noursei.* Nystatin, U.S.P. (Mycostatin, Nilstat).	Cream or ointment 100,000 U./Gm. 500,000 U. Once or twice a day. Oral. 100,000 U. Vaginal tablets. 100,000 U./Gm. Topical powder. 100,000 U./ml. suspension.	Antifungal; effective against intestinal moniliasis, vulvovaginal candidiasis, cutaneous or mucocutaneous infections caused by Candida.	Mechanism of action is believed to be by binding to sterols in the cell membrane with resultant change in membrane permeability.	Rare, but sensitivities have occurred. Stop drug and treat symptoms.	

Name, Source, Synonyms, Preparations	Dosage and Administration	Uses	Action and Fate	Side Effects and Contraindications	Remarks
ANTIFUNGAL POLYENES (Continued)					
AMPHOTERICIN B. *Bacterial. Streptomyces nodosus.* Amphotericin B, U.S.P. (Fungizone).	Begin with 0.25 mg./kg./day, increase to 1 mg./kg./day when possible. Available in 50 mg. vial. I.V. Topical, lotion.	Used to treat deep-seated mycotic infections.	Exact mechanism of action not known. Effective against fungal infections, but of no value in bacterial infections. Excreted slowly by kidneys.	Toxicity not yet clearly established, but anorexia, headache, chills, fever may occur. Treatment: palliative.	Should be given systemically only to hospitalized persons.
ORAL ANTIFUNGAL PREPARATION FOR SYSTEMIC FUNGAL INFECTIONS					
Flucytosine (Ancobon).	50-150 mg./kg./day at 6-hour intervals. Oral.	Used only in the treatment of serious infections caused by susceptible strains of *Candida* and/or *Cryptococcus.*	Mode of action is not known, but has in vitro and in vivo activity against *Candida* and *Cryptococcus.* It is not metabolized significantly when given orally and is excreted primarily by the kidneys.	Nausea, vomiting, diarrhea, rash, anemia, leukopenia, thrombocytopenia, elevation of hepatic enzymes, BUN and creatinine have been reported. Also seen: confusion, hallucinations, headache, sedation and vertigo.	Nausea and vomiting may be reduced if capsules are given a few at a time over a 15 minute period. Must be used with extreme caution in patients with impaired renal function. Drug can affect hepatic and hematologic systems and these must be monitored during therapy. Renal function should be determined before treatment is started.
ORAL ANTIFUNGAL PREPARATION FOR FUNGAL INFECTIONS OF SKIN, NAILS, HAIR					
GRISEOFULVIN. *Fungal. Penicillium griseofulvin* or *nigricans.* Griseofulvin, U.S.P. (Fulvicin U/F, Grifulvin, Grisactin) (Grisovin, Likuden [C]).	125-250 mg.-500 mg. Two to four times a day. Oral. Usually given four times a day in adult.	For treatment of mycotic infections by dermatophytes in hands, feet, nails, and scalp.	Deposited in precursor cells that form the keratin layer, rendering the keratin layer resistant to fungal infections. Bulk of oral dose excreted in feces.	Claimed to be mild and transient; heartburn, nausea, epigastric discomfort, diarrhea, headache. Discontinue if drug rash occurs. Patient's blood should be tested regularly for signs of leukopenia with prolonged therapy. Blood levels of griseofulvin may be lowered clinically to ineffective levels by concurrent or recent administration	Treatment usually prolonged (several months), owing to the mechanism of action involved.

				of phenobarbital, other barbiturates such as amobarbital, butabarbital, pentobarbital, secobarbital, and talbutal. If patient is on anticoagulants, the prothrombin times should be performed weekly until a stable level is found. This interaction does not occur in all patients.	
RESERVE GROUP. USED ONLY WHEN NECESSARY					
NOVOBIOCIN. *Bacterial. Streptomyces spheroides.* Novobiocin calcium or sodium (Albamycin).	0.25-0.5 Gm. q. 12 h. Oral.	Used mainly in infections caused by various penicillin resistant staphylococci and Proteus organisms.	Mechanism is not known, but organisms have been able to develop resistance rapidly. Well absorbed. Excreted mainly in bile. Crosses the placental barrier and has caused hyperbilirubinemia of the fetus.	Rare, but a yellow pigment has been found in the plasma of patients receiving the drug. This does not indicate liver damage. Treatment: none usually required. Leukopenia has been seen in patients receiving novobiocin.	Also available as a syrup, which is useful for children, and in preparations for parenteral use.
RISTOCETIN. *Fungal. Nocardia lurida.* Ristocetin (Spontin, Riston).	25-50 mg./kg. of body weight b.i.d. I.V.	Most effective against gram-positive cocci. Especially useful in bacterial endocarditis and staphylococcal septicemia.	Exact mechanism is not known but thought to be similar to that of vancomycin. Excreted mainly in urine.	Some allergic reactions and gastrointestinal symptoms may occur. Reduce dosage or stop drug.	Irritating to the tissues, so that care must be taken to prevent leakage. Frequent blood and urine tests should be made.
VANCOMYCIN. *Bacterial. Streptomyces orientalis.* Vancomycin, U.S.P. (Vancocin).	0.5 Gm. q.i.d. I.V. Given with I.V. infusions.	Effective against infections caused by strains resistant to other antibiotics.	Mechanism of action is not known. Half-life in circulation 6 hours. Excreted mainly by kidneys.	Toxicity usually low but may cause eighth cranial nerve damage, renal disorders, or both. Stop drug and treat symptoms. Contraindicated in reduced renal function.	

Name, Source, Synonyms, Preparations	Dosage and Administration	Uses	Action and Fate	Side Effects and Contraindications	Remarks
THE FOLLOWING ARE USED MAINLY IN TUBERCULOSIS OR AS RESERVE ANTIBIOTICS IN RESISTANT CASES					
Capreomycin sulfate (Capastat Sulfate) A polypeptide antibiotic obtained from *Streptomyces capreolus.*	1 Gm. daily, I.M. (not to exceed 20 mg./kg. per day) for 60 to 120 days followed by 1 Gm. 2 or 3 times a day for 18-24 months.	To be used with other anti-tuberculosis drugs in pulmonary infections caused by strains of *M. tuberculosis* sensitive to capreomycin when primary agents have been ineffective or cannot be used because of toxicity or resistant organisms.	Not absorbed in appreciable amounts from gastrointestinal tract. Must be given by injection. In patients with normal renal function 52% of a 1 Gm. dose can be recovered unchanged in the urine in 12 hours.	Shows some or all of the following in varying degrees: nephrotoxicity, ototoxicity, hepatotoxicity. Leucocytosis and leucopenia have been reported, as have urticaria and other skin rashes. Sterile abscess and excessive bleeding at point of injection have occurred. Use in patients with renal insufficiency or pre-existing auditory impairment must be undertaken with great caution. Safety for use during pregnancy or for infants and children has not been established.	Cross resistance occurs between capreomycin and viomycin and some has been reported with kanamycin and neomycin. After reconstitution, it may be stored for 48 hours at room temperature or for 14 days under refrigeration. Audiometric and renal function tests should be done before and during therapy.
Cycloserine, U.S.P. (Oxamycin, Seromycin). *Bacterial. Streptomyces orchidaceus* or *S. garyphalus.*	0.25-0.5 Gm. t.i.d. Oral.	Used mainly in severe pulmonary tuberculosis.	Competes with D-alanine as a cell wall precursor. Body distribution good. Excreted mainly in urine.	Neurotoxic. Mental confusion, convulsions. Reduce dosage or stop. Contraindicated in epilepsy and severe renal insufficiency.	Safe use during pregnancy has not been established. Concurrent excessive use of alcoholic beverages should be avoided.
Rifampin (Rifadin, Rimactane).	600 mg. daily. Oral. For children: 10-20 mg./kg. daily. Oral. Not to exceed 600 mg. daily. Given once daily on an empty stomach.	For tuberculosis. Should not be given without at least one other antitubercular agent such as isoniazid or ethambutol or both.	Rifampin is believed to inhibit DNA-dependent RNA polymerase activity in susceptible cells (bacterial), but does not affect mammalian cells.	The drug may cause liver damage, especially in patients with impaired liver function. Should not be used with other hepatotoxic drugs for such patients. Liver function tests should be done frequently in such cases. Animal experimentation has shown the drug to be teratogenic; the effect in	
	600 mg. daily for 4 consecutive days. Oral. For children: 10-20 mg./kg. daily for 4 consecutive days. Oral.	For meningococcal carriers.	Peak blood levels vary with individuals, but are usually reached in 2-4 hours after a 600 mg. dose. Half-life is about 3 hours.		The use of rifampin in meningococcal carriers should be limited to situations in which the risk of meningococcal meningitis

	Dosage for children under 5 years of age has not been established.		Elimination is mainly through bile, a very little in urine.	man is not known. Use in women of child-bearing age or during pregnancy should be carefully weighed—benefits against possible dangers. Contraindication: The only known contraindication is sensitivity to the drug.	is high.
VIOMYCIN SULFATE. *Bacterial. Streptomyces puniceus.* Viomycin sulfate, U.S.P. (Vinactane, Viocin).	1-2 Gm. I.M. b.i.d. every third day or b.i.s.	Effective against acid-fast organisms. Used mainly in the treatment of tuberculosis.	Bacteriostatic. Resembles streptomycin in its action but is a basic polypeptide. Good distribution. Excreted mainly by kidneys.	Allergic reactions, signs of renal disturbances, edema, dizziness, hearing loss. Change drug and treat symptoms. Contraindicated in known renal disorders.	
ANTIBIOTICS WITH VARIOUS USES					
FUMAGILLIN. *Fungal. Aspergillus fumigatus.* Fumagillin (Fugillin, Fumidil).	10-60 mg. Daily in divided doses. Oral.	Used mainly in amebic dysentery. Also used in the treatment of certain neoplasms.	Has direct action on the amebae without effect on other intestinal flora.	Gastrointestinal disturbances, headache, rash. Effect upon blood not yet determined. Stop drug and treat symptoms.	Frequent blood tests should be done.
LINCOMYCIN. *Bacterial. Streptomyces lincolnensis var.* Lincomycin hydrochloride (Lincocin).	500 mg. Three to four times a day. Oral. 600 mg. q. 12-24 h. I.M. 600 mg.-1 Gm. Given in 250 or more ml. of 5% glucose solution q. 8-12 h. I.V.	Used mainly in penicillin resistant gram-positive infections, and in patients who are allergic to penicillin.	Interferes with protein synthesis of bacterial organism. Distributed in all body tissues except central nervous system. Good absorption and distribution. Body half-life about 6 hours. Excreted in bile and urine.	Loose stools or diarrhea, sometimes severe and persistent, with blood and mucus; nausea, vomiting, abdominal cramps, skin rash, rectal irritation, vaginitis, urticaria, and pruritus have occurred. Neutropenia, leukopenia, agranulocytosis and thrombocytopenic purpura have been reported. Abnormal liver function tests, jaundice and hypotension following parenteral use, especially, rapid I.V. administration. Also, cardiopulmonary arrest has occurred after rapid I.V. infusion.	Lincomycin must not be administered at same time as kaolin-containing products since it may reduce as much as 90% absorption. Lincomycin should be given 1 hour before or 2 hours after eating.

Name, Source, Synonyms, Preparations	Dosage and Administration	Uses	Action and Fate	Side Effects and Contraindications	Remarks
ANTIBIOTICS WITH VARIOUS USES (Continued)					
LINCOMYCIN (Continued)				Known *Candida* (monilial) infections should be treated concurrently with an anti-fungal agent such as nystatin.	
Clindamycin hydrochloride hydrate. *Synthetic.* (Cleocin) (Dalacin [C]).	150-600 mg. q. 6 h. (average 150 mg. q. 6 h.). Oral. 300-600 mg. I.M. or I.V. For children: 4-10 mg./lb./day in 4 divided doses. Oral.	See lincomycin. For beta-hemolytic streptococcal infections, treatment should be continued at least 10 days to diminish the likelihood of subsequent rheumatic fever or glomerulonephritis.	50% of oral dose is absorbed. Widely distributed in body fluids and tissues. Biological half-life is 2.4 hours. 10% of bioactive drug is excreted in the urine and about 3% in the feces. The remainder is excreted as bio-inactive metabolites.	See lincomycin. It is said to have more in vivo potency, better oral absorption and fewer gastrointestinal side effects than the parent drug. Safe use during pregnancy has not been established.	A synthetic derivative of lincomycin. Because of antagonism shown in vitro, clindamycin and erythromycin should not be administered simultaneously.
Rifomycin B. *Bacterial. Streptomyces mediterranei.*	1-2 Gm. I.M.	Effective mainly against gram-positive organisms and mycobacteria.	Exact mechanism of action not known.	Toxicity very low.	
Spectinomycin dihydrochloride pentahydrate (Trobicin). Derived from *Streptomyces spectabilis.*	2 Gm. single dose I.M. for male patients. 4 Gm. for retreatment.	Acute gonorrheal urethritis and proctitis in males. Acute gonorrheal cervicitis and proctitis in females when due to susceptible strains of *N. gonorrhea.*	Good absorption following I.M. injection giving peak concentration after 1 to 2 hours.	During single dose therapy, soreness at injection site, urticaria, dizziness, nausea, chills, fever and insomnia may occur.	Can mask symptoms of developing syphilis. Serologic study should be done monthly for 3 months if syphilis is suspected. Safety in pregnancy not established.
SPECIFIC ANTI-INFECTIVES					
ANTIVIRAL					
PROPHYLAXIS FOR ASIAN INFLUENZA					
Amantadine hydrochloride, N.F. (Symmetrel).	200 mg. o.d. or b.i.d. capsule or syrup. Oral. Children: 1-9 yrs. 2-4 mg./lb. not to exceed	Used in the prophylaxis of Asian (A_2) influenza. For parkinsonism.	Appears to act by preventing penetration of the virus into the host cell rather than as a viricide. 90% of oral dose excreted	Contraindications: used with caution if at all in central nervous system disorders, geriatric patients with arteriosclerosis or patients	Not to be used in active cases of influenza or other respiratory disease. Do not give concurrently with psychopharmacologic agents or

	150 mg./day in divided doses t.i.d.; 9-12 yrs. 200 mg./day in divided doses t.i.d. 100 mg. up to b.i.d. Oral.		unchanged in urine, half within the first 20 hours.	with epilepsy or history of other seizures. Side effects: ataxia, nervousness, insomnia, inability to concentrate and some psychic reactions have occurred. Dry mouth, gastrointestinal disturbances and skin rashes have been reported.	with central nervous system stimulants. Safety during pregnancy and lactation has not been established.
HERPETIC KERATITIS					
IDOXURIDINE. *Synthetic.* Idoxuridine (Dendrid, Herplex, Stoxil).	0.1% solution or ointment. 1 gtt. q. 1 h. during day q. 2 h. during night in acute stage. Topical.	Used for herpes simplex of the eyes.	Irritation, pain, pruritus, edema of eye or lids, or photophobia may occur. Not used with steroids.	Mechanism of action is not known.	
ANTIBACTERIAL					
TUBERCULOSIS. See also antibiotics and antileprosy drugs.					
AMINOSALICYLIC ACID (PAS). *Synthetic.* Aminosalicylic acid, U.S.P. (p-aminosalicylic acid, Pamisyl, Parasal, PAS).	Daily doses total 12-16 Gm. as one dose or divided two to five times per 24 hours. Oral.	Used as adjunctive treatment with streptomycin or isoniazid in certain types of tuberculosis or alone when streptomycin is contraindicated.	Effective only against *Mycobacterium tuberculosis.* Exact mode of action not known. Most effective in pulmonary tuberculosis. Delays emergence of resistant bacterial strains. Excreted by kidney mostly in acetylated form which is not bacteriostatic. Action on cerebrospinal tuberculosis is erratic.	Anorexia, nausea, vomiting, abdominal discomfort, and diarrhea may occur. Treatment: symptomatic.	Available as several salts.

Name, Source, Synonyms, Preparations	Dosage and Administration	Uses	Action and Fate	Side Effects and Contraindications	Remarks
TUBERCULOSIS (Continued)					
Ethambutol Hydrochloride (Myambutol).	Initial treatment: 15 mg./kg. as a single dose daily. Oral. Retreatment: 25 mg./kg. as a single dose. Oral. After 60 days reduce to 15 mg./kg.	Used in the treatment of tuberculosis.	Good oral absorption and distribution. Appears to inhibit the synthesis of one or more metabolites in growing bacterial cells causing impairment of cell metabolism, arrest of multiplication and cell death. No cross resistance with other available antimycobacterial agents has been demonstrated. Does not show any activity against fungi, viruses or other bacteria. 75-80% of oral dose absorbed. Has good distribution. Excreted in urine and feces.	May cause decrease in visual acuity, uni- or bilateral. Eyes should be tested before use and for several months thereafter. Other adverse reactions include anaphylactoid reaction, headaches, malaise, anorexia, dizziness, fever, nausea, gastrointestinal disturbances, dermatitis, pruritus, numbness, and tingling of extremities due to peripheral neuritis. Contraindicated in patient with optic neuritis. Cautions: Effect on fetus of this drug alone or in combinations is not known. Dosage should be reduced in patients with decreased renal function. With long-term therapy, renal, hepatic and hematopoietic tests should be routinely done.	Drug should not be used alone. Usually combined with isoniazid or isoniazid and streptomycin.
ETHIONAMIDE. *Synthetic.* Ethionamide (Trecator S.C.).	0.25-1 Gm. Daily. Oral.	Used to treat pulmonary tuberculosis in patients with organisms resistant to isoniazid.	Mechanism is believed to be similar to that of isoniazid. Readily absorbed and distributed in body. Rapidly excreted by kidneys but less than 1% still in unchanged form.	Gastrointestinal disturbances may occur. Renal, hepatic, and blood tests should be done during administration. Reduce dosage or stop drug if toxic reactions occur. Used with caution, if at all, in children under 12 years.	Used in conjunction with other antituberculosis drugs. This drug can potentiate psychotoxic effects of alcohol.
ISONIAZID. *Synthetic.* Isoniazid, U.S.P. (Hyzyd, Isonico, Laniazid, Niconyl, Nicozide,	50-200 mg. t.i.d. or b.i.d. Oral.	Used as adjunctive treatment with streptomycin, PAS, or both in the treatment of	Bacteriostatic to *Mycobacterium tuberculosis.* Enters cerebrospinal fluid	Constipation, difficulty in voiding, postural hypotension, dizziness, low	Patients who are genetically slow inactivators of isoniazid may experience

Nydrazid, Rimifon, Teebaconin) (I.N.H.) (isonicotinic acid hydrazid, Isozide, [C]).		certain types of tuberculosis. Also used to prevent development of active tuberculosis in recently converted tuberculin positive persons.	in therapeutic amounts; also therapeutic in urine. Excreted by kidneys, 50-70% within 24 hours.	hemoglobin, and eosinophilia may occur. Decrease or stop drug and alkalinize patient. Contraindicated when adrenergic drugs are being given, as well as in older patients and coexisting renal damage. Isoniazid crosses the placental barrier and can cause retarded psychomotor activity in the fetus.	diphenylhydantoin toxicity when taken concurrently. When given with PAS, isoniazid blood levels are increased due to competition for the same pathway of excretion.
PYRAZINAMIDE. *Synthetic.* Pyrazinamide (Aldinamide) (Tebrazid [C]).	35-50 mg./kg. of body weight. Three grams daily for 2 weeks before and after surgery. Oral.	Potent antituberculosis drug. Because of toxicity used for short-term therapy such as presurgery.	Bacteriostatic. Organism develops resistance relatively fast. Thought to have action similar to that of isoniazid. Well absorbed after oral dose; primarily excreted by the kidneys.	May cause liver damage. Stop drug or reduce dosage and treat symptoms. Frequent tests for liver function should be made.	
LEPROSY. See also drugs used in the treatment of tuberculosis.					
SULFONE SERIES. *Synthetic.* Acetosulfone (Promacetin).	0.5-2 Gm. Oral.	Anti-infective. Especially effective in leprosy and tuberculosis.	Bacteriostatic. Slow acting. Slow excretion. Continued use will usually arrest disease and control symptoms. Good oral absorption. Distributed to all body tissues. Excreted slowly in the urine.	Nausea and vomiting, mental confusion, headache, hepatitis, cyanosis, drug fever, allergic reactions, and blood dyscrasias may occur. Dapsone is excreted very slowly, thus cumulative poisoning may occur, but it is less toxic than most of the sulfone drugs.	Several of these compounds are being tried; their exact value has not been determined. Dapsone blood levels may be increased by as much as 50% by concurrent administration of probenecid so, if possible, these two drugs should not be given at the same time.
Dapsone, U.S.P. (Avlosulfon) (diaphenylsulfone [C]).	0.1-0.4 Gm. Twice weekly. Oral.	As above.			
Glucosulfone sodium, U.S.P. (Promin).	1-5 Gm. Daily 6 days a week with rest periods. I.V.	As above.			
Sulfoxone sodium, U.S.P. (Diasone).	0.165-1.0 Gm. One dose daily. Oral.	For maintenance in dermatitis herpetiformis.			
Thiazolsulfone (Promizole).	0.5-2 Gm. Daily in divided doses. Oral. 0.33 Gm. I.M. daily.	Also indicated for the treatment of dermatitis herpetiformis.			

Name, Source, Synonyms, Preparations	Dosage and Administration	Uses	Action and Fate	Side Effects and Contraindications	Remarks
ANTISPIROCHETAL AND ANTIPROTOZOAL DRUGS (These drugs have largely been replaced by penicillin in the treatment of syphilis.) See also drugs used for amebiasis.					
ARSENIC. *Mineral.* Oxophenarsine hydrochloride, U.S.P.	40-60 mg. q. 4 to 7 days. I.V.	Anti-infective, especially useful in protozoal infections.	Arsenicals act as protoplasmic poison by their affinity for sulfhydryl groups. They are not used widely since the introduction of penicillin and other antibiotics which are effective and less toxic for treatment of treponemal infections. Distributed widely after I.V. injection, but not into central nervous system. Excreted mainly by the kidneys.	Immediate or nitritoid reactions: flushing of face, edema of lips, profuse diaphoresis, fall in blood pressure, feeling of anxiety. Stop drug, give adrenalin, treat symptoms. Intermediate or Herxheimer reaction: chills, fever, headache, malaise, nausea. Treatment: symptomatic. Delayed reaction: dermatitis (may be exfoliative) hepatitis, blood dyscrasias, hemorrhagic encephalitis. Treatment: symptomatic. For dermatitis, give sodium thiosulfate; for blood dyscrasias, give BAL (British antilewisite).	
ARSTHINOL (Mercaptoarsenol). *Synthetic. Trivalent arsenical.* Arsthinol (Balarsen).	10 mg./kg. Daily. 50-100 mg. After breakfast for 5 days. Oral. Caution: Not over 500 mg. daily.	Effective in amebiasis and in yaws.	As above.	May cause abdominal cramps, diarrhea, skin eruptions. Reduce dosage or stop drug and treat symptoms.	Combination of arsenoxide and dimercaprol (BAL).

ANTIMONY POTASSIUM TARTRATE. *Mineral. Synthetic.* Antimony potassium tartrate, U.S.P. (tartar emetic).	40-140 ml. as a 0.5% solution. I.V. on alternate days. Usually given with sterile water or glucose. 8 ml. of 0.5% solution initially, increase dose given on alternate days by 4 ml. until maximum dose of 28 ml. has been reached.	Anti-infective. Especially effective in schistosomiasis, kala-azar and granuloma inguinale. Also used as expectorant and emetic.	The exact mechanism of action is not known, but is thought to be similar to that of the arsenicals. Excreted very slowly, primarily by the kidneys.	Coughing, muscular stiffness, and severe symptoms similar to arsenic poisoning. Treatment: symptomatic.
BISMUTH. *Mineral.* Glycobiarsol, N.F. (Amoebicon, Broxolin, Milibis) (bismuth glycollylarsanilate [C]). 15% arsenic 42% bismuth	0.5 Gm. t.i.d. for 7-10 days. Oral or topical. One vaginal suppository daily for 10 days.	Mainly used in amebiasis and in trichomonas vaginitis as vaginal suppositories.	Poor oral absorption limits its use in amebiasis to intestinal organisms.	
HYDROXYSTILBAMIDINE ISETHIONATE. *Synthetic.* Hydroxystilbamidine isethionate, U.S.P. (Stilbamidine).	2 mg./kg. Daily for 8 days. I.V. Occasionally I.M.	Used to treat protozoal infections such as leishmaniasis and some fungal infections such as North American blastomycosis. Also used in the palliative treatment of multiple myeloma.	As antifungal and antiprotozoal. Exact mechanism is not known but is thought to be due to enzyme inhibition. It does not enter CNS and is too irritating if given intrathecally.	Fall in blood pressure, tachycardia, nausea, dyspnea, syncope, etc. Stop drug temporarily and proceed very slowly. Best prevented by giving the solution very slowly.
LUCANTHONE. *Synthetic.* Lucanthone hydrochloride, U.S.P. (Miracil D).	0.2 Gm. Usually given 15 mg./kg. daily in divided doses for 7 to 20 days. Oral.	Used for oral treatment of schistosomiasis. Most effective against *S. haematobium.*	Has been said to react with nucleoprotein and to inhibit mitosis. Readily absorbed orally. Most is degraded in body. About 10% appears in urine.	Side effects may include anorexia, nausea, vomiting, vertigo, or tremor. Convulsions may result from overdosage. Chronic toxicity may result in liver and kidney degeneration. Use with caution in cases of liver damage or impaired kidney function.

Name, Source, Synonyms, Preparations	Dosage and Administration	Uses	Action and Fate	Side Effects and Contraindications	Remarks
ANTISPIROCHETAL AND ANTIPROTOZOAL DRUGS (Continued)					
MERCURY. *Mineral.* Mild mercurous chloride ointment (calomel ointment).	30% in oily base. Topical.	For venereal prophylaxis.			
STIBOPHEN. *Antimony compound. Synthetic.* Stibophen, U.S.P. (Fuadin).	7% solution 0.1-0.3 Gm. Daily for about 2 weeks. I.V.	Especially effective in schistosomiasis, kala-azar, granuloma inguinale.	Anti-infective. Action believed to be similar to that of arsenic.	Coughing, muscular stiffness, and severe symptoms similar to those of arsenic poisoning. Treatment: symptomatic.	Less toxic and easier to administer than tartar emetic.
ANTIAMEBIC DRUGS					
ARSENIC COMPOUNDS. *Synthetic, mineral.* Carbarsone, N.F.	0.1-0.25 Gm. Oral. Given b.i.d. for 7-10 days; also rectally as enema, followed by alkaline enema. 0.13 Gm. Vaginal.	Especially effective in amebiasis, balantidiasis, and trichomoniasis.	Anti-infective. See under Arsenic. Well absorbed orally. Slowly excreted in urine, so oral therapy should be interrupted.	May cause gastrointestinal disorders, hepatitis, skin rashes, or visual disturbances. Reduce dosage or stop drug and treat symptoms.	
BIALAMICOL HYDROCHLORIDE. *Synthetic.* Bialamicol hydrochloride (diallylamicol hydrochloride, Camoform Hydrochloride) (biallylamicol [C]).	250-500 mg. t.i.d. Oral.	Used to treat amebic infections.	A substituted cresol which has amebicidal activity. Rapid oral absorption stored in high concentration in liver and lungs. Slowly excreted mainly in bile which gives prolonged fecal levels.	Relatively nontoxic but some nausea, vomiting, and abdominal distress reported at high doses; skin rashes also have been reported.	
GLAUCARUBIN. *Plant. Glycoside of Simarouba glauca.* Glaucarubin (Glarubin).	3 mg./kg. of body weight daily for 5-10 days. Maximum dose of 200 mg./day should not be exceeded. Oral.	Used in the treatment of intestinal amebiasis.	Has amebicidal action.	Anorexia, nausea, vomiting, abdominal pain, bloody stools, giddiness, difficulty in urination. Treatment: symptomatic.	

IPECAC. *Plant. Ipecacuanha, emetine, cephaeline.*		Especially effective in amebiasis. Also used as expectorant and emetic.	Anti-infective. Directly kills motile forms of *Entamoeba histolytica* but does not affect cysts.	Rare in therapeutic dosage. Sweating and depression may occur. Watch for cumulative action.	Emetine bismuth iodide is less reliable than the hydrochloride.
Emetine-bismuth-iodide.	0.2 Gm. Oral.				
Emetine hydrochloride, U.S.P.	30-60 mg. O.D. for 6-10 days. I.M. Bed rest essential during treatment.	Emetine is effective in amebic abscess.	Absorbed readily but excreted slowly. May cause cumulative symptoms.	Ipecac is contraindicated in cardiac and metabolic diseases.	
Ipecac.	0.3 Gm. enteric capsules. Oral.				
Metronidazole (Flagyl). *Synthetic.*	250 mg. b.i.d. X 10 days. Oral.	For trichomoniasis (male).	Has direct trichomonicidal and amebicidal activity. Well absorbed orally, reaches peak serum concentration in about 1 hour. Excreted mainly in urine—unchanged or as various metabolites. Low concentrations are found in saliva and breast milk during therapy.	Side effects are mainly gastrointestinal—anorexia, nausea, vomiting, diarrhea, epigastric distress. An unpleasant metallic taste is not uncommon. Monilial overgrowth may occur giving a furry tongue, glossitis and stomatitis. A moderate leukopenia may occur, but usually returns to normal when drug is stopped. Contraindications: patients with history of blood dyscrasia or active organic disease of the central nervous system. Should not be given during the first trimester of pregnancy, since drug crosses the placental barrier. For use later in pregnancy, the doctor must weigh advantages against possible adverse effects.	Patients taking metronidazole should be advised not to drink any alcoholic beverages, since they may experience a disulfiram-like reaction. Urine may be darkened in color, believed to be caused by the metabolites.
	250 mg. t.i.d. X 10 days. Oral.	For trichomonase (female).			
	500 mg. vaginal tablets 1 daily X 10.	Reduce oral to b.i.d. when using vaginal tablets concurrently.			
	750 mg. t.i.d. for 5 to 10 days. Oral.	For intestinal amebiasis in adults.			
	500-750 mg. t.i.d. for 5 to 10 days.	For amebiasis with liver abscess.			
	35-50 mg./kg. of body weight per 24 hours divided t.i.d. for 10 days.	For children.			
OXYQUINOLINE-IODINE COMPOUNDS. *Synthetic.* Diodohydroxyquin, U.S.P. (Diodoquin) (diiodohydroxyquin, direxiode [C]).	0.2 Gm. Give 3 tablets t.i.d. for 20 days. Oral.	Especially effective in intestinal amebiasis and trichomoniasis.	Anti-infective. Exact mode of action not understood. Is not effective in amebic abscesses. Very little absorbed. Most passes unchanged in feces.	Gastrointestinal disorders. Treatment symptomatic.	Diiodohydroxyquin is less toxic and more effective than Chiniofon or Vioform.

Name, Source, Synonyms, Preparations	Dosage and Administration	Uses	Action and Fate	Side Effects and Contraindications	Remarks
ANTIAMEBIC DRUGS (Continued)					
Iodochlorhydroxyquin, N.F. (Vioform) (iodochlorohydroxyquine, clinquinol, Domeform [C]).	0.25 Gm. Give 3 tablets t.i.d. for 20 days.		Little if any absorption.		
Sodium iodohydroxyquinoline sulfonate (Chiniofon).	1.0 Gm. Given daily for 10 days. Oral. 2.5% solution 200 ml. Rectal.		About 15% absorbed after oral dose. Most of absorbed drug eliminated in urine.		
ANTIMALARIAL DRUGS. These are all synthetic drugs unless otherwise indicated.					
Amodiaquine hydrochloride.	0.2-0.4 Gm. o.d. Oral. 0.5 Gm. Daily for suppressive therapy.	To treat malaria. Also used to treat rheumatoid arthritis and lupus erythematosus.	Similar to chloroquine. Most effective against estivo-autumnal malaria.	Nausea, vomiting, salivation, diarrhea, and melanosis. Treatment: symptomatic.	
Chloroguanide hydrochloride (Guanatol, Paludrine).	0.3 Gm. weekly as a suppresant. Oral. 0.1 Gm. daily for 10 days. Therapeutic.	To treat malaria.	Anti-infective. Especially effective in malaria caused by *Plasmodium falciparum*. Destroys parasites in the asexual-erythrocytic stage. Slowly absorbed after oral dose approximately 70-90%. Rapidly excreted in urine. 60% unchanged.	Nausea, vomiting, diarrhea, Treatment: symptomatic.	Tends to cause resistant strains to develop.
Chloroquine phosphate, U.S.P. (Aralen, Nivaquine) (Quinachor [C]).	0.25-0.6 Gm. t.i.d. first day then o.d. or alt. d. Oral.	Used to treat malaria and amebiasis. Also used to suppress lupus erythematosus.	Anti-infective. Especially effective in malaria caused by *Plasmodium vivax* and *P. falciparum*.	Similar to quinacrine. May cause pruritus. Treatment: symptomatic. Chloroquine crosses the placenta and can cause thrombocytopenia in the fetus.	Also available as the diphosphate. Does not discolor skin.
Chloroquine hydrochloride.	160-200 mg. daily for 10-12 days. I.M.	Used for patients unable to tolerate oral therapy.	Destroys parasites in the asexual-erythrocytic stage. Complete absorption following oral dose. Widely distributed in body but concentrated by certain tissues such as liver, spleen, kidneys, lung and leukocytes. Most degraded by body. Slowly excreted by the kidneys.		

Hydroxychloroquine sulfate, U.S.P. (Plaquenil).	0.8 Gm. initially, then 0.4 Gm. in 6-8 hours; follow with 0.4 Gm. on 2 successive days for total of 2.0 Gm. Oral.	Antimalarial.	Effective against both intestinal and abscess forms of amebic dysentery. Absorption and excretion similar to chloroquine.		Also used to suppress lupus erythematosus.
	0.4-0.6 Gm. Daily initially, then reduced gradually to 0.2-0.4 Gm. daily to weekly. Oral.	For maintenance in collagen diseases.			
Pamaquine naphthoate. (Plasmochin).	20 mg. daily. Oral.	To treat tertian malaria.	Anti-infective. Especially effective in malaria caused by *Plasmodium vivax.* Destroys exoerythrocytic forms and is effective against gametocytes.	Anorexia, nausea, epigastric tenderness, diarrhea, cardiac arrhythmia, headache, pallor, subnormal temperature, and blood changes. Treatment: symptomatic. Watch for cyanosis.	This drug has largely been replaced by pentaquine phosphate.
Pentaquine phosphate. (Isopentaquine).	13.3 mg. t.i.d. for 14 days. Oral.	To treat tertian malaria.	Destroys exoerythrocytic forms and is effective against gametocytes.	Nausea, abdominal pain, anorexia, anemia, leukopenia, fever, cyanosis, jaundice. Treatment: symptomatic.	Usually given with quinine. More toxic when given with sulfonamides.
Primaquine phosphate, U.S.P.	17.5-26.5 mg. q.i.d. Oral.	Used to treat malaria, especially relapses.	Considered more effective than most antimalarial drugs. Since it destroys the sexual exoerythrocytic forms, it therefore aids in clearing blood of parasites. Rapidly absorbed and most metabolized by the body.	Toxicity low, but nausea and vomiting may occur. In susceptible individuals renal and blood disorders have been reported. Stop drug and treat symptoms. More toxic in dark than in light skinned persons in regard to the hemolytic anemias.	Has largely replaced pamaquine.
Pyrimethamine, U.S.P. (Daraprim).		Used mainly to treat toxoplasmosis. Sulfadiazine is usually given at the same time. Also used as a malarial preventive, and to treat chronic malaria.	Similar to Primaquine in preventing relapses. Causes patient's blood to become noninfective to mosquito. Absorption and excretion data variable, but compound has been found in body up to 30 days following a single 100 mg. dose.	Cumulative: anorexia, diarrhea, bad taste, headache, weakness, gingivitis, rash, convulsions, and blood dyscrasias. As this is a folic acid antagonist, frequent blood checks are advised.	This drug has produced anomalies in experimental laboratory animals. Its use during pregnancy must be weighed against possible risk to the fetus from the drug or from active toxoplasmosis in the mother.
	50-75 mg. daily. Oral.	For toxoplasmosis.			
	25-50 mg. weekly. Oral.	For malaria prevention.			

Name, Source, Synonyms, Preparations	Dosage and Administration	Uses	Action and Fate	Side Effects and Contraindications	Remarks
ANTIMALARIAL DRUGS (Continued)					
Quinacrine hydrochloride, U.S.P. (Atabrine) (mepacrine hydrochloride [C]).	0.1 Gm. q.d. Suppressive. Oral.	Used to treat and to prevent malaria, and to treat giardiasis and tapeworm infestations. Also used to suppress lupus erythematosus and to treat rheumatoid arthritis.	Anti-infective. Especially effective in malaria and giardiasis. Similar to quinine but considered to be more effective and less toxic. Rapidly absorbed, widely distributed in body and strongly tissue bound. Slowly excreted from body, found in urine up to 2 months following therapy for malaria.	Dizziness, headache, gastrointestinal disturbances. Has cumulative action. Treatment: symptomatic. Causes a temporary yellowish, harmless discoloration of skin; also discolors urine.	Has been largely replaced by chloroquine and amodiaquine. With alkaline urine, the excretion of the drug is slowed.
	50-100 mg. initially intracavitary to test sensitivity and tolerance. Then 200-400 mg. intracavitary daily.	Used for symptomatic relief of malignant tumors, mainly intrapleural and intraperitoneal.	Exact action not known, but it does control effusions and ascites. It is believed to produce serositis and have direct cytotoxic action on the tumor cells contained in or bathed by the effusions.	Simultaneous bilateral intrapleural injections are not advised as this may be hazardous. Concomitant use with steroids has caused convulsive seizures. May cause fever, pain at site of injection. Some transient central nervous system symptoms have been reported.	
QUININE. *Active principle of Cinchona succirubra. Other active principles: quinidine, cinchonines, cinchonidine.*		Especially effective in malaria. Also used as a bitter tonic, antipyretic, analgesic, oxytocic, and emmenagogue.	Anti-infective. Destroys the asexual forms of the malarial organism, but not the sexual. Most effective in tertian and least effective in estivoautumnal malaria. Rapidly absorbed. Metabolically degraded in body. Less than 5% excreted unchanged in urine. Excretion is twice as fast with acid as with alkaline urine.	Fullness in head, ringing in ears, slight impairment in hearing, heart and respiratory weakness. May cause skin eruption, visual disturbances, vertigo, gastric pain, and vomiting. Quinine crosses the placenta and has been associated with deafness and thrombocytopenia of the newborn.	Quinidine is used as a heart depressant.
Quinine bisulfate (Dentogel [C]).	1 Gm. o.d. Oral } Suppresive				
Quinine dihydrochloride, N.F.	1 Gm. o.d. Oral } Suppresive				
Quinine ethylcarbonate (Euquinine).	1 Gm. o.d. Oral } Suppresive				
Quinine hydrochloride.	0.6 Gm. o.d. Oral } Suppresive 0.2 Gm. I.M.				
Quinine phosphate.	0.3 Gm. o.d. Oral.				
Quinine sulfate, U.S.P. (quinine acid sulfate). (Novoquinine [C]).	0.6 Gm. o.d. Oral.				
Totaquine.	0.6 Gm. o.d. Oral.				Contains a mixture of cinchona alkaloids.

HELMINTHICS. All these drugs are synthetic unless otherwise indicated.

Oleoresin of *Aspidium.* *Rhizomes of aspidium (Dryopteris filixmas).*	3-5 Gm. one dose. Oral. Follow with a saline cathartic.	Especially effective in tapeworm infestations.	Anthelminthic. Aids by paralyzing the muscles of the worm. Try to limit absorption by reduction of lipids in intestinal tract. Absorbed aspidium is excreted by the kidneys, but is irritating to them.	Heart depression, colic, diarrhea, headache, dizziness, yellow vision, dyspnea, temporary blindness. Treat with evacuants, then demulcents. Non-stimulating emetics, saline cathartics. Treat for shock. Contraindicated in debilitated patients, in disease of heart, liver, or kidney, or during pregnancy.	Avoid oils, fats, and alcohol. Save all stools for examination. If not effective, do not repeat for at least 3 weeks.
Bephenium hydroxynaphthoate (Alcopara) (benphenium embonate, Alcopar [C]).	2-5 Gm. one dose. Oral.	Used to treat hookworm and roundworm infestations.	Anthelminthic. Not absorbed in any appreciable amounts.	Toxic symptoms rare, but some nausea, vomiting, and soft stools have been reported.	No purge necessary following drug. Especially useful in severe infestations.
Carbon tetrachloride (Benzinoform).	2.5-3 ml. Before breakfast with water or low fat milk followed in 2 hours with saline cathartic. Oral.	Effective in most infestations except tapeworm.	Anthelminthic.	Headache, insomnia, nausea, vomiting, colic, diarrhea, convulsive seizures may occur. May cause liver, kidney, or heart damage. Treatment: symptomatic.	Avoid oils, fats, and alcohol. May be repeated after 3 weeks.
Chenopodium oil. *Chenopodium ambrosioides vasanthelmiticum.*	1 ml. one dose. Oral.	Anthelminthic. Especially effective in hookworm, pinworm and roundworm infestations.	Thought to cause direct paralysis of the worm's muscles.	Irritation of the mucous membranes, circulatory depression, dizziness, nausea; sometimes vomiting, deafness, albuminuria, and hematuria. Treatment: symptomatic. Contraindicated in nephritis, cardiac disorders, hepatic dysfunction, gastrointestinal ulcers, and pregnancy.	
Diphenan (p-amino-benzyl-phenyl carbamate chloride).	0.5-1 Gm. t.i.d. p.c. for 1 week. Oral.	Anthelminthic. Especially effective in pinworm infestations.	Hydrolyzed to p-benzyl phenol which is said to produce extreme contraction that kills the worms.	Toxic symptoms rare. Treatment: none usually required.	

Name, Source, Synonyms, Preparations	Dosage and Administration	Uses	Action and Fate	Side Effects and Contraindications	Remarks
HELMINTHICS (Continued)					
Hexylresorcinol, N.F. (Caprokol, Crystoids).	1 Gm. One dose to fasting patient and follow in 2 hours with saline purge. Oral.	Anthelminthic. Effective in most infestations. Less potent but also less toxic than most drugs of this group.	Directly vermicidal to hookworms, ascarides, and trichiuris. Approximately 1/3 absorbed after oral dose. Rapidly excreted in urine as ethereal sulfate, unabsorbed hexylresorcinol appears in feces unchanged.	Irritation of the mucous membrane. Treatment: none usually required. Capsules must be swallowed whole to avoid burning mouth.	Also an intestinal and urinary antiseptic. May be repeated in 3 days if needed. Can be used for debilitated patients and children unable to take far more potent drugs.
Methylrosaniline chloride.	60 mg. t.i.d. p.c. for 1-2 weeks. Oral.	Anthelminthic. Especially effective in strongyloidosis.	Exact mechanism of action not established.	Nausea, vomiting, diarrhea, constipation, abdominal pain. Reduce or stop drug and treat symptoms. Contraindicated in heart, liver, or kidney damage or during pregnancy.	
Methylrosaniline chloride solution (crystal violet, gentian violet, methyl violet).	1:1000 1% solution by duodenal intubation. Rectal.	For pinworms.			
Diethylcarbamazine citrate, U.S.P. (Hetrazan).	2.0 mg./kg. of body weight. Oral. 100 mg. t.i.d. for 21 days. Oral.	Especially valuable in the treatment of filariasis. Inhibits microfilaria but has little effect on adult worm.			
Piperazine calcium edathamil (Perin).	75 mg./kg. of body weight. Oral.	Used in treatment of pinworm and roundworm infestations.	Readily absorbed from gastrointestinal tract. Partly excreted in urine. Piperazine also inhibits growth of ascarides and pinworms.	Rare in therapeutic dosage. May cause urticaria, vomiting, blurred vision, and weakness. Stop drug and treat symptoms.	No starvation or purging required.
Piperazine citrate, U.S.P. (Antepar, Anthecole, Ascarex, Multifuge, Oxucide, Parazine, Ta-Verm, Vermago).	50 mg./kg. of body weight. Oral.				
Piperazine tartrate (Piperate) (Various salts of piperazine: Ancazine, Entacyl, Piperinal [C]).	50 mg./kg. of body weight. Usually given O.D. for 5-7 days. Repeat after 7 days if needed. Oral.				
Pyrantel pamoate (Antiminth).	11 mg./kg. of body weight. Oral. 200 mg. total maximum dosage. 50 mg./ml. liquid form.	Used in the treatment of ascariasis and enterobiasis.	The anthelmintic activity is probably due to the neuromuscular blocking property of the drug. It is partially absorbed with about 7%	Side effects: nausea, vomiting, gastralgia, abdominal cramps, diarrhea and tenesmus. A transient elevation of SGOT may occur. Head-	This drug is non-staining.

			of the single dose found in the urine unchanged or as metabolites. More than 50% is recovered unchanged in in the feces.	ache, dizziness, drowsiness, insomnia and rashes have been reported. Safe use in pregnancy has not been established.	
Pyrvinium pamoate, U.S.P. (Povan) (viprynium, Vanquin [C]).	50 mg./10kg. single dose. Oral.	An anthelminthic of value in the treatment of pinworm infestation.	In low concentrations inhibits oxygen uptake by parasites; in higher concentrations inhibits anaerobic metabolism of parasite. No appreciable absorption.	Toxicity is low, but nausea and vomiting may occur.	May stain stool a reddish-brown.
Infusion quassia. *Plant. Quassia.*	Varied. Topical. Given as enema.	Anthelminthic.	Action is not well understood.	Nontoxic.	
Tetrachloroethylene, U.S.P.	2-4 ml. Administered in morning in fasting state. Oral.	Anthelminthic. Especially effective in hookworm infestation.	Mechanism of action is not known.	Drowsiness, dizziness. Treatment: usually none required. Can cause hepatitis.	Avoid oils, fats, and alcohol. May be repeated after 7-10 days.
Thiabendazole, U.S.P. (Mintezol).	10 mg./lb. b.i.d. Oral. Repeat in 7 days. 10 mg./lb. b.i.d. Oral on 2 successive days. As above and repeat after 2 days. Doses given preferably p.c. Recommended maximum dose 3 Gm.	Enterobiasis. Intestinal parasites. Larva migrans. Used for many conditions such as the above and uncinariasis, trichinosis and trichuriasis.	Broad spectrum anthelminthic. Exact mechanism of action is not known. Reaches maximum blood levels 1-3 hours after oral dose.	Side effects include nausea, vomiting, dizziness, diarrhea, epigastric distress and many more. May impart odor to the urine; also crystalluria and hematuria and transient leukopenia have been reported. Stevens-Johnson syndrome has been observed following use of thiabendazole. Patient should be warned not to operate machinery or drive a car during therapy, since this drug causes drowsiness.	See commercial brochure for further information. Safety for use in pregnancy and lactation has not been established.
Thymol. *Plant. Thymol camphor.*	2 Gm. Administered in morning in fasting state; follow in 2 hours by a saline cathartic. Oral.	Anthelminthic. Especially effective in hookworm infestation. Sometimes used for pinworm and whipworm infestations.	Action similar to that of hexylresorcinol.	Central nervous system depression; later, spinal cord may be affected. Treatment: evacuants; and symptomatic.	Avoid oils, fats, and alcohol. May be repeated after 3 weeks.

BIOLOGICALS

Biologicals are attenuated or killed suspensions of microorganisms (vaccines), products of microorganisms (extracts, toxoids), or antibodies stimulated by microorganisms or their products (antitoxins, immune serum globulins). The term also applies to antigenic extracts of materials known to be allergenic (allergens), and solutions of antibodies to the venom of snakes and spiders (antivenoms). They are used for prevention or modification of diseases (vaccines, toxoids, antitoxins, immune serum globulins, allergens, antivenoms) and detection of susceptibility to or possible presence of disease agents (allergens, extracts).

BIOLOGICALS USED FOR THE PREVENTION OR MODIFICATION OF MICROBIAL DISEASES

Name, Source, Synonyms, Preparations	Dosage and Administration	Uses	Action and Fate	Side Effects and Contraindications	Remarks
Botulism antitoxin polyvalent. *Plasma of immunized animals.*	10,000 units of each type at 4-hour intervals.	Treatment of suspected botulism.	Neutralizes the toxin. Passive immunity.	Anaphylaxis or serum sickness may result in sensitive patients.	Test for sensitivity according to manufacturer's instructions before administering.
Cholera vaccine, U.S.P. *Killed bacteria.*	0.5-1.0 ml. 1-4 weeks apart. Subcutaneous.	Cholera prophylaxis for travelers to endemic areas.	Active immunity. Booster dose of 0.5 ml. every 6 months required.	Soreness, fever, malaise and headache may occur.	
Diphtheria antitoxin, U.S.P. *Plasma of immunized animals.*	1000-5000 U, I.M. 10,000-20,000 U, I.V.	For prophylaxis after exposure when immune status is uncertain or unknown. For treatment.	Passive immunity.	As with botulism antitoxin.	As with botulism antitoxin.
Diphtheria and tetanus toxoids and pertussis vaccine, U.S.P. (Triogen, Tri-Solgen, Adsorbed, DTP). *Killed bacteria and toxoids of diphtheria and tetanus.*	Three doses at 4-6 week intervals and another one year after the third dose.	For primary immunization of infants.	Booster doses when beginning school, at exposure and every 10 years. Active immunity.		Volume of dose varies with the manufacturer.
Tetanus and diphtheria toxoids (Td), U.S.P. Adult type. *Mixed toxoids.*	One dose I.M. every 10 years or on exposure.	Maintenance of active immunity and booster effect in potential exposure.	Active immunity.		Volume of dose varies.
Tetanus antitoxin (TAT), U.S.P. *Plasma of immunized animals.*	3000-5000 U, I.M. 20,000-50,000 U, I.M. or I.V.	For prophylaxis when immune status is uncertain or unknown. For treatment.	Passive immunity.	Serum sickness or anaphylaxis may result in sensitized patients.	As with botulism antitoxin. Use only if Tetanus Immune Globulin (Human) is not available.
Tetanus and gas gangrene antitoxin, N.F. *Plasma of immunized animals.*	Dosage varies. Parenteral.	As above.	Passive immunity.	As above.	As above.
Tetanus immune globulin (human), U.S.P. (Homo-Tet, Hyper-Tet, IMMU-tetanus, Pro-Tet, TIG). *Plasma of immunized humans.*	250 U, I.M.	Prophylaxis when immune status is absent or uncertain.	Passive immunity lasting longer than with TAT.		This is the passive immunity of choice; usually free of side effects of TAT.

Tetanus toxoid (T), U.S.P.	One dose I.M.	In case of predisposing wounds. Booster effect upon exposure.	Active immunity.		Used in wound prophylaxis only with history of prior immunization.
Immune serum globulin, U.S.P. (Gamasta, Gamulin, ISG). *Pooled human plasma.*	0.1 ml./lb. 0.02 ml./lb. 0.01-0.02 ml./lb. 10 ml. followed in 1 month by a second 10 ml. 0.3-0.45 ml./lb.	Prophylaxis of measles. Modification of measles. Prophylaxis of viral hepatitis. Prophylaxis of serum hepatitis. Treatment of agammaglobulinemia.	Passive immunity lasting 6-12 weeks.	Rare serum sickness type reaction may occur.	
Influenza virus vaccine, Bivalent. (Flu-Immune, Fluogen). *Inactivated virus from chick embryo.*	Two doses given 6 weeks apart. Subcutaneous.	Prophylaxis for persons at "high risk" from influenza, especially the chronically ill and aged.	Active immunity. Requires annual booster.	Contraindicated in patients known to be sensitive to eggs.	See manufacturer's instructions for dose volume and for children's doses.
Measles virus vaccine, live, attenuated, (Attenuvac, M-Vac). *Attenuated virus from chick embryo or dog kidney cell culture.*	One dose at approximately 1 year of age.	For lasting protection.	Active immunity.	15% of vaccinees have rectal temperatures of 103° beginning 6 days post-vaccination and lasting up to 4 days. Contraindicated in conditions of altered immune states, pregnancy, and hypersensitivity to eggs or dog dander.	Check manufacturer's instructions for dose volume. Also available in combination with mumps and rubella vaccines for multiple immunization (MMR).
Mumps immune globulin (human), (Hyparotin). *Plasma of immunized humans.*	2-10 ml. I.M. 1.5-4.5 ml. I.M.	For prophylaxis following exposure. For modification or treatment of mumps.	Provides passive immunity lasting for 6-12 weeks.	Rare serum sickness type reaction occurs.	
Mumps virus vaccine, *Live attenuated virus from chick embryo.*	One dose subcutaneously.	For lasting protection.	Active immunity.	Contraindicated during acute febrile illness, sensitivity to eggs, neomycin, depressed immune states or pregnancy.	May be administered at any age after 12 months. Also available in combination with measles and rubella vaccines (MMR).
Pertussis immune globulin (human), U.S.P. (Hypertussis). *Plasma of immunized humans.*	1.25 ml. I.M.	Prophylaxis or treatment of pertussis when immune status is absent or uncertain.	Passive immunity.	Rare serum sickness type reaction occurs.	
Pertussis vaccine. See Diphtheria and tetanus toxoid and pertussis vaccine (page 44).					

BIOLOGICALS (Continued)

BIOLOGICALS USED FOR THE PREVENTION OR MODIFICATION OF MICROBIAL DISEASES *(Continued)*

Name, Source, Synonyms, Preparations	Dosage and Administration	Uses	Action and Fate	Side Effects and Contraindications	Remarks
Plague vaccine, U.S.P. *Killed suspension of bacteria.*	Two doses of 0.5 ml. at 4 or more week intervals and 0.2 ml. 4-12 weeks after second dose.	Prevention for travelers and people working with the bacteria or living in enzootic areas.	Active immunity. Boosters needed every 6-12 months.	Mild pain, reddening and swelling at injection site. Fever, headache, malaise occur more often with repeated doses.	See manufacturer's instructions for children under 10 years of age.
Poliomyelitis vaccine (Salk vaccine). *Inactivated virus.*	Two doses of 1 ml. 4 weeks apart, followed by one dose 6-7 months later and another 12 months after that. Subcutaneous.	Prevention of poliomyelitis.	Active immunity.		Has largely been replaced by the oral type vaccine.
Poliovirus vaccine, live, oral, trivalent, U.S.P. (Sabin vaccine). *Attenuated virus.*	Two doses 6-8 weeks apart, followed by one dose 8-12 months after second dose.	Polio prevention against all three types of polio virus.	Lasting active immunity.	Contraindicated in conditions resulting in altered immune states.	Usually started at 6-12 weeks of age but is effective in children and adults. Available also as monovalent vaccine for each type.
Rabies vaccine, U.S.P. (duck embryo vaccine, DEV) *Inactivated virus from duck embryo culture.*	Pre-exposure: two doses of 1 ml. I.M., 1 month apart and one dose 6-7 months later or three doses of 1 ml. at weekly intervals and one dose 3 months later. Post-exposure: 14-21 doses as determined by the physician.	Rabies prophylaxis. Pre-exposure immunization recommended only for high risk personnel.	Active immunity.	Erythema, pruritus, pain and tenderness at injection site are common. Low-grade fever and rarely shock may occur late during treatment. Neuroparalytic reactions are rare with DEV.	DEV has largely replaced the Semple type which was of nervous tissue (rabbit brain) origin and caused a higher incidence of neuroparalytic reactions. Corticosteroids may interfere with development of immunity and should be avoided during vaccination.
Antirabies serum (equine origin), U.S.P. *Plasma of immunized horses.*	40 U/kg. subcutaneous or I.M.	Post-exposure rabies prophylaxis used in conjunction with rabies vaccine.	Passive immunity.	Serum sickness or anaphylactic reaction may occur.	Package instructions for sensitivy testing must be followed before administration.
Rocky Mountain spotted fever vaccine, U.S.P. *Inactivated rickettsiae from chick embryo culture.*	Adults: three 1.0 ml. doses at 7-10 day intervals. Children under 12 years: 0.5 ml. as above.	Pre-exposure prophylaxis.	Active immunity.	Pain, tenderness and erythema at injection site. Contraindicated in sensitivity to eggs.	Recommended only for high-risk personnel, such as laboratory workers, and those risking exposure due to occupations which take them into infected tick areas.
Rubella virus vaccine. *Live, attenuated virus from duck embryo, dog or rabbit kidney cell culture.*	One dose subcutaneously between 1 year of age and puberty.	Rubella prophylaxis.	Lasting active immunity.	Rash, lymphadenopathy and joint pains occur in about 5% of vaccinees.	Also available in combination with measles and mumps vaccines (MMR).

				Contraindicated in pregnancy, altered immune states, severe febrile illness or sensitivity to vaccine components.	
Smallpox vaccine, U.S.P. *Glycerinated or lyophilized vaccinia virus.*	One dose by multiple pressure, multiple puncture or jet injection.	Smallpox prophylaxis of hospital and medical personnel at high risk and travelers to endemic areas.	Active immunity. Requires revaccination at 3 year intervals for maintenance.	Rare encephalitis, vaccinia necrosum, eczema vaccinatum. Contraindicated in skin disorders, pregnancy and altered immune states.	No longer recommended as a routine pediatric immunization in the United States.
Tetanus. See Diphtheria and Tetanus Toxoids and Pertussis Vaccine (page 44).					
Typhoid vaccine, U.S.P. *Suspension of killed bacteria.*	0.25 ml. subcutaneously for ages 6 mo. to 10 years, 0.5 ml. subcutaneously for ages over 10 years; two doses at 4 week intervals. 0.5 ml. subcutaneously or 0.1 ml. intradermally every 3 years as booster or on exposure.	Prophylaxis of typhoid fever. Given to persons traveling in endemic regions and in high-risk occupations.	Active immunity.	Local erythema, tenderness at site of injection, malaise, myalgia, headache and fever. Contraindicated in acute illness, debilitating disease, tuberculosis, agammaglobulinemia, or patients receiving corticosteroids, antineoplastic or immusuppressive drugs.	Routine immunization is not recommended. Should be given to contacts of carriers, or on exposure or possible exposure.
Typhus vaccine, U.S.P. *Inactivated rickettsiae from chick embryo culture.*	Two doses 4 or more weeks apart.	Typhus prophylaxis for travelers to endemic areas and high-risk personnel.	Active immunity. Booster required every 6-12 months for maintenance.	Contraindicated in patients sensitive to eggs.	See manufacturer's instructions for dose volume.
Vaccinia immune globulin, (VIG). *Plasma from immunized humans.*	0.6 ml./kg. I.M.	Treatment of complications resulting from smallpox vaccination.	Passive immunity.	Rare serum sickness.	Distributed only by the United States Public Health Service.
Yellow fever vaccine, U.S.P. *Attenuated virus from chick embryo culture.*	0.5 ml. subcutaneously.	Yellow fever prophylaxis for high-risk personnel and travelers to endemic areas.	Long-term active immunity.	Contraindicated in pregnancy, altered immune states and sensitivity to eggs.	Also available from the United States Public Health Service.

BIOLOGICALS USED FOR TESTING PRESENCE OF OR SUSCEPTIBILITY TO MICROBIAL DISEASE AGENTS

Blastomycin, U.S.P. *Extract of Blastomyces.*	0.1 ml. of 1:100 dilution. Intradermal.	Diagnostic test for blastomycosis.		Erythema and induration in positive test.	
Coccidioidin, U.S.P. *Extract of Coccidioides immitis.*	0.1 ml. of 1:100 or 1:10 dilution. Intradermal.	Diagnostic test for coccoidioidomycosis (coccidioidal granuloma).		As above.	

BIOLOGICALS (Continued)

BIOLOGICALS USED FOR TESTING PRESENCE OF OR SUSCEPTIBILITY TO MICROBIAL DISEASE AGENTS *(Continued)*

Name, Source, Synonyms, Preparations	Dosage and Administration	Uses	Action and Fate	Side Effects and Contraindications	Remarks
Diphtheria toxin, U.S.P. *Active toxin from bacterial culture.* (Schick test).	0.1 ml. intradermally.	The Schick test is for susceptibility to the toxin of diphtheria.		As above.	A negative test is an indication that the patient has sufficient circulating antibodies to neutralize the toxin and is thus immune.
Histoplasmin, U.S.P. *Extract of Histoplasma capsulatum.*	0.1 ml. of a 1:100 dilution. Intradermal.	Diagnostic test for histoplasmosis.			
Frei Antigen, (Lygranum). *Extract from chick embryo culture of the specific strain of Chlamydiae.*	0.1 ml. intradermally.	Diagnostic test for lymphogranuloma venerum.			
Tuberculin, old, U.S.P. (Mantoux test, Mono-Vaco test, Tine test). *Products of bacterial growth.*	5 TU, intradermally.	Determining sensitivity to the causative agent.		Induration at site 48-72 hours after inoculation in positive test.	A positive tuberculin test indicates sensitivity to the bacterium. Sputum and/or chest examination may be required to rule out active disease. TU means "tuberculin units."
Tuberculin, PPD, U.S.P. *Purified protein derived from bacterial cells.*	1, 5, 250 TU, intradermally.	As above.		As above.	As above
AGENTS USED FOR PREVENTION OR MODIFICATION OF NON-MICROBIAL CONDITIONS					
Allergens (Anergex, Allpyral). *Extracts or suspensions of allergenic materials.*	Individually determined.	Single small doses used as test for sensitivity. A series of larger doses is used for desensitization.	Requires annual desensitization.	Severe allergic or anaphylactoid reactions may occur.	
Antivenom Crotalidae, polyvalent. *Plasma of immunized horses.*	15-75 ml. initially dependent on size of snake and size and condition of patient. Parenteral.	Treatment for bite of rattlesnake, copperhead, moccasin, fer-de-lance and bushmaster.	Neutralizes the venom.	Serum sickness or anaphylaxis may occur in patients sensitive to horse serum.	Package instructions for sensitivity testing must be followed before administration.
Antivenom (Lacrodectus mactans). *Plasma of immunized horses.*	2.5 ml. I.M.	Treatment for bite of the black widow spider.	As above.	As above.	As above.
Bothrops antitoxin. *Plasma of immunized horses.*	Dosage varies. Parenteral.	Treatment for bite of a South American snake.	As above.	As above.	As above.
Poison oak-ivy extracts. *Extracts of the plant material.*	Dosage varies. Oral or I.M.	Prevention and treatment of poison oak or ivy.	Requires annual doses for prophylaxis.	Allergic type reactions may occur.	

Rh (D) immune globulin, (human). *Plasma of immune humans.*	300 mcg. I.M. within 72 hours after delivery.	Prevents development of Rh antibodies by Rh negative mothers delivering Rh positive infants.	Neutralizes Rh antigen.	Infrequent slight soreness at injection site and/or slight fever.	Should be administered within 72 hours after delivery or abortion. Is given to mother only, never to the father or infant. Effective only if the mother has not already built up antibodies.

DRUGS AFFECTING THE AUTONOMIC NERVOUS SYSTEM

SYMPATHOMIMETICS (SYMPATHETIC STIMULANTS, ADRENERGIC AGENTS)

Sympathetic stimulants act through what has been called adrenergic effector cells. In the late 1940's, it was shown that these effectors were made up of two distinct receptor types which were given the names of alpha (α) receptors and beta (β) receptors. The alpha responses are mainly 1) vasoconstriction of the arterioles of the skin and splanchnic area which results in an increase in blood pressure, 2) relaxation of the gastrointestinal tract and 3) dilation of the pupils. The beta responses include 1) cardiac acceleration and increased contractility, 2) bronchial relaxation, 3) vasodilation of the arterioles supplying the skeletal muscles and 4) uterine relaxation. These responses cannot be totally separated, but some agents can be classified primarily as alpha effectors (norepinephrine), beta effectors (isoproterenol) and those which affect both the alpha and the beta receptors (epinephrine). The heart and lungs contain primarily beta receptors, whereas the arterioles have both alpha and beta receptors.

The sympathomimetic drugs act in a manner somewhat similar to that of the parasympathetic depressants. In certain specific instances they are more effective. In some respects, these drugs have actions similar to the antihistamines, and they are sometimes used for the same purposes. Some act systemically as central nervous system stimulants.

NATURAL SYMPATHETIC AMINES					
EPINEPHRINE. *Animal glands.* *Synthetic.* Ephinephrine bitartrate, U.S.P. (Adrenatrate, Epitrate, Mytrate) (Epifrin, Lyophrin [C]). Epinephrine hydrochloride, U.S.P. (Adrenalin, Sus-Phrine, Adrenatrate, Epifrin, Intranefrin, Lyophrin [C]).	0.1 ml. of a 2% solution. Topical in eyes. 0.06-1 ml. of a 1:1000 solution. Parenteral. 1:100 solution. Topical as spray. 0.2-1 ml. I.M. and topical as spray. 1:10,000 solution for intracardial use.	Used in number of conditions such as bronchial asthma, urticaria and other allergic conditions, shock, cardiac and respiratory failure, congestion of mucous membranes, and to prolong action of local anesthetics.	Main action is vasoconstriction of peripheral blood vessels. There is usually a temporary rise in blood pressure. In large doses there is stimulation of the myocardium with increased cardiac output. Rapidly inactivated by enzymes catechol orthomethyl transferase and monoamine oxidase. Most excreted by kidneys after inactivation as metanephrine and 3 methoxy-4 hydroxy	Tremors, nervous apprehension, palpitation, precordial distress. Severe symptoms may include acute cardiac dilation, pulmonary edema. Treatment: symptomatic. Cardiac and respiratory stimulants may be ordered. Epinephrine and some other sympathomimetics (levarterenol, metaraminol, methoxamine, ephedrine, mephentermine, and phenylephrine) can interact with	Epinephrine hydrochloride cannot be given orally, as it is inactivated by the digestive juices. There is a warning on most sympathomimetic drugs that they should not be used for patients with heart disease, high blood pressure, diabetes or thyroid disease unless closely supervised by a physician.

Name, Source, Synonyms, Preparations	Dosage and Administration	Uses	Action and Fate	Side Effects and Contraindications	Remarks
NATURAL SYMPATHETIC AMINES (Continued)					
Epinephrine hydrochloride (Continued)			mandelic acid. Very short acting; extended by delaying absorption by making a suspension "Sus-Phrine" or putting it in oil, "Adrenalin in oil."	cyclopropane and other halogenated hydrocarbon anesthetics to give cardiac arrhythmias. This interaction is dependent on the amount of sympathomimetic agent used and mode of administration. Epinephrine, when given with the tricyclic antidepressants, antihistamines or sodium 1-thyroxin will give an enhanced adrenergic effect. When given to patients taking azapetine there is a reversal of the pressor effect of epinephrine. This hypertensive effect of epinephrine is antagonized by the phenothiazines and butyrophenones. Some sympathomimetic drugs, when given to patients receiving a monoamine oxidase inhibitor, may cause a hypertensive crisis.	
LEVARTERENOL BITARTRATE. *Synthetic.* Levarterenol bitartrate, U.S.P. (noradrenaline, norepinephrine, Levophed).	1-10 micrograms p.r.n. I.V.	Used for acute hypotension.	A potent vasoconstrictor which raises blood pressure markedly with increased cardiac output. Pulse rate is usually slowed. It is the salt of norepinephrine. Excretion data similar to epinephrine.	Tremors, nervous apprehension, palpitation, precordial distress. Severe symptoms may include acute cardiac dilation, pulmonary edema. Treatment: symptomatic, antihypertensive drugs. Contraindicated with cyclopropane anesthesia or when myocardial ischemia is suspected. See epinephrine for	Blood pressure should be checked every 5 to 15 minutes.

				interactions. Also the thiazide diuretics antagonize the hypertensive effect of this drug. Toxic to subcutaneous tissues. Avoid infiltration.	
ETHYLNOREPINEPHRINE HYDROCHLORIDE. *Synthetic.* Ethylnorepinephrine hydrochloride (Bronkephrine).	2 mg. q. 3-4 minutes. Parenteral.	Used for severe asthma.			
Isoetharine (Dilabon–a component of Bronkosol).	By inhalation usually q. 4 h. is sufficient. Used full strength or diluted with three parts saline or other suitable solution.	Treatment of bronchial asthma and bronchospasm, associated with emphysema, bronchitis and chronic broncho-pulmonary disorders.	Acts as a bronchodilator.	Same as for others of this group. Should not be used with epinephrine but can be used alternately.	
SYNTHETIC SYMPATHETIC AGENTS. Sympathetic agents used as pressor agents. These are all synthetic preparations.					
Also see under natural amines. Angiotensin amide, N.F. (Hypertensin).	2.5 mg. in at least 250 ml. infusion. I.V.	Used for treatment of shock and collapse when blood pressure must be restored quickly.	Produces rise in blood pressure owing to constriction of peripheral blood vessels with increased peripheral resistance. Agent degraded by peptidases present in serum and plasma. Has mainly alpha response.	Too rapid or too great a rise in blood pressure. Use antihypertensive medication. Not given in myocardial infarction.	Check blood pressure every 1 to 5 minutes until stabilized.
Mephentermine sulfate, (Wyamine [C]).	12.5-25 mg. b.i.d. or t.i.d. Oral. 15-35 mg. p.r.n. I.V. or I.M.	Used mainly to raise blood pressure in shock and hemorrhage, but also used as decongestant.	Constricts the peripheral blood vessels. Causes rise in blood pressure due to peripheral resistance. For fate see ephedrine.	Toxicity rare in therapeutic dosage. Treatment: none usually required. When patients have been receiving reserpine or guanethidine there is a diminished response to this drug.	
Metaraminol bitartrate, U.S.P. (Aramine, Pressonex).	2-10 mg. p.r.n. Subcutaneous or I.M. 15-100 mg. Usually given in dextrose. p.r.n. I.V.	Used mainly in postsurgical or other pathologically induced hypotension. It is not very effective in idiopathic hypotension.	It has a powerful and prolonged vasopressor action. As with most of these drugs action is mainly due to constriction of peripheral blood vessels. Excretion similar to ephedrine.	Severe hypertension. Give antihypertensive drugs. When patient is on reserpine or guanethidine, metaraminol can give a diminished response from what is expected.	

Name, Source, Synonyms, Preparations	Dosage and Administration	Uses	Action and Fate	Side Effects and Contraindications	Remarks
SYNTHETIC SYMPATHETIC AGENTS (Continued)					
Methoxamine hydrochloride, U.S.P. (Vasoxyl).	5-20 mg. p.r.n. I.M.	Used to raise blood pressure in shock and collapse.	Strong vasopressor action due to constriction of peripheral blood vessels with increased blood pressure. Excretion similar to ephedrine. Can be used during surgery with cyclopropane as it does not increase irritability of the cyclopropane sensitized heart.	Rare, but watch for too high blood pressure. Stop drug and give antihypertensive drugs.	
Sympathetic stimulants with local vascular and bronchial effect, and used mainly for local or systemic vasoconstriction or bronchial dilation. These are all synthetic preparations except as noted.					
Cyclopentamine hydrochloride, N.F. (Clopane).	0.5% solution. Topical.	Used for nasal congestion as vasoconstrictor and vasopressor.	Stimulation of the sympathetic nervous system. Vasoconstriction, especially of superficial blood vessels; dilation of bronchial tubes; hemostatic when applied locally.	Headache, dizziness, palpitation, anxiety. Severe symptoms include cardiac depression, tremors, diaphoresis, fainting. Treatment: symptomatic. Should be used with caution in patients with cardiac disorder.	
EPHEDRINE. *Active principle of Ephedra vulgaris and E. equisetina (ma huang). Synthetic.*					
Ephedrine hydrochloride, N.F. (Ephedra, Neo-Fedrin [C]). Ephedrine sulfate, U.S.P. Etafedrine hydrochloride (Nethamine) (Acepifylline [C]).	15-25-50 mg. q. 3-4 h. Oral. p.r.n. as nasal jelly. Topical. 25-50 mg. q. 3-4 h. p.r.n. Oral. 3% solution. Topical. 12-24 mg. q. 3-4 h. p.r.n. Oral.	Used in hypotension, asthma and other allergies, narcotic poisoning, narcolepsy; as a mydriatic, and with neostigmine in myasthenia gravis.	In small dosage stimulates the heart, increasing rate and force of beat. Raises blood pressure by constriction of muscles and blood vessels. Ephedrine and most other noncatechol amines are effective orally and are longer acting than the catecholamines. They resist	Headache, dizziness, palpitation, anxiety. Severe symptoms include cardiac depression, tremors, diaphoresis, fainting. Treatment: symptomatic. Patients on long-term reserpine therapy may not respond adequately to normal pressor doses of ephedrine.	Ephedrine, unlike ephinephrine, can be given orally since it is not destroyed by the digestive juices. Available in preparations for topical and parenteral use.

			inactivation by enzymes—monoamine oxidase and catechol orthomethyl transferase. They are widely distributed in body and 50-75% are excreted unchanged by the kidneys.	See epinephrine for interaction with anesthetic agents and the monoamine oxidase inhibitors. Ephedrine interferes with the hypotensive effect of guanethidine.	
Hydroxyamphetamine hydrobromide U.S.P. (Paredrine hydrobromide).	0.25-1% solution, p.r.n. Topical. 20-400 mg. daily in divided doses. Oral.	Used to relieve congestion of mucous membranes, as a mydriatic, and as a vasoconstrictor. Orally for postural hypotension, carotid sinus syndrome and heart block.	Action same as that of cyclopentamine. See ephedrine for excretion data.	Toxic symptoms are rare in therapeutic dosage. Treatment: none usually needed.	
Pseudoephedrine hydrochloride (Isophedrine, Sudafed).	30-60 mg. q. 3-4 h. p.r.n. Oral.	Used to relieve congestion of the mucous membranes and for bronchodilator properties.			Often given in combination with phenobarbital and antihistamines.
Isoproterenol hydrochloride U.S.P. (Aludrin, Isuprel, Norisodrine-H) (isoprenaline, isopropylnoradrenaline, isopropylarterenol, Iso-Intranefrin, Isovon [C]).	10-15 mg. Oral; sublingual. q.i.d. but not more than 60 mg. in one day. 1:200-1:100 solution. p.r.n. Topical or by inhalation.	Used in a number of conditions, such as bronchial asthma, shock, urticaria and other allergic conditions, cardiac and respiratory failure, congestion of mucous membranes, and to prolong action of local anesthetics.	A strong bronchodilator. Has direct action on the myocardium. Increases cardiac output by increasing strength of contraction and, to a lesser degree, the rate of contraction. It facilitates expectoration of pulmonary secretions. Topically, a decongestant. This is a catechol amine. Absorption and excretion similar to epinephrine.	Tremors, nervous apprehension, palpitation, precordial distress. Severe symptoms may include acute cardiac dilation, pulmonary edema. Treatment: symptomatic. The effect of isoproterenol can be blocked by propranolol, so patients on propranolol will not receive the desired effects from the drug.	Should not be administered simultaneously with epinephrine.
Isoproterenol sulfate, N.F. (Isonorin, Norisodrine-S).	0.2-1 mg. I.M. or I.V. 10% solution. p.r.n. Topical by nebulizer. 5 mg. Rectal.				
Methoxyphenamine hydrochloride (Orthoxine).	50-100 mg. q. 4 h. p.r.n. Oral.	Used as a bronchodilator and antiallergic agent. Has minimal vasopressor effect.	See Uses. Absorption and excretion similar to ephedrine.	Rare in therapeutic dosage. Treatment: none usually required.	Also added to cough syrups.
Methylaminoheptane hydrochloride (Oenethyl).	50-100 mg. p.r.n. I.M. or I.V.	Used mainly to treat hypotension.	Vasoconstriction, with resulting rise in blood pressure.	Rare, but watch for too high blood pressure. Stop drug and give antihypertensive drugs.	
Methylhexaneamine (Forthane).	Dosage varies. By inhalation (inhaler) p.r.n. not more often than q. 1 hr.	Used to shrink mucous membranes in rhinitis and sinusitis.	Decongestant due to local vasoconstriction.	Toxicity low, but headache, nervousness, tremors, and mental stimulation may occur. Stop drug and treat symptoms.	Caution against too frequent use.

Name, Source, Synonyms, Preparations	Dosage and Administration	Uses	Action and Fate	Side Effects and Contraindications	Remarks
SYNTHETIC SYMPATHETIC AGENTS (Continued)					
Naphazoline hydrochloride, N.F. (Privine) (Albalon, Vasocon [C]).	0.05-0.1% solution. p.r.n. Topical as drops or nebulae. 0.05% jelly. p.r.n.	Used locally to reduce nasal congestion.	Decongestant due to local vasoconstriction.	Occasionally causes too much blanching of the mucous membrane. Stop drug.	Do not put in aluminum container. Caution against too frequent use.
	0.012% solution eye drops. Topical.	For relief of red, irritated eyes.			
Oxymetazoline hydrochloride, N.F. (Alfrin hydrochloride) (Nafrine, Drixine, Hazol [C]).	1:2000 solution. Topical, either 2-4 gtt. or as nasal spray.	Main use is in allergic rhinitis.	Decongestant.	Side effects rare, but temporary nasal irritation may occur.	
Phenylephrine hydrochloride, U.S.P. (Almefrin, Isophrin, Neo-Synephrine) (Deca-Nephrine, Isoptofrin, Prefrin [C]).	10 mg. q. 3-4 h. p.r.n. Oral. 1-10 mg. p.r.n. Parenteral. 0.25-0.5% solution. q. 3-4 h. p.r.n. Topical. 2-10% solution drops in eye q.i.d. As a mydriatic p.r.n. q. 1 h.	Used as a decongestant in vasomotor rhinitis, sinusitis, and hay fever. Used to prolong action of spinal anesthetics and to maintain blood pressure. Also used in eye with other agents when mydriasis is desired without cycloplegia or when local vasoconstriction is desired.	Like all these preparations it is a decongestant locally but a stimulant and vasoconstrictor systemically. See ephedrine for excretion data. Acts primarily on alpha receptors.	Rare, but watch for too high blood pressure. Stop drug and give antihypertensive drugs. For eye, use with caution in patients with glaucoma. Also use with caution in diabetes or known hypertension.	
Phenylpropanolamine hydrochloride, N.F. (Propadrine).	0.5-1% solution. p.r.n. Topical. 25-50 mg. q. 3-6 h. p.r.n. Oral.	Used as a mucous membrane decongestant and to treat allergic conditions.	Topical decongestant due to vasoconstriction. Systemic vasoconstrictor.	Rare in therapeutic dosage. Does not have the untoward effect of ephedrine.	
Phenylpropylmethylamine (Vonedrine).	0.5% solution. Topical by inhaler p.r.n.	Used mainly as a local decongestant.	Topical decongestant due to vasoconstriction.	Rare in therapeutic dosage. Treatment: none usually required.	
Propylhexedrine, N.F. (Benzedrex).	Dosage varies. Topical by inhaler.	Used as a local decongestant.	Topical decongestant due to vasoconstriction.	Rare in therapeutic dosage.	
Protokylol hydrochloride.	2-4 mg. t.i.d. with meals and h.s. Oral.	Used as a bronchial dilator in asthma.	Local decongestant. Systemic action: vasoconstriction and bronchial dilation.	May cause palpitation, tachycardia, tremors, tension, insomnia, dizziness, nausea, and vomiting. Adjust dosage.	Can be used for long-term treatment of asthma. Often effective when other drugs fail.

Tetrahydrozoline hydrochloride, N.F. (Tyzine, Visine).	0.05-1% solution. Topical in nose or eyes.	Used as a topical decongestant.	Vasoconstriction with resulting decongestion.	Same as for others of this group.	
Tuaminoheptane sulfate, N.F. (Tuamine sulfate) (Rhinosol [C]).	1.0% solution. Topical and inhalational.	Used mainly as a local decongestant.	Vasoconstriction with resulting decongestion.	Rare in therapeutic dosage. Treatment: none usually required.	Safe use during pregnancy has not been established.
Xylometazoline hydrochloride (Otrivin).	0.1% solution q. 3-4 h. Topical in nose.	Used mainly as a local decongestant.	Vasoconstriction with resulting decongestion.	Rare in therapeutic dosage.	
Sympathetic amines whose main use is in treatment of bladder spasm.					
Isometheptene hydrochloride (Octin hydrochloride) (methylisooclenylamine [C]).	50-100 mg. stat and repeat in 4-6 h. I.M.	Used mainly to relax muscles of the urinary and gastrointestinal tracts.	Antispasmodic and vasoconstrictor.	Toxicity low, but there may be a slight rise in blood pressure, light-headedness, nervousness, and nausea. Adjustment of dosage is usually sufficient.	Must *not* be administered I.V.
Isometheptene mucate (Octin mucate).	0.12-0.25 Gm. q. ½ hr. Not more than four doses or q.i.d. Oral.	Used also for migraine headaches.			
Sympathetic amines which produce peripheral vasodilation by relaxation of the smooth muscles of the arterioles. Increases rate and force of heart and may relax uterus.					
Isoxsuprine hydrochloride (Vasodilan).	10 mg. Three to four times daily, oral, or two to three times daily I.M. I.M. doses greater than 10 mg. are not recommended.	For symptoms due to peripheral and cerebral arterial insufficiency or cerebral vascular disease associated with arteriosclerosis and hypertension. Also for uterine hypermotility, primary dysmenorrhea, threatened abortion, and premature labor.	Vasodilator and uterine relaxant. Acts directly on smooth muscles of blood vessels and uterus.	May cause palpitation, vomiting, dizziness, weakness, tachycardia, and hypotension. Adjust dosage or change to another drug. Treat symptoms.	
Nylidrin hydrochloride, N.F. (Arlidin) (buphenine hydrochloride, Pervadil [C]).	6-12 mg. Three to six times daily. Oral.	Peripheral vasodilator used to lower blood pressure.	A sympathomimetic drug whose main clinical action is peripheral vasodilation.	Toxicity apparently low.	

DRUGS AFFECTING THE AUTONOMIC NERVOUS SYSTEM (Continued)

SYMPATHOLYTICS (SYMPATHETIC DEPRESSANTS, ADRENOLYTIC AGENTS)

Name, Source, Synonyms, Preparations	Dosage and Administration	Uses	Action and Fate	Side Effects and Contraindications	Remarks
	These drugs are antagonistic to epinephrine and similar drugs. They cause vasodilation and increase tone of alimentary tract muscles and of other smooth muscle tissue. They vary in their effects and some will be discussed in areas of important therapeutic activity. These are synthetic preparations except as noted.				
Azapetine phosphate (Ilidar) (azepine [C]).	25 mg. t.i.d. individually adjusted. Oral.	Used in peripheral vascular disease in which vasospasm is predominant.	Adrenergic blocking agent similar to tolazoline hydrochloride. It can reverse the pressor effect of epinephrine and reduce the vasoconstrictor effect of norepinephrine.	Rare in therapeutic dosage but may cause drug fever, nausea, vomiting, postural hypotension, and syncope. Dosage adjustment is usually sufficient treatment. Contraindicated when fall in blood pressure is dangerous and in coronary disorders.	Safe use in pregnancy has not been established.
Phenoxybenzamine hydrochloride (Dibenzyline).	10-20 mg. q.d. or b.i.d. Dosage individually adjusted. Oral.	Used to treat peripheral vascular diseases.	Alpha adrenergic blocking agent.	Nasal congestion, miosis, tachycardia, postural hypotension. Reduce dosage or stop drug. Contraindicated when sudden fall in blood pressure might be dangerous.	
Phentolamine hydrochloride, N.F. (Regitine hydrochloride) (Rogitine [C]).	50 mg. Four to six times a day. Dosage individually adjusted Oral.	Used to treat peripheral vascular disease and to control hypertension caused by pheochromocytoma.	Same as azapetine.	Side effects are rare. Tachycardia has been reported. Myocardial infarction, cerebrovascular spasm and cerebrovascular occlusion have been seen, usually in association with marked hypotensive episodes with shock-like states which follow parenteral administration.	As above.
Phentolamine, mesylate, U.S.P. (Regitine methanesulfonate).	3 mg. I.M. 1 mg. I.V.	Mainly used to test for pheochromocytoma and for control during surgery.	As above.	As above.	Also used in small amounts with norepinephrine to reduce damage from extravasation when this cannot be avoided.
Tolazoline hydrochloride (Priscoline, Tazol, Tolavad, Tolpol).	25-75 mg. q.i.d. Oral or parenteral.	Used in spastic peripheral vascular disorders including acrocyanosis, acroparesthesia,	Adrenergic blocking agent causing dilation of peripheral arterioles, presumably	Rare in therapeutic dosage. When toxic symptoms do occur they are similar to the	

		arteriosclerosis obliterans, Buerger's disease, causalgia, diabetic arteriosclerosis, gangrene, endarteritis, frostbite (sequelae), thrombophlebitis, Raynaud's disease and scleroderma.	from competitive interference at the pressor receptor.	mild toxic symptoms of the nitrites. Stop drug and treat symptoms. Contraindicated in collapse or shock. Given cautiously, if at all, in cases of coronary disease or peptic ulcers.	
ERGOT. *Claviceps purpurea.* *Semisynthetic and synthetic.* Dihydroergotamine mesylate (DHE45).	1 ml. at onset of headache then q. 1 h. up to 3 ml. I.M. Or 2 ml. in buffered solution. I.V.	Used to treat migraine syndrome and various types of vascular headache. Also for postherpetic pain.	Various active principles produce different results. Ergotamine and ergotoxine stimulate smooth muscle tissue, and tend to raise blood pressure. Ergotoxine has greater ecbolic action than ergotamine. Both are adrenergic blocking agents. Ergonovine has greater ecbolic action and does not tend to raise blood pressure. It does not act as an adrenergic blocking agent but rather appears to stimulate the effector cells connected with adrenergic nerves; it does not paralyze them.	Acute: nausea, vomiting, thirst, tingling of extremities, uterine bleeding, and abortion if patient is pregnant. Late: face and limbs swell, abnormal skin sensation occurs, and there is pallor. Terminal: temperature falls, convulsions, coma and death occur due to cardiac and respiratory failure. Treatment: lavage, enemas, purgation, central nervous system stimulants. Toxic symptoms: chronic—dry gangrene may occur, and cataracts may form. Spasmodic—vertigo, tinnitus, headache, muscle tremors, and abnormal skin sensations occur. Treatment: symptomatic, but prognosis is poor.	
Dihydrogenated ergot alkaloid mixture (Hydergine).	0.1 mg. I.M., 0.5 mg. sublingual, 4-6 tablets daily.	Used to treat peripheral vascular disease.			
Ergonovine maleate, U.S.P. (Ergotrate, ergosterine, ergometrine).	1-2 mg. Two to three times daily. Oral. 2 mg. once for uterine bleeding. I.M. or I.V. Severe hemorrhage may require more than one dose.	Mainly used as an ecbolic.			
Ergot.	150 mg.-1 Gm. Maximum dose 5-6 Gm. in 24 hours. Oral.	As above.			
Ergot aseptic.	1-2 ml. I.M.	As above.			Ergot aseptic and extract are rarely used at present.
Ergot extract.	0.5 Gm. Oral.	As above.			
Ergot fluid extract.	2 ml. Usually once daily; not over 5 ml. in 24 hours. Oral.	As above.			
Ergotamine tartrate, U.S.P. (Femergin, Gynergen, Ergomar).	0.25-0.5 mg. and repeat in 40 minutes if not relieved. I.M. or I.V. Not more than 2 mg. weekly. 2-6 mg. (two to six 1 mg. tablets) used per attack. Oral.	Used to treat vascular headaches.		Ergotamine and dihydroergotamine are contraindicated in peripheral vascular diseases, angina pectoris, and hepatic or renal dysfunction.	Also available as inhaler: Medihaler—ergotamine.

Name, Source, Synonyms, Preparations	Dosage and Administration	Uses	Action and Fate	Side Effects and Contraindications	Remarks
ERGOT (Continued)					
Methylergonovine maleate, U.S.P. (Methergine).	0.2 mg. Three or four times daily for postpartum bleeding. Oral. 0.2 mg. after third stage of labor. I.M. or I.V. 0.2 mg. I.M. or I.V.	Used mainly for postpartum hemorrhage.		Methylergonovine should not be administered I.V. routinely because of the possibility of inducing sudden hypertensive and cerebrovascular accidents. In emergency, it can be given slowly over a 60-second duration with careful monitoring of blood pressure. Warning: retroperitoneal fibrosis, pleuropulmonary fibrosis and fibrotic thickening of cardiac valves may occur in patients on long term therapy.	These preparations are semisynthetic.
Methysergide maleate (Sansert).	2-4 mg. t.i.d. with meals. Oral. For each 6 months' period of taking drug, there should be a 3 or 4 week rest period.	Used prophylactically in vascular headaches in patients whose headaches are frequent and/or severe and uncontrollable and who are under close medical supervision.	A potent antiserotonin agent. Inhibits vasoconstrictor and pressor effects of 5-Ht but mechanism of action unknown.	Mild nausea, heartburn, and occasional vomiting have been reported. Contraindicated or used with caution in pregnancy, coronary artery disease, severe hypertension, peripheral vascular disease, arteriosclerosis, collagen diseases, fibrotic diseases, valvular heart disease or impaired renal or hepatic function.	
SYNTHETIC PREPARATIONS					
Bretylium tosylate (Darenthin).	0.1-0.3 Gm. t.i.d. Oral.	Used in hypertension and peripheral diseases.	An antihypertensive agent that acts by blocking sympathetic nerve impulses beyond their ganglia. It is not an adrenolytic agent.	Toxicity low, but nasal stuffiness, pupillary constriction, and irregularity of pulse have been reported. Reduce dosage.	

Guanethidine sulfate, U.S.P. (Ismelin).	10-50 mg. Dosage individually adjusted. Oral.	For treatment of moderate to severe and malignant hypertension and to treat peripheral vascular diseases. Is a strong hypotensive agent.	Appears to interfere with the release of the chemical mediator (presumably norepinephrine) at the sympathetic neuroeffector junction. Tends to reduce orthostatic blood pressure more than recumbent blood pressure. Action long lasting.	Side effects similar to those of other potent antihypertensives; usually controlled by reduction or interruption of dosage. May inhibit ejaculation in males. Contraindicated in pheochromocytoma. Safe use during pregnancy has not been established. When used with amphetamine or other sympathetic agents such as ephedrine or methylphenidate, the effectiveness of guanethidine in reducing blood pressure can be severely antagonized. The same effect takes place with desipramine and probably with imipramine, amitriptyline and nortriptyline. The thiazide diuretics enhance the hypotensive effect of guanethidine and may allow a reduction of dosage so there may be fewer adverse effects.	Patients should be cautioned to avoid strenuous exercise during administration for fear of severe hypotension.
Methyldopa, U.S.P. (Aldomet) (Presinal, Sembrina [C]). Methyldopa hydrochloride U.S.P. (Aldomet ester hydrochloride).	0.5-2 Gm. Given daily in divided doses. Oral. 250-500 mg. q. 6 h. I.V.	An antihypertensive drug used in patients with sustained moderate to severe hypertension.	Produces orthostatic hypotension as a result of a reduction of brain serotonin and peripheral norepinephrine. Maximum lowering appears by second day. Half oral dose absorbed and excreted unchanged and as its mono-o-sulfate. Therapeutic dose has maximal effect in 6-8 hours.	Hemolytic anemia has occurred. Some patients develop a positive direct Coombs' test when on continued therapy. This disappears in weeks to months after discontinuing the drug. Sedation, anxiety, apprehension, dizziness, and postural hypotension. Contraindicated in pregnancy, pheochromocytoma, acute hepatitis and active cirrhosis.	Liver and blood tests should be done during therapy.

DRUGS AFFECTING THE AUTONOMIC NERVOUS SYSTEM (Continued)

PARASYMPATHOMIMETICS (PARASYMPATHETIC STIMULANTS, CHOLINERGIC AGENTS)

Drugs which stimulate the parasympathetic divisions of the autonomic nervous system all to a greater or lesser degree decrease the rate of the heart, contract smooth muscle tissue, contract the pupils of the eye, and increase the secretions of most of the glands. Since the two divisions of the autonomic nervous system work mainly in opposition to each other, the stimulation of one division will usually depress the other and vice versa. The drugs have been classified for their main therapeutic activity.

Name, Source, Synonyms, Preparations	Dosage and Administration	Uses	Action and Fate	Side Effects and Contraindications	Remarks
CHOLINE DERIVATIVES. *Synthetic.*					
Acetylcholine chloride (Miochol).	½ to 2 ml. (20 mg. per 2 ml.) instilled into the anterior chamber of the eye.	To obtain complete miosis in seconds. Used in cataract surgery or in iridectomies.	Rapid miotic. Deactivated by acetylcholine esterases and other esterases.	Note: in cataract surgery use only after delivery of the lens.	Prepare immediately before use and discard unused portion as solutions are unstable.
Bethanechol chloride, U.S.P. (Urecholine chloride).	2.5-5 mg. t.i.d. or q.i.d. Subcutaneous. 10-30 mg. t.i.d. or q.i.d. Oral.	Used in peripheral vascular diseases, rheumatoid arthritis, paroxysmal tachycardia. Also used in postoperative retention, occasionally as a miotic or as a diaphoretic.	These preparations act in the body as does the endogenous acetylcholine, but are usually not inactivated as rapidly by cholinesterase.	Dyspnea, disturbances of vision, and cardiac failure. Place patient in Fowler's position. Treat symptoms. Atropine is usually ordered.	Bethanechol chloride is not given intramuscularly or intravenously. Less toxic and less effective than methacholine.
Carbachol, U.S.P. (Carcholin, Carbamylcholine chloride) (IsoptoCarbachol [C]).	0.75-2.25% solution. q. 8-12 h. Topical in eyes.	Used to relieve intraocular tension in glaucoma.	As above.	As above. Contraindicated in asthma and hypertension.	Carbachol is not given systemically because of toxicity.
Methacholine bromide, N.F. (Mecholyl bromide). Methacholine chloride, N.F. (Mecholyl chloride).	50-600 mg. Oral. 10-25 mg. Subcutaneous. 1:200-1:500 solution for iontophoresis.	Same as bethanechol; also used to treat chronic ulcers, overcome vascular spasms due to moderate exposure to cold, and scleroderma.	As above.	As above.	
CHOLINESTERASE INHIBITORS. *Synthetic.*			These act by blocking the action of cholinesterase and thus prolong the action of acetylcholine. Some have an irreversible effect.		The safety of use of the cholinesterase drugs during pregnancy has not been established, nor has the absence of adverse effects on the fetus or on the respiration of the neonate.
Ambenonium chloride, N.F. (Mytelase, Mysuran).	5-25 mg. t.i.d. or q.i.d. Oral.	A cholinesterase inhibitor used in myasthenia gravis.	Good oral absorption and longer duration of action than with neostigmine.	Similar to neostigmine bromide but is considered less toxic.	
Demecarium bromide (Humorsol).	0.25% solution. 1-2 gtt. Dosage individually adjusted. Topical.	A cholinesterase inhibitor used to treat glaucoma.	As above.	As with Ambenonium chloride.	

Echothiophate iodide (Phospholine iodide).	0.03-0.25% solution. 1-2 gtt. in eyes once or twice daily. Individually adjusted. Topical.	Acetylcholinesterase inhibitor for treatment of glaucoma.	As above.	Include gastrointestinal disturbances. For severe conditions, atropine is usually ordered. Use with extreme care in patients with history of retinal detachment or in closed angle glaucoma.	
Isoflurophate, N.F. (D.F.P., Floropryl) (difluorophate, Dyflos [C]).	0.1% solution. Topical. 0.25% ophthalmic ointment.	Used in glaucoma and occasionally in myasthenia gravis.	Long acting due to irreversible inactivation of cholinesterase.	Similar to neostigmine but more toxic.	Rarely used systemically owing to toxicity.
Neostigmine bromide, U.S.P. (Prostigmin bromide). Neostigmine methylsulfate, U.S.P. (Kirkstigmine, Neostigmeth, Prostigmin methylsulfate).	15 mg. Oral. 0.25-1 mg. Parenteral. 5% ophthalmic solution.	Used mainly as a miotic and a diaphoretic. It is also an antipruritic and antipyretic but does not reduce temperature except when fever exists. Used to increase urinary and intestinal peristalsis, and in the treatment of myasthenia gravis. Used as an antidote for tubocurarines following surgery and to counteract the neuromuscular blockage seen when neomycin is given with tubocurarines and/or ether. Since it has the same properties as physostigmine and pilocarpine it can be used for the same purposes.	See Ambenonium chloride. Oral dose, much is destroyed in intestines so much larger dose required. Exact fate in man is not known.	Toxicity relatively low, but may cause any of the following: cholinergic crisis, myasthenia crisis, weak, slow heart action, decreased blood pressure, increased bronchial secretions, may produce pulmonary edema. Other symptoms include nausea, vomiting, and muscular twitching. Contraindicated in mechanical intestinal or urinary blockage. Treatment: symptomatic; atropine is drug of choice to reverse effects in cholinergic crisis. Treat for shock. Artificial respiration may be needed. Treat symptoms.	
Pyridostigmine bromide, U.S.P. (Mestinon).	0.6 to 1.5 Gm. daily in divided doses. Oral.	Main use in myasthenia gravis.	For action see Ambenonium chloride. Fate in body is not known.	See above.	

Name, Source, Synonyms, Preparations	Dosage and Administration	Uses	Action and Fate	Side Effects and Contraindications	Remarks
OTHER CHOLINERGIC DRUGS					
DEXPANTHENOL. *Synthetic.* Dexpanthenol (Alco-pan, Ilopan, Motilyn, d-pantothenyl alcohol) (dexpanthenol, panthenol [C]).	0.25-0.5 Gm. I.M. or I.V. diluted and given slowly. q. 2-6 h.	Used to increase peristalsis in atony and paralysis of the lower bowel.	Alcoholic analog of D-pantothenic acid which is converted in body to D-pantothenic acid; this is claimed to be a precursor of coenzyme A.	Toxicity apparently low. Is used in place of, but not with the prostigmine-like drugs. Should wait 12 hours after neostigmine and 1 hour after succinylcholine before starting dexpanthenol. Its use is contraindicated in hemophilia.	
PHYSOSTIGMINE. *Physostigma venenosum* or *Calabar bean.* Physostigmine salicylate, U.S.P. (Antilirium, Eserine salicylate) (eserine, Isopto-Eserine [C]).	1-2 mg. t.i.d. Oral. 0.5-1 mg. Subcutaneous. 0.2-1% solution. Topical in eyes.	It is an antipruritic and antipyretic but does not reduce temperature except when fever exists. Used as a miotic and a diaphoretic and also to increase peristalsis. Stimulates respiration. Used as an antidote to the toxic effects of belladonna alkaloids and to reverse effects of atropine and scopolamine.	Postganglionic stimulant of parasympathetic system with direct action; causes miosis, bradycardia, increased intestinal motility. Rapidly absorbed from gastrointestinal tract, subcutaneous tissues and mucous membranes. Thought to be degraded in body by cholinesterase. After subcutaneous injection duration of effect approximately 2 hours.	Weak heart action, abdominal cramps, diarrhea, excessive perspiration, salivation, muscular twitching, pinpoint pupils, shock, and collapse. Treatment: atropine and caffeine may be used. Treat for shock. Artificial respiration as indicated. Watch for asthmatic attack. Contraindicated in known asthmatic patients, gangrene, diabetes, cardiovascular disease, mechanical obstruction of the intestinal or urinary tract or in patients receiving neuromuscular blocking agents such as decamethonium or succinylcholine.	Also available as the sulfate.
PILOCARPINE. *Pilocarpus jaborandi. Synthetic.* Pilocarpine hydrochloride, U.S.P. (Almocarpine, Isopto-Carpine, Miocarpine, Pilomiotin [C]).	5-20 mg. p.r.n. Oral or parenteral.	Used mainly as a miotic and a diaphoretic. It is also an antipruritic and antipyretic but does not reduce temperature except when	Has direct action on cholinergic receptors and produces strong postganglionic and some ganglionic stimulation when acetylcholine is the	Weakens and slows heart action, lowers blood pressure, increases bronchial secretion, may produce pulmonary edema. Other	Action is similar to that of the choline derivatives.

Pilocarpine hydrochloride solution, U.S.P. Pilocarpine nitrate, U.S.P. (Carpine nitrate [C]). Pilocarpine nitrate solution, U.S.P. Pilocarpus fluid extract.	0.25-10.0% solution. Up to q.i.d. Topical in eye. 5-20 mg. p.r.n. Oral or parenteral. 0.5-6% solution. Up to q.i.d. Topical in eye. 0.5-2 ml. p.r.n. Oral.	fever exists.	mediator. Stimulates salivation and bronchial secretion, produces sweating, and increases peristalsis. May improve drainage from anterior chamber of eye in glaucoma. Little is known of fate of pilocarpine in body. Some degradation but most is excreted in urine in combined form.	symptoms include nausea, vomiting, and muscular twitching. Treatment: atropine, caffeine, and camphor may be used. Treat for shock. Artificial respiration may be needed. Treat symptoms.	

PARASYMPATHOLYTICS
(PARASYMPATHETIC DEPRESSANTS, CHOLINERGIC BLOCKING AGENTS)

The general effects of these drugs are opposite to those of the parasympathetic stimulants but similar to those of the sympathetic stimulants. They produce mydriasis, cycloplegia, reduced secretion of certain glands, relaxation of smooth muscle tissue, and increased heart action. Most of these drugs are derived from various plants of the Solanaceae family. Each plant yields all or most of the alkaloids. Many of the drugs have been synthesized, and many synthetic preparations similar to the natural alkaloids are available. These drugs are *contraindicated in glaucoma* and used with caution in patients with prostatic hypertrophy or pyloric obstruction.

BELLADONNA. *(atropine, hyoscine, hyoscyamine). Atropa belladonna. Synthetic.* Atropine methylnitrate (Ekomine, Harvatrate, Metanite, Metropine) (atropine methonitrate [C]). Atropine sulfate, U.S.P. (Isopto-atropine [C]).	1 mg. Oral. 1% solution. Topical. 0.25-0.6 mg. Oral or parenteral. 0.5-1% ophthalmic ointment.	Used in a wide variety of conditions; to decrease secretions, relax smooth muscle tissue, dilate pupils, increase heart rate, increase rate of respirations, for general cerebral stimulation, and locally as an anodyne. Used with many other drugs in various combinations, as with phenobarbital in the treatment of gastrointestinal disorders.	These compounds of the belladonna group interfere with transmission of postganglionic parasympathetic impulses and this action is thought to be due to receptor site attachment. Most belladonna alkaloids are rapidly absorbed orally and can also enter circulation from mucosal surfaces. They are widely distributed in the body. The quaternary derivatives are only about one quarter absorbed and they do not cross the blood-brain barrier and so are lacking in central effects.	Excessive dryness of mouth and throat, dysphagia, intense thirst, impaired vision, red and dry skin, delirium, convulsions, tachycardia, and increased blood pressure. Treatment: symptomatic. Parasympathetic stimulants such as pilocarpine are usually ordered, as are cardiac and respiratory stimulants. Use with caution in cardiovascular disease. Contraindicated with gastrointestinal or genitourinary obstruction, glaucoma, prostatic hypertrophy or during pregnancy.	Preparations of mixtures of belladonna alkaloids are also available, such as Bellafoline.
Atropine sulfate solution (Atropisol).	0.5-2% solution. Topical.	As a mydriatic.			Times of administration of these products vary with use and gravity of the situation.
Atropine tartrate.	2 mg. I.M. or I.V.	To combat paralyzing action of nerve gas.			

Name, Source, Synonyms, Preparations	Dosage and Administration	Uses	Action and Fate	Side Effects and Contraindications	Remarks
BELLADONNA (Continued)					
Belladonna tincture, U.S.P. (Taladonna).	0.3-0.6 mg. Oral.	Also available as an extract for oral administration and as an ointment for topical use.			
Genatropine (Atropine-N-Oxide, Xtro) (hyoscine aminoxide [C]).	0.5-1 mg. two or three times a day. Oral.	See atropine.	See atropine.	See atropine.	
HYOSCYAMINE. *Active principle of Hyoscyamus niger.*		General uses same as those of belladonna.	Similar to belladonna but affects the peripheral organs more and the internal organs less than atropine.	Excessive dryness of mouth and throat, dysphagia, intense thirst, impaired vision, red and dry skin, delirium, convulsions, tachycardia, and increased blood pressure. Treatment: symptomatic. Parasympathetic stimulants such as pilocarpine are usually ordered, as are cardiac and respiratory stimulants. For contraindications, see above.	See above.
Hyoscyamine hydrobromide, N.F. (Daturine).	0.25-1 mg. Oral or parenteral.	Available also as extract, fluid extract, and tincture.			
Hyoscyamine sulfate, N.F.	0.25-1 mg. Oral or parenteral.				
Levohyoscyamine sulfate (Anaspaz, Levsin).	0.125-0.250 mg. 3 to 4 times daily. Oral.	Antispasmodic, antisecretory.			
SCOPOLAMINE *(Hyoscine* [C]). *Active principle of Scopolia atropoides. Synthetic.*		General uses same as those of belladonna. The synthetic product is used for paralysis agitans, delirium tremens, and drug addiction.	Similar to belladonna. It exerts a depressant action on brain, heart, and respiration.	Excessive dryness of mouth and throat, dysphagia, intense thirst, impaired vision, red and dry skin, delirium, convulsions, tachycardia, and sometimes increased blood pressure. The heart action may initially be temporarily slowed and the blood pressure lowered. Occasionally severe depression occurs.	
Methscopolamine bromide, N.F. (Pamine, Scoline, Tropane) (hysocine methobromide, scopolamine methobromide [C]).	2.5-5 mg. t.i.d. and h.s. Oral. 0.5 mg. parenteral up to q.i.d.				
Methscopolamine nitrate (Epoxytropine tropate methylnitrate).	2-4 mg. t.i.d. and h.s. Also prepared for subcutaneous and I.M. use and in delayed action tablets.				
Scopolamine aminoxide hydrobromide (Genoscopolamine) (hyoscine aminoxide [C]).	0.5 mg. Oral or parenteral.				Scopolamine aminoxide hydrobromide is less apt to produce tolerance than scopolamine.

Scopolamine hydrobromide, U.S.P. (hyoscine hydrobromide) (Isopto-Hyoscine [C]).	0.2-0.5% solution. Topical. 0.3-0.6 mg. Oral or parenteral.				Scopolamine hydrobromide as a preoperative medication produces less tenacious sputum than atropine.
STRAMONIUM. *Datura stramonium.* Stramonium leaves.	None specified. Inhalation.	General uses same as those of belladonna. Used mainly in bronchial asthma.	Similar to belladonna.	Toxic symptoms rare but are the same as for atropine.	Leaves are burned and the smoke inhaled as a palliative treatment for asthma.

SYNTHETIC PARASYMPATHOLYTIC DRUGS

These drugs resemble the natural alkaloids in general structure or are simple bases with a trivalent nitrogen. They have a central nervous system effect as well as a ganglionic effect. These are all synthetic preparations.

Adiphenine hydrochloride (Trasentine).	50-75 mg. q. 3 h. Oral.	Used in gastric ulcers, colitis, etc.	Adiphenine HCl has selective action in relaxation of smooth muscle tissues.	Toxicity similar to that of atropine.	A number of drugs similar to atropine are listed here. Since lack of space prohibits inclusion of much detailed information, this list is not comprehensive. Almost all members of this group are available in combination with a barbiturate.
Dicyclomine hydrochloride, N.F. (Bentyl) (dicycloverine, Bentylol [C]).	5-20 mg. t.i.d. or q.i.d. Individually adjusted. Oral. I.M.	General uses same as those of belladonna. Used mainly as an antispasmodic.	Similar to atropine, but it is not a secretory depressant.	Toxicity rare, but similar to that of atropine when it occurs.	
Octatropine methylbromide (Valpin) (anisotropine methylbromide [C]).	10 mg. a.c. tablets or elixir. Oral.	Similar to atropine.	Similar to atropine.	Toxicity similar to that of atropine.	Safe use during pregnancy has not been established.
Oxyphencyclimine hydrochloride, N.F. (Daricon, Vio-Thene).	10 mg. Usually given b.i.d. Oral.	Anticholinergic used similarly to methantheline.	Similar to methantheline.	Toxicity similar to that of methantheline.	
Piperidolate hydrochloride (Dactil).	50 mg. q.i.d. Oral.	Used as an antispasmodic, especially to control spasms of the stomach, upper intestinal tract, and gall bladder. Not used to treat gastric ulcers.	Similar to the peripheral action of atropine. Depresses muscular action but not secretion.	Toxicity rare in therapeutic dosage.	

Name, Source, Synonyms, Preparations	Dosage and Administration	Uses	Action and Fate	Side Effects and Contraindications	Remarks
SYNTHETIC PARASYMPATHOLYTIC DRUGS (Continued)					
This group contains a quaternary nitrogen and has lessened central nervous system effect and accentuated ganglionic effects, but absorption after oral use is usually incomplete. These are all synthetic preparations. Many members of this group are available in combination with a barbiturate.					
Diphemanil methylsulfate, N.F. (Prantal) (diphenmethanil [C]).	0.1-0.2 Gm. q. 4-6 h. between meals. Oral.	General uses same as those of belladonna. Used mainly as an anticholinergic agent to control peptic ulcers. Reduces pain, pyrosis, and nausea. Also used to treat hyperhidrosis and as an antipruritic.	Similar to atropine.	Toxic symptoms rare, but similar to those of atropine when they occur.	The effects last longer than those of methantheline bromide.
Glycopyrrolate, N.F. (Robinul), (glycopyrronium bromide [C]).	1-2 mg. t.i.d. Oral. 0.2 mg./kg. s.q., I.M. 0.1-0.2 mg. I.V. t.i.d. or q.i.d.	An anticholinergic with uses and actions similar to those of others of this group; management of gastric and duodenal ulcers.	Similar to others of this group.	Similar to others of this group.	
Hexocyclium methylsulfate (Tral).	25-50 mg. q.i.d. Oral. Also available as sustained release tablets given b.i.d.	As above.	As above.	Toxicity similar to that of atropine.	
Isopropamide iodide, N.F. (Darbid).	5 mg. Usually q. 12 h. Individually adjusted. Oral.	Used for gastric ulcers and for hypermotility of the gastrointestinal tract.	Similar to hyoscyamine. Inhibits gastric secretion and motility.	Toxicity similar to that of hyoscyamine.	
Mepenzolate methylbromide, N.F. (Cantil) (glycophenylate bromide [C]).	25 mg. Usually q.i.d. Individually adjusted. Oral.	Used mainly in conditions in which hypermotility of the lower bowel is a problem.	Similar to others of this group.	Toxicity similar to that of atropine. Reduction of dosage is usually sufficient treatment.	
Methantheline bromide, N.F. (Banthine).	50-100 mg. q.i.d. Individually adjusted. Oral, I.V., or I.M.	General uses same as those of belladonna. Used mainly as an anticholinergic agent to control peptic ulcers.	Similar to belladonna. Reduces both motility and hyperacidity.	Rare, but similar to those of atropine when they occur. Occasionally, urinary retention in prostatic hypertrophy. Treatment: none usually required, but when needed is the same as for atropine.	
Oxyphenonium bromide (Antrenyl).	5-10 mg. q.i.d. Oral. 1-2 mg. p.r.n. Subcu-	Used in gastric ulcers and similar conditions, also	Similar to atropine.	Toxicity similar to that of atropine.	

	taneous or I.M.	in place of atropine or scopolamine in preoperative medications.			
Pentapiperide methylsulfate (Quilene).	10-20 mg. q.i.d. Oral. As much as 30 mg. q.i.d. may be used. Best given a.c. and h.s.	Used for the treatment of peptic ulcers.	Similar to atropine.	See atropine.	
Penthienate bromide, N.F.	5-10 mg. q.i.d. Oral.	Used mainly in the management of peptic ulcers.	Similar to atropine.	Usually mild, but similar to atropine.	
Pipenzolate bromide (Piptal).	5-10 mg. q.i.d. Oral.	Similar to atropine and used for the same purposes.	Similar to atropine.	Toxicity lower than that of atropine.	
Poldine methylsulfate (Nacton).	5-10 mg. Three to four times daily. Oral.	Main use is to reduce gastric acidity and motility in peptic ulcers.	Similar to atropine.	Large doses may cause xerostomia, dysuria, tachycardia. Reduction of dosage is usually sufficient.	
Propantheline bromide, U.S.P. (Pro-Banthine) (Banlin, NeoBanex, Novopantheline [C]).	15 mg. q.i.d. Oral. 30 mg. p.r.n. I.M. or I.V. A powder to be dissolved in a suitable diluent.	General uses same as those of belladonna. Used mainly as an anticholinergic agent to control peptic ulcers. Reduces both motility and hyperacidity.	Similar to atropine.	Toxic symptoms rare but similar to those of atropine when they occur. Occasional urinary retention in prostatic hypertrophy. There are fewer side effects than with Banthine. Treatment: none usually required, but when needed is the same as for atropine.	
Tricyclamol chloride.	50-100 mg. q.i.d. Oral.	Similar to others of this group.	Similar to others of this group.	Toxicity similar to that of atropine.	
Tridihexethyl chloride, N.F. (Pathilon).	5-25 mg. t.i.d. or q.i.d. Oral or parenteral.	Similar to others of this group.	Similar to others of this group.	Toxicity similar to that of atropine.	
Valethamate bromide, N.F. (Murel).	10-20 mg. t.i.d. or q.i.d. Oral, I.M., or I.V.	Similar to the atropine-scopolamine drugs.	An anticholinergic, musculotropic, ganglionic blocking agent.	Toxicity similar to that of atropine.	

Parasympatholytics primarily used in treatment of Parkinson's disease, acting mainly on central nervous system. Contain tertiary nitrogen instead of quaternary, and are well absorbed after oral administration.

Benztropine mesylate, N.F. (Cogentin).	0.5-2 mg. Doses individually adjusted. Oral or parenteral.	Used in the treatment of parkinsonism. Also with phenothiazines to decrease extrapyramidal effects.	Has both anticholinergic and antihistaminic action.	Toxicity usually low but drug has cumulative action. Side effects may be those of either the cholinergic or antihistamine drugs.	Usually started with small dose h.s. and increased as required.

Name, Source, Synonyms, Preparations	Dosage and Administration	Uses	Action and Fate	Side Effects and Contraindications	Remarks
SYNTHETIC PARASYMPATHOLYTIC DRUGS (Continued)					
Biperiden, N.F. (Akineton).	1-2 mg. Three to four times daily. Dosage individually adjusted. Oral. Occasionally given I.M. or I.V.	Used in treatment of Parkinson's disease and certain forms of spasticity. Also with phenothiazines to decrease extrapyramidal effects.	Claimed to have greater myospasmolytic effect and less drying effect on salivary glands than atropine.	Side effects include blurring of vision, drowsiness, nausea, and vomiting. Reduce and treat symptoms. Contraindicated in all forms of epilepsy, and caution should be observed in patients with glaucoma.	
Caramiphen hydrochloride.	12.5-50 mg. Dosage individually adjusted.	Used mainly in the treatment of Parkinson's disease.	Exact mode of action is not known.	Rare in therapeutic dosage, but nausea, epigastic burning, and mild sedation have been reported.	
Cycrimine hydrochloride, N.F. (Pagitane hydrochloride).	1.25-2.5 mg. Dosage individually adjusted up to 15 mg. daily. Oral.	As above.	As above.	Avoid using in patients with glaucoma, urinary retention, or tachycardia.	
Procyclidine hydrochloride (Kemadrin).	5-10 mg. Three to four times daily. Oral.	Used mainly in the palliative treatment of Parkinson's syndrome.	Similar to atropine.	Toxicity similar to that of atropine.	Safe use during pregnancy or for children has not been established.
Trihexyphenidyl hydrochloride, U.S.P. (Artane, Pipanol, Tremin) (benzhexol, Novohexidyl, Trinexy [C]).	2-5 mg. t.i.d. or q.i.d. Oral.	General uses same as those of belladonna. Used mainly as an antispasmodic in such conditions as parkinsonism.	Similar to others of this group.	Toxic symptoms are rare.	
Several antihistamine agents are also used in the treatment of Parkinson's disease, such as chlorphenoxamine hydrochloride (Histol, Phenoxene), ethopropazide hydrochloride (Parsidol), and orphenadrine hydrochloride (Disipal).					
Anticholinergic drugs which are used primarily for local effects in the eye. These are synthetic or semisynthetic drugs.					
Cyclopentolate hydrochloride, U.S.P. (Cyclogyl) (Mydplegic [C]).	0.5-2% solution. Topical.	Used as a cycloplegic and mydriatic.	Action is that of mydriatic and cycloplegic.	Nontoxic in topical use.	
Eucatropine hydrochloride, U.S.P. (Euphthalmine).	2% solution. Topical.	As a mydriatic.	Action is mydriatic.	Toxicity low.	
Homatropine hydrobromide, U.S.P.	2-5% solution. Topical.	As a mydriatic.	Action is that of mydriatic and cycloplegic.	Toxicity similar to that of atropine is rare.	
Homatropine methylbromide, N.F. (Homapin, Malcotran, Mesopin, Novatropin) (Isopto-Homatropine [C]).	10 mg. Oral.	Similar to atropine. Used in gastric ulcers, colitis, and as a mydriatic.	Action similar to that of atropine.		

Tropicamide (Mydriacyl).	0.5-1% solution. Topical for use in eyes.	Used as a mydriatic and cycloplegic.	As above.	None unless ingested.	

DRUGS AFFECTING THE CENTRAL NERVOUS SYSTEM

STIMULANTS

AMMONIA. *Chemical.* Aromatic ammonia spirits.	2 ml. Oral; also administered by inhalation.	Used as an emergency cardiac and respiratory stimulant, especially in fainting.	Acts as a reflex stimulant by irritation of nerve endings.	Rare in therapeutic dosage. Treatment: none usually needed.	Alcohol is also a reflex stimulant of nerve endings but is a depressant after absorption.
AMPHETAMINE. *Synthetic.* Amphetamine phosphate (Bar-Dex, Dietamine).	10 mg. Daily in divided doses. Oral or parenteral.	Used systemically to stimulate the nervous system in narcolepsy, postencephalitic parkinsonism; to increase peristalsis, and to raise blood pressure. Used as an anorexic agent and in hyperkinetic behavior disorders.	Stimulates the cerebral cortex, and if respiratory depression is present, this will be improved. After an oral dose, the individual is more alert and better able to work, and has a general feeling of euphoria. After a large dose physical exertion may be much increased, but when it has worn off, there is greater fatigue and depression than before and a longer period of rest is required. Readily absorbed and widely distributed in body fluids. Some is excreted unchanged by the kidneys. Fate of remainder not well understood.	Restlessness and insomnia, with severe overstimulation, cardiaç failure. Treatment: symptomatic, and includes rest, quiet, and sedation. Contraindicated in hypertension. Used with caution in thyrotoxicosis, acute coronary disease, or cardiac decompensation. Amphetamines should not be given concurrently with the monoamine oxidase inhibitors as it can cause a hypertensive crisis. The therapeutic effectiveness of guanethidine is antagonized by the concurrent use of the amphetamines. Amphetamines and chlorpromazine are antagonistic to their effects on noradrenergic and dopaminergic receptors. This can be used to advantage in poisoning of amphetamine-like drugs but concurrent therapeutic use is not pharmaceutically sound.	In most cases should not be given after 4:00 P.M. to avoid insomnia. Although amphetamine causes central nervous stimulation it should not be used by normal individuals to induce capacity for extra work. Amphetamines have a significant potential for abuse. In view of their short term anorectic effect and rapid development of tolerance, they should be used only for limited periods and with extreme caution in weight reduction programs.
Amphetamine solution.	1% solution. Topical.				
Amphetamine sulfate, N.F. (Amphedrine, Benzedrine).	10-20 mg. Daily in divided doses. Oral.				
Benzphetamine hydrochloride, N.F. (Didrex).	25-150 mg. Daily in divided doses. Oral.				
Dextroamphetamine elixir.	5 mg./ml. b.i.d. Oral.				
Dextroamphetamine phosphate, N.F. (Dextro-Profetamine)	5 mg. b.i.d. Oral.				
Dextroamphetamine sulfate, U.S.P. (dexamphetamine, d-amphetamine, Dexellets, Novamphene [C]).	5 mg. b.i.d. Oral.				
Dextroamphetamine tannate (Tanphetamine) (Synatan [C]).	17.5 mg. Oral.				
Levamphetamine (Ad-nil) (levanfetamine, Cyril [C]).	5 mg. b.i.d. Oral.				

Name, Source, Synonyms, Preparations	Dosage and Administration	Uses	Action and Fate	Side Effects and Contraindications	Remarks
AMPHETAMINE (Continued) Methamphetamine hydrochloride, U.S.P. (Desoxedrine, Desoxyephedrine, Desoxyn, Phedrisox, Semoxydrine, Neodrine [C]).	2.5-7.5 mg. b.i.d. or t.i.d. Oral. 15-30 mg. I.M. or I.V. Often given with methylcellulose in reducing diets; similar to amphetamine.	Mild stimulant and biochemical corrective for treating metabolic deficiencies of the brain. Used in chronic headaches of psychogenic origin, and in control of obesity.	See amphetamine.	See amphetamine.	
CAFFEINE. *Active principle of Thea sinensis, Coffea arabica, kola nut, guarana, and yerba. Other active principles: theobromine, theophylline.* Caffeine citrated, N.F. Caffeine and sodium benzoate, U.S.P. Caffeine and sodium salicylate.	 0.2-0.3 Gm. p.r.n. Not over 2.5 Gm. daily. Oral. 0.5 Gm. p.r.n., usually not over 2.5 Gm. daily. Oral or I.M. 0.2 Gm. p.r.n. Oral.	Used as a general cerebral stimulant. Valuable in shock and collapse. It is an antidote for narcotic poisoning, radiation sickness, and heat exhaustion. It is a diuretic and general body stimulant. Will help relieve certain types of headache.	Is a descending central nervous system stimulant. Small doses affect the cerebrum mainly; larger doses, the brainstem, including the medulla. Large doses increase heart action and cause peripheral vasodilation. Absorption of caffeine is erratic. Salts of caffeine are more readily absorbed. Excreted by kidneys as l-methy uric acid and 1-methyl xanthine, about 10% unchanged.	Rarely severe; mild symptoms include insomnia, restlessness, nervousness, palpitation, nausea, vomiting. Functional cardiac symptoms may occur. Treatment: stop drug and give evacuants and sedatives.	Caffeine is one of the xanthine drugs. The others are theobromine and theophylline (refer to Diuretics). Since most people drink either coffee or tea they are used to receiving a daily dose of caffeine; hence, they have a tolerance for the drug and do not usually develop toxic symptoms from using it as a drug.
DEANOL. *Synthetic.* From acetylcholine. Deanol Acetamidobenzoate (Deaner).	25-100 mg. q.i.d. Oral.	Possibly effective in the following: to increase attention span and to improve behavior in children with various problems.	Exact mechanism not known, but claimed to enhance action of an acetylcholinic precursor and make it more readily available in the cortex.	Toxicity relatively low. Contraindicated in convulsive states, such as grand mal epilepsy.	
METHYLPHENIDATE HYDROCHLORIDE. *Synthetic.* Methylphenidate hydrochloride, U.S.P. (Ritalin hydrochloride).	5-20 mg. Two or three times daily. Oral.	Used systemically to stimulate the nervous system in narcolepsy and postencephalitic parkinsonism. Also used in the treatment of hyperkinetic children.	Action somewhat like that of amphetamine and caffeine. Affects heart and blood pressure less. Does not affect appetite. Given I.V. it markedly stimulates	Side effects usually mild; not used alone in agitated patients. Anorexia, dizziness, nausea, headache, palpitation, drowsiness. Treatment: reduce dosage	Methylphenidate can be abused and patients on long-term therapy must be closely monitored. Safe use during pregnancy has not been established.

		Used primarily for the psychoneuroses of senility.	depressed respiratory function. Absorption and excretion similar to ephedrine.	or discontinue. Rarely causes insomnia. May lower the convulsive threshold. Should be used with caution in patients with hypertension. For interactions see under amphetamines. Can raise serum levels of diphenylhydantoin, but this is rare. May affect warfarin levels when the last two are given together. Patients should be closely monitored for toxic side effects.	
NIKETHAMIDE. *Synthetic.* Nikethamide, N.F. (Coramine, Nikorin) (Cardiamine, Kardonyl, [C]).	1-5 mg. Oral or parenteral.	Used mainly in respiratory and circulatory failure.	Main action is stimulation of the medullary centers. Causes increase in respiration, and peripheral vasoconstriction. There is some cortical stimulation and usually a rise in blood pressure.	Rare in therapeutic dosage. Excessive dosage may produce convulsions and death. Treatment: symptomatic.	A dependable stimulant, usually given I.V. or I.M. Related chemically to nicotinic acid.
NUX VOMICA. *Strychnos nux-vomica.* Strychnine, brucine. Nux vomica tincture Strychnine nitrate Strychnine phosphate (Anoro). Strychnine sulfate	 1 ml. Oral. 2 mg. Oral. 2 mg. Oral. 2 mg. Oral.	Used mainly to increase muscle tone in conditions such as gastrointestinal stasis, paralysis, and debility.	An ascending stimulant affecting the spinal cord first and the cerebrum last. The margin between therapeutic and toxic action is narrow. Readily absorbed and widely distributed. Rapidly inactivated by kidneys, within 10 hours.	Stiffness of neck muscles, risus sardonicus, tetanic convulsions. Treatment: early–lavage, chemical antidotes (charcoal, potassium permanganate, tannic acid); later–hypnotics, sedatives (barbiturates), artificial respiration.	Strychnine is the active principle of nux vomica. Its therapeutic value has been questioned but it is still used, especially in many proprietary "tonics." These drugs have largely been replaced by less toxic drugs.
PENTYLENETETRAZOL. *Synthetic.* Pentylenetetrazol, N.F. (Metrazol, Pentrazol, Petrolone) (pentetrazol [C]).	0.1-0.3 Gm. Three to four times daily. Oral or parenteral.	Used mainly as a respiratory and cardiac stimulant in shock and collapse, asphyxia neonatorum, and as an antidote in depressant drug poisoning.	Stimulates cerebral medullary centers and increases spinal reflexes, especially if depressed. Does not appear to stimulate the myocardium or the blood vessels. Readily absorbed, widely and evenly distributed throughout body fluids. Inactivated by the liver and excreted by the kidneys. Exact form when excreted is not known.	Burning sensation in mouth, esophagus and stomach; salivation, nausea, vomiting, colic, and diarrhea. Other symptoms that may occur include diaphoresis, pallor, headache, palpitation, shallow respirations, convulsions, and lockjaw. Treatment: emetics, chloroform; also for shock.	Was used to induce convulsions in treatment of psychoses; largely replaced by electric therapy. General use limited, due to toxicity.

ANTIDEPRESSANTS

Name, Source, Synonyms, Preparations	Dosage and Administration	Uses	Action and Fate	Side Effects and Contraindications	Remarks
These are synthetic drugs. **TRICYCLIC ANTIDEPRESSANTS**					
Amitriptyline (Elavil) (Elatrol, Levate, Mareline, Novotriptyn [C]).	10-50 mg. t.i.d. Oral. 20-30 mg. q.i.d. I.M.	Antidepressant for depression resulting from psychoses or neuroses; also has a tranquilizing action.	Acts to relieve mental depression by unknown mechanism. It is not an amine oxidase inhibitor. Amitriptyline inhibits the membrane pump mechanism responsible for re-uptake of norepinephrine into the adrenergic neurons. Readily absorbed. Rapidly disappears from circulating blood. Probably metabolized or conjugated. Exact fate is not known.	May cause dizziness, nausea, excitement, hypotension, fine tremor, jitteriness, headache, heartburn, anorexia, diaphoresis, numbness and tingling, activation of latent schizophrenia, rare epileptiform seizures in chronic schizophrenia. Temporary confusion or impaired concentration may occur with high dosage. Reduce or interrupt dosage. Contraindicated in glaucoma and urinary retention. Not recommended during acute recovery phase following myocardial infarction.	The tricyclic compounds can block the antihypertensive effects of guanethidine. Alcohol toxicity is potentiated especially during first few days of therapy. When used with chlordiazepoxide, impairment of motor function can occur. However, with close monitoring, they can be used together. The use of the tricyclic antidepressants with monoamine oxidase inhibitors should be avoided, but with close monitoring they may be used concurrently.
Desipramine hydrochloride, N.F. (Norpramin, Pertofrane) (desmethylimipramine [C]).	25-50 mg. t.i.d. Oral. (150 mg./day is maximum).	Main use is in depression of a psychogenic origin.	Relatively quick antidepressant that does not produce euphoria. Exact mode of action is not known. Absorption and excretion similar to amitriptyline.	Contraindicated in glaucoma, urinary or gastric retention, epilepsy, or when the monoamine oxidase inhibitors are used. Side effects include dry mouth, constipation, sweating, agitation, dizziness, tachycardia, jaundice.	Liver and blood tests should be done during prolonged therapy even though toxicity has not been observed in respect to liver and blood. Safe use during pregnancy has not been established.
Imipramine hydrochloride, N.F. (Presamine, Tofranil) (Chem-Ipramine, Impamine, Impram, Impranil, Impril, Novopramine [C]).	Dosage should be determined for individual patient. Maintenance dose usually 50-150 mg. daily. Oral and parenteral.	Main use as an antidepressant in psychoses and non-psychotic conditions with depressed emotional tone. Used in the treatment of enuresis.	Mechanism of action is not known. See amitriptyline.	Effects similar to those of atropine; also dizziness, weight gain, skin rash, tremors, transient hypotension. Reduce dosage and if this not enough, stop drug. Treat symptoms. Use with caution in patients with increased intraocular pressure.	Caution: should not be given concurrently with or for 14 days after treatment with monoamine oxidase inhibitors. Safe use during pregnancy has not been established.

<u>Nortriptyline hydrochloride,</u> N.F. (Aventyl) (Acetexa, Avantyl [C]).	25 mg. t.i.d. Adjusted to suit patient's response. Oral.	Used in depression, anxiety, and psychosomatic disorders.	Exact mode of action not well established. See amitriptyline.	Contraindicated with monoamine oxidase inhibitors. 10-20 days should be allowed between the use of this drug and the monoamine oxidase inhibitors. Used with caution in glaucoma and urinary retention, hypotension, or convulsive states. Should not be used during pregnancy. May cause dry mouth, drowsiness, constipation, dizziness, confusion, restlessness, weakness, and blurred vision. Adjustment of dosage will usually suffice.
<u>Protriptyline hydrochloride</u> (Vivactil) (Triptil [C]).	15-40 mg. daily in divided doses t.i.d. or q.i.d. Oral.	Relief of symptoms of depression in the depressed patient who is under close medical supervision.	This drug is chemically related to amitriptyline. Rapid onset of antidepressant action usually without tranquilizing or sedative effects often within one week. Has autonomic effects, including potentiation or prolonged effects of norepinephrine and by stimulation of sympathetic nerves. It reduces or blocks the effects of indirect sympathetic amines such as amphetamine, tyramine or phenethylamine. It antagonizes the prolonged depletion of tissue catecholamines by quanethirine and alpha-methylmetatyrosine. It has relatively weak anticholinergic properties.	Contraindicated in glaucoma, stenosis, urinary retention. Do not give with monoamine oxidase inhibitors, guanethidine and similar compounds. Not recommended for children under 12 years of age or for women of child bearing age unless risks are outweighed by benefits. Side effects are very numerous (see commercial brochure for side effects and precautions). Some of the side effects are: tachycardia, postural hypotension, drowsiness (occasionally) and such things as bad taste, dry mouth, dystonia, tremors, fatigue, weakness, blurring of vision, mental confusion, and many others. Exposure to sunlight should be avoided during treatment with protriptyline.

Name, Source, Synonyms, Preparations	Dosage and Administration	Uses	Action and Fate	Side Effects and Contraindications	Remarks
MONOAMINE OXIDASE INHIBITORS					
Isocarboxazid, N.F. (Marplan).	Initially 30 mg. daily (10 mg. t.i.d.); then reduce to 10-20 mg. daily. Doses over 30 mg. daily are not recommended. Oral.	Used as psychic energizer.	This is a monoamine oxidase inhibitor and raises both the serotonin and norepinephrine levels. Readily absorbed. Thought to be rather rapidly excreted, but it takes some time for enzyme to be reactivated. Exact fate not known.	Drugs of this class may induce postural hypotension, transient impotence, nausea, ankle edema, delayed micturition, constipation, dizziness, overactivity, insomnia, dry mouth, blurred vision, skin rashes. Control with adjunctive therapy or reduce dosage. Watch for signs of liver damage with all these drugs.	The monoamine oxidase inhibitors can produce severe hypertensive crisis when food containing large amounts of tyramine is eaten. These monoamine oxidase inhibitors can cause hypertension when used with tricyclic antidepressants, sympathetic amines and levodopa. Meperidine should not be used for patients on the monoamine oxidase inhibitors since the combination can have catastrophic results.
Phenelzine dihydrogen sulfate (Nardil).	15 mg. t.i.d. for treatment; maintenance dose 15 mg. once daily. Oral.	Use and action similar to those of isocarboxazid.	Monoamine oxidase inhibitor. See isocarboxazid for absorption data.	Side effects similar to those of isocarboxazid.	
Tranylcypromine sulfate, N.F. (Parnate).	20 mg. given 10 mg. twice daily to start. May increase to a total of 30 mg. per day. Oral.	Used to treat various states of depression.	Monoamine oxidase inhibitor. See isocarboxazid for absorption data.	Restlessness, insomnia, postural hypotension, headache, dizziness, and anorexia. Many contraindications; see manufacfacturer's pamphlet.	Caution: Use only in hospitalized patients or patients in whom all other drugs have been ineffective; do not use in patients over 60 or those with a history of hypertension.
OTHER ANTIDEPRESSANTS					
Pipradrol hydrochloride, N.F. (Meratran).	1-2.5 mg. Morning and noon. Oral.	Used mainly to counteract depression.	A mild cerebral stimulant producing elevation of mood, increased ability to work and to concentrate, and increased confidence. Has little effect on pulse, blood pressure or respirations.	Side effects rare and mild. May produce insomnia, excitability, and anorexia.	

INTOXICANTS

ALCOHOL. *Synthetic.* Absolute alcohol (dehydrated alcohol). Alcohol, U.S.P. (ethyl alcohol, ethanol).	99% by volume. Rarely used. 95% by volume. Rarely used.	Used for temporary reflex stimulation in certain cases of shock. Used to increase appetite. Ninety-nine per cent alcohol is injected into the fifth cranial nerve in the treatment of tic douloureux.	Initial effects: increased heart and respiratory rate, superficial vasodilation, rise in blood pressure, increase in flow of digestive juices. Later effect: depression. Many authorities feel no effective stimulation is secured from alcohol. Absorption from the stomach varies with the amount of food it contains. Rapid if empty. From the intestines absorption is rapid with or without food. Widely distributed throughout the body. Most is oxidized by liver or other tissues. About 2-10% is excreted unchanged by the kidney.	Progressive descending depression starting with the higher cerebral centers, gradually descending to the brainstem medulla and in large dose to the spinal cord. Alcohol can interact with a large number of compounds. These include the following. With the tricyclic antidepressants, there is an impairment of motor function, especially in the first few days of antidepressant therapy. Alcohol can accentuate occult blood loss and damage to gastric mucosa induced by aspirin. This is important clinically in patients taking 2 to 3 Gm. of aspirin daily. With the barbiturates or chloral hydrate, the depressant action of each drug is increased over its action if taken alone. This can be very serious. With chlordiazpoxide, there is some enhancement. With diazepam or meprobamate, the potential for central nervous system depression is in proportion to the alcoholic intake. With the monoamine oxidase inhibitors, there is a possible interaction with alcohol other than the reaction with the high tyramine	Nongrain alcohols such as methyl, denatured, isopropyl, butyl, etc., are never used for internal administration because of toxicity.

Name, Source, Synonyms, Preparations	Dosage and Administration	Uses	Action and Fate	Side Effects and Contraindications	Remarks
INTOXICANTS (Continued)					
ALCOHOL (Continued)				beverages, wine and beer. If the diabetic patient treated with phenformin drinks alcohol, he can have a hypoglycemic reaction which will lead to lactic acidosis and shock. Patients treated with tolbutamide and who regularly consume considerable alcohol will metabolize the tolbutamide at a much more rapid rate than is usual. The half life may be reduced 50% of the expected time.	
Brandy (spiritus vini vitis).	51% by volume. Oral.				Brandy and whiskey must be aged in wood at least 4 years.
Diluted alcohol.	49% by volume. Rarely used.				
Whiskey (spiritus frumenti).	50% by volume. Oral.				
Wines.	Concentration varies. Oral.				Many types and strengths of wines are used medicinally, especially to increase appetite.
ANALGESICS—Narcotics, Opium.		Used to relieve pain, to induce sleep (especially when sleep is prevented by pain), to check peristalsis, to suppress cough, to relieve dyspnea. Also used as preoperative medication, to check diarrhea and reduce excitement and convulsions. Morphine, codeine, and thebaine affect the cerebral cortex mainly. Morphine relieves pain, and codeine reduces cough; thebaine has same effect but to a minor	The exact method of action is not known, but it depresses the cerebral cortex and probably the thalami. Opium (morphine) produces mood elevation, euphoria, and relief of fear and apprehension. Slows both mental and physical activity. It is a strong respiratory depressant, but affects heart and blood pressure to only a minor degree. The cough center is depressed and gastrointestinal motility	Acute poisoning. Early symptoms include mental stimulation, physical ease, rapid pulse. Later symptoms are dizziness, nausea, languor, slow weak pulse, pinpoint pupils, slow respirations, cyanosis. Terminally there is Cheyne-Stokes respiration, coma, and death. Treatment: naloxone (Narcan) given parenterally, lavage, colon flush, purgation, central nervous stimulants.	
OPIUM. *(Morphine, codeine, thebaine, narcotine, papaverine). Papaver somniferum.*					
Opium compound and glycyrrhiza mixture (brown mixture).	4 ml. p.r.n. for cough. Oral.				
Opium powdered, U.S.P.	60 mg. p.r.n. for pain. Oral or rectal.				
Opium tincture (laudanum).	0.6 ml. p.r.n. for pain or diarrhea. Oral.				
Opium powdered and ipecac (Dover's powders).	0.3 Gm. Oral.				
Paregoric, U.S.P. (opium camphorated tincture).	2-10 ml. Oral. p.r.n. for diarrhea and dysmenorrhea.				

		degree. Papaverine relaxes muscle tissue, especially smooth muscles. Narcotine (noscopine, nectadon) also relaxes smooth muscle tissue and reduces cough.	decreased. Other effects include increase in perspiration, contraction of pupils, and relaxation of muscle tissues. The fate of the different alkaloids varies. Morphine is absorbed from the gastrointestinal tract, but the rate and amount are unpredictable. Morphine is widely distributed throughout the body and though its main effect is in the central nervous system, most of the drug is not concentrated in the cerebrospinal fluid. It is taken up mainly by the spleen, liver, lungs and kidneys. Morphine is conjugated with glucuronic acid and excreted mainly in conjugated form by the kidneys. About 90% is excreted in 24 hours after usual dose. Other alkaloids such as codeine, heroin and the morphine surrogates are metabolized by the liver and excreted by the kidneys.	A respirator and intravenous drugs such as nikethamide or doxapram (Dopram) may be ordered. Chemotherapeutic drugs and antibiotics may be used to combat pneumonia. Undesirable side effects of opium and particularly of morphine are common and include constipation, nausea, vomiting, itching, diaphoresis.	
Pantopium hydrochloride, (Pantopon).	5-20 mg. q. 3-4 h. p.r.n. for pain. Oral or parenteral.				Pantopon is a mixture of the purified alkaloids of opium in the same proportions as in crude opium.
ANTISPASMODIC PREPARATIONS DERIVED FROM OPIUM					
Ethaverine hydrochloride (Ethaquin, Harverine, Neopavrin A, Papertherine, Verina) (ethylpapaverine [C]).	100 mg. Oral. 15-100 mg. I.V.	An antispasmodic similar to but more effective than papaverine. Used in peripheral or cerebral vascular insufficiency associated with arterial spasm.	The tetraethyl analog of papaverine.	Toxicity similar to that of papaverine but not as severe. Use with caution in glaucoma. Its use is contraindicated in complete arterio-ventricular dissociation.	Not a narcotic drug.

Name, Source, Synonyms, Preparations	Dosage and Administration	Uses	Action and Fate	Side Effects and Contraindications	Remarks
ANALGESICS (Continued)					
Papaverine hydrochloride, N.F. (Pavabid).	30-60 mg. I.M. or slowly I.V. 100-200 mg. Three to five times daily. Oral.				Papaverine is an antispasmodic and not an analgesic. See under spasmolytics.
Preparations from or similar to opium. Morphine and morphine type: some derived directly from opium, some semisynthetic, others entirely synthetic.					
Apomorphine. See under Emetics.					
Morphine hydrochloride.	8-15 mg. q. 3 h. p.r.n. Oral or parenteral.	See opium.	See opium. Morphine crosses the placenta and can cause neonatal addiction, respiratory depression and has been responsible for some neonatal deaths.	See opium.	
Morphine sulfate, U.S.P.	8-15 mg. q. 3 h. p.r.n. Oral or parenteral.				
Codeine phosphate, U.S.P.	15-30-60 mg. q. 3-4 h. p.r.n. Oral or parenteral.				
Codeine sulfate, N.F.	15-30-60 mg. q. 3-4 h. p.r.n. Oral or parenteral.				
Dextromethorphan hydrobromide, N.F. (Romilar, Tussade).	5-15 mg. p.r.n. for cough. Oral.	A morphine derivative used mainly in the control of cough.	Depresses the cough center mainly. Does not have analgesic property.	Similar to other narcotics. Toxicity low.	
Diamorphine hydrochloride (diacetyl-morphine, heroin).		See opium.	See opium.	See opium.	Heroin is not legally available in the United States or Canada.
Ethylmorphine hydrochloride, N.F. (Dionin).	16 mg. p.r.n. Oral or I.M. 1-5% solution. Topical.	As an expectorant. As an anodyne for ophthalmic use.			
Fentanyl (Sublimaze).	Given I.M. or I.V. Brochure should be consulted for specific dosage which varies from 0.025-0.1 mg.	Narcotic analgesic; main use is in anesthesia.	With I.V. use full effect in 3-5 minutes, lasts 30-60 minutes. With I.M. onset in 7-8 minutes, duration 1-2 hours. For further action see narcotic analgesics.	Contraindicated in children under 2 or women during pregnancy as safety has not been demonstrated. Main toxic effect is respiratory depression. Not recommended for use with monoamine oxidase inhibitors. When used with other depressants dose should be reduced. For further information see narcotic analgesics.	Drug also available in combination with droperidol (Innovar).

Hydrocodone bitartrate, N.F. (Dicodid, Mercodinone) (dihydrocodeinone bitartrate, Hycodan [C]).	5-15 mg. p.r.n. Oral or parenteral.	Uses and action similar to those of codeine.	Similar to codeine.	Similar to codeine.	
Hydromorphone hydrochloride, N.F. (Dilaudid, Hymorphan) (dihydromorphinone hydrochloride [C]).	2.0-3.0 mg. p.r.n. Oral or parenteral.	For pain.	Similar to morphine.	Similar to morphine.	
Levorphanol tartrate, N.F. (Levo-Dromoran) (levorphan [C]).	2-3 mg. q. 3-4 h. p.r.n. Oral or parenteral.	Use is similar to that of morphine when given parenterally and to methadone when administered orally.	Analgesic action similar to that of morphine. Has less effect on smooth muscle tissue than morphine.	Same as for morphine, but much less severe. Treatment same as for morphine. Can cross placenta and cause neonatal respiratory depression.	Tolerance is developed with long usage.
Methorphinan (Dromoran)	2.5-5 mg. q. 3-4 h. p.r.n. Oral or parenteral.				
Metopon hydrochloride.	3 mg. p.r.n. Oral.	Used mainly in cancer, as it relieves pain when taken orally.	Similar to morphine.	Rare in therapeutic dosage. Treatment: none usually required. Has few side effects.	Does not produce tolerance quickly.
Oxymorphone, N.F. (Numorphan).	1-15 mg. q. 4-6 h. I.M. or subcutaneously. 2-5 mg. q. 4-6 h. Rectal.	A potent analgesic.	Similar to morphine in analgesic effect but with less respiratory depression, nausea, and constipation.	Relatively low, but respiratory depression, nausea, and constipation may occur. Treatment: symptomatic.	May be habit forming.
Phenazocine (Prinadol) (Xenagol [C]).	2 mg. q. 4-6 h. p.r.n. I.M.	A synthetic narcotic used as adjunct to anesthesia, for postoperative pain, obstetrics, and acute and chronic pain of all kinds, including cancer.	Synthetic molecule similar to morphine; claimed to have fewer sedative and hypotensive effects.	Watch for respiratory depression which can be corrected with levallorphan or nalorphine. Contraindications: hepatic disorders, coma, increased intracranial pressure, convulsions, acute alcoholism, myxedema.	
MEPERIDINE GROUP. *Synthetic narcotic preparations.* Meperidine hydrochloride, N.F. (Demerol, Dolosal), (isonipecaine, pethidine, Phytadon [C]).	25-100 mg. q. 3-4 h. p.r.n. Oral or parenteral.	Widely used as an analgesic and sedative. Used to produce analgesia in obstetrics.	A descending central nervous system depressant. It is analgesic and sedative, but does not cause constipation or pupillary constriction as does morphine. May produce temporary euphoria. Respiratory depression occurs only with very high dosage.	Lowering of blood pressure, bradycardia, shock, vasodilation (nitritoid reaction), dizziness, nausea, vomiting. Treatment: symptomatic. Meperidine should not be given to patients taking monoamine oxidase inhibitors because of possible catastrophic results which	Can be given orally but is less effective. May cause habituation or addiction.

Name, Source, Synonyms, Preparations	Dosage and Administration	Uses	Action and Fate	Side Effects and Contraindications	Remarks
ANALGESICS (Continued) Meperidine hydrochloride (continued)			These drugs are readily absorbed from most routes. They are demethylated and conjugated by the liver and excreted by the kidneys. Very little is excreted unchanged.	include convulsions, excitation, hypertension and, less often, hypotension and hallucinations.	
Alphaprodine hydrochloride, N.F. (Nisentil).	40-60 mg. q. 3-4 h. p.r.n. for pain. Subcutaneous or I.V.	Used for quick short-duration analgesia.	Produces mild euphoria, sedation, dizziness, itching, and sweating. Has little or no cumulative action. Duration of action less than meperidine.	Rare in therapeutic dosage. Treatment: none usually required. Can cross placenta and cause neonatal respiratory depression, if given late in labor.	Tolerance may develop. Addiction is rare.
Anileridine, N.F. (Leritine).	25-50 mg. q. 3-4 h. p.r.n. for pain. Oral or parenteral.	Uses much like those of other synthetic narcotics, especially meperidine.	Similar to meperidine.	Similar to other synthetic narcotics.	The drug comes as several salts: phosphate salt for oral use, hydrocloride for parenteral.
Ethoheptazine citrate, N.F. (Zactane).	75 mg., 1-2 tablets. Three to four times daily. Oral.	Uses similar to those of aspirin.	The analgesic action is similar to that of synthetic analgesics of the meperidine group but it is much less potent and is said not to have the addiction property.	Side effects similar to meperidine, but usually are less severe and occur less often.	
Methadone hydrochloride, U.S.P. (Adanon, Dolophine, Miadone, Polamidon).	5-10 mg. q. 3-4 h. p.r.n. Parenteral. 5-10 mg. q. 3-4 h. p.r.n. Oral. Dose for maintenance and withdrawal is quite variable.	Used to relieve pain in trauma, myalgia, dysmenorrhea, and cancer. Also used in opium withdrawal and in maintenance programs.	Similar to morphine. Less euphoria occurs. Respiratory depression occurs except in low dosage. Does not cause constipation. Readily absorbed. Concentrated mainly in liver, spleen, lungs and kidneys. Degraded mainly by the liver and excreted by the kidneys. Excretion is relatively slow. Less than 10% is excreted unchanged.	Nausea, vomiting, dizziness, and drowsiness may occur. Treatment: symptomatic.	

				Drug crosses placenta and can cause respiratory depression in fetus and also dependence if mother is dependent.	
ANALGESICS. Miscellaneous. *Synthetic.* Mefenamic acid (Ponstel) (Ponstan [C]).	250 mg. Oral. p.r.n.	Relief of pain. Short term analgesia.	For complete action see commercial brochure. Action differs in quality from the anti-inflammatory effects of the glucocorticoids. It is independent of the pituitary adrenal system and is not associated with depression of general growth.	For side effects, see commercial brochure. Contraindicated in intestinal ulceration, children, and women of child-bearing potential. Used with inflammatory diseases of the gastrointestinal tract, known asthma and renal dysfunction. If rash or diarrhea occurs, drug should be stopped.	
Methotrimeprazine, N.F. (Levoprome) (levomepromazine, Nozinan [C]).	5-40 mg. at intervals of q. 1-24 h. Usual dosage 10-20 mg. q. 4-6 h. Deeply I.M.	Relief of pain in chronic illness. For obstetric and pre- and postoperative analgesia.	Analgesia. 10-20 mg. said to be as effective as 10-15 mg. morphine or 50-100 mg. meperidine. This is a phenothiazine derivative and has antiemetic and tranquilizing action.	Contraindications: addiction to drugs, coma, overt or incipient uropathy, hypotension, severe cardiac or renal disease. Side effects: main side effect is orthostatic hypotension, which usually clears after a few doses. Other side effects: amnesia, disorientation, dizziness, drowsiness, weakness, slurring of speech, gastrointestinal disturbances, nasal congestion, chills, difficulty in urination, uterine inertia. Pain may occur at site of injection. With prolonged use jaundice and agranulocytosis may occur.	Do not give I.V. or subcutaneously. Has been shown to have additive effect and dosage should be reduced with antihypertensive drugs, barbiturates, atropine, reserpine and meprobamate. If a vasopressor is required, phenylephrine is preferred. Epinephrine may cause a paradoxical lowering of the blood pressure. Has not been shown to be addictive. Do not give to children under 14 years of age.

Name, Source, Synonyms, Preparations	Dosage and Administration	Uses	Action and Fate	Side Effects and Contraindications	Remarks
ANALGESICS (Continued)					
Pentazocaine, N.F. (Talwin).	30-60 mg. Oral. Subcutaneous, I.M. or I.V. q. 3-4 h.	Nonaddicting, narcotic type analgesic. However, special care must be exercised in prescribing this drug for emotionally unstable patients and those with a history of drug abuse, since there have been cases of psychological and physiological dependence in such patients.	Congeners similar to nalorphine and levallorphan. Analgesia usually occurs within 15-20 minutes after I.M. or subcutaneous injection, 2-3 minutes after I.V. and 15-20 minutes after an oral dose. Pentazocine has about 1/50 of the effect of nalorphine as an antagonist.	Contraindicated in patients with head injury, or pathologic brain condition in which clouding of sensorium is undesirable and in children under 12 years of age. Used with caution in pregnant women or women delivering premature infants, respiratory depression (e.g., from other drugs, uremia or severe infection), cyanosis, obstructive respiratory conditions, patients dependent upon narcotics, patients with myocardial infarction who have nausea and vomiting, or patients who are to have biliary surgery. Side effects include nausea, vertigo, dizziness, lightheadedness, vomiting and respiratory depression; occur in about 1% of patients; more rarely constipation, circulatory depression, diaphoresis, urinary retention, alteration in mood, hypertension, sting on injection, headache, dry mouth, flushed skin, altered uterine contractions, dermatitis, paresthesia, dyspnea. For further information see commercial brochure.	30 mg. of drug is said to be as effective as 10 mg. morphine or 75 to 100 mg. of meperidine. Duration of action may be less than morphine. In case of overdosing, use the narcotic antagonist naloxone (Narcan) only. The others are not effective and can increase respiratory depression. Do not mix in syringe with soluble barbiturates as a precipitate will occur. Can be used for those patients taking oral anticoagulant drugs and needing short-term analgesic therapy.

Propoxyphene, N.F. (Darvon) (dextropropoxyphene, Depronal, Levodal, Neo-Mal, Progesic, Proxyphene [C]).	30-60 mg. q. 4-6 h. p.r.n. Oral.	A non-narcotic analgesic used in all mild to moderate pain. Not useful in severe pain.	Similar to codeine. Does not suppress cough. Has little effect on the gastrointestinal tract.	It is apparently nonaddictive and of low toxicity.	Claimed to be devoid of any antipyretic activity. Often combined with other analgesic drugs. The levisomer is claimed to have antitussive effect.
NARCOTIC ANTAGONISTS *Synthetic* or *Semisynthetic.*					
Levallorphan tartrate (Lorfan).	0.3-1.2 mg. Parenteral.	Used to lessen respiratory depression occurring from narcotic drugs.	Like nalorphine.	Like nalorphine.	
Nalorphine hydrochloride, U.S.P. (Nalline, Lethidrone). Synthetic from morphine.	Adult 5-10 mg. Parenteral. Infant, 0.2 mg. Parenteral.	Used as a narcotic antidote and to combat extreme narcosis. It is not used in drug addiction but only in acute poisoning. It is also a powerful emergency respiratory stimulant when cause of depression is the narcotic analogs. Addicts may be detected by rapid appearance of withdrawal symptoms following its administration.	Acts as an antagonist of morphine and similar drugs. Is a powerful respiratory stimulant when cause of depression is the narcotic analogs. Readily absorbed after subcutaneous injection but poorly absorbed from gastrointestinal tract. It is inactivated by the liver.	Large doses cause lethargy, drowsiness, sweating, and dysphoria. In morphine addicts rapid withdrawal symptoms occur.	Is not effective in treating barbiturate poisoning.
Naloxone (Narcan).	0.4 mg. I.V., repeat in 2-3 minutes X 3. If no improvement, probably condition will not respond to this drug.	Used to reverse the respiratory depression induced by natural or synthetic narcotics or by pentazocine.	A pure narcotic antagonist, it does not possess any morphine characteristics, as do other antagonists. Does not produce respiratory depression, psychotomimetic effects or pupillary constriction. In absence of narcotic drugs, exhibits no pharmacologic activity. Will produce withdrawal symptoms in those who are physically dependent upon narcotics. Onset of action given I.V. is about 2 minutes.	Side effects: in rare instances nausea and vomiting have been reported in postoperative patients after receiving higher than recommended doses. Contraindications: Caution. This drug is not effective when respiratory depression is caused by nonnarcotic drugs. Not recommended for use with neonates or during pregnancy except during labor.	

Name, Source, Synonyms, Preparations	Dosage and Administration	Uses	Action and Fate	Side Effects and Contraindications	Remarks
COMPOUNDS USED TO POTENTIATE ANALGESIA					
Synthetic preparations.					
Promethazine hydrochloride, U.S.P. (Ganphen, Phenergan) (Histaritil [C]).	25-50 mg. q. 3-4 hr. p.r.n. I.M. or I.V.	See page 123 for other uses.	Readily absorbed, inactivated by liver and excreted by kidneys.	See page 123.	See under Antihistamines.
Propiomazine hydrochloride, N.F. (Largon).	10-30 mg. q. 3-4 h. p.r.n. I.M. or I.V.	For pre- and postoperative sedation and to potentiate analgesic and hypnotic action in obstetric and surgical patients.	Phenothiazine derivative with antihistamine and sedative properties that enhance the action of analgesic.	Causes irritation if extravasation occurs. Contraindications as for other phenothiazine antihistamines.	Doses of hypnotics should be reduced by one-half and naroctics by one-fourth or one-half.
ANALGESICS–ANTIPYRETICS					
Synthetic phenol derivatives.					
Acetaminophen, N.F. (Anapap, Apamide, Febrolin, Fendon, Nasprin, Nebs, Pyrapap, Sk-Apap, Tempra, Tylenol, Valadol) (APAP, Atasol, Chem-Cetaphen, Dymadon, NAPAP, paracetimid, Paralgin [C]).	0.3-0.6 Gm. p.r.n. Oral or rectal.	Used as an analgesic for relief of headache, myalgia, and arthralgia and to reduce fever.	Similar to acetanilid but less toxic.	Toxicity apparently low. Very little gastric irritation and does not affect prothrombin time. It can be used for patients on anticoagulants and those patients who are allergic to aspirin.	Also prepared in flavored liquid for children.
Acetanilid (Acetylaniline, Antifebrin).	0.2 Gm. q. 4 h. p.r.n. Oral.	Used for the relief of pains such as headache, neuralgia, dysmenorrhea, etc. Also used to reduce fever.	Decreases activity of brain. Relieves various pains and nervous irritability. If fever is present, it will be reduced owing to peripheral vasodilation and perhaps action on hypothalami. Sweating is increased. Readily and almost completely absorbed from gastrointestinal tract. Peak plasma level reached in ½-2 hours. Rapidly diffused throughout tissue. Degraded by liver and excreted by kidneys about 30 minutes later.	Acute: cyanosis, weakness, sweating, weak pulse and respirations, dyspnea, delirium, convulsions. Treatment: lavage, evacuants, central nervous system stimulants. Chronic: weakness, palpitation, anorexia, dizziness, nausea, numbness of extremities. Withdraw drug, substitute barbiturates, aspirin, or codeine if needed. Antianemia treatment is indicated.	Habituation may occur.

Phenacetin, U.S.P., (Acetophenetidin).	0.3 Gm. q. 4 h. p.r.n. Oral.	Used for the relief of pains such as headache, neuralgia, dysmenorrhea, etc. Also used to reduce fever.	Similar to acetanilid. Somewhat less analgesic but less toxic.	Similar to acetanilid but is less toxic. Skin eruptions occasionally occur. Treatment: same as for acetanilid, and symptomatic.	Same as for acetanilid. Has been implicated in some blood dyscrasias and may be harmful to the kidneys on long-term use.
Synthetic pyrazolone derivatives.					
Aminopyrine (Amidofebrin, Amidopyrazoline, Novamidon, Pyradone).	0.3 Gm. q. 4 h. p.r.n. Oral.	Used mainly as an analgesic but is also antipyretic and antispasmodic. Acts slowly, but longer-lasting than antipyrine.	Action similar to acetanilid. The pyrazolones are readily and almost completely absorbed. Peak blood levels in 1-2 hours. Slowly metabolized mainly by the liver and excreted by kidneys. About 2-5% excreted unchanged.	Same as antipyrine but is more apt to cause toxic symptoms. Drug is said to cause granulocytopenia. Treatment: same as antipyrine, and symptomatic.	Habituation may occur. Formerly a common ingredient in many "headache" remedies in combination with other drugs. This is now prohibited by law without a prescription.
Antipyrine, N.F. (Analgesine, Anodynine, Parodyne, Phenylone, Pyrazoline, Sedatine).	0.3 Gm. q. 4 h. p.r.n. Oral.	Used mainly as an antipyretic but has analgesic and antispasmodic action.	Similar to others of this group, but more antipyretic and less analgesic.	Depression, rapid pulse, collapse, cyanosis, diaphoresis, fall in temperature. Convulsions and delirium may occur. Treatment: lavage, evacuants, central nervous system stimulants, artificial respiration.	An ingredient of some analgesic ear drops.
Dipyrone (Dimethone, Diprone, Methapyrone, Novaldin, Pyralgin).	0.3-0.6 Gm. t.i.d.-q.i.d. Oral. 0.5-1 Gm. q. 3 h. p.r.n. Parenteral.	An analgesic, antipyretic, and antirheumatic agent. Used for all types of pain amenable to such a drug.	Similar to others of this group.	Skin rashes, dizziness, chills have been reported. This drug should not be given in large doses for prolonged periods unless leukocyte and differential counts are done frequently.	An aminopyrine derivative, and has been reported to cause agranulocytosis.

Name, Source, Synonyms, Preparations	Dosage and Administration	Uses	Action and Fate	Side Effects and Contraindications	Remarks
SALICYLIC ACID. *Synthetic from willow and poplar.*		Used as an analgesic, antirheumatic, diaphoretic, antiseptic, and cholagogue. Some derivatives have anodyne action and some are anthelminthics.	Tends to raise blood pressure. Most of these drugs given in correct dosage will reduce pain and swelling in arthritis. They do not remove the cause. Exact mode of action is not clearly understood.	Toxic symptoms–severe (relatively uncommon): heart depression, polyuria, impairment of hearing and vision, and skin eruptions. Stop drug and treat symptoms.	Patients should be cautioned against too high a dosage as well as indiscriminate use of these drugs.
Aspirin, U.S.P. (acetylsalicylic acid, A.S.A.) (Acetal, Acetophem, Acetyl-Sal, Ancasol, Cetasal, Ecotrin, Entrophen, Monasalyl, Neopirine, Novo-Phase, Novasen, Rhonal, Supasa, Tolerin [C]).	0.3-0.6 Gm. q. 3-4 h. p.r.n. (not more than 3 Gm. in 24 hours). Oral.	An extremely common analgesic and antirheumatic drug alone and in many combinations.	Readily and almost completely absorbed from gastrointestinal tract. Peak blood levels in 1-2 hours. Widely distributed throughout body with lowest concentration in brain. Aspirin is rapidly hydrolyzed to salicylic acid, mainly in liver. Excreted by the kidneys as salicylates and salicyluric acid. Salicylates cross the placental barrier and have been associated with neonatal bleeding.	Toxic symptoms–severe (relatively uncommon): heart depression, polyuria, impairment of hearing and vision, and skin eruptions. Stop drug and treat symptoms. Aspirin and other salicylates in large doses (6 Gm. or more) daily, may significantly increase prothrombin time and, in lower doses (1-3 Gm.), can cause gastric blood loss and prolonged bleeding time.	
Aluminum aspirin, N.F. (aluminum acetylsalicylate).	0.67 Gm. q. 4 h. p.r.n. Oral.	As above.			
Methyl salicylate (oil of wintergreen).	Dosage varies. Topical.	As an anodyne in lotions or ointments in arthritis.			
Salicylamide, N.F. (Amid-Sal, Liquiprin, Salicim, Salrin) (Chem-Sal [C]).	0.3-2 Gm. q. 3-4 h. p.r.n. (not more than 3 Gm. in 24 hours). Oral.	Uses are similar to those of aspirin.			
Salicylic acid, U.S.P. (psoriacide [C]).	Dosage varies. Topical.	As an anodyne in lotions or ointments in arthritis. Also is keratolytic.			
Sodium salicylate, U.S.P.	0.3-1 Gm. q. 4 h. Oral. 6-8 Gm. Rectal.	Mainly used as an antirheumatic.			
Ammonium salicylate (Armyl).	1 Gm. Oral.	Antirheumatic.			
Calcium acetylsalicylic carbamide (Calurin).	0.3 Gm. Oral.	Antirheumatic.			
Choline salicylate (Actasal, Arthropan)	0.87 Gm. Oral.	Antirheumatic.			
Ethylsalicylate (Sal-Ethyl).	0.3-0.6 Gm. Oral.	Antirheumatic.			
Gentisate sodium (Gentasol).	0.5 Gm. Oral.	Antirheumatic.			
Salicylsalicylic acid (Sulysal).	0.3 Gm. Oral.	Antirheumatic.			

ANALGESICS—ANTIRHEUMATICS. See also miscellaneous analgesics, especially the salicylates.					
CINCHOPHEN. *Synthetic.* Neocinchophen (Novatophan).	0.3 Gm. t.i.d. Oral.	Used in the treatment of gout, arthritis, and similar conditions. Acts as an analgesic, antipyretic, and cholagogue.	Analgesic, antipyretic, and uricosuric. Causes a marked increase in quantity of uric acid secreted by kidneys. Adequately absorbed from gastrointestinal tract. Widely distributed mainly in the extracellular fluid. Almost completely metabolized. Only about 2% excreted unchanged by the kidneys.	Anorexia, nausea, vomiting, skin eruptions; liver damage may occur. Stop drug, force fluid (oral and I.V.) and treat symptoms.	Neocinchophen is less effective and also less toxic than cinchophen.
COLCHICUM. *Meadow saffron, Colchicine.* Colchicine, U.S.P. (Novocolchine [C]). Colchicum glucoside colchicoside. Colchicum seed, fluid extract. Colchicum seed, tincture.	 0.5-0.6 mg. Oral. 10-20 mg. I.V. 0.2 ml. Oral. 2.0 ml. Oral.	Used in the treatment of gout, arthritis, and similar conditions. Action is mainly analgesic.	Action not well understood. It relieves the pain of gouty arthritis, but does not reduce the level of uric acid. It is thought, however, to decrease lactic acid production by leukocytes and thereby decrease depositing of urate crystal and subsequent inflammatory response. It also arrests cell division by preventing spindle formation in metaphase in numerous plant and animal cells. Readily absorbed. Transported to liver, excreted in bile and some is reabsorbed. Concentrated in kidneys, liver, spleen, and intestines. Some is deacetylated by the liver. In normal persons 28% of a given dose is excreted as colchicine and 8% as metabolites within 48 hours. In patients with gout the percentages are 3.5 and 12. Reason for this difference is not known.	Nausea, vomiting, diarrhea, abdominal pain, diaphoresis, rapid thready pulse, slow shallow respirations. Treatment: lavage or emetics, external heat, stimulants, and symptomatically. Prolonged administration may cause bone marrow depression with agranulocytosis, thrombocytopenia, and/or aplastic anemia.	Considered very toxic; watch carefully. Times and dosage individually adjusted.

Name, Source, Synonyms, Preparations	Dosage and Administration	Uses	Action and Fate	Side Effects and Contraindications	Remarks
ANALGESICS–ANTIRHEUMATICS (Continued)					
SYNTHETIC PREPARATIONS					
Oxyphenbutazone, N.F. (Oxalid, Tandearil).	100 mg. Oral. Usually given 300-600 mg./day in divided doses with reduction to minimum required for maintenance.	Uses and action similar to those of phenylbutazone.	Similar to phenylbutazone.	Similar to phenylbutazone. Same interactions as under phenylbutazone.	Similar to phenylbutazone.
Phenylbutazone, N.F. (Azolid, Butazolidin) (Anevral, Butagesic, Eributazone, Intrabutazone, Malgesic, Nadozone, Phenbutazol [C]).	0.1-0.2 Gm. Usually t.i.d. Individually adjusted. Give with meals or glass of milk. Oral.	Used in the treatment of gout, arthritis, and similar conditions.	Acts as analgesic, antipyretic, anti-inflammatory agent. In gout, uric acid is reduced in blood. Renal excretion of sodium and chloride occurs. Rapid and complete absorption. Slowly metabolized by the liver, some to oxyphenbutazone. Slowly excreted in the urine.	Gastrointestinal irritation, edema, rash, anemia. Has caused agranulocytosis. Reduce or stop drug and treat symptoms. Contraindicated in edema, renal, cardiac, or hepatic damage; also in marked hypertension or in patient who has peptic ulcers. This drug can potentiate the effect of the warfarin type anticoagulants. When used in patients taking these drugs, care should be taken to adjust the dose of the anticoagulant. Phenylbutazone enhances the hypoglycemic effects of acetohexamide, and the dose of acetohexamide should be adjusted downward. The other sulfonureas may give the same reaction and should be closely watched. Phenylbutazone may diminish the effects of the steroids by enzyme induction. This drug can cross the placental barrier and has been implicated in neonatal goiter.	Low sodium diet is often recommended. Sodium free antacid aids in preventing gastric irritation. Use with caution during pregnancy, especially in the 1st trimester, weighing possible risks against benefits.

Sulfinpyrazone (Anturane) (sulphinpyrazone, Anturan [C]).	100 mg. b.i.d. or q.i.d. Individually adjusted. Administer with food or milk in case of gastrointestinal disturbance. Oral.	For treatment of chronic gout, especially with joint involvement.	Interferes with the tubular transport of uric acid and thereby increases the excretion of uric acid. Not useful in relieving an acute attack of gout. Readily absorbed. Highly bound to plasma proteins. Most excreted unchanged by the kidneys.	May include upper gastrointestinal disturbance and skin rash. Patient's blood picture should be watched. Citrates and salicylates are contraindicated since they antagonize its ability to increase renal excretion of uric acid, and they can reduce renal clearance of nitrofurantoin and lead to toxic blood levels while decreasing the effectiveness of the anti-infective agent in urinary tract infections. Caution: do not give to patients with peptic ulcers. Interactions same as for phenylbutazone.	Insure adequate fluid intake and alkaline urine to prevent urolithiasis or renal colic.
OTHER SYNTHETIC PREPARATIONS Indomethacin, N.F. (Indocin) (Indocid [C]).	25 mg. two or three times a day. If necessary, dose may be increased to 200 mg. in divided doses daily. Larger doses than this probably will not be more effective. Oral.	Antirheumatic drug with anti-inflammatory, analgesic, and antipyretic actions. Used to treat rheumatoid arthritis, rheumatoid spondylitis, degenerative joint disease of the hip (osteoarthritis), and gout.	Anti-inflammatory agent unlike the corticosteroids, as it has no effect on pituitary or adrenal function. Well absorbed orally. Peak plasma levels in about 2 hours. Eliminated by kidneys as the glucuronide.	May mask the signs and symptoms of peptic ulcer, or cause peptic ulceration or irritation of the gastrointestinal tract. Should not be given to patients with active peptic ulcer, gastritis, or ulcerative colitis for this reason. Side effects include dizziness and lightheadedness; feeling of detachment; gastrointestinal disturbances such as nausea, vomiting, epigastric distress, abdominal pain, and diarrhea. Aspirin and other salicylates decrease and delay the gastrointestinal absorption of indomethacin. When indomethacin is given concurrently with probenecid, it	Renal function should be checked in individuals receiving long-term therapy.

Name, Source, Synonyms, Preparations	Dosage and Administration	Uses	Action and Fate	Side Effects and Contraindications	Remarks
ANALGESICS–ANTIRHEUMATICS (Continued)					
Indomethacin (Continued)				can cause a rise in serum level, since excretion is blocked. Dose of indomethacin should be adjusted. Indomethacin may potentiate the effects of warfarin-type anticoagulants. A few cases of psychic disturbances, blurred vision, stomatitis, pruritus, urticaria, angioneurotic edema, skin rashes, and edema have been reported. Manufacturer does not recommend use in pediatric age groups until indications for use and dosage have been established for these groups.	
SEDATIVES–HYPNOTICS. See also general anesthetics. *Synthetic.*					
Acetylcarbromal (Acetyl adalin, Abasin, Sedamyl).	0.25 Gm. 1 or 2 tablets t.i.d. Oral.	Used mainly for daytime sedation.	Relieves tension and anxiety with little effect on perception and alertness.	Does not have undesirable side effects. Toxicity rare in therapeutic dosage.	
Bromisovalum (Bromural).	0.3 Gm. Three to four times daily as sedative. Oral. 0.6 Gm. h.s. as hypnotic. Oral.	Used as a sedative-hypnotic.	A gentle quick-acting hypnotic for persons who are restless or excited. Action lasts only 3 to 4 hours.	On long-term use can cause bromide toxicity.	
Carbromal (Adalin).	0.3 Gm. 1 or 2 tablets h.s.	Used as a sedative-hypnotic.	Fate of these 3 drugs is similar to that of bromide, which they liberate.	Carbromal can decrease the duration of activity of dexamethasone by liver enzyme induction.	

BARBITURATES. Salts and derivatives of barbituric acid. *Long Duration–Slow Action.*		Used for sedation, hypnosis, suppression of convulsions, partial and complete anesthesia, amnesia and analgesia (especially in obstetrics); for analgesia in migraine headaches, neuritis, and neuralgia, and to reduce peristalsis. These drugs have a wide and expanding field of effectiveness. Barbiturates are often added to analgesic drugs to produce sedation as well as relief of pain. Various combinations with amphetamine derivatives have been used for their euphoric effect.	Depression of the central nervous system, beginning usually with the diencephalon; certain preparations affect the motor centers mainly. Therapeutic doses have little effect on the visceral organs, but heavy doses cause respiratory and cardiac depression. Most of the barbiturates tend to lower blood pressure. Barbiturates are well absorbed and are rapidly distributed to all tissues and fluids and they cross the placenta. After initial distribution, they are concentrated in certain tissues, dependent upon which compound is used and the time elapsed after administration. Three factors affecting distribution and fate are lipid solubility, protein binding and extent of ionization. The ultra short acting have the greatest lipid solubility, then progressively less from short to long acting compounds. The barbiturates are redistributed in the body. The oxybarbiturates are metabolically degraded by the enzymes of the liver. The thiobarbiturates are degraded mainly by the liver and to a small degree by the enzymes in the kidneys and brain. They are excreted by the kidneys.	Acute mental confusion, drowsiness, fall in blood pressure, coma, rapid pulse, moist skin, pulmonary edema, collapse. Treatment: lavage, oxygen, cardiac stimulants, intravenous glucose. Chronic: habituation is easily acquired. Anorexia, headache, weakness, psychoses, visual disturbances, anemia, renal damage, amnesia. Stop drug and treat symptoms. The barbiturates, especially the short acting ones such as pentobarbital and secobarbital, may cause dependency. If this occurs, withdrawal may have serious effects. The barbiturates significantly reduce the effectiveness of the oral anticoagulants. Phenobarbital and possibly other barbiturates will significantly reduce the effectiveness of griseofulvin. The monoamine oxidase inhibitors and the sulfonylureas enhance the central nervous system effects of the barbiturates. Antacids may decrease the absorption of the barbiturates by raising the pH of the gastric contents and by reducing their solubility. The barbiturates can reduce or shorten the effect of cortisone derivatives by enzyme induction.	Act slowly (30-60 minutes) but effects are of relatively long duration (6-8 hours). Tablet preparations are given orally. Ampule preparations (sodium salts) may be administered parenterally. Dosage given is for one dose. Repeated dosage is individually adjusted. The use of barbiturates with alcohol should be avoided since these drugs reinforce each other with serious, even fatal, results.
Barbital (Veronal, Barbitone)	0.3 Gm. Oral.				
Barbital sodium (Medinal) (barbitone sodium [C]).	0.3 Gm. Oral.				
Mephobarbital, N.F. (Mebaral) (methylphenobarbital [C]).	30-200 mg. Oral. 400-600 mg. daily in divided doses. Oral.	Used as a sedative in neuroses and in treating epilepsy.			
Metharbital (Gemonil)	100 mg. Oral.				
Phenobarbital, U.S.P. (Barbipil, Barbita, Eskabarb, Lixophen, Luminal) (phenobarbitone, Epilol, Epsylone, Fenosed, Gardenal, Hypnotone, Novo-Pheno, Novo-Rectal Phenocaps, PEBA, Phen Bar, Sedabar, Sedlyn [C]).	15-100 mg. Oral.	Relatively nontoxic. May be given over a long period of time. Widely used for many purposes.			
Phenobarbital, elixir, U.S.P., (Barbilixis [C]).	5 ml. (5 ml. contains 20 mg.) Oral.				
Phenobarbital sodium, U.S.P. (Luminal Sodium).	15-100 mg. Oral or parenteral.				
Intermediate					
Amobarbital, U.S.P. (Amospan, Amytal) (amylbarbitone, Isonal [C]).	20-40 mg. Oral.	Used as hypnotic or sedative.			Action and duration of moderate effect.
Amobarbital sodium, U.S.P. (Amytal sodium) (amylbarbitone sodium, Novomobarb, Intrased sodium [C]).	60-100 mg. Oral. 250-500 mg. Parenteral.				

DRUGS AFFECTING THE CENTRAL NERVOUS SYSTEM (Continued)

DEPRESSANTS *(Continued)*

Name, Source, Synonyms, Preparations	Dosage and Administration	Uses	Action and Fate	Side Effects and Contraindications	Remarks
BARBITURATES (Continued)				Concurrent use of the antihistamines with the barbiturates can give additive central nervous system depression. They can increase the orthostatic hypotension which occurs with the phenothiazines. The barbiturates can cross the placental barrier and can depress neonatal respiration.	
Aprobarbital, N.F. (Alurate).	60 mg. Oral.	As a hypnotic.			
Aprobarbital sodium (Alurate sodium).	10 mg. Oral.	As a sedative.			
Butabarbital sodium (Bubartal, Butak, Butezem, Butisol, Insolat, Mebutal) (Buta-Barb, Interbarb, Neo-Barb, Neurosidine [C]).	15-60 mg. Oral. 45-100 mg. Oral.	As a sedative. As a hypnotic.			
Butethal (Neonal) (butabarbital, butabarbitone, Soneryl [C]).	50-100 mg. Oral.	Often given in small doses over several hours for sedation.			
Cyclopentenyl barbituric acid (Cyclopal, Cyclopen).	50-100 mg. Oral.	As a quick-acting sedative.			
Diallylbarbituric acid (Allobarbital, Allobarbitone, Diadol) (allobarbitone, Analgyl [C]).	100-300 mg. Oral.	Sedative effects last 18-24 hours.			
Probarbital calcium (Ipral calcium).	100-200 mg. Oral.	Sedative effects often last into second night.			
Short Acting					
Cyclobarbital calcium (Cyclobarbitone, Phanodorn).	200 mg. Oral.	Mainly used for hypnosis.			Short acting. Acts quite rapidly, but effects not prolonged.
Hexethal sodium (Ortal).	200-400 mg. Oral.	As above.		Absolute contraindications: latent or manifest porphyria or a familial history of intermittent porphyria. Relative contraindication: impaired hepatic or renal function.	
Hexobarbital sodium (Sombucaps).	250-500 mg. Oral. p.r.n. 3-6 ml. of a 10% solution I.V.	Pre- and postanesthesia sedation, hypnosis. For induction or short anesthesia.			
Pentobarbital sodium, U.S.P. (Nembutal, Penta) (pentobarbitone sodium, Butylova, Hypnotol, Hypnol, Ibalal, Novopentobarb, Pentanca, Pentogen, Somnotol [C]).	100 mg. 1 or 2 h.s. Oral, rectal or parenteral.	As above.			
Secobarbital sodium, U.S.P. (Evronal, Seconal, Synate) (quinalbarbitone, Secolone, Hyptrol, Secogen, Secobal, Notrium, Seotal, Secotabs [C]).	50-100 mg. Oral, rectal or parenteral.	As above.			
Talbutal (Lotusate).	30-120 mg. Oral.	As above.			
Vinbarbital sodium, N.F.	100-200 mg. Oral or parenteral.	As above.			

Very Short Acting					
Methitural sodium (Neraval).	3-6 ml. I.V.	Used for induction anesthesia and for short anesthesia.		Respiratory depression and laryngospasm may occur. May cause hypotension and tachycardia. There are many contraindications. See manufacturer's pamphlets for details.	Very short acting: quick acting but effects of short duration. Dose is repeated as is deemed advisable. All dosages subject to individual patient's reaction.
Methohexital sodium (Brevital) (methohexitone, Brietal [C]).	5-12 ml. of a 1% solution. I.V.	As above.			
Thiamylal sodium, N.F. (Surital).	3-6 ml. of a 2.5% solution. I.V.	As above.			
Thiopental sodium, U.S.P. (Pentothal sodium).	2.3-3 ml. I.V.	As above.			
BROMIDES. *Synthetic* from bromine.		Used for sedation and hypnosis; as an antiemetic, aphrodisiac, and anticonvulsant; in some cases in pyelography.	Depress the central nervous system, including the spinal cord, but have little or no effect on the medullary centers. Produce drowsiness, some loss of muscle coordination and reflexes, decreased reception of sensory stimuli. Do not markedly affect cardiac, respiratory, or gastrointestinal activity. Hypnotic action is indirect, owing to lessened sensations and mental activity. Readily absorbed and widely distributed in extracellular fluid. The distribution of the bromide ion is dependent upon the concentration of the chloride ion as they are somewhat interchangeable. Excreted by the kidneys.	Acute: sweet odor to breath, coated tongue, slurred speech, ataxia, dilated pupils, tachycardia, and sometimes acute bromoderma. Stop drug, force fluids (I.V. if necessary), give sodium chloride. Chronic: mental depression, foul breath, coated tongue, slow pulse, slow speech, skin lesions, and ataxia. Stop drug, give sodium chloride and vitamin B (niacinamide). Bromides cross the placental barrier and have caused neonatal skin eruptions.	Individual tolerance to bromides varies greatly.
Ammonium bromide, N.F.	1 Gm. t.i.d. Oral.				
Bromide 5 elixir.	4 ml. h.s. Also available as tablets. Oral.				Bromide 5 contains ammonium, sodium, calcium, lithium, potassium bromide.
Bromide 3 elixir.	4 ml. As above. Oral.				Bromide 3 contains ammonium, sodium, potassium bromide.
Calcium bromide.	1 Gm. t.i.d. Oral.				For hypnosis, bromide is given in one dose h.s. For sedation and as an anticonvulsant, usually t.i.d. or q.i.d.
Lithium bromide.	1 Gm. t.i.d. Oral.				
Potassium bromide.	1 Gm. t.i.d. Oral.				
Sodium bromide.	0.3-1 Gm. t.i.d. Oral.				
Sodium bromide elixir, N.F.	4 ml. h.s. Oral.				
Syrup of bromides.	4 ml. h.s. Oral.				

Name, Source, Synonyms, Preparations	Dosage and Administration	Uses	Action and Fate	Side Effects and Contraindications	Remarks
SEDATIVES (Continued)					
CHLORAL HYDRATE. *Synthetic.* Chloral hydrate, U.S.P. (Aquachloral, Felsules, Hydral, Lycorol, Noctec, Rectules, Somnos) (Cloralixir, Cloratol, Chloralvan, Novochlorhydrate [C]).	0.25-0.6 Gm. h.s. Available as liquid and capsules. Oral or rectal.	Used as sedative, hypnotic, analgesic, and antispasmodic. Chloral derivatives are used locally as antipruritics.	Depresses central nervous system and decreases the reception of sensory stimuli. Therapeutic doses produce little effect on cardiovascular or respiratory action. Good absorption and distribution. Degraded by the liver mainly to trichloroethanol and other products. Degraded products excreted by the kidneys and in bile.	Coma, muscle relaxation, cold extremities, low blood pressure, convulsions, delirium. Treatment: lavage, oxygen, artificial respiration, central nervous system stimulants. When given to patients on oral anticoagulants, chloral hydrate can cause transient potentiation of hypoprothrombinemia. Concurrent ingestion of chloral hydrate and alcohol results in greater central nervous system depression than when either is taken alone.	Usually given one dose, h.s., but may be given in smaller dose t.i.d. May be habit forming. Do not give with alcohol. Chloral hydrate can cross the placental barrier and in large doses can cause death of the fetus.
Chloral betaine, N.F. (Beta Chlor).	0.44-0.87 Gm. 1 or 2 tablets h.s. (Equals 0.25-0.5 Gm. chloral hydrate). Oral.	Sedative.	Same as choral hydrate but said to cause less gastric distress.		
Chlorobutanol, U.S.P. (Chloretone).	0.6 Gm. Oral.	Can be given subcutaneously; preserves injectables. Mild local anesthetic (dentistry).			
Petrichloral (Periclor).	0.3-0.6 Gm. h.s. Oral.				
Triclofos sodium (Triclos).	1500 mg. h.s. Oral.	Used to induce sleep.	Triclofos is dephosphorylated in the gut, mainly yielding trichlorethanol, which is the same active metabolite of chloral hydrate. Peak serum levels reached in one hour. Has a half-life in the body of about 11 hours.	Side effects: headache, "hang-over," drowsiness, gastrointestinal disturbances (gas, flatulence, nausea, vomiting, bad taste), staggering gait, ataxia, ketonuria, relative eosinophilia, urticaria, lightheadedness, vertigo, nightmares, malaise, and reduction in total white blood cell count. Contraindications: in renal or hepatic impairment and in patients known to be sensitive to chloral hydrate. Triclofos will increase the effects of other central	Caution. May be habit forming. Safety for use during pregnancy and lactation has not been established. Should be used with caution in patients with cardiac arrhythmias or any severe cardiac disease.

				nervous system depressants such as alcohol and the tranquilizers.	
OTHER SYNTHETIC PREPARATIONS. Ectylurea (Levanil, Nostyn).	0.15-0.3 Gm. t.i.d. Oral.	As a sedative in mild anxiety-tension states.	Produces mild depression of central nervous system. Hypnosis occurs only with very high doses.	Skin rashes, cholestatic jaundice, dizziness, nausea, vomiting, and headache.	Is said to be of little value in overexcited or overagitated patients.
Ethchlorvynol, N.F. (Placidyl).	0.5-0.75 Gm. Hypnotic h.s.; sedative 0.1-0.5 Gm. two to three times daily. Oral.	A nonbarbiturate sedative hypnotic.	Central nervous system depressant producing sedation and hypnosis if pain is not a factor. Is not analgesic. Acts quickly, within 15-30 minutes. Effects last 5-6 hours. Readily absorbed orally, but exact fate not known.	Low toxicity, though it may cause drowsiness, fatigue, and some "hang-over." Overdose gives symptoms similar to those of barbiturates. Not recommended during the 1st and 2nd trimesters of pregnancy. Can reduce the effectiveness of the oral anticoagulants.	
Ethinamate, N.F. (Valmid)	0.5-2 Gm. h.s. Oral.	A mild sedative hypnotic which is effective when deep hypnosis is not needed.	Central nervous system depression with mild sedation and light hypnosis. Acts quickly, within 15-30 minutes. Lasts 4-5 hours. Good absorption. Believed to be inactivated by the liver and excreted in the urine.	Safe use during pregnancy has not been established. Rare cases of thrombocytopenia, purpura and oral idiosyncrasies with fever have been reported. Mild gastrointestinal disturbances and skin rashes have occurred. Concurrent use of alcohol, especially in overdosage, can increase potential hazards.	Habituation, addiction, and tolerance have been reported.

Name, Source, Synonyms, Preparations	Dosage and Administration	Uses	Action and Fate	Side Effects and Contraindications	Remarks
SEDATIVES (Continued)					
Flurazepam (Dalmane)	15-30 mg. h.s. Oral.	Used for insomnia.	Exact mode of action is not known. However, animal studies indicate it reduces the pressor response to electrical stimulation of the hypothalamus and increases the arousal threshold to stimulation of the amygdala and the hypothalamus. It is rapidly absorbed from the gastrointestinal tract and rapidly metabolized.	Side effects most commonly seen include: dizziness, drowsiness, lightheadedness, staggering, ataxia and falling. These latter have occurred mostly in elderly or debilitated patients. For other side effects, toxicity, etc., see brochure. Contraindications: sensitivity to the drug. This drug has similar interactions to chlordiazepoxide (page 110). This drug does not appear to interact with the oral anticoagulants.	Use during pregnancy or for persons under 12 years of age is not recommended, as studies with these groups have not been completed.
Glutethimide, N.F. (Doriden) (Somide [C]).	0.25 Gm. t.i.d. p.c. as a sedative. Oral. 0.5-1 Gm. h.s. For preoperative sedation or hypnosis. Oral.	Used for sedation and hypnosis, as are the barbiturates.	Central nervous system depression producing sedation or hypnosis according to dosage. Poor and irregular oral absorption. Well distributed throughout body. Degraded by the liver, excreted in bile. Some reabsorbed. Some excreted by the kidneys.	Rare in therapeutic doses, but nausea and skin rashes have occurred. Stop drug; use evacuants, if indicated, and treat symptoms. Glutethimide interacts with the oral anticoagulants to decrease their effectiveness.	
Methaqualone (Quaalude, Parest) (Hyptor, Mequelon, Pexaqualone, Rouqualone, Somnofax, Tiqualoine, Tualone [C]).	75 mg. p.c. and h.s. 150-400 mg. h.s.	For sedation and sleep.	Same as others of this group.	Used with caution in impaired hepatic function and the anxiety states, especially if there is evidence of impending depression or when suicidal tendencies exist.	
Methylparafynol (Dormison, Somnesin) (methylpentynol, Oblivan [C]).	0.25-0.5 Gm. h.s. Oral.	Used for sedation and hypnosis in the same situations as the barbiturates, but does not contain any barbituric acid.	Produces hypnosis by action thought to be similar to that of amylene hydrate. Does not cause respiratory depression or have antispasmodic action.	Toxicity low. Probably due to rapid metabolism of the drug, but hallucinations and gastrointestinal disburbances have occurred.	

Methyprylon, N.F. (Noludar).	50-100 mg. Three to four times daily for sedation. Oral. 200-400 mg. h.s. for hypnosis. Oral.	Produces good sedation and hypnosis.	Action similar to that of the barbiturates but it is unrelated chemically. Produces less respiratory depression.	Rare; occasional vertigo, nausea, and vomiting occur.	
PARALDEHYDE. *Synthetic.* Ethane derivative. Paraldehyde, U.S.P. (Paral).	4 ml. Oral. 32 ml. Rectal. 4 ml. I.M. (maximum dose by injection should not exceed 0.2 ml./kg.) 1 ml. I.V.	Used for sedation, hypnosis, and as an anticonvulsant. It has antiseptic properties. Mainly used in status epilepticus, delirium tremens, and tetanus.	Depresses central nervous system, but not the medullary centers (in therapeutic dosage). Produces sleep in 10-15 minutes which lasts 6-8 hours. It is not an analgesic. Rapid absorption from gastrointestinal tract or parenteral site. Some excreted unchanged by lungs. Remainder metabolized, probably by liver. End products believed to be carbon dioxide and water.	Nausea, headache, dizziness, and unconsciousness may occur. Fatalities are rare. Treatment: lavage, external heat, central nervous system stimulants. Contraindicated in lung congestion. Paraldehyde crosses the placental barrier and, in large doses, can depress neonatal respiration.	Give ice cold or with cold drink. May be habit forming. Gives bad odor to breath.
ANTISPASMODICS–ANTI-CONVULSANTS *Synthetic Hydantoin Derivatives*	Interactions: Diphenylhydantoin can diminish the effect of dexamethasone and may impair therapeutic response. When it is given to patients who are genetically slow inactivators of isoniazid, diphenylhydantoin toxicity can occur. Methylphenidate may raise the sensitivity levels of diphenylhydantoin. It is not common, but if ataxia appears, the dose of diphenylhydantoin should be lowered. Phenobarbital can affect the blood levels of diphenylhydantoin in any of three ways–increase, decrease or cause no change. Probably this is not clinically significant with the usual dosage used for anticonvulsive therapy. Diphenylhydantoin may be expected to cause some elevation in glucose tolerance, especially in the older age groups owing to suppression of endogenous insulin secretion. Diphenylhydantoin can potentiate the anticoagulant effects, probably because of displacement of the anticoagulant from protein binding sites in the plasma. The possibility that all hydantoin derivatives can react as does diphenylhydantoin should be considered.				
Diphenylhydantoin, N.F. (Dantoin, Dilantin, Diphenlyn) (phenyltoin, Divulsan, Novodiphenyl, Orlan [C]). Diphenylhydantoin sodium, U.S.P. (Denyl sodium, Dilantin sodium, Diphentoin, Diphenylan sodium, Kessodanten) (See above [C]).	30-100 mg. Up to four times daily. Oral. 30-100 mg. Dosage regulated to suit patient. Available in flavored tablets and suspension for children. Oral, I.M. or I.V.	Used mainly as an anticonvulsant in epilepsy. Its action is highly selective, affecting only motor centers and not the remainder of the cerebral cortex.	Action is through selective depression of motor center in brain. Has little or no sedative or hypnotic action. Readily but slowly absorbed. The sodium salts are rapidly absorbed, widely distributed, slowly detoxified by the liver, and excreted in the urine.	Tremors, ataxia, blurring of vision, loss of taste, insomnia, irritability, gastric irritation, gingivitis, and hyperplasia of the gingiva.	Safe use of the antispasmodic anticonvulsant drugs during pregnancy has not been established. When tolerated, the total daily dose may be given at one time.

Name, Source, Synonyms, Preparations	Dosage and Administration	Uses	Action and Fate	Side Effects and Contraindications	Remarks
ANTISPASMODICS (Continued)					
Mephenytoin (Mesantoin) (methoin [C]).	0.2-0.6 Gm. Dosage regulated to suit patient. Oral.	Used mainly as an anticonvulsant in grand mal epilepsy and in psychomotor equivalent. Also used in chorea.	Similar to diphenylhydantoin. Somewhat less potent and more sedative than diphenylhydantoin.	Rare, but may cause morbilliform rash and pruritus. Stop drug and treat symptoms. Some patients develop tolerance or blood damage.	
OTHER SYNTHETIC ANTICONVULSANTS					
Ethosuximide (Zarontin).	0.25-1 Gm. Dosage individually adjusted. Oral.	For treatment of petit mal epilepsy.	Similar to diphenylhydantoin, but exact mechanism is not known.	Similar to other drugs of this type.	
Ethotoin (Peganone).	0.5-3 Gm. Dosage individually adjusted. Oral.	Similar to hydantoin. Used alone or with other drugs to treat grand mal epilepsy.	Same as above.	Toxicity is low but is similar to that of diphenylhydantoin.	Somewhat slower acting, but fewer side effects than with other similar drugs.
Metharbital, N.F. (Gemonil).	100 mg. Up to t.i.d. Oral.	Used in the treatment of all types of epilepsy.	Similar to phenobarbital in action, fate and distribution.	Similar to phenobarbital. See phenobarbital for interactions.	Use during pregnancy can cause a reduction of vitamin K-dependent clotting factors in the infant. It has been suggested that vitamin K be given prophylactically to such infants at birth.
Methsuximide, N.F. (Celontin) (mesuximide [C]).	0.15-0.3 Gm. Dosage individually adjusted. Oral.	Used for petit mal and psychomotor attacks.	Similar to diphenylhydantoin.	Rare in therapeutic dosage.	
Paramethadione, U.S.P. (Paradione).	0.3-0.9 Gm. Dosage regulated to suit patient. Oral.	Used mainly as an anticonvulsant in petit mal, myoclonic, and akinetic epilepsy. It is also used with other drugs in grand mal epilepsy, and as a sedative.	Depresses the cerebral cortex, including the motor centers. Acts as an anticonvulsant; gives some analgesia. Exact action is not clearly understood.	Mistiness of vision, skin rash, gastric disturbances. Aplastic anemia has been reported after its use. Much less toxic than trimethadione. Contraindicated in severe renal or hepatic disorders.	
Phenacemide (Phenurone) (phenacetylcarbamide [C]).	0.5 Gm. Dosage individually adjusted. Oral.	Used mainly as an anticonvulsant in petit mal, myoclonic, and akinetic epilepsy. It is also used to treat grand mal epilepsy and as a sedative.	Exact mechanism is not known, but it is thought to act similarly to the hydantoins, and is effective against psychic and psychomotor types of epilepsy. Well absorbed orally, slowly changed by liver. Little if any excreted unchanged.	Personality changes, signs of hepatic disorder, depression of blood count, and drug rash may occur. Stop drug and treat symptoms.	Used only when other anticonvulsants are ineffective.

Phensuximide, N.F. (Milontin).	250-500 mg. Dosage individually adjusted. Oral.	Used to treat petit mal epilepsy.	Similar to diphenylhydantoin.	Drowsiness, nausea, vertigo occur. Adjust dosage.	
Primidone, U.S.P. (Mysoline).	0.05-0.25 Gm. Dosage individually adjusted. Oral.	Used mainly in grand mal epilepsy and psychomotor equivalent.	Pyrimidine derivative similar to phenobarbital. Absorbed from gastrointestinal tract. Exact fate unknown, but it is thought that both liver and kidneys act to metabolize it.	Toxicity may cause nausea, vomiting, drowsiness, headache, ataxia, lethargy, and malaise. Adjustment of dosage usually suffices. Emotional disturbances, skin rash, and megaloblastic anemia have been reported infrequently.	Blood picture should be checked with prolonged use.
Trimethadione, U.S.P. (Tridione) (troxidone, Trimedone [C]).	0.1-0.3 Gm. Dosage regulated to suit patient. Oral.	Used mainly as an anticonvulsant in petit mal, myoclonic, and akinetic epilepsy. It is also used with other drugs in grand mal epilepsy, and as a sedative.	Similar to paramethadione. Readily absorbed, widely distributed. Changed mainly by liver, but other tissues may aid in its degradation.	Mistiness of vision, skin rash, gastric disturbances. Aplastic anemia has been reported after its use. Stop drug and treat symptoms.	
ANTISPASMODICS–SKELETAL MUSCLE RELAXANTS					
SYNTHETIC PREPARATIONS					
Carisoprodol (Rela, Soma) (isomeprobamate [C]).	350 mg. Usually given q.i.d. Oral.	Muscle relaxant and analgesic for back pain, sprains, and traumatic injuries.	Similar to meprobamate but said to have a greater skeletal muscle relaxant effect. Carisprodol is metabolized by the liver and excreted by the kidneys.	May cause drowsiness and other central nervous system effects or skin rashes of the allergic-reaction type. See meprobamate for interactions.	
Chlormezanone (Chlormethazanone, Trancopal).	100-200 mg. Usually given q.i.d. Oral.	Treatment of mild anxiety and tension states.	Exact mechanism is not known.	May cause drug rash, dizziness, flushing, nausea, weakness, anorexia, or voiding difficulties.	
Chlorphenesin carbamate (Maolate).	400 mg. q.i.d. to 800 mg. t.i.d. Oral.	As an adjunct in short-term therapy of inflammatory and traumatic conditions of skeletal muscles when relief of discomfort is desired.	Said to have selective internuncial blocking action. It antagonizes the convulsions produced by strychnine or electroshock, but not those produced by pentylenetetrazol.	Drowsiness, dizziness, nausea, insomnia, increased nervousness and headache. If skin rash or other signs of sensitivity occur the drug should be stopped. Chlorphenesin is not recommended for patients with hepatic dysfunction.	Safety for use during pregnancy and lactation or for children has not been established. Patients should be cautioned about driving a motor vehicle or using dangerous mechanical apparatus.

Name, Source, Synonyms, Preparations	Dosage and Administration	Uses	Action and Fate	Side Effects and Contraindications	Remarks
ANTISPASMODICS (Continued)					
Chlorzoxazone (Paraflex).	250 mg. Usually given three to four times daily. Oral.	Uses as for carisoprodol.	Similar to mephenesin in ability to interrupt nervous impulses in polysynaptic pathways of spinal cord.	Anorexia, headache, weakness, drowsiness, and skin rash. Impaired liver function and jaundice have been reported.	
Mephenesin (Daserol, Myanesin, Romeph, Tolsil) (Tolserol [C]).	0.25-1 Gm. Individually adjusted. Oral.	Used to relax muscles in conditions such as parkinsonism, hemiplegia, spastic paralysis, choreoathetosis, choreiform types of cerebral diplegia. Also used in various conditions in which tension is a problem.	Depresses the basal ganglia, brainstem, and synaptic connections in the spinal cord. Some sedation also occurs. Good absorption and distribution by all routes. Higher concentration found in brain than in plasma. Metabolic degradation occurs in liver, products of which are excreted in urine.	Rare in therapeutic dosage. Treatment: none usually required. Lassitude occasionally occurs, and leukopenia has been reported but rarely.	
Meprobamate, N.F. (Equanil, Meprospan, Meprotabs, Miltown, Vio-Bamate) (Gene-Bamata, LanDel, Meditran, Mep-E, Meprox-400, Novomepro, Neo-Tran, Proboson, Quietal, Tranquate, Tranquiline, Tranquinal, Trelmar, Wescomep [C]).	400 mg. t.i.d. or q.i.d. Oral and I.M.	Used in treatment of neuroses and as a muscle relaxant. Especially valuable in emotional disturbances. Used as a tranquilizer alone and in various combinations. The only indication for intramuscular meprobamate is in tetanus.	Acts as a skeletal muscle relaxant and ataractic. It is said to block interneural synaptic passage of impulse and to reduce sensitivity of the thalami. Good oral absórption and uniform distribution throughout body. Some excreted unchanged but most as hydroxymeprobamate and as the glucuronide.	Rare in therapeutic dosage. Allergic reactions have been reported. Dosage adjustment, antihistamine, or both usually suffice. When taken concurrently, meprobamate and alcohol give an additive or synergistic increase in central nervous system depression. Meprobamate is capable of inducing hepatic microsomal enzymes which metabolize warfarin, but it has been shown in animals only, not in man.	

Metaxalone (Skelaxin).	400-800 mg. Oral.	A skeletal muscle relaxant for treatment of acute muscle spasms caused by traumatic injuries.	Drug blocks synaptic pathways in the spinal cord.	Nausea, vomiting, dizziness, headache, nervousness, and skin rash. Blood changes may occur in some patients. Contraindicated during pregnancy or in patients with a tendency to drug-induced leukemia or anemia.	Should not be given longer than 10 days.
Methocarbamol, N.F. (Robaxin) (glyceryl guaiacolate carbamate, [C]).	0.5-2 Gm. Usually given q.i.d. Oral. 1 Gm. I.V. or I.M.	Uses as for carisoprodol. Low therapeutic index.	Similar to mephenesin.	May cause lightheadedness, drowsiness, mental confusion. Nausea, flushing, and dizziness have been reported with I.V. administration.	
Orphenadrine citrate, N.F. (Norflex).	100 mg. b.i.d. or t.i.d. Oral.	Used for acute spasm of voluntary muscles, regardless of location. Especially for post-traumatic, discogenic, and tension spasms.	Relieves skeletal muscle spasm and associated pain through centrally mediated action.	Side effects are due mainly to anticholinergic action of drug. Orphenadrine can cause lightheadedness and syncope and may impair ability of patient to engage in potentially hazardous activities. It should not be used in patients with glaucoma, pyloric or duodenal ulcer, prostatic hypertrophy, obstruction of bladder neck, or myasthenia gravis.	The hydrochloride salt, Disipal, is used in Parkinson's disease. See pages 123 and 67.
MUSCLE RELAXANTS (Strong, Surgical Adjunct Drugs)					
Hexafluorenium bromide (Mylaxen) (hexaflurenium bromide [C]).	Adjusted according to amount of succinylcholine administered. See package insert. Parenteral.	Used to prolong and potentiate the relaxing action of succinylcholine during surgery.	Neuromuscular blocking agent with action similar to that of curare, when given to an anesthetized subject.		A synthetic preparation.

Name, Source, Synonyms, Preparations	Dosage and Administration	Uses	Action and Fate	Side Effects and Contraindications	Remarks
MUSCLE RELAXANTS (Continued)					
CURARE. *Species of Strychnos and synthetic.*	Interactions: The use of quinidine in the immediate postoperative period following use of tubocurare can result in recurarization and can lead to respiratory paralysis. Tubocurare, when used concurrently with the following antibiotics, neomycin, streptomycin, kanamycin, polymyxin-B, bacitracin, viomycin, colistin, and gentamycin, can result in a significant incidence of prolonged respiratory failure. The neuromuscular block of tubocurare can be augmented, both in magnitude and duration, by the concurrent use of propranolol. The action of all non-depolarizing muscle relaxants may be enhanced by the thiazide diuretics, chlorthalidone, furosemide and ethacrynic acid.				
Dimethyl tubocurarine iodide, N.F. (Metubine). Tubocurarine chloride, U.S.P. (Delacurarine) (Tubarine [C]).	1.5-6 mg. I.V. 6-9 mg. I.V.	Used to relax the skeletal muscles in surgery, tetanus, encephalitis, poliomyelitis, and in any condition in which a strong muscle relaxant is needed. Used also to lessen the convulsions in shock therapy.	Blocks passage of nerve impulse at the myoneural junctions. Action starts in muscles of eye, finger, and toes and then spreads. Respiratory muscles are affected last. A less pronounced action is the blocking of the impulse in the autonomic ganglia. Widely distributed with concentrations at neuromuscular junction. After intravenous administration, effects begin to wear off in 20 minutes, with residual effect for 2 to 4 hours. Approximately half is excreted unchanged by the kidneys; remainder probably metabolized by the liver. Dimethyl tubocurarine has a shorter duration of action.	Respiratory and cardiac paralysis may occur. Treatment: artificial respiration. Neostigmine (Prostigmin) and edrophonium are the physiologic antidotes.	Dosage of curare or curare-like drugs varies with individual cases.
Pancuronium bromide (Pavulon).	Individualized. Adults usually 0.04 to 0.1 mg./kg. initially. For endotracheal intubation 0.06 to 0.1 mg./kg. I.V.	Used to induce skeletal muscle relaxation during surgery or for endotracheal intubation.	Has all the characteristics of curare-like drugs on the myoneural junctions. Approximately 5 times as potent as d-tubocurarine chloride, mg. for mg. basis. Major portion is excreted unchanged in the urine.	Side effects: main side effect is duration of action which is longer than usually required for surgery, and can leave skeletal muscle weakness for prolonged periods, resulting in respiratory insufficiency or apnea.	Caution: Should be used only by physicians thoroughly prepared to handle this type of medication and having facilities to deal with any complication. Safe use in pregnancy has not been established.

				Also, there is inadequate reversal by anticholinesterase agents requiring manual or mechanical ventilation until the dose wears off. Slight increase in pulse rate, salivation and a transient rash have been seen.	Patients with a history of myasthenia gravis can suffer profound effects from very small doses of the drug.
Decamethonium bromide (Syncurine). Gallamine triethiodide, U.S.P. (Flaxedil). Succinylcholine chloride, U.S.P. (Anectine, Quelicin, Sucostrin, Suxinyl) (suxamethonium chloride, Scoline, Sux-Cert [C]).	2-25 mg. I.V. 1 mg./kg. of body weight. I.V. 10-30 mg. I.V.		Decamethonium bromide and succinylcholine chloride act by persistent depolarization of motor end plate. Decamethonium and gallamine are excreted by the kidneys unchanged. Succinyl choline is rapidly hydrolized by the pseudocholine esterases to succinic acid and choline which are naturally occurring body constituents. About 10% excreted unchanged by the kidneys.	Decamethonium bromide or succinylcholine chloride is never counteracted with neostigmine or endrophonium, as either of these will enhance the depolarizing effect of the drugs.	The action resulting from the use of decamethonium bromide and gallamine iodide is similar to that of curare. However, gallamine is a non-depolarizing type of muscle relaxant. Succinylcholine chloride is similar to curare and does not have cumulative action.

TRANQUILIZERS AND SIMILAR DRUGS. (Refer also to antiemetics, antihistamines, antihypertensives, skeletal muscle relaxants, and central nervous system depressants.) With many of these drugs, drowsiness or delayed reflexes may occur. Patients should be cautioned on initiation of drug about driving or operating machinery. These are all synthetic preparations unless otherwise noted.

INTERACTIONS OF PHENOTHIAZINES, BUTYROPHENONES AND THIOTHEXENES.

The phenothiazines and the barbiturates interact in a number of ways. The phenothiazines can potentiate the central nervous system depressant effect of the barbiturates. The barbiturates can increase the risk of increased orthostatic hypotension, especially when given intravenously. When barbiturates are given concurrently with the phenothiazines, both in large doses, the barbiturates can cause an increase in metabolic inactivation of the phenothiazines.

Adrenergic blocking agents such as propranolol and phentolamine should be used in lower dosage when given concurrently with the phenothiazines.

Phenothiazines can enhance the hypotensive effects of some antihypertensive drugs, but with guanethedine the opposite appears to be true.

Concurrent use of phenothiazines and amphetamines, except in amphetamine overdosage, is not pharmacologically sound owing to their antagonistic effects. The reverse may also be true.

Epinephrine should not be given to patients who are taking phenothiazines, since it may result in a fall in blood pressure. However, levarterenol and phenylephrine can be used.

Haloperidol may reduce the prothrombin time when given concurrently with phenindiones or indandiones.

The phenothiazine derivatives all have similar actions, but vary as to degree. All exert a depressant action on selective portions of the brain, probably the hypothalamus. They tend to make patients more cooperative, less anxious, etc. They all are to some extent antiemetic, antihistaminic, weak beta-adrenergic blockers, antispasmodic, hypotensive, and hypothermic. These drugs all potentiate other depressant drugs, but amount of depression varies.

Name, Source, Synonyms, Preparations	Dosage and Administration	Uses	Action and Fate	Side Effects and Contraindications	Remarks
PHENOTHIAZINE DERIVATIVES					
Acepromazine (Atravet, Plegicil).	10-30 mg. Oral. 0.15-0.2 Gm. Oral.	As a tranquilizer and anti-emetic. In treating psychoses.	Readily absorbed from gastrointestinal tract and parenteral sites. Widely and rapidly distributed with highest concentration	Central nervous system depression, hypotension, epileptoid reactions. Stop or reduce dosage and treat symptoms.	Periodic blood checks are advised.
Acetophenazine maleate, N.F. (Tindal).	20-40 mg. t.i.d. Oral.	Use in the control of anxiety and tension states. Aids in overcoming insomnia.	in lungs and in following organs in decreasing order: liver, adrenal glands, spleen,	Oversedation, dizziness, increase in dreaming.	Watch blood picture and liver function.
Butaperazine (Repoise).	Up to 100 mg. per day, Start with 5-10 mg. t.i.d. and increase as indicated.	Management of chronic schizophrenic patients under close medical supervision.	brain and plasma. Metabolic degradation occurs in the liver. Metabolites excreted by kidneys. Unchanged drug found about equally in urine and stools. Excretion is relatively slow. Some found in body for days or weeks.	Side effects as with others of this group. Contraindicated in comatose patients, especially those whose depression is due to drugs, in the presence of circulatory collapse, bone marrow depression, in patients with history of jaundice, blood dyscrasias or hypersensitivity to phenothiazines.	For further information see commercial brochure.
Carphenazine maleate, N.F. (Proketazine).	12.5-50 mg. Dosage individually adjusted. Oral.	An ataractic and tranquilizing agent used to treat certain schizophrenic reactions in hospitalized patients.	Similar to other phenothiazine drugs.	Alteration in cephalin flocculation; extrapyramidal and peripheral reactions; somnolence, weakness, dizziness, hypotension have been reported. With prolonged use, blood, urine, and liver function tests should be checked. Contraindicated in excessive psychomotor agitation, in comatose states, and during pregnancy. Used with caution if central nervous system depressants are being used.	

Chlorpromazine hydrochloride, U.S.P. (Promapar, Thorazine) (Chlor-Promanyl, Chlorpromazine, Chlorprom, Chlorprom-Ez-Ets, Elmarine, Largactil, Onazine, Promosol [C]).	10-200 mg. t.i.d. Oral or I.M., depending on condition being treated.	Used as an antiemetic, to overcome motion sickness, as a mild sedative, to reinforce the action of other drugs, and as a tranquilizer.	As with others of this group.	Usually slight. May cause drowsiness, postural hypotension, and tachycardia.	If patient is ambulatory, watch for signs of overdepression; with prolonged therapy, watch for jaundice.
Chlorprothixene, N.F. (Taractan) (Tarasan [C]).	10-100 mg. Daily. Oral. 25-50 mg. I.M. Dosage individually adjusted.	A calming agent used to treat tension, agitation, anxiety (pre- and postoperatively), some schizophrenia, and alcoholic psychoses.	Is a thioxanthene derivative and has action similar to that of the phenothiazines.	Drowsiness, dermatitis, tachycardia, and postural hypotension.	Hematologic studies advised with prolonged use.
Fluphenazine enanthate (Prolixin enanthate). Fluphenazine hydrochloride, N.F. (Permitil, Prolixin, Trancin) (Moditen [C]).	25 mg. every 2 weeks. I.M. or subcutaneous. 0.25-5 mg. Three times daily. Dosage individually adjusted. Oral, I.M.	For treatment of anxiety states and psychoses.	As other phenothiazine derivatives.	Watch for evidence of bone marrow depression. Side effects: hypotension and dermatitis have been reported rarely; edema, nasal congestion, polyuria, perspiration, flushing, lethargy, blurred vision, "jitteriness," insomnia, or fatigue may develop. Reduce dosage or withdraw drug. Contraindicated in comatose states resulting from use of central nervous system depressants. Use with caution in patients with history of convulsive disorders.	
Fluphenazine decanoate (Prolixin Decanoate Inj.).	Dosage individually adjusted. Usually 25-50 mg. every 2 or 3 weeks. I.M. or subcutaneously.	See fluphenazine enanthate for details.		See phenothiazines for side effects, etc.	
Mepazine (Pacatal)	25-50 mg. b.i.d. or t.i.d. Oral or I.M.	A tranquilizer used mainly in the treatment of psychoneuroses but also as pre- or postoperative sedative.	Like others of this group.	Apparently low.	The drug comes as several salts.
Mesoridazine besylate (Serentil)	10-400 mg. daily. Oral or I.M. Dosage individually adjusted.	Used the same as other phenothiazine derivatives, such as for schizophrenia, alcoholism, psychoneurotic manifestations, behavioral problems in mental deficiency and chronic brain syndrome.	Action as with others of this group. Well absorbed orally; biological half-life between 24 and 48 hours; excreted mainly in urine, but there is some via biliary tract.	As with others of this group. Safe use of this drug during pregnancy or for children under 12 years of age has not been established.	A phenothiazine tranquilizer chemically related to thioridiazine.

Name, Source, Synonyms, Preparations	Dosage and Administration	Uses	Action and Fate	Side Effects and Contraindications	Remarks
PHENOTHIAZINE DERIVATIVES (Continued)					
Methoxypromazine maleate (Tentone).	10-50 mg. t.i.d. Dosage individually adjusted to a total of 30-500 mg./day in divided doses. Oral.	For treatment of anxiety states, psychoneurotic affective disorders, and tension states.	As above.	May produce drowsiness with large doses. Watch blood picture for signs of liver or bone marrow damage.	
Perphenazine, N.F. (Trilafon).	2-16 mg. t.i.d. Oral. 5 mg. I.M. Repeat in 6 hours if required. Dosage should be individually adjusted.	Uses similar to those of others of this group.	As above.	Similar to others of this group.	
Piperacetazine (Quide).	10-160 mg. daily. Oral. Dosage individually adjusted. Starting dose not to exceed 40 mg./day.	Same as other piperidine phenothiazine derivatives.	Same as other piperidine phenothiazine derivatives.	Same as other piperidine phenothiazine derivatives.	Safe use during pregnancy or for children has not been established.
Prochlorperazine, N.F. (Compazine) (Stemetil [C]).	5-25 mg. Three to four times a day. Rectal.	As above.	As above.	As above.	
Prochlorperazine edisylate, U.S.P. (Compazine edisylate).	5-10 mg. Oral or I.M.	As above.	As above.	As above.	
Prochlorperazine maleate, U.S.P. (Compazine dimaleate).	10-75 mg. b.i.d. Sustained-release capsules. Oral. 5-25 mg. Three to four times a day. Dosage should be individually adjusted. Oral.	As above.	As above.	As above.	
Promazine hydrochloride, N.F. (Sparine) (Atarzine, Intrazine, Promagen, Promanyl, Promwill, Promazettes, Premegerine [C]).	25-100 mg. q. 4-6 h. Oral and parenteral.	Used as an antiemetic, to overcome motion sickness, as a mild sedative, and to reinforce the action of other drugs. Used mainly as an ataractic agent.	As above.	Similar to others of this group.	
Thiopropazate dihydrochloride, N.F.	5-10 mg. Three to four times daily. Oral.	A tranquilizer whose use is the same as that of others of this group.	This is said to be hydrolyzed to perphenazine.	Apparently low.	
Thioridazine (Mellaril) (Novoridazine, Thioril [C]).	10-200 mg. Three to four times daily. Oral.	Indicated in mental and emotional disturbances,	Potentiates action of hypnotics and narcotics.	Watch for possible hematopoietic or hepatic depression.	

		intractable pain, and alcoholism.		Yellow vision with later eye damage may occur. Eye damage is usually due to excessive dosage. May cause postural hypotension.	
Thiothixene (Navane).	Initial 5 mg. b.i.d., then adjust to suit response. Maximum 60 mg. daily. Oral. Up to 30 mg. daily I.M. Usually 2 to 4 mg. q.i.d.	Management of schizophrenia and in anxiety, manifest psychosis with secondary symptoms of schizophrenia such as hallucinations, tensions, suspiciousness.		Side effects as with other phenothiazine drugs. Contraindications: patients with respiratory collapse, comatose states, central nervous system depression due to any cause, blood dyscrasias. Not recommended for children under 12 years of age.	
Trifluoperazine (Stelazine) (Chem-Flurazine, Clinazine, Fluazine, Novoflurazine, Pentazine, Solazine, Triflurin, Terfluzine, Trifluoper-Ez-Ets, Triperazine [C]).	1-10 mg. three to four times daily. Dose individually adjusted. Oral or I.M.	For treatment of psychopathic patients, such as withdrawn apathetic schizophrenics, chronic patients refractory to other therapies, patients with delusions and hallucinations.	As above.	Similar to others of this group. Contraindicated in patients with impaired cardiovascular systems.	
Triflupromazine hydrochloride, N.F. (Vesprin).	10-50 mg. t.i.d. to q.i.d. Oral. 2-20 mg. t.i.d. to q.i.d. Parenteral. 35-70 mg. One b.i.d. Suppository.	An antiemetic, tranquilizing, and psychopharmaceutical agent. Use same as that of others of this group.	As above.	Similar to others of this group.	
Tybamate, N.F. (Solacen).	250-500 mg. t.i.d. or q.i.d. Dosage individually adjusted. Not more than 3 gm. in any one day. Oral.	Used to treat a variety of psychoneurotic conditions, especially when anxiety and tension are the predominant symptoms.	Appears to exert its action on the hippocampal and limbic structures of the brain. Does not seem to affect cerebral cortical activity to any appreciable extent. Fate in body similar to meprobamate.	Adverse symptoms are usually mild and require only dosage adjustment. However, many symptoms have been reported, including drowsiness, dizziness, nausea, insomnia, euphoria, pruritus, skin rash, ataxia, confusion, headache, fatigue, and gastrointestinal disturbances. Contraindicated, at present, during pregnancy, when the phenothiazine preparations are being used, and in children under 6 years of age.	This is not a phenothiazine but is included here because of its action.

Name, Source, Synonyms, Preparations	Dosage and Administration	Uses	Action and Fate	Side Effects and Contraindications	Remarks
BUTYROPHENONE DERIVATIVES					
Droperidol (Inapsine).	2.5-10 mg. I.M. or I.V. 30-60 minutes prior to induction. 2.5 mg./20-25 lb., usually I.V. 1.25-2.5 mg. I.V. 1.0-1.5 mg./20-25 lb. for children 2-12 years of age.	As premedication, before surgery. For induction anesthesia. Maintenance of anesthesia. Drug is sedative, tranquilizer, has antianxiety activity, and will reduce nausea and vomiting.	See haloperidol.	See haloperidol. Use with caution in patients with liver or kidney dysfunction and those with parkinsonism. Safe use during pregnancy has not been established.	
Haloperidol, N.F. (Haldol).	Initial 1-5 mg. b.i.d. Adjust individually. Oral, I.M.	Control of psychomotor agitation, mania, aggressiveness, assaultiveness, hostility, hallucinations and delirium associated with acute or chronic psychoses. All types of schizophrenia. Psychotic reactions in adults with organic brain damage and mental deficiency.	This is a butyrophenone with chemical structure similar to meperidine but with action similar to the piperazine substituted phenothiazines.	Side effects as with others of this group. Contraindications: Comatose patients, those depressed by alcohol or other centrally acting agents, patients with parkinsonism, those under 12 years of age and during pregnancy. Caution: potentiates primary effects of anesthetic agents, analgesics and central nervous system depressants such as barbiturates, but not the anticonvulsants. Can cause transient hypotension, and, if possible, precipitation of anginal pain.	See above.
RAUWOLFIA DERIVATIVES	Interactions: Concurrent use of rauwolfia alkaloids and cardiac glycosides can increase the likelihood of cardiac arrhythmias, even though in most cases they can be used without adverse effects. Patients on long-term rauwolfia (reserpine) therapy may require larger than normal pressor doses of ephedrine and related drugs. In patients on rauwolfia (reserpine) therapy, the dose of quinidine used to convert atrial fibrillation to normal sinus rhythm should be considerably decreased or, if given together, the initial dose of quinidine should be lower than normal. The use of rauwolfia (reserpine) with the tricyclic antidepressants has been effective in tricyclic-refractory endogenous depression, but the hazard of reserpine reversal and resultant mania that can be produced suggests caution in using this combination.				

RAUWOLFIA SERPENTINA *Rauwolfia.*		Used as an antihypertensive agent in essential hypertension and as a general tranquilizer.	Has a calming action, probably owing to depression of central nervous system at the hypothalamic level. It releases serotonin and tends to suppress the sympathetic branch of the autonomic system centrally, thus allowing the parasympathetic system to predominate. Results include calming without analgesia or true sedation, lowering of blood pressure, increased motility and secretion of the gastrointestinal tract, slowing of the heart rate, and constriction of the pupils. It does not potentiate other central nervous system depressants.	Sedation, nasal congestion, weight gain, and varied gastrointestinal symptoms. Reduce dosage or stop drug and treat symptoms. Safety of the rauwolfia preparations for use during pregnancy has not been established; therefore, these drugs should be used only when in the judgment of the doctor their use is essential for the welfare of the patient.	Reserpine crosses the placental barrier and can cause nasal block and respiratory obstruction in the fetus. *Rauwolfia serpentina* contains the whole root with all the alkaloids.
Alseroxylon (Koglucoid, Raudolfin, Rautensin, Rauwiloid, Vio-Serpine).	2-4 mg. These are all given orally two to four times daily according to conditions being treated and response of patient.				
Deserpidine (Harmonyl).	0.1-1 mg.				
Rauwolfia serpentina, N.F. (Ekans, Hyperloid, Raudixin, Rauserfia, Rauserpa, Rautina, Rauwoldin) (Novoralfia, Raufonol, Rausenal-S1, Rautabs [C]).	50-300 mg.				
Rescinnamine, N.F. (Moderil) (Anaprel-500 [C]).	0.25-0.5 mg.				
Reserpine, U.S.P. (Anquil, Key-Serpine, Lemiserp, Rau-Sed, Reserpoid, Sandril, Serpanray,	0.25-1 mg. b.i.d. to q.i.d. Oral or parenteral.				Reserpine was one of the first tranquilizers to be used.
Serpasil, Sertina, Vio-Serpine) (Alserin, Ebserpine, Eskaserp, Neo-Serp, Resercine, Reserpanca, Serpone, Sertens [C]).	0.1-0.5 mg. Daily. Oral.	To lower blood pressure.	Rapid absorption from gastrointestinal tract or parenteral site. Widely distributed in body. Exact method of degradation and excretion not known but many metabolites have been identified.		
Syrosingopine, N.F. (Singoserp).	0.5-1 mg. Two to three times daily. Oral.				Syrosingopine is partially synthetic. It is derived from reserpine.
VARIED. *Synthetic* preparations.					
Buclizine hydrochloride.	50 mg. t.i.d. Oral.	Used to treat mild anxiety states, tension, and for sedation.	An antihistamine with prominent sedative powers.	Said to be relatively nontoxic, but excessive drowsiness may occur.	Available as ingredient in combination products. (Ex. Bucladin).
Captodiamine hydrochloride (Suvren).	50-100 mg. t.i.d. or q.i.d. Given with meals. Oral.	A tranquilizer similar to others of this group but whose action is cumulative, not immediate.	Reduces emotional states without excessive drowsiness. Is mildly stimulating. Causes reduced spasticity in smooth muscle tissue.	Apparently similar to other drugs of this group.	

Name, Source, Synonyms, Preparations	Dosage and Administration	Uses	Action and Fate	Side Effects and Contraindications	Remarks
VARIED. *Synthetic* preparations. (Continued)					
Clorazepate dipotassium (Tranxene).	15-30 mg. daily in divided doses. Elderly or debilitated start with 7.5-15 mg. daily in divided doses. Oral.	Anxiety associated with neuroses or psychoneuroses when anxiety is a prominent symptom. In any disease state in which anxiety is manifested.	Similar to other benzodiazepines. Primary metabolite nordiazepam. Peak blood level in about 1 hour. Plasma half-life about 24 hours. Metabolized in liver; excreted mainly in urine.	Side effects: drowsiness most common. Others: dizziness, gastrointestinal disturbances, dry mouth, blurred vision, nervousness, headache and mental confusion. Contraindications: narrow angle glaucoma, nursing mother, pregnancy.	Caution. Due to drowsiness, operating machinery or driving should not be done. Concurrent use of alcohol or central nervous system depressants should only be under direct medical supervision. Use for children under 18 years of age not advised.
Chlordiazepoxide, N.F. (Librium) (Chem-Dipoxide, Corax, C-Tran, Diapox, Gene-Poxide, Medilium, Methaminodiazepoxide hydrochloride, Nack, Novopoxide, Protensin, Quiecil, Solium, Sterium, Via-Quil [C]).	5-10-25 mg. t.i.d. or q.i.d. Oral. 100 mg. q. 4-6 h. I.M. or I.V. Dosage individually adjusted.	Used to reduce tension, fears, and anxiety in simple and severe forms. For alcoholism and acute anxiety.	Sedative-tranquilizer with muscle relaxant properties. Acts by unknown mechanism. It is slowly absorbed. Does not reach peak blood levels for several hours and is excreted slowly. Plasma levels may last several days after discontinuance of the drug.	Occasional nausea, constipation, skin rashes, or ataxia may occur. Reduce dosage. Withdrawal symptoms have been seen 7-8 days following high doses (300 to 600 mg. daily). Can enhance central nervous system depression, seen with alcohol and barbiturates. With the monoamine oxidase inhibitors an additive effect may occur, both depressive and excitatory. With the phenothiazines, the central nervous depression can be potentiated and an atropine-like effect can result. Safety for use during pregnancy has not been established.	
Diazepam, N.F. (Valium).	2.5-10 mg. t.i.d. or q.i.d. Oral. 2-10 mg. I.M. or I.V. q. 3-4 h.	See Librium. Also used as adjunct in skeletal muscle spasm and convulsive diseases.	See chlordiazepoxide.	Fatigue, drowsiness, ataxia, following cessation of drug after very large doses. Withdrawal symptoms have been observed for long periods. Safe use during pregnancy has not been established.	

Doxepin hydrochloride (Sinequan)	75-300 mg. daily. Oral. Dosage individually adjusted.	Used for anxiety and depression such as occur in alcoholism, psychotic disorders, involutional depression and manic-depressive reactions.	Well absorbed orally and rapidly metabolized. Has tranquilizing and antidepressant effects. Has interactions similar to the tricyclic antidepressants.	Drowsiness, dry mouth, blurred vision, tachycardia, and hypotension. For other side effects and toxicity refer to brochure. Contraindications: glaucoma, tendency to urinary retention and sensitivity to the drug.	Safe use during pregnancy has not been established. Monoamine oxidase inhibitor drugs should be discontinued for two weeks before starting this drug.
Hydroxyzine hydrochloride, N.F. (Atarax, Vistaril) (Pas-Depress [C]).	10-100 mg. Oral. 25-100 mg. I.M. Available as a syrup, 10 mg./5 ml.	Used as an antiemetic, to overcome motion sickness, as a mild sedative, and to reinforce the action of other drugs. It is a good antihistamine. Used mainly in senility and to relieve headaches and muscle spasms. Given with other drugs in the treatment of arthritis and angina pectoris. Is best used in acute conditions.	Relaxing, mildly sedative action. Action seems best in the nonpsychotic patient who is emotionally disturbed.	Postural hypotension may occur, and decrease in granulocytes has been reported. Reduce dosage or stop drug as conditions indicate. Treat symptoms. If a vasopressor is needed, norepinephrine is preferred over epinephrine. Contraindicated in early pregnancy.	The injection should never be given subcutaneously. Use I.M. route only.
Hydroxyzine pamoate, N.F. (Vistaril).	25-100 mg. Dosage individually adjusted. Oral.	As above.	As above.	As above.	
Lithium carbonate (Eskalith, Lithane, Lithonate).	Dosage individually adjusted to maintain serum level of lithium between 0.5 and 1.5 mEq./L.	Used in the control of the manic episodes of manic-depressive psychoses.	Lithium alters the transport in nerve and muscle cells and effects a shift toward intraneural metabolism of catecholamines, but the exact biochemical mechanism of lithium action is not known. Acetazolamide may cause increased excretion of lithium.	There are many adverse reactions to lithium therapy. The brochure should be studied in detail before administering the drug. Contraindicated in persons with significant cardiovascular or renal disease or evidence of brain damage. Lithium toxicity is closely related to its serum level and can occur at doses close to therapeutic levels.	The adequate intake of sodium and fluid must be maintained while lithium is being given, and the use of diuretics should be avoided. Facilities for prompt and accurate serum determinations should be available before initiating therapy. Lithium carbonate has been implicated in cases of neonatal goiter.

Name, Source, Synonyms, Preparations	Dosage and Administration	Uses	Action and Fate	Side Effects and Contraindications	Remarks
VARIED. *Synthetic* preparations. (Continued)					
Mephenoxalone (Methoxydone, Tranpoise).	400 mg. Given 100-200 mg. q.i.d. Oral.	Used like others of this group, especially when accompanied by muscle spasm associated with trauma or musculoskeletal disease.	Mild tranquilizer and skeletal muscle relaxant with action similar to that of meprobamate.	Skin rash, dizziness, nausea, and drowsiness occur infrequently and may be controlled by reduction or discontinuance of dosage.	Blood picture should be watched with prolonged dosage.
Oxazepam, N.F. (Serax).	10-30 mg. Three or four times daily. Oral.	See chlordiazepoxide.	See chlordiazepoxide.	Drowsiness, dizziness, vertigo, headache, and syncope have been reported. Instances of minor diffuse skin rashes (morbilliform, urticarial, and maculopapular) have occurred. Nausea, lethargy, edema, slurred speech, tremors, altered libido, and ataxia have been reported, but rarely. When excessive dosage is continued for weeks or months, dosage should be reduced gradually rather than abruptly. Patients should be told that they may have a lowered tolerance to alcohol.	Caution: Administer with caution to patients in whom a drop in blood pressure might lead to cardiac complications. Safety for use during pregnancy has not been established. During prolonged therapy periodic blood counts and liver function tests are advisable.
Phenaglycodol (Ultran).	0.2-0.3 Gm. t.i.d. Oral.	Used as a tranquilizer in various neurologic and emotional disorders.	Mild sedating and relaxing agent.	Rare in therapeutic dosage, but drowsiness and dizziness occur.	
GENERAL ANESTHETICS. See also local anesthetics and sedatives-hypnotics. These are synthetic preparations.					
Chloroform, N.F. (Trichloromethane).	Dosage varies. Inhalation.	Used as a general anesthetic and also as an anodyne, carminative, sedative, antispasmodic, and as a counterirritant.	Descending, progressive central nervous system depressant. Produces surgical anesthesia in a very short time. Gives good muscle relaxation; tends to produce a steadily decreasing blood pressure.	Local irritation, cardiac paralysis during anesthesia, acidosis during recovery. Treatment: symptomatic. Toxic symptoms: (delayed) hepatotoxic, progressive weakness, cyanosis, restlessness, vomiting, delirium,	Use limited owing to toxicity. Not used for long anesthesia. Not flammable. Easy to administer, relatively pleasant to take. Chloroform can interact with sympathomimetics to produce cardiac arrhythmias.

Other Chloroform Preparations That Are Not Anesthetics.			Induction fairly rapid. Rapidly passes lung barriers. Carried mainly by red blood corpuscles rather than plasma. Excreted largely unchanged by the lungs.	coma. Death may occur. Treatment: symptomatic. Contraindicated in cardiac disorders.	
Chloroform liniment.	Dosage varies. Topical.	As a counterirritant.			
Chloroform spirits.	2 ml. Oral.	As a carminative, antispasmodic, and sedative.			
Chloroform water.	15 ml. Oral.				
GENERAL ANESTHETICS (Continued)					
Cyclopropane, U.S.P. (Trimethylene).	Dosage varies. Inhalational. 10-20% with oxygen 80-90% will maintain surgical anesthesia.	Used as a general anesthetic. Depth sufficient for major surgery, and recovery rapid without adverse effects, except occasional nausea.	A potent central nervous system depressant, producing anesthesia with relatively low dosage. Sufficient oxygen can be given and still maintain adequate anesthesia. Muscle relaxation moderate. Induction about 5 minutes. Readily absorbed and excreted mostly unchanged by the lungs. A small amount is metabolized by the body into carbon dioxide and water.	Rarely sensitizes myocardium to epinephrine. Cardiac arrhythmia and failure may occur. Stop anesthesia and treat symptoms. Cyclopropane can interact with the sympathomimetics to produce cardiac arrhythmias. Also, in high dosage it can interact with the antibiotics–streptomycin, kanamycin, polymyxin-B, colistimethate, viomycin and paromomycin to give neuromuscular blockage and can cause respiratory arrest.	Is highly explosive; must be given in a closed circuit with pure oxygen, and where sparks cannot occur. Widely used in elderly and poor-risk patients. Cyclopropane can cross the placenta and cause neonatal respiratory depression.
Enflurane (Ethrane) *(a fluorinated ether).*	3.5-4.5% to induce surgical anesthesia. Maintenance, 1.5-3.0%.	Inhalation anesthesia. Induction in 7-10 minutes.	Induction and recovery fairly rapid. Levels of anesthesia change rapidly. Heart rate remains relatively constant, but there is an increase in amount of hypotension with increased level of anesthesia. Depth of ventilation is reduced as anesthesia is increased.	The nondepolarizing muscle relaxants are markedly potentiated and neostigmine does not reverse the direct effect of enflurane. Contraindicated in certain seizure disorders and in patients sensitive to the halogenated anesthesias. Motor activity shown by movement of various muscle groups and/or seizures may be encountered with deep levels of anesthesia. Hypotension and respiratory depression have occurred. Arrhythmias,	Must be used only with equipment that can measure concentration. Safety for use in pregnancy has not been established.

Name, Source, Synonyms, Preparations	Dosage and Administration	Uses	Action and Fate	Side Effects and Contraindications	Remarks
GENERAL ANESTHETICS (Continued)					
Enflurane (Continued)				shivering, nausea and vomiting have been reported and elevation of white blood cell count has been seen. This may be due to factors other than the anesthesia.	
Ether, U.S.P. (diethyl ether).	Dosage varies. Inhalational.	Used mainly for general anesthesia, especially when muscular relaxation is essential. Also used as an anodyne, carminative, sedative, and antispasmodic.	Progressive, descending central nervous system depressant. Gives good muscle relaxation. Somewhat slow induction and recovery. Absorbed through lung mucosa. About 90% excreted by the same route. It can be detected in expired air up to several hours later. A small amount is metabolized by the body. Some is excreted unchanged in urine, perspiration and other body fluids.	Local irritation, especially of mucous membranes; respiratory paralysis and circulatory involvement may occur. Stop drug, give artificial respiration. Epinephrine and caffeine may be used. Toxic symptoms: (delayed) symptoms of liver and kidney damage. Similar to vinyl ether. Treatment: symptomatic.	Ether is usually contraindicated in respiratory diseases. Ether vapor is explosive in some concentrations with oxygen. The fluid is not explosive. Ether can cross the placenta and cause apnea in the neonate.
Ethyl vinyl ether (Vinamar).	Dosage varies. Inhalational.	Inhalational general anesthesia.	As above.		
Vinyl ether, N.F. (Vinethene, divinyl ether).	Dosage varies. Inhalational.	Mainly used for minor surgery.	Somewhat less irritating than ether; quicker induction. Gives good muscle relaxation.	Contraindicated in cardiovascular disease, renal insufficiency, and hepatic damage.	May be given by open drop method. More volatile than ether and equally explosive.
Ethylene, N.F. (Ethene).	Dosage varies. Inhalational.	Used as a general anesthetic.	Induction short, depth sufficient for major surgery, and recovery rapid without adverse effects.	Rare in therapeutic dosage. Treatment: symptomatic, if needed.	Has an unpleasant odor. Is highly explosive; must be given in a closed circuit with pure oxygen and where sparks cannot occur.
Fluroxene (Fluoromar).	Dosage varies. Inhalation.	A general anesthetic agent used for all types of surgery and obstetrics.	If muscle relaxation under moderate anesthesia is inadequate, muscle relaxants should be used, especially in abdominal surgery.	This drug does not appear to alter liver function as measured by conventional tests. Levels of anesthesia can be changed very easily and rapidly. With deep	Chemically fluroxene is trifluoroethyl vinyl ether. It is flammable above 4% concentration with O_2; therefore cautery should not be used when

				anesthesia, marked hypotension and respiratory depression are encountered. Guedel pupillary signs for depth of anesthesia are not reliable with fluroxene.	fluroxene is being given. Same interactions as halothane.
Halothane, U.S.P. (Fluothane).	Dosage varies. Inhalational.	Liquid anesthetic agent that can be used in either open or closed method.	Complete anesthetic causes continuous respiratory depression; is a bronchodilator and myocardial depressant; sensitizes myocardium to epinephrine, so that ventricular arrhythmias may occur. Absorbed through lung mucosa. About 60% excreted by lungs.	Cases of hepatic necrosis and dysfunction have been reported. Nausea and vomiting rare. Heavy dosage may cause cardiac arrest, severe hypotension or both. Treatment: amphetamine or similar drugs; usual emergency treatment.	It has not been shown that the use of this anesthetic will not have an adverse effect upon the fetus. Epinephrine, levarterenol and other sympathomimetics can cause cardiac arrhythmias. Halothane can interact with the antibiotics streptomycin, kanamycin, polymyxin-B, viomycin, colistimethate and paromomycin to give reduced neuromuscular blockage and can cause respiratory arrest.
Ketamine hydrochloride (Ketaject, Ketalar).	1-4.5 mg./kg. I.V. anesthesia in 30 seconds, lasts 5-10 min. 6.5-13.0 mg./kg. I.M. anesthesia in 3-4 minutes, lasts 12-25 min.	Used for short anesthesia when muscle relaxation is not required, for induction and to supplement low potency agents such as nitrous oxide.	Rapid acting agent, produces good analgesia without muscle relaxation. Skeletal cardiac and respiratory muscles have slightly increased tone. Rapid administration may cause respiratory depression. Blood pressure is increased. Rapidly absorbed, widely distributed throughout the body, undergoes metabolic degradation. The degradation products are excreted in the urine, a small amount in feces.	Though toxicity is low, there are many warnings and precautions. Rapid administration may cause respiratory depression requiring resuscitative measures. Emergence reactions (anything from a dream-like state to hallucinations, confusion or excitement) are not uncommon. Contraindications: drug should not be used for the hypertensive patient. It is not used for an acute or chronic alcoholic patient.	Commercial brochure should be consulted before administering this drug. Ketamine should not be administered by the same equipment used for the barbiturates since a precipitate will be formed. Safe use during pregnancy or delivery has not been established.

Name, Source, Synonyms, Preparations	Dosage and Administration	Uses	Action and Fate	Side Effects and Contraindications	Remarks
GENERAL ANESTHETICS (Continued)					
Methoxyflurane, N.F. (Penthrane) (Methofane [C]).	Dosage varies. Inhalational.	General inhalational anesthetic agent used chiefly for maintenance.	Complete anesthetic with moderate skeletal relaxation. Also lowers blood pressure.	Respiratory and circulatory depression. Treatment: symptomatic. Epinephrine and levarterenol are contraindicated. See specific contraindications and interactions under halothane.	Used either in open or closed technique. Central nervous system depressant; dosage should be reduced. Usual eye signs do not apply.
Nitrous oxide, U.S.P. (nitrogen monoxide).	Dosage varies. Inhalational.	Used alone as a short general anesthetic, with oxygen for longer periods, and with oxygen and ether for prolonged anesthesia.	Small amounts mixed with air act as an intoxicant; patient feels happy, laughs, is loquacious. If mixed with oxygen alone, patient loses consciousness rapidly. Is a relatively weak anesthetic at atmospheric pressure. Combination with other agents is required for deeper anesthesia.	Slow pulse; cyanosis; irregular rate, depth, and rhythm of respiration. Stop drug and treat symptoms. See interactions under Ether, page 114.	Unless ether is added there is little muscle relaxation. "Laughing gas" is the common name.
Trichloroethylene, U.S.P. (Trilene)	1 ml. Inhalational.	Used as a general and specific anesthetic agent. Main use is in obstetrics for pain after cervix is dilated at least 3 cm. Is also used for minor surgery.	Produces a light plane of anesthesia. Does not produce muscle relaxation in usual dosage.	Cardiac arrhythmias, increasing muscular activity. Stop drug and treat symptoms. Trichloroethylene alone is not recommended for anesthesia or the induction of anesthesia. Epinephrine should not be used at the same time. Interactions same as for chloroform.	May be habit forming; apt to be dangerous. Should never be used in closed system with soda lime. Has been used in tic douloureux.

DEPRESSANTS

LOCAL ANESTHETICS AND ANODYNES. See also general anesthetics.					
AMOLANONE HYDROCHLORIDE. *Synthetic.* Amolanone hydrochloride (Amethone).	9% solution (concentrated). Diluted to 0.33%. Topical.	A local anesthetic used mainly for urologic surgery.	Produces insensitivity of nerve endings in mucous membranes.	Toxic symptoms rare.	
BENZYL ALCOHOL (Phenylcarbinol). *Synthetic.* Benzyl alcohol, N.F.	Dosage varies. Topical and subcutaneous.	Used mainly for local and block anesthesia.	Produces insensitivity by blocking nerve impulses. If absorbed, it is converted to hippuric acid by the body.	Very rare. No treatment required.	Also used as a preservative.
COCAINE. Active principle of coca shrub. *Synthetic.* Amylocaine hydrochloride (Stovaine).	5-10 Gm. vial diluted as needed. Spinal.	Used for surface, infiltration, conduction and regional, paravertebral, sacral, and spinal anesthesia. Cocaine in pure form is limited in use, but derivatives have wide usage. All are used in dilute solutions.	In surface anesthesia, the nerve endings are rendered incapable of receiving and transmitting impulses. With other anesthetics of this type the conducting nerve fibers are rendered incapable of transmitting impulses. Some anesthetics have both types of action.	Excitement, anxiety, dizziness, severe headache, convulsions, fall in blood pressure. Death may occur from cardiovascular and respiratory failure. Treatment (prophylactic): barbiturates before surgery, slow administration of the local anesthetic agent, use of dilute solution, caution to prevent intravenous administration, use of epinephrine hydrochloride to delay absorption. Treatment (active): stop drug, give barbiturates, treat symptoms. If area of administration allows, use tourniquet. Idiosyncrasy is common even with small doses.	Epinephrine hydrochloride is often added to a local anesthetic to prolong its action.
Benoxinate hydrochloride (Dorsacaine).	0.4% solution. Topical.	Ophthalmic.			
Benzocaine, N.F. (Americaine).	5% ointment. Topical.				

Name, Source, Synonyms, Preparations	Dosage and Administration	Uses	Action and Fate	Side Effects and Contraindications	Remarks
LOCAL ANESTHETICS (Continued)					
Bupivaine hydrochloride (Marcaine hydrochloride).	0.25-0.75% solution.	Local anesthetic agent used for peripheral nerve block, infiltration, sympathetic block, caudal or epidural block.	Duration of action is significantly longer than with other commonly used local anesthetics.	Safe use in pregnancy or for children under 12 years of age has not been established.	Parenteral administration stabilizes the neuronal membrane and prevents initiation and transmission of nerve impulses. Warning. Resuscitative equipment and drugs should be available when any local anesthetic is used parenterally.
Butacaine sulfate (Butyn) (Amolyn, Optyn [C]).	2% solution. Topical.	Main use: eye, ear, nose, and throat surgery.			
Butethamine formate (Monacaine).	100-150 mg. Spinal.	Similar to procaine but more toxic. Main use in dentistry.			
Butethamine hydrochloride, N.F. (Monocaine hydrochloride) (Novocol [C]).	1-2% solution. Regional.				
Butyl aminobenzoate, N.F. (Butesin) (Planolorn [C]).	Dosage varies. Topical.				
Chloroprocaine hydrochloride, N.F. (Nesacaine) (Versacaine [C]).	1-3% solution. Injection.				
Cocaine hydrochloride, N.F.	1-5% solution. Topical.		Cocaine, local vasoconstriction limits absorption. That which is absorbed is detoxified by the liver and excreted unchanged by kidneys.		Cocaine comes under the jurisdiction of Drug Enforcement Agency. Surface anesthesia only. Action is prolonged.
Cyclomethycaine sulfate (Surfacaine).	0.5-1% solution, ointment, and cream. Topical.				
Dibucaine hydrochloride, U.S.P. (Nupercainal, Nuperlone, Nupercaine) (cinchocaine [C]).	0.5-2% solution or ointment. Topical.			Very toxic.	
Dimethisoquin hydrochloride, N.F. (Quotane).	0.5% lotion or ointment, Topical.			Too toxic for injection.	
Diperodon hydrochloride (Diothane).	19% ointment or cream. Topical.				
Dyclonine hydrochloride, U.S.P. (Dyclone).	0.5% solution. Topical. 1% cream. Topical.				

Ethyl aminobenzoate (Anesthesin, Anesthaone, Benzocaine, Orthesin, Parathesin).	5% solution. Topical.				
Eucaine or betaeucaine hydrochloride.	Dosage varies. Topical.				Weaker and slower acting than cocaine.
Hexylcaine hydrochloride, N.F. (Cyclaine).	2-10% solution or jelly. Topical or parenteral.				
Lidocaine hydrochloride, U.S.P. (Xylocaine) (lignocaine, Octocaine, Topilidon [C]).	0.5-5.0% solution. Topical, subcutaneous, spinal. 2.5-5% ointment. Topical.	This drug is used I.V. in the treatment of cardiac arrhythmias.			See page 134 for other information and interactions.
Mepivacaine hydrochloride, N.F. (Carbocaine).	1-2% solution. Parenteral.	For infiltration and nerve block.			Mepivacaine can cross the placenta and cause fetal bradycardia and neonatal depression.
Naepaine hydrochloride (Amylsine, Amylcaine).	2-4% solution. Topical.	Local anesthetic for eye when mydriasis is not desired.			
Oxethazine (Oxaine).	0.2% solution. Topical.	Mainly for gastric distress.			
Parethoxycaine hydrochloride (Diethozin, Intracaine).	2-5% solution. Topical, and subcutaneous.				About twice as effective as procaine.
Phenacaine hydrochloride, N.F. (Holocain, Holocaine).	1% solution. Topical.	Main use as local anesthetic for eye.			
Piperocaine hydrochloride (Metycaine).	1-10% solution. Topical. 0.13-0.5% solution. Subcutaneous.				
Pramoxine hydrochloride, N.F. (Tronothane) (pramocaine [C]).	1% cream, jelly, lotion or solution. Topical.				
Prilocaine hydrochloride (Citanest) (Xylonest [C]).	1%, 2%, 3% solution infiltration.	Therapeutic nerve block.	Same as others of this group.	Contraindications: patients hypersensitive to local anesthetic agents of the amide type. Also in congenital and idiopathic methemoglobinemia. Side effects: syncope, hypotension, headache, backache, apnea, nausea, vomiting and drowsiness.	Not recommended for spinal anesthesia.
Procaine hydrochloride, U.S.P. (Novocain, Syncaine) (Westocaine [C]).	0.25-2% solution. All routes except topical.		Readily absorbed from parenteral sites. Broken down both in liver and plasma and excreted in urine.		Most widely used local anesthetic.

Name, Source, Synonyms, Preparations	Dosage and Administration	Uses	Action and Fate	Side Effects and Contraindications	Remarks
LOCAL ANESTHETICS (Continued)					
Proparacaine hydrochloride (Ophthaine) (proxymetacaine, Ophthetic [C]).	0.5% solution. Topical.	In eyes.			
Propoxycaine hydrochloride, N.F. (Blockain, Ravocaine).	0.5% solution. Topical or subcutaneous.				
Propylaminobenzoate (Propaesin).	Dosage varies. Topical as ointment.				
Quinocaine.	Dosage varies. Topical and subcutaneous.	Used for prolonged local anesthesia, 2-7 days.			
Tetracaine, N.F.					
Tetracaine hydrochloride, U.S.P. (Amethocaine, Pontocaine, Tetracel) (amethacaine, Anethaine [C]).	Maximum 20 mg. Topical and spinal.	Main use: eye, ear, nose, and throat surgery and spinal anesthesia.			
Tutocaine hydrochloride (Butamin).	Maximum, 200 mg. Topical and subcutaneous.	Main use: on mucous membranes.			
ETHYL CHLORIDE. *Synthetic.*		Used for short topical anesthesia.	Acts by freezing area.	Nausea, vomiting, cardiac failure, prostration. Stop drug and treat symptoms.	
Ethyl chloride, N.F.	Dosage varies. Topical and inhalational.	Used by inhalation for short general anesthesia and as an induction anesthetic agent.		Interactions as with chloroform when administered by inhalation.	
QUININE AND UREA HYDROCHLORIDE. *Cinchona and synthetic.*					
Quinine and urea hydrochloride, U.S.P.	Dosage varies. Topical and subcutaneous	Used for local and block anesthesia.	Painful, but then produces anesthesia lasting several days; also used as sclerosing agent.	Mainly local irritation, may cause sloughing. Treatment: symptomatic.	Solutions must be very dilute.

ANTIHISTAMINES

Name, Source, Synonyms, Preparations	Dosage and Administration	Uses	Action and Fate	Side Effects and Contraindications	Remarks
SYNTHETIC PREPARATIONS					
Antazoline hydrochloride, U.S.P. (Antastan, Antistin [C]).	100 mg. Up to q.i.d. Oral.	Used to relieve the symptoms of allergic reactions, especially nasal and conjunctival allergy. Also for treatment of allergic manifestations	These drugs block the action of the normal body enzyme, histamine, which is present in excess in the blood of patients suffering from	Drowsiness, dizziness, dryness of mouth and throat, disturbed coordination, lassitude, muscular weakness, gastrointestinal disturbances,	Dosage individually adjusted. As with some other drugs, patients should be cautioned about driving or operating machinery.

Antazoline phosphate, N.F. (Nasocon).	0.5% solution. Inhalational in nebulizer. 0.5% solution. Topical as eye drops.	such as dermatitis, urticaria, angioneurotic edema, occupational allergies; drug, food, and cosmetic allergies; serum sickness; some are used in Parkinson's disease; some are used as sedative or hypnotic agents, or both.	various allergies and hypersensitivities. Some have antinauseant action, others aid in motion sickness, and still others have sedative-hypnotic action. Most are readily absorbed from the gastrointestinal sites. Most reach a peak level in 30-60 minutes and effects last for 3-6 hours. Concentration in tissues is greatest in lungs with progressively less in spleen, kidneys, brain, muscle and skin. Most metabolic transformation occurs in liver, but some also in lungs and kidneys. Most excreted by the kidneys as various metabolic degradation products.	nervousness, insomnia, xerostomia, nausea, vomiting. Reduce dosage or stop drug and treat symptoms. These drugs can increase central nervous system depression when given simultaneously with other central nervous system depressants such as alcohol, narcotics, barbiturates, tranquilizers, anesthetics and reserpine. They give additive effects when used concurrently with anticholinergic drugs. They can reduce the effects of hormones if given repeatedly by enzyme induction. This property varies with the different classes of antihistamines. Persons whose occupations expose them to halogenated insecticides have a diminished effect from this class of drugs and need larger doses for therapeutic response. Antihistamines with phenothiazines or nylidin should probably not be used concurrently, since the action of both appears to be potentiated.	Many of these drugs are prepared in both quick acting and delayed action tablets. The delayed action tablets are given once or twice daily, the others more often.
Bromodiphenhydramine hydrochloride, N.F. (Ambodryl) (bromazine [C]).	5-25 mg. Up to q.i.d. Oral or parenteral.				
Brompheniramine maleate, N.F. (Dimetane) (parabromdylamine [C]).	4-12 mg. 4 mg. q.i.d. Oral. Or 8-12 mg. b.i.d. Oral. 5-20 mg. b.i.d. Parenteral.				
Carbinoxamine maleate, N.F. (Clistin) (paracarbinoxamine, [C]).	4-8-12 mg. 4 mg. q.i.d. Oral. 8-12 mg. b.i.d. Oral.				
Chlorcyclizine hydrochloride, N.F. (Peracil [C]).	50 mg. Up to q.i.d. Oral.	Slower acting, but longer duration than most antihistamines.			
Chlorothen citrate, N.F. (chlorothenylpyramine, Tagathen [C]).	25 mg. q.i.d. Oral.				
Chlorpheniramine maleate, U.S.P. (Chlor-Trimeton, Histaspan, Teldrin) (chlorphenamine, chlorprophenpyridamine, Histalon, Chlor-Tripolon, Chlortrone, Novo-pheniran [C]).	4-12 mg. 4 mg. q.i.d. Oral. 8-12 mg. b.i.d. Oral.				Chlorpheniramine is contraindicated in severe cardiac conditions.
Chlorpheniramine maleate injection, N.F. (Pheneton, Chlor-Trimeton).	10 mg. Parenteral.				
Chlorphenoxamine (Phenoxene).	20-40 mg. q.i.d. Oral. 10 mg. I.M. or I.V.	Used to treat local and systemic allergies and Parkinson's disease.			
Clemizole hydrochloride (Reactrol).	20 mg. q.i.d. Oral.	Used especially for skin allergies; drug, food and cosmetic hypersensitivity; and serum sickness.			
Cyclizine hydrochloride, U.S.P. (Marezine) (Marzine [C]).	50 mg. Up to q.i.d. Oral or rectal.	Used also as antiemetic and a tranquilizer.			Doctor should weigh potential of use as an antiemetic during pregnancy against the possible teratogenic effect of the drug.
Cyclizine lactate (Harezene).	50 mg. Up to q.i.d. Parenteral.				

Name, Source, Synonyms, Preparations	Dosage and Administration	Uses	Action and Fate	Side Effects and Contraindications	Remarks
SYNTHETIC ANTIHISTAMINE PREPARATIONS (Continued)					
Cyproheptadine hydrochloride, N.F. (Periactin).	4 mg. t.i.d. or q.i.d. Oral.	An antihistamine similar to atropine for treatment of allergy and pruritus. Antagonist against both histamine and serotonin.			Has been said to increase appetite.
Dexbrompheniramine maleate, N.F. (Disomer).	2 mg. q.i.d.; 4-6 mg. b.i.d. Oral.				
Dexchlorpheniramine maleate, N.F. (Polaramine) (d-chlorpheniramine [C]).	2-6 mg. q.i.d. Oral.				Also available in a sustained release form.
Dimethindene maleate, N.F. (Forhistal, Triten) (dimethpyrindine maleate [C]).	1 mg. q.i.d. Oral. 2.5 mg. b.i.d. delayed release. Oral.			Causes some sedation.	
Diphenhydramine hydrochloride, U.S.P. (Benadryl) (Benhydramil [C]).	25-50 mg. q.i.d. Oral, parenteral, topical.	Uses same as those of others of this group. Also useful in asthma. Causes some muscular relaxation.		Causes more sedation than most antihistamines.	
Diphenylpyraline (Diafen, Hispril) (Dorahist, Neo-Lergic [C]).	2 mg. t.i.d. Oral. 5 mg. sustained release capsules. Two or three times a day. Oral.				
Doxylamine succinate, N.F. (Decapryn).	12.5-25 mg. t.i.d. Oral.			Effectiveness limited because of sedative action.	
Ethopropazine (Parsidol) (profenamine, Parsitan [C]).	50 mg. q.i.d. Oral.	Main use is in treatment of Parkinson's disease.			
Isothipendyl.	4 mg. t.i.d. Oral.				
Methapyrilene hydrochloride, N.F. (Allergin, Histadyl, Histafed, Lullamin, Pyrathyn, Somnicaps) (Norbarbitate [C]).	50-100 mg. Usually h.s. Oral. 2% cream p.r.n. Topical.	Used for insomnia because of its sedative action.			
Methdilazine hydrochloride (Tacaryl) (Dilosyn, Disyncran [C]).	4-8 mg. Two to four times daily. Available as 8 mg. tablets and syrup containing 4 mg./5 cc. Usually given b.i.d.; also chewable tablet 3.6 mg. Oral.	Used mainly in allergic pruritus.			Methdilazine hydrochloride potentiates the action of hypnotics.

Orphenadrine hydrochloride (Dispal).	50 mg. t.i.d. Oral.	Main use in treatment of Parkinson's disease.			
Phenyltoloxamine dihydrogen citrate (Floxamine).	25-50 mg. t.i.d. Oral.				
Promethazine hydrochloride, U.S.P. (Phenergan) (Histantil [C]).	6-50 mg. p.r.n. Oral. Also available in cough medications. 25-50 mg. p.r.n. Rectal or parenteral.	Used for preoperative sedation, to control post-operative nausea, and to potentiate action of analgesics.			
Pyrathiazine hydrochloride (Pyrrolazote).	25-50 mg. o.d. or t.i.d. Oral.			With pyrathiazine hydrochloride, agranulocytosis has been reported.	
Pyrilamine maleate, N.F. (Histalon, Neopyramine, PYMA, Pyramaleate, Pyristan) (mepyramine maleate, pyranilamine, pyranisamin, Neo-Antergan [C]).	25 mg. Up to q.i.d. Oral.				
Pyrrobutamine phosphate, N.F.	15 mg. t.i.d. Oral.				
Rotoxamine tartrate (Twiston).	2 mg. Three or four times a day, 4-6 mg. b.i.d. Oral.				
Thenyldiamine hydrochloride, N.F.	15-30 mg. t.i.d. Oral.				
Tripelennamine citrate, U.S.P. (Pyribenzamine citrate).	25-75 mg. t.i.d. Oral.				More palatable than the hydrochloride.
Tripelennamine hydrochloride, U.S.P. (Pyribenzamine hydrochloride) (Benzoxal, Pyrizil [C]).	50-100 mg. t.i.d. Available for topical use and as an ingredient of cough mixtures. Oral.				Available in sustained release form.
Trimeprazine tartrate, N.F. (Temaril) (alimemazine, Panectyl, Theralene, Vallergan [C]).	2.5-5 mg. Oral.	An oral dermatologic and systemic antipruritic.	A phenothiazine derivative with antipruritic action.	Mild drowsiness may occur. Stop drug. A few cases of jaundice and blood dyscrasias have been reported.	
Triprolidine hydrochloride (Actidil).	2.5 mg. t.i.d. or q.i.d. Oral.				

HISTAMINES

SYNTHETIC PREPARATIONS					
Histamine azoprotein (Hapamine).	0.01-0.02 ml. Subcutaneous.	Used to desensitize in cases of hypersensitivity.	Does not stimulate secretion of gastric juice.	May cause local and systemic reactions similar to those of hypersensitivity. Treatment: antihistaminic.	

Name, Source, Synonyms, Preparations	Dosage and Administration	Uses	Action and Fate	Side Effects and Contraindications	Remarks
SYNTHETIC PREPARATIONS (Continued)					
Histamine phosphate, U.S.P. (Histapon).	0.3-1.0 mg. Subcutaneous.	Used to desensitize in cases of hypersensitivity, as a diagnostic aid to stimulate secretion of the glands of the gastric mucosa, and in the treatment of peripheral vascular diseases.	Does stimulate secretion of gastric juice. Readily absorbed from parenteral sites but poorly absorbed from gastrointestinal tract. It diffuses rapidly into tissues and is metabolized. Metabolic products are excreted by the kidneys.	Rare in therapeutic dosage. Epinephrine is used if needed.	For further information see Diagnostic Drugs.

DRUGS ACTING ON THE CIRCULATORY SYSTEM

Name, Source, Synonyms, Preparations	Dosage and Administration	Uses	Action and Fate	Side Effects and Contraindications	Remarks
HEMATINICS (hematopoietic agents). See also Vitamins.					
COPPER, MANGANESE. *Mineral.*	These are added to other hematopoietic preparations. No specific preparation or dosage given for these.	Cobalt may be included in this group. These and possibly zinc and nickel are used with iron to treat iron deficiency anemia.	Believed to act as catalytic agents in the utilization of iron.	Rare in minute amounts used. Treatment: none usually required.	
IRON. *Mineral.*		Used to stimulate the hematopoietic system and to increase hemoglobin. There is a general tonic effect upon the entire body which is probably due to better blood supply (better oxygen carrying ability). Used locally as a styptic. Especially valuable in treating iron deficiency anemia.	Iron is contained in all hemoglobin as well as in other parts of the body. It is absorbed in the small intestines. Average daily excretion is about 1 mg. If not replaced by the diet, the reserve is depleted. About 80% of iron from disintegrated red blood cells is retained and reused. Iron to be absorbed from the gastrointestinal tract must be in the soluble ferrous form. Many factors are involved in the absorption. But once absorbed it is transported in the blood	Disorders of the gastrointestinal system. Pasty, black stools are common. Fullness in the head, insomnia, tachycardia, and skin eruptions may occur. The latter symptoms are most apt to occur after a single large dose. Treatment: (for severe symptoms) gastric lavage, emetics, tannic acid solutions orally, and treat symptoms: (for mild symptoms) decrease or stop drug, give a laxative, and treat symptoms. Ingestion of liquid or tablets by children (overdose) can be *very toxic.* Mothers	Give extra laxative foods during iron therapy. Give fluid preparations through a tube to protect teeth. Give with food (milk or fruit juice) if diet allows. Iron is commonly given in combination with other drugs such as vitamins (especially B), liver, and stomach extract. Products containing iron and an organic compound are available, but their effectiveness is open to question, hence they are not in common use.
Ferric ammonium tartrate.	0.5-1 Gm. t.i.d. Oral.	For iron deficiency anemia.			
Ferric chloride.	Dosage varies. Topical.	Astringent for skin disorders.			
Ferric subsulfate solution (Monsel's solution).	Dosage varies. Topical.	Use undiluted as a styptic.			

Ferrocholinate (Chel-Iron, Ferrolip).	0.3-0.6 Gm. Given as a solution or tablet, usually t.i.d. Oral.	For iron deficiency anemia.	to certain organs with a high concentration of iron. These are liver, spleen and marrow. The body excretes small amounts in the feces, urine and bile. The amount of iron is controlled through limited absorption and not by excretory processes.	should be warned to keep out of child's reach. Avoid infiltration. Do not give subcutaneously. Many side effects and contraindications.	
Ferroglycine sulfate complex (Ferronord).	40 mg. (40 mg. of ferrous iron in each dose) b.i.d. (between meals). Oral.	As above.			
Ferrous carbonate pills (Blaud's pills).	0.3 Gm. t.i.d. Oral.	As above.			
Ferrous fumarate, U.S.P. (C-Ron, Fumasorb, Ircon, Prematinic, Toleron) (Feroton, Ferrofume, Fumiron, Irofume, Novofumar, Palafer, Tolifer [C]).	0.2 Gm. t.i.d. Oral.	As above.			Also available in saccharated form.
Ferrous gluconate, N.F. (Fergon) (Novoferroglue [C]).	0.3 Gm. t.i.d. Oral.	As above.			
Ferrous iodide syrup (Genofer [C]).	1 ml. t.i.d. Oral.	As above.			
Ferrous sulfate, U.S.P. (Feosol, Ferralyn) (Fer-in-Sol, Fesofor, Ferro-Gradumet, Novoferrosulf, Ferrosulph [C]).	0.06-0.3 Gm. t.i.d. with meals or p.c. Available as tablets, solution, delayed action capsules. Oral.	As above.			
Iron-dextran injection, U.S.P. (Imferon).	50-250 mg. Dosage and times individually adjusted. I.M. or I.V.	For treatment of iron deficiency anemia when oral administration is not advisable.		Local irritation and staining may occur. Other side effects same as with any iron preparation. Sarcomata have been reported in experimental animals but not in man. Allergic or anaphylactoid reactions are not common, but have occurred, including 3 fatalities.	
Iron sorbitex, U.S.P. (Jectofer) (iron-sorbital citric acid complex [C]).	100 mg. of iron (1 ampule) 10 to 20 injections as indicated by condition. I.M.	As above.		As above.	
Polyferose iron carbohydrate complex (Jefron [C]).	4-8 ml. t.i.d. Oral.	See ferrous sulfate.		As above.	

Name, Source, Synonyms, Preparations	Dosage and Administration	Uses	Action and Fate	Side Effects and Contraindications	Remarks
LIVER AND STOMACH PREPARATIONS. *Animal.* Liver injection (Bexiver, Foli-Brumin). Liver injection, crude (Campolon, Pernaemon). Liver extract with stomach extract (Extralin).	1-15 micrograms of B_{12} q. 1-3 weeks. I.M. 1-2 micrograms of B_{12} q. 1-3 weeks. I.M. 1 U. o.d. Oral.	Used to stimulate the production of red blood cells. Owing to increased oxygen carrying power of the blood, these preparations also cause an increase in the activity of all the body organs.	Increase the activity of the hematopoietic organs.	Probably none in therapeutic dosage. May cause local irritation. Change site of injections regularly.	Liver extract is often added to other tonic and anti-anemic drugs.
VASODILATORS–ANTI-HYPERTENSIVES. See also drugs affecting the central and autonomic nervous systems, intoxicants, histamines, and diuretics.					
GANGLIONIC BLOCKING AGENTS. These are synthetic quaternary ammonium compounds unless otherwise stated.			These drugs all block passage of impulses of both the sympathetic and parasympathetic ganglia and produce symptoms similar to those of the sympatholytic and parasympatholytic drugs. When given orally they are (except mecamylamine) only incompletely and erratically absorbed from the gastrointestinal tract. Drugs are mainly confined to the extracellular fluids. Penetration of the blood-brain barrier is limited. Most are excreted unchanged by the kidneys.		
Azamethonium bromide (Pentiomide, Pentamin).	25-50 mg. I.V.	Ganglionic blocking agent used mainly for controlled hypotension during surgery and as an emergency anti-hypertensive agent.		May produce cardiovascular collapse. Treatment: epinephrine, levarterenol, or phenylephrine.	
Hexamethonium bromide (Bistrium bromide).	25-50 mg. Parenteral. 125 mg. q.i.d. Oral.	Used in severe hypertension and in peripheral vascular	See azamethonium.	Rare in therapeutic dosage. When toxic symptoms occur	This drug has largely been replaced by more

	Dosage varies with the condition of the patient.	disease.		they are similar to the mild toxic symptoms of the nitrites. Stop drug and treat symptoms. Contraindicated in coronary disease, renal disorders, and recent blood loss.	effective medicines.
Hexamethonium chloride.	0.125-0.25 Gm. Usually started q.i.d. Dosage is established individually. Oral.	Used for reduction of blood pressure.	See azamethonium.	Same as for others of this group. Contraindications same as for hexamethonium bromide.	Can be used for long-term administration. If patient is constipated, this should be corrected before drug is used. Also prepared for parenteral administration.
Mecamylamine hydrochloride, U.S.P. (Inversine) (dimecamine [C]).	2.5-10 mg. Dosage individually adjusted. Oral.	Exerts a strong hypotensive action. Usually used only in severe cases of hypertension.	Completely absorbed from the gastrointestinal tract. Widely distributed. Found in high concentration in liver and kidneys. It penetrates the blood-brain barrier. Slowly excreted unchanged by the kidneys.	Toxicity, side effects, and contraindications are the same as for other ganglionic blocking agents.	Not a quaternary.
Pentolinium tartrate (Ansolysen) (pentolonium [C]).	20-200 mg. Usually started q. 8 h. Individually adjusted. Oral, subcutaneous, or I.M. Not given I.V.	A potent ganglionic blocking agent whose main use is for hypertension. It is also useful in some peripheral vascular disorders.	See azamethonium.	Side effects are the same as for other ganglionic blocking agents.	
Trimethaphan camsylate, U.S.P. (Arfonad) (trimetaphan [C]).	1-4 mg./minute. Usually given in 1 mg./cc. concentration in 5% dextrose or normal saline as continuous drip until blood pressure has reached desired level. I.V.	Ganglionic blocking agent with direct vasodilating action. Main use for controlled hypotension during neurosurgery. Also used in hypertensive crisis.	Lowers both diastolic and systolic pressure in normotensive and hypertensive patients.	Toxicity low, but is similar to that of the nitrites.	Not a quaternary ammonium compound.
OTHER ANTIHYPERTENSIVE AND SIMILAR DRUGS. *Synthetic preparations unless otherwise noted.*					
Nicotinyl alcohol (Roniacol).	25-50 mg. t.i.d. Oral.	Used for vasodilation: peripheral vascular disease, migraine headache, neuralgia, and other conditions in which vasodilation of the superficial blood vessels is desired.	Vasodilation of superficial blood vessels.	Similar to the mild toxic symptoms of the nitrites, but rare in therapeutic dosage.	Also prepared in a delayed release tablet (150 mg. o.d.)

Name, Source, Synonyms, Preparations	Dosage and Administration	Uses	Action and Fate	Side Effects and Contraindications	Remarks
VASODILATORS (Continued)					
Cyclandelate (Cyclospasmol).	0.1-0.2 Gm. q.i.d. Oral.	A vasodilator used mainly in peripheral vascular diseases.	A spasmolytic agent with action similar to that of papaverine.	Toxicity low, but flushing and nausea may occur. Adjust dosage.	Safe use during pregnancy has not been established.
Diazoxide (Hyperstat).	300 mg. in 20 ml. given undiluted, rapidly, intravenously. Do not give I.M., subcutaneously or into body cavity. Use a superficial vein. May be repeated in 30 minutes, if required. Can be repeated in 4 to 24 hours to maintain reduction.	For the reduction of malignant hypertension in hospitalized patients, when rapid reduction of diastolic pressure is essential. Used as a temporary expedient. Orally effective drugs should be started as soon as possible.	Pressure usually reduced to lowest level in 5 minutes. Increases fairly rapidly for next 10 to 30 minutes, slowly for next 2 to 12 hours. Rarely reaches pretreatment level. Acts by relaxing smooth muscle tissue in peripheral arterioles. Cardiac output is increased as pressure is reduced. Renal blood flow is increased.	Side effects are frequent and serious: sodium and water retention after repeated injections, especially in patients with impaired cardiac reserve. Hyperglycemia is frequent, but usually requires treatment only in patients with diabetes mellitus. Infrequent but serious: hypotension to shock levels, myocardial and/or cerebral ischemia, atrial or ventricular arrhythmias, marked changes in ECG, unconsciousness, convulsions, paralysis, confusion, persistent retention of nitrogenous wastes in the blood stream after repeated injections, many other adverse reactions. Most are transient in nature.	Should be administered only to hospitalized patients where close monitoring of electrolytes, glycemic levels, cardiac and renal functions is possible. This drug is not effective against hypertension caused by pheochromocytoma.
Dioxyline phosphate (Paveril phosphate) (dimoxyline, Paverone [C]).	0.2-0.5 Gm. Once or twice daily. Oral.	Mainly used for muscle relaxation.	Action similar to that of papaverine.	Rare in therapeutic dosage.	
Dipyridamole (Persantine).	25-50 mg. Before meals t.i.d. Oral.	Used to treat coronary insufficiency and to prevent coronary and myocardial insufficiency. Improves the hypoxic heart.	A spasmolytic agent with special action on the myocardium. It is metabolized in the liver and excreted in the feces, either unchanged or as the glucuronide.	Headache, dizziness, nausea, flushing, mild gastrointestinal disturbances, syncope, and weakness. Reduce dosage or stop drug. Used with caution in hypotensive states. Not advised for acute phase of myocardial infarction.	

Hydralazine hydrochloride, N.F. (Apresoline) (hydralazine [C]).	25-50-100 mg. Oral. 20 mg. I.M. or I.V. Dosage individually adjusted.	Used to treat hypertension.	Acts chiefly on the midbrain, produces both adrenolytic and sympatholytic action. Blood flow through kidneys is increased. Well absorbed from gastrointestinal tract or parenteral sites. After oral dose maximum blood levels reached in 3 to 4 hours. Fate and excretion not well understood.	Rare in therapeutic dosage. When toxic symptoms do occur, they are similar to the mild toxic symptoms of the nitrites. There have been reports of cases resembling acute systemic lupus erythematosus and rheumatoid arthritis, which usually disappear when drug is withdrawn. Contraindications: coronary artery disease and mitral valvular rheumatic heart disease.	With high dosage arrhythmias are seen.
Mebutamate (Capla).	0.3 Gm. three or four times daily. Oral.	Mildly tranquilizing, antihypertensive agent. Used alone or in conjunction with other hypertensive drugs.	Said to act centrally to reduce the hypertensive effect of the stimulated vascular control centers in the hypothalamus, medulla and spinal vasomotor areas. It is metabolized by the liver and excreted by the kidneys.	Occasional drowsiness and lightheadedness have been reported. Contraindicated in persons with acute intermittent porphyria. Can have additive central nervous system depressant effects when used with other central nervous system depressants or psychotropic drugs. It is capable of inducing the hepatic microsomal enzymes which metabolize warfarin and other drugs.	Safe use in pregnancy and lactation has not been established.
NITRITES. *Salts and esters of nitrous acid and organic nitrates.* Amyl nitrite, N.F. (isoamylnitrate).	0.2 ml. inhalation. Comes prepared in perles, ready for crushing and inhaling.	Used for vasodilation, to lower blood pressure. Used in variety of conditions such as angina pectoris, chronic hypertension, asthma, pylorospasm, and certain forms of nervous disorders.	The nitrite ion relaxes smooth muscle tissue, especially of the coronary vessels. Antihypertensive action is less potent than that of some other drugs, but action on coronary vessels is stronger. These drugs also increase pulse rate, increase the rate and depth of respirations, and are antispasmodic in action.	Irregular pulse, headache, dizziness, rise in intraocular pressure, blurred vision, flushed face, palpitation, vomiting, diarrhea, mental confusion, muscular weakness, cyanosis, slowing of heart rate and respiratory rate. Any or all symptoms may occur. Deaths are rare. Stop drug and give evacuants. Cold applications	All these substances become nitrites in the body. Tolerance may occur, requiring change in form or dosage.
Erythrityl tetranitrate, N.F. (Cardilate) (erythrol tetranitrate [C]).	5-30 mg. p.r.n. Oral. 5-15 mg. p.r.n. Sublingual.				
Ethyl nitrite spirits (sweet spirits of niter, spirits of nitrous ether).	1-2 ml. p.r.n. Oral.				

DRUGS ACTING ON THE CIRCULATORY SYSTEM (Continued)

Name, Source, Synonyms, Preparations	Dosage and Administration	Uses	Action and Fate	Side Effects and Contraindications	Remarks
VASODILATORS (Continued)					
NITRITES (Continued)			Amyl nitrate is absorbed through the lungs. Nitroglycerin and others such as isorbide dinitrate and erythrityl tetranitrate are best absorbed sublingually. Other nitrates such as pentaerythritol tetranitrate, trolnitrate, sodium nitrite and mannitol hexanitrate are readily absorbed from the gastrointestinal tract. Some nitrate preparations can be absorbed through the skin. Both nitrite ions and organic nitrates disappear rapidly from the blood stream. The blood concentration from a single dose does not appear to be directly correlated with the therapeutic effects. About 2/3 of the nitrite ions disappear in the body and the exact fate and excretion are not well known.	to the head, artificial respiration, and shock therapy as indicated. Digitalis, strychnine, and sodium sulfate should be available.	
Glyceryl trinitrate spirit (nitroglycerin spirit).	0.06 ml. p.r.n. Oral.				Both nitroglycerin and pentaerythritol are available in sustained release form.
Isosorbide dinitrate (Isordil, Sorbitrate) (Coronex [C]).	2.5-10 mg. q. 4 h. or p.r.n. Oral or sublingual.				
Mannitol hexanitrate (Maxitate, Nitranitol).	15-60 mg. q. 4-6 h. Oral.				Mannitol hexanitrate is used cautiously in anemia as it tends to produce methemoglobin.
Nitroglycerin, U.S.P. (glyceryl trinitrate).	0.1-0.6 mg. p.r.n. Oral or sublingual.				
Pentaerythritol tetranitrate, N.F.	5-20 mg. One or 2 tablets as needed for anginal attacks. t.i.d. or q.i.d. for prophylaxis. Oral.				There are any number of proprietary names for nitroglycerin and pentaerythritol in the United States and Canada. Space does not permit their inclusion.
Sodium nitrite, U.S.P. (Anti-Rust, Filmerine).	30-60 mg. p.r.n. Oral.				Main use now is in instrument sterilizing solutions as an antirust agent.
Trolnitrate phosphate (Metamine, Nitretamin).	2-4 mg. t.i.d. p.c. and h.s. Oral.				
PAPAVERINE. *Active principle of the opium poppy.*		Used for vasodilation and as an antispasmodic to relieve gastric, intestinal, bronchial, biliary, and urethral colic. Also used in peripheral vascular disease and pulmonary embolism. It produces some sedation (mild), some coronary dilation, and some hypotension.	Smooth muscle tissue relaxant. Acts more on muscles in spasm than on those with normal tonus. Well absorbed from all routes. Some is localized in the fat tissue of the liver. A considerable amount is bound to plasma proteins. The exact extent of therapeutic effectiveness is not known,	Rare in therapeutic dosage. However, hepatic hypersensitivity has been reported with gastrointestinal symptoms, jaundice, and altered liver function tests.	No tolerance or habituation has been demonstrated. The sedative effect of papaverine is very limited and probably due to its antispasmodic action.
Papaverine hydrochloride, N.F.	0.03-0.1 Gm. Three to four times daily. Oral or parenteral.				

			but every 6 hour dosage appears adequate. It is excreted in an inactivated form by the kidneys.		
PARGYLINE HYDROCHLORIDE. *Synthetic.* Pargyline hydrochloride, N.F. (Eutonyl).	10-50 mg. Daily. Oral.	Antidepressant and antihypertensive agent used to treat most types of hypertension, but not recommended for labile hypertension or patients amenable to treatment with sedatives and the thiazide diuretics.	Monoamine oxidase inhibitor mainly used in the treatment of hypertension, but exact mechanism is not known.	Postural hypotension, gastrointestinal disturbances, insomnia, urinary frequency, dry mouth, nightmares, impotence, and edema have been reported. Congestive failure may occur in patients with reduced cardiac reserve. Used with caution if at all in labile or malignant hypertension, pregnancy, pheochromocytoma, renal failure, paranoid schizophrenia, and hyperthyroidism. Pargyline is a monoamine oxidase inhibitor. For interactions, see under Monoamine oxidase Inhibitors, page 74. Meperidine is contraindicated in patients taking pargyline. This drug should be discontinued 2 weeks before elective surgery.	Blood and liver tests should be done frequently. Patients should be warned against the taking of the following: over-the-counter cold preparations or antihistamines, alcoholic beverages, certain types of cheese.
VERATRUM. *Veratrum viride (green hellebore).* Alkavervir (Veriloid, Rauvera).	3-5 mg. t.i.d. q. 6-8 h. Oral. 1-3 mg. q. 2-3 h. I.M. 1-3 mg. in 10 ml. saline or dextrose. Given slowly. I.V.	Used as a vasodilator in the treatment of hypertension, angina pectoris, some cases of asthma. It is also used to treat emergency conditions such as toxemia of pregnancy, acute glomerulonephritis, and hypertensive encephalopathy. Sometimes used as a uterine sedative and general tranquilizer.	The hypotensive action is due chiefly to direct central nervous system action resulting in vasodilation. It reduces both the systolic and the diastolic pressure. It produces some bradycardia through reflexes in heart and lungs. It tends to reduce urinary output.	Substernal or epigastric burning sensation, anorexia, nausea, vomiting. Reduce dosage or stop drug and treat symptoms. In acute poisoning there may be cardiovascular collapse. Epinephrine or similar drug is used in treatment.	Varied preparations of *Veratrum* differ in their hypotensive effect. Their generally low toxicity allows prolonged usage. Dosage is individually adjusted. With continued use there is a tendency to gain weight. All preparations listed are a mixture of alkaloids.

DRUGS ACTING ON THE CIRCULATORY SYSTEM (Continued)

Name, Source, Synonyms, Preparations	Dosage and Administration	Uses	Action and Fate	Side Effects and Contraindications	Remarks
VASODILATORS (Continued)					
VERATRUM (Continued)			Only 5-20% of these alkaloids is absorbed from the gastrointestinal tract. The absorption is not only limited but variable. Little is known of the fate of these drugs in the body. Only a very small percentage is excreted unchanged by the kidneys.		
Cryptenamine acetate (Unitensin acetate).	1-2 mg. Used in emergencies. Repeated at 1-2 h. intervals until desired pressure is secured. I.M. or I.V.				
Cryptenamine tannate (Unitensin tannate) (Unitensyl [C]).	1-2 mg. Two or three times a day. Oral.				
Protoveratrine A (Protalba).	0.1-0.2 mg. Two or three times a day. Oral.				
Protoveratrine A & B (Veralba).	0.1-0.5 mg. Two or three times a day. Oral. 0.1-0.5 mg. q. 1-3 h. (See Cryptenamine acetate) I.V.				Protoveratrine A & B is a potent drug. I.V. administration is used only in hypertensive emergencies.
Protoveratrine A & B maleates (Provell maleate).	0.5-2.5 mg. Two or three times a day. Oral.				
CARDIOTONICS (Indirect Heart Stimulants).					
DIGITALIS *(glycosides, digitoxin). Digitalis purpurea and lanata.*	Dosages listed are maintenance doses, usually o.d.	Main use is to treat cardiac decompensation. Also used for other cardiac conditions. Used as an emergency drug and also for maintenance of the chronic patient. Preparations from *Digitalis purpurea* (primarily digitoxin) have slower and more prolonged action than those from *Digitalis lanata* (primarily digoxin). One unit of digitalis is equal to 0.1 gm. (100 mg.) of the powdered leaves. It is frequently used	Stimulates the vagus nerve, thus increasing the strength of the heart beat while decreasing its rate. The pulse is slower and stronger. Improvement in heart action relieves cyanosis, dyspnea, and cardiac edema. It also benefits all body processes by improving blood supply. Reduces high blood pressure and increases low blood pressure caused by circulatory disorder. Urinary output is increased in individuals with edema of cardiac origin.	Cumulative: slow pulse (below 60), anorexia, vomiting, irregular and intermittent pulse. Rapid change in pulse rate, diarrhea, abdominal pain, weakness, headache, vertigo, and visual disturbances may occur. Treatment: withhold further digitalis until the physician is notified. Keep patient quiet. Apply ice bag to precordium. Atropine and caffeine should be available. Other drugs that may be required include	Digitalis and similar products are given in a number of circumstances. Emergency: usually one large dose given intravenously to cover immediate needs. Rapid digitalization. One large dose or several doses given close together to produce desired effect in a few hours. Gradual digitalization: given in lesser doses and over a longer time so that digitalization takes several days. Digitalis products are irritating
Acetyldigitoxin, N.F. (Acylanid).	1-2 mg. Oral.				
Deslanoside, U.S.P. (Cedilanid-D).	0.3-0.8 mg. Oral.				
Digitalis powdered, U.S.P. (Digitora).	0.1 Gm. Oral.				
Digitalis tincture, N.F.	0.75-1.5 ml. Oral.				
Digitoxin, U.S.P. (Crystodigin, Digitaline-Nativelle, Myodigin, Purodigin, Unidigin) (digitoxoside [C]).	0.1-0.2 mg. Acetyl salt also available. Oral.				
Digitoxin injection, N.F.	0.2 mg. I.V.				
Digoxin, U.S.P. (Lanoxin) (Natigoxin, Nativelle, Reugoxin, Winoxin [C]).	0.125-0.5 mg. Oral.				

Digoxin injection, U.S.P., N.F. Gitalin amorphous, N.F. (Gitaligin). Lanatoside C, N.F. (Cedilanid). Lanatoside C injection.	0.1-0.5 mg. I.V. 0.3-0.8 mg. Oral. 0.5 mg. Oral. 0.5 mg. I.V.	to establish relative doses.	Most glycosides are absorbed from the intestinal tract, a little from the stomach. Absorption from parenteral sites, subcutaneous or intramuscular, is irregular and uncertain. Lanatoside C is absorbed only about 10%, digitalis, digilanid and digifolin about 20%, digoxin 50% and digitoxin 100%. Much of these drugs is bound to plasma protein, but this does not appear to greatly decrease their effectiveness. Ouabain is unbound and lanatoside C only slightly bound. Digoxin, more active than digitoxin, is excreted much more rapidly. Digoxin and lanatoside C are excreted by the kidneys largely unchanged. Digitoxin is broken down by the liver and the degradation products are excreted by the kidneys.	epinephrine, sodium phenobarbital, bromide, or the opiates. Drugs which can markedly increase plasma levels of calcium and those that decrease the plasma calcium level diminish effective use of digitalis preparations. The increase of calcium enhances the digitalis preparations. Thiazide diuretics, ethacrynic acid and furosemide can lead to hypercalcemic and hypomagnesic states. In these states, the digitalis glycosides are more apt to cause cardiac arrhythmias which are usually seen with high blood levels of these preparations.	to the tissues and are never given subcutaneously and rarely intramuscularly. Since drug is apt to cause cumulative poisoning, patients on long-term use should skip an occasional dose as directed by the physician. Many plants contain glycosides which act similarly to digitalis. However, digitalis, digitoxin, digoxin, and either strophanthin or ouabain are the drugs most commonly used. If one of these preparations is not effective, usually another will be. The other glycosides are not considered reliable.
STROPHANTHUS *(Strophanthin, Ouabain). Strophanthus bispidus* and *kombe.* Ouabain, U.S.P. (injection). Ouabain, U.S.P. Strophanthin-K (ampul) (K-Strophanthin).	As with digitalis, these are maintenance doses, and are usually given o.d. 0.5 mg. I.V. or I.M. 0.25-0.5 mg. b.i.d. Oral. 0.5 mg. I.V.	Used mostly for patients who need digitalis but do not respond to that drug. It is sometimes used to sustain a patient who has cumulative toxic symptoms from digitalis and cannot use that drug for a time.	Similar to digitalis but less reliable. The active principles act quickly.	Similar to digitalis but not so severe. Stop drug and treat symptoms.	Ouabain and strophanthin-K act somewhat faster than digitalis and are often used intravenously in emergencies.

DRUGS ACTING ON THE CIRCULATORY SYSTEM (Continued)

Name, Source, Synonyms, Preparations	Dosage and Administration	Uses	Action and Fate	Side Effects and Contraindications	Remarks
CARDIAC DEPRESSANTS					
Lidocaine hydrochloride 2% solution (Xylocaine 2%).	50-100 mg. I.V. under electrocardiographic monitoring at a rate of approximately 25-30 mg./min. If initial dose does not give desired response, dose may be repeated in 5 minutes. No more than 200-300 mg. should be given in a one-hour period. For a continuous infusion the rate is from 1-4 mg./min. under electrocardiographic monitoring.	Used in the management of acute ventricular arrhythmias.	Has been reported to exert antiarrhythmic effect by increasing the electrical stimulation threshold of the ventricles during diastole. Ninety per cent of dose is metabolized by the liver and 10 per cent is excreted unchanged by the kidneys.	Contraindicated in patients with a history of sensitivity to local anesthetics of the amide type, in patients with Adams-Stokes syndrome or with a severe degree of sino-atrial, atrioventricular or intraventricular block. Use with caution in the following: repeated use for patients with severe renal or liver disease, as it can induce toxic phenomena as a result of accumulation of the drug; patients with sinus bradycardia in whom this drug is used to eliminate ventricular ectopic beats if patient has had prior accelerated heart rate since it may provoke more frequent and serious ventricular arrhythmias.	Constant monitoring with the electrocardiograph is essential for the proper administration of this drug.
PROCAINAMIDE HYDROCHLORIDE *Synthetic* from procaine. Procainamide hydrochloride, U.S.P. (Pronestyl).	0.25-0.5 Gm. q. 4-6 h. Oral. 0.2 Gm. to 1 Gm. (100 mg./ml.) I.V. Dosage regulated to suit patient and condition.	Used in the treatment of ventricular tachycardia and atrial arrhythmias.	Decreases the irritability of the ventricular muscles, thus slowing pulse. Rapid and almost complete absorption after oral dose. Maximum blood level is reached in about 1 hour, after I.M. dose about 15 minutes. Widely distributed and except for brain, tissue concentrations are higher than plasma	May cause agranulocytosis in susceptible individuals. Hypotension may occur. Stop drug and treat symptoms. Contraindicated in kidney or liver disorders. When used shortly after surgery or in the immediate post-surgical period in which a polarizing or non-polarizing muscle relaxant has been given,	Check blood pressure frequently.

			concentrations. Most is excreted unchanged by the kidneys.	procainamide can cause a recurarization to occur.	
<u>Propranolol hydrochloride (Inderal)</u>. *Synthetic.*	10-30 mg. 3-4 times a day a.c. and h.s. 20-40 mg. 3-4 times a day a.c. and h.s. 60 mg. oral in divided doses for 3 days. 30 mg. daily in divided doses. 1-3 mg. I.V. given under ECG monitoring. Not to exceed 1 mg. per minute. Once an alteration is noted no more should be given until full effect is observed. A second dose may be given in 2 minutes, but no additional for 4 hours.	For cardiac arrhythmias. For hypertrophic subacute stenosis. Preoperatively for pheochromocytoma. Used concomitantly with an alpha adrenergic blocking agent for inoperable tumor. If excessive bradycardia occurs, atropine 0.5-1.0 mg. should be given I.V.	This is a beta adrenergic blocking agent. Blockage with this drug produces a decrease in heart rate, reduction in cardiac output, a reduction in resting stroke volume, a reduction in oxygen consumption and an increase in left ventricular end diastole pressure. This drug reduces pressor response to norepinephrine, potentiates that to epinephrine hydrochloride but has no effect on response to phenylephrine. It is widely distributed in the body, with the highest concentration in lungs, spleen and kidneys. After intravenous dose, the metabolic half-life is approximately 1 hour.	Side effects include nausea, vomiting, mild diarrhea, lightheadedness, mental depression, skin rash, paresthesia of hands, fever combined with sore throat, visual disturbances and hallucinations. Contraindications: bronchial asthma, allergic rhinitis during hay fever season, sinus bradycardia and greater than second degree or total heart block, cardiogenic shock, right ventricular or failure secondary to pulmonary hypertension, congestive heart failure, in patients receiving anesthetic agents that produce myocardial depression, and in patients receiving adrenergic augmenting psychotropic drugs (including the monoamine oxidase inhibitors) and during the two weeks withdrawal period from such drugs. Propranolol can increase the acute central nervous system toxicity of hexobarbital. Propranolol and quinidine have synergistic effects and the dose of both drugs can be reduced when they are given concurrently.	Commercial brochure should be consulted before giving this drug. Indications for the use of this drug are paroxysmal atrial tachycardia, sinus tachycardia and extra systoles (atrial and ventricular), atrial flutter and fibrillation, tachyarrhythmia of digitalis intoxication, ventricular tachycardias (when cardioversion technique is not available) in the management of hypertropic subaortic stenosis and pheochromocytoma. Safe use during pregnancy has not been established.

DRUGS ACTING ON THE CIRCULATORY SYSTEM (Continued)

Name, Source, Synonyms, Preparations	Dosage and Administration	Uses	Action and Fate	Side Effects and Contraindications	Remarks
QUINIDINE. *Active principle of cinchona.* Quinidine gluconate, U.S.P. (Quinaglute) (Quinate [C]). Quinidine hydrochloride, U.S.P. Quinidine polygalacturonate (Cardioquin). Quinidine sulfate, U.S.P. (Quinidate, Quinidex, Quinora) (Kinidine, Novoquinidin, Quincardine [C]).	0.3-0.5 Gm. I.M. or I.V. 0.2-0.4 Gm. q. 12 h. Oral. 0.2-0.4 Gm. p.r.n. Oral, I.M. or I.V. 275 mg. two to three times daily. Oral. 0.2-0.4 Gm. Two or three times a day. Oral. 300-500 mg. I.M. or I.V.	Used to decrease pulse rate in many cardiac and cardiovascular disorders.	Slows rate of impulses of the sinoauricular node. Depresses all activity of the heart muscle. There is reduced force, reduced tonus, and a prolonged refractory period. Produces a lessened heart rate. Rapidly and completely absorbed from the gastrointestinal tract. Maximum effects occur in 1-3 hours and last 6-8 hours. After I.M. dose, maximum effect in 1-1½ hours. An appreciable amount is bound to plasma protein. About half of the quinidine is excreted unchanged by the kidneys within 24 hours. The remainder is excreted as metabolic degradation products.	Same as quinine: ringing in ears, nausea, vomiting, dizziness, headache. Reduce or stop drug and treat symptoms. Antiarrhythmic effects of quinidine are enhanced in the presence of reserpine. When given together, the dose should be reduced. Quinidine, like procainamide, can cause recurarization in the immediate postoperative period. See page 134. Quinidine exerts a mild hypoprothrombinemic effect which can potentiate the action of warfarin-like compounds. Aluminum hydroxide and related antacids can cause a delay in the absorption of quinidine.	
BLOOD SUBSTITUTES (Blood Replacement). See also biologicals.		Used as substitutes for blood plasma; especially valuable in the control of shock resulting from hemorrhage. They are called plasma expanders.	These preparations maintain blood volume until nature can replenish it or whole blood or plasma can be secured.	Varied: drug may stay in the organs and act as a foreign body, but this is relatively rare. Treatment: symptomatic.	
COLLOIDAL SOLUTIONS. *Animal* and *vegetable.* Dextran (Expandex, Gentran, Plavolex) (Dextraven, LMD 10 per cent, Macrodex, Rheomacrodex [C]).	These are all given p.r.n. 6-12% solution. 250-500 ml. I.V.	A glucose polymer used to expand plasma and to maintain blood pressure in emergencies.	They remain in the body for 12-24 hours, are partly metabolized, and usually excreted by the kidneys.		
Dextran-40 (Rheomacrodex).	10-20 ml./kg. as sole primer or additive varying with volume of perfusion circuit. 10% solution added to normal saline or 5% dextrose I.V.	Used as a priming fluid, either as sole primer or an additive in pump oxygenator during extracorporeal circulation. Flow improver for cardiopulmonary bypass.	See uses.	Contraindications: thrombocytopenia, hypofibrinogenemia, renal disease with anuria or severe oliguria. Use with caution in poorly hydrated patients.	Dosage should not exceed 20 ml./kg. With dosage over recommended limits prolongation of bleeding time may occur.

PLASMA AND SERUM. *Human blood.*		General use same as for whole blood.	These contain all blood factors except cells, thus they do not produce any additional oxygen-carrying ability. Serum does not contain the clotting elements.	Rare: allergic reaction if any. Treatment: if needed, is anti-allergic. Since this is made from pooled human blood, it could contain the causative agent of serum hepatitis. This should be considered when it is administered.	
Albumin, normal human serum, U.S.P. (Albumisol, serum albumin).	2.2 ml. (cc)/kg. body weight. Given slowly, usually 250-500 ml. I.V.				
Antihemophilic human plasma, U.S.P.	50 ml. in 250 ml. diluent I.V.	Contains clotting factors. Used in hemorrhagic conditions.			
Antihemophilic factor (Factor VIII, AHF, AHG).	Varies with circumstances and with different patients. Parenteral.	Used in the treatment of hemophilia.	A stable dried preparation of human antihemophilic factor in concentrated form with minimal quantities of other protein. Action is substitutive.		Expiration date should be carefully checked.
Citrated normal human plasma.	250-1000 ml. I.V. Occasionally given in small doses I.M.				
Fibrinogen, U.S.P. (Parenogen).	1-2 Gm. with 50-200 ml. of diluent. I.V.	Used in hemorrhagic conditions.			
Plasma, normal human, U.S.P.	250-1000 ml. I.V. Occasionally given in small doses I.M.				
Plasma protein fraction, U.S.P. (Plasmanate).	5% solution, 250 ml. I.V.	Used to combat hypoproteinemia and in same conditions as albumin.			
Salt poor serum albumin 25%.	50-100 ml. Usually given every 24 hours until symptoms subside. I.V.	Used in nephrosis and other conditions in which there is hypoproteinemia.			
SALINE SOLUTIONS. *Water and various salts.*		Used to restore blood volume in hemorrhage and blood pressure in shock, and to compensate for fluid loss from burns, dehydration, and many similar conditions. Also as a means of giving needed I.V. medications.	Electrolyte solutions given to maintain balance. The type used depends upon the needs of the patient. Isotonic sodium chloride is used if sodium is depleted, potassium preparations in potassium depletion. Other solutions contain several electrolytes and are used as general replacement.	Rare in therapeutic use.	
Sodium chloride solution isotonic, U.S.P. (normal saline solution).	100-1000 ml. I.V. or subcutaneous.				
Sodium chloride solution (0.45 per cent) (one-half isotonic).	100-1000 ml. I.V.				
Sodium chloride solution (0.2 per cent).	100-1000 ml. I.V.				
Lactated Ringer's solution, U.S.P., (Hartmann's solution).	100-1000 ml. I.V. or subcutaneous.				

DRUGS ACTING ON THE CIRCULATORY SYSTEM (Continued)

Name, Source, Synonyms, Preparations	Dosage and Administration	Uses	Action and Fate	Side Effects and Contraindications	Remarks
SALINE SOLUTIONS (Continued)					
Multiple (balanced) electrolytes (Butler's solution, Ionosol MB, Talbot's solution, Travert's solution).	100-1000 ml. I.V. or subcutaneous.				
Potassium acetate, bicarbonate and citrate solution.	100-1000 ml. I.V. or subcutaneous.				
Potassium chloride injection, U.S.P.	0.3% solution 1000 ml. I.V. (over 4 hour period).				
Potassium chloride in dextrose (Kadalex).	100-1000 ml. I.V. or subcutaneous.				
Potassium lactate solution (Darrow's solution, Potassic saline, Ionosol P.S.L.).	40-100 ml./kg. of body weight. I.V. or subcutaneous.				
Ringer's solution, N.F. (3 Chlorides, Triple Chloride).	100-1000 ml. I.V. or subcutaneous.				
Sodium lactate, injection, U.S.P.	1000 ml. 1/6 molar solution. I.V.				
SUGAR SOLUTIONS. *Water and various monosaccharides and disaccharides.*		Used for the same purposes as the saline solutions, with added nutrients. Strong solutions are diuretic in action and reduce edema, especially meningeal.	Dextrose is prepared in isotonic sodium chloride and also in distilled water for use as patient's condition indicates. These solutions provide an easily metabolized source of calories.	Rare in therapeutic use.	
Dextrose solution, U.S.P.	100-1000 ml. Dextrose is used in strengths varying from 2 to 50%. I.V.				
Fructose injection (Levugen) N.F.	10% solution. 100-1000 ml. I.V.				
WHOLE BLOOD. *Human blood.*					
Citrated whole human blood, U.S.P.	200-1000 ml. I.V.	Used to replace blood. Also used in the treatment of shock, burns, debility, and certain diseases (especially diseases of the blood).	If blood is compatible, action is same as that of patient's blood.	If blood is compatible there is usually no toxic reaction. Otherwise, chills, anxiety, back pain, flushing of the face, tachycardia, dyspnea, and allergic symptoms may occur. Treatment: anti-allergic and symptomatic.	Blood may be obtained from public or private donors or from blood banks. The possibility of the transfer of viral diseases such as serum hepatitis or of protozoal infections such as malaria should not be overlooked. Typing and cross matching are required.
Packed human blood cells, U.S.P.	Equivalent of 1 unit (500 ml.) of whole blood. I.V.	As above.			

CHEMOTHERAPY OF NEOPLASTIC DISEASES. See also hematinics and radioactive drugs.		Used, occasionally, as an ingredient in "tonic" proprietary preparations as a general tonic or alterative. Previously it was thought to increase the number of red blood cells; this is not generally accepted. Used as a specific in certain diseases, as a white blood cell depressant in certain leukemias, and in certain skin disorders.	Depresses cell respiration. Readily absorbed from all mucous membranes and parenteral sites. Some lipid preparations of arsenic are at least partially absorbed through the skin. Rapidly leaves the blood stream and deposits in the tissues, probably as protein thioarsenite. It is stored mainly in the liver, kidneys, walls of the intestinal tract, spleen and lungs. Much smaller amounts are in muscle and nervous tissue. Arsenic is slowly excreted in the urine and feces. Excretion starts within 2-8 hours, but may take as long as 10 days for elimination to be complete after a single dose.	Anorexia, nausea, and other gastrointestinal disorders may occur. Acute poisoning: nausea, vomiting, diarrhea, neuritis, uremia, and death. Have BAL (British antilewisite) available for use if needed. Treat symptoms. Chronic poisoning: swelling of eyelids, injection of conjunctiva, nausea, vomiting, diarrhea, skin rashes. Stop drug and treat symptoms.	
ARSENIC. *Mineral.*					
Arsenic trioxide (arsenous acid, white arsenic).	2 mg. Oral.				
Arsenous acid solution (hydrochloric solution of arsenic, arsenic chloride solution).	0.2 ml. Usually given t.i.d. p.c. and increased 0.06 ml. per day until a stated amount (0.55 ml.) is reached, then reduced 0.06 ml. each day or stopped for a period of 10-14 days. Oral.				
Potassium arsenite solution (Fowler's solution).	0.2 ml. Same as above. Oral.				
Sodium cacodylate.	60 mg. weekly. I.M.				
DACTINOMYCIN. *Streptomyces parvelbus.*		Used only in palliative treatment of hospitalized patients with Wilms's tumor, rhabdomyosarcoma and carcinoma of the testis and uterus.	Exact mechanism is not known. It is believed that this drug concentrates in the submaxillary glands, liver and kidneys. About half is excreted unchanged in the bile, about 10% in the urine.	Toxic reactions are frequent and may be severe. This is not dose dependent.	Commercial brochure should be consulted before administering this drug.
Dactinomycin, U.S.P. (Cosmogen) (Actinomycin D [C]).	0.5 mg. daily for a maximum of 5 days. I.V. Children: 15 micrograms/kg. daily for a maximum of 5 days. I.V.				

DRUGS ACTING ON THE CIRCULATORY SYSTEM (Continued)

Name, Source, Synonyms, Preparations	Dosage and Administration	Uses	Action and Fate	Side Effects and Contraindications	Remarks
SYNTHETIC PREPARATIONS.					
Busulfan, U.S.P. (Myleran) (busulphan [C]).	2-4 mg. Dosage adjusted individually. Oral.	Used in the treatment of chronic myelocytic leukemia.	Depresses bone marrow but not lymphoid tissue. Produces remissions of a few weeks to several months. May depress thrombocytes. Well absorbed orally. Found mainly in the nuclei of the myelocytic cells. It is excreted almost entirely as methanesulfonic acid in the urine.	After small or average doses, nausea and vomiting may occur. After heavy doses, bone marrow depression has been reported. Reduce dosage or stop drug and treat symptoms.	The doctor should weigh potential benefits of the use of these drugs during pregnancy or in women of child-bearing age against the possible teratogenic effects. Frequent blood counts, including platelets (at least weekly), should be done during therapy.
Chlorambucil, U.S.P. (Leukeran) (Leukran [C]).	0.1-0.2 mg./kg. of body weight. Dosage individually adjusted. Oral.	Used for the treatment of chronic lymphatic leukemia and malignant lymphomas, including Hodgkin's disease.	A derivative of nitrogen mustard drugs which is cytotoxic. Gives symptomatic relief and general remissions of varying lengths. Produces a rapid reduction in total white blood cell count. Good oral absorption, but fate in body is not known.	Small or average doses may produce nausea and vomiting. After heavy doses, bone marrow depression has been reported. Reduce dosage or stop drug and treat symptoms.	See above.
Cyclophosphamide, N.F. (Cytoxan) (Procytox [C]).	25-50 mg. Oral. 100-500 mg. into tumor. Dosage individually adjusted. I.V., I.M., I.P.	Used for palliative treatment of Hodgkin's disease, lymphomas, acute and chronic leukemias, multiple myeloma, mycosis fungoides, neuroblastoma, adenocarcinoma of ovary, retinoblastoma.	A nitrogen mustard derivative with similar but more prolonged action. Readily absorbed after oral dose. Maximum plasma levels in about 1 hour. A large part of an oral dose excreted in stools, a small part in the urine. Exact fate in body is not well known, but it concentrates in neoplastic tissue.	Toxicity similar to that of the nitrogen mustard drugs, but somewhat less toxic. When used in nephrotic syndrome and arthritis, sterility in the male and the female must be considered. Adequate fluid intake and frequent voiding will help prevent the development of cystitis. Dosage must be reduced in adenocarcinoma of ovary,	See package insert for details of administration, toxicity, etc. Cytoxin should not be stored at temperatures above 90° F.

Cytarabine (Cytosar) (cytosine arabinoside [C]).	Dosage individually adjusted. For induction of therapy the I. V. route is usually best, with subcutaneous for maintenance. 1 mg./kg. weekly or semiweekly subcutaneously has been found satisfactory for maintenance in the majority of patients.	Used for the induction of remission of acute granulocytic leukemia and secondarily for other acute leukemias in adults and children.	This drug is cytotoxic to a variety of mammalian cells in tissue culture. It is believed to exert its primary effect by inhibition of deoxycytidine synthesis. After I.V. administration only 5-8% is excreted unaltered in the urine after 24 hours. It is deaminated to arabinofuranosyl uracil (an inactive metabolite) by the liver and possibly by the kidneys. 15 minutes after a single high I.V. dose, the blood level falls to unmeasurable amounts in most patients. The drug is excreted by the kidneys as the above mentioned metabolite.	Leukopenia, thrombocytopenia, bone marrow suppression, megaloblastosis, anemia, nausea, vomiting, diarrhea, oral inflammation or ulceration, thrombophlebitis, hepatic dysfunction and fever occur most often. For other side effects and the drug's use for children, see package insert. Contraindications: patients with pre-existing drug-induced bone marrow suppression, unless the physician feels that such management offers the most helpful alternative.	When this drug is used, the patient should be under close medical supervision, and during induction therapy should have daily leukocyte and platelet counts. In patients with poor liver function, dosage should be reduced. In use of this drug during pregnancy or in women of child-bearing age, the potential hazards must be weighed against possible benefits. Safe use in infants has not been established.
5-Fluorouracil (Fluorouracil, Efudex).	Dosage individually adjusted. I.V. but no more than 800 mg. daily.	Used in the palliative treatment of carcinoma of breast, colon, rectum, stomach and pancreas.	It is believed to block the methylation reaction of deoxyuridilic acid to thymidylic acid. It then interferes with the synthesis of DNA.	Bone marrow depression, stomatitis, diarrhea, gastrointestinal ulcerations and bleeding, and hemorrhage may occur. Relatively toxic drug.	Not an antileukemic drug.
	Solution 2-5% or cream 5% b.i.d. Topical.	Used to treat solar keratoses.	The drug is administered I.V. since the oral route attenuates its effectiveness. It is reduced in the body to urea and CO_2. The former is excreted in the urine, the latter through the lungs.	Given with caution in patients considered poor risks. Local adverse reactions include: dermatitis, scarring, soreness and tenderness.	With topical use, if an occlusive dressing is applied, there may be an increase in the incidence of inflammatory reactions. During therapy, prolonged exposure to ultraviolet light should be avoided.

DRUGS ACTING ON THE CIRCULATORY SYSTEM (Continued)

Name, Source, Synonyms, Preparations	Dosage and Administration	Uses	Action and Fate	Side Effects and Contraindications	Remarks
SYNTHETIC PREPARATIONS (Continued)					
Floxuridine (FUDR).	0.1-0.6 mg./kg. daily. Intra-arterial infusion only. (Higher doses usually used hepatic artery infusion, since liver metabolizes drug. Less risk of toxicity.)	Palliative management of carcinoma by regional, intra-arterial infusion in patients considered incurable by surgery or other means. Best results are achieved by use of pump to overcome pressure in large arteries.	It is rapidly metabolized to 5-fluorouracil. Its action is to interfere with the synthesis of DNA. After it is metabolized, it acts mainly on RNA to inhibit its formation.	Has all the toxic manifestations of 5-fluorouracil. Side effects: nausea, vomiting, diarrhea, enteritis, stomatitis and localized erythema. Laboratory abnormalities include anemia, leukopenia, elevations of alkaline phosphatase, serum transaminase, serum bilirubin and lactic dehydrogenase. See brochure for others.	Therapy is continued until adverse symptoms occur. May be restarted as they subside. Floxuridine is a highly toxic drug with a narrow margin of safety. For this reason, close supervision is required, since therapeutic response is unlikely to occur without some evidence of toxicity. Caution. Therapy should be discontinued at first signs of stomatitis, pharyngitis, leukopenia (WBC below 3500) or a rapidly falling WBC, vomiting, intractable diarrhea, gastrointestinal ulceration, thrombocytopenia, platelet count below 100,000 or hemorrhage.
Melphalan, U.S.P. (Alkeran).	6 mg. daily for 2-3 weeks; discontinue for up to 4 weeks; then start maintenance dose of 2 mg. daily.	Used in the treatment of multiple myeloma.	Alkylating agent consisting of phenylalanine nitrogen mustard which has been found useful in multiple myeloma. Good oral absorption. Exact fate in body is not known, but it is believed the metabolic products are excreted through the kidneys.	Nausea and vomiting, depression of the bone marrow. Should not be given concurrently with radiation treatment.	
Mercaptopurine, U.S.P. (Purinethol).	50 mg. Oral.	Used to reduce the white blood cell count, especially in leukemia.	Depresses bone marrow. Reduces white cell count. Causes temporary remission. Readily absorbed from the	Nausea, vomiting, moderate lymphopenia, neutropenia, anemia, and thrombocytopenia may occur. Occasionally bleeding occurs. Stop	Also available as the methyl derivative. Frequent blood counts should be done. If a sudden large reduction in white

			intestinal tract. Plasma half-life about 1½ hours. Rapidly metabolized. Metabolites excreted by the kidneys.	drug and treat symptoms. When mercaptopurine and allopurinol are given concurrently, the dose of mercaptopurine must be reduced to as little as ⅓ to ¼ of the usual dose.	blood cells occurs, stop drug.
Methotrexate, U.S.P. (amethopterin).	5-30 mg. Dosage individually adjusted. Oral or parenteral.	Used in the treatment of acute leukemia. Also used to treat uterine choriocarcinoma and testicular tumors. Chemotherapy of psoriasis.	A folic acid antagonist which often produces remissions. Well absorbed from the gastrointestinal tract. Part is rather rapidly excreted in the urine. Significant amounts of the drug are retained in the body, particularly in the liver and kidneys, for long periods (sometimes for months).	As with all such drugs, hemopoietic system depression may occur. Leucovorin is an effective antidote if given soon enough after dose of methotrexate. When given concurrently with sulfisoxazole, methotrexate is replaced from plasma binding sites, and this can raise the levels of methotrexate to possible toxic amounts.	Blood counts twice weekly recommended. Citrovorum factor I.M. aids in avoiding damage to such structures as intestinal mucosa and bone marrow. The patient should be fully informed of the risks involved and should be under the constant supervision of the physician.
Mithramycin (Mithracin).	25-30 mcg./kg. daily for 8-10 days. Dose not to exceed 30 mcg./kg. Drug should be diluted in 5% glucose in water and given slowly. I.V. over a 4-6 hour period. 25 mcg./kg. for 3-4 days. If desired reduction is not secured, course may be repeated in one week or more to achieve normal calcium levels in serum and urine. A single weekly dose may maintain normal levels once they are obtained.	Used for certain inoperable testicular malignancies. In patients with hypercalcemia and hypercalciuria associated with a variety of advanced neoplasms.	The exact mechanism of action is not known, but it has been shown to form a complex deoxyribonucleic acid (DNA) and to inhibit cellular ribonucleic acid (RNA) and enzymic synthesis. The binding of the DNA (in presence of divalent cation) is responsible for inhibition of DNA-dependent or DNA-directed RNA synthesis.	The most important side effect is a bleeding syndrome. For others refer to package insert. Contraindications: thrombocytopenia, thrombocytopathy, any coagulation disorder or an increased susceptibility to bleeding due to other causes, in patients with bone marrow impairment or in patients who are not hospitalized.	

DRUGS ACTING ON THE CIRCULATORY SYSTEM (Continued)

Name, Source, Synonyms, Preparations	Dosage and Administration	Uses	Action and Fate	Side Effects and Contraindications	Remarks
SYNTHETIC PREPARATIONS (Continued)					
Pipobroman, N.F. (Vercyte).	Initial dose 1 mg./kg./day. Larger doses up to 1.5-3.0 mg./kg./day may be used. Not to exceed 30 days. When hematocrit is 50-55% maintenance dose is 0.1-0.2 mg./kg./day. Oral.	To treat polycythemia vera.	This is classified as an alkylating agent. Exact mechanism of action is not known.	Should not be given to patients with bone marrow depression following x-ray or cytotoxic chemotherapy.	Not recommended for children or during pregnancy.
	1.5-2.5 mg./kg./day initial dose. Oral. Maintenance dosage individually adjusted.	To treat chronic granulocytic leukemia.			
Procarbazine (Matulane) (Natulan [C]).	100-200 mg. daily for 1st week, then 200 mg. daily until white count falls below 4000 per cu. mm. or the platelet count is below 100,000 per cu. mm. or until maximum response is obtained. For children the dose is highly individualized, and very close monitoring is essential because of possible adverse side effects. Dosage is usually started with 50 mg. daily for one week, then maintained at 100 mg./sq. m. of body surface (to the closest 50 mg.) until leukopenia, thrombocytopenia or maximum response is reached.	Indicated for the palliative treatment of generalized Hodgkin's disease and for those patients who have become resistant to other forms of therapy.	The exact mode of action has not been clearly defined but it is believed the drug may act by inhibition of protein, DNA and RNA synthesis. No cross-resistance with other chemotherapeutic agents, radiotherapy or steroids has been demonstrated.	Occurring frequently: leukopenia, anemia, thrombocytopenia, nausea and vomiting. There are many other less common side effects; refer to package insert. Contraindications: in patients known to be hypersensitive or those with inadequate bone marrow reserve. This should be considered in patients who have leukopenia, thrombocytopenia and/or anemia. Use during pregnancy or for women of childbearing age should be carefully weighed, potential benefits against possible hazards. Meperidine should not be used in patients taking procarbazine.	Alcoholic intake should be stopped when this drug is given, as it can possibly give a disulfiram-like reaction. Procarbazine has some monoamine oxidase inhibitor activity. Foods high in tyramine content should be avoided, as should sympathomimetic drugs and the tricyclic antidepressants. One month interval should be allowed following termination of therapy with radiation or with drugs with bone marrow depressant action before starting this drug.

NITROGEN MUSTARDS Mechlorethamine hydrochloride, U.S.P. (Mustargen) (Methyl bis beta chloroethylamine hydrochloride) (chlomethine, mustine [C]).	Dosages individually adjusted. 10 mg. in 20 ml. I.V. 0.1 mg./kg. of body weight given in isotonic saline solution. Do not give into tissues, as severe damage may occur. I.V.	Used to reduce the white blood cell count, especially in leukemia. Also used in lymphosarcoma, Hodgkin's disease, lymphoblastoma of the skin, and mycosis fungoides.	A polyfunctional alkylating agent cytotoxic to cell tissue; affects the mitotic cells first, thereby destroying malignant tissue before normal tissue. Readily absorbed, but usually given I.V. Rapidly metabolized. Little or none is excreted unchanged by the kidneys.	Nausea, vomiting, moderate lymphopenia, neutropenia, anemia, and thrombocytopenia may occur. Occasionally bleeding occurs. Stop drug and treat symptoms. Toxic to tissue, vesicant to skin; avoid infiltration; margin of safety small.	The doctor should weigh potential benefits of use of these drugs during pregnancy or in women of childbearing age against the teratogenic effects. Frequent blood counts, including platelets, should be done during therapy. Use only freshly prepared solutions.
Uracil mustard.	1-2 mg. As much as 5 mg. given in one day. Oral.	Mainly used in chronic leukemia, lymphosarcoma, and Hodgkin's disease.	Quickly but incompletely absorbed orally. Rapidly disappears from the circulation. Drug is almost completely metabolized by the body.		
PHENYLHYDRAZINES.	Dosages individually adjusted	Used to reduce the red blood cell count, especially in polycythemia vera. It depresses the erythropoietic activity of the red bone marrow.	Depresses red cell count without appreciably changing white count.	Hypoplastic anemia and liver damage may occur. Stop drug and treat symptoms.	Watch hemoglobin and stop drug when it reaches 100% or goes below this figure. Radioactive phosphorus has largely replaced this drug.
Acetylphenylhydrazine.	0.1 Gm. Oral.				
Phenylhydrazine.	0.1-0.26 Gm. Three times weekly. Oral.				
OTHER SYNTHETIC PREPARATIONS. Hydroxyurea (Hydrea).	80 mg./kg. every third day, orally, or 20-30 mg./kg. daily, orally (each based on actual or ideal weight, whichever is less). 20-30 mg./kg. daily (single dose), orally.	Solid tumors. Until intermittent therapy can be evaluated. Myelocytic leukemia (resistant chronic).	Mechanism of action is not known. It is believed to act by inhibition of the synthesis of DNA without affecting RNA or protein synthesis.	Side effects: bone marrow depression (leukopenia, thrombocytopenia, anemia), gastrointestinal symptoms (stomatitis, nausea, vomiting, diarrhea), some dermatological reactions (maculopapular rash), alopecia and some neurological symptoms have been reported. Contraindications: marked bone marrow depression (below 2500 WBC), thrombocytopenia (below 100,000) or severe anemia and in women of child-bearing age.	Precautions: complete blood picture including bone marrow examination and liver function tests should be done prior to—and repeatedly during—treatment with this drug. Hemoglobin, leukocyte and platelet counts should be done weekly.

Name, Source, Synonyms, Preparations	Dosage and Administration	Uses	Action and Fate	Side Effects and Contraindications	Remarks
OTHER SYNTHETIC PREPARATIONS (Continued)					
Megestrol acetate (Megace).	40 mg. daily in divided doses. Oral. Given as long as beneficial results are seen. Adequate trial period is 2 months of continuous therapy.	Used as adjunct or palliative treatment of recurrent or metastatic endometrial carcinoma.	Mechanism of action is not known but it is thought to act by an antiluteinizing effect mediated through the pituitary gland. The compound possesses biological properties similar to progesterone.	Side effects: feeling of coldness. Caution. Used with caution in patients with a history of thrombophlebitis.	
Testolactone (Teslac).	100 mg. three times a week I.M. 50 mg. t.i.d. Oral. However, up to 2000 mg./day has been given.	Used as adjunctive therapy in the palliative treatment of advanced disseminated breast cancer in postmenopausal women when hormone therapy is indicated. It may be used for premenopausal women in whom ovarian function has been terminated.	The precise mechanism of action is not known. The chemical configuration is similar to that of the androgens, but it is devoid of androgenic activity in the commonly employed dosage.	Maculopapular erythema, increased blood pressure, paresthesia, aching and edema of extremities, nausea, vomiting and hot flashes; however, some of the adverse symptoms could be due to the disease and cannot always be attributed to the drug. Pain and local inflammation at site of injection is seen. Contraindicated in the treatment of breast cancer in men.	Treatment should be continued for at least 3 months in order to evaluate the response unless there is active progression of the disease. The drug has been found to be effective in about 15% of the patients. treated. Warning: Calcium levels should be monitored routinely, especially during times of active remission of bony metastases. If hypercalcemia occurs, steps should be taken to lower this level.
Thioguanine, N.F.	Dosages individually adjusted. Usually, initial dose is 2 mg./kg./day. If not effective after 14-21 days, 3 mg./kg./day may be tried. Effective maintenance dose is usually 2 mg./kg./day.	Used to treat acute leukemia. Has been used in chronic granulocytic leukemia. This may provide sustained remission and avoid early relapse.	Causes a depletion of bone marrow with neutropenia, reticulopenia, anemia, thrombocytopenia and prolonged clotting time.	Nausea, vomiting, anorexia and stomatitis may occur. Toxic hepatitis may be related to this drug. If jaundice appears drug should be stopped. Dosage should be reduced if used concurrently with allopurinol.	Not used in chronic lymphocytic leukemia. Not advised during the first trimester of pregnancy. Weekly blood counts are recommended. Drug should be discontinued at first signs of abnormal bone marrow depression.
Triethylenemelamine, N.F. (Tretamine, TEM) (tetramine, triethanomelamine [C]).	0.5-5 mg. Usually given daily 1-2 hours before breakfast with sodium	Used to reduce the white blood cell count, especially in leukemia. Also used in	Polyfunctional alkylating agents similar to nitrogen mustard.	May cause nausea and vomiting. Reduce dosage or stop drug and treat symptoms.	Parenteral solutions must be prepared fresh for each administration. As with all

	bicarbonate, orally. Individually adjusted I.V., I.M., intra-tumor, intraserosal.	Hodgkin's disease, lympho-sarcoma, polycythemia vera, mycosis fungoides, carcinoma of lung and ovaries, metastatic cancer of ovary or breasts, epithelial carcinoma, and cutaneous melanoma.	Absorbed orally. Converted to ethylenimonium quaternary compound which reacts with functional groups of many cell protein enzyme systems. Very little excreted unchanged in the urine.	If used during pregnancy, this drug can cause congenital anomalies.	these drugs, frequent blood counts should be done.
Triethylene-thio-phosphoramide (Thio-Tepa).	0.2 mg./kg. daily for no more than 5 days. I.M. 40-50 mg. intracarotid q. 6-8 weeks. 10-60 mg. intratumor. 10-50 mg. intraserosal.	Used in the palliative treatment of a number of diseases.	See above. Usually given by injection because of erratic oral absorption. It rapidly acts with cellular elements. About half of the drug is eliminated unchanged in the urine. The remainder is metabolized, but the metabolites have not been identified.	Nausea, vomiting, anorexia, and headache may occur. Hemopoietic depression (all formed elements) mild to severe has been reported. This drug is actively teratogenic.	See above.
VINBLASTINE. *Alkaloid of Vinca rosea linn.* Vinblastine sulfate, U.S.P. (Velban) (Velbe [C]).	0.1-0.15 mg./kg. of body weight I.V.	Used to treat Hodgkin's disease and choriocarcinoma that are resistant to other therapy, histiocytosis, lymphosarcoma and reticulum cell sarcoma.	It is believed to interfere with metabolic pathways of amino acids, leading from glutamic acid to the citric acid cycle and to urea. Also, vinblastine has an effect on cell energy production required for mitosis and interferes with nucleic acid synthesis.	Not well established, but apparently similar to other drugs used for these conditions. Contraindicated if W.B.C. count is under 4000/cu. mm. and in bacterial infections.	These drugs may possibly have teratogenic effects. Consult commercial brochure for more complete details.
Vincristine sulfate, U.S.P. (Oncovin).	Dose in children 0.05 to 0.15 mg./kg. Weekly. I.V.	Acute leukemia in children.	Mechanism of action is not known. Drug leaves blood stream rapidly after infusion. Most is excreted through the bile and feces, only a small amount by way of the kidneys.		

DRUGS ACTING ON THE CIRCULATORY SYSTEM (Continued)

Name, Source, Synonyms, Preparations	Dosage and Administration	Uses	Action and Fate	Side Effects and Contraindications	Remarks
SCLEROSING AGENTS					
QUININE HYDROCHLORIDE AND URETHANE. *Synthetic and from cinchona.* Quinine and urea hydrochloride, U.S.P.	0.5-5 ml. Into varicosities.	Used to produce sclerosing, thrombosis, and obliteration of varicose veins and hemorrhoids.	Action of these solutions varies slightly, but most destroy the endothelium and set up a fibrosing (scarring) process, which eventually obliterates the vein.	Drowsiness and gastrointestinal distrubances may occur. Severe symptoms are rare. Treatment: none usually required. Contraindicated in pregnancy, during menstruation, or in the presence of cardiac diseases, nephritis, diabetes, upper respiratory infections, phlebitis, or suppurative ulceration, or incompetence of the deep veins.	
SODIUM MORRHUATE. *Cod liver oil.* Sodium morrhuate injection, U.S.P.	0.5-5 ml. of a 5% solution into varicosities. Used with vein ligation in large veins and without ligation in small veins.	See above.	See above.	Rare in therapeutic usage. Treatment: none usually required.	
SODIUM TETRADECYL. *Synthetic.* Sodium tetradecyl sulfate (Sotradecol, Trombovar [C]).	1-5% solution. Injection into varicosities.	See above.	See above.	As above. This drug is contraindicated during pregnancy.	
ANTICOAGULANTS. (Prothrombin time should be checked regularly when giving any of these drugs.)					
In Vitro					
SODIUM CITRATE AND SIMILAR PREPARATIONS. *Chemical, Food, Synthetic.*		Used to prevent blood clotting outside the blood vessels, as in indirect transfusions.	Prevents clotting in vitro but does not prevent clotting in vivo.	None.	

Sodium citrate solution, anti-coagulant, N.F.	For whole blood. 50 ml. will prevent coagulation of 450 ml. of whole blood.				
In Vivo BISHYDROXYCOUMARIN. *Spoiled sweet clover hay. Synthetic.*	Dosages are adjusted daily as indicated by the prothrombin time.	Used to prolong the clotting time of blood and to treat thrombophlebitis, pulmonary embolism, certain cardiac conditions, or any disorder in which there is excessive or undesirable clotting. It is especially valuable in thrombosis and embolism, except in cases of bacterial endocarditis.	Prolongs the clotting time of blood by preventing the production of prothrombin in the liver. The action of these drugs is slower but more prolonged than that of heparin. They are often given with heparin to secure both immediate and delayed action. Coumarin products are used for maintenance. Oral absorption is slow and erratic and varies widely with the individual. Most is bound to plasma proteins, widely distributed throughout the body, but little reaches the brain. Slowly metabolized by the body, but a small percentage is excreted by the kidneys. Plasma levels may be maintained for up to 5 days.	Not common, but hemorrhage may occur. either as one large local hemorrhage or as a number of smaller bleeding points. Stop drug, give whole blood or coagulants. Phytonadione (vitamin K_1) may be ordered. Cumulative action may occur. Also seen are alopecia, urticaria, dermatitis, fever, nausea, diarrhea and hypersensitivity reactions. Oral anticoagulants cross the placental barrier and danger of fatal hemorrhage in the fetus in utero may exist even within the accepted therapeutic range of maternal prothrombin level. The doctor must determine if potential benefits outweigh possible risks.	Many factors can influence the prothrombin time of people on anticoagulant therapy. Among these are: diet, environment, physical state and other medications. The patient should understand that other drugs should be added or stopped only under the physician's direct observation so that additional prothrombin times can be taken to determine the effect. See brochure for the endogenous and exogenous factors which may influence the prothrombin time response.
Acenocoumarol (Sintrom) (acenocoumarin, nicoumaline [C]).	4-16 mg. Oral.				
Bishydroxycoumarin, U.S.P. (Dicumarol) (dicoumarin, Dufalone [C]).	50-200 mg. q.d. Oral.				
Phenprocoumon, N.F. (Liquamar) (Marcumar [C]).	0.75-4.5 mg. Oral.				
WARFARIN SODIUM. *Synthetic.* Sodium warfarin, U.S.P. (Athrombin, Coumadin, Panwarfin) (Warfilone, Warnerin [C]).	2-25 mg. Dosage is adjusted as indicated by prothrombin time. Oral, I.V. or I.M.		Action: similar to that of bishydroxy coumarin. Fate: after oral dose, absorption is practically complete. Maximal plasma concentration reached in 2-12 hours. It is largely bound to plasma protein. Maximal effects in 36-72 hours. Blood levels effective 4-5 days.	Aspirin, phenylbutazone, or C-17-alkylated androgens can increase the hypoprothrombinemic effect of coumarins and warfarin. Their action is antagonized by the barbiturates, glutethimide and griseofulvin. Quinidine exerts a mild direct hypoprothrombinemic effect and can potentiate the action of the anticoagulants. Their concurrent use with tolbutamide can cause a hypoglycemic effect.	

DRUGS ACTING ON THE CIRCULATORY SYSTEM (Continued)

Name, Source, Synonyms, Preparations	Dosage and Administration	Uses	Action and Fate	Side Effects and Contraindications	Remarks
ANTICOAGULANTS (Continued)					
FIBRINOLYSIN. *Naturally derived fraction of human plasma.* Fibrinolysin (Actase, Hydrolysin, Thrombolysin).	50,000 to 100,000 U. q./h. for 1 to 6 hours per day. Given as I.V. infusion.	For I.V. dissolution of thrombi, thrombophlebitis and pulmonary embolism.	Normal blood plasma fraction which causes lysis of blood clots.	Precautions as for any anticoagulant. Contraindicated in hemorrhagic disorders, fibrinogen deficiency, or major liver dysfunction.	
HEPARIN SODIUM. *Liver or lungs of animals.* Depo-heparin sodium, U.S.P. (contains heparin, gelatin, dextrose, and water) (Depo-Heparin). Heparin Sodium, U.S.P., (Hepathrom, Lipo-Hepin, Liquaemin, Panheprin) (Hepalean [C]).	20,000-40,000 U. I.M. 5000-30,000 U. May be intermittent, or in continuous drip with saline or dextrose solution. I.V. or subcutaneous.	Used to prolong the clotting time of blood and to treat thrombophlebitis, pulmonary embolism, certain cardiac conditions, or any disorder in which there is excessive or undesirable clotting.	Action not fully understood but believed to inhibit conversion of prothrombin to thrombin and also fibrinogen to fibrin. It does not dissolve clots but it does prevent extension of old clots and formation of new ones. After injection it slowly disappears from the blood. The larger the dose, the longer levels can be seen in the plasma. Most is metabolized by the liver and excreted by the kidneys. With large doses as much as 50% may be excreted unchanged.	Not common, but hemorrhage may occur, either as one large hemorrhage or as a number of smaller bleeding points. Stop drug. Vitamin K_1 may be ordered. Toluidine blue is sometimes used, as is protamine. I.M. administration may cause local irritation and ecchymosis.	During heparin therapy, clotting time should be checked frequently. Watch closely for any signs of hemorrhage, external or internal.
PHENINDIONE AND SIMILAR DRUGS. *Synthetic.*	All doses individually adjusted.	As above.	Action same as coumarin.	Side effects similar to those of coumarin, but considered less toxic.	
Anisindione, N.F. (Miradon). Diphenadione, N.F. (Dipaxin). Phenindione (Danilone, Hedulin) (Phenylendanedione [C]).	50 mg. Oral. 20-30 mg. Initial. Oral. 3-5 mg. Maintenance. Oral. 0.2-0.3 Gm. Daily in divided doses in acute conditions. Oral. 0.05-0.1 Gm. Daily in divided doses for maintenance. Oral.		Well absorbed from the gastrointestinal tract. Therapeutic effectiveness reached in 24-48 hours and lasts 1-4 days. Exact fate in the body is not known, but a metabolic product produces a red-orange color in alkaline urine.		Anisindione is chemically related to phenindione; claimed to give greater control because of speed and uniformity of response and absence of accumulation.

COAGULANTS. See also vitamins. *Topical.*					
ABSORBABLE GELATIN. *Gelatin.*					
Absorbable gelatin sponge, U.S.P. (Gelfoam).	Size and amount used varies.	Used as a local hemostatic agent.	Gives a good surface for and aids in clot formation.	None.	
CELLULOSE, OXIDIZED. *Vegatable.*					
Cellulose, oxidized, U.S.P. (Hemo-Pak, Oxycel).	Size and amount used varies	Used as a local hemostatic agent.	As above.	None.	An absorbable oxidized cellulose in sterile gauze or cotton-like form.

Many other preparations are used to stop bleeding locally. They are mainly from animal sources, although some are mineral or synthetic. Some of these preparations from animal sources (in addition to those given above) are brain lipoid (impure, cephalin), brain and lung extract, thromboplastin, thrombin, blood fractions, and fibrinogen. Ferropyrin (antipyrine and ferric chloride), ferric chloride, alum, burnt alum, chromium trioxide, silver nitrate, and cotarnine biphthalate (Styptol) are made from chemical sources. The following are synthetic preparations unless otherwise noted.

Aminocaproic acid, N.F. (Amicar).	4-5 Gm. first hour followed by 1 Gm./h. for up to 8 hours or until bleeding is controlled. Oral or I.V.	Used in hemorrhage resulting from overactivity of the fibrinolytic system.	Inhibits both plasminogen activator substances and to a lesser degree plasmin activity. Good absorption orally. Peak plasma levels in about 2 hours. Excreted rapidly in urine, mostly unchanged.	Nausea, cramps, diarrhea, dizziness, tinnitus, malaise, conjunctival suffusion, nasal stuffiness, headache, and skin rash have been reported. Contraindicated when there is evidence of an active intravascular clotting process during the first and second trimesters of pregnancy, unless the need outweighs possible hazards.	
Calcium chloride, U.S.P. (Calcivitam [C]). Calcium lactate, N.F. (Novocalcilac [C]).	1 Gm. p.r.n. Oral. 1 Gm. Oral or subcutaneous.	Used to control bleeding in such conditions as purpura, intestinal bleeding, and any multiple small hemorrhages.	Calcium salts are essential for clot formation and if blood level is low, bleeding is apt to occur.	Rare in therapeutic dosage.	The chloride is more irritating than the lactate when given parenterally.
Carbazochrome salicylate (Andrenosem) (Adrestat, Statimo [C]).	Surgical use: 10 mg. preoperatively. Oral or I.M. 10 mg. q. 2 h. p.r.n. postoperatively. Oral or I.M. Nonsurgical use: 2.5 mg. t.i.d. Oral or I.M.	For control of capillary oozing and bleeding and to prevent capillary permeability.	Action not completely understood.	Low.	

DRUGS ACTING ON THE CIRCULATORY SYSTEM (Continued)

Name, Source, Synonyms, Preparations	Dosage and Administration	Uses	Action and Fate	Side Effects and Contraindications	Remarks
COAGULANTS (Continued)					
Protamine sulfate, U.S.P.	5-8 mg./kg. of body weight. Dosage should not exceed 50 mg. at any one time or 300 mg. in any one day. I.V. or I.M.	Used as a heparin antagonist and for irradiation hemorrhage. Also used in hemorrhagic diseases.	Protamine by itself is an anticoagulant and will cause an increase in clotting time. When given with heparin the drugs are attracted to each other instead of the blood factors.	Rare in therapeutic dosage, but extravascular bleeding may occur from large dosage. Stop drug and treat symptoms.	Protamine solution should be stored under refrigeration.

DIAGNOSTIC DRUGS

These are all synthetic preparations, except as noted.

Name, Source, Synonyms, Preparations	Dosage and Administration	Uses	Action and Fate	Side Effects and Contraindications	Remarks
Azuresin, N.F. (Quinine carbocrylic resin) (Diagnex Blue [C]).	2 Gm. given with 0.59 Gm. caffeine and sodium benzoate. The caffeine may be ordered ½ to 1 hour before the Azuresin. Oral.	As indicated for the determination of achlorhydria.	It depends upon a process of cation exchange. Eliminates need for intubation and gastric expression.	Usually none.	Examination of the urine indicates the amount of hydrochloric acid in the stomach.
ETHYL ALCOHOL. *Grain.* Alcohol, ethyl, U.S.P. (Ethanol).	7% solution. Amount individually determined. Oral.	Used for the same purpose as histamine, when measuring gastric secretion.	A gastric stimulant which indicates the ability of the mucosa to secrete hydrochloric acid. 90-98% of ingested alcohol is metabolized by the body. Only 2-10% is excreted unchanged chiefly in the urine and to a lesser extent in expired air.	May cause symptoms of intoxication. Treat symptoms. Has a large number of drug interactions. See page 75.	
FLUORESCEIN PREPARATIONS. Fluorescein (Fluorescite) (Fluor-I-Strip [C]).	See circular for various doses depending on use.	Determine circulation time, determine if tissue is viable. String test.	It is a strongly fluorescent dye that can readily be seen under ultraviolet light.	Nausea.	

Sodium fluorescein ophthalmic solution, U.S.P.	0.1 ml. of a 2% solution. Topical in conjunctival sac.	Used to reveal ulcers and foreign bodies in the eyes.	Outlines the foreign body or lesion, making it easier to locate.	Rare in therapeutic dosage.	
HISTAMINE PREPARATIONS. *Animal, synthetic.*		Used to test secretion of gastric juice and the amount of acid secreted by the gastric mucosa.	Similar to ethyl alcohol, but is a stronger stimulant.	Urticaria, severe dyspnea, bronchial spasms, severe vasomotor reactions. Treatment: epinephrine (1 mg. will neutralize 10 mg. of histamine). Ephedrine and aminophylline will help to relieve symptoms. Use with care, especially in cases of allergy. Have epinephrine ready.	
Histamine phosphate injection, U.S.P. (Histapon).	0.3 mg. Subcutaneous.				
Betazole hydrochloride, U.S.P. (Histalog).	50 mg. I.M. or subcutaneous.				
Indocyanine green, U.S.P. (Cardio-Green).	1.25 to 5 mg. I.V.	Test cardiac function.	A dye that is easily measured to derive the dilution curve to determine cardiac output.	None noted as yet.	Use the day it is reconstituted.
MANNITOL. *Vegetable. A form of sugar.*					
Mannitol, N.F. (d-Mannitol, Mannite, Manna Sugar).	25% solution. Amount determined individually. I.V.	Used to measure glomerular filtration.	A hexahydric alcohol which is neither absorbed nor secreted by the kidney tubule. Thus the amount excreted gives an accurate estimation of glomerular filtration.	Relatively nontoxic.	Also see under Diuretics (page 208).
Metyrapone, U.S.P. (Metopirone) (methapyrapone [C]).	Usual dosage is 750 mg. q. 4 h. for six doses. Oral. 100 mg. I.V.	Used to test for residual pituitary function.	Selectively inhibits 11-B-hydroxylation in the biosynthesis of the three main corticosteroids—cortisol, corticosterone, and aldosterone.	Transient vertigo or dizziness. Treat symptoms. Adrenal insufficiency may develop in patients with minimal adrenal function.	Refer to package for complete dosage schedule.
Phenolsulfonphthalein injection, U.S.P.	6 mg. Exact dosage and directions vary. I.M. or I.V.	Used to test kidney function.	A dye which is excreted by the kidneys after I.V. administration. 25-45% should be eliminated in 15 minutes. After I.M. administration 40-50% should be eliminated the first hour.	Rare in therapeutic dosage. Safe use during pregnancy has not been established.	

DIAGNOSTIC DRUGS (Continued)

Name, Source, Synonyms, Preparations	Dosage and Administration	Uses	Action and Fate	Side Effects and Contraindications	Remarks
DIAGNOSTIC DRUGS (Continued)					
Phentolamine hydrochloride, N.F. (Regitine) (Rogitine [C]).	5 mg. I.M. or I.V.	Test for pheochromocytoma. Also administer small amounts with norepinephrine I.V. to combat tissue if extravasation is found to occur.	Adrenalytic and sympatholytic.	Tachycardia, weakness, dizziness, orthostatic hypotension, nasal stuffiness and gastrointestinal disturbances.	
Sodium aminohippurate, U.S.P.	20% solution. Amount individually determined. I.V.	Used to test renal plasma flow and to determine tubular excretory capacity.	See circular for calculations and method of determination.	With rapid administration, nausea, vomiting, and sensation of warmth may occur. Reduce rate of infusion.	
SODIUM RADIOIODINE (I^{131}). *Mineral, synthetic.*		Used to diagnose and to treat certain malignant tumors, especially those of the thyroid gland.	Since the thyroid cells have a definite affinity for iodine, the radioactive form affects these cells (normal or malignant) first; thus, by using a scanner, the area of the gland, metastatic tumor, or both may be determined and treated. The iodine is converted to iodide in the gastrointestinal tract and absorbed as such. Widely distributed in the extracellular fluid, but mainly concentrated in the thyroid tissue with lesser amounts in saliva gastric secretions. Most iodine is excreted in the urine.	As for both iodine and radiation. Treat symptoms as they occur.	
Sodium iodide (I^{131}), U.S.P. (Iodotrope, Oriodide, Radiocaps, Theriodide, Tracervial).	1-100 microcuries. Oral or I.V. 1-100 millicuries. Oral or I.V.	As a diagnostic aid. For treatment of malignant lesions.			
Sodium sulfobromophthalein, U.S.P. (Bromsulphthalein).	See circular (2-5 mg./kg.) I.V.	To determine hepatic function.	Bromsulphthalein (BSP) when injected is removed by the liver and excreted in the bile. The amount removed from the blood gives a measure of hepatic function.	Anaphylactic reactions have occurred. Use with caution in patients with allergic history or bronchial asthma.	Check brochure for drugs that interfere with test.

DRUGS ACTING ON THE GASTROINTESTINAL SYSTEM

STOMACHICS, BITTERS, APPETIZERS

The therapeutic value of these drugs has never been proved, and they are not now used to any great extent. Sometimes they are added to other drugs, or used alone for the psychologic effect only. Unless otherwise ordered, all these drugs are given ½ hour before meals, diluted only slightly.

CINCHONA. *Bark of any species of Cinchona.* Compound tincture of cinchona.	4 ml. t.i.d. a.c. Oral.	Used to increase appetite and to stimulate the secretion of the digestive juices.	The bitter taste is thought to stimulate the flow of the digestive juices.	Rare in therapeutic dosage. In excessive amounts will cause the same symptoms as quinine (page 40). Treatment: see Quinine.	Contains cinchona, serpentaria, bitter orange peel.
GENTIAN. *Gentina Intea.* Compound tincture of gentian.	4 ml. t.i.d. a.c. Oral.	Used to increase appetite and to stimulate the secretion of the digestive juices.	See above.	None.	Contains gentian, cardamom, bitter orange peel.
IRON, QUININE, AND STRYCHNINE. *Mineral, vegetable.* Elixir of iron, quinine, and strychnine.	4 ml. t.i.d. a.c. well diluted and through a straw or tube. Oral.	Used to increase appetite and to stimulate the secretion of the digestive juices. Also used as a general alterative.	As above.	Rare in therapeutic dosage. In excessive amounts same as for drugs, mainly strychnine. Pasty, dark stools may result.	

ALKALINE DRUGS (antacids, carminative drugs)

These are all mineral preparations unless otherwise noted. There are many combinations of these drugs. They are all used for the treatment of peptic ulcers and other gastric disorders.

ALUMINUM PREPARATIONS Aluminum hydroxide gel, suspension, U.S.P. (Al-U-Creme, Co-Lu-Gel, Creamalin, Gelumina, Hartgel, Hydroxal).	4-8 ml. Given between or before meals with generous amount of water. All q.i.d. or p.r.n. Oral.	Used as an antacid in the treatment of gastric ulcers and any gastric hyperacidity. Also used as a carminative, protective, and astringent.	Aluminum hydroxide acts as an antacid by combination with hydrochloride of the stomach acid to give $AlCl_3$ (aluminum chloride) and H_2O. Acts more slowly	Rare in therapeutic dosage since it is not absorbed to any appreciable extent. These compounds have been shown to reduce the absorption of tetracycline,

Name, Source, Synonyms, Preparations	Dosage and Administration	Uses	Action and Fate	Side Effects and Contraindications	Remarks
ALUMINUM PREPARATIONS (Continued)					
Aluminum hydroxide gel, dried, N.F. (Adsogil, Co-Lu-Gel, Creamalin) (A-H-Gel, Amphojel, Alocol, Alugel, Chem-Gel [C]).	0.3-0.6 Gm. Oral.		than soluble alkalies but there is much less incidence of acid rebound. Dried aluminum hydroxide gel is less antacid than the fluid.	and concurrent use should be avoided or the tetracycline given one hour before or two hours after the aluminum-containing preparation.	
Aluminum phosphate gel, N.F. (Phosphajel) (Uigel [C]).	15 ml. Oral.		Aluminum phosphate gel is less antacid than the hydroxide but more demulcent and adsorbative.		
Basic aluminum carbonate (Basaljel).	30 ml. Oral.		Little if any absorption occurs.		
Dihydroxy aluminum aminoacetate, N.F. (Alglyn, Alkam, Robalate).	0.5 Gm. Oral.				Dihydroxy aluminum aminoacetate is a combination of aluminum hydroxide and glycine. Less apt to cause constipation than the hydroxide.
Monalium hydrate (Riopan) (magaldrate [C]).	0.4-0.8 Gm. Oral.				
ALKALINE BISMUTH SALTS					
Bismuth, milk of, N.F. (Cremo-Bismuth, Lac-Bismo).	4 ml. q.i.d. Oral.	Used to decrease gastric acidity and as a demulcent in gastric ulcers. Also used as a carminative, antiemetic, and antacid.	They are demulcent, astringent, and mildly antiseptic. They tend to coat irritated or denuded surfaces, as in peptic ulcers. Being basic, they also help neutralize excess gastric acidity. Not absorbed to any degree because of insolubility.	Rare except in presence of a large raw surface, in which case the bismuth may be absorbed, causing such toxic symptoms as black gums, swelling of the tongue, dysphagia, salivation, gastrointestinal disorders. Stop drug and treat symptoms.	
Bismuth subcarbonate, U.S.P. (Cremo-Carbonate).	1 Gm. q.i.d. Oral.				
Bismuth subgallate.	1 Gm. q.i.d. Oral.				
ALKALINE CALCIUM SALTS.					
Precipitated calcium carbonate, (precipitated chalk) (Calcibarb [C]). Calcium carbonate tablets, N.F.	1-2 Gm. q.i.d. Oral.	Used mainly as an antacid and protective for raw surfaces.	Good long acting antacid with less chance of alkalosis or rebound because it is relatively insoluble.	Rare in therapeutic dosage, but may cause constipation. Stop drug and treat symptoms.	Releases carbon dioxide in the stomach; is not absorbed.
MAGNESIUM PREPARATIONS					
Magnesia, milk of, U.S.P. (magnesia magma, magnesium hydroxide).	4 ml. q.i.d. as antacid. Oral.	Used mainly as an antacid and as a laxative.	Acts as antacid, and in sufficient dose following interaction with stomach	Rare in therapeutic dosage. Interaction with the tetracyclines same as aluminum	Magnesia magma also comes in tablet form.

Magnesium carbonate, N.F. Magnesium oxide, U.S.P. Magnesium trisilicate, U.S.P. (Trisomin) (Neutrasil [C]).	0.6 Gm. } q.i.d. as antacid. 0.25 Gm. } Oral. 1 Gm. p.r.n. Oral.		acid acts as saline laxative. Little if any absorption occurs.	compounds.	Magnesium trisilicate is a rapid powerful adsorbent used in toxic conditions; gives slow long-continued action but is not systemic.
PHOSPHATE PREPARATIONS.					
Calcium phosphate tribasic, N.F. Magnesium phosphate, N.F.	1 Gm. q.i.d. or p.r.n. Oral. 1 Gm. q.i.d. or p.r.n. Oral.	Used mainly as an antacid and as a laxative.	Similar to others of this group. Tribasic calcium phosphate tends to cause systemic action. Raises blood calcium. Tribasic magnesium phosphate is similar to magnesium trisilicate.	Same as the constituent drugs. May cause mild constipation and acid rebound.	
ALKALINE SODIUM SALTS.					
Sodium acetate, N.F. Sodium bicarbonate, U.S.P. (baking soda). Sodium citrate, U.S.P.	1.5 Gm. p.r.n. Oral. 1-2 Gm. p.r.n. Oral. 44.6 mEq. ampul. I.V. 1 Gm. p.r.n. Oral.	Used for many purposes, such as to decrease gastric acidity, to reduce acidity systemically, and locally as an antipruritic. The citrate also is used to prevent blood clotting in blood to be used for transfusions.	Alkaline salts which act as antacid because of their basic nature. These salts are soluble and are widely distributed. They are excreted by the kidneys and will cause the urine to be alkaline.	Rare in therapeutic dosage. Excessive amounts may cause alkalosis. Stop drug and give mild acids. Sodium salts, especially the bicarbonates, are more apt to cause alkalosis. Sodium bicarbonate may cause acid rebound and increase in CO_2 in the stomach.	Sodium bicarbonate is used intravenously to combat metabolic acidosis especially in cardiac arrest. When sodium citrate is given to alkalinize the urine, the patient should be on a low-calcium diet, (no milk or milk products) since calcium will precipitate in an alkaline urine.
Polyamine-methylene resin (Exorbin, Resinat). *Synthetic from resin.*	0.5-1 Gm. q. 2 h. p.r.n. Oral.	Used to lessen gastric hyperacidity.	Causes temporary binding of hydrochloric acid. Later released in intestines, not absorbed. Has no systemic action. Does not affect electrolyte balance.	Rare in therapeutic dosage. Excessive dosage may cause nausea and vomiting.	

DRUGS ACTING ON THE GASTROINTESTINAL SYSTEM (Continued)

EMETICS

Name, Source, Synonyms, Preparations	Dosage and Administration	Uses	Action and Fate	Side Effects and Contraindications	Remarks
ALUM. *Mineral.* Alum, N.F.	1-2 Gm. Oral.	Used as an emetic and locally as an astringent.	Powerful astringent and styptic with irritant qualities; if taken in sufficient quantities is an emetic and purgative.	Rare in therapeutic dosage. If taken in large quantities can cause gastrointestinal irritation.	Do not use in cases of corrosive poisoning.
ANTIMONY AND POTASSIUM TARTRATE (*tartar emetic*). *Mineral and vegetable.* Antimony potassium tartrate, U.S.P.	0.03-0.12 Gm. Oral.	Used as an emetic and expectorant. It is also used as an anti-infective. Used more frequently as an expectorant than as an emetic.	It acts as an emetic, due to its irritating effect.	Rare in therapeutic dosage. Treatment: see antimony poisoning.	
APOMORPHINE HYDROCHLORIDE. *Synthetic derivative of opium (morphine).* Apomorphine hydrochloride, N.F.	5 mg. Subcutaneous.	Used as an emetic and expectorant. May produce mild hypnosis. Occasionally used as a hypnotic in asthma, in delirium tremens, and to control paroxysmal tachycardia.	Acts as a direct stimulant on the vomiting center in the medulla. It is metabolized mainly by the liver and degradation products are excreted in the urine.	Salivation, lacrimation, weakness, dizziness, convulsions. Stop drug, treat symptoms, maintain respiration.	
COPPER SULFATE. *Mineral.* Copper sulfate.	0.3-1 Gm. Either one dose or 0.3 Gm. q. 15 minutes for three doses. Oral.	Used as an emetic and as a catalyst with iron given for anemia. Also acts as an antidote in phosphorus poisoning.	Acts as an irritant to mucous membranes.	Rare in therapeutic dosage.	Do not use in cases of corrosive poisoning.
IPECAC (emetine, cephaeline). *Cephaelis ipecacuanha.* Ipecac, U.S.P. Ipecac syrup, U.S.P.	0.5 Gm. Oral. 8 ml. Oral.	Used as an emetic and expectorant, but more frequently as an expectorant.	Vomiting is slower than with apomorphine, but ipecac produces less depression.	Rare in therapeutic dosage. Sweating and depression may occur. Stop drug and treat symptoms.	Action of these preparations as emetics is uncertain.

MUSTARD. *Spinapis nigra.* Ground mustard.	4-10 Gm. Dissolve in warm water. Oral.	Used as an emetic and locally as a counterirritant.	Action uncertain but often effective; frequently used in emergencies, especially in the home.	Rare in therapeutic dosage.	Safe, but not very effective.
ZINC SULFATE. *Mineral.* Zinc sulfate, U.S.P.	0.6-1 Gm. Give well diluted. Oral. 220 mg. t.i.d. Oral.	Used as an emetic and also general treatment with trace elements. Treatment of leg ulcer in diabetic patients.	Same as copper sulfate.	Rare in therapeutic dosage.	Do not use in cases of corrosive poisoning. Said to help increase the ability to taste in patients shown to have lower than normal serum levels of zinc.

ANTIEMETICS—ANTINAUSEANTS

See also antacids, antihistamines, tranquilizers, and vitamins. Patients should be warned about operating machinery and driving car when taking these drugs (especially for the first time) or upon initiation of treatment. These are all synthetic preparations.

Dimenhydrinate, U.S.P. (Dramamine, Reioamine) (Dramavol, Dymenol, Gravol, Neo-Matic, Novodimenate, Travamine, Traveller's Friend [C]).	50-100 mg. q. 4 h. p.r.n. Oral or parenteral.	Used as an antiemetic, to overcome vertigo and dizziness, and for motion sickness, labyrinthitis, and nausea.	Exact nature of action is uncertain but it appears to depress the central nervous system and reduce reaction of sensory stimuli, expecially from the labyrinth. The fate of this drug is the same as that of the antihistamines. They are readily absorbed and widely distributed. They are of short duration of action since they are rapidly metabolized. The degradation products are usually eliminated in the urine.	Rare in therapeutic dosage.	

ANTIEMETICS–ANTINAUSEANTS *(Continued)*

Name, Source, Synonyms, Preparations	Dosage and Administration	Uses	Action and Fate	Side Effects and Contraindications	Remarks
Diphenidol (Vontrol).	25-50 mg. q. 4 h. p.r.n. Oral. 50 mg. q. 4 h. p.r.n. Rectal. 20-40 mg. q. 4 h. p.r.n. I.V. or I.M. Children's dosage: 0.4 mg./lb. Oral or rectal. 0.2 mg./lb. by injection.	Antiemetic and antivertigo.	Apparently acts on vestibular apparatus to control vertigo and on the chemoreceptor trigger zone to control nausea and vomiting.	Contraindications: Safety for nausea of pregnancy has not been established. Side effects: dry mouth, drowsiness, gastrointestinal irritation, blurred vision, dizziness, skin rashes, malaise, headache, slight transient lowering of blood pressure.	Cautions: Do not inject subcutaneously. Drug may mask overdose of drugs and may obscure the diagnosis of other conditions (such as intestinal obstruction or brain tumor).
Meclizine hydrochloride, U.S.P. (Antivert-25, Bonine) (histamethizine, Bonamine, Meclozine, Mecazine, Nauzine [C]).	25 mg. t.i.d. p.r.n. Oral.	Used as an antiemetic, to overcome vertigo, dizziness, motion sickness, labyrinthitis, and nausea.	See dimenhydrinate.	Rare in therapeutic dosage.	Not for use in women who are pregnant or may become pregnant. Drug has possible teratogenic effects.
Thiethylperazine maleate, N.F. (Torecan).	10-30 mg. Daily. Oral. 10-20 mg. Daily. I.M.	Antiemetic and antinauseant for the treatment of all forms of nausea and vomiting.	As above. Same fate as that of the phenothiazines.	Drowsiness, dry mouth, orthostatic hypotension. Contraindicated in severely depressed or comatose patients.	
Trimethobenzamide, N.F. (Tigan).	100-250 mg. q.i.d. p.r.n. Oral, parenteral, rectal.	Used like thiethylperazine and also for motion sickness.	As dimenhydranate.	Incidence of drowsiness claimed to be rare.	

SUBSTITUTIVE AGENTS (Digestants. See also Acidifiers.)

Name, Source, Synonyms, Preparations	Dosage and Administration	Uses	Action and Fate	Side Effects and Contraindications	Remarks
BILE AND BILE SALTS. *Animal.*					
Cholic acid and ketocholanic acid (Chodile).	0.1 Gm. t.i.d. Oral.	Used to aid digestion of fats. Also increases peristalsis and aids absorption of fat-soluble vitamins. Replacement therapy.	These preparations act in the body like the natural bile salts.	Rare in therapeutic dosage but may cause mild diarrhea if taken in excessive amounts. Stop drug and treat symptoms.	
Dehydrocholic acid, N.F. (Cholan-D H, Decholin, Ketacholanic acid) (Biocholin, Dehydrocholin, Dycholium, Idrocrine, Novodecholin, Transibyl [C]).	0.25-0.5 Gm. t.i.d. Oral.	Used to test circulation time in cholecystography and cholangiography.			
Desiccated whole bile (Desicól).	0.325 Gm. t.i.d. Oral.				
Florantyrone (Zanchol).	0.25-1 Gm. t.i.d. Oral.				Florantyrone is a synthetic preparation with action similar to that of dehydrocholic acid.
Ox bile extract.	0.3 Gm. t.i.d. Oral.				

Sodium dehydrocholate injection, N.F. (Decholin sodium, Dilabil sodium).	5-10 ml. of a 20% solution. Usually given daily for 3 days. I.V.				
DILUTE HYDROCHLORIC ACID. *Chemical.*					
Hydrochloric acid, diluted, N.F.	0.6-1 ml. t.i.d. a.c. Should be given well diluted through a straw to protect teeth. Oral.	To aid in gastric digestion when there is insufficient hydrochloric acid.	Aids in protein digestion in cases of achlorhydria.	Rare in therapeutic dosage.	
DRIED DUODENUM. *Animal.*					
Dried duodenum (Viodenum) Desiccated and defatted.	0.5-1.0 gm. t.i.d. a.c. Oral.	Used in the treatment of gastric and duodenal ulcers.	Hormone-like substance, whose exact mechanism of action is not known.	None.	Similar to urogastrone.
GLUTAMIC ACID HYDROCHLORIDE. *Chemical.*					
Glutamic acid hydrochloride, N.F. (Acidoride, Acidulin, Glutan, Hydrionic) (Acidogen, Antalka [C]).	1-2 capsules before meals. Oral.	To aid in gastric digestion when there is insufficient hydrochloric acid.	Action same as that of hydrochloric acid.	Rare in therapeutic dosage.	Not unpleasant to take, and does not injure teeth.
MALT. *Vegetable.*					
Malt extract.	15 Gm. With meals. Oral.	Used to aid digestion of carbohydrates, and as a nutrient.	Is able to convert at least five times its weight of starch into sugar.	None.	
PANCREATIN. *Animal.*					
Pancreatin, N.F. (Panopsin, Stamyl 1). Lipancreatin (Cotazym B).	0.5 Gm. With meals. Oral. 2000 U. With meals. Oral.	Used to assist digestion of protein and carbohydrate foods and to aid digestion of fats, especially in pancreatic insufficiency. Used also to peptonize milk.	Action is the same as that of the enzymes of the pancreatic juice.	None.	May be given in enteric-coated pills or capsules; each is sufficient to digest 34 Gm. dietary protein and 40 Gm. dietary starch.
PANCRELIPASE. *Animal; concentrated pancreatic enzyme.*					
Pancrelipase (Cotazym) (lipanereatin [C]).	1-3 capsules. With meals. Oral.	Used to treat pancreatic insufficiency.	As above.	Rare, but sensitivity may occur.	Each capsule contains digestive enzymes, sufficient to digest, as follows: lipase, 17 Gm. fat; trypsin, 34 Gm. protein; amylase, 40 Gm. starch.

DRUGS ACTING ON THE GASTROINTESTINAL SYSTEM (Continued)

SUBSTITUTIVE AGENTS *(Continued)*

Name, Source, Synonyms, Preparations	Dosage and Administration	Uses	Action and Fate	Side Effects and Contraindications	Remarks
PEPSIN. *Animal.*					
Pepsin.	0.5 Gm. With meals. Oral.	Used to aid digestion of proteins.	Supposed to replace depleted pepsin and to increase the digestion of proteins.	None.	Value appears questionable. Acts only in an acid medium, so additional acid may be indicated.
Pepsin elixir.	8 ml. With meals. Oral.				
SACCHARIN. *Synthetic.*					
Saccharin, U.S.P. (Benzosulfimide, Gluside, Saxin).	15-60 mg. With food. Oral.	Used as a sugar substitute in diabetes, reducing diets, and other conditions in which sugar is not allowed.	A sweetening agent with no caloric value.	None.	
Sodium saccharin, N.F. (sodium benzosulfimide, Sweeta) (Crystallose, Hermesetas [C]).	15-60 mg. With food. Oral.				
TAKA-DIASTASE. *Proprietary from enzyme of Aspergillus oryzae.*					
Taka-Diastase, Elixir.	4 ml. With meals. Oral.	Used to aid digestion of carbohydrates and to relieve indigestion.	A mixture containing the active enzymes of malt.	Rare in therapeutic dosage.	
Taka-Diastase (aspergillus oryzae enzyme [C]).	1 Gm. With meals.				
ANTISEPTIC (See also Anti-infectives and Urinary Antiseptics.)					
FURAZOLIDONE. *Synthetic.*					
Furazolidone, N.F. (Furoxone).	50-100 mg. q.i.d. Oral.	Used as an anti-infective for the intestinal tract.	Action and use are similar to those of the poorly absorbed sulfonamides.	Toxicity usually low, but sensitivity reactions may occur. Hypertensive crisis can occur. Safe use during pregnancy has not been established.	Has effects similar to disulfiram (Antabuse), so alcohol must not be used. Also acts as a monoamine oxidase inhibitor. The usual precautions and interactions prevail. See page 74.
ADSORBENTS (ABSORBENTS), PROTECTIVES, ANTIDIARRHEICS (See also Antacids and Astringents.)					
ACTIVATED CHARCOAL *(purified organic charcoal).*					
Activated charcoal.	1-8 Gm. p.r.n. Oral.	Mainly used to treat flatulence.	An adsorbent, especially of gases.	Drugs of this type, when given concurrently with other medication, can significantly reduce absorption of the drug.	An ingredient of many proprietary preparations.

BENTONITE *(hydrous aluminum silicate). Earth (clay).*					
Bentonite magma, U.S.P.	Dosage varies. p.r.n. Oral.	Used to treat flatulence and nonspecific diarrhea.	Acts as an adsorbent and protective.	As above.	Often used in combination with other drugs.
DIATOMACEOUS EARTH *(purified siliceous earth). Earth (clay).*					
Purified siliceous earth.	Dosage varies. Oral or topical.	Also used to treat flatulence and nonspecific diarrhea.	Acts as an adsorbent and protective.	As above.	
DIPHENOXYLATE. *Synthetic.*					
Diphenoxylate hydrochloride, N.F. (Lomotil).	2.5 mg. Three or four times daily. p.r.n. Tablets or liquid.	Used in diarrhea or any condition in which there is hypergastrointestinal motility.	Chemically related to narcotic drugs but no addiction has been reported. Not analgesic. Only important action appears to be decreased intestinal peristalsis.	Toxicity apparently low. Constipation may result and require mild laxatives. Use with caution in patients with glaucoma or advanced liver disease.	Contains a subtherapeutic amount of atropine sulfate.
GASTRIC MUCIN. *Animal.*					
Gastric mucin.	2.5 Gm. q. 2 h. Oral.	Mainly used in the treatment of gastric ulcers.	Acts as a demulcent and adsorbent. Does not produce alkalosis.	Rare in therapeutic dosage.	
KAOLIN *(aluminum silicate). Earth (clay, china clay).*					
Kaolin, N.F. (Collo-Kaolin [C]).	50-100 Gm. p.r.n. Oral.	Used to treat dysentery, food poisoning, nonspecific diarrhea.	Acts as a protective and adsorbent.	Kaolin should not be given concurrently with lincomycin, since the absorption of lincomycin can be reduced by as much as 90 per cent.	
Kaolin mixture with pectin, N.F. (Kao-con, Kaopectate, Kalpec, Ka-Pek, Paocin, Pargel, Pektamalt).	4-30 ml. p.r.n. Oral.				
Kaomagma (kaolin and magnesia).	4-15 ml. p.r.n. Oral.				
MISCELLANEOUS					
SIMETHICONE. *Synthetic.*					
Simethicone (Antiform, Mylicon, Silain).	40-50 mg. p.c. and h.s. Oral.	Used to relieve flatulence due to functional or organic disease.	Physiologically inert. Changes surface tension.	None.	

CATHARTICS

Name, Source, Synonyms, Preparations	Dosage and Administration	Uses	Action and Fate	Side Effects and Contraindications	Remarks

The use of cathartic drugs should be confined to such conditions as relief of temporary constipation, presurgery or prediagnostic procedures, relief of edema, to lessen the work of the kidneys, and in treatment of disorders and diseases of the gastrointestinal tract. Other measures should be used for the treatment of chronic or persistent constipation. Cathartics may be classified in a variety of ways. The more common classifications are as follows: According to degree of action–laxative, mild; purgative, more severe; drastic purgative, very severe. According to method of action–increase bulk of intestinal content; lubrication; chemical irritation of the mucosa; selective action. Varying the amount of the drug or the type of drug will produce different degrees of action.

Name, Source, Synonyms, Preparations	Dosage and Administration	Uses	Action and Fate	Side Effects and Contraindications	Remarks
SALINE CATHARTICS AND ANTACID MINERAL SALTS					
MAGNESIUM, SODIUM, POTASSIUM SALTS. *Mineral.*		Used to increase the intestinal content by "salt action," producing fluid or semifluid stools. Used also to reduce edema, obesity, milk secretion, and intracranial pressure. Most of the cathartics are given at bedtime. Liquid saline preparations are given early in the morning, usually before breakfast and, except in edema, with ample fluid.	The carbonate or hydroxide derivatives of these salts have an antacid action. These preparations withdraw fluid from the blood and the tissues. Some diuresis usually results.	Nausea, colic, and polyuria may occur. Force fluids, if indicated, otherwise no treatment is needed. See interactions under magnesium compounds, page 156.	Compound effervescent powders contain potassium and sodium tartrate 7.5 Gm. and sodium bicarbonate 2.5 Gm. in the blue paper. Tartaric acid 2.2 Gm. in the white paper. Dissolve separately in about one-fourth glass of water, mix at bedside, and administer as soon as possible.
Compound effervescent powders (Seidlitz powders).	See last column. Oral.				
Magnesium carbonate, N.F.	8 Gm. Oral.				
Magnesium citrate solution, N.F.	200 ml. Oral.				
Magnesia, milk of, U.S.P. (magnesia magma).	15 ml. Also comes in tablet form, often given h.s. Oral.				
Magnesium oxide, U.S.P. (calcined magnesia).	4 Gm. Oral.				
Magnesium sulfate, U.S.P. (Epsom salts).	15 Gm. Oral.				
Potassium sodium tartrate, N.F. (Rochelle salts).	10 Gm. Oral.				
Sodium phosphate, N.F.	4 Gm. Oral.				
Sodium phosphate, dried, N.F.	2 Gm. Oral.				
Sodium phosphate, effervescent, N.F.	10 Gm. See last column. Oral.				Effervescent sodium phosphate contains sodium phosphate, citric and tartaric acid, and sodium bicarbonate.
Sodium sulfate (Glauber's salt).	15 gm. Oral.				
BULK LAXATIVES					
AGAR *(agar-agar). Dried seaweed.*	These drugs are often added to food.	Used in both temporary and chronic constipation. Especially valuable in spastic conditions.	Produce colloidal bulk in the intestines, thus promoting peristalsis and formation of soft stools. Slow acting.		Copious amounts of water must be given with the colloidal bulk laxatives to prevent the formation of hard dry stools. Obstruction may occur if sufficient fluid is not administered.
Agar, U.S.P. (Agar-agar, Benzal gelatin).	Dosage varies. Oral.				

BASSORAN. *Proprietary compound from Sterculia gum, bassorin and magnesium sulfate.*					
Bassoran.	Dosage varies. Oral.	As above.	As above.	None.	Sterculia gum granules coated with magnesium trisilicate.
BRAN. *Outer covering of cereal grain.*					
Bran.	Dosage varies. Oral.	As above.	As above.	None.	Usually added to food, as are many of the bulk laxatives. Bran is not a lubricant, as are most of the bulk laxatives.
FLAXSEED *(linseed) Flax.*					
Oxyphenisatin acetate (Acetphenolisatin, Bisatin, Endophenolphthalein, Isocrin, Phenylisatin) (acetphenolisan, Lavema, Normalax [C]).	5 mg. Oral.	As above.	As above.	None.	A constituent of many bulk laxatives.
Linseed, N.F.	Dosage varies. Oral.				
METHYLCELLULOSE. *Cellulose.*					
Methylcellulose, U.S.P. (Cellothyl, Cologel, Hydrolose, (Isopto-Plain [C]) Melozets, Methocel, Nicel) (conjunctival lubricant; Gonioscopic fluid, Isopto-Alkaline, Isoptotears, Isopto-Plain, Lacril, Methocel, Methulose, Tearisol).	1.5 Gm. p.r.n. Oral.	Used as a bulk laxative as is agar; also as an anorexic agent and for conjunctival lubrication.	As above.	None.	There are several proprietary preparations that contain either methylcellulose or vegetable gums, such as Imbicoll, Saraka, Serutan, Effergel.
PSYLLIUM SEED. *Plantago psyllium.*					
Plantago ovata coating (Betajel, Konsyl, Metamucil, L.A. formula).	5-10 Gm. p.r.n. Oral.	See Agar.	As above.	None.	Metamucil contains psyllium and other ingredients.
Plantago seed, N.F. (Psyllium, Plantain seed).	7.5 Gm. p.r.n. Oral.				
TRAGACANTH. *Astragalus gummifer.* See agar.					
Tragacanth.	Dosage varies. p.r.n.	See agar.	As above.	None.	

CATHARTICS *(Continued)*

Name, Source, Synonyms, Preparations	Dosage and Administration	Uses	Action and Fate	Side Effects and Contraindications	Remarks
LUBRICANTS					
LIQUID PETROLATUM *(Mineral oil.)*		Used for the same purpose as olive oil.	Action similar to that of olive oil, but it is less demulcent and is not absorbed. Has been thought to prevent the absorption of some of the fat-soluble vitamins.	None.	Liquid petrolatum in large doses tends to "seep" through the rectum and soil the clothes.
Mineral oil, emulsion (Milkinol).	15-30 ml. Oral.				
Mineral oil, light, N.F. (Nujol, Albolene).	15 ml. Oral.				
Petrogalar, plain (Agoral, Kondremul).	15-30 ml. Oral.				
OLIVE OIL. *Vegetable. Olive fruit.*					
Olive oil.	30 ml. Usually given in divided doses during the day and at bedtime. Oral.	Used to lubricate the intestinal tract and to produce soft stools. Useful in certain types of chronic constipation.	Acts as a demulcent. Tends to empty the gallbladder. Some of the oil is absorbed and acts as any fat.	None.	
IRRITANT CATHARTICS. (Anthracene, Emodin or Anthraquinone). This group of cathartics includes rhubarb, senna, aloe, cascara, and related substances.			These drugs act after partial hydrolysis as irritants of the large bowel.		
ALOE *(aloin). Aloe vera and similar plants.*		Used as a purgative–mild to moderate–according to dosage. Used to relieve temporary constipation, atonic chronic constipation or both.	Acts as a stomachic if not given in pill or tablet form.	Rare in therapeutic dosage. Causes congestion of pelvic organs and is therefore contraindicated in pregnancy, during menstruation, or when hemorrhoids are present.	
Aloe, U.S.P.	0.25 Gm. Oral.				
Aloin.	15 mg. Oral.				
Aloin, belladonna, cascara, podophyllin pills (Hinkle pills).	1 pill. Oral. These should be given at bedtime because of their action on colon.				
CASCARA SAGRADA. *Rhamnus purshiana.*					
Casanthranol (Peristim).	30 mg. Oral. Should be given at bedtime because of its action on the colon.	Used as a purgative–mild to moderate–according to dosage. Most useful in chronic constipation to improve tone of intestinal muscles. Does not cause increased constipation.	Action as with others of this group.	Rare in therapeutic dosage.	Casanthranol contains cascara and glycyrrhiza.
Cascara sagrada tablets, N.F.	Dosage varies. Oral.				
Cascara sagrada aromatic fluid extract, U.S.P.	4-5 ml. Oral.				

Cascara sagrada elixir. Cascara sagrada extract, N.F. Cascara sagrada fluid extract, N.F.	4 ml. Oral. 0.3 Gm. Oral. 1 ml. Oral.				
DANTHRON. *Synthetic from vegetable.* Danthron, N.F. (Dionone, Dorbane, Istizin) (dioxyanthraquinone, Danthrone [C]).	0.15 Gm. h.s. Oral.	Use is much the same as for aloe.	As above.	Rare in therapeutic dosage.	
SENNA. *Cassia acutifolia and C. angustifola.* Compound senna powder Senna, N.F. (Aperens, Senokot).	4 Gm. Oral. 0.6-2 Gm. Best given as a tea with manna. Oral.	Use is much the same as for aloe.	As above.	Rare in therapeutic dosage. Some griping may occur. The fluid extract does not cause griping.	Compound senna powder contains senna, sulfur, fennel, glycyrrhiza.
Senna fluid extract, N.F. Senna syrup, N.F. Sennosides A and B (Glysennid).	2 ml. Oral. 8 ml. Oral. 12 mg. Oral. These should be given at bedtime because of their action on colon.				Sennosides A and B are the purified senna principles.
IRRITANT OILS					
CASTOR OIL. *(oleum ricini) Ricinus communis.* Castor oil, U.S.P. Castor oil aromatic, N.F. (Neoloid).	15 ml. Oral. 15 ml. Oral. Usually given before breakfast in fruit juice or soft drinks. Ice held in the mouth before taking it will help prevent tasting the drug.	Used to secure rapid catharsis, Especially valuable to remove toxic substances and to clear the intestinal tract before surgery or diagnostic tests.	Acts on the small intestine and produces soft watery stools.	Nausea is not uncommon. Excessive purgation may occur. May cause constipation after catharsis.	Has an unpleasant odor and taste.

Name, Source, Synonyms, Preparations	Dosage and Administration	Uses	Action and Fate	Side Effects and Contraindications	Remarks
MERCURIALS					
MERCURY. *Mineral.*					
Mercurous chloride, mild (Calomel).	0.12 Gm. Usually given in divided doses, h.s. Oral.	Used to increase peristalsis and glandular secretions, especially bile. Also used as an intestinal antiseptic and to reduce edema.	Decreased absorption of food and food products. Causes soft dark green stools.	Griping, colic, severe diarrhea, metallic taste, oliguria, anuria, and hematuria may occur. Treatment: saline cathartics are given to remove drug. Treat for shock and treat symptoms. Dimercaprol (British Antilewisite, BAL) is used in chronic poisoning. Mercurial cathartics should be used with caution in anemia, cachexia, nephritis, pulmonary tuberculosis, scurvy, dysentery, severe heart disorders, or when iodides are being given.	May destroy needed intestinal bacteria. Mercurous chloride mild compound pills contain calomel and a number of drastic purgatives.
MISCELLANEOUS					
BISACODYL. *Synthetic.*					
Bisacodyl, N.F. (Dulcolax) (Bisacolax, Laco, Sogalax [C]).	5 mg. h.s. Oral. 10 mg. p.r.n. Suppositories.	A contact laxative for the relief of all types of constipation.	Acts as a stimulant to the mucosa of the colon, and initiates a reflex peristalsis. No appreciable absorption.	Abdominal cramping can occur.	Do not chew or crush tablets. Do not use within 1 hour of ingestion of an antacid.
DIOCTYL SODIUM SULFOSUCCINATE. *Synthetic.*					
Dioctyl calcium sulfosuccinate, N.F. (Surfak). Dioctyl sodium sulfosuccinate, N.F. (Colace, Diomedicone, Diosuccin, Doxinate, Duosol, Kosate, Laxinate, Parlax, Regutol, Revac) (Bantex, Constiban, Octyl-softener, Regulex [C]).	50-240 mg. h.s. or more often p.r.n. Oral. 60-250 mg. As above. Oral.	Used any time a laxative is indicated. Especially valuable when a soft stool is desired.	Acts as a wetting agent. Does not cause any intestinal irritation or increase in bulk, but makes stools soft.	Rare in therapeutic dosage.	Preparations are available for infants and children.

PHENOLPHTHALEIN. *Phenol and phthalic anhydride.* Phenolphthalein, N.F. (Thalinol) (Fractineb, Laxatabs [C]).	60 mg. h.s. Oral.	Used as a purgative or laxative according to dosage.	Action is similar to that of the anthracene cathartics. Mildly irritating to mucous lining of both large and small intestines, especially the former. It is excreted in the bile and exerts action over a longer period than most purgatives.	Skin rashes, renal irritation, especially if taken over a period of time. Stop drug and treat symptoms.	This drug is the active ingredient found in many proprietary cathartic preparations.
POLOXALKOL. *Synthetic.* Poloxalkol (Polykol).	0.25 Gm. h.s. Oral.	Similar to dioctyl sodium sulfosuccinate.	See dioctyl sodium sulfosuccinate.	Toxicity apparently low.	
SULFUR. *Mineral.* Washed sulfur (Bensulfoid).	Dosage varies. p.r.n. Oral.	Used in the relief of constipation, especially when soft stools are desired.	Forms gas, which permeates the stool and makes it soft.	Rare in therapeutic dosage.	

Suppositories, especially glycerin, cause catharsis by irritation of the lower bowel. Also available for securing evacuation of the lower bowel are enema solutions such as sodium biphosphate and sodium phosphate (Phospho-Soda, Fleet), sodium dihydrogen phosphate (anhydrous) and sodium citrate (dihydrous) (Travad). See also drugs acting on the smooth muscle tissue, for other drugs that act as cathartics.

METABOLIC DRUGS

HORMONES (See also Miscellaneous drugs)

All hormones are secured from either animal or synthetic sources; all hormones are relatively nontoxic except in large doses; many hormones, especially new ones, are experimental. Many changes occur in the use, dosage, etc., of these drugs as their clinical significance and usefulness become better known. See also other biologic and metabolic drugs such as vitamins, serums, and drugs acting on the reproductive organs.

Name, Source, Synonyms, Preparations	Dosage and Administration	Uses	Action and Fate	Side Effects and Contraindications	Remarks
GONADAL HORMONES COMBINED					
Tylosterone (diethylstilbestrol, methyltestosterone).	1 tablet o.d. Oral. 0.5-1 ml. p.r.n. I.M.	The use of the gonadal hormones in groups of two or three is not unusual, especially in the treatment of the symptoms of the climacteric in both sexes and in cancer of the genitals.	See estrogenic substances and testosterone.	Toxicity does not usually occur, since one hormone tends to counteract the effect of the other.	Contains 0.25 mg. diethylstilbestrol and 5 mg. methyltestosterone. Many such products are marketed. The physician often uses one or two preparations at the same time.
OVARIAN HORMONES					
ESTROGENS. *Synthetic, animal.*		Used for many purposes such as relief of the symptoms of menopause, as an antilactagogue, to relieve the symptoms of prostatic cancer, as a palliative treatment for breast cancer in women. Also used for vaginitis in children, senile vaginitis, and pruritus vulvae. Estrogens may increase or decrease uterine bleeding, according to conditions.	Estrogens act as do the natural hormones. They tend to inhibit pituitary activity, cause hyperplasia of the endometrium, and to bring about breast development. They also tend to cause closure of the epiphyseal diaphyseal junction in youth; conversely, they cause bone development in adult women, thereby preventing and correcting osteoporosis. The estrogens have some tendency to cause sodium and fluid retention, but less than the adrenal hormones.	It has been shown statistically that women on progestin-estrogen birth control pills have a higher incidence of the following serious reactions than women not taking the "pill": thrombophlebitis, pulmonary embolism and cerebral thrombosis. Long continued use may produce sclerosis of the ovaries, and may also disturb the calcium metabolism, increased blood sugar levels and decreased glucose tolerance, an increase in blood pressure and an aggravation of migraine. Excessive doses may cause nausea, vomiting, headache, dizziness. These may occur even from therapeutic dosage. Reduce dosage or change to another preparation. Because of possible adverse reaction on the fetus, the	The time for the use of various estrogen substance varies widely according to condition of patient, and use for which drug is given. Synthetic estrogens: there are a large number of such products which have very similar names and uses. Can be used alone or in combination with progestational agents for breast engorgment.
Benzestrol, N.F. (Octofolin)	1-25 mg. Oral. (synthetic sources)				
Chlorotrianisene, N.F. (Tace).	12-72 mg. Oral. (synthetic sources)				
Dienestrol, N.F. (Dienoestrol, Synestrol) (dienoestral, Willnestrol [C]).	0.1-10 mg. Oral topical, as vaginal cream or suppository. (synthetic sources)				
Diethylstilbestrol, U.S.P. (DES, Stilbestrol, Synestrin) (diethylstilbestrol, Honvol, Stilbilium [C]).	0.1-100 mg. Oral, I.M. or vaginal suppository. (synthetic sources)				
Diethylstilbestrol dipropionate, N.F. (Dibestil) (Orestrol [C]).	0.5-5 mg. I.M. (synthetic sources)				
Estradiol, N.S. (Aquadiol, Aquagen, Femogen, Microdial, Progynon).	10-25 mg. Implant. 1-10 mg. Parenteral. (animal sources)				
Estradiol benzoate, N.F. (Estrobev-E, Ovacylin-B).	1 mg. I.M. (animal sources)				
Estradiol cypionate, N.F. (Depo-Estradiol, Estromed-P.A., Spendepiel).	1-15 mg. I.M. synthetic				

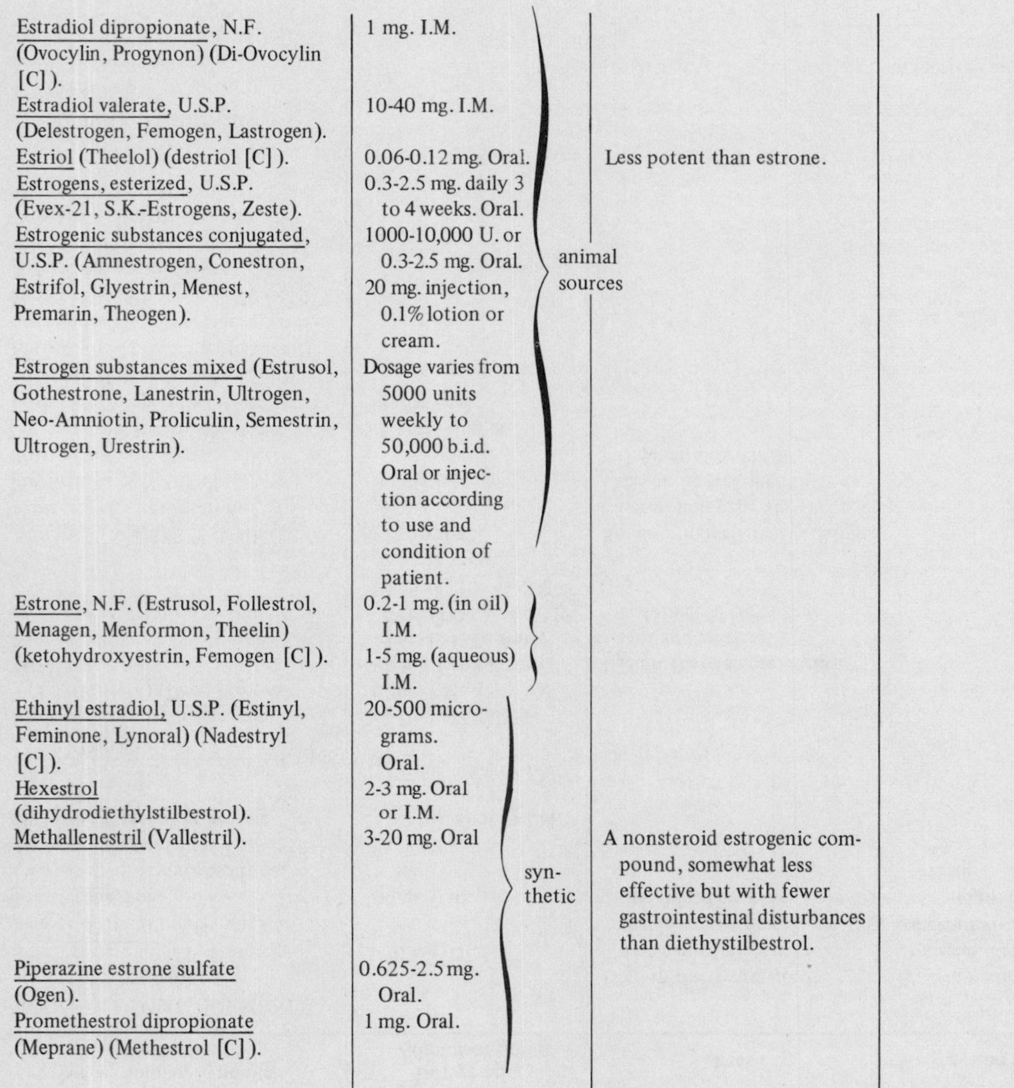

Drug	Dosage	Source	Remarks		Precautions	Uses
Estradiol dipropionate, N.F. (Ovocylin, Progynon) (Di-Ovocylin [C]).	1 mg. I.M.	animal sources			risk of estrogen therapy should be weighed against possible benefits when used during a known pregnancy.	
Estradiol valerate, U.S.P. (Delestrogen, Femogen, Lastrogen).	10-40 mg. I.M.	animal sources				In combination with progestational agents it can be used in habitual or threatened abortion, or alone for breast engorgment.
Estriol (Theelol) (destriol [C]).	0.06-0.12 mg. Oral.	animal sources	Less potent than estrone.			
Estrogens, esterized, U.S.P. (Evex-21, S.K.-Estrogens, Zeste).	0.3-2.5 mg. daily 3 to 4 weeks. Oral.	animal sources				
Estrogenic substances conjugated, U.S.P. (Amnestrogen, Conestron, Estrifol, Glyestrin, Menest, Premarin, Theogen).	1000-10,000 U. or 0.3-2.5 mg. Oral. 20 mg. injection, 0.1% lotion or cream.	animal sources				
Estrogen substances mixed (Estrusol, Gothestrone, Lanestrin, Ultrogen, Neo-Amniotin, Proliculin, Semestrin, Ultrogen, Urestrin).	Dosage varies from 5000 units weekly to 50,000 b.i.d. Oral or injection according to use and condition of patient.	animal sources				
Estrone, N.F. (Estrusol, Follestrol, Menagen, Menformon, Theelin) (ketohydroxyestrin, Femogen [C]).	0.2-1 mg. (in oil) I.M. 1-5 mg. (aqueous) I.M.					
Ethinyl estradiol, U.S.P. (Estinyl, Feminone, Lynoral) (Nadestryl [C]).	20-500 micrograms. Oral.	synthetic				
Hexestrol (dihydrodiethylstilbestrol).	2-3 mg. Oral or I.M.	synthetic				
Methallenestril (Vallestril).	3-20 mg. Oral	synthetic	A nonsteroid estrogenic compound, somewhat less effective but with fewer gastrointestinal disturbances than diethystilbestrol.			
Piperazine estrone sulfate (Ogen).	0.625-2.5 mg. Oral.	synthetic				
Promethestrol dipropionate (Meprane) (Methestrol [C]).	1 mg. Oral.	synthetic				

Name, Source, Synonyms, Preparations	Dosage and Administration	Uses	Action and Fate	Side Effects and Contraindications	Remarks
PROGESTATIONAL HORMONES. *Animal or Synthetic.*					
Dydrogesterone, N.F. (Isopregnenone, Duphaston, Gynorest).	5-20 mg. Oral.	Used in the treatment of dysmenorrhea, menorrhagia, metrorrhagia, and threatened abortion.	Tend to relax the uterine muscles. Prepare endometrium for pregnancy and aid in maintaining this state.	Rare in therapeutic dosage.	Most progestational hormonal drugs are prepared synthetically, although originally they were obtained from animal corpus luteum or placenta. Time of administration varies according to purpose, use, duration of action of various products, and condition of patient.
Ethisterone, N.F. (anhydrohydroxyprogesterone, Lutocyl, Progestelets [C]).	10 mg. Oral.				
Hydroxyprogesterone acetate (Prodox).	25-50 mg. Oral or I.M.				
Hydroxyprogesterone caproate, U.S.P. (Delalutin).	25-50 mg. Oral or I.M.				
Medroxyprogesterone acetate, U.S.P. (Provera) (Depo-Provera [C]).	2.5-10 mg. Oral. 50 mg. I.M. 400 mg./ml. for injection. I.M. To start, 400-1000 mg. weekly, then as little as 400 mg. per month.	Used for inoperable, recurrent and metastatic endometrial carcinoma.			
Norethindrone, U.S.P. (Norlutin, Norlutate) (Norethisterone [C]).	5-20 mg. Oral.	See also under Tissue-building hormones, page 185.			Norlutate is norethindrone acetate.
Pregnenolone (Natolone, Sharmone).	100 mg./cc. I.M.	Used in the treatment of rheumatoid arthritis.			
Progesterone, N.F. (Colprosterone, Corlutone, Corpomone, Gesterol, Glanestin, Lingusorbs, Lipo-Lutin, Lucorteum, Lutocylin, Lutocylol, Lutromone, Lutrone, Macrogestin, Membrettes, Migestrone, Myosol-P, Nalutin, Progelan, Progesteroid, Progestin, Progestone, Progestronol, Progestron, Prolutin) (Luteinol, Progestilin [C]).	5-50 mg. Oral or parenteral.				
OTHER OVARIAN HORMONES. *Animal and synthetic.*					
Lututrin (Lutrexin).	2000-4000 U. Oral.	Used mainly in dysmenorrhea.	A luteal extract which acts as a uterine relaxant.	Rare in therapeutic dosage.	From animal source.

NORETHYNODREL. *Synthetic.* Norethynodrel, U.S.P. (Enovid).	5-10 mg. Oral.	Main use is to control menstrual disorders, and as an oral contraceptive.	Suppresses ovulation.	Rare, but nausea may occur.	Enovid is a combination of norethynodrel and ethynyl estradiol.

There are several drugs similar to Norethynodrel used as oral contraceptives. They are all combined hormonal drugs. Some of the major ones are Demulen, Enovid, Norinyl, Norlestrin, Ortho-Novum, Ovral, Ovulen.

The sequential type of oral contraceptive agents is also available. Examples of this type are Norquen, Oracon and Ortho-Novum SQ. With agents of this kind a tablet containing an estrogenic substance is taken for 14 to 15 days, beginning on the fifth day of the menstrual cycle, then a progestational agent is taken for the next 5 or 6 days. These agents are said to be more like the normal cycle than the other agents. However, greater care must be taken to be sure to take the tablets on a daily basis or there is much greater chance of an unwanted pregnancy.

The third type of oral contraceptives involves the use of a small amount of a progestational agent on a continual daily basis. There is a greater chance of pregnancy with this type. If two consecutive days are missed, the manufacturers state that other means of contraception should be employed until the next menstrual period. An example follows.

Norethindrone (Micronor).	0.35 mg./tablet One tablet daily on a continuous basis.	Contraceptive.	Effectiveness less than with the combination and sequential drugs.	Side effects, contraindications, etc., same as with the others.	Safety during pregnancy or lactation has not been established.
PANCREAS. (Islets of Langerhans).					
INSULIN. *Animal.*	All insulin is given in units. Actual dosage varies widely from 1-100 units. Insulin is given subcutaneously. Regular (unmodified) insulin is also given I.V.	Used as a specific in the treatment of diabetes mellitus. Also used to produce unconsciousness in shock therapy, to stimulate the appetite, and in cases of hyperglycemia not directly caused by diabetes mellitus.	Tends to lower blood sugar by increasing the metabolism of sugar. One unit of insulin will metabolize 1.5 Gm. of dextrose. Insulin is secreted by the beta cells (Islets of Langerhans) of the pancreas.	Excessive doses may cause hypoglycemia (insulin shock) with weakness, sweating, nervousness, anxiety, pallor, or flushing. Later symptoms of insulin shock include aphasia, convulsive seizures, coma, and even death. Give soluble sugar orally or I.V. Orange juice, if given early, will relieve the symptoms. Care must be taken to rotate areas of injection to prevent skin reactions and infection.	Insulin is available in vials (usually 10 ml.) containing 40, 80 or 100 U./ml. Vials of 20 U./ml. are also prepared but not commonly used. Since insulin is a protein molecule, it is destroyed by the digestive juices and hence must be given parenterally. Non-protein hypoglycemic agents are available for specific uses. See below.

Name, Source, Synonyms, Preparations	Dosage and Administration	Uses	Action and Fate	Side Effects and Contraindications	Remarks
PANCREAS (Continued)	**Type of Action**	**Onset of Action**	**Height of Action**	**Duration of Action**	
Insulin injection, U.S.P. (regular, unmodified) (Iletin).	Quickest acting.	20-30 minutes.	1-2 h.	5-8 h.	When mixed with other insulins (except Lente), time and duration can be affected.
Insulin zinc suspension, prompt, U.S.P. (Semi-Lente Iletin).	Quick acting.	50-60 minutes	2-3 h.	6-8 h.	Main use is for patients allergic to regular insulin.
Globin insulin with zinc, U.S.P.	Medium acting.	1-2 h.	8-16 h.	18-24 h.	
Insulin isophane suspension, U.S.P. (NPH Iletin).	Medium acting.	1-2 h.	10-20 h.	28-30 h.	
Insulin zinc suspension, U.S.P. (Lente Iletin).	Medium acting.	1-2 h.	10-20 h.	20-32 h.	Lente insulins can be mixed with each other or with any insulin as their action depends on the size of the particle, rather than additives.
Insulin zinc suspension, extended, U.S.P. (Ultra-Lente Iletin).	Long acting.	4-6 h.	16-24 h.	24-36 h.	
Insulin protamine zinc suspension, U.S.P. (Protamine Zinc and Iletin).	Long acting.	4-6 h.	16-24 h.	24-36 h. or longer.	

NONHORMONAL DRUGS USED IN THE TREATMENT OF DIABETES MELLITUS. SYNTHETIC HYPOGLYCEMIC DRUGS.

Synthetic preparations used chiefly in treatment of older diabetics. Not usually recommended for juvenile or ketotic diabetic. All dosages are individually adjusted. The safe use of these drugsduring pregnancy has not been established. Their use in women of child-bearing age should be carefully weighed by the physician, hazards against benefits. The sulfonylurea compounds interact with a number of drugs. With phenylbutazone, oxyphenylbutazone and sulfinpyrazone, there can be an increased hypoglycemic effect, and the dose of the sulfonylurea drug should be adjusted downward if given concurrently with any of these drugs. Chloramphenicol increases the half-life of the sulfonylurea compounds, and this can cause a hypoglycemic reaction. Patients who regularly take alcohol in quantity will metabolize tolbutamide at an accelerated rate and will require larger than usual doses.

Name, Source, Synonyms, Preparations	Dosage and Administration	Uses	Action and Fate	Side Effects and Contraindications	Remarks
Acetohexamide, N.F. (Dymelor) (Dimeler [C]).	250-500 mg. o.d. to q.i.d. Oral.	Used in stable, mild, adult diabetes. Occasionally used in moderately severe diabetes in conjunction with insulin.	A sulfonylurea drug; tends to increase the secretion of endogenous insulin.	Usually mild, such as gastro-intestinal disturbances, skin rash, headache, nervousness, etc. Jaundice has been reported infrequently. Hypoglycemia may appear in those patients who do not eat regularly or who exercise without caloric supplementation. Contraindicated in juvenile or severe diabetes and during pregnancy. Used with caution in debilitated patients or in	

				patients known to have liver damage.	
Chlorpropamide, U.S.P. (Diabinese) (Chlorolase, Chloromide, Diazene, Novoproamide, Stabinol, Melinase [C]).	100-250 mg. Oral. Up to 750 mg. daily for maintenance.	Use and indications similar to those for tolbutamide.	See tolbutamide. Rapidly absorbed. Is bound to plasma proteins. Is slowly excreted by the kidneys largely unchanged. Half-life is about 36 hours.	Similar to tolbutamide. Contraindicated in patients with impairment of hepatic, renal, or thyroid function.	
Phenformin, U.S.P. (DBI, Meltrol).	25 mg. Usually given b.i.d. or t.i.d. after stabilization. Also available in 50-100 mg. sustained release capsule. Oral.	Use and precautions similar to those for tolbutamide. May prove useful in children.	The exact action of this drug is not well understood. Unrelated to tolbutamide or chlorpropamide in activity and chemical structure. Adequately absorbed from the gastrointestinal tract. Duration of action is from 6 to 14 hours.	May cause gastrointestinal irritation. Phenformin and alcohol can cause a hypoglycemic reaction, so patients taking phenformin should avoid or restrict their intake of alcohol.	This is not a sulfonylurea compound.
Tolazamide, U.S.P. (Tolinase).	Individually adjusted. Oral. If more than 500 mg. is required daily, it should be divided 250 mg. b.i.d. More than 1000 mg. per day will probably not result in better control.	Used to treat stable or maturity onset diabetes	Appears to act on endogenous insulin secretion.	Contraindicated in juvenile diabetes, severe trauma, impending surgery, ketosis, acidosis, coma or history of these complications.	Available in 100-250 mg. tablets. Not recommended for patients with concurrent liver, renal or endocrine disease or during pregnancy.
Tolbutamide, U.S.P. (Orinase) (Hypoglymid, Mobenol, Tolbugen, Tolbutol, Tolbutone, Willbutamide [C]). (Other Canadian trade names include: Chem-Butamide, Glycemex, Mallitol, Neo-Dibetil, Novobutamide, Oramide, Wescotol.	0.5-3 Gm. Oral.	Used in the treatment of diabetes mellitus in the adult whose condition is stabilized.	Appears to stimulate the beta cells to secrete insulin, hence is valuable only in patients who retain some functioning cells. It is chemically related to the sulfonamide drugs. Rapidly absorbed from gastrointestinal tract; peak concentration in 3-5 hours. Bound to plasma proteins and metabolized. Half-life in body about 5 hours.	Nausea and other gastric disturbances and skin eruptions. Reduce dosage or stop drugs and treat symptoms. Contraindicated in juvenile or severe diabetes mellitus.	

Name, Source, Synonyms, Preparations	Dosage and Administration	Uses	Action and Fate	Side Effects and Contraindications	Remarks
PARATHYROID. *Animal.*					
Parathyroid injection, U.S.P. (Para-Thor-mone).	25-50 U. o.d. Parenteral.	Used as a specific in hypoparathyroidism and hypocalcemia (tetany). Paratyroid injection is used in acute conditions, since vitamin D and calcium are more valuable in chronic disorders.	Parathyroid hormone raises the blood calcium level from a tetanic level of 5-7 mg./100 ml. of blood to the normal of 10-12 mg./100 ml. in about 9-18 hours. However, this effect lasts only 12-36 hours.	Rare in therapeutic dosage.	
PITUITARY					
ANTERIOR. *Animal.*			Several hormones secreted by this gland control growth and development, stimulation of the various other glands, and general regulations of many body functions.		
Anterior pituitary extract.	0.5-5 ml. t.i.s. I.M.	Anterior pituitary extract is said to contain the growth promoting factor and gonadotropic and thyrotropic factors.			
Cosyntropin (Cortrosyn).	0.25-0.75 mg. I.M. or I.V.	For a rapid screening test of adrenal function and can be used to differentiate between some types of primary and secondary insufficiency.	Cosyntropin exhibits the full corticosteroidogenic activity of natural ACTH. Cosyntropin contains 24 of the 39 amino acids of natural ACTH starting from the N terminus. In activity, 0.25 mg. of cosyntropin has the activity of 25 units of natural ACTH. It also possesses the extra-adrenal effects of natural ACTH which include increased melanotropic activity, increased growth hormone secretion and an adipokinetic effect. It has been shown that with the 24 amino acid chain length there is much less antigenicity than with the 39 chain natural substance.	Side effects and contraindications: it has slight immunologic activity and is not completely devoid of hypersensitivity reactions. There have been only three such reactions, and in all three cases, the patients had a pre-existing allergic disease and/or a previous reaction to natural ACTH.	

Corticotropin injection, U.S.P. (adrenocorticotropin, ACTH, Acthar, Action-X, Cortrophin, Duraction [C]).	10-100 U. o.d. I.M., S.Q., or I.V.	Corticotropin is used to treat various conditions such as arthritis, allergy, and hypersensitivity, and experimentally in a large number of disorders.	Corticotropin stimulates the adrenal cortex to secrete its hormones. It is useful only if the adrenal cortex is able to respond to the stimulation.	Use of corticotropin may result in a rounded contour of the face, mild hirsutism, mental disorders, transient retention of salt and water with edema, restlessness, insomnia, euphoria, and hyperglycemia. Contraindicated in tuberculosis (active, healed or questionably healed), ocular herpes simplex, and acute psychosis. Relative (possible) contraindications: diverticulitis, active or latent peptic ulcer, osteoporosis, diabetes mellitus, myasthenia gravis, severe hypertension, thromboembolic phenomena first trimester of pregnancy and any serious, acute or chronic infection if antibodies are unavailable or ineffective.	Corticotropin depresses the activity of the anterior pituitary substance, with atrophy from prolonged use. For interactions, see under suprarenal, page 179.
Corticotropin injection repository, U.S.P. (Acthar-Gel-HP, ACTH-Gel, Corticotropin-Gel, Cortropin-Gel).	10-80 U. U.S.P. units. o.d. Entire daily dose may be given at one time. Individually adjusted. The gel delays absorption and prolongs the action. I.M.				
Corticotropin zinc hydrochloride suspension, U.S.P. (Cortropin-Zinc).	40-80 U. U.S.P. units. o.d. Dosage individually adjusted. I.M.				
Chorionic gonadotropin (Antuitrin, A.P.L., Apestrin, Follutein, Pregnyl, Riogon, Tropigon).	200-500 U. Parenteral. Two or three times weekly (q. 2-3 s.).	Chorionic gonadotropin is used to stimulate gonadal secretion of sex hormones in treatment of cryptorchidism, hypogonadism, uterine bleeding, amenorrhea, functional sterility, acne vulgaris, dysmenorrhea, threatened abortion, Frohlich's syndrome, and impotence.			These preparations have properties similar to those of anterior pituitary hormone. They are obtained from blood serum or from urine of pregnant mares.
CLOMIPHENE CITRATE. *Synthetic.*					
Clomiphene citrate (Clomid).	50 mg. o.d. oral for 5 days. May increase to 100 mg. o.d. for 5 days if 50 mg. is not effective. Increasing dose or duration of therapy beyond 100 mg. for 5 days should not be done. Three courses of 5 days each constitutes an adequate trial and treatment. Use beyond this is not recommended.	Used to induce ovulation in appropriately selected cases. (See brochure).	Action appears to be mediated through increased output of pituitary gonadotropins, which in turn stimulates the maturation and endocrine activity of the ovarian follicle and the subsequent development and function of the corpus luteum. The pituitary role is indicated by increased urinary excretion of gonadotropins and the response of the ovary is shown by increased urinary estrogen excretion.	Contraindications: pregnancy, liver disease, abnormal bleeding of undetermined origin, ovarian cyst. Side effects: visual symptoms (if they occur, stop drug and have complete ophthalmologic evaluation), multiple births, ovarian enlargement. Also hot flashes and abdominal discomfort.	Great care should be taken in the selection of the patients to be put on this drug. (See brochure.) This drug is not a hormone, but is placed here because it appears to act on the pituitary gland.

Name, Source, Synonyms, Preparations	Dosage and Administration	Uses	Action and Fate	Side Effects and Contraindications	Remarks
PITUITARY (Continued) POSTERIOR. *Animal and synthetic.*					
Lypressin. *Synthetic.* (Diapid).	Nasal spray (one spray approximately 2 U.S.P. posterior pituitary [pressor] units) (0.185 gm./ml. equivalent to 50 units). 1-2 sprays in one or both nostrils q.i.d. and h.s. If patient needs more than this, results are better if the time interval is reduced rather than increasing the number of sprays per dose.	Used for the control of diabetes insipidus due to a deficiency of endogenous posterior pituitary antidiuretic hormone.	This is a synthetic product which takes the place of the endogenous antidiuretic hormone. Absorption is fairly good from the nasal mucosa. It is not effective orally. Duration of action is 3-8 hours.	Cardiovascular effects are minimal when used nasally as directed. But it should be used with caution in patients in whom such effects are undesirable. Large doses may cause coronary artery constriction.	This drug is synthetic lysine-8-vasopressin. The effectiveness may be lessened with nasal congestion, allergic rhinitis and upper respiratory infection.
Oxytocin injection, U.S.P. (Pitocin, Syntocinon, Uteracon).	0.3-1 ml. p.r.n. Subcutaneous, I.V. or I.M.	An oxytocic agent.	Oxytocin is specifically oxytocic and is devoid of most pressor activity.	Rare in therapeutic dosage. Should not be used early in labor as trauma to mother or child may result.	
Sparteine sulfate (Spartocin, Tocosamine) (Tocine [C]).	75-150 mg. up to a total not to exceed 600 mg. I.M.	Oxytocic for the induction of labor and for the treatment of uterine inertia.	Oxytocic.	Contraindications: heart disease, normal labor, when there is evidence of hypertonic or tumultuous uterine contractions, cephalopelvic disproportion, previous abdominal deliveries, abdominal scar, placentae praevia, abruptio placentae, grand multiparity, elective induction of labor when obstretrical conditions are not favorable.	WARNING: This drug, as with other oxytocic agents, may cause tetanic uterine contractions and in multiparous patients can cause uterine rupture. If drug is not effective and oxytocin is to be used, several hours should elapse between drugs because of their synergistic action. Sparteine sulfate is not a hormone, but is placed here because of the similarity of use and action with oxytocin.
Posterior pituitary, N.F., B.P. Posterior pituitary injection, N.F. (Infundin, Pituitrin).	5-20 mg. Snuffed. 10 U. Subcutaneous.	Used to treat diabetes insipidus and to stimulate smooth muscle tissue.	See oxytocin and vasopressin.	Rare in therapeutic dosage.	Contains complete posterior pituitary hormone.

Vasopressin injection, U.S.P. (Pitressin).	0.3-1 ml. p.r.n. Subcutaneous.	As above.	Vasopressin is a vasopressor and an antidiuretic agent. It raises blood pressure and stimulates smooth muscle tissue, thus increasing peristalsis and decreasing the flow of urine.	As above.	
SUPRARENAL (Adrenal) CORTEX		Used as a specific in the treatment of Addison's disease and in all conditions in which corticotropin is used.	The adrenal glands appear to be concerned mainly with stress conditions: the medulla with acute stress, the cortex with chronic or prolonged stress. There are several active steroids secreted by the adrenal cortex. Aldosterone and desoxycorticosterone are concerned primarily with electrolyte balance. They tend to increase the retention of sodium and the excretion of potassium. These are sometimes called mineral corticoids. Cortisone and hydrocortisone are concerned primarily with glucose metabolism and are called glucocorticoids. Aldosterone and hydrocortisone have more selective action. Cortisone and desoxycorticosterone have more general action. Most of the synthetic products are used for their anti-inflammatory properties, both systemic and local.	Same contraindications and toxicity as those listed under corticotropin. Toxicity of individual preparations may vary somewhat in kind and extent; thus, aldosterone may cause excessive loss of potassium, etc. Also contraindicated in systemic fungal infections. Safe use of these drugs during pregnancy has not been established. Interactions: diphenylhydantoin, barbiturates and antihistamines decrease the pharmaceutical and physiological effect of the steroids by enzyme induction. Salicylates and phenylbutazone displace the steroids from plasma protein binding sites and give enhanced steroid effects so that lower doses will be effective. Steroids antagonize the hypoglycemic action of the oral agents and insulin, because of their gluconeogenic and glycogenolytic activity in the liver.	Many of these preparations are combined with other drugs such as the antibiotics, especially the topical preparations. Check blood pressure frequently and watch for edema. The dose range is very great. Strengths shown are those available and do not necessarily constitute actual dosage administered.
Adrenal cortex (Eschatin, Recortex).	2-10 ml. (50 dog U./ml.) Parenteral. 0.5-1 U. Oral.				
Aldosterone (Aldocertin, Electrocortin).	0.1-0.3 mg. Oral or I.M.	Action similar to that of desoxycorticosterone.			
Betamethasone, N.F. (Celestone), (Betnelan, Betnesol, Betnovate [C]).	0.6-4.8 mg. Oral.	Use and action similar to those of prednisolone and derivatives.			
Betamethasone 17 valerate (Valisone) (Celestoderm [C]).	0.1% cream and ointment. Topical.				
Cortisone acetate, N.F. (Cortone acetate) (Novocort [C]).	5-300 mg. Oral or I.M. 0.25-2.5% ointment. Topical.	Cortisone primarily affects protein, fat, and carbohydrate metabolism. Used in the treatment of a variety of conditions such as asthma, other allergies, some infections, arthritis, etc.			

Name, Source, Synonyms, Preparations	Dosage and Administration	Uses	Action and Fate	Side Effects and Contraindications	Remarks
SUPRARENAL (Continued)					
Desonide (Tridesilon).	0.05% ointment. Topical.	Same as other topical steroids.	This is a nonfluorinated corticosteroid. Same as other topical steroids.	Same as other topical steroids.	
Desoxycorticosterone acetate, N.F. (Cortate, Deoxycortone Acetate, DOCA-acetate, Percorten) (desoxycortone [C]).	2-5 mg. Oral or parenteral. 75-125 mg. Tablet implants.	Desoxycorticosterone primarily affects water and salt metabolism.			Warning: Do not administer more than 10 mg. desoxycorticosterone acetate in oil at any one time.
Desoxycorticosterone pivalate, N.F. (Percorten trimethylacetate).	25-100 mg. I.M. monthly.				
Dexamethasone, N.F. (Decadron, Deronil, Dexameth, Gamma-corten, Hexadrol, Maxidex).	0.5-0.75 mg. Oral. 0.1% ophthalmic solution.	See cortisone.	It is almost devoid of any mineralocorticoid effects.		
Dexamethasone phosphate sodium, U.S.P. (Decadron phosphate, Hexadrol) (Dexamethadrone, Maxidex, Novo-Methasone [C]).	4-20 mg. I.M. or I.V. 0.8-4 mg. Intra-articular. 0.05-0.1% solution.				
Dichlorisone acetate (Diloderm).	0.18-0.25% Aerosol and cream. Topical.	Used for treatment of allergic or pruritic inflammations.			
Flumethasone pivalate (Locorten) (Locacorton [C]).	0.03% cream. Apply 3 to 4 times a day. Topical.	A topical corticosteroid. Used as others of this group.	As with others of this group.	As with others of this group. Contraindications: as with others and hypersensitivity—vaccinia and varicella.	
Fluocinolone acetonide, N.F. (Synalar) (Synamel [C]).	0.01-0.02% cream. Topical. 0.1% suspension for eyes.				
Fluocinonide (Lidex).	0.05% cream. Topical.	As adjunct therapy for relief of inflammatory manifestations of acute and chronic corticosteroid responsive dermatoses.		See flucinolone.	21 acetate ester of fluocinolone acetonide.
Fluorocortisone acetate (Cortef-F acetate, Florinef acetate) (Fluorocortone [C]).	0.1-0.5 mg. Oral.	Mainly used for its effect on electrolytes as in Addison's disease.			

Fluorometholone, N.F. (Oxylone).	0.025% cream or ointment. Topical.				
Fluorometholone (FML).	0.1% solution. Topical in eyes. 1-2 gtts. b.i.d. to q.i.d. May be used as much as gtt. q. 2 h.	For inflammation of palpebral and bulbar conjunctiva, cornea and anterior segment of the globe.	Same as others of this group.	As with others of this group.	
Fluprednisolone, N.F. (Alphadrol).	0.75-1.5 mg. Oral.			Edema and hypertension rarely occur.	
Flurandrenalide (Cordran) (Drenison [C]).	0.025-0.05% cream or ointment. Topical. 4 mcg./sq. cm. tape. Topical.			Contraindicated with tubercular or secondary bacterial skin infections.	
Hydrocortamate hydrochloride (Ulcort) (ethamicort [C]).	0.5% ointment. Topical.	As for cortisone.			
Hydrocortisone or Cortisol, U.S.P. (Compound F, Cortdome, Cortef, Domolene-HC, Heb-Cort, Hydrocortone). (Bio-Cort, Cortanal, Cort-Dome, Corticreme, Cortiment, Cremocort, Hycortol, Manticor [C]).	5-20 mg. Oral. Also prepared for topical use.	Uses same as for cortisone.	Concerned primarily with glucose metabolism.		
Hydrocortisone acetate, U.S.P. (Cortef acetate, Cortril-A, Hydrocortone Acetate) (Emo-Cort, Hytone, Ipso-Hydrocortisone, Microcort, Novohydrocort, Sterocort, Surfa-Cort, Texacort, Unicort, Wincort [C]).	5-20 mg. Intra-articular. 1-2.5% solution or ointment. Topical.				
Hydrocortisone phosphate.	50-500 mg. Parenteral.				
Hydrocortisone sodium succinate, U.S.P. (Solu-Cortef).	50-1000 mg. Parenteral. Also available in preparations for topical use.				
Lipo-adrenal cortex extract.	1-2 ml. (40-80 U.) I.M.				
Medrysone (HMS).	1% solution eye drops. One drop in conjunctival sac q.i.d.	Used for allergic conjunctivitis, episcleritis and epinephrine sensitivity.	Has topical anti-inflammatory and antiallergic action.	Transient burning and stinging or instillation. Contraindications: untreated purulent ocular infections, acute herpes simplex keratitis, viral diseases of conjunctiva and cornea, ocular tuberculosis and fungal diseases of the eye.	This is an anti-inflammatory agent related to progesterone. There is less sodium retention than with some others such as prednisone.
Meprednisone (Betapar).	Up to 60 mg. daily. Oral. Available as 4 mg. tablets.				
Methylprednisolone, N.F. (Medrol, Wyacort).	2-16 mg. Oral.				

METABOLIC DRUGS (Continued)

HORMONES *(Continued)*

Name, Source, Synonyms, Preparations	Dosage and Administration	Uses	Action and Fate	Side Effects and Contraindications	Remarks
SUPRARENAL (Continued)					
Methylprednisolone acetate, N.F. (Depo-Medrol, Medrol, Wyacort).	20-40 mg. I.M. 20-120 mg. Intra-articular.				
Methylprednisolone sodium succinate, N.F. (Solu-Medrol).	10-1000 mg. I.M. or I.V.				
Paramethasone acetate, N.F. (Haldrone, Stemex).	1-12 mg. Oral. Also prepared for aerosol use.	Use and action similar to those of prednisolone and derivatives.			
Prednisolone, U.S.P. (Delta-Cortef, Meticortelone, Paracortol, Prednis, (metacortandrolone, Cormalone, Inflamase, Isopto-prednisolone [C]).	1-5 mg. Oral. 0.5% cream. Topical.	These are cortisone derivatives with greater activity than cortisone, thus allowing lower dosage and less toxicity. Used topically for anti-inflammatory action, as are many corticosteroids.			
Prednisolone acetate, U.S.P. (Nisolone, Sterane acetate).	1-5 mg. I.M.				
Prednisolone and metacortandracin (Meticortelone).	5-30 mg. Oral and topical.				
Prednisolone butylacetate.	4-30 mg. Subcutaneous or intrasynovial.				
Prednisolone phosphate sodium, U.S.P. (Hydeltrasol, PSP I.V.).	2-30 mg. Subcutaneous, I.M., intrasynovial, I.V. 0.25-0.5% cream. Topical.				
Prednisone, U.S.P. (Delta-Dome, Deltasone, Deltra, Meticorten, Paracort) (metacortandracin, Colisone, Decortancyl, Prednisol, Wescopred, Winpred [C]).	1-20 mg. Oral.				
Triamcinolone acetonide, U.S.P. (Aristocort-acetonide, Aristoderm, Kenalog) (Triamalone [C]).	0.025-0.05% cream, ointment or lotion. Topical.				
Triamcinolone diacetate, N.F. (Aristocort, Diacetate).	1-16 mg. Oral. 10-25 mg. Intra-articular or intralesonial.				
Triamcinolone, U.S.P. (Aristocort, Kepacort).	1-16 mg. Oral.	A derivative of prednisolone that is said to have fewer side effects.			

MEDULLA. For uses of the adrenal medullary hormone, refer to Drugs acting on the autonomic nervous system—epinephrine. (See page 49.)

TESTICULAR					
Calusterone (Methosarb).	50 mg. q.i.d. (range 150-300 mg./day).	Only for palliative therapy of inoperable or metastatic carcinoma of the breast in postmenopausal women when hormonal therapy is indicated.	Biochemical mechanism by which calusterone produces its effects is at present unknown.	Side effects: hypercalcemia may occur, drug related edema, PSP retention and increases in SGOT have been observed. Others are those usually seen with the androgen drugs: deepening of voice, acne, facial hair growth. Nausea and vomiting is also a common side effect. Contraindicated in carcinoma of the male breast and premenopausal women.	Should be given a minimum of 3 months to evaluate the response unless there is active progression of the disease.
Fluoxymesterone, U.S.P. (Halotestin, Ora-Testryl, Ultrandren) (Oratestin [C]). *(A halogenated androgen similar to testosterone, but more potent.)*	4-10 mg. Oral.	Used in the treatment of male hypogonadism, climacteric, and cryptorchidism. Also used to treat symptoms of menopausal state in females, menorrhagia, and other gynecologic conditions.	The secretion of the testes whose primary function is the maintenance of the secondary male characteristics. Performs the same function in the male as estrogen does in the female.	Patient should be watched for elevated blood calcium, exacerbation of condition being treated, edema, flushing or acne of face, and—in the female—hirsutism and deepening of voice, as well. Reduce or stop drug. In males, the following postpubertal adverse reactions have occurred: inhibition of testicular function, testicular atrophy, oligospermia, impotence, chronic priapism, gynecomastia, epididymitis and bladder irritation.	Fluoxymesterone is also used as an anabolic agent. Times for all these drugs vary with the use and the condition of the patient. Contraindicated in female patients during pregnancy and lactation.
Methyltestosterone, N.F. (Metandren, Neo-Hombreal-M, Oreton-M) (Andrhormone-M, Testostelets [C]).	5-20 mg. Oral.	Also used to treat breast cancer in female.		Contraindicated in patients with severe liver damage and in male patients with prostate or breast cancer.	
Testosterone Cypionate, U.S.P. (Depo-Testosterone).	50-100 mg. I.M.			Also in patients with nephrosis or the nephrotic phase of nephritis.	A long acting form of testosterone.
Testosterone enanthate, U.S.P. (Delatestryl, Reposo-TE) (Melogex [C]).	0.2 Gm. in oil. I.M.				As above.

Name, Source, Synonyms, Preparations	Dosage and Administration	Uses	Action and Fate	Side Effects and Contraindications	Remarks
TESTICULAR (Continued)					
Testosterone pellets, N.F. (Oreton micro pellets).	0.3 Gm. Subcutaneous implants.				
Testosterone propionate, U.S.P. (Androlin, Neo-Hombreol, Oreton) (Andr-hormone-P, Testavirol [C]).	10-75 mg. in oil. I.M.				
Testosterone suspension, N.F. (Andronaq, Malestrone, Neo-Hombrel-F, Oreton Sterotate).	25 mg. Aq. I.M.				
THYROID		Used as a specific in hypothyroidism, which produces conditions such as goiter, myxedema (adult) or cretinism (child), mental and physical retardation, gonadal disorders, and obesity.	The thyroid hormone is reciprocal with the thyrotropic hormone of the anterior pituitary. An increase in one causes a decrease in the other. The thyroid hormone is also related to the normal functioning of the gonads, the involution of the thymus, carbohydrate metabolism, and proper calcium level. There are, perhaps, other functions. It increases the rate of body metabolism.	Thyroid preparations may cause excessive weight loss, tachycardia, excessive nervvousness, tremors, visual disturbances, hypertension, and other symptoms of excessive metabolism. May have cumulative action. Interactions: thyroid appears to enhance the effects of the tricyclic antidepressants, especially in patients with depressed or abnormal thyroid function. Thyroid absorption is hindered by the concurrent administration of cholestyramine. It is recommended that 4 to 5 hours should elapse between oral doses of these two drugs. Patients treated with thyroid compounds will require a lower dose of oral anticoagulants when the drugs are given concurrently.	Skipping an occasional day's dosage is advised by some physicians. All doses of thyroid preparations are individually adjusted. Total dose may be taken at one time (o.d.) or in divided doses. It should not be given too late in the day as it may cause insomnia.
Sodium levothyroxine, U.S.P. (Letter, Synthroid) (Eltroxin [C]).	0.05-0.3 mg. Oral. 0.05 mg. injection.				
Sodium liothyronine, U.S.P. (Cytomel, Trionine) (tertroxin [C]).	5-50 micrograms. Oral.				
Thyroglobulin (Endothyrin Proloid, Thyrar, Thyroprotein).	60 mg. Oral.				
Thyroid, U.S.P. (Thyronol [C]).	60 mg. Dosage may vary from 15 to 300 mg. daily. Oral.				
Thyrotropin (Thytropar) (Thyrotron [C]).	5-10 U. I.M. or subcutaneous.	Diagnostic and therapeutic agent. Thyrotropic hormone from anterior pituitary (TSH).	Acts to stimulate the thyroid gland.		
dl-Triiodothyronine sodium (dl-Liothyronine, Trinone).	5-50 micrograms. Oral.		See thyroid.		
Sodium dextrothyroxine, N.F. (Choloxin) (d-thyroxine sodium [C]).	1.0-2.0 mg. o.d. Oral first day. Increase 1.0-2.0 mg. and hold	Used to treat hypercholesteremia in euthyroid patients. May also be used	Thought to stimulate normal catabolism of cholesterol and its degradation products	Contraindications: known organic heart disease, hypertensive states, advanced	This drug may potentiate the effect of anticoagulants. Dose should be reduced

	this daily dose 2.0-4.0 mg. for one month. Increase in this manner until controlled. Do not increase beyond 6.0-8.0 mg. daily. Maintenance dose is usually 4.0-8.0 mg. daily. Children: 0.05 mg./kg. daily. May increase 0.05-0.1 mg. monthly per kg. to 4.0 mg. daily if needed to control.	to treat hypothyroidism in patients with cardiac disease who cannot tolerate other types of thyroid medication. Main use is to lower blood cholesterol.	in the body with subsequent increase in excretion of cholesterol and its degradation products via the biliary route. Absorbed orally, metabolized by body. Small amounts not metabolized are excreted in urine and feces in about equal amounts.	liver or kidney disease, pregnancy, during lactation, history of iodism. Side effects: mainly those of increased metabolism: insomnia, nervousness, tremors, palpitation, loss of weight, lid lag, sweating, flushing, hyperthermia, loss of hair, diuresis, menstrual disorders, abdominal disorders.	by one third on initiation of therapy and readjusted on the basis of prothrombin times. Has been shown to decrease concentration of blood factors VII, VIII and IX and platelet activity in some people.
TISSUE-BUILDING HORMONES. These are semisynthetic or synthetic preparations.		Used to promote growth and repair of body tissues in senility, chronic illness, convalescence, and prematurity.	Tissue building steroids. May also stimulate erythropoiesis in certain types of anemia.	Toxicity low but edema may occur in malnourished patients with cardiac or renal impairment. The following adverse effects have been seen with the use of anabolic steroids: increased or decreased libido, flushing of the face, acne, habituation, excitation, sleeplessness, chills, leukopenia and bleeding in patients on concomitant anticoagulant therapy. These drugs are used with caution, if at all, in prostatic cancer and severe renal and hepatic disorders, some cardiac disorders, and during pregnancy. Menstrual disturbance may occur during therapy.	Methandrostenolone potentiates warfarin and indondione anticoagulants, so prothrombin time should be closely monitored. Methandrostenolone and norethandrolone are said to be free of gonadal action.
Ethylestrenol (Orgabolin, Maxibolin).	2-8 mg. Daily. (0.1 mg./kg. to start, increasing as required). Oral.				
Methandrostenolone, N.F. (Dianabol) (methandienone, Danabol [C]).	5 mg. q.d. Oral.				
Methandriol (Methyltestediol [C]).	5-10 mg. Oral.				
Nandrolone decanoate, N.F. (Deca-Durabolin).	50 mg. Monthly. I.M.				
Nandrolone phenpropionate, N.F. (Durabolin).	25 mg. Once a week. I.M.				
Norethandrolone, N.F. (Nilevar [C]).	30-50 mg. q.d. Oral or I.M.				
Norethindrone, N.F. (Norlutin, Norlutate, Norethisterone).	5 mg. Up to 20 mg. q.d. daily. Oral.	Used for gynecological symptoms associated with pregnancy and menstruation.			Norethindrone is similar to norethandrolone in structure and action.
Oxandrolone (Anavar) (Protivar [C]).	2.5 mg. daily. Two to four times daily. Oral.				
Oxymetholone, N.F. (Anadrol, Adroyd tablets) (Anapolon [C]).	2.5-5 mg. Given in divided doses for 4-6 week period. Oral.	See above.	See above.	See above.	

Name, Source, Synonyms, Preparations	Dosage and Administration	Uses	Action and Fate	Side Effects and Contraindications	Remarks
TISSUE-BUILDING HORMONES (Continued)					
Stanozolol, N.F. (Winstrol).	2 mg. t.i.d. Oral.	Used for debilitated, underweight, and catabolic patients.	A steroidal anabolic agent used to produce positive nitrogen balance.	As above. Increased retention of sulfobromophthalein has been reported.	Androgenicity low; mild virilizing effects may occur with long use, especially in young women.

VITAMINS

FAT SOLUBLE

Since vitamins A and D are usually found in the same preparations, they will be listed together. Petroleum oil should not be given with the fat-soluble vitamins as it delays or prevents absorption of some of them. Dosages of vitamins vary according to purpose. In most cases, dosage given is average daily dosage. May be divided or given at one time according to circumstances.

Name, Source, Synonyms, Preparations	Dosage and Administration	Uses	Action and Fate	Side Effects and Contraindications	Remarks
VITAMIN A. Precursors are carotene (alpha, beta, gamma) and cryptoxanthin. *Preformed vitamin A is secured from animal sources (fish liver oil, milk, fortified margarine, liver, egg yolk). Precursors are secured from vegetables (yellow fruits and vegetable and dark green vegetables). Only about 50% of the precursors taken are absorbed.*		Used to treat xerophthalmia, nyctalopia, retarded growth, and susceptibility of the mucous membranes to infection.	Deficiency produces xerophthalmia, nyctalopia, hyperkeratosis of the skin, and increased susceptibility to colds, influenza, and similar conditions. Recommended daily allowance (not yet satisfactorily determined) about 1.5 mg. (5000 U.S.P. units). Protective for children and for lactating mothers, possibly 5000-8000 U.S.P. units. For treatment: 7.5-60 mg. (25,000 U.S.P. units). Vitamin A is readily absorbed from gastrointestinal tract. Most carotenes are changed to vitamin A in the intestinal wall and absorption is incomplete. It is widely distributed but stored in the liver. Almost completely metabolized to carbon dioxide, fatty acids, and water-soluble derivatives.		
Carotene (Caritol).	5000-7500 U. Oral.				
Vitamin A, U.S.P. (Oleovitam A) (Anatola, Vi-Alpha) (Afraxin, Alphalin, Aquasol, Aret-A, Arovite, Viatate, Vita-A, Win-Vite-A [C]).	25,000-50,000 U. Oral.				
Vitamin A water-miscible, U.S.P. (Acon, Aquamic Aleum A, Aquasol, A-Visol, Sol-A-Caps, Vi-Dom-A).	25,000-50,000 U. Oral.				

Tretinoin (retinoic acid, Vitamin A acid) (Retin-A, Aberel).	Topical application to skin lesions once daily for 2-3 weeks or as long as 6 weeks. Then dose usually may be reduced.	Treatment of acne vulgaris when comedones and pustules predominate. Not effective in severe cases with pustules and deep cystic nodules.	Results may be seen in 2-3 weeks, but may not be optimal until 6 weeks.	During early treatment exacerbation may occur, but is due to revealing of deep pustules not previously seen. Can cause severe local erythema and peeling at site of application. If severe enough, use should be discontinued. Contraindicated for patients with eczematous skin.	Should not be used with other agents containing peeling agents such as sulfur, resorcinol, benzoyl peroxide or salicylic acid. If these drugs have been used, it is best to wait for their effects to subside before using tretinoin.
VITAMIN D. Precursors are calciferol D_2, 7-dehydrocholesterol (irradiated D_3). *Fish liver oil, egg yolk, ergosterol.* Ergocalciferol, U.S.P. (Deltalin, Deratol, Drisdol, Ertron, Hi-Deratol, Infron) (Ostoforte, Ostogen, Radiostol [C]). Ergosterol (Drisdol) (solution of irradiated ergosterol). Oleovitamin D synthetic (viosterol in oil).	 50,000-500,000 U. Oral. 50,000-500,000 U. Oral. 10-37.5 micrograms. Oral.	Used to treat rickets, bone fracture (especially in older people), infantile tetany, osteomalacia, arthritis, diarrhea, psoriasis, and lupus vulgaris (the last four conditions with varying degrees of success).	Deficiency produces rickets, infantile tetany, osteomalacia, and other conditions in which bone and tooth development is delayed or abnormal. Recommended daily allowance (not yet satisfactorily determined) about 800-1200 U.S.P. units. Protective: for child, 3000 U.S.P. units may be required. Especially needed during pregnancy. Vitamin D is absorbed from the gastrointestinal tract. Widely distributed; some is stored in the liver. Slowly metabolized and excreted, mostly by kidneys.	Excessive vitamin D may cause nausea, vomiting, diarrhea, lassitude, and urinary infrequency in adults. It may also cause untoward symptoms in children.	Dosage of vitamin D should be carefully regulated to suit the individual, and the patient should be under the care of the physician at all times.
BOTH VITAMINS A AND D Cod liver oil, N.F. Cod liver oil, N.F. (nondestearinated) Cod liver oil concentrate. Oleovitamin A and D, N.F. (A-D Percomorph, Alpha-Deltalin, Super-D).	 4 ml. Oral. 4 ml. Oral. Dosage varies. Oral. Dosage varies. Oral.				

Name, Source, Synonyms, Preparations	Dosage and Administration	Uses	Action and Fate	Side Effects and Contraindications	Remarks
VITAMIN E. Tocopherol (alpha, beta, gamma). *Wheat germ, vegetable oils, leafy vegetables, milk, eggs, whole grains, legumes.*		Used to treat sterility, muscular dystrophy, thrombosis, abortion, abruptio placentae, symptoms of menopause, and other conditions.	Deficiency in animals produces sterility, loss of embryo, muscular dystrophy, paralysis, and signs of nervous disorders. Research has not shown specific results of deficiency in man. Recommended daily allowance has not been established. Readily absorbed from the gastrointestinal tract via lymph. Widely distributed. Very slowly excreted. Excretion is in bile and urine. Some is metabolized, some is excreted unchanged.	Rare in therapeutic usage.	
dl-alpha-Tocopherol (Alfacol, Aquasol E, Denamone, Ecofrol, Eprolin-S, Epsilan-M)	10-200 mg. Oral.				
Tocopherols, mixed concentrate (Eprolin Gelseals, Tofaxin, Vitamin E Concentrate).	10-200 mg. Oral or I.M.				
d-alpha-Tocopheryl acetate concentrate, N.F. (Ecofrol, Econ, E-Ferol, Natopherol-A_2, Pletocol, Tocopherox, Tocopherol, Tokols, Vi-Dom-E, Vi-E).	10-200 mg. Oral or I.M.				
d-alpha-Tocopheryl acetate (E-Hart, Ephynal acetate, Tocophrine, Vi-Ea).	10-200 mg. Oral or I.M.				
d-alpha-Tocopheryl acid succinate, N.F. (E-Ferol Succinate). Canadian trade names for various vitamin E preparations: Aquasol-E, Daltose, Ephynal, Eprolin, Phytoferol, Tocopherex, Tofaxin, Vita-E.	10-200 mg. Oral.				
VITAMIN K. *Pork liver, green vegetables, cereals, vegetable oils, synthetic.*		Used to treat hemorrhagic conditions, especially when associated with low prothrombin, liver and biliary disturbances, or both.	Deficiency produces delayed bleeding time, low prothrombin, delayed clotting time. Most commonly seen with disturbances of the liver and biliary tract. Recommended daily allowance has not been established.	Toxicity generally considered low, but menadione should be used with caution during pregnancy.	Vitamin K_5 is a vitamin K analogue.
Vitamin K-5 (Synkamin).	5 mg. Oral. 1 mg. Parenteral.				
Menadiol sodium diphosphate, N.F. (Kappadione, Synkayvite) (Vitamin K_4, Synkavite [C]).	5 mg. Oral. 5-75 mg. Parenteral.				
Menadione, N.F. (menaphthone, [C]).	1 mg. Oral.				

Menadione sodium bisulfite, N.F. (Hykinone) (Vitamin K_3, [C]). Phytonadione, U.S.P. (Vitamin K_1) (AquaMephyton, Konakion, Mephyton) (phytomenadione [C]).	2-5 mg. Oral or parenteral. 1-100 mg. I.V. or subcutaneous. 5 mg. Oral.	A recognized antidote for Dicumarol or warfarin toxicity.	Natural forms absorbed from gastrointestinal tract via lymph, water soluble forms via blood. Not stored to any great extent. Completely metabolized by the body. The vitamin K found in stools is apparently produced by intestinal bacteria.		

WATER SOLUBLE

Since vitamin B consists of many different factors which have different uses, each factor will be considered as a separate vitamin. It is common practice to give two or more factors at the same time; often the entire B-complex is given because deficiency in one B-fraction is usually associated with deficiency in other B-fractions. It is often wise not to give one factor alone, since this produces a lessening of the absorption of the other B-fractions from the food. Research is being done on many B-factors whose therapeutic value has not been established. Among these are biotin (vitamin H), choline, and inositol. There are too many multivitamin compounds to permit all of them to be considered here. Many combinations of two or three vitamins are available, as well as innumerable preparations that include most of the known vitamins. Vitamin preparations also often include essential minerals.

B COMPLEX. *Liver, yeast, and other foods as listed under the various B-factors.* Brewer's yeast. Yeast, dried, N.F. Liver B-vitamin concentrate.	 10 Gm. Oral. Dosage varies. Oral. Dosage varies. Oral or parenteral.	Used to treat all the conditions listed under the various factors and to aid in building the body generally (as a "tonic").	See various individual fractions. Recommended daily allowances are listed under the various factors. B-vitamins are essential for general health, especially concerned with nerve functioning and cell metabolism.	Rare.	There are numerous proprietary B-complex preparations.
CYANOCOBALAMIN, VITAMIN B_{12}. *Mainly from liver, organs, and muscles of animals and commercially from Streptomyces fermentation.*		Used to treat pernicious anemia, other macrocytic anemias, and sprue.	Deficiency produces pernicious anemia; other conditions produced by deficiency not yet satisfactorily determined.		Combinations of vitamin B_{12} with "intrinsic factor" are available. Radiocyanocobalamin, U.S.P., also available for diagnosis of pernicious anemia.

Name, Source, Synonyms, Preparations	Dosage and Administration	Uses	Action and Fate	Side Effects and Contraindications	Remarks
CYANOCOBALAMIN, VITAMIN B_{12} (Continued)					
Vitamin B_{12}, U.S.P. (Cyanocobalamin) (cobalamin, cobalamine) (Berubigen, Betolin-12, Bevidox, Docibin, Dodecavite, Dodex, Ducobee Hepcovite, Redisol, Rubramin, Sytobex, Vi-Twel) (Anacobin, Bedox, Cyanabin, Duodebex, Nova-Rudi, Pinkamin, Rubexin [C]).	10 micrograms to 1 mg. Oral or parenteral.		Daily allowance probably about 1-2 micrograms. Oral absorption, except in extremely high doses, is dependent upon gastric intrinsic factor. Readily absorbed from parenteral sites. Bound to plasma proteins; fairly widely distributed. Some stored in the liver.		
Hydroxocobalamin (alpha-Redisol) (Vitamin B_{12a}, Sytobex-H Rubranova [C]).	10 micrograms-1 mg. I.M.				
FOLIC ACID, VITAMIN M. *Yeast, liver, and organs and muscles of animals.*		Used to treat sprue, macrocytic anemia, and other anemic conditions.	Deficiency produces macrocytic anemia; other conditions produced by deficiency not yet established. Recommended daily allowance not yet satisfactorily determined.		Folic acid is usually given in combination with other drugs. It alone is not sufficient to control pernicious anemia. It may mask symptoms of pernicious anemia until nerve damage has occurred.
Folic acid, U.S.P. (Folvite, L. casei factor, Pteroylglutamic acid, vitamin Bc) (Novofolacid [C]).	1-5 mg. p.r.n. Oral or parenteral.				
NICOTINIC ACID. *Yeast, liver, organs and muscles of animals, rice polishings, and bran.*		Used to treat pellagra, dermatitis, glossitis, and gastrointestinal and nervous system distrubances, and to aid in the treatment of many other diseases and conditions. Used to depress serum cholesterol. Also used for peripheral vasodilation.	Deficiency produces pellagra, dermatitis, glossitis, and gastrointestinal and nervous system disturbances. Recommended daily allowance not yet satisfactorily determined. Recommended amount for adults is 15-20 mg. Readily absorbed, widely distributed. Most is metabolized, excess excreted by the kidneys as are the metabolites.	Large doses of nicotinic acid cause transitory flushing and other unpleasant symptoms.	
Aluminum nicotinate (Nicalex).	0.5-1 Gm. Oral.				
Niacin, N.F. (Naotin, Nicosode, Nicotinic acid) (Efacin, Nico-Span) (Nioforte [C]).	20-50 mg. Oral or parenteral. Three to 10 times daily.				
Niacinamide, U.S.P. (Aminicotin, Dipegyl, Nicamindon, Nicotamide, Nicotilamide, Nicotinic acid amide, Pelonin Amide.)	50 mg. Oral or parenteral.	Does not produce flushing.			

PANTOTHENIC ACID. *Yeast, liver, rice, bran, wheat germ, organs and muscles of animals, tikitiki (rice polishings).* Calcium pantothenate, U.S.P. Racemic calcium pantothenate, U.S.P. (Pantholin).	 250-500 mg. p.r.n. I.M. 20-100 mg. Oral.	Used to treat certain dermatoses.	Deficiency symptoms not determined. Readily absorbed. Wide distribution with highest concentrations in the liver. Excreted unchanged, about 70% in urine, 30% in feces.	Rare.	Pantothenyl alcohol (panthenol) has been used in treating postoperative paralytic ileus.
VITAMIN B_1. *Egg yolk, bran and wheat germ, whole grains, and tikitiki (rice polishings). Synthetic.* Thiamine hydrochloride, U.S.P. (anuerin hydrochloride, thiamine, thiamine chloride, vitamin B_1) (Apatate, Betalin S, Bethiamin, Bewon) (Betaxin [C]). Thiamine mononitrate (Thiamine nitrate).	 1-100 mg. Oral or I.M. 1-15 mg. Oral.	Used to treat beriberi, gastrointestinal disturbances, visual phenomena, polyneuritis (especially that associated with alcoholism), pregnancy, pellagra, and arrested growth in infancy and childhood. It produces a feeling of well-being and is helpful in many diseases and conditions.	Deficiency produces beriberi, gastrointestinal disturbances, visual phenomena, polyneuritis of alcoholism, pellagra, arrested growth in children. Recommended daily allowances: adults, 1-2.5 mg.; children, 0.03 mg. for each 100 calories of food intake; infants, 0.15-0.5 mg. Poorly absorbed from gastrointestinal tract, but large doses allow for ample absorption of required amounts. Widely distributed with highest concentration in liver, brain, kidneys and heart. Some is split by the body to pyrimidine. This and excess thiamine are excreted by the kidneys.	Rare.	Rarely given alone; more often with other B-fractions.
VITAMIN B_2. *Yeast, liver, organs and muscles of animals, eggs, some vegetables, whole grains, and synthetic.* Riboflavin, U.S.P. (lactoflavin, vitamin B-2, vitamin G, Riboderm) (Flamotide [C]).	 1-5 mg. Oral. 1-10 mg. Parenteral.	Used to treat cheilosis, glossitis, seborrheic lesions, loss of weight, and photophobia. It produces a feeling of well-being and is used to treat a variety of diseases and conditions.	Deficiency produces cheilosis, glossitis, seborrheic lesions, loss of weight, and photophobia. Recommended daily allowances: adults, 1.8 mg.; children, 1 mg. Good absorption and wide distribution with highest concentration in kidneys, liver and heart. Very little is stored. With normal intake only about 9% is excreted in urine. Fate of remainder is not known.	Rare.	

METABOLIC DRUGS (Continued)

VITAMINS *(Continued)*

Name, Source, Synonyms, Preparations	Dosage and Administration	Uses	Action and Fate	Side Effects and Contraindications	Remarks
VITAMIN B_6. *Yeast, liver, lean meats, whole grains, legumes, egg yolk, and fish.*		Used to treat gastrointestinal disturbances, neuromuscular pains, nausea and vomiting, pernicious vomiting, neuritis, herpes zoster, irradiation sickness, and many other conditions.	Deficiency produces gastrointestinal disturbances and neuromuscular pains. Recommended daily allowance not yet satisfactorily determined. Recommended amount for adults is 1.5 mg. Readily absorbed. Well distributed. Metabolized in liver and degradation products excreted by the kidneys.	Rare.	
Pyridoxine hydrochloride, U.S.P. (Bedoxine, Beesix, Hexa-Betalin, Hydoxin) (Hexavibex, Winvite-6 [C]).	5-100 mg. Oral or parenteral.				
VITAMIN C. *Oranges, lemons, limes, tomatoes, raw cabbage, onions, peppers, turnips, grapefruit.*		Used to treat and prevent scurvy and similar conditions. Valuable in any condition in which there is an increased tendency to bleed or tendency toward capillary fragility. Also used to acidify the urine.	Deficiency produces scurvy, defective teeth, and prescorbic conditions. Minimum daily requirements: adults 50-70 mg., children, 10-50 mg. Readily absorbed from the gastrointestinal tract. Widely distributed. Most is utilized by body. Excretion via urine, occurs mainly when there is excess intake.	Rare.	
Ascorbic acid, U.S.P. (cevitamic acid) (Cecon, Cevalin, C-Quin, Ce-Vi-Sol, Lequi-Cee) (Adenex, C-Vita, C-Vite, Erivit-C, Redoxon, Scortab, Vitascorbol [C]).	0.1-1 Gm. Oral.				
Ascorbic acid injection, U.S.P. (Ascorbin, Cantaxin, Cenolate, Cevalin, Vicin).	0.1-1 Gm. Parenteral.				
VITAMIN P. *Rind of lemons, paprika.*		Used to treat conditions in which there is increased capillary permeability.	Deficiency produces increased permeability of the capillaries with plasma loss, hypoproteinemia, edema, and interstitial bleeding. Recommended daily allowance not determined.	None has been determined.	There are no official preparations of vitamin P. Its uses and properties are controversial. Rutin is a similar product. Rutin is a glycoside of quercetin and aids in restoration of normal capillary tonus.
Bioflavonoids (Koracitin).	Usually added to other antihemorrhagic drugs.				
Rutin	25-50 mg. Oral.				
VITAMIN COMPOUNDS. *Synthetic.*					
Decavitamins, U.S.P.	Dosage varies.	Widely used as a vitamin supplement.	See individual vitamins.	See individual vitamins.	General vitamin products containing several different vitamins. There are many proprietary preparations.
Hexavitamin, N.F.	Dosage varies.	Widely used as a vitamin supplement.	See individual vitamins.	See individual vitamins.	

MINERALS

NON-NUTRIENT

Certain minerals are used directly to change body metabolism. These are usually considered with the metabolic drugs. Other minerals are used to treat specific conditions alone or in various combinations; these are discussed with the areas involved. Considerable attention is now focused on the so-called trace elements–those elements that occur in the body in minute amounts but seem to play a very important part in body metabolism. As research in this field continues there will, no doubt, be significant developments.

CALCIUM AND PHOSPHORUS. *Mineral.*		Used to treat disorders of bones and teeth and to aid in the proper growth and development of bones and teeth. Also used to treat tetany, various disorders of the nervous system and mucous membranes, and as a dietary supplement during pregnancy.	Calcium and phosphorus are essential elements. They affect the proper functioning and metabolism of bones, teeth, nerves, muscles, and glands, and calcium is needed for proper blood clotting.	Rare in therapeutic dosage. Low calcium may produce relaxation of the heart, while excess may cause a prolonged state of contraction. Stop drug and treat symptoms. Interactions: an increase in plasma calcium concentration markedly enhances the action of digitalis and a decrease diminishes its effect. This fact should be remembered when giving calcium I.V. to patients on digitalis therapy. For interaction with the tetracyclines see page 21.	
Calcium carbonate, U.S.P. (Calabarb [C]).	1 Gm. q.i.d. Oral.				
Calcium chloride, U.S.P.	1 Gm. p.r.n. I.V.				Calcium chloride must not be given into the tissues as it is irritating.
Calcium gluconogalactogluconate (Neo-Calglucon)	1-3 Gm. t.i.d. Oral. 1 Gm. I.V. p.r.n.				1.395 Gm. is equivalent to 1.0 Gm. calcium gluconate.
Calcium gluconate, U.S.P. (Calglucon) (Glucaloids [C]).	5 Gm. t.i.d. Oral. 1 Gm. p.r.n. I.V.				
Calcium glycerophosphate.	0.3 Gm. Usually given in solution up to q.i.d. Oral.				
Calcium lactate, N.F. (Novocalcilate [C]).	5 Gm. t.i.d. or q.i.d. Oral.				
Calcium oxalate.	Dosage varies. Oral.	Used to treat infantile tetany.			
Calcium tartrate.	Dosage varies. Oral.	Used to treat infantile tetany.			
Compound hypophosphites syrup.	8 ml. t.i.d. Oral.				
Dibasic calcium phosphate, U.S.P. (Calphate, DCP).	1-5 Gm. Daily. Oral.				
COLLOIDAL SULFUR. *Mineral.*		Used in the treatment of certain types of arthritis.	Nonspecific therapy used in treatment of arthritis.	Rare in therapeutic dosage.	
Colloidal sulfur (Sulphocol).	0.3-0.6 Gm. t.i.d. p.c. Oral. 2-3 ml. at 2-7 day intervals. Courses of 15-20 doses are suggested. I.M.				
IODINE. *Seaweed.*		Used for various conditions such as disorders of the thyroid gland, as a specific, and as an antiseptic. For the last two usages see page 184 and page 2. Also used	The primary function of iodine in the body is in the production of thyroglobin. However, iodine performs many medicinal functions (see uses).	Refer to page 2.	
Iodobrassid (Lipodine, Lipiodine).	0.3-0.6 Gm. Up to q.i.d. Oral.				Iodobrassid is also used in cough medications.
Potassium iodide, U.S.P. (KI-N-tabs).	0.3 Gm. Up to q.i.d. Oral.				

Name, Source, Synonyms, Preparations	Dosage and Administration	Uses	Action and Fate	Side Effects and Contraindications	Remarks
IODINE (Continued)					
Sodium iodide, U.S.P.	0.1-0.3 Gm. Up to q.i.d. Oral. 1 Gm. I.V. every other day.	to cause liquefaction and aid removal of abnormal tissue.			
Strong iodine solution, U.S.P. (Lugol's solution, capu-Lugols, (Lugol Caps).	0.1-1 ml. Up to t.i.d. Give in a bland medium.	Used to prepare patients for thyroid surgery.			
POTASSIUM. *Mineral.*					
Potassium acetate, bicarbonate, and citrate (Potassium Triplex Elixir).	15-30 ml. Daily. Oral.	Used during convalescence from debilitating diseases. Also used to aid in control of sodium retention edema.	Potassium is a constituent of all cells. It should be in balance with sodium, which is primarily intercellular. This balance prevents edema and dehydration.	Rare in therapeutic dosage, but patients on thiazide diuretics, furosemide, ethacrynic acid or digitalis should be closely followed. Contraindicated in renal disorders.	
Potassium chloride, U.S.P. (Kaochlor, Kay Cel, K-10, Slow-K [C]).	1 Gm. Up to t.i.d. Oral. 0.25-2 Gm. p.r.n. given slowly. I.V.				Potassium chloride is available in various forms: liquids 10-20%, effervescent tablets and powders. 5.0 ml. of a 10% solution of potassium chloride = 6.7 mEq. of potassium.
Potassium gluconate, N.F. (Kaon).	15-30 ml. daily. Oral. 5 mEq. tablets, 8 daily. Oral.				
SODIUM. *Mineral.*					
Sodium fluoride (Flura, Flursol, Karidium, Luride, Pediaflor, Pergantene, So-Flo) (Fluordrops, Fluorotabs, Pre-Care [C]).	0.25-0.5 mg. daily. Oral. Dosage is adjusted to suit fluoride content of drinking water.	Prophylaxis against dental caries.	Fluoride decreases the formation of dental caries.	In patients hypersensitive to fluoride, skin reaction such as eczema, dermatitis and urticaria may occur.	Do not use if drinking water contains more than 0.7 parts of fluoride per million. 2.2 mg. of sodium fluoride = 1.0 mg. of fluoride.

NUTRIENTS

NUTRIENT (see also circulatory drugs).

There are many preparations containing amino acids, easily absorbed carbohydrates, vitamins, and needed minerals. These are available in various combinations for oral or intravenous administration. They are especially valuable in debilitating diseases and during convalescence.

Name, Source, Synonyms, Preparations	Dosage and Administration	Uses	Action and Fate	Side Effects and Contraindications	Remarks
Balanced diet. *Low residue.* (Jejunal, Vivonex, W-T Low Residue).	Varies with requirements of the patient. Oral.	To provide nutrients for patients on low residue diets. To aid in preventing or overcoming a negative nitrogen balance.	Provides calories, essential amino acids and other nutrients such as carbohydrates, fats, vitamins and minerals.	May cause nausea and/or diarrhea. Adjustment of dosage and/or times of administration usually is all that is required.	Consult manufacturer's brochure before administering these products. Osmolality of the various preparations and flavors varies considerably and some patients react unfavorably (diarrhea).

GLUTAMIC ACID and related amino acids. *Synthetic.*					
Arginine glutamate (Modumate).	25-50 mg. in 500-1000 ml. I.V.	Used for ammonia intoxication.	These all supply arginine, which is an intermediate in the Krebs urea cycle and is used to reduce the blood ammonia level by conversion to urea.	None unless used to excess.	
Arginine hydrochloride (Argivene, R-Gene).	20 Gm. in 500-1000 ml. I.V.				
Sodium glutamate (Glutavene).	29 Gm. in 1000 ml. I.V.				Glutavene-K also contains potassium.
Medium chain triglycerides oil (MCT). *A lipid fraction of coconut oil.*	15 ml. 3 or 4 times daily. Oral.	Special dietary supplement for use in nutritional management of children and adults who cannot efficiently digest and absorb long chain food fats.	Consists of medium length (C-6 to C-8) chains of fats. 15 ml. weighs 14 grams and contains 115 K calories.	In persons with advanced cirrhosis of the liver, large amounts of medium chain triglycerides in the diet may result in elevated blood and spinal fluid levels. These elevated levels have been associated with precoma and hepatic coma in some patients.	
METHIONINE. *Synthetic.*					
Methionine, N.F. (Amurex, Meonine, Oradash, Pedameth) (dl-methionine, Methurine, Ninol [C]).	3-6 Gm. Daily. Oral.	Used to provide needed body material. Used orally to treat diaper rash when it is thought to be due to ammoniacal urine.	An essential amino acid for which lipotropic activity has been suggested. Acts by lowering the pH of urine.		
PROTEIN HYDROLYSATE. *Water and protein products.*					
Protein hydrolysate, U.S.P. (Amigen, Aminogen, Aminonat, Aminosol, Lofenalac).	5% solution. 250-1500 ml. I.V. 15 Gm. In easily assimilated form. Oral.	Used to replace body proteins when depleted for any reason. To provide protein when intake, digestion, or absorption is interfered with, as after operation or in severe illness.	To provide a readily available source of amino acids.	Rare in therapeutic dosage.	
Crystalline amino acid mixture (Freamine 8.5% solution). *Isolated and purified from edible soybean hydrolysate or synthesized.*	Varies with requirement of patient. Parenteral hyperalimentation.	As an adjunct in prevention of nitrogen loss or in the treatment of negative nitrogen balance, when oral alimentation is not feasible and/or there is impaired gastrointestinal absorption of protein.	Provides all essential nutrients when given with sufficient dextrose.	Contraindicated in anuria or hepatic coma.	Consult manufacturer's brochure before administering this product.

DRUGS ACTING ON THE RESPIRATORY SYSTEM

STIMULANTS (See also Nalorphine, Naloxone and Levallorphan.)

Name, Source, Synonyms, Preparations	Dosage and Administration	Uses	Action and Fate	Side Effects and Contraindications	Remarks
CARBON DIOXIDE. *Gas.* Carbon dioxide with oxygen, U.S.P. (Carbogen) (carbon dioxide 5%, oxygen 95%).	Dosage varies. Inhalational.	Used to increase depth and rate of respiration in such conditions as asphyxia, postanesthesia, carbon monoxide poisoning.	Direct stimulant to the respiratory center in the medulla. Other effects include pulmonary hyperventilation and increased muscle tone.	Rare in therapeutic dosage, but excessively deep and rapid respirations may occur. Stop drug and give oxygen. Carbon dioxide is contraindicated in pulmonary edema, cardiac decompensation, and pulmonary collapse (except for very brief administration).	Hyperventilation may be obtained by breathing into a closed space (a paper or plastic bag) for 5 minutes.
Doxapram hydrochloride, N.F. (Dopram).	0.5-1.0 mg./kg. I.V.	Used to stimulate respiration in patients with postanesthetic respiratory depression or apnea other than that due to muscle relaxant drugs.	Acts as a respiratory stimulant.	Contraindications: Epilepsy and other convulsive states, incompetence of the ventilatory mechanism due to muscle paresis, flail chest, pneumothorax, airway obstruction, extreme dyspnea, severe hypertension, and cardiovascular accidents. Not recommended for children under 12 years of age or for women during pregnancy.	
ETHAMIVAN. *Synthetic.* Ethamivan, N.F. (Emivan).	100-500 mg. p.r.n. I.V.	Used to treat hypoventilation due to many causes such as allergy, emphysema, chronic bronchitis; chest cage abnormalities; cardiopulmonary disease; central nervous system and respiratory involvement in elderly. Used as adjunct therapy in depressant drug intoxication.	Principal action is central respiratory stimulation associated with medullary respiratory centers. Increases the depth of respiration and to a lesser extent the rate.	Rare. If insomnia occurs, reduce dosage. Contraindicated in epilepsy.	An open airway is essential for the drug to be of value.

LOBELIA. *Lobelia inflata.*					
Alpha lobeline hydrochloride (Lobeline).	3-10 mg. Parenteral.	Used to increase the depth and the rate of respiration. Especially used in emergencies when respiration is failing. It is sometimes used in asphyxia neonatorum.	Acts as carotid sinus stimulant.	Nausea, vomiting, collapse, convulsions, Cheyne-Stokes respirations. Treat symptoms.	Rarely used now as it is unreliable, and toxic symptoms occur from therapeutic doses.
Lobeline sulfate (Lobelcon, Kiloban, No-Kotin) (Fumaret [C]).	1 mg. Oral.	Used to help reduce or stop smoking.	As above.	As above.	

SMOOTH MUSCLE RELAXANT (BRONCHIAL DILATOR) (See also sympathomimetics)

AMINOPHYLLINE (theophylline ethylenediamine). *Synthetic.* Aminophylline, U.S.P. (Aminocardol, Ammophyllin, Cardophyllin, Carena, Diophyllin, Genophyllin, Inophylline, Metaphyllin, Phylliden, Rectalad-Amino-phylline, Theolamine, Theophyldine) (Aminophyl, Corophyllin, Ethophylline [C]).	0.1-0.2 Gm. t.i.d. or q.i.d. Oral.	Widely used for many conditions. Mainly used to relax smooth muscle tissue and to dilate the bronchial tubes in asthma, emphysema and similar conditions. Also used to increase the flow of urine, especially when edema is present, as in cardiac or renal insufficiency, to relax coronary vessels in angina pectoris, and to treat pulmonary edema.	Causes increased renal output, especially water, in the presence of edema. Increases the output of sodium. Tends to relax smooth muscle tissue, hence causes coronary vessel relaxation and peripheral vasodilation. However, it tends to stimulate skeletal and cardiac muscle. It increases cardiac output, thus giving all organs better blood supply. Causes some central nervous stimulation but much less than caffeine.	Rare in therapeutic dosage, but may cause gastric and urinary irritation and occasionally fullness in the head, and headache. Stop or reduce dosage and treat symptoms. With I.V. administration watch for signs of cardiovascular distress. I.M. administration is not advised since drug is irritating to the tissues.	Aminophylline is synthetic theophylline. It is one of the xanthine preparations. The others are caffeine, used mainly as a central nervous system stimulant, and theophylline and theobromine, used mainly as diuretics. All these drugs cause central nervous system stimulation, increased urinary output and smooth muscle relaxation. However, degree of action varies with each drug. Aminophylline is widely used for so many conditions that it could be placed in many categories.
Aminophylline injection, U.S.P.	0.2-0.5 Gm. I.M. or I.V. Given very slowly, often added to I.V. infusions.				
Aminophylline suppositories, U.S.P. (neutraphylline) (Suppophylline [C]).	0.25-0.5 Gm. Rectal suppository usually h.s.				

NEBULAE AND SPRAYS

These preparations are usually combinations of several drugs. See also drugs acting on the skin and mucous membranes and those acting on the nervous system. Since most of these preparations are compounds, the sources are varied according to content.

Aromatic spray.	Dosage varies. Given through an atomizer or nebulizer. Inhalational.	Used to relieve irritation of the mucous membranes of the respiratory tract.	Most of these sprays contain antiseptic, demulcent, or emollient drugs. They are soothing, and decrease infection. They also may have sedative and decongestant action.	If prepared in oil may cause lipoid pneumonia; otherwise toxic symptoms are rare.	Contains phenol, menthol, thymol, camphor, benzoic acid, eucalyptol, methyl salicylate, oil of cinnamon, and oil of clove.

NEBULAE AND SPRAYS *(Continued)*

Name, Source, Synonyms, Preparations	Dosage and Administration	Uses	Action and Fate	Side Effects and Contraindications	Remarks
Cyclopentamine and aludrine compound (Aerolone).	Dosage varies. Given through an atomizer or nebulizer. Inhalational.	Used to relieve irritation of the mucous membranes of the respiratory tract. It is also a decongestant.	See above.	If used too freely, dryness of the nose and throat may result. Stop drug. No actual treatment is required.	Contains cyclopentamine (Clopane), Aludrine, atropine sulfate, and procaine hydrochloride.
Compound ephedrine spray.	Dosage varies. Given through an atomizer or nebulizer Inhalational.	Used to relieve irritation of the mucous membranes of the respiratory tract. It is also a decongestant.	See above, and also ephedrine, under autonomic nervous system drugs.	If used too freely, symptoms of ephedrine poisoning may occur. (See autonomic nervous system drugs for details.) Stop drug and treat symptoms.	Compound ephedrine spray contains ephedrine, methyl salicylate, camphor, and oil of thyme. Ephedrine spray contains ephedrine 1% and methyl salicylate 0.2%.
Ephedrine spray.	Dosage varies. Given through an atomizer or nebulizer. Inhalational.				
Isoproterenol sulfate, U.S.P. (Isonorin, Medihaler-Iso, Norisodrine) (isoprenaline, Iso-Intraefrin, Isovon, Isuprel, Vapo-N-Iso [C]).	Dosage varies. Given through an atomizer. or nebulizer. Inhalational.	Used for bronchial dilation.	Relaxes bronchial spasms and facilitates expectoration of pulmonary secreta. It is primarily a beta adrenergic stimulator.	Rare in therapeutic dosage, but tachycardia, palpitation, nervousness, nausea, and vomiting may occur.	Dosage must be carefully regulated in patients with hyperthyroidism, acute coronary disease, and cardiac asthma. Isoproterenol hydrochloric, U.S.P., is also available as a spray.
Menthol nebulae.	Dosage varies. Given through an atomizer or nebulizer. Inhalational.	Used to relieve irritation of the mucous membranes of the respiratory tract. It is not a decongestant.	See aromatic nebulae.	If prepared with oil it may cause lipoid pneumonia, otherwise toxic symptoms are rare. Stop drug and treat symptoms.	Contains menthol, camphor, methyl salicylate, and eucalyptol.
Tyloxapol (Alevaire, Macilose-Super, Superinone, Triton-WR).	Dosage varies. Given through nebulizer or with a stream of oxygen. Inhalational.	Used to aid liquefaction and removal of mucopurulent material from the respiratory tract.	A detergent, used to help liquefy mucus.	Rare in therapeutic dosage. However, patients should be watched for signs of pulmonary edema. Treatment: none is usually required, but if signs of edema develop, stop drug and treat symptoms.	

GASES USED MEDICINALLY (See also General anesthetics and Respiratory stimulants.)

Name, Source, Synonyms, Preparations	Dosage and Administration	Uses	Action and Fate	Side Effects and Contraindications	Remarks
HELIUM. *Gaseous element.* Helium, U.S.P.	Dosage varies. p.r.n. Inhalational.	Used as a vehicle for the administration of other gases. It is especially useful with	An inert gas which, because of its lightness, allows greater distribution of the	None when administered with oxygen.	Helium 75-80% and oxygen 20-25% is the combination most frequently used.

		oxygen in the treatment of laryngeal stridor, acute pulmonary edema, emphysema, and pulmonary fibrosis. Helium is also used as a vehicle for general anesthetics.	other gases than does the atmospheric nitrogen.		
OXYGEN. *Gaseous element.* Oxygen, U.S.P. (Lif-O-Gen, Oxy Swig).	Dosage varies. p.r.n. Inhalational.	Used in any case of anoxemia, such as pulmonary edema, cardiac disorders, carbon monoxide poisoning, asthma, lung collapse, migraine headache, shock and many other conditions. It effects a general improvement in the patient's condition, as all the organs receive more oxygen.	Oxygen by inhalation increases the available amount of oxygen to the blood. Relieves anoxia when processes for oxygen absorption, conveyance, and utilization are not unduly impaired.	None in therapeutic dosage. However, should be used with caution in the premature infant to avoid retrolental fibroplasia.	Widely used in the treatment of many disorders. The exact method of administration varies greatly.

COUGH MEDICATIONS (ANTITUSSIVE AGENTS)

Many preparations could be considered under the heading "cough medications." Three groups will be discussed: (1) demulcents and emollients; (2) expectorants; (3) sedatives. See also nervous system drugs and drugs acting on the skin and mucous membranes. Many cough preparations include two or more of the different groups of cough drugs. Since it is impossible to include all the ingredients, only the important main constituents will be considered.

DEMULCENTS AND EMOLLIENTS

Demulcents and emollients are usually combined with other drugs. Preparations such as vegetable oils, psyllium seeds, flaxseed, methylcellulose, tragacanth, and similar substances are used in combination with other drugs in various cough medications as demulcents or emollients.

ACACIA. *Acacia tree.* Acacia, U.S.P. Acacia mucilage, N.F.	Dosage varies. p.r.n. Oral or topical. 15 ml. p.r.n. Oral.	Used to reduce cough.	A demulcent which coats and protects the mucous membranes.	None in therapeutic dosage.	
GLYCERIN. *Synthetic.* Glycerin, U.S.P. (Glyrol [C]).	Dosage varies. p.r.n. Oral. 2-3 ml./kg. body weight. Oral.	As above. Used presurgically in glaucoma to help to lower intraocular pressure.	An emollient used to coat and protect the mucous membrane.	As above.	

COUGH MEDICATIONS *(Continued)*

Name, Source, Synonyms, Preparations	Dosage and Administration	Uses	Action and Fate	Side Effects and Contraindications	Remarks
GLYCYRRHIZA. *Licorice root.*					
Glycyrrhiza, U.S.P.	Dosage varies. p.r.n. Oral.	As above.	A demulcent used to coat and protect the mucous membrane.	As above.	
EXPECTORANTS Drugs which aid in the removal of respiratory secretions and excretions.					
AMMONIA. *Mineral.*					
Ammonium carbonate, N.F.	0.3 Gm. Oral.	Used to treat acute and chronic bronchitis and similar conditions.	Increases the liquefaction and removal of mucus from the lungs.	Rare in therapeutic dosage, but nausea may occur. Treatment: none usually required.	
Ammonium chloride, U.S.P. (Amchlor, Ammoneric).	0.3-1 Gm. Oral.				
BALSAM. *Myroxylon Sp.:*		Used to treat irritated or denuded conditions of skin and mucous membranes.	These induce repair of mucous membranes, reduce inflammation, and decrease bronchial secretions. They act as irritants, astringents, and to a certain extent as antiseptics.	Rare in therapeutic dosage.	
Benzoin, U.S.P.	30% tincture p.r.n. Topical. 10% compound tincture p.r.n. Topical.	Used topically to increase the rate of healing and to cover denuded areas.			
Peruvian balsam.	Dosage varies. Oral.	An ingredient in many cough syrups.			
	Topical.	To aid in the healing of wounds or lesions.			
Tolu balsam, U.S.P.	Dosage varies. Oral.	Same as above.			
CREOSOTE (Cresols phenols). *Wood.*		Used to treat coughs from many causes.	See above.	Rare in therapeutic dosage.	
Creosote.	0.25 ml. p.r.n. Oral.	Ingredients in many cough syrups.			
Creosote carbonate.	1 Gm. p.r.n. Oral.				
Glyceryl guaiacolate, N.F. (Dilyn, Glycotuss, Robitussin) (methphenoxydiol, glyceryl, guaiacol ether, Resyl, Balminil, Motussin, Pectus-Sachets, Tussanca [C]).	100 mg. in 5 ml. of syrup p.r.n. Oral.	Antitussive agent.		With glyceryl guaiacolate nausea and drowsiness occur, but rarely.	
Guaiacol.	0.5 ml. p.r.n. Oral.	See above.	See above.		

CUBEB. *Piper cubeba.*					
Cubeb.	2 Gm. Oral.	Used in some cough syrups.	See above.	Rare in therapeutic dosage.	
EUCALYPTUS. *Eucalyptus globulus.*					
Eucalyptol.	0.3 ml. p.r.n. Oral.	See above.	See above.	Rare in therapeutic dosage.	
Eucalyptus oil, N.F.	0.5 ml. p.r.n. Oral.				
IODIDES. *Seaweed, minerals.*					
Hydriodic acid syrup (Hyodin).	5 ml. Oral.	Used as an expectorant.	Exact mode of action not determined.	Rare in therapeutic dosage. Contraindicated in thyroid disturbances or tuberculosis, and not advised in acute inflammatory conditions.	Potassium and sodium iodide are also used in hyperthyroidism.
Potassium iodide solution, N.F.	0.3 Gm. Oral.				
Sodium iodide, U.S.P.	0.3 Gm. Oral.				
Syrup of calcidrine.	5 ml. Oral.				
SQUILL. *Urginea martima (sea-onion).*					
Squill compound syrup.	2 ml. p.r.n. Oral.	Used mainly as an expectorant.	Aids in removal of mucus.	Rare in therapeutic dosage.	Has been used for the same purpose as digitalis but is not as reliable.
Squill fluid extract.	0.1 ml. p.r.n. Oral.				
TURPENTINE. *Pine tree.*					
Rectified oil of turpentine.	0.3 ml. p.r.n. Oral.	See creosote.	Induces repair of mucous membrane, reduces inflammation, and decreases bronchial secretions. It acts as an irritant, astringent, and to a certain extent as an antiseptic.	Rare in therapeutic dosage.	
Terpin hydrate, N.F.	Dosage varies, q. 4 h. p.r.n. Oral.				Usually given in combination with other drugs. Not a true expectorant since it does not increase secretion.
Terpin hydrate elixir, N.F.	5 ml. q. 4 h. p.r.n. Oral.				
Terpin hydrate and codeine elixir, N.F.	5 ml. q. 4 h. p.r.n. Oral.				
Terpin hydrate and dextromethorphan elixir, N.F.	5 ml. q. 4 h. p.r.n. Oral.				

SEDATIVES.

These are all synthetic preparations, unless otherwise noted. These preparations aid in reducing the tendency to cough.

Benzonatate, N.F. (Tessalon). (benzononatine [C]).	50-100 mg. t.i.d. Oral. Capsules should not be allowed to dissolve in mouth.	Used to treat coughs from many causes.	A selective antitussive agent which depresses cough without depressing respiration.	Mild drowsiness, nausea, nasal congestion, dizziness have been reported. Decrease dosage.

Name, Source, Synonyms, Preparations	Dosage and Administration	Uses	Action and Fate	Side Effects and Contraindications	Remarks
SEDATIVES (Continued)					
Caramiphen ethanedisulfonate (ingredient in Dondril and Tuss-Ornade).	10-20 mg. p.r.n. Oral.	See carbetapentane citrate.	Antitussive agent similar to carbetapentane.	Rare in therapeutic dosage. Contraindicated in glaucoma.	
Carbetapentane citrate, N.F. (Loucarbate) (clofedanol, Ulone [C]).	15-30 mg. Usually given t.i.d. Oral.	For acute cough associated with upper respiratory infections.	An antitussive agent. Also has slight atropine-like antisecretory action.	A low order of toxicity is claimed. Contraindicated in glaucoma.	
Chlophedianol hydrochloride (Bayer-BL 86, Detigon, ULO).	10-25 mg. Syrup. t.i.d. Oral.	Used to suppress excessive and undesirable coughing.	A non-narcotic cough depressant.	Rare in therapeutic dosage.	
CODEINE. *Active principle of opium.*					
Codeine syrups (Broncho-Tussin, Cheracol, Citro-Cerose, Citro-Codea, Cobenzil, Codahist, Cotussis, Daldrin, Ephedrol, Histussin, Prunicodeine, Respi-Sed, Senodin, Tussadine, Tussi-Organidin).	5 ml. q. 4-6 h. Oral.	See above.	Has sedative action on the cough reflex.	Rare in therapeutic dosage but similar to opium if they occur. Treatment: if required, same as that for opium.	All contain several other ingredients. Other opium derivatives are also used in various cough preparations.
Dimethoxonate hydrochloride (Cothera).	25 mg./5 ml. syrup. 5-10 ml. t.i.d. p.r.n. Oral.	Used like other antitussive agents.	Depresses cough.	Drowsiness and nausea have been reported. Treatment: none usually required.	
Homarylamine hydrochloride.	20-40 mg. t.i.d. p.r.n. Oral.	Used in mild or acute cough.	Sympathomimetic. An antitussive agent with weak anticholinergic and antihistamine effects.	Rare, but nausea, vomiting, and drowsiness may occur. Contraindicated in glaucoma.	
HYDROCODONE. *Synthetic codeine derivative.*					
Hydrocodone bitartrate syrup, U.S.P. (Dicodethal, Dicodid, Dicodrine, Hycodan, Mercodinene, Stodcodon) (dihydrocodeinone bitartrate [C]).	5 ml. Not more than q. 4 h. Oral.	See codeine.	See codeine.	None, though some depression may occur. Reduce dosage.	
Levopropoxyphene napsylate, N.F. (Novrad).	50-100 mg. t.i.d. p.r.n. Available in 50-100 mg. capsules and syrup 50 mg./5 ml. Oral.	For the control of cough in acute, chronic and allergic respiratory tract diseases and various conditions causing cough.	An antitussive agent.	Nausea, drowsiness, dizziness, and skin rash or urticaria have been reported.	

NOSCAPINE. *Isoquinolin alkaloid of opium.*		Used as a cough suppressant in acute and chronic respiratory disorders.	Action similar to that of papaverine; smooth muscle relaxant and antitussive agent. Primarily used for antitussive effect.	Rare in therapeutic dosage.	Formerly called narcotine.
Noscapine, N.F. (Nectadon) (narcotine, Oscotabs [C]).	15-30 mg. Oral.				
Noscapine hydrochloride (Nectadon-H).	15-30 mg. Oral.				
Pipazethate hydrochloride (Theratuss).	10 mg. Oral.	A non-narcotic antitussive agent for suppression of cough from various causes.	Thought to depress cough centers in medulla without any sedative effect, and is nonaddicting.	Nausea and vomiting occur, but rarely. Not given to children under 7 years of age.	

There are any number of drugs used in cough medications. Space does not permit the inclusion of all these preparations.

DRUGS ACTING ON THE URINARY SYSTEM

ACIDIFIERS–ALKALINIZERS

These drugs increase the general acid or alkaline content of the body but they are usually given to increase the acidity or alkalinity of the urine. Many foods also increase the body acids or alkalis. See also drugs acting on the gastrointestinal and circulatory systems. Some of these are also diuretic in action.

INORGANIC ACIDS AND SALTS. *Mineral, synthetic.*	Most of these drugs are best given after meals to prevent gastric irritation. All the purely acid preparations should be given well diluted through a straw or tube. Rinse mouth with an alkaline solution after use.	Used to replace the acid in the gastric juice and to increase general body and urine acidity. The diuretic effect of acid-producing salts depends upon large doses. These salts are usually used with other diuretics to enhance their action.	Acid-producing salts cause a shift in the acid base equilibrium to the acid side and the specific action of the acid radical. The nitrate radical has the most marked diuretic effect, while the chloride radical produces the most marked shift in acid-base balance to the acid side.	Rare in therapeutic dosage. May cause local burning sensation. Excessive dosage may cause acidosis. Stop drug and give alkalinizer.	Diluted nitrohydrochloric acid, phosphoric acid, and sulfuric acid have been largely replaced by other preparations. Potassium chloride and nitrate are also available in solutions and in enteric coated tablets. These are "low kidney threshold diuretics."
Ammonium chloride, U.S.P. (Amchlor, Ammoneric).	1 Gm. q.i.d. Oral.	Ammonium chloride is also used as an expectorant.			
Calcium chloride.	1 Gm. q.i.d. Oral or I.V.	Diluted hydrochloric acid is mainly used to increase gastric acidity. Calcium chloride, sodium biphosphate, and sodium phosphate are mainly used to acidify urine.			
Hydrochloric acid, diluted, N.F.	0.3-4 ml. Oral.				
Nitrohydrochloric acid, diluted.	1 ml. Oral.				
Phosphoric acid, diluted, N.F.	1 ml. Oral.				

ACIDIFIERS–ALKALINIZERS *(Continued)*

Name, Source, Synonyms, Preparations	Dosage and Administration	Uses	Action and Fate	Side Effects and Contraindications	Remarks
INORGANIC ACIDS AND SALTS (Continued)					
Potassium chloride, U.S.P. (Hypomal, Kaochlor, K-Lyte, Kluride, K-Ciel, Slow-K [C]).	1 Gm. Up to six times daily. Oral.			Enteric-coated potassium tablets may cause irritation, even ulceration or perforation, of the intestinal mucosa, especially in the elderly or debilitated patient.	
Potassium nitrate (Crataganite).	1 Gm. Up to nine or 12 times daily. Oral.				
Diluted sulfuric acid.	0.3-4 ml. Oral.				
Sodium biphosphate (Betaphos).	0.6 Gm. q.i.d. Oral.				
ORGANIC ACID SALTS. *Various plants.*		Used mainly when an alkaline urine is desirable.	Most alkaline metal and alkaline earth metal salts of organic acids act as alkalinizers after absorption and various metabolic processes.	Rare in therapeutic dosage. Excessive use may cause mild adverse symptoms, but this is rare. Stop drug and treat symptoms.	
Potassium acetate, N.F.	1 Gm. Up to q.i.d. Oral. 2-4 Gm. q.i.d. Oral.	As diuretic.			
Potassium citrate, N.F.	1 Gm. t.i.d. Oral.				
Sodium acetate, N.F.	1.5 Gm. Oral. q.i.d. 2-4 Gm. Oral. q.i.d.	As diuretic.			
Sodium citrate, U.S.P.	1 Gm. Oral. q.i.d.	Also used to prevent coagulation of blood for indirect transfusions.			
Sodium chloride, U.S.P.	0.2, 0.45, 0.9% I.V.	Varied uses.			

ANTISEPTICS (See general anti-infective drugs.)

Name, Source, Synonyms, Preparations	Dosage and Administration	Uses	Action and Fate	Side Effects and Contraindications	Remarks
ETHOXAZENE HYDROCHLORIDE. *Synthetic.*					
Ethoxazene hydrochloride (Serenium) (Diamazol, Diaphenyl [C]).	100 mg. q.i.d. Usually given in enteric-coated tablets. Oral.	Used as urinary analgesic and antiseptic in nephritis, pyelitis, and cystitis.	Action similar to that of pyridium.	Low, but gastrointestinal disturbances may occur. Contraindicated or used with caution in pyelonephritis of pregnancy, severe liver disease, uremia, or parenchymatous nephritis with poor renal function.	Colors urine orange or red.
MANDELIC ACID. *Synthetic.*		Used as a urinary antiseptic in nephritis, pyelitis, and cystitis. Especially valuable in enterococcal infections.	This is a keto acid which is bacteriostatic. It is excreted unchanged.	Nausea, vomiting, diarrhea, dysuria, hematuria, and ringing in ears with lessened auditory acuity may occur. Stop drug, force fluids, and treat symptoms.	Effective only in strongly acid urine, therefore fluids are restricted and an acidifying agent given. Citrus fruits may be restricted. Urine should be tested regularly.
Ammonium mandelate.	0.3-0.5 Gm. q.i.d. Oral.				
Ammonium mandelate syrup (Amdelate).	5 ml. q.i.d. Oral.				
Calcium mandelate (Urisept).	4 Gm. q.i.d. Oral.				
Mandelic acid.	2-3 Gm. q.i.d. Oral.				

METHENAMINE. *Synthetic compound of ammonia and formaldehyde.*					
Methenamine, N.F. (Cystamin, Cystogen, Uritone, Urotropin) (hexamine, Uroformine [C]).	0.5-1.5 Gm. q.i.d. Oral.	Used as a urinary antiseptic in nephritis, pyelitis, and cystitis.	A compound of ammonia and formaldehyde. The latter is liberated in an acid medium and acts as a bacteriostatic agent. Readily absorbed and rapidly excreted by kidneys.	Rare in therapeutic dosage, but dysuria, hematuria, bladder pain, and albuminuria may occur. Stop drug and treat symptoms.	Effective only in acid urine. An acidifying drug should be given with this, and the urine tested regularly.
Methenamine anhydromethylenecitrate (Formanol, Helmitol, Neo-Urotropin, Uropurgol).	0.6-1 Gm. Oral.				
Methenamine and sodium biphosphate, N.F. (Hexosed).	0.3 Gm. q.i.d. Oral.				
Methenamine with ammonium chloride (Uro-Chor).	1-1.3 Gm. q.i.d. Oral.				
Methenamine hippurate (Hiprex).	1 Gm. b.i.d. Oral.	See methenamine mandelate.	Same as others of this group.		
Methenamine mandelate, U.S.P. (Mandelamine) (Mandelurine, Methadine, Sterine [C]).	0.25-1.5 Gm. q.i.d. Oral.	Effective against *E. coli, S. aureus, S. Albus,* and some streptococci. Effectiveness approximately that of the sulfonamides or streptomycin.	Readily absorbed and rapidly excreted by the kidneys.		Methenamine mandelate, U.S.P., yields methenamine and mandelic acid.
NALIDIXIC ACID. *Synthetic.*					
Nalidixic acid, N.F. (NegGram).	0.25-1 Gm. q.i.d. Oral.	Used for the treatment of acute and chronic infections caused by one or more species of sensitive organisms. Most effective in gram-negative infections of the genitourinary tract.	Anti-infective effective against *E. coli, Aerobacter aerogenes, Klebsiella pneumoniae Shigella Flexneri,* and *Salmonella typhimurium.* Good oral absorption and rapid excretion by kidneys.	Gastrointestinal disturbances, occasional drowsiness, fatigue, pruritus, rash, urticaria, and a mild eosinophilia have occurred.	
NITROFURANTOIN. *Synthetic.*					
Nitrofurantoin, U.S.P. (Cyantin, Furadantin, N-Toin) (Furanex, Furanite, Furantine, Nephronex, Novofuran, Nifuran, Urex, Urofuran [C]).	50-100 mg. q.i.d. Best given with or following ingestion of food. Oral. 180 mg. p.r.n. I.V.	Used as a urinary antiseptic in nephritis, pyelitis, and cystitis.	A nitrofurantoin derivative with a wide range of antibacterial activity against both gram-negative and gram-positive organisms. It is both bacteriostatic and bactericidal. It is not effective against viruses or fungi.	Usually mild, but nausea, vomiting, and skin sensitivity may occur. Reduction of dosage is usually sufficient for these.	
Nitrofurantoin macrocrystals (Macrodantin).	50-100 mg. q.i.d. Oral. 180 mg. b.i.d. I.M. for patients 120 lb. and over. 3 mg./kg. b.i.d. I.M. for patients under 120 lb. Should not be used longer than 5 days when given I.M.	As above.		Hemolytic anemia and neuropathies have been reported. When used in patients on probenecid there is increased renal clearance of nitrofurnantoin and this may lead to nitrofurantoin toxicity and decreased efficacy as urinary tract anti-infective owing to lower levels of drug in urine.	Nitrofurantoin macrocrystals are less irritating to gastrointestinal tract. Use with caution, if at all, during pregnancy and lactation and in women of child-bearing age. Not used for infants under 1 year. Safe use for these patients has not been established.

Name, Source, Synonyms, Preparations	Dosage and Administration	Uses	Action and Fate	Side Effects and Contraindications	Remarks
PHENAZOPYRIDINE. *Synthetic coal tar derivative.* Phenazopyridine hydrochloride, N.F. (Phenylazo, Pyridium).	0.1-0.2 Gm. q.i.d. Usually given in enteric-coated tablets. Oral. 1% solution. Topical.	Used as urinary antiseptic in nephritis, pyelitis, and cystitis. It also has an analgesic effect upon the urinary mucosa.	An azo dye, it is mildly antiseptic. Exerts a definite analgesic effect upon the urinary mucosa.	Low toxicity, but sensitivity may occur. Contraindicated in conditions producing poor renal function and in severe hepatitis.	Causes orange colored urine. Combinations with sulfonamide preparations are also used (Azo-Gantrisin, Thio-sulfil-A).

DIURETICS

Diuretics are drugs used to reduce the volume of extracellular fluid by increasing the output of water and certain electrolytes, mainly sodium, but also chloride and potassium. The various compounds differ in the amount and kinds of electrolytes excreted. Patients on long-term use of diuretics should have serum electrolyte determinations at intervals during therapy.

Diuretics are contraindicated in most renal disorders, except the nephrotic syndrome, since they would increase the severity of the condition. One of the most important functions of diuretics is in the control of edema accompanying cardiac disorders, especially cardiac decompensation. They are also used in the management of certain types of hypertension.

The interaction of diuretics with other medicinal agents will vary somewhat with the specific diuretic drug, but some are the same for most of the drugs. Some of the more important interactions include the following.

1. When diuretics are given to patients taking any of the digitalis glycosides, there can be an increase in the possibility of digitalis toxicity, owing to lower levels of serum potassium and higher levels of calcium. The higher levels of calcium are seen especially when the thiazide diuretics are being given.

2. The thiazide compounds as well as ethacrynic acid and furosemide may, because of their hypoglycemic effect, result in loss of control in the diabetic patient using the oral hypoglycemic agents. Those requiring insulin may need to increase the amount of insulin used.

3. With the non-depolarizing muscle relaxants, the hypokalemia produced by most diuretics may result in loss of deep tendon reflexes and can progress to paralysis.

4. When diuretics are given concurrently with antihypertensive agents such as methyldopa, guanethidine or a ganglionic blocking agent, orthostatic hypotension can result. The dose of the antihypertensive drugs should be lowered to avoid this possibility.

5. The use of ethacrynic acid or furosemide with any of the amnioglycoside antibiotics, especially if given intravenously, should be avoided, because of the increased possibility of ototoxicity seen with such combinations. With cephaloridine and these diuretics, there may be nephrotoxicity due to additive action.

6. The thiazide diuretics can cause an elevation of the serum level of uric acid. This can disrupt the control of the patient with gout or gouty arthritis who is being treated with probenecid or sulfinpyrazine. It can also increase the uric acid level in other patients.

7. Diuretics can replace warfarin from plasma protein binding sites, and this may require an adjustment of the dosage of the anticoagulant agent.

Drug	Dosage	Uses	Action	Side effects	Remarks
XANTHINES (See also caffeine, under central nervous system stimulants).					
THEOPHYLLINE. *Active principle of Theosinensis. Synthetic.*		Used mainly to increase the flow of urine; especially when there is edema present. May be used alone or in conjunction with other diuretics such as the mercurials. Also used in the treatment of asthma and certain cardiac conditions. Main use is in the treatment of asthma.	Causes increased renal output, especially water, in the presence of edema. Increases the output of sodium. Tends to relax smooth muscle tissue, hence causes coronary vessel relaxation and peripheral vasodilation. However, it tends to stimulate skeletal and cardiac muscle. It increases cardiac output, thus giving all organs better blood supply. Causes some central nervous stimulation but much less than caffeine.	Rare in therapeutic dosage, but may cause gastric and urinary irritation and occasionally fullness in the head, and headache. Stop or reduce dosage and treat symptoms. With I.V. administration watch for signs of cardiovascular distress.	Theophylline and theobromine are xanthine preparations. The others are caffeine, used mainly as a central nervous system stimulant, and aminophylline (theophylline ethylenediamine), used mainly as a smooth muscle relaxant in various respiratory conditions and other conditions for which this type of action is desirable. All the xanthine drugs cause central nervous system stimulation, increased urinary output and relaxation of smooth muscles. However, degree of action varies with the different drugs.
Dyphylline (Neothylline) (diprophylline, Protophylline, Coeurophilline, Dilin, Neuphylline, Neutraphylline [C]).	0.1-0.2 Gm. t.i.d. Oral.				
Magnesium theophylline.	0.1-0.2 Gm. t.i.d. or q.i.d. Oral.				
Oxtriphylline, N.F. (Choledyl) (choline theophyllinate [C])	0.1-0.4 Gm. t.i.d. or q.i.d. Oral.				
Theophylline, U.S.P. (Acrolate, Elixophyllin, Theocin) (Theofin [C]).	0.2-0.3 Gm. t.i.d. or q.i.d. Oral.				
Theophylline and calcium salicylate (Phyllicin) (Theocalcin [C]).	0.2-0.3 Gm. t.i.d. or q.i.d. Oral.				
Theophylline sodium acetate, N.F. (Theacitin).	0.2-0.3 Gm. t.i.d. or q.i.d. Oral.				
Theophylline methylglucamine (Glucephylline).	0.15-0.75 Gm. t.i.d. or q.i.d. p.c. Oral. 0.75 Gm. p.r.n. I.M. 0.36-0.75 Gm. in 10-20 ml. slowly p.r.n. I.V.				
Theophylline monethanolamine (Clysmathane).	0.1-0.2 Gm. Three to six times a day. Oral. 0.4-0.8 Gm. Daily in divided doses. Oral.	For heart conditions. For asthma.			
Theophylline sodium glycinate, N.F. (Synophylate, Theoglycinate) (Corivin, Theocyne [C]).	0.3-1 Gm. q. 4-6 h. Oral. 0.87 Gm. q. 4-6 h. Rectal. 0.4 Gm. in 10 ml. slowly p.r.n. I.V.				

Name, Source, Synonyms, Preparations	Dosage and Administration	Uses	Action and Fate	Side Effects and Contraindications	Remarks
XANTHINES (Continued)					
THEOBROMINE. *Active principle of Theobroma cacao.*					
Theobromine and sodium acetate (Thesodate).	0.5-1 Gm. Oral.	Used to increase the flow of urine, especially when edema is present, as in cardiac and renal insufficiency.	Decreases the reabsorption of water in the renal tubules. It tends to dilate the coronary vessels and to improve the general circulation, giving all the organs a better blood supply. Also stimulates cardiac and skeletal muscles. The action of theobromine is weaker than that of theophylline or aminophylline, but its effects are more lasting.	Toxicity low, but gastric and urinary irritation, fullness in the head, and headache all have been reported. If symptoms persist, reduce dosage or stop drug and treat symptoms.	
Theobromine and sodium salicylate (Diuretin).	0.5-1 Gm. Oral.				
Theobromine calcium gluconate.	0.5-1 Gm. Oral.				
Theobromine calcium salicylate (Theocalcin) (contains theobromine, calcium, and calcium salicylate).	0.5-1 Gm. Oral.				
OSMOTIC DIURETICS					
Dextrose, U.S.P.	10-50% solution. p.r.n. I.V.	Dextrose (glucose) is also used to treat cerebral edema as well as other edema.			
Mannitol, N.F. (Osmitrol).	5-10-20% concentration. p.r.n. I.V. infusion.	Used to increase urinary output in oliguria, anuria, edema, ascites, intoxications, and to aid in lowering intraocular pressure in acute glaucoma prior to surgery.	Mannitol increases the osmotic pressure in the urinary tubules, thus preventing reabsorption of water.	Mannitol may produce such side effects as thirst, headache, chills, constrictive feeling in chest. In large dosage patients may show signs of water intoxication, including pulmonary edema. Contraindicated in severe renal impairment and some cases of metabolic edema.	Avoid infiltration. Check response and stop I.V. if urinary response is inadequate.
Urea, U.S.P. (Carbamide) (Ureaphil [C]).	8 Gm. p.c. Oral.	Used for the same purposes as the mercurial diuretics.	A normal constituent of blood resulting from the deamination of amino acids. It is excreted along with water.	Rare in therapeutic dosage but may cause anorexia and nausea. Treatment: symptomatic.	Urevert is a solution of urea 90 Gm. in 210 ml. of 10% invert sugar solution.

Urevert.	90 gtt. 1 minute. I.V.	Used to reduce intracranial pressure.		Contraindicated in impaired renal function.	
MERCURIAL DIURETICS. *Mineral, vegetable, synthetic.* Chlormerodrin, N.F. (Mercloran, Neohydrin).	18.3 mg. o.d. Oral.	Mainly used to reduce edema in cardiac decompensation. Also used to treat ascites associated with liver disorders, nephrotic edema, and occasionally in certain related cases of subacute and chronic nephritis. Most effective if given with a xanthine diuretic–usually theophylline–and by simultaneous use of acid-producing salts such as ammonium chloride.	These preparations act by irritation of the renal tubules. This is a toxic effect and may be too severe. It prevents the reabsorption of certain electrolytes, especially the chloride ion, and thus increases the excretion of sodium chloride and water.	May cause stomatitis, gingivitis, salivation, diarrhea, nausea, vomiting, albuminuria, hematuria, and cardiac failure. For mild symptoms no treatment is required. For severe symptoms stop drug and treat as indicated by symptoms.	
Mercaptomerin sodium, U.S.P. (Thiomerin sodium) (40 mg. mercury).	1 ml. o.d. Irritating if given too deeply. Subcutaneous.				Mercaptomerin and mercumatilin appear to be less toxic than other mercurial diuretics.
Mercurophyllin (Mercupurin) (80 mg. mercury, 30 mg. theophylline).	0.2 Gm. o.d. Oral.				
Mercurophyllin injection (100 mg. mercury, 40 mg. theophylline).	1 ml. I.M. o.d., t.i.s., b.i.s., or o.s.		Rapid absorption from parenteral sites, but absorption from gastrointestinal tract is slow and unpredictable. Excreted by kidneys, 50% within 3 hours, 95% within 24 hours.		
Merethoxylline procaine (Dicurin Procaine) (39.3 mg. mercury ml.).	0.05-0.2 Gm. (2 ml.) o.d. Subcutaneous or I.M.				
Mersalyl and theophylline (100 mg. mersalyl, 50 mg. theophylline) (Diursol, Merphylline, Mersalyn) (Merraluril, Salangan-Theophylline, Theo-Syl [C]).	1-2 ml. o.d. I.M. or I.V.				
CARBONIC ANHYDRASE INHIBITORS. *Synthetic.* *Zolamide Series.* Acetazolamide, U.S.P. (Diamox).	Most of these are given o.m. to avoid interference with sleep. 0.25-0.5 Gm. o.d. Oral. Tablets and Spansules.	Used mainly to reduce edema of cardiac origin. Also used to lessen intraorbital pressure in glaucoma, intracranial pressure from trauma or neoplasm, in migraine headache, to reduce premenstrual tension, and in epilepsy.	Inhibit the action of the enzyme carbonic anhydrase which acts to convert carbon dioxide and water to carbonic acid. Some of these drugs also appear to have additional diuretic action in addition to carbonic anhydrase inhibition. These drugs decrease the reabsorption of sodium and chloride ions and to a lesser extent that of potassium.	Usually slight, but with continued use patient should be watched for signs of electrolyte imbalance. Potassium depletion may occur. There may be drowsiness, mild paresthesia (especially with the "zolamide" preparations), confusion, loss of appetite, urticaria, melena, hematuria, glycosuria, hepatic insufficiency or convulsions.	Most of these drugs are chemically related to the sulfonamides. Some may not be carbonic anhydrase inhibitors technically, but all have similar action. All dosages are individually adjusted for maintenance. Acetazolamide should not be used during pregnancy, especially in the 1st trimester, unless the physician feels that the benefits
Acetazolamide sodium, U.S.P. (Diamox sodium).	0.25-0.5 Gm. o.d. I.M. or I.V.				
Dichlorphenamide, U.S.P. (Daranide, Oratrol).	0.1-0.2 Gm. Initial dose o.d. Oral. 25-50 mg. maintenance o.d. Oral.	Used mainly in glaucoma.			

Name, Source, Synonyms, Preparations	Dosage and Administration	Uses	Action and Fate	Side Effects and Contraindications	Remarks
CARBONIC ANHYDRASE INHIBITORS (Continued) *Zolamide Series (Continued)*			Readily absorbed orally. Peak plasma levels in approximately 2 hours. Tightly bound to carbonic anhydrase, especially in the erythrocytes and renal cortex. It is excreted unchanged within 24 hours.	Contraindicated in renal hyperchloremic acidosis, Addison's disease, when severe sodium or potassium loss has been previously encountered, or in conditions with low sodium or potassium blood levels.	outweigh possible adverse effects.
Ethoxzolamide, U.S.P. (Cardrase, Ethamide).	62.5-125 mg. o.d. Oral.	Used mainly in edema, glaucoma, or epilepsy.			
Methazolamide, U.S.P. (Neptazane).	50 mg. o.d. Oral.	Used mainly in glaucoma.			
Thiazide Series. Synthetic.	Dosage individually adjusted.	Indicated in the management of conditions involving retention of fluid; congestive heart failure, renal edema, edema associated with hepatic disease, edema and toxemia of pregnancy, and fluid retention occurring in premenstrual tension and obesity.	Enhances the excretion of sodium, chloride and potassium. Onset of action following oral administration is usually within 2 hours, with maximal effects in 6 to 12 hours. The thiazides are rather rapidly absorbed from the gastrointestinal tract. Diuretic effect may appear in as little as 1 hour. Widely distributed in the extracellular fluid. They are concentrated only in the kidneys. Excretion is usually complete in 6 hours. Some are excreted unchanged, others are metabolized.	Side effects include the following: early signs of electrolyte imbalance such as dryness of mouth, thirst, weakness, lethargy, drowsiness or restlessness, muscle pains or cramps, muscular fatigue, hypotension, oliguria, gastrointestinal disturbances, azotemia, hyperglycemia and glycosuria. Thrombocytopenia, leukopenia, agranulocytosis, and aplastic anemia have been reported as rare side reactions. Photosensitivity, purpura, rash, and other dermatologic manifestations have been reported. Contraindicated in patients with anuria or oliguria.	Patients using these diuretics should have a serum electrolyte determination in order to protect against a possible depressed potassium or other electrolyte imbalance. Hypochloremic alkalosis or hypokalemia may occur. Potassium supplements should be administered during use in digitalized patients and in patients with cardiac arrhythmias or if secondary aldosteronism is suspected. The thiazide compounds should be used with caution during pregnancy and lactation since these drugs cross the placental barrier and also appear in the milk. This may result in fetal or neonatal hyperbilirubinemia, thrombocytopenia, altered carbohydrate metabolism and possibly other adverse reactions which have been seen in the adult patient.
Bendroflumethiazide, N.F. (Naturetin) (benzydroflumethiazide [C]).	2.5-5 mg. o.d. Oral.				
Benzthiazide, N.F. (Edenex, Exna, NaClex) (ExNa [C]).	25-100 mg. o.d. Oral.				
Chlorothiazide, N.F. (Diuril) (Chlorthiazidex [C]).	0.5 Gm. o.d. Oral. 0.25 Gm. o.d. Oral.	As a diuretic. For hypertension.			
Chlorothiazide sodium (Lyovac Diuril).	0.5 Gm. o.d. or p.r.n. I.V.				
Cyclothiazide, N.F. (Anhydron).	1-2 mg. daily. Oral.				
Hydrochlorothiazide, U.S.P. (Aquarius, Esidrix, Hydro-Diuril, Oretic) (Edemol, Fluvin, Hydrozide, Hydril, Hydro-Aquil, Neocodema, Novohydrozide, Urozide [C]).	25-50 mg. o.d. Oral.				
Hydroflumethiazide, N.F. (Saluron).	50 mg. o.d. Oral.				
Methyclothiazide, N.F. (Enduron) (Duretic [C]).	2.5-5 mg. o.d. Oral.				
Polythiazide, N.F. (Renese) (Lotense [C]).	1-4 mg. o.d. Oral.				
Trichlormethiazide, N.F. (Flutra, Metahydrin, Naqua).	2-4 mg. o.d. Oral.				

MISCELLANEOUS. These are all synthetic preparations unless otherwise stated.					
Aminometradine (Nictine, Mincard).	0.2-0.8 Gm. o.d. Oral.	A nonmercurial diuretic used mainly in edema due to mild cardiac decompensation, cirrhosis of the liver, nephrosis, pregnancy, and for premenstrual tension.	Mode of action not entirely clear, but apparently due to lessened reabsorption of the sodium ion.	Little toxicity has been noted. Not recommended in severe congestive heart failure.	
Chlorazinil hydrochloride (Daquin).	0.15 Gm. Oral.	Similar to the thiazide drugs.	Similar to the thiazide drugs.	Rare in therapeutic dosage. Watch for signs of potassium depletion.	
Chlorthalidone (Hygroton) (chlorphthalidone, Uridon [C]).	50-100 mg. Three times weekly. Oral.	As above.	As above.		See thiazides for side effects, contraindications and warnings.
COPAIBA. *Balsam of Copaifera officinalis* and *C. langsdorffi.* Copaiba.	1 ml. Oral.	Used mainly in chronic urinary conditions.	Is a diuretic with some antiseptic action.	May cause anorexia, colic, diarrhea, and occasionally skin rash. Stop drug and treat symptoms.	Copaiba is an ingredient in some non-prescription (OTC) diuretic preparations. Similar products include buchu, from a species of Barosma and juniper, from *Juniperus communis.*
Ethacrynic acid, U.S.P. (Edecrin).	Dosage varies with situation and condition of patient. Refer to manufacturer's brochure for details. 25-50 mg. Oral or I.V.	Congestive heart failure, acute pulmonary edema, renal edema, hepatic cirrhosis with ascites and edema due to other causes. Useful in children with nephrotic syndrome and congenital heart disease when a diuretic is indicated. Not recommended for infants.	Thought to act on both proximal and distal segments of the renal tubules. Also believed to act in the ascending limb of the loop of Henle. Readily absorbed. Accumulates only in the liver. Some excreted in bile. Some undergoes degradation. The acid and metabolites are excreted in urine.	Hyperuricemia and decreased urinary urate excretion. See manufacturer's brochure for the description of the numerous other side effects. Use in pregnancy is not recommended.	Can precipitate an attack of gout. Drug may augment effects of alcohol. Dosage of coadministered antihypertensive drugs may require adjustment. Frequent serum CO_2, electrolyte and blood urea nitrogen checks are desirable. Use of this drug I.V. with kanamycin should be avoided. See kanamycin.

Name, Source, Synonyms, Preparations	Dosage and Administration	Uses	Action and Fate	Side Effects and Contraindications	Remarks
MISCELLANEOUS (Continued)					
Furosemide, U.S.P. (Lasix).	40-80 mg. o.m. Depending upon response a second dose may be given 4-6 hours later. Oral. 20-40 mg. parenterally. Dosage may be titrated up to 600 mg. daily, and higher doses are under investigation.	Edema associated with congestive heart failure, cirrhosis of the liver, renal disease and the nephrotic syndrome.	Primarily inhibits the reabsorption of sodium in the proximal and distal tubule and in the loop of Henle. Action is independent of any inhibitory action of carbonic anhydrase and aldosterone. Onset of action, 1 hour; height, 1-2 hours; duration, 6-8 hours. Appears to have a blood pressure lowering effect similar to the thiazides.	Contraindications: anuria, if azotemia and oliguria increase during use in renal disease drug should be stopped or in hepatic coma or in a state of electrolyte imbalance. Increase in blood glucose and alteration of glucose tolerance tests have been reported with the use of furosemide. Not recommended in hypertension, for children or during pregnancy and lactation. Side effects: skin rashes, pruritus, paresthesia, blurred vision, postural hypotension, nausea, vomiting, diarrhea, fatigue, weakness, lightheadedness, dizziness, muscle cramps, thirst, urinary frequency.	Excessive diuresis may cause dehydration and reduction in blood volume with circulatory collapse. In patients taking digitalis excessive potassium loss may precipitate digitalis toxicity. Serum electrolyte, CO_2 and blood urea nitrogen should be checked frequently, especially during first few months of therapy.
Quinethazone, U.S.P. (Hydromox) (Aquamox [C]).	50 mg. q.d. or b.i.d. Oral.	Used to treat edema and hypertension.	A nonmercurial diuretic whose action is similar to that of the thiazide diuretics.	Increase in serum uric acid, photosensitivity, skin rash, and gastrointestinal disorders. Hypokalemia may require potassium supplementation.	Drug not related chemically to the thiazide series.
Spironolactone, U.S.P. (Aldactone).	25-100 mg. t.i.d. Oral.	Similar to other synthetic diuretics.	An aldosterone-blocking agent, interfering with sodium retention and potassium excretion effects of natural and synthetic mineralocorticoids. Indications and uses as for other diuretics.	Contraindicated in anuria. Low, but electrolyte imbalance may occur. Drowsiness, ataxia, and skin rashes have been reported with high dosage.	Patients with impaired renal function should be checked for hyperkalemia. For pregnancy warning, see thiazide series.

Triamterene, U.S.P. (Dyrenium).	100 mg. Up to b.i.d. Oral.	Used in edema associated with congestive heart failure, cirrhosis of the liver, nephrotic syndrome, late pregnancy, steroid induced edema, idiopathic edema, and due to secondary hyperaldosteronism.	Has two distinct actions: 1. Aldosterone antagonizing effect. 2. A direct effect on the transfer of sodium and other ions in the distal renal tubules.	Nausea, vomiting, gastrointestinal distress, weakness, headache, dry mouth, rash, and in rare instances electrolyte imbalance.

MISCELLANEOUS DRUGS

DRUGS USED FOR ALCOHOLISM

DISULFIRAM. *Synthetic.* Disulfiram (Alcophobin, Antabuse).	2 Gm. first day (do not give in divided doses). 1.5 Gm. second day. 1 Gm. third day. 0.5 Gm. fourth through eighth days. Oral. 0.125-0.5 Gm. maintenance. Oral.	Used to discourage the intake of alcohol so that supportive treatment and psychotherapy can be given.	Disulfiram alone has no effect, but in the presence of alcohol it produces very distressing symptoms. Disulfiram blocks the oxidation of alcohol at the acetaldehyde stage. This accumulates in the body, producing unpleasant symptoms. As small an amount as ½ ounce of whiskey will produce any or all of the following: flushing, palpitation, dyspnea, hyperventilation, tachycardia, nausea and vomiting, cyanosis, lowered blood pressure, and occasionally profound collapse. Readily absorbed. It tends to accumulate in the fat. Action is relatively slow. Reaches peak in about 12 hours. Some is oxidized by liver and some excreted unchanged by the kidneys.	Rare in absence of alcohol; mild drowsiness, fatigue, and headache may occur. Treat symptoms. Many drug interactions with this drug occur since it decreases the rate at which some drugs are metabolized. Examples: diphenylhydantoin blood level is increased; with the oral anticoagulants, the prothrombin time is increased; patients on isoniazid should be closely observed for changes in gait or marked changes in mental status due to increased serum levels of isoniazid. This drug should be used with caution in patients with the following conditions: diabetes mellitus, hyperthyroidism, epilepsy, cerebral damage, chronic or acute nephritis, hepatic cirrhosis or insufficiency. Its safe use during pregnancy has not been established.

Name, Source, Synonyms, Preparations	Dosage and Administration	Uses	Action and Fate	Side Effects and Contraindications	Remarks
ANOREXIC DRUGS These are all synthetic preparations.					
Chlorphentermine hydrochloride (Pre-Sate).	65 mg. each morning after breakfast.	For the treatment of obesity.	Similar to amphetamine, but claimed to have little or no effect on blood pressure.	Mydriasis, nausea, constipation, dry mouth, nervousness, insomnia, drowsiness, sedation, headache, urticaria, and dizziness may occur. Contraindicated in glaucoma and in patients receiving monoamine oxidase inhibitors. Safety for use during pregnancy has not been established. Not recommended for use by lactating women.	The use of these drugs, as with the amphetamines, concurrently with the phenothiazines is not pharmaceutically sound as they are antagonistic relative to their effects on noradrenergic and dopaminergic receptors in the nervous system.
Diethylpropion hydrochloride, N.F. (Naterexic, Tenuate, Tepanil, Regenon) (amfepramone [C]).	25 mg. Usually given t.i.d. ½ hour before meals. Oral. 75 mg. sustained release o.m.	Used to control appetite.	Similar to amphetamine but claimed to be devoid of central nervous system stimulation.	Rare, but oral dryness and constipation have been reported. Reduce dosage. Contraindicated in patients on monoamine oxidase inhibitors.	
Fenfluramine hydrochloride (Pondimin).	20-40 mg. t.i.d. a.c. Oral.	Short term adjunct therapy for weight control.	Sympathomimetic amine but appears to produce more central nervous system depression than stimulation.	Side effects. Most common: drowsiness, diarrhea and dry mouth. Drug can impair the ability of the patient to engage in potentially hazardous activities such as operating machinery or driving a motor vehicle. Contraindications: glaucoma, during or for 14 days following the use of monoamine oxidase inhibitors. Interactions: this drug can cause diarrhea and central nervous system depression	This drug is related chemically to the amphetamines and should be used cautiously, if at all, in persons with a history of drug abuse and tolerance. Safe use in pregnancy and in children under 12 years of age has not been established.

				unlike most other anorexic drugs. Therefore, other central nervous system depressants should be used concurrently with caution, if at all. Fenfluramine can increase slightly the effect of antihypertensive drugs such as guanethidine reserpine and methyldopa.	
Phendimetrazine bitartrate (Plegine) (Dietrol [C]).	35 mg. Usually given b.i.d. or t.i.d. Oral.	For appetite control in treatment of obesity.	Similar to amphetamine.	Occasional insomnia and nervousness. Rarely may cause dryness of mouth, nausea, blurred vision, dizziness, constipation, and stomach pain. Treatment: reduce or interrupt dosage. Contraindicated in presence of coronary disease, hypertension, thyrotoxicosis. Use with caution in highly nervous or agitated patients.	
Phenmetrazine hydrochloride, N.F. (Preludin) (Anorex, Metrabese, Neo-zine, Phenmetrazinal, Phentrol, Probese, Willpower [C]).	25 mg. b. or t.i.d. ½ hour a.c. Oral. 75 mg. Sustained release o.m.	Used mainly in obesity and as an euphoriant.	Similar to amphetamine.	Same as amphetamine but said to be less toxic and to have fewer side effects.	
Phentermine (Ionamin, Wilpo)	15-30 mg. o.m. Oral.	Anorexic agent used to treat obesity.	Similar to amphetamine.	Rare, but dryness of mouth, insomnia, and mild central nervous system stimulation may occur. Adjust dosage.	

ANTIRHEUMATIC DRUGS (See also Analgesic drugs, especially salicylates and phenylbutazone.)

These are all synthetic drugs, except as indicated.

Allopurinol, U.S.P. (Zyloprim) (Bloxanth [C]).	100 mg. b.i.d. or t.i.d. Oral. 200 mg. b.i.d. or t.i.d. Oral. 200 mg. t.i.d. or q.i.d. Oral.	For mild gout. For moderately severe tophaceous gout. For the prevention of uric acid nephropathy during antineoplastic therapy.	Inhibits uric acid production, reducing both serum and urinary uric acid levels. Said to prevent the formation of tophi in gout and the reduction in size of tophi already present.	Contraindications: Not used for other types of hyperuricemia than those listed. Give to children only as indicated. Not advised for women of child-bearing age or during pregnancy.	Should not be given with iron salts or if the immediate relatives of patient have idiopathic hemochromatosis. Maintenance doses of colchicine should be used when allopurinol is started to

Name, Source, Synonyms, Preparations	Dosage and Administration	Uses	Action and Fate	Side Effects and Contraindications	Remarks
Allopurinol (Continued)	For children: 6-10 yrs. 100 mg. t.i.d. Oral. Under 6 years 50 mg. t.i.d. Oral.	Used only for children if hyperuricemia is secondary to malignancy.	Acts on purine catabolism without disrupting the biosynthesis of purines. It does this by inhibiting the enzyme xanthine oxidase.	Side effects: skin rashes, gastrointestinal disturbances, occasionally chills, fever and blood dyscrasias.	prevent increased attacks of gout. Fluid intake should assure at least 2 liters of urine per day. The urine should be kept neutral or slightly alkaline. Liver and kidney function tests should be done early in therapy. If Purinethol is being given, dosage should be reduced one fourth to one third.
Glucurolactone.	0.2 Gm. q.i.d. Oral.	Used to treat various forms of arthritis.	An antiarthritic drug which appears to reduce joint inflammation.	There may be some flushing and mild gastrointestinal symptoms. Reduction of dosage will usually be effective.	
GOLD. *Mineral.*		Used in the treatment of lupus erythematosus, acute rheumatoid arthritis, and other similar conditions.	Mechanism unknown. Water soluble salts are rapidly absorbed from intramuscular sites. If suspended in oil, absorption is much slower. It is bound to plasma proteins and is very slowly excreted by the kidneys.	Urticaria, dermatoses, transient albuminuria, gastrointestinal disturbances, and agranulocytosis. Stop drug and treat symptoms.	All dosages individually adjusted; usually started low and increased gradually.
Aurothioglucose, U.S.P. (Gold thioglucose, Solganal).	25-50 mg. Weekly. I.M.				
Gold sodium thiomalate (Myochrysine) (sodium authiomalate [C]).	25-50 mg. Weekly. I.M.				
Gold sodium thiosulfate (Auricidine, Aurocidin, Aurolin, Aurosan, Auropin, Novacrysin, Solfocrisol, Thiochrysine).	25-50 mg. Weekly. I.M.				
Probenecid, U.S.P. (Benemid).	0.5-1 Gm. One to three times daily. Oral.	Used mainly in the treatment of chronic gout. Also used for other forms of arthritis and to delay the excretion of penicillin and some other drugs so as to maintain higher blood levels.	Depresses renal secretion of certain organic compounds. Well absorbed orally. Body half-life 6 to 12 hours. Largely bound to plasma proteins. Excreted in urine. More rapidly excreted in alkaline than in acid urine.	Rare, but skin rashes have occurred. Stop drug or reduce dosage and treat symptoms. Interactions: probenecid competes with various drugs for the same renal tubular excretory mechanism and can potentiate the effect of these drugs, sometimes requiring a reduction in the	Should not be used with the salicylates as their action is antagonistic.

				dose of the drug. Examples include indomethacin, penicillin and some penicillin derivatives such as ampicillin, the cephalosporin-type antibiotics, sulfonamides, aminosalicylic acid and dapsone. For interaction with nitrofurantoin, see page 205.	
Sulfinpyrazone, U.S.P. (Anturan).	400-800 mg. o.d. Oral.	Used in the palliative treatment of chronic gout.	Lessens crystal masses in joints. Increases uric acid excretion. Readily absorbed orally. Bound to plasma proteins. Usually excreted, largely unchanged, in 24 hours.	Can precipitate occurrence of acute gout. May cause epigastric distress or activate a peptic ulcer. Leukopenia and thrombocytopenia may occur.	Same as above.

DRUGS USED FOR BIOLOGICAL DEBRIDEMENT

ACETYLCYSTEINE. *Synthetic.* Acetylcysteine (Mucomyst) (Airbron, NAC [C]).	20% or more dilute solution by inhalation.	Adjunct therapy in bronchopulmonary disorders when mucolysis is desirable.	Acts by breaking the disulfide bonds of the mucus and in this way reduces the viscosity and facilitates its removal.	Untoward reactions are rare. Warning: after administration the liquefied secretions must be removed. If cough is inadequate to clear the airway, mechanical suction might be indicated.	If bronchospasms in asthmatic patients progress, this drug should be discontinued.
ALPHA-AMYLASE. *Synthetic.* alpha-Amylase (Buclamase, Fortizyme).	10-20 mg. Administered as buccal tablets t.i.d. or q.i.d. Sublingual.	For management of inflammation, edema, and pain in traumatic athletic injuries, surgical conditions, allergic states, connective tissue disorders, dental disorders and ear, eye, nose and throat disorders.	Claimed to initiate physiologic compensatory response to inflammation.	None reported.	

Name, Source, Synonyms, Preparations	Dosage and Administration	Uses	Action and Fate	Side Effects and Contraindications	Remarks
BROMELAINS. *Plant proteolytic enzyme from pineapple.* Bromelains (Ananase, plant protein concentrate).	50,000-100,000 U. Oral.	Used to treat traumatic injuries, cellulitis, furunculosis, ulcerations, and any condition requiring enzymic action.	A proteolytic enzyme which tends to dissolve fibrin and acid. Reduces inflammation.	Rare, but sensitivity may be a factor. Used with caution in blood clotting disorders and renal or hepatic disease.	
Collagenase (Santyl). Derived from *Clostridium histolyticum.*	250 units of collagenase per gram ointment. Topical. Apply once a day.	Used for debriding of dermal ulcers and burned areas.	Has ability to digest native collagen as well as denatured collagen. Optimal pH range for enzyme is 7-8.	Enzymatic action is adversely affected by detergents, hexachlorophene, heavy metal ions and by acidic solutions such as Burow's solution.	The action of the enzyme may be stopped by application of Burow's solution (pH 3.6 to 4.4). The commercial brochure should be consulted before using this product.
HYALURONIDASE. *Enzyme.* Hyaluronidase, N.F. (Alidase, Diffusin, Enzodase, Hyazyme, Infiltrase, Wydase).	150 T.R.U. dissolved in 1 ml. Added to fluid or drug or injected at the site.	Used to aid absorption of fluids and drugs given interstitially.	It acts on hyaluronic acid, hydrolyzing and depolymerizing it; thus acting as a spreading factor. Action entirely local.	Tissue damage may occur. Treatment symptomatic. Should not be used when there is infection.	T.R.U. is abbreviation for turbidity reducing units.
PANCREATIC DORNASE. *Biological.* Pancreatic dornase (Dornavac).	Varied. Inhalational.	Used in the treatment of various lung diseases.	The enzyme deoxyribonuclease derived from beef pancreas. Tends to dissolve and loosen mucus, making it easier for the patient to expectorate it.	Apparently low. Sensitivity may be a factor.	
PAPASE. *Extract of proteolytic enzyme of Carica papaya.* Papase (Papain) (papayatin, Caroid [C]).	10,000 U. Oral or Sublingual.	Use similar to that of other proteolytic enzymes, to treat hematoma, inflammation, and edema resulting from injury or allergy and various chronic respiratory conditions.	Same as other proteolytic enzymes.	Rare, but possibility of sensitivity should be kept in mind.	Contraindicated in severe systemic infections or blood clotting disorders. Do not use with an anticoagulant.
Subtilains (Travase). Derived from *Bacillus subtilis.*	82,000 units per gram ointment. Topical. Apply once daily.	For biochemical debridement of wounds (burns, decubitus, incisional, traumatic or	Proteolytic enzyme.	Contraindications and precautions: do not let ointment come in contact with	Wounds must be cleansed of antiseptics or heavy-metal antibacterials such as

		pyogenic wounds or ulcers secondary to peripheral vascular disease.		the eyes. Do not apply to wounds communicating with major body cavities or those containing exposed major nerves or nervous tissue, or fungating neoplastic ulcers. It should not be used on wounds in women of childbearing age because of lack of information concerning its effect on the fetus.	silver nitrate, hexachlorophene, benzalkonium, chloride, nitrofurazone, etc., which may denature enzymes or alter the substrate characteristics.
STREPTOKINASE-STREPTODORNASE. *Bacterial enzymes.* Streptokinase-Streptodornase (Varidase) (Bistreptase, Dornokinase [C]).	10,000 U. Streptokinase 2500 U. Streptodornase Oral or buccal tablets. 20,000 U. Streptokinase 5000 U. Streptodornase Powder for injection. I.M.	Used as physiologic agent to remove necrotic tissue, pus, blood, and such material from areas of burns, infected wounds, gangrene, empyema, abscesses, and similar conditions. Also used to reduce inflammation and edema.	Streptodornase depolymerizes extra cellular desoxyribonucleic acid and desoxyribonucleoprotein. Streptokinase activates a plasma factor called plasminogen which is the precursor of plasmin; this promotes lysis of fibrin. These two promote the liquefaction and removal of clots and pus.	None except that allergic reactions may occur. Usual anti-allergic treatment. Contraindicated in patients with reduced plasminogen or fibrinogen.	
TRYPSIN. *Mammalian pancreas (crystalline trypsin).* Chymotrypsin, N.F. (Alpha-Chymar, Avazyme, Chymar, Chytryp, Enzeon, Quimotrase, Zolyse) (Alfapsin, Catarase, Chymolin, Chymar, Chymetin, Zonulyn [C]).	5000-10,000 U. Oral, I.M. 750 U. application to eye.	Used as physiologic agent to aid in removal of necrotic tissue, pus, blood and such material from areas of burns, infected wounds, gangrene, empyema, abscesses, and similar conditions. Also used to reduce inflammation and edema. Used for enzymatic zonulysis for intracapsular lens extraction.	Trypsin digests protein material but does not affect protoplasm.	None except that allergic reactions may occur. Usual antiallergic treatment. Contraindicated in severe hepatic disorders. Use with caution if blood clotting disorders exist.	Do not give intravenously.
Trypsin and chymotrypsin (Chymolase, Chymoral, Orenzyme).	50,000-100,000 units total activity of trypsin and chymotrypsin. Oral. Ratio varies from 6:1 to 3:1 trypsin and chymotrypsin.	Used following traumatic injury.			
Trypsin crystallized, N.F. (Tryptar, Tryptest) (Parenzymol [C]).	5 mg. I.M. Also available in topical form.				

MISCELLANEOUS DRUGS (Continued)

DETOXIFYING AGENTS (See also Nalorphine and Levallorphan.)

Name, Source, Synonyms, Preparations	Dosage and Administration	Uses	Action and Fate	Side Effects and Contraindications	Remarks
CALCIUM DISODIUM EDETATE. *Synthetic.* Calcium disodium edetate, U.S.P. (Calsol, Edathamil, Endrate, EDTA, Sequestrene, Versenate) (Mesatil, Sormetal [C]).	1-2 Gm. In saline or dextrose solution. I.V. 30 mg./kg. of body weight. Oral.	Used mainly in the treatment of lead poisoning. It is also used in the treatment of scleroderma.	Acts as chelating agent for the removal of metals, mainly lead. Poor oral absorption. After I.V. administration about 50% is excreted by the kidneys in the first hour, 95% in the first 24 hours.	Possible kidney damage.	Available as edetate, edetate disodium, and calcium disodium edetate. The latter is the most commonly used form.
Deferoxamine (Desferal).	1 Gm. I.M. followed by 0.5 Gm. q. 4 h. for 2 doses depending upon response. 0.5 Gm. q. 4-12 h. Total not to exceed 6 Gm. in 24 hours. I.V. but at a rate not to exceed 15 mg./kg./hr. Used only for patients in cardiovascular collapse. Same doses as I.M.	Adjunct therapy for iron intoxication.	Deferoxamine complexes with iron to form ferrioxamine, a stable chelate that prevents the iron from entering into further chemical reactions. This chelate is readily soluble in water and passes easily through the kidneys, giving the urine a characteristic reddish color.	Contraindicated in renal disease or anuria. Side effects include erythema, urticaria and hypotension. Warning: Patients on long term therapy should have periodic eye examinations as cataracts have been seen in patients on long term therapy.	Only slightly absorbed orally. Should not be used in women of childbearing age or during early pregnancy unless in the doctor's judgment benefits outweigh possible hazards.
DIMERCAPROL. *Synthetic.* Dimercaprol, U.S.P. (BAL, British antilewisite).	0.25-0.3 ml. (cc.) of a 10% solution/10 kg. of body weight. I.M.	Used in the treatment of heavy metal poisoning. Also in the palliative treatment of multiple neuritis.	Forms a relatively stable compound with arsenic, mercury, and gold, thus preventing their metabolizing with body chemicals. After intramuscular injection peak systemic concentration is reached in 30 minutes.	Tachycardia, hyperpnea, tremors, nausea, and vomiting. Stop drug; the barbiturates are usually ordered.	Has a very unpleasant odor. Avoid spilling.
EDROPHONIUM CHLORIDE. *Synthetic.* Edrophonium chloride, U.S.P. (Tensilon).	10 mg. I.V.	Used as a specific anticurare agent to terminate the action of curare. Also used in the diagnosis of myasthenia gravis.	Apparently acts by displacing curare at the myoneural junction, allowing normal reflexes to pass. Acts in 30-60 seconds and action lasts about 10 minutes.	Rare in therapeutic dosage, but may cause some lacrimation, salivation, nausea, colic, and perspiration. Stop drug and treat symptoms.	

LEUCOVORIN CALCIUM. *Biological.* Leucovorin calcium (folinic acid [C]).	3-6 mg. o.d. I.M.	Used to counteract the toxic effects of the folic acid antagonists when too much is given.	Known as citrovorum or folinic acid. It reverses the action of folic acid antagonists such as methotrexate or aminopterin.	No adverse reactions reported with recommended dosages.	
METHYLENE BLUE (Methylthionine chloride). *Synthetic coal tar derivative.*		Used as a urinary antiseptic in nephritis, pyelitis, and cystitis. Also used to treat methemoglobinemia.	Acts as a bacteriostatic agent. It appears to be most effective in urinary tuberculosis. It reduces methemoglobin. Most effective in small doses I. V. Excessive doses may reverse this and turn hemoglobin to methemoglobin.	Rare in therapeutic dosage.	Causes urine to turn greenish.
Methylene blue, U.S.P. (Hexalol, Urised).	0.15 Gm. q.i.d. Oral. 0.06-0.13 Gm. q. 4 h. Oral. 1-2 mg./kg. of body weight. I.V.	As urinary antiseptic. For methemoglobinemia For methemoglobinemia.			
PENICILLAMINE. *Synthetic.* Penicillamine, U.S.P. (Cuprimine).	Starting dose for adults and children: 250 mg. q.i.d. 1-½ hours a.c. and h.s. Thereafter dosage individually adjusted. Infants over 6 months and small children 250 mg. daily. Given dissolved in fruit juice. Oral.	Used to reduce blood copper level in Wilson's disease (symptomatic and asymptomatic). Best used with a regimen designed to reduce absorption of copper through the intestinal tract. Also used to treat cystinuria.	A chelating agent which increases the renal excretion of copper.	Localized ecchymosis in skin, maculopapular rash, lymphadenopathy may occur. Reduce dosage or stop drug temporarily. Patients taking penicillamine may require supplemental pyridoxine.	Frequent blood and urine examinations advised. Review of manufacturer's pamphlet is advised.
PENICILLINASE. *Biological.* Penicillinase (Neutrapen).	800,000-1,000,000 U. I.M. or I.V.	Used to treat hypersensitivity reactions to penicillin. More effective for pruritus than for other symptoms.	One unit of penicillinase will inactivate 1 unit of penicillin. Designed to counteract the sensitivity reactions to penicillin. It is not effective for acute emergency reactions, but does aid in delayed reactions.	Can induce sensitivity.	

Name, Source, Synonyms, Preparations	Dosage and Administration	Uses	Action and Fate	Side Effects and Contraindications	Remarks
PRALIDOXIME CHLORIDE. *Synthetic.* Pralidoxime chloride, U.S.P. (Protopam chloride) (2 PAM chloride [C]).	Adjusted to suit indivi-ual case.	Antitoxicant against organic phosphate pesticides.	Antagonist to certain cholines-terase inhibitors.	Rare in therapeutic usage.	

PYRETICS (Drugs used to induce fever)

Fever is also induced by means of diathermy and electric cabinets (hyperthermia cabinets). Except in specific cases drugs are rarely used to produce fever.

Name, Source, Synonyms, Preparations	Dosage and Administration	Uses	Action and Fate	Side Effects and Contraindications	Remarks
MALARIAL PARASITES. *Biological.* (pure viable strains of the organisms must be used). Malarial parasites.	Dosage varies. I.V.	Used mainly to induce hyper-pyrexia in tertiary syphilis and in certain other condi-tions in which an excessively high fever tends to destroy the infecting agent.	A predetermined number of malarial paroxysms are in-duced, then antimalarial treatment is instituted.	The usual toxic effects of malaria occur, as well as the usual effects of high fever. Treatment: as for any high fever or for malaria.	
TYPHOID VACCINE. *Biological.* (pure killed vaccine must be used). Typhoid vaccine.	Dosage varies. I.V.	Use same as for malarial parasites.	The effects of the vaccine occur rapidly and last only a short time. Dosage of vaccine is repeated as indicated.	None, other than those of high fever. Treatment: same as for high fever.	

THYROID INHIBITORS (See also Radioactive iodine, page 228.)

These are all synthetic drugs.

Name, Source, Synonyms, Preparations	Dosage and Administration	Uses	Action and Fate	Side Effects and Contraindications	Remarks
Methimazole, U.S.P. (Tapazole) (thiamazole [C]).	5-10 mg. q. 8 h. Oral.	See the following.	Its action is more potent but less consistent than that of thiouracil preparations.	Patients on methimazole may have a decreased response to warfarin and other anti-coagulants. Also see the following.	Consult brochure for possible use during pregnancy and for other pertinent information.
Iothiouracil sodium (Itrumil).	50-300 mg. Divided doses. Oral.	Used in the treatment of hyperthyroidsim. It inhibits	These preparations interfere with the production of the	Sore throat, malaise, coryza, drug fever, leukopenia,	The protein bound iodine test is invalid for patients

Methylthiouracil, N.F. (Antibason, Methiacil, Muracil, Thimecil). Propylthiouracil, U.S.P. (Propyl-Thyracil [C]). Thiouracil.	50 mg. Divided doses. Oral. 0.1 Gm. q.i.d. Oral. 0.1 Gm. Up to q.i.d. Oral.	the activity of the thyroid gland. All these drugs are used to prepare patients for thyroid surgery and to maintain those who are poor surgical risks.	thyroid hormone. This decreases the symptoms of hyperthyroidism. After discontinuance of the drug, the gland quickly regains its ability to secrete the hormone. Rapid and adequate absorption from gastrointestinal tract. Duration of action only 2-3 hours. With large doses may last up to 8 hours. Exact fate is not known.	agranulocytosis, and dermatitis may occur. Stop drug and treat symptoms. The antibiotics, especially penicillin, are usually used.	receiving iothiouracil sodium. Methylthiouracil and propylthiouracil are less apt to cause toxic symptoms than thiouracil.

VARIOUS DRUGS NOT EASILY CLASSIFIED

These are all synthetic preparations unless otherwise noted.

Azathioprine (Imuran).	3-5 mg./kg. daily. Oral.	Adjunct therapy for the prevention of rejection in renal homograft. Other uses are investigational.	This is an antimetabolite and interferes at the enzyme level with purine metabolism. The drug is well absorbed orally and is metabolized in the body to mercaptopurine. It is oxidized and methylated to give various degradation products. Small amounts are excreted unchanged in the urine and also small amounts of 6-mercaptopurine.	Side effects: hypersensitivity, anemia, leukopenia, thrombocytopenia and bleeding, oral lesions, skin rashes, drug fever, alopecia, pancreatitis, arthralgia and steatorrhea. Jaundice has been seen in some patients and with this extremely high alkaline phosphatase levels with slightly elevated bilirubin. A patient taking allopurinol will have a significant rise in the blood level of mercaptopurine as allopurinol inhibits the enzymatic oxidation of mercaptopurine.	

Name, Source, Synonyms, Preparations	Dosage and Administration	Uses	Action and Fate	Side Effects and Contraindications	Remarks
Carbamazepine (Tegretol).	200-1200 mg. every 24 hours. Initial 100 mg. b.i.d. 1st day, then increase 100 mg. q. 12 h. until control of pain is achieved. At least every 3 months attempts should be made to reduce or stop the drug altogether.	Treatment of pain associated with true trigeminal neuralgia (tic douloureux).	Serum half-life is usually greater than 14 hours.	Contraindications: patients sensitive to tricyclic compounds such as amitriptyline, desipramine, and imipramine; patients on monoamine oxidase inhibitors unless 7 days have elapsed from last dose; pregnancy (at least first 3 months) and then only if clinical conditions warrant it; and nursing mothers. Used with caution in patients with history of coronary heart disease or congestive heart failure or increased intraocular pressure. There are many other precautions and multiple side effects, see commercial brochure. Patients should be cautioned about driving a car or operating machinery during therapy because of tendency to dizziness and drowsiness.	The commercial brochure should be thoroughly read before administering this drug. The following warning appears on it: "Following treatment with carbamazepine, deaths from agranulosis, thrombocytopenia and transitory leukopenia have been observed. In order to detect serious bone marrow injury *early* complete blood and platelet counts should be done at frequent intervals."
Cholestyramine resin, U.S.P. (Cuemid, Questran).	4 Gm. t.i.d. Oral.	Relief of pruritus associated with cholestasis as occurs in biliary cirrhosis with incomplete biliary obstruction and other forms of partial obstructive jaundice.	Acts by combining with the bile salts, which are eliminated in the feces. Removal of these salts reduces the pruritus, although the underlying cause is not corrected. Aids in excretion of cholesterol.	Chronic use may be associated with increased bleeding tendency, and hyperchloremic acidosis may occur. Safe use of drug in pregnancy has not been established.	Should be given at least 4 hours after other oral medications.
Clofibrate, N.F. (Atromid-S).	500 mg. q.i.d. Oral.	Used to reduce serum lipids (cholesterol).	Good oral absorption. Extensively bound to plasma proteins. Distribution in body limited mainly to plasma and extra cellular fluid. Half-life in man approximately 12 hours.	Side effects: most commonly nausea; also vomiting, loose stools, dyspepsia, flatulence and abdominal distress. Other side effects include headache, dizziness, fatigue, skin rash, urticaria, pruritus	When used in conjunction with an anticoagulant drug, the dose of the anticoagulant should be reduced 1/3 to 1/2, depending upon *individual response*, to maintain

			Action: it is believed to inhibit cholesterol biosynthesis in the liver in a manner similar to that of physiologic control mechanism.	and stomatitis.	the desired prothrombin time. Frequent prothrombin time determinations should be made until it has stabilized.
Chloresium. *Vegetable.*	Dosage varies. Topical.	Used to stimulate cell growth and to deodorize wounds, burns, and skin ulcers.	Mechanism has not been established.	None.	
Cromolyn sodium (Intal, Aarane).	20 mg. powder by inhalation. 4 times a day at regular intervals.	Used as adjunct therapy in the treatment of patients with severe perennial bronchial asthma. It is not used for acute attacks especially status asthmaticus.	Cromolyn inhibits the degranulation of sensitized mast cells which occurs after exposure to specific antigens. It also inhibits the release of histamine and SRS-A. It has no intrinsic bronchodilator, antihistaminic or anti-inflammatory activity. It is poorly absorbed orally. After inhalation of the powder, about 8% is absorbed from the lungs and rapidly excreted unchanged in urine and bile. The remainder is deposited in the oropharynx, swallowed and excreted via the alimentary tract.	Side effects: maculopapular rash and urticaria have been reported. Cough and/or bronchospasm can occur. The latter may be serious enough to require discontinuation of the drug. Eosinophilic pneumonia has been reported. If this occurs, drug should be stopped.	One capsule contains 20 mg. Comes with special inhalator and patient must be carefully instructed as to its use.
Flavoxate (Urispas).	100-200 mg. t.i.d. or q.i.d. Oral.	Used as an antispasmodic for the urinary system.	This drug has direct spasmolytic effect on the smooth muscle of the lower urinary tract.	Nausea and vomiting, dry mouth, nervousness, vertigo, headache, drowsiness, blurred vision, increased ocular tension, disturbances in eye accomodation, urticaria, mental confusion (especially in the elderly patient), dysuria, tachycardia and palpitation. Contraindicated in patients with the following: obstructive conditions, pyloric, duodenal intestinal lesions	Use with caution in patients with glaucoma. Safe use during pregnancy or in children under the age of 12 years has not been established.

Name, Source, Synonyms, Preparations	Dosage and Administration	Uses	Action and Fate	Side Effects and Contraindications	Remarks
Flavoxate (Continued)				or ileus; achalasia; gastrointestinal hemorrhage; obstructive uropathies of the lower urinary tract.	
Flurothyl, N.F. (Indoklon).	Dosage varies. Inhalational.	Treatment of psychotic patients in whom convulsive therapy is indicated, as in depressive disorders, schizoid-affective disorders, and paranoid schizophrenia.	Acts as a convulsant. It is rapidly excreted by the lungs.	Mild: upper respiratory disturbances. Severe: cardiovascular, hepatic, or renal disease. Marked increase in intraocular or intraspinal pressure. Not used in patients with abnormal temperature. Should not be used during pregnancy, as no data are available to establish safety.	
Glucagon, U.S.P. (pancreatic polypeptide [C]). *Glandular extract.*	0.5-2 mg. Dosage individually adjusted. Parenteral.	For use in hypoglycemic coma resulting from any cause.	A crystalline polypeptide pancreatic extract. Causes increased blood glucose concentration.	Excessive dosage may cause hyperglycemia. Treatment: insulin administration.	
Levodopa (Dopar, Larodopa).	Dosage is individually adjusted. Initial dose usually 0.5-1.0 Gm. daily. Slowly increased until optimal effect is obtained. The usual daily dose is from 4-6 Gm. in divided doses 3 or more times a day. Not more than 8 Gm. a day should be given. The optimal therapeutic range is usually reached in 6-8 weeks after institution of therapy.	Indicated for Parkinson's disease or syndrome. It relieves the symptoms, particularly rigidity and bradykinesis. It is sometimes helpful in tremors, dysphagia, sialorrhea and postural instability.	The symptoms of parkinsonism are believed to be associated with a depletion of striatal dopamine. Since dopamine does not cross the blood-brain barrier, it is ineffective. Levodopa, which is the precursor of dopamine in the body, does cross the barrier; it is believed to have its effect by being converted to dopamine after crossing the barrier.	Because of the high incidence of adverse reactions and the necessity for individualization of therapy, the physician should be thoroughly familiar with the brochure before beginning therapy. This drug should not be given to patients with clinical or laboratory evidence of the following conditions: uncompensated endocrine, renal, hepatic, cardiovascular or pulmonary diseases; narrow angle glaucoma; blood dyscrasias.	Levodopa should not be used when a sympathomimetic amine is contraindicated. Monoamine oxidase inhibitors should be discontinued at least 2 weeks before the institution of levodopa therapy. Doses of 10-15 mg. of pyridoxine appear to reverse the effects of levodopa, so use of multivitamin compounds with this drug is not recommended unless pyridoxine can be removed.
Monobenzone, N.F. (Alba-Dome, Benoquin).	20% ointment. 5% lotion. Topical.	Used to reduce excessive pigmentation.	A melanin inhibiting agent.	Can cause irritation and dermatitis.	In non-caucasian individuals can cause unattractive depigmentation.

Phosphentaside (Cardiomone, My-B-Den)	20 mg. Sublingual or I.M.	Used for the systemic treatment of pruritus and for angiospastic conditions.	Mechanism is not understood.	Rare in therapeutic dosage.	
Surgibone (Bo-Plant). *Animal.*	Amount indicated by condition.	Bone or cartilage implants used in orthopedic surgery, rhinoplasty, and maxillofacial surgery.	Surgibone is sterile processed heterogeneous bone or cartilage obtained from bovine embryos, or young calves. Forms a base upon which new bone grows.		
Trimethylsporalen (Trisoralen).	10 mg. daily 2-4 hours before exposure to ultraviolet or fluorescent black light.	Used to facilitate repigmentation in vitiligo, increase tolerance to solar exposure, and enhance pigmentation.	Exact mode of action has not been established.	Gastric discomfort has been reported. The drug is contraindicated in diseases associated with photosensitivity (porphyria, acute lupus erythematosus, or leukoderma of infectious origin). To date safety of drug has not been established in young children (2 years or under) aphakic people, pregnant women, or young women of child-bearing age.	
Tromethamine, N.F. (Tham).	Least amount of 0.3 M solution required to bring the blood to the normal pH levels.	Correction of systemic acidosis or acidity in whole blood during cardiac bypass surgery. Metabolic acidosis associated with cardiac arrest.	Increases blood pH. Dosage should be adjusted so that blood pH does not increase above normal, approximately pH 7.4.	Anuria and uremia. Used only in lifethreatening cases during pregnancy. Do not use more than one day. Used cautiously in patients with renal disease and/or reduced renal output.	

RADIOACTIVE DRUGS

The dosage of all these drugs is individually adjusted. Toxicity of all drugs includes the toxic symptoms of radiation and of the specific chemical.

RADIOACTIVE ISOTOPES USED TO TREAT DISEASE					
RADIOACTIVE GOLD (AU^{198}) (Radio-Gold Collid, Auroloid, Aureotope).	35-20 mc. Intracavitary.	Used for intracavitary injection to reduce effusions due to malignant neoplasms.	Reduce fluid accumulation.	See above.	Fluid is first withdrawn from the cavity.

Name, Source, Synonyms, Preparations	Dosage and Administration	Uses	Action and Fate	Side Effects and Contraindications	Remarks
RADIOACTIVE ISOTOPES (Continued)					
RADIOACTIVE IODINE. *Seaweed and fission products.* Sodium iodide I^{131}, U.S.P. (radioactive iodine, Iodotope, Oriodide, Radiocaps, Theriodide, Tracervial).	1-100 microcuries. 1-100 micrograms (non-radioactive iodine). Oral. Given together as a tracer. Doses vary according to condition.	Used in the diagnosis and treatment of malignant diseases of the thyroid. Also used to treat non-malignant thyroid conditions in older people, especially those who are poor surgical risks.	Because of the affinity of thyroid tissue for iodine, the material is concentrated in the gland or, in cases of metastatic cancer, in the metastases as well. The radioactive iodine has a half life of 8.08 days and liberates beta particles and gamma rays.	See above.	Dosage for treatment individually adjusted.
Radioactive phosphorus (P^{32}) (Phosphotope, Sodium Radio-Phosphate).	2.5-5 mc. Oral, I.V., topical.	Used in the palliative treatment of blood dyscrasias, especially polycythemia vera and chronic adult leukemia. Used topically for skin cancer, keloids, keratoses.	Decreases production of red blood cells. May bring about remissions which leave patient symptom-free for months. Has preferential uptake by neoplastic tissue.	See above.	
Radio-chromated serum albumin (Cr^{51}) (Chromalbin).	30-50 mc. I.V.	Used in the detection and quantitation of gastro-intestinal protein loss with hypoproteinemia associated with a variety of diseases.	See uses.	See above. Should not be administered to pregnant women or to persons under 18 years of age, unless clinical condition warrants it.	
Technetium sulfate 99m (Pertechnetate Tc 99m). Derived from molybdenum technetium 99m generators. (See column 6.)	0.5-20.0 mc (millicuries) I.V.	Used primarily for diagnosis of disorders of the brain (brain scans). Can also be used for liver and spleen scans when prepared in colloidal form.	Half-life of 6 hours.	Usual precautions and side effects of radiation. However, since half-life is so short, adverse results are rare.	Molybdenum has a half-life of 80 hours. Since the half-lives of both mother and daughter isotopes are so short, this isotope must be produced where and when it is to be used. Generator kits are available from several sources. Some of these are Pertgen-99m, Technetope, and Ultratechnekow.

Many isotopes are used for diagnosis and research. Among these are: Radioiodinated serum albumin, U.S.P. (Albumotope I^{131}, Risa), human serum albumin tagged with I^{131} (I^{125} U.S.P. is also used in research), used to determine blood and plasma volume, Radioactive chromium, U.S.P. (Cr^{51}) (Chromitope Sodium Cr^{51}, Rachromate-51), used to test for red blood cell survival, red cell volume, and fecal blood loss determination. Radioactive cobalt (Co^{57} and Co^{60}) tagged vitamin B_{12} is used to test for pernicious anemia. Radioactive Fe^{59}, as the citrate, is used to determine erythropoiesis (iron turnover). I^{131} tagged Rose Bengal is used in liver scanning. Chlormerodrin tagged with Hg^{203} and Hg^{197} is used in renal scanning and in tumor localization (brain). $Selenium^{75}$ as selemethionine is used in pancreatic scanning. I^{131} as iodohippurate is used to determine renal clearance. I^{131} as iodinated triolein is used to determine fat absorption and as iodinated oleic acid to determine fatty acid absorption. $Krypton^{85}$ as a dissolved gas is used to determine cardiac output, cerebral blood flow and pulmonary blood flow. Other isotopes used include iridium, calcium, cesium, copper, potassium, sodium, sulfur and technetium, and this list is constantly being expanded.

INDEX

A

C

D

E

F

G

H

I

J

K

N

O

P

Q

R

S

T

U

V

W

X

Y

Z

TABLE OF METRIC AND APOTHECARIES' SYSTEMS

(Approved *approximate* dose equivalents are enclosed in parentheses. Use *exact* equivalents in calculations.)